SPINE SECRETS

THIRD EDITION

SPINE SECRETS

EDITOR:

VINCENT J. DEVLIN, MD, FAAOS
Orthopaedic Surgeon
Fulton, Maryland

ELSEVIER

1600 John F. Kennedy Blvd.
Ste 1800
Philadelphia, PA 19103-899

Notices

Practitioners and researchers must always rely on their own experience and knowledge in evaluating
and using any information, methods, compounds or experiments described herein. Because of rapid
advances in the medical sciences, in particular, independent verification of diagnoses and drug dosages
should be made. To the fullest extent of the law, no responsibility is assumed by Elsevier, authors,
editors or contributors for any injury and/or damage to persons or property as a matter of products
liability, negligence or otherwise, or from any use or operation of any methods, products, instructions,
or ideas contained in the material herein.

ISBN: 978-0-323-63662-9

Content Strategist: Marybeth Thiel
Content Development Manager: Ellen Wurm-Cutter
Content Development Specialist: Sara Watkins
Publishing Services Manager: Deepthi Unni
Project Manager: Janish Ashwin Paul
Design Direction: Bridget Hoette

Printed in the United States of America

Last digit is the print number: 9   8   7   6   5   4   3   2

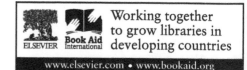

Working together
to grow libraries in
developing countries

www.elsevier.com • www.bookaid.org

To my wife, Sylvia.
Without her support and encouragement,
completion of this book would not have been possible.

CONTRIBUTORS

Owoicho Adogwa, MD, MPH
Spine Fellow
Orthopaedic Surgery
Washington University
St. Louis, MO

Bradley Anderson
Syracuse University
New York, NY

D. Greg Anderson, MD
Orthopaedic Surgeon
Rothman Orthopaedics
Bensalem, PA

Professor
Departments of Orthopaedic and Neurological Surgery
Thomas Jefferson University
Philadelphia, PA

Paul A. Anderson, MD
Professor
Orthopaedic Surgery and Rehabilitation
University of Wisconsin
Madison, WI

Mundeep S. Bawa, BS
Department of Orthopaedic Surgery
Rush University Medical Center
Chicago, IL

Andrew M. Block, BS
Department of Orthopacdic Surgery
Rush University Medical Center
Chicago, IL

Christopher R. Brigham, MD, MMS
Consultant
Hilton Head Island, SC and Portland, ME;
Editor, Guides Newsletter;
Senior Contributing Editor, AMA Guides to the Evaluation
   of Permanent Impairment, Sixth Edition
Author, Living Abled and Healthy: A Guide to Injury and
   Illness Recovery

Thomas N. Bryce, MD
Professor
Rehabilitation and Human Performance
Icahn School of Medicine at Mount Sinai
New York, NY

Alejandro Carrasquilla, MD
Resident
Neurosurgery
Icahn School of Medicine at Mount Sinai
New York, NY

R. Carter Cassidy, MD
Associate Professor
Orthopaedic Surgery
UK Healthcare
Lexington, KY

Jens R. Chapman, MD
Orthopaedic Spine Surgeon
Orthopaedic and Neurosurgery
Swedish Hospital, Seattle, WA

Stephen L. Demeter, MD, MPH
Private Practice
Las Vegas, NV;
Retired Professor and former Head of Pulmonary and
   Critical Care Medicine, Northeastern Ohio College of
   Medicine
Past President of the International Academy of
   Independent Medical Evaluators (IAIME; formerly
   the American Academy of Disability Evaluating
   Physicians)
Editor of Disability Evaluation Editions 1 & 2

Vincent J. Devlin, MD, FAAOS
Orthopaedic Surgeon
Fulton, MD

Doniel Drazin, MD, MA
Neurosurgeon
Neurosurgery
Evergreen Health
Kirkland, WA

Mostafa H. El Dafrawy, MD
Fellow-Spine Surgery
Orthopaedic Surgery
Washington University in St. Louis
St. Louis, MO

Benjamin D. Elder, MD, PhD
Assistant Professor
Neurosurgery
Mayo Clinic
Rochester, MN

Winston Fong, MD
Chief
Department of Spine Surgery
McBride Orthopaedic Hospital
Oklahoma City, OK

Munish C. Gupta, MD
Chief of Spine, Professor of Orthopaedics
Department of Orthopaedic Surgery
Washington University in St. Louis
St. Louis, MO

Robert Hart, MD
Spine Surgeon
Orthopaedic Surgery, Spine Surgery
Spine Specialists at SNI
Seattle, WA

Vincent Huang, MD
Assistant Professor
Department of Rehabilitation and Human Performance
Icahn School of Medicine at Mount Sinai
New York, NY

Nikhil Jain, MD
Fellow
Department of Neurosurgery
University of Louisville
Louisville, KY

José H. Jiménez-Almonte, MD, MS
Orthopaedic Surgery
University of Kentucky
Lexington, KY

Lawrence I. Karlin, MD
Associate Attending
Orthopaedic Surgery
Boston Children's Hospital
Boston, MA

Floreana N. Kebaish, MD
Professor
Orthopaedic Surgery
Johns Hopkins University
Baltimore, MD

Khaled, M. Kebaish, MD, FRCSC
Professor
Orthopaedic Surgery
Johns Hopkins University
Baltimore, MD

Benjamin Khechen, BA
Department of Orthopaedic Surgery
Rush University Medical Center
Chicago, IL

Terrence Kim, MD
Co-Medical Director
Spine Education
Cedars Sinai Medical Center
Los Angeles, CA

Paul M. Kitei, MD
Attending Physician
Rothman Institute
Philadelphia, PA

Brian H. Kopell, MD
Director, Center for Neuromodulation
Neurosurgery
The Icahn School of Medicine at Mount Sinai
New York, NY

Mohammad E. Majd, MD
Orthopaedic Surgery
Baptist Health Medical Group New Albany, IN

Scott C. McGovern, MD
Spine Surgeon
Orthopaedic Surgery
Peninsula Orthopaedic Associates
Salisbury, MD

Michael J. Moses, MD
Orthopaedic Surgery
NYU Langone Medical Center
New York, NY

Ronald Moskovich, MD, FRCS Ed
Assistant Professor
Orthopaedic Surgery
NYU Langone Health
New York, NY

Justin Munns, MD
Orthopaedic Surgeon
Private Practice
ORA Orthopaedics
Moline, IL

Rod J. Oskouian, MD
Neurosurgeon, Spine Specialist
Swedish Neuroscience Institute
Seattle, WA

David C. Ou-Yang, MD
Orthopaedic Surgery
University of Colorado
Aurora, CO

Fedor E. Panov, MD
Assistant Professor
Neurosurgery
Mount Sinai Health System
New York, NY

Daniel K. Park, MD
Attending Spine Surgeon
Orthopaedic Surgery
William Beaumont Hospital
Royal Oak, MI

Dil B. Patel, BS
Department of Orthopaedic Surgery
Rush University Medical Center
Chicago, IL

Preston Phillips, MD
Orthopaedic Surgery
Warren Clinic Orthopaedic Surgery and Sports Medicine
Tulsa, OK

Jonathan Ramin, DO
Resident
Department of Rehabilitation Medicine
Icahn School of Medicine Mount Sinai
New York, NY

Jonathan J. Rasouli, MD
Neurosurgery Resident
Icahn School of Medicine at Mount Sinai
Mount Sinai Health System
New York, NY

Thomas A. Schildhauer, MD, PhD
Professor
Department of General and Trauma Surgery
BG University Hospital Bergmannsheil, Ruhr-University
 Bochum
Bochum, Germany

Adam L. Shimer, MD
Associate Professor
Orthopaedic Surgery
University of Virginia
Charlottesville, VA

Kern Singh, BS, MD
Associate Professor
Orthopaedic Surgery
Rush University Medical Center
Chicago, IL

John C. Steinmann, DO
Medical Director
Spine and Joint Institute (SJI)
Redlands Community Hospital
Redlands, CA

Mark A. Thomas, MD
Associate Professor of Physical Medicine and
 Rehabilitation; Program Director of Physical Medicine
 and Rehabilitation Residency
Montefiore Medical Center
Bronx, NY

Eeric Truumees, MD
Professor
Surgery and Perioperative Care
University of Texas, Dell Medical School
Austin, TX

Alexander R. Vaccaro, MD, PhD
President
Orthopaedics
Rothman Orthopaedic Institute
Philadelphia, PA

Eric S. Varley, DO
Complex Adult and Pediatric Spine Surgeon
Orthopaedic and Neurological Surgery
Spine Institute of Idaho
Boise, ID

Vikas V. Patel, MD
Professor
Department of Orthopaedic Surgery
University of Colorado
Denver, CO

Sayed E. Wahezi, MD
Associate Professor of Physical Medicine and
 Rehabilitation and Anesthesiology; Program Director
 of Interventional Pain Management Fellowship
Montefiore Medical Center
Bronx, NY

Jeffrey C. Wang, MD
Chief, Orthopaedic Spine Service; Co-Director USC
 Spine Center; Professor of Orthopaedic Surgery and
 Neurosurgery
USC Spine Center
University of Southern California Spine Center
Los Angeles, CA

Robert G. Watkins III, MD
Co-Director
Marina Spine Center
Cedars-Sinai Marina del Rey Hospital
Marina del Rey, CA

Robert G. Watkins IV, MD
Co-Director
Marina Spine Center
Cedars-Sinai Marina del Rey Hospital
Marina del Rey, CA

Philip J. York, MD
Resident
Department of Orthopaedic Surgery
University of Colorado
Aurora, CO

PREFACE

Although spinal disorders are among the most common conditions requiring medical care, identification of the optimal pathways for evaluation and management remains a challenge. Rapid advances related to the field of spinal disorders have opened new avenues for evaluation and treatment of affected patients. A wide range of medical specialties, including but not limited to orthopaedic surgery, neurological surgery, anesthesiology, physical medicine and rehabilitation, pain medicine, radiology, internal medicine, family medicine, critical care medicine, pediatrics, neurology, emergency medicine, rheumatology, infectious disease, medical oncology, pathology, and psychiatry, are involved in the evaluation and treatment of patients with spinal problems on a daily basis. Knowledge of current concepts relating to spinal disorders is crucial in order to provide appropriate evaluation, referral, and treatment.

The goal of *Spine Secrets* is to provide broad-based coverage of the diverse field of spinal disorders at an introductory level, using the proven and time-tested question-and-answer format of the Secrets Series. The book covers the common conditions encountered during evaluation and treatment of spinal patients. Topics are arranged to provide the reader with a sound knowledge base in the fundamentals of spinal anatomy, clinical assessment, spinal imaging, and nonoperative and operative management of commonly encountered spinal disorders. The full spectrum of disorders affecting the cervical, thoracic, and lumbar spine in pediatric and adult patients is covered, including degenerative spinal conditions, fractures, spinal deformities, tumors, infections, and systemic problems, such as osteoporosis and rheumatoid arthritis. This information will benefit the reader during patient rounds, as well as in the clinic and the operating room. The book is not intended to provide comprehensive coverage of specific topics, which is more appropriately the domain of major textbooks and specialty courses. However, it is hoped that readers will be stimulated to further their knowledge of spinal disorders through additional study, as directed by the internet resources and references listed at the end of each chapter.

The intended audience for this book is wide ranging and includes any health care provider interested in furthering their knowledge and understanding of spinal disorders: medical students, residents, orthopaedic and neurosurgery spinal fellows, nurses, physician assistants physical therapists, and chiropractors, and practicing physicians. The book may also be of interest to biomedical engineers, medical researchers, hospital administrators, attorneys, worker compensation professionals, medical-device and regulatory professionals, as well as patients with spinal problems.

I wish to acknowledge the innumerable people who have provided guidance over the years and contributed to my development as a physician and spinal surgeon. I also thank the staff at Elsevier, especially Marybeth Thiel and Sara Watkins, for bringing this project to completion. Finally, I thank my patients and practice colleagues for their confidence and support of my clinical work, which has focused on providing the best care possible for challenging spinal problems. This book is dedicated to the medical trainees, nurses and allied health professionals I have been honored to work with and I sincerely hope this new edition will be of value to all interested in increasing their knowledge regarding spinal disorders.

Vincent J. Devlin, MD

CONTENTS

IV NONSURGICAL MANAGEMENT OF SPINAL DISORDERS

V SURGICAL INDICATIONS AND PERIOPERATIVE MANAGEMENT OF THE SPINE PATIENT

VI BASIC SPINAL PROCEDURES, SURGICAL APPROACHES, AND SPINAL INSTRUMENTATION

VII   PEDIATRIC SPINAL DEFORMITIES AND SPINAL DISORDERS

VIII   DEGENERATIVE DISORDERS OF THE ADULT SPINE

TOP 100 SECRETS

These secrets are 100 of the top board alerts. They summarize the concepts, principles, and most salient details of spinal disorders.

REGIONAL SPINAL ANATOMY

1. The **typical spinal column** is composed of 33 vertebrae: 24 presacral vertebrae (7 cervical, 12 thoracic, and 5 lumbar); the sacrum (5 fused vertebrae); and the coccyx (4 fused vertebrae).
2. There are eight pairs of cervical **nerve roots** but only seven cervical **vertebrae**. The cervical nerve roots exit the spinal canal above the pedicle of the corresponding vertebrae. The thoracic and lumbar nerve roots exit beneath the pedicle of the corresponding vertebrae.
3. The **thoracic spinal cord** between T4 and T9 is poorly vascularized. This region is termed the critical vascular zone of the spinal cord and corresponds to the narrowest region of the spinal canal.
4. The spinal cord normally terminates as the **conus medullaris** at the L1–L2 level in adults. The **cauda equina** occupies the thecal sac distal to the L1–L2 level.
5. The **posterior spinal musculature** functions to maintain normal sagittal spinal alignment through application of dorsal tension forces against the intact anterior spinal column. The posterior spinal musculature is able to function as a tension band only if the anterior spinal column is structurally intact and able to resist compression and axial loading. Approximately 70%–80% of axial load is carried by the **anterior spinal column** and the remaining 20%–30% is transmitted through the posterior spinal column.
6. **Pedicle dimensions** are narrowest in the midthoracic region (T4–T6), widen slightly in the upper thoracic region (T1–T3), and widen markedly in the lower thoracic region (T10–T12). The lower thoracic pedicles are typically larger than the upper lumbar pedicles. L1 is generally the narrowest pedicle in the lumbar spine. Pedicle dimensions gradually increase between L2 and S1.

CLINICAL EVALUATION OF THE SPINE PATIENT

7. The most **common cervical diagnoses** evaluated for nonsurgical management in an outpatient clinic or office setting include axial neck pain, radiculopathy, and myelopathy. These conditions may present singly or in combination.
8. **Thoracic spine pain** may arise from a variety of sources, including thoracic and cervical spinal structures, chest wall structures, as well as referral from cardiopulmonary, gastrointestinal, and miscellaneous causes.
9. The most common reason for referral for outpatient evaluation of the lumbar spine is **axial low back pain with or without lower extremity pain**. Conditions to consider in the **differential diagnosis** include: lumbar strain or lumbar sprain, discogenic pain, zygapophyseal (facet) joint pain, sacroiliac joint (SIJ) pain, radiculopathy due to a herniated lumbar disc, lumbar spinal stenosis, lumbar spondylolysis/spondylolisthesis, osteoporotic compression fracture, scoliosis, spine infection, spine tumors, hip joint pathology, rheumatologic disorders, and referred pain from visceral or vascular structures.
10. A comprehensive patient history and physical examination is the first step in diagnosis of a spine complaint. It is critical to identify and distinguish **urgent and emergent spinal conditions** such as tumor, infection, fracture, and progressive neurologic loss from common **nonemergent spinal conditions** such as nonspecific axial pain.
11. Multiple facets of human disease may be associated with a spinal deformity depending on its etiology. A **spinal deformity** may be only one manifestation of an underlying systemic disorder that may affect multiple organ systems. The etiology of spinal deformities is wide ranging and includes congenital disorders, developmental disorders, degenerative disorders, trauma, infection, tumors, metabolic disorders, neuromuscular disorders, and conditions whose precise etiology remains incompletely defined such as idiopathic scoliosis.
12. The **supine straight-leg raise test** and its variants increase tension along the sciatic nerve and are used to assess the L5 and S1 nerve roots. The **reverse straight-leg raise test** increases tension along the femoral nerve and is used to assess the L2, L3, and L4 nerve roots.
13. Identification of **clinical characteristics associated with decreased satisfaction and persistent pain and disability** in the treatment of chronic spinal pain syndromes is important. Some key characteristics to assess during the patient's history include psychosocial factors, employment status, tobacco use, and chronic opioid use.
14. **Impairment** reflects an alteration from normal bodily functions, can be assessed using traditional medical means, and can be objectively determined. **Disability** results from impairment, is task specific, and is measured in the context of the system to which an injured worker has applied for relief. Disability determination is an administrative determination that uses both medical and nonmedical information.

SPINAL IMAGING

15. Imaging tests are appropriate when the information obtained from the test will affect medical decision making.
16. One of the major challenges encountered in the evaluation of patients with spinal conditions is **determination of the clinical relevance of abnormalities detected on spinal imaging tests** since these tests are extremely sensitive but relatively nonspecific. It is important to order the imaging study best suited to evaluate the suspected pathologic process based on the clinician's working diagnosis, as well as the sensitivity, specificity, and accuracy of each imaging modality.
17. When ordering spinal imaging studies, health care providers should consider the **relative radiation exposures for various imaging studies** that use ionizing radiation and balance the medical benefit to the patient versus potential radiation risks associated with each examination.
18. **Plain radiographs** are inexpensive, widely available, involve relatively low radiation exposure, and provide valuable information about spinal alignment and bone structure, but are unable to define soft tissue and neural structures.
19. **Magnetic resonance imaging** (MRI) is the best initial advanced spinal imaging study to evaluate nontraumatic spinal conditions because it provides the greatest amount of information regarding a single spinal region. MRI provides excellent visualization of pathologic processes involving the disc, thecal sac, epidural space, neural elements, paraspinal soft tissue, bone, and bone marrow.
20. **Multiplanar computed tomography** (CT) is the imaging study of choice for evaluating the osseous anatomy of the spine and is the preferred initial advanced imaging study for evaluation of spinal trauma. The radiation dosage associated with CT is an important concern and may be minimized by following appropriate protocols.

ASSESSMENT AND NONSURGICAL MANAGEMENT OF SPINAL DISORDERS

21. Initial management of **acute cervical pain** begins with an evaluation to rule out major structural pathology. If there are no findings suggesting serious pathology, the patient should be reassured that recovery is likely within 2–3 months. The patient should be encouraged to stay active and return to normal activities. A home exercise program with stretching, strengthening, and aerobic exercise is initially recommended. Referral to physical therapy is considered based on patient preference, for patients with barriers to recovery, or if symptoms persist despite initial self-treatment. Structured patient education combined with exercise, as well as multimodal care, is advised. It is recommended that nonoperative treatment of acute neck pain emphasize patient education and active treatments over passive modalities. Nonnarcotic medications such as nonsteroidal antiinflammatory drugs (NSAIDs) or short-term use of a nonbenzodiazepine muscle relaxant may be considered.
22. Treatment of **chronic neck pain** should address both the biomechanical issues and the psychosocial factors that contribute to the patient's pain and disability. Evidence-based treatment for chronic neck pain includes active rehabilitation therapy with supervised exercise. This may include stretching, strengthening with isometric and/or dynamic exercises, cervicothoracic stabilization, and aerobic conditioning. Multimodal care (exercise in conjunction with manipulation or mobilization) is an additional treatment option. Pharmacologic treatment options include NSAIDs or serotonin-norepinephrine reuptake inhibitors (SNRIs) such as duloxetine. Alternatively, a short course (few weeks) of a nonbenzodiazepine muscle relaxant may be considered. Opioid medications are not indicated for treatment of chronic musculoskeletal cervical pain. Alternative therapies supported by randomized controlled evidence include qigong (a holistic system of coordinated body posture and movement) and Iyengar yoga (emphasizes precision and alignment in all postures). Select patients may benefit from cognitive behavioral therapy or a functional restoration program. For patients in whom zygapophyseal joint pain is considered, diagnosis is confirmed with nerve blocks performed by anesthetizing the medial branch nerves innervating the target facet joint(s). Anesthetic agents of varying duration of effect are utilized during two separate injection sessions. If the diagnosis is confirmed, percutaneous radiofrequency neurotomy to ablate the medial branch nerves innervating the target facet joint(s) is a treatment option. Although cervical disc degeneration is a cause of neck pain in some patients, distinguishing painful from nonpainful cervical discs remains challenging.
23. Studies have described a favorable history for most patients with **cervical radiculopathy**. The majority of patients with cervical radiculopathy improve within several weeks. Longer term follow-up (2–19 years) has shown that the majority of patients experience no, mild, or intermittent symptoms. Patients who experience progressive or persistent neurologic weakness, myelopathy, or intractable pain should be referred for surgical evaluation.
24. Nonsurgical management of **degenerative cervical myelopathy** (DCM) does not alter the natural history of the disease. Surgical intervention is the only treatment that can arrest the progression of DCM and is recommended for patients with moderate or severe DCM. Nonsurgical management may be considered for patients with mild myelopathy. However, it is unclear which types of nonoperative treatment provide benefit when compared with the natural history of DCM.
25. **Musculoskeletal thoracic pain** occurs in the absence of significant pathologies such as infection, neoplasm, metastatic disease, osteoporosis, inflammatory arthropathies, fractures, or pain referred from abdominal or pelvic viscera. Limited evidence exists to guide nonoperative treatment of musculoskeletal thoracic pain. Active interventions, including stretching, postural, strengthening, and stabilization exercises are the most commonly recommended treatments. Passive interventions, including mobilization, soft tissue massage, acupuncture, and

electrotherapy, are also commonly prescribed but supporting evidence is limited. A multimodal program of care with manual therapy, soft tissue therapy, exercises, heat/ice, and education is recommended by many providers. A limited course of NSAIDs or acetaminophen may provide benefit.

26. Recommendations for initial management of patients with **acute lumbar pain without radiation** include education and reassurance. In the first several days following pain onset, cold packs may provide relief of acute pain, and may be followed by use of alternate heat and/or cold depending on patient preference. NSAIDs or a short-term course of a muscle relaxant may be considered. Patients should be advised to stay active and continue usual activities as pain permits, including work.

27. Patients with **chronic low back pain** are more challenging to treat than those with acute or subacute low back pain and require different treatment strategies. Multiple factors may contribute to development of chronic low back pain including biophysical, psychologic, social, and genetic factors. Generalized treatment recommendations for chronic low back pain include a graded activity or exercise program directed toward improvement in function, psychologic therapies such as cognitive behavioral therapy and mindfulness-based stress reduction, adjunctive interventions including tai chi, yoga, acupuncture, and manipulation as second-line treatment options. Pharmacologic treatment is recommended only following inadequate response to nonpharmacologic therapy (avoid use of paracetamol and routine use of opioids). Spinal fusion surgery and disc replacement demonstrate marginally improved outcomes compared with the results of multidisciplinary rehabilitation, but surgery is associated with a greater risk of adverse events.

28. Management of an acute episode of **sciatica** focuses on identifying positions of comfort, which result in decreased leg pain. Lying supine with the lower legs on a chair (Z-position) or side lying are suggested, but alternative positions may be effective. First-line medications prescribed to decrease pain intensity are NSAIDs. The acute pain phase resolves in many patients over 4–6 weeks as patients become more mobile and gradually return to daily activities. Referral to physical therapy for instruction in a home or supervised exercise program is an option. Patients who continue to experience severe radicular pain after initial nonoperative treatment may benefit from epidural steroid injections. Patients who present with or develop symptoms and physical examination findings consistent with cauda equina syndrome or a progressive neurologic deficit require urgent evaluation with MRI and surgical consultation. The natural history of an acute lumbar disc herniation is quite favorable. Gradual improvement in symptoms over several weeks is noted in the majority of patients. Comparison of nonsurgical and surgical treatment has shown that surgically treated patients recover more quickly from sciatic pain symptoms, report better long-term functional status and higher satisfaction. Both nonsurgical and surgical treatments are associated with clinically significant improvement over time and the differences between treatment groups narrows over time.

29. Symptoms of **neurogenic claudication** are generally relieved with sitting in a forward flexed posture. It is important to distinguish neurogenic claudication from vascular claudication, which is unrelieved with positional change. Nonoperative treatments for neurogenic claudication secondary to lumbar spinal stenosis include education, active physical therapy, transfer and gait training, manual therapy, and NSAIDs. Epidural injections are frequently performed but limited evidence supports this practice. For patients with symptoms of neurogenic claudication that limit function, surgical treatment has been demonstrated to provide substantially greater improvement in pain and function compared with continued nonoperative treatment. The natural history of symptomatic lumbar spinal stenosis is favorable in approximately 50% of patients, regardless of initial or subsequent treatment. Significant deterioration in symptoms with nonsurgical treatment is uncommon. Surgery has been shown to be more effective than nonoperative management in patients with symptomatic lumbar spinal stenosis, as well as degenerative spondylolisthesis associated with spinal stenosis in short- to medium-term follow-up (2–4 years). At long-term follow-up (8–10 years), certain outcome parameters were noted to converge between operative and nonoperative treatment groups, but the overall benefit of surgical treatment appeared to be maintained.

30. Treatment of radicular symptoms secondary to disc herniation is the most common and most well-supported indication for **epidural steroid injections**. Epidural steroid injections are also a treatment option for patients with radicular symptoms due to neuroforaminal stenosis or central canal stenosis. Limited evidence supports the role of epidural injections for treatment of axial pain. Access options for epidural injections include translaminar, transforaminal, and caudal approaches.

31. **Medial branch nerve blocks** are the most reliable test for diagnosis of facet-related pain.

32. An analgesic response to a properly performed **diagnostic SIJ block** is considered the most reliable test to diagnose SIJ-mediated pain.

33. **Provocative discography** is a diagnostic test performed to identify patients with discogenic pain. Patient selection for this test is critical as false-positive results are reported in a high percentage of patients with psychologic distress, chronic pain syndromes, and litigation or workers' compensation issues.

34. The **electrodiagnostic examination** is an extension of the history and physical examination. Its goal is to help differentiate the variety of causes for numbness, weakness, and pain. The standard examination consists of two parts: **electromyography** (EMG) and **nerve conduction studies** (NCS). EMG is the most useful diagnostic test to establish and/or confirm a clinical diagnosis of radiculopathy. EMG has limited usefulness in the evaluation of spinal stenosis and postlaminectomy syndrome or when the diagnosis of radiculopathy is already certain. NCS are most useful for diagnosis of peripheral entrapment neuropathy and peripheral neuropathy but are generally normal in patients with radiculopathy.

35. **Spinal orthoses** are classified according to the region of the spine immobilized by the orthosis: cervical orthosis (CO), cervicothoracic orthosis (CTO), thoracolumbosacral orthosis (TLSO), lumbosacral orthosis (LSO), and sacroiliac orthosis (SIO).
36. A **TLSO** provides effective motion restriction between T8 and L4 but paradoxically increases motion at the L4–L5 and L5–S1 levels. If motion restriction is required above T8, a cervical extension is added. If motion restriction is required at L4–L5 and L5–S1, a thigh cuff is necessary.

SURGICAL INDICATIONS AND PERIOPERATIVE MANAGEMENT OF THE SPINE PATIENT

37. Inappropriate **patient selection** guarantees a poor surgical result despite how expertly a surgical procedure is performed.
38. General **indications for surgical intervention** for spinal disorders include decompression, stabilization, deformity correction, and motion preservation following intervertebral disc excision.
39. **Risk stratification strategies** help to inform decision making regarding the benefits and risks of spine surgery and to guide strategies directed toward minimization of medical and surgical complications.
40. Successful outcomes for complex spine procedures are dependent on the implementation of **standardized and co-ordinated team-based approaches** to optimize care and minimize intraoperative and postoperative adverse events.
41. **Multimodality, intraoperative neurophysiologic monitoring** permits assessment of the functional integrity of the spinal cord, spinal nerve roots, brachial plexus, lumbosacral plexus, and peripheral nerves during spinal surgery. Intraoperative assessment of spinal cord function is optimally achieved with a combination of transcranial electric motor-evoked potentials (tceMEPs) and somatosensory-evoked potentials (SSEPs). Intraoperative assessment of nerve root function is achieved with electromyographic (EMG) monitoring techniques and monitoring of tceMEPs from specific myotomes. The optimal anesthesia maintenance protocol for successful intraoperative neurophysiologic monitoring of spinal cord function is a total intravenous anesthesia (TIVA) regimen with avoidance of muscle relaxation, nitrous oxide, and inhalational agents.
42. **Adverse events** following spine surgery are unavoidable, but their negative effects can be lessened by prompt diagnosis followed by appropriate and expedient treatment. Adverse events at the operative site may be related to the surgical approach, neural decompression, or spinal instrumentation. Systemic adverse events after spine surgery may involve the entire spectrum of body organ systems.
43. **Cauda equina syndrome** manifests as a constellation of signs and symptoms including low back pain, bilateral lower extremity pain and/or weakness, saddle anesthesia, and varying degrees of bowel and/or bladder dysfunction resulting from a space-occupying lesion (e.g. disc herniation) within the lumbosacral spinal canal. Treatment is prompt surgical decompression.

BASIC SPINAL PROCEDURES, SURGICAL APPROACHES, AND SPINAL INSTRUMENTATION

44. Selection of an appropriate procedure for **spinal decompression** depends on a variety of factors, including clinical symptoms, spinal level, location of compression, number of involved levels, and the presence/absence of spinal instability or spinal deformity.
45. **Spinal arthrodesis and spinal instrumentation** are indicated in conjunction with decompression in the presence of spinal deformity or spinal instability or when decompression results in destabilization at the surgical site.
46. The **transoral approach to the craniocervical junction** is indicated for fixed deformity causing anterior midline neural compression.
47. The **posterior midline cervical approach** is extensile and provides access from the occiput to the thoracic region.
48. A key to the **anterior approach to the cervical spine** is an understanding of the **anatomy of the fascial layers of the neck**. The superficial cervical fascia lies between the dermis and the deep cervical fascia and blends with the platysma muscle. The deep cervical fascia consists of three layers. The most superficial or investing layer surrounds all of the structures in the neck and splits to encircle the trapezius and sternocleidomastoid muscles. The middle layer consists of the pretracheal or visceral fascia, which encloses the trachea, esophagus, and thyroid gland and blends laterally with the carotid sheath. The deep or prevertebral layer surrounds the cervical vertebral column.
49. The **posterior surgical approach to the thoracic and lumbar spine** is the most utilized approach and provides extensile surgical access for spinal decompression, fusion, and instrumentation from T1 to the sacrum.
50. The key to avoiding complications during **surgical exposures of the anterior spinal column** is a detailed knowledge of the relationship of the vascular, visceral, and neurologic structures to the anterior and lateral aspects of the spine.
51. **Minimally invasive spine (MIS) procedures** intend to limit approach-related surgical morbidity through use of smaller skin incisions and targeted muscle dissection but do not eliminate the potential for serious and life-threatening complications. Use of MIS techniques is widespread, but claims that MIS procedures are more effective than traditional spine procedures await validation in the current medical literature.

52. **Posterior cervical instrumentation** most commonly involves use of screw-rod systems. Screws may be placed in the occiput, C1 (lateral mass), and C2 (pedicle, pars, or translaminar screws). In the subaxial cervical region, lateral mass screws or pedicle screws may be used at the C3–C6 spinal levels, whereas pedicle screws are used at C7 and distally in the thoracolumbar region.

53. **Anterior cervical plates** may be classified as static or dynamic fixation devices. Anterior cervical plates are used in conjunction with a structural allograft or fusion cage to reconstruct the load-bearing capacity of the anterior spinal column.

54. Contemporary **posterior thoracolumbar spinal instrumentation systems** attach to the spine at multiple anchor points throughout the instrumented spinal segments. Pedicle screws are the most commonly used anchor type, but hooks, wires, cables, and bands also play a role in specific clinical scenarios. A complete implant assembly is termed a spinal construct. A spinal instrumentation construct consists of longitudinal members on each side of the spine, which may be connected transversely by cross-linking devices to increase construct stability.

55. **S1 pedicle fixation** is the most common sacral anchor point utilized when performing posterior fusions to the sacrum. Some form of **sacropelvic fixation** should be used to supplement S1 pedicle screws whenever the biomechanical forces across the lumbosacral junction are expected to exceed the ability of the S1 pedicle screws to provide the stable biomechanical environment needed to achieve solid arthrodesis. S2 alar-iliac and iliac screw are the most protective and stable forms of sacropelvic fixation. Structural interbody support at the L4–L5 and L5–S1 levels increases fusion rates and decreases the risk of construct failure when performing fusion to the sacrum.

56. **Graft material options for use in spinal arthrodesis** include autograft bone, allograft bone, demineralized bone matrix, ceramics, bone marrow aspirate, and osteoinductive proteins. Graft materials may function as bone graft extenders, enhancers, or substitutes. An ideal graft material for use in spinal fusion possesses osteoinductive, osteoconductive, and osteogenic properties. Grafts material may be classified as structural or nonstructural depending on whether mechanical support is provided by the material during fusion consolidation.

57. Options for use in **anterior spinal column reconstruction** include structural autogenous bone graft (iliac or fibula), structural allograft bone graft, or synthetic materials (e.g., titanium mesh, carbon fiber, and polyetheretherketone [PEEK] cages).

58. **Spinal fusion cages** are devices that contain graft material and provide structural support to the anterior spinal column and promote fusion following removal of an intervertebral disc (i.e., **intervertebral body fusion device**) or vertebral body (**vertebral body replacement device**).

59. Selection of appropriate candidates for **revision spinal surgery** depends on comprehensive assessment to determine the factors that led to a suboptimal outcome following the prior surgical procedure. For poor surgical outcomes due to errors in surgical strategy or technique, appropriate revision surgery may offer a reasonable chance of improved outcome. For surgical failures due to errors in diagnosis or inappropriate patient selection for initial surgery, revision surgery may offer little chance for improved outcome. In the absence of relevant and specific anatomic and pathologic findings, pain itself is not an indication for revision surgery.

60. **Explantation of a failed lumbar total disc arthroplasty** is a complex and high-risk procedure in comparison with revision surgery for a failed cervical total disc arthroplasty.

61. **Spinal cord stimulation** is a minimally invasive treatment appropriate for select patients with persistent pain following spinal surgery, chronic regional pain syndromes, and other neuropathic pain syndromes. **Implantable drug delivery systems** are considered for patients with nociceptive and/or neuropathic pain syndromes who do not experience relief with medication, spinal cord stimulation, or neuroablative procedures.

PEDIATRIC SPINAL DEFORMITIES AND SPINAL DISORDERS

62. Unique **anatomic features of the immature spine** lead to different **traumatic injury** patterns in pediatric and adult patients. Odontoid fractures are the most common pediatric cervical spine fracture. Children younger than 8 years of age are predisposed to upper cervical injury due to their high head-to-body ratio, which must be taken into account when these patients are immobilized on a spine board. Elevation of the thorax or use of a pediatric spine board with an occipital recess is recommended to prevent excessive cervical flexion. After 8 years of age, traumatic injuries most commonly involve the subaxial cervical, thoracic, and lumbar spinal regions. Due to the elasticity of the spinal column in children, forces applied to the spine may be accommodated by the spinal column but exceed the elastic limit of the spinal cord and result in a stretch injury to the spinal cord without observable findings on plain radiographs or CT, referred to as a **spinal cord injury without radiographic abnormality** (SCIWORA). Skeletally immature patients who sustain a spinal cord injury require surveillance for the development of spinal deformities.

63. Traditionally, **back pain in children** was considered uncommon, and was thought to be associated with a definable cause. Current data show that back pain is a frequent complaint in the pediatric population and that the probability of identifying a specific cause is low. Back pain is much less common before age 10, increases during adolescence, and approaches adult population rates by age 18 years. Diagnosis of a definable cause of back pain symptoms is possible in less than 20% of pediatric patients. Spinal pain in adolescence is considered to be a risk factor for spinal pain as an adult. Initial evaluation of the pediatric patient presenting with back pain

consists of a detailed history, physical examination, and spinal radiographs. Spinal MRI is obtained for pediatric patients with abnormal neurologic findings, constant pain, night pain, or radicular pain. Although no diagnosis is unique to a single age group, some generalizations regarding the likely diagnosis according to age include: **younger than 10 years of age**: disc space infection, vertebral osteomyelitis, and tumors such as Langerhans cell histiocytosis, leukemia, astrocytoma, and neuroblastoma; **older than 10 years of age**: nonspecific back pain, spondylolysis, spondylolisthesis, Scheuermann kyphosis, fractures, lumbar disc herniation, apophyseal ring injury, osteoid osteoma, tumors, and spinal infections.

64. **Thoracic insufficiency syndrome (TIS)** is defined as the inability of the thorax to support normal respiration or lung growth. TIS develops in skeletally immature patients due to a wide range of conditions that restrict lung volume, lung expansion, and postnatal lung growth. These conditions include hypoplastic thorax syndromes such as Jeune syndrome, spinal dysplasias, including spondylocostal and spondylothoracic dysplasia, congenital scoliosis with fused ribs and various etiologies responsible for early onset spinal deformities associated with distortion of the rib cage.

65. **Early onset scoliosis (EOS)** is defined as scoliosis with an onset prior to 10 years of age. Patients with EOS are at risk for developing progressive deformity involving the spine and thorax, which has the potential to adversely impact normal growth and development of the spinal column, thoracic cavity, and lung parenchyma leading to TIS and early mortality. The **four main etiologic categories** of EOS are congenital-structural, neuromuscular, syndromic, and idiopathic. Surgical implants used to treat EOS are referred to as "growth-friendly" implants as they are intended to control spine and chest deformities and maximize function, thoracic volume, and spinal column growth without requiring spinal fusion. **Growth-friendly spinal implants** are classified into three main types based on the corrective forces exerted by the implants on the spine and thoracic cage: (1) distraction-based systems, such as the vertical expandable prosthetic titanium rib (VEPTR), traditional and hybrid growing rods, and magnetically controlled growing rods; (2) guided growth systems such as Shilla; and (3) compression-based systems such as spinal tethers.

66. **Idiopathic scoliosis**, the most common type of pediatric scoliosis, is defined as a spinal deformity characterized by lateral bending and fixed rotation of the spine in the absence of a known cause. The criterion for diagnosis of scoliosis is a coronal plane spinal curvature of 10° or more as measured by the Cobb method. Traditionally, idiopathic scoliosis patients were classified according to age at onset as infantile (birth–3 years), juvenile (4–10 years), and adolescent (after 10 years). Current terminology classifies idiopathic scoliosis that is present before 10 years of age as EOS and idiopathic scoliosis that develops after 10 years of age as **late-onset scoliosis**. Progressive EOS curves are treated initially with bracing or serial casting. Curves that continue to progress despite nonoperative treatment are treated surgically using posterior growth-friendly instrumentation. Treatment options for late-onset idiopathic scoliosis patients include observation (curves <20°–25°), orthoses (curves 25°–45° in patients who are Risser stage 0, 1, or 2; and, for female patients <1 year postmenarche), and operations. For skeletally immature adolescents, posterior spinal fusion and instrumentation is indicated for curves greater than 40°–45° that are progressive despite brace treatment. In the mature adolescent, surgery is considered for curves approaching or greater than 50°. Recently, nonfusion options for surgical treatment of skeletally immature patients with idiopathic scoliosis have been introduced and include vertebral body tethering and posterior minimally invasive deformity correction.

67. **Congenital scoliosis** is a lateral curvature of the spine caused by vertebral anomalies that produce a frontal plane growth asymmetry. The anomalies are present at birth, but the curvature may take years to become clinically evident. The **main categories** of congenital scoliosis are **failures of vertebral formation, failures of vertebral segmentation,** and **mixed types of anomalies**. As development of the spine occurs at the same time as other organ systems, patients with vertebral malformations often have associated anomalies within or outside the spinal column, including cardiac and renal anomalies.

68. **Neuromuscular spinal deformities** develop in patients with underlying neuropathic or myopathic disorders due to trunk muscle weakness, spasticity, or spinal imbalance, which compromise the ability to maintain normal alignment of the spine and pelvis. Common etiologies include cerebral palsy, Duchenne muscular dystrophy, spinal muscular atrophy, myelodysplasia, posttraumatic deformities, and Rett syndrome. Asymmetric spinal column loading of the immature spine leads to asymmetric vertebral body growth due to the Hueter-Volkmann principle, which states that increased loading across an epiphyseal growth plate inhibits growth, while decreased loading accelerates growth. The severity of a deformity is influenced by a range of patient-specific factors, including the underlying diagnosis, the type and extent of neuromuscular involvement, ambulatory status, and skeletal maturity. A broad spectrum of spinal deformities may develop including scoliosis, hyperkyphosis, hyperlordosis, and complex multiplanar deformities. The decision to intervene surgically for treatment of a neuromuscular spinal deformity depends on a range of factors, including etiology of the underlying neuromuscular disorder, deformity magnitude, skeletal maturity, and associated medical comorbidities. The operative treatment options for neuromuscular spinal deformities include both nonfusion and fusion surgical techniques.

DEGENERATIVE DISORDERS OF THE ADULT SPINE

69. Degenerative changes involving the intervertebral discs and zygapophyseal joints are not a disease in the traditional sense, but rather the natural consequences of mechanical stresses applied to the spine throughout life and

subject to influence by traumatic, nutritional, biochemical, and genetic factors. Although disc and facet joint degeneration are universal in the aging spine, these changes are inconsistently and only occasionally associated with pain and functional limitation. There is concern that labeling patients with a diagnosis such as **"degenerative disc disease"** may have a negative impact on certain patients who may perceive their diagnosis as a progressive, irreversible disease that may not improve over time. Caution is recommended in interpreting the clinical relevance of spinal degeneration features noted on imaging studies due to the high prevalence of imaging findings of spinal degeneration in asymptomatic subjects.

70. The **clinical manifestations of degenerative spinal disorders** include axial pain syndromes, radiculopathy, myelopathy, spinal instabilities, and spinal deformities.

71. Self-reported **neck pain** is very common and is experienced by 30%–50% of the adult population annually. The precise location and source of neck pain is often unidentified. Half to three-quarters of patients with neck pain continue to report neck pain 1–5 years later. Risk factors for neck pain are multifactorial in nature and include genetic factors, advanced age, female gender, physical activity participation, poor psychologic health, tobacco use, history of neck or low back pain, and rear-end automobile accidents. The presence of cervical spinal degeneration on imaging studies is not considered a risk factor for neck pain. The natural history of neck pain in adults is favorable overall, but pain recurrence and chronicity are reported in a substantial number of patients.

72. Surgical treatment options for patients with **cervical radiculopathy** secondary to cervical disc herniation at one or two contiguous levels include posterior foraminotomy with discectomy, anterior cervical discectomy and fusion, cervical total disc arthroplasty, and hybrid procedures.

73. **Degenerative cervical myelopathy** is the most common cause of spinal cord dysfunction in patients older than age 55. Diagnosis is based on a history of myelopathic symptoms, the presence of myelopathic signs or neurologic deficits on physical examination, and imaging findings that demonstrate cervical cord compression. Surgical treatment is indicated for moderate or severe cervical spondylotic myelopathy unless medically contraindicated, because no good nonsurgical treatment exists. Factors that are considered in selection of the optimal surgical approach include sagittal alignment, anatomic location of compressive pathology, number of levels of spinal cord compression, type of compressive pathology (spondylosis, ossification of the posterior longitudinal ligament [OPLL]), presence of spinal instability or deformity, and bone quality. Surgical options include posterior procedures (laminoplasty, laminectomy, or laminectomy in combination with instrumented posterior fusion), anterior procedures (discectomy, corpectomy, or hybrid procedures), and circumferential procedures. Cervical disc arthroplasty is an option for treatment of cervical degenerative myelopathy involving one or two spinal levels where stenosis is limited to the level of the disc space.

74. A high prevalence of anatomic abnormalities is noted on thoracic spine MRI studies in asymptomatic patients. **Thoracic disc herniations** associated with neurologic deficit are rare lesions with an estimated incidence of one per million population and occur most commonly in the lower third of the thoracic spine. An anterior transthoracic surgical approach is preferred for central thoracic disc herniations, especially if the herniation is large and calcified. Posterolateral surgical approaches are an option for paracentral and lateral thoracic disc herniations. Thoracic spinal stenosis is increasingly recognized and occurs most frequently at the thoracolumbar junction. Posterior thoracic decompression, posterior decompression and fusion in combination with segmental pedicle screw-rod fixation, and circumferential decompression and fusion with instrumentation from an entirely posterior approach are options for treatment of thoracic stenosis.

75. Evidence-based treatment options for symptomatic **lumbar degenerative disc disease** include a structured outpatient physical rehabilitation program, spinal fusion, and lumbar disc arthroplasty.

76. **Lumbar disc herniations** most commonly occur at the L4–L5 and L5–S1 levels. Diagnosis is based on clinical assessment and confirmed with MRI. Standard **terminology** used to describe lumbar disc pathology on MRI includes **degeneration, bulge, protrusion, extrusion, and sequestration**. The location of disc pathology is described in terms of location within the spinal canal and relationship along the circumference of the annulus fibrosus (central, posterolateral, foraminal, or extraforaminal). A **central** disc herniation compresses the thecal sac and one or more of the caudal nerve roots. A **posterolateral** disc herniation compresses the traversing nerve root of the motion segment. A **foraminal** or **extraforaminal** disc herniation compresses the exiting nerve root of the motion segment. The majority of patients with a lumbar disc herniation improve with nonoperative treatment. Appropriate criteria for surgical intervention include: functionally incapacitating leg pain extending below the knee within a nerve root distribution, nerve root tension signs with or without neurologic deficit, failure to improve with 4–8 weeks of nonsurgical treatment, a confirmatory MRI study that correlates with the patient's physical findings and pain distribution. Additional criteria include a progressive neurologic deficit or cauda equina syndrome. Open lumbar discectomy using microsurgical techniques remains the gold standard for the treatment of a symptomatic lumbar disc herniation.

77. **Lumbar spinal stenosis** is defined as any type of narrowing of the spinal canal, nerve root canals, or intervertebral foramen. The two main types of lumbar spinal stenosis are congenital-developmental and acquired spinal stenosis. Patients with symptomatic lumbar spinal stenosis present with symptoms of **neurogenic claudication**, which include tiredness, heaviness, and discomfort in the lower extremities with ambulation. The distance walked until symptoms begin and the maximum distance that the patient can walk without stopping varies from day to day, and even during the same walk. Patients report that leaning forward relieves symptoms, while activities performed in extension (e.g., walking down hill) exacerbate symptoms. In contrast, patients with **vascular claudication** describe cramping or tightness in the calf region associated with ambulation. The distance walked

before symptoms occur is constant and is not affected by posture. Surgical treatment options for lumbar spinal stenosis include insertion of an interspinous spacer, lumbar decompression (laminotomy or laminectomy), and lumbar decompression combined with fusion with or without the use of spinal instrumentation.

78. As **SIJ pain** presents with symptoms similar to hip and lumbar spine pathology, the SIJ is often overlooked as a pain generator. The diagnosis of SIJ pain is based on physical examination of the SIJ and confirmatory diagnostic injections. During physical examination, the diagnosis of SIJ pain is supported by localization of pain immediately inferomedial to the posterior superior iliac spine (Fortin finger test) and reproduction of symptoms with three or more provocative maneuvers, which include the Gaenslen test, pelvic distraction, pelvic compression, sacral thrust, thigh thrust, and Patrick or FABER (flexion-abduction-external rotation) tests. Image-guided diagnostic intraarticular SIJ injections are used to confirm the diagnosis of SIJ pain in patients with a history and physical findings consistent with SIJ pathology. Nonoperative treatment is initially indicated and may include physical and manual therapy, medications, and pelvic belts or supports. For patients who fail to improve with nonoperative treatment, SIJ fusion through a minimally invasive or open surgical approach is an option.

ADULT SPINAL DEFORMITIES

79. **Spondylolisthesis** refers to anterior displacement of the cranial vertebral body in relation to the subjacent vertebral body. The deformity not only involves the olisthetic vertebra but affects the entire spinal column above the level of slippage as the entire trunk moves forward with the displaced vertebra. The **degree of slippage** is measured as the amount of anterior translation of the displaced vertebra relative to the superior aspect of the inferior vertebra and is expressed as a percentage according to the **Meyerding Classification**: grade 1, 1%–25%; grade 2, 26%–50%; grade 3, 51%–75%; grade 4, 76%–100%; and grade 5, slippage of the L5 vertebra anterior and distal to the superior S1 endplate, referred to as spondyloptosis. Slippages <50% are referred to as low grade spondylolisthesis, while slippages ≥50% are referred to as high grade spondylolisthesis. The **Wiltse Classification** identifies **types of lumbar spondylolisthesis** based on a combination of etiologic and anatomic features as dysplastic, isthmic, degenerative, traumatic, pathologic, or postsurgical.

80. **Isthmic spondylolisthesis** most commonly occurs at the L5–S1 level, while **degenerative spondylolisthesis** most commonly occurs at the L4–L5 level. Radiculopathy most commonly involves the exiting nerve root in isthmic spondylolisthesis, while the traversing nerve root is most commonly involved in degenerative spondylolisthesis.

81. The two most **common types of scoliosis in adults** are **degenerative** and **idiopathic**. Degenerative scoliosis, also called *de novo* scoliosis, develops after age 40 in patients with previously straight spines as the result of multilevel asymmetric disc and facet joint degeneration. The second type of scoliosis presenting in adulthood is idiopathic scoliosis, which most commonly develops in adolescence and is unrecognized or left untreated. Nonoperative treatment is appropriate for patients without disabling spine-related symptoms but is unlikely to provide significant long-term improvement in pain and function. Surgical indications for adult scoliosis include progressive deformity, pain, and symptomatic neural compression.

82. The various types of **spinal osteotomies** that play a role in the surgical correction of spinal deformities include Smith-Petersen osteotomy, Ponte osteotomy, pedicle subtraction osteotomy, combined anterior and posterior osteotomy, and vertebral column resection.

83. There is an interrelationship between the orientation of the distal lumbar spine, sacrum, and the pelvic unit, which influences sagittal alignment of the spine. Three **pelvic parameters** are measured: pelvic incidence (PI), sacral slope (SS), and pelvic tilt (PT). PI is a fixed anatomic parameter unique to the individual. SS and PT are variable parameters. The relationship among the parameters determines the overall alignment of the sacropelvic unit according to the formula $PI = PT + SS$.

SPINAL TRAUMA

84. Patients with a traumatic spinal cord injury are assessed according to the **International Standards for Neurological Classification of Spinal Cord Injury** (ISNCSCI). The **skeletal level of injury** is defined as the level in the spine where the greatest vertebral damage is found on radiographic examination. The **neurologic level of injury** is defined as the most caudal segment of the spinal cord with normal sensory function and antigravity (grade 3 or more) motor function bilaterally, provided there is intact sensory and motor function proximal to this segment.

85. The **American Spinal Injury Association Impairment Scale**, a component of the ISNCSCI, is a five-category scale used to specify the severity of neurologic injury: **A = Complete:** No sensory or motor function is preserved in the sacral segments S4–S5; **B = Sensory Incomplete:** Sensory but not motor function is preserved below the neurologic level and includes the sacral segments S4–S5; **C = Motor Incomplete:** More than half of key muscles below the neurologic level have a muscle grade less than 3; **D = Motor Incomplete:** At least half of key muscles below the neurologic level have a muscle grade 3 or greater; and **E = Normal.**

86. **Incomplete spinal cord syndromes** include: cruciate paralysis, central cord syndrome, anterior cord syndrome, Brown-Séquard syndrome, conus medullaris syndrome, and cauda equina syndrome. **Cruciate paralysis** results from damage to the anterior spinal cord at the C2 level (level of corticospinal tract decussation) with greater loss of motor function in upper extremities compared with lower extremities, variable sensory loss, and variable

cranial nerve deficits. **Central cord syndrome** results from damage to the central spinal cord below the C2 level with greater loss of motor function in upper extremities, especially in the hands, compared with lower extremities with variable sensory loss, at least partial sacral sparing, and variable bowel and bladder involvement. **Anterior cord syndrome** results from damage to the anterior spinal cord with relative preservation of proprioception and variable loss of pain sensation, temperature sensation, and motor function. **Brown-Séquard syndrome** results from damage to the lateral half of the spinal cord with relative ipsilateral proprioception and motor function loss and contralateral pain and temperature sensation loss. **Conus medullaris syndrome** results from damage to the sacral segments of the spinal cord located in the conus medullaris, which typically results in an areflexic bowel and bladder, lower extremity sensory loss, and incomplete paraplegia. **Cauda equina syndrome** results from damage to lumbosacral nerve roots within the neural canal, which results in variable lower extremity motor and sensory function, bowel and bladder dysfunction, and saddle anesthesia.

87. **The AOSpine Trauma Classification** subdivides the spinal column into **four major regions**: upper cervical spine (occiput-C2), subaxial cervical spine (C3–C7), thoracolumbar spine (T1–L5), and sacral spine (S1–S5, coccyx). Injuries are classified based on **fracture morphology** (A, B, C), **neurologic status** (N), and **region-specific clinical modifiers** (M), which influence treatment decision making. **Three main injury morphologies** are identified: **Type A,** compression injuries; **Type B,** tension band injuries; **Type C,** translational injuries. In the subaxial cervical region only, when the dominant injury involves the facet joints, this is classified as **Type F.** Neurologic status is identified as: N0: neurologically normal; N1: transient neurologic deficit; N2: nerve root injury, cranial nerve injury, or radiculopathy; N3: incomplete spinal cord, conus or cauda equina injury; N4: complete spinal cord injury; Nx: unexaminable patient; and, N+: ongoing spinal cord compression.

88. **Upper cervical spine injuries** occur in a bimodal distribution. The first spike involves younger, mainly male patients aged 25–40 years, and is caused by road traffic accidents and falls from a height. The second spike affects patients aged 65 and older and mainly results from ground-level falls. In patients over age 65, odontoid fractures are the most common isolated spine fracture, and have the highest morbidity and mortality of any spine fracture—up to 50% depending upon age and comorbidities. The **AOSpine upper cervical injury classification** categorizes injuries into **three anatomic regions**: (1) Occipital condyle and craniocervical junction: occipital condyle fractures, atlanto-occipital dislocation; (2) Atlas and atlantoaxial joints: atlas fractures, transverse ligament injuries, atlantoaxial dislocation; and (3) Axis and C2–C3 joints: odontoid fractures, traumatic spondylolisthesis of the axis, axis body fractures, and C2–C3 dislocations. **Clinical modifiers** for upper cervical injuries are M1: injury at high risk of nonunion with nonoperative treatment; M2: injury with significant potential for instability; M3: patient-specific factors adversely affecting healing potential; and, M4: vascular injury or abnormality affecting treatment.

89. **Subaxial cervical injuries** are responsible for two-thirds of all cervical injuries and may be stratified as Type A, B or C injuries according to the **AOSpine subaxial cervical classification**. For **Type A injuries**, A0 injuries (minor injuries such as isolated lamina or spinous process fractures) are treated nonoperatively with a rigid cervical orthosis. A1 (compression fracture, single endplate involvement) and A2 injuries (coronal split or pincer fracture involving both endplates) lack posterior vertebral body wall involvement and are treated initially with a rigid orthosis in most cases. Patients with A1 and A2 injuries who fail nonoperative treatment or present with extensive osseous involvement or traumatic disc herniation are treated with anterior decompression, fusion, and plate stabilization. Burst fractures involving one (A3) or both (A4) endplates, with posterior vertebral body wall involvement but without disruption of the posterior tension band, often require surgical treatment due to neurologic injury and/or extensive osseous disruption. For **Type B injuries**, B1 injuries (distraction injuries through the posterior osseous structures) are treated nonoperatively in neurologically intact patients, while surgical stabilization is performed for patients with displaced injuries, neurologic deficits, or those who fail nonoperative treatment. B2 injuries (flexion-distraction injuries that disrupt the posterior tension band and involve capsular or ligamentous structures and possibly the anterior spinal column) and B3 injuries (disruption of the anterior tension band) usually require surgical treatment. **Type C injuries** (translational) are highly unstable injuries and require surgical treatment. **Facet injuries** may occur as the primary component of an injury or in association with other A, B, or C injury types. When the dominant injury involves the facet joints, this is classified as a **Type F injury** according to the AOSpine classification. F1 injuries (unilateral nondisplaced facet fractures involving either the superior or inferior facet with a fragment size <1 cm, or fractures involving <40% of the lateral mass) are treated initially with a rigid collar in the absence of radiculopathy, listhesis, or fracture comminution. F2 injuries (unilateral facet injuries with displacement or a fracture fragment size >1 cm, or injuries involving >40% of the lateral mass) are treated operatively. F3 injuries (ipsilateral disruption of the pedicle and lamina with dissociation of the superior and inferior articular processes from the vertebral body), also referred to as a fracture-separation of the lateral mass, are treated surgically with anterior or posterior instrumentation and fusion over two motion segments. F4 injuries (subluxed, perched or dislocated facets, unilateral or bilateral) require reduction, decompression, and surgical stabilization. **Clinical modifiers** for subaxial cervical injuries are M1: posterior capsuloligamentous complex injury without complete disruption; M2: critical disc herniation; M3: stiffening or metabolic bone diseases such as ankylosing spondylitis; and, M4: signs of vertebral artery injury.

90. **Thoracolumbar injuries** may involve the thoracic region (T1–T9), thoracolumbar junction (T10–L2), or lumbar region (L3–L5). More than 50% of these injuries involve the thoracolumbar junction. Recognizable categories of injuries include compression fractures, burst fractures, flexion-distraction injuries, fracture-dislocations, and

extension injuries. The **AOSpine thoracolumbar classification** identifies three main injury morphologies. **Type A injuries** are compression injuries with an intact tension band and include fractures commonly described as compression fractures and stable burst fractures. **Type B injuries** are anterior or posterior tension band injuries, which occur through distraction and include fractures commonly described as unstable burst fractures, Chance fractures, flexion-distraction injuries, and extension injuries. **Type C injuries** are associated with translation along any axis and include injuries described as fracture-dislocations. **Clinical modifiers** for thoracolumbar injuries are M1: indeterminate injury to the posterior tension band based on clinical examination or imaging studies, and, M2: patient-specific comorbidities that influence surgical decision making such as metabolic bone diseases, ankylosing disorders, or burns or abrasions involving skin across the injured spinal levels.

91. **Sacral fractures** may occur as the result of high-energy or low-energy injury mechanisms and include insufficiency or stress fractures in specific subgroups such as endurance athletes, patients with osteoporosis, and following instrumented lumbosacral fusion surgery. The **AOSpine sacral classification system** stratifies injuries into three main groups. **Type A injuries** involve the lower sacrococcygeal region below the level of the SIJ and do not impact posterior pelvic or spinopelvic stability. However, some Type A injuries may have adverse outcomes due to associated pain and neurologic dysfunction. **Type B injuries** impact posterior pelvic ring stability but do not impact spinopelvic stability. These are osteoligamentous injuries that unilaterally disrupt the posterior pelvic ring in a longitudinal fashion but do not impact spinopelvic instability as the ipsilateral superior S1 facet is continuous with the medial portion of the sacrum. **Type C injuries** are sacral injuries such as bilateral longitudinal fractures or U- or H-type fractures, which dissociate the lower appendicular skeleton from the pelvis and result in spinopelvic instability. **Clinical modifiers** for sacral fractures are M1: soft tissue injury; M2: metabolic bone disease; M3: anterior pelvic ring injury; and M4: SIJ injury.

92. **Sports-related injuries** may involve the muscles, ligaments, intervertebral discs, osseous structures, and neural elements. Common athletic-related **cervical spine injuries** include muscular strains, intervertebral disc injuries, major and minor cervical spine fractures, "stinger" or "burner" injuries, and cervical cord neuropraxia. A **stinger** is a peripheral nerve injury involving individual cervical nerve roots or a portion of the brachial plexus associated with unilateral burning arm pain or paresthesias, and may be accompanied by weakness, most often in the muscle groups supplied by the C5 and C6 nerve roots (deltoid, biceps, supraspinatus, infraspinatus) on the affected side. Bilateral symptoms suggest a different etiology, such as a neurapraxic injury of the spinal cord. **Cervical cord neuropraxia** is a temporary neurologic episode following cervical trauma and is characterized by sensory symptoms with or without motor changes involving at least two extremities in the absence of cervical instability. The most commonly described mechanism of injury is axial compression with a component of either hyperflexion or hyperextension. **Lumbar spine injuries** are also commonly encountered in athletes. In adolescents, the most common lumbar conditions diagnosed following an athletic-related injury are lumbar strain, spondylolysis/spondylolisthesis, lumbar disc injuries, and overuse syndromes. In adults, the most common conditions diagnosed following an athletic-related injury are lumbar strain, discogenic pain syndromes, disc herniations, and spinal stenosis.

SYSTEMIC PROBLEMS AFFECTING THE SPINAL COLUMN

93. The **differential diagnosis of a spinal tumor** is determined by the anatomic compartment in which it occurs: extradural, intradural-extramedullary, or intramedullary. **Extradural tumors** may be primary spinal tumors (benign or malignant) or secondary tumors (due to metastatic disease). The most common extradural spinal tumor is a metastatic tumor. **Intradural-extramedullary tumors** arise within the dura but outside the spinal cord. The most common tumors occurring in the intradural-extramedullary compartment are schwannomas, neurofibromas, and meningiomas. If the tumor arises as the nerve root leaves the dural sac, it may possess both an intradural and extradural component (dumbbell-shaped tumor). **Intramedullary tumors** originate from the parenchyma of the spinal cord. The most common types of intramedullary tumors are ependymomas, astrocytomas, and hemangioblastomas.

94. **Primary tumors** of the spine arise *de novo* in the bone, cartilage, neural or ligamentous structures, and are classified as extradural or intradural. Primary spine tumors are extremely rare. The most common primary osseous malignant process is multiple myeloma. Secondary tumors are either metastatic to the spine from distant origins or grow into the spine from adjacent structures (e.g., Pancoast tumor from the upper lobe of the lung). **Metastatic lesions** involving the spine are the most common type of spinal tumor and account for 95% of all spinal tumors. The malignancies which most commonly metastasize to the spine in descending order of frequency are: breast (21%), lung (14%), prostate (7.5%), renal (5%), gastrointestinal (5%), and thyroid (2.5%). A useful mnemonic to aid recall of common malignancies that metastasize to the spine is **P T B**arnum **L**oves **K**ids (prostate, thyroid, breast, lung, kidney).

95. **Osteoporosis** is the most prevalent metabolic bone disease and is characterized by a decreased amount of normally mineralized bone per unit volume. Osteoporosis may be diagnosed based on a T-score less than or equal to −2.5 on dual energy x-ray absorptiometry (DEXA) and by clinical factors. Half of all osteoporotic-related fractures occur in patients with bone mineral density (BMD) values classified as low bone mass (osteopenia). Assessment of the probability for fracture using the Fracture Risk Assessment (FRAX) tool can be used to determine the 10-year probability of major osteoporotic fracture and identify patients with low bone mass who could potentially

benefit from pharmacologic treatment. Preventative measures include counseling patients to maintain adequate dietary calcium and vitamin D intake and a routine of weight-bearing and muscle-strengthening exercise to reduce the risk of falls and fractures. Options for pharmacologic therapies include various antiresorptive and anabolic medications.

96. **Vertebral compression fractures** are the most common type of fracture related to osteoporosis. Vertebral fractures are two to three times more prevalent than hip or wrist fractures. A person who develops an osteoporotic vertebral compression fracture is five times more likely to develop an additional fracture when compared with a control patient without a fracture. As many as two-thirds of fractures are asymptomatic and diagnosed incidentally on radiographs. Initial treatment options for acute osteoporotic vertebral compression fractures include analgesics, activity modification, bracing, physical therapy, and injections. Percutaneous vertebral augmentation procedures such as vertebroplasty or kyphoplasty are considered for patients with inadequate pain relief with initial nonsurgical care or when persistent pain adversely affects quality of life.

97. **Spinal infection** should be suspected in patients who present with nonmechanical back pain symptoms and risk factors for infection such as diabetes, immunosuppression, advanced age, intravenous drug use history, travel history to endemic areas, or recent surgical procedures. Organisms responsible for spinal infections include bacteria, which cause pyogenic infections; tuberculosis or fungi, which are responsible for granulomatosis infections; or parasites, which are the least common etiology. Evaluation should begin with a detailed history and physical examination and initial lab tests, including blood and urine cultures and C-reactive protein levels. MRI with gadolinium contrast is the most reliable imaging study for diagnosis and determination of the extent of spinal infections. Identification of the responsible organism(s) and determination of antibiotic sensitivities, most commonly obtained through CT-guided needle biopsy and culture, are necessary to guide medical treatment. Note that the disc is nearly always involved in pyogenic vertebral infections, while granulomatous infections often do not involve the disc space. Initial treatment is nonsurgical in most cases and consists of antibiotic therapy and immobilization. Surgery is indicated for open biopsy in cases where closed biopsy is negative, for persistent or recurrent infection despite appropriate medical management, for drainage of clinically important abscesses, and for treatment of neurologic deficit, spinal instability, or progressive spinal deformity due to extensive disc and/or vertebral body destruction.

98. **Rheumatoid arthritis** is a chronic, systemic inflammatory disorder of uncertain etiology that affects the synovium of joints. It is an immunologically mediated systemic disorder that affects articular and nonarticular organ systems. The articular involvement is a symmetrical peripheral joint disease affecting large and small joints. Axial involvement predominantly affects the cervical region, especially the upper cervical spine. Three types of cervical deformities may develop secondary to rheumatoid disease, and may present singularly or in combination: atlantoaxial subluxation, atlantoaxial impaction (vertical migration of the odontoid), and subaxial subluxation.

99. **Ankylosing spondylitis (AS)** and **diffuse idiopathic skeletal hyperostosis (DISH)** are the most commonly encountered ankylosing spinal disorders. **AS** is a seronegative rheumatic disease, or axial spondyloarthropathy, which presents with inflammatory arthritic pain that involves the SIJs and other spinal regions. A classic feature of AS is inflammation at the attachments of ligaments, tendons, and joint capsules to bone, referred to as enthesopathy. Reactive bone formation characteristically involves the outer layers of the annulus fibrosus of the intervertebral disc and leads to formation of marginal syndesmophytes that may progress to a characteristic appearance described as "bamboo spine." Ossification often involves the facet joints and spinal ligaments. **DISH** is a proliferative bone disease of unknown etiology and is associated with type 2 diabetes, cardiac disease, and obesity. DISH is often asymptomatic and diagnosed as an incidental finding on imaging studies. The radiographic hallmark of DISH is the presence of asymmetric, nonmarginal syndesmophytes, which appear as flowing anterior ossification originating from the anterior longitudinal ligament, typically involving four or more vertebrae in the thoracic region. The intervertebral discs, facet joints, and SIJs are not involved in DISH. Patients with ankylosed spines secondary to AS and DISH are at increased risk of spine fractures and their clinical outcomes are worse compared with the general spine trauma population. Low energy trauma may lead to highly unstable three-column injuries whose diagnosis is often delayed and is not infrequently associated with secondary neurologic deterioration. The long rigid lever arms of stiff spine segments above and below the level of injury magnify spinal instability and make treatment challenging. Nonoperative management is associated with a high complication rate and prompt surgical stabilization is recommended.

EMERGING SPINAL TECHNOLOGIES

100. A wide range of **assistive technologies** have been introduced for use in spinal surgery. These include advanced intraoperative imaging systems such as three-dimensional fluoroscopy and intraoperative CT, surgical navigation, and robotics. Each technology or combination of technologies offers potential advantages compared with traditional surgical techniques, including increased procedural accuracy, precise orientation to unexposed spinal anatomy, limitation of radiation exposure, and reduction in operative time. Obstacles to widespread adoption of these technologies include cost considerations, learning-curve issues, and limited high-quality data to support improved clinical outcomes associated with their use.

REGIONAL SPINAL ANATOMY

I

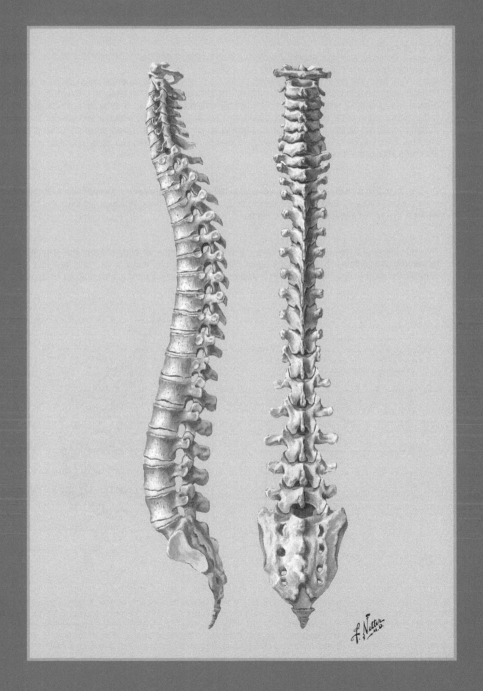

CLINICALLY RELEVANT ANATOMY OF THE CERVICAL REGION

Vincent J. Devlin, MD and Darren L. Bergey, MD

OSTEOLOGY

1. Describe the bony landmarks of the occiput.

   The occiput forms the posterior osseous covering for the cerebellum. The **foramen magnum** is the opening through which the spinal cord joins the brainstem. The anterior border of the foramen magnum is termed the **basion** (clivus), and the posterior border is termed the **opisthion**. The **inion** or **external occipital protuberance** is the midline region of the occiput where bone is greatest in thickness. The **superior and inferior nuchal lines** extend laterally and distally from the inion. The transverse sinus is located in close proximity to the inion (Fig. 1.1). The area in the midline below the inion is an ideal location for screw insertion for occipital fixation as it is the thickest portion of the occiput.

2. What is meant by typical and atypical cervical vertebrae?

   C3, C4, C5, and C6 are defined as **typical cervical vertebrae** because they share common structural characteristics. In contrast, C1 (atlas), C2 (axis), and C7 (vertebra prominens) possess unique structural and functional features and are therefore termed **atypical cervical vertebrae**.

3. Describe a typical cervical vertebra.

   The components of a typical cervical vertebra (C3–C6) include an **anterior body** and a **posterior arch** formed by **laminae** and **pedicles**. Posteriorly, the lamina blends into the **lateral mass**, which comprises the bony region between the superior and inferior articular processes. The paired superior and inferior articular processes from

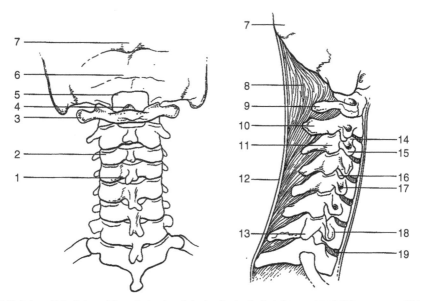

Fig. 1.1 Posterior and lateral views of the occiput and cervical spine showing the basic bony anatomy. *1*, Spinous process; *2*, lateral articular process or lateral mass; *3*, transverse process of C1; *4*, odontoid process of C2; *5*, foramen magnum; *6*, inferior nuchal line; *7*, inion; *8*, ligamentum nuchae; *9*, posterior arch of C1; *10*, spinous process of C2; *11*, lateral mass; *12*, supraspinous ligament; *13*, lateral articular process; *14*, uncinate process; *15*, anterior tubercle of transverse process; *16*, neural foramen; *17*, transverse foramen; *18*, carotid tubercle; *19*, intervertebral disc. (From An HS, Simpson JM. Surgery of the Cervical Spine. Baltimore: Williams & Wilkins; 1994, with permission.)

adjacent vertebrae form the **facet joint**. Anteriorly, the **uncovertebral (neurocentral) joints** are formed by bony ridges that extend upward from the lateral margin of the superior surface of the vertebral body and articulate with a corresponding shallow concavity of the vertebra above to form the anterior border of the intervertebral foramen. The **intervertebral foramina** protect the exiting spinal nerves and are located behind the vertebral bodies between the pedicles of adjacent vertebrae. The **transverse processes** of the lower cervical spine are directed anterolaterally and composed of an anterior costal element and a posterior transverse element. The **transverse foramen**, located at the base of the transverse process, permits passage of the vertebral artery. The **spinous process** originates in the midsagittal plane at the junction of the laminae and is bifid between C2 and C6 (Fig. 1.2).

4. **What are the distinguishing features of C1 (atlas)?**
The ring-like atlas (C1) is unique because during development its body fuses with the axis (C2) to form the odontoid process. Thus the atlas has no body. The atlas also lacks a spinous process. It is composed of two thick, load-bearing lateral masses, with concave superior and inferior articular facets. Connecting these facets are a relatively straight, short anterior arch and a longer, curved posterior arch. The anterior ring has an articular facet on its posterior aspect for articulation with the dens. The posterior ring has a groove on its posterior-superior surface for the vertebral artery. The weakest point of the ring is at the narrowed areas where the anterior and posterior arches connect to the lateral masses (location of a Jefferson fracture). The transverse process of the atlas has a single tubercle, which protrudes laterally and can be palpated in the space between the tip of the mastoid process and the ramus of the mandible (Fig. 1.3).

5. **What are the distinguishing features of C2 (axis)?**
The axis (C2) receives its name from its **odontoid process (dens)**, which forms the axis of rotation for motion through the atlantoaxial joint (Fig. 1.4). The dens is a bony process extending cranially from the body of C2, formed from the embryologic body of the atlas (C1). The dens has an anterior hyaline articular surface for articulation with the anterior arch of C1, as well as a posterior articular surface for articulation with the transverse ligament. The C2 superior articular processes are located anterior and lateral to the spinal canal, while the C2 inferior articular processes are located posterior and lateral to the spinal canal. The superior and inferior articular processes on each side are connected by the **pars interarticularis**. Hyperflexion or hyperextension injuries may subject the axis to shear stresses, resulting in a fracture through the pars region (termed a *hangman's fracture*). The **C2 pedicle** is defined as that portion of the C2 vertebra connecting the posterior osseous structures with the vertebral body. This is a narrow area located between the vertebral body and the pars interarticularis. The

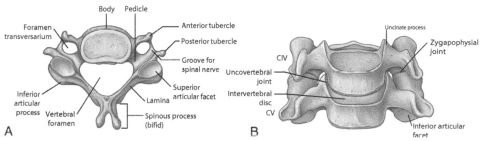

Fig. 1.2 Typical cervical vertebra. (A) Superior. (B) Anterior. (From Drake R, Vogl AW. Mitchell AW. Gray's Atlas of Anatomy. 2nd ed. Philadelphia, PA: Elsevier; 2014.)

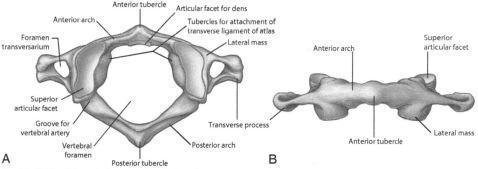

Fig. 1.3 (A) Atlas (C1 vertebra) superior view. (B) Atlas (C1 vertebra) anterior view. (From Drake R, Vogl AW, Mitchell AWN. Gray's Atlas of Anatomy. 2nd ed. Philadelphia, PA: Elsevier; 2014.)

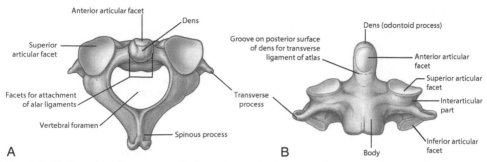

Fig. 1.4 (A) Axis (C2 vertebra) superior view. (B) Axis (C2 vertebra) anterior view. (From Drake RL, Vogl W, Mitchell AWN. Gray's Atlas of Anatomy. 2nd ed. Philadelphia, PA: Elsevier; 2014.)

atlantodens interval (ADI) is the space between the hyaline cartilage surfaces of the anterior tubercle of the atlas and the anterior dens. Normal adult and childhood ADI measurements are 3 mm and 5 mm, respectively.

6. What are the distinguishing features of C7 (vertebra prominens)?
   The unique anatomic features of the C7 vertebra reflect its location as the transitional vertebra at the cervicothoracic junction:
   - Long, nonbifid spinous process, which provides a useful landmark
   - Its foramen transversarium usually contains vertebral veins but usually does not contain the vertebral artery, which generally enters the cervical spine at the C6 level
   - The C7 transverse process is large and possesses only a posterior tubercle
   - The C7 lateral mass is the thinnest lateral mass in the cervical spine
   - The inferior articular process of C7 is oriented in a relatively perpendicular direction (similar to a thoracic facet joint)

ARTICULATIONS, LIGAMENTS, AND DISCS

7. Describe how normal range of motion is distributed across the cervical region.
   Facet joint orientation, bony architecture, intervertebral discs, uncovertebral joints, and ligaments all play a role in determining range of motion at various levels of the cervical spine. Approximately 50% of cervical flexion-extension occurs at the occiput–C1 level. Approximately 50% of cervical rotation occurs at the C1–C2 level. Lesser amounts of flexion-extension, rotation, and lateral bending occur segmentally between C2 and C7.

8. What are the key anatomic features of the atlanto-occipital (O–C1) articulation?
   The atlanto-occipital joints are synovial joints comprised of the convex occipital condyles that articulate with the concave lateral masses of the atlas. Motion at the O–C1 segment is restricted primarily to flexion-extension due to bony and ligamentous constraints and absence of an intervertebral disc. The most important ligaments are the paired **alar ligaments** (extend from the tip of the dens to the medial aspect of each occipital condyle and restrict rotation of the occiput on the dens). The **tectorial membrane** is also important (continuous with the posterior longitudinal ligament and extends from the posterior body of C2 to the anterior foramen magnum and occiput). Less important ligaments include the anterior and posterior atlanto-occipital membrane, the O–C1 joint capsules, and the apical ligament (Fig. 1.5).

9. What are the key anatomic features of the atlantoaxial (C1–C2) articulation?
   The atlantoaxial articulation is composed of three synovial joints—paired lateral mass articulations and a central articulation between the dens and the anterior C1 arch and transverse ligament (see Fig. 1.5). The primary motion at the atlantoaxial joint is rotation; approximately 50% of cervical spine rotation occurs at the C1–C2 joints. The approximation of the odontoid against the anterior arch of C1 resists translation of C1 relative to C2.
   The **transverse atlantal ligament**, the major stabilizer at the C1–C2 level, attaches to the medial aspect of the lateral masses of the atlas (see Fig. 1.5). This ligament has a wide middle portion where it articulates with the posterior surface of the dens. Superior and inferior longitudinal fasciculi extend to insert on the anterior foramen magnum and the posterior body of the axis respectively. These structures are collectively named the **cruciform ligament**. This ligament holds the dens firmly against the anterior arch of the atlas. Other important ligaments attaching to C2 include:
   - **Anterior atlantoaxial ligament:** continuous with the anterior longitudinal ligament in the lower cervical spine
   - **Posterior atlantoaxial ligament:** continuous with the ligamentum flavum in the subaxial spine
   - **Apical ligament:** extends from the tip of the dens to the foramen magnum
   - **Alar ligaments:** extend from the lateral dens and attach to the medial border of the occipital condyles

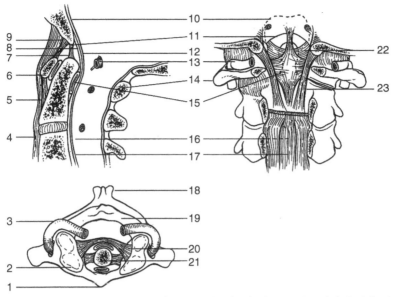

Fig. 1.5 Ligamentous and bony anatomy of the upper cervical region. *1*, Anterior tubercle; *2*, superior articular facet; *3*, vertebral artery; *4*, anterior longitudinal ligament; *5*, anterior atlas-axis membrane; *6*, anterior arch of atlas; *7*, apical ligament; *8*, vertical cruciform ligament; *9*, anterior atlas–occipital membrane; *10*, attachment of tectorial membrane; *11*, anterior edge of foramen magnum; *12*, tectorial membrane; *13*, vertebral artery; *14*, atlas; *15*, transverse ligament; *16*, origin of tectorial membrane; *17*, posterior longitudinal ligament; *18*, spinous process (axis); *19*, atlas; *20*, transverse ligament; *21*, dens (odontoid process); *22*, alar ligament; *23*, deep tectorial membrane. (From An HS, Simpson JM. Surgery of the Cervical Spine. Baltimore: Williams & Wilkins; 1994, with permission.)

10. Name the arrangement of ligaments at the craniovertebral junction as the spine is sectioned in an anterior to posterior direction.
    1. Anterior atlanto-occipital membrane (continuous with anterior longitudinal ligament)
    2. Apical ligament (extends from tip of the dens to anterior edge of foramen magnum)
    3. Alar ligaments (extend from the tip of the dens to the medial aspect of each occipital condyle)
    4. Cruciform ligament
    5. Tectorial membrane (continuous with the posterior longitudinal ligament)
    6. Posterior atlanto-occipital membrane (continuous with the ligamentum flavum)

11. Describe the ligament anatomy of the subaxial spine.
    The major ligaments of the subaxial cervical spine are:
    - **Anterior longitudinal ligament (ALL):** This strong ligament extends from the body of the axis to the sacrum, binding the anterior aspect of the vertebral bodies and intervertebral discs together. It resists hyperextension of the spine and gives stability to the anterior aspect of the disc space. It is continuous with anterior atlanto-occipital membrane.
    - **Posterior longitudinal ligament (PLL):** This is a weaker ligament, which extends from the axis to the sacrum. It is thicker and wider in the cervical spine than in the thoracolumbar segments. It serves to protect from hyperflexion injury and reinforces the intervertebral discs from herniation. It is continuous with tectorial membrane.
    - **Ligamentum flavum:** This structure may be considered to be a segmental ligament, which attaches to adjacent laminae. This structure attaches to the ventral aspect of the superior lamina and the dorsal aspect of the inferior lamina. Laterally, the ligamentum flavum is in continuity with the facet capsules.
    - **Ligamentum nuchae, supraspinous ligament, and interspinous ligament:** These ligaments lie dorsal to or between the spinous processes, respectively. The supraspinous ligament extends from the sacrum to C7 and is in continuity with the ligamentum nuchae. The ligamentum nuchae extends from C7 to the occiput and forms a sheet-like structure that serves as an attachment for neighboring muscles and acts as a posterior tension band to maintain an upright neck posture.

12. Describe the articulations between vertebrae in the subaxial cervical spine (C3–C7).
    The anatomy of the lower cervical spine (C3–C7) can be described in terms of a functional spinal unit consisting of two adjacent vertebrae, an intervertebral disc, and related ligaments and facet joint capsules. The anterior

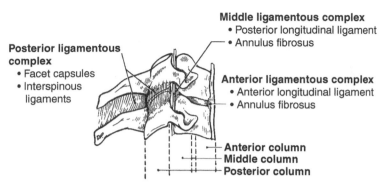

Middle ligamentous complex
• Posterior longitudinal ligament
• Annulus fibrosus

Posterior ligamentous complex
• Facet capsules
• Interspinous ligaments

Anterior ligamentous complex
• Anterior longitudinal ligament
• Annulus fibrosus

Anterior column
Middle column
Posterior column

Fig. 1.6 Components of the three columns of the cervical spine. (From Stauffer ES, MacMillan M. Fractures and dislocations of the cervical spine. In: Rockwood CA, Green DP, Bucholz RW, et al., editors. Fractures in Adults, vol. 2. 4th ed. Philadelphia, PA: Lippincott-Raven; 1996, pp. 1473–1628, with permission.)

elements include the vertebral body and intervening intervertebral disc. Paired lateral columns consist of pedicles, lateral masses, and facet joints. The posterior structures include the laminae, spinous processes, and posterior ligamentous complex. Various theories have conceptualized the functional anatomy of the cervical spine in terms of a columnar structure (Fig. 1.6).

13. **What are the unique features of the subaxial cervical facet joints?**
At each cervical level (C3–C7) there are paired superior and inferior articular processes. The superior articular process is positioned anterior and inferior to the inferior articular process of the adjacent cranial vertebra. These articulations are covered with hyaline cartilage and form synovial zygapophyseal (facet or Z) joints. The orientation of the facet joints is a major factor in the range of motion of the cervical spine. The typical cervical facet joints are oriented 45° in the sagittal plane and 0° in the coronal plane. These are the most horizontally oriented regional facet joints in the spinal column. Laxity of the joint capsule permits sliding motion to occur and explains why unilateral or bilateral dislocation without fracture may occur. The orientation of these facets allows flexion and extension, lateral bending, and rotation of the lower cervical spine. Flexion and extension in the subaxial cervical region are greatest at the C5–C6 and C6–C7 levels. This has been postulated to be responsible for the relatively high incidence of degenerative changes noted at these two cervical levels.

14. **What are the uncovertebral joints (joints of Luschka)?**
When viewed anteriorly, the lateral margin of the superior surface of each subaxial cervical vertebral body extends cranially as a bony process called the **uncinate process**. These processes articulate with a reciprocal convex area on the inferolateral aspect of the next cranial vertebral body. This articulation is named the **uncovertebral joint** or **neurocentral joint of Luschka**. It is believed to form as a degenerative cleft in the lateral part of the annulus fibrosus. The uncinate process, unique to the cervical spine, serves as a "rail" to limit lateral translation or bending and as a guiding mechanism for flexion and extension.

15. **What are the components of the intervertebral disc?**
Each intervertebral disc is composed of a central gel-like nucleus pulposus surrounded by a peripheral fibrocartilaginous annulus fibrosus. The endplates of the vertebral bodies are lined with hyaline cartilage and bind the disc to the vertebral body. The **annulus fibrosus** (predominantly type 1 collagen) attaches to the cartilaginous endplates via collagen fibers, which run obliquely at a 30° angle to the surface of the vertebral body and in a direction opposite to the annular fibers of the adjacent layer. The **nucleus pulposus** is composed primarily of glycosaminoglycans and type 2 collagen, which have the capacity to bind large amounts of water. In a normal healthy disc, loads acting on the disc are transferred to the annulus by swelling pressure (intradiscal pressure) generated by the nucleus. With aging, biochemical changes occur that limit the ability of the nucleus pulposus to bind water. Dehydration of the nucleus and increased loading of the annulus occurs. Fissuring and disruption of the annulus develops and migration of nuclear material through the annulus may occur.

NEURAL ANATOMY

16. **Describe the regional anatomy of the spinal cord, meninges, and adjacent structures.**
In the adult, the spinal cord occupies the upper four-fifths of the vertebral canal. It extends from the foramen magnum and ends distally at the level of the L1–L2 disc space where it tapers to form the **conus medullaris** (Fig. 1.7). Distal to the termination of the spinal cord (conus), the lumbar, sacral, and coccygeal roots continue as a leash of nerves termed the **cauda equina**. The **filum terminale** is a fibrous band that extends from the distal tip

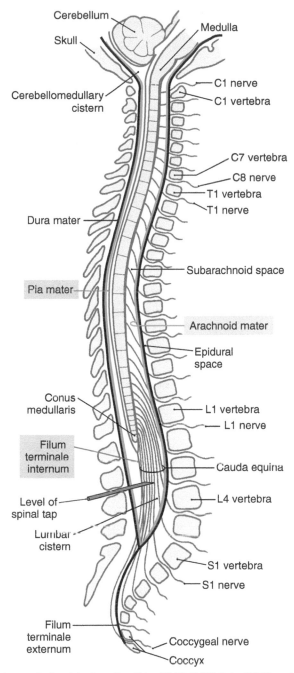

Fig. 1.7 Spinal cord, meninges, and adjacent structures. (From Haines DE, Mihailoff GA, Yezierski RP. The spinal cord. In: Fundamental Neuroscience for Basic and Clinical Applications. 5th ed. Chapter 9. Philadelphia, PA: Elsevier; 2018, pp. 138–151.)

of the spinal cord and attaches to the first coccygeal segment. Enlargements of the spinal cord between C3 and T2 (cervical enlargement) and between T9 and T12 (lumbar enlargement) correlate with the origin of nerves supplying the upper and lower extremities.

The spinal cord possesses a trilayered covering termed **meninges**. The **dura mater** is the outermost meningeal layer and extends the entire length of the vertebral column from the foramen magnum to S2, where it tapers to cover the filum terminale. The layer underneath the dura mater is the **arachnoid mater**, which forms a thin membrane adjacent but not adherent to the dura mater and extends to S2. The **pia mater** is the meningeal layer closest to the spinal cord and adheres to its surface.

Between the arachnoid and pia mater is the **subarachnoid space**, a large interval filled with **cerebrospinal fluid (CSF)** and is continuous with the subarachnoid space surrounding the brain. **Denticulate ligaments**, comprised of longitudinally oriented fibers of pia mater, extend from the spinal cord surface to the dura mater and position the spinal cord centrally within the subarachnoid space. CSF is predominantly produced in the choroid plexus, located in the lateral and fourth ventricles. The rate of CSF production is approximately 25 mL per hour (approximately 500 mL per day). The average adult has 100–150 mL of CSF. CSF returns to the vascular system and is renewed three to four times daily. Lumbar puncture (spinal tap) for removal of CSF is safely performed without endangering the spinal cord by entering the subarachnoid space in the lower lumbar region.

The **epidural space** is located between the dura mater and the vertebral column. Contents of this space include semiliquid fat, lymphatics, arteries, loose areolar connective tissue, spinal nerve roots, and venous plexuses. Pathologic processes involving this space include hematoma, abscess, and lipomatosis.

17. Describe the cross-sectional anatomy of the spinal cord and the location and function of the major spinal cord tracts.

A cross-sectional view of the spinal cord demonstrates a central butterfly-shaped area of gray matter and peripheral white matter (Fig. 1.8, Table 1.1). The central gray matter contains the neural cell bodies. The peripheral white matter contains the axon tracts. Tracts are named with their point of origin first. Ascending (afferent) tracts carry impulses toward the brain, whereas descending (efferent) tracts carry nerve signals away from the brain. The axon tracts may receive and transmit signals to the same side of the body (uncrossed tracts) or may transmit or receive signals from the opposite side (crossed tracts). The major spinal tracts important to the spine clinician include:

- **Corticospinal tracts:** The lateral corticospinal (pyramidal) tract is a descending tract located in the lateral portion of the cord that transmits ipsilateral motor function. The tract is anatomically organized with efferent motor

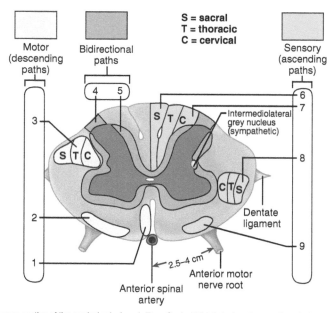

Fig. 1.8 Schematic cross-section of the cervical spinal cord. (From Gardocki RJ. Spinal anatomy and surgical approaches. In: Azar FM, Beaty JH, Canale ST, editors. Campbell's Operative Orthopaedics.13th ed. Philadelphia, PA: Elsevier; 2017, Fig. 37.3; Modified from Patton HD, Sundsten JW, Crill WE, et al., editors. Introduction to Basic Neurology. Philadelphia, PA: WB Saunders; 1976.)

Table 1.1 Ascending and Descending (Motor) Tracts

NUMBER	SPINAL CORD TRACT	FUNCTION	SIDE OF BODY
1	Anterior corticospinal tract	Skilled movement	Opposite
2	Vestibulospinal tract	Facilitates extensor muscle tone	Same
3	Lateral corticospinal (pyramidal) tract	Skilled movement	Same
4	Dorsolateral fasciculus	Pain and temperature	Bidirectional
5	Fasciculus proprius	Short spinal connections	Bidirectional
6	Fasciculus gracilis	Position/fine touch	Same
7	Fasciculus cuneatus	Position/fine touch	Same
8	Lateral spinothalamic tract	Pain and temperature	Opposite
9	Anterior spinothalamic tract	Light touch	Opposite

From Gardocki RJ. Spinal anatomy and surgical approaches. In: Azar FM, Beaty JH, Canale ST, editors. Campbell's Operative Orthopaedics. 13th ed. Philadelphia, PA: Elsevier; 2016, Table 37.1; Modified from Patton HD, Sundsten JW, Crill WE, et al., editors. Introduction to Basic Neurology. Philadelphia, PA: WB Saunders; 1976.

axons to the cervical area located medially and sacral efferent axons located laterally. The anterior corticospinal tract is a crossed tract, which facilitates skilled movements.
- **Spinothalamic tracts:** Ascending tracts located in the anterior and lateral portion of the cord that transmit sensations of pain, temperature, and light touch. Light touch sensation is carried primarily in the anterior spinothalamic tract. Pain and temperature sensation are carried primarily in the lateral spinothalamic tract. These tracts cross shortly after entering the spinal cord and therefore transmit sensations from the contralateral side of the body.
- **Dorsal column tracts:** Ascending tracts (fasciculus gracilis, fasciculus cuneatus) that convey proprioception, vibration, and discriminative touch sensation from the ipsilateral side of the body.

18. How many spinal nerves exit from the spinal cord?
The spinal nerves exit from the spinal cord in pairs. There are 31 pairs of spinal nerves: 8 cervical, 12 thoracic, 5 lumbar, 5 sacral, and 1 coccygeal.

19. What structures contribute to the formation of a spinal nerve? What are the branches of a spinal nerve?
Each spinal nerve (Fig. 1.9) is composed of both sensory and motor fibers. The collection of sensory fibers is termed the **dorsal root**. The cell bodies for these sensory fibers are located in the **dorsal root ganglion**. The collection of motor fibers is termed the **ventral or anterior root**. The cell bodies for these motor fibers are located in the anterior horn of the gray matter of the spinal cord. A **mixed spinal nerve** is formed by the union of the dorsal and ventral roots, which occurs just distal to the dorsal root ganglion. The spinal nerve becomes covered by a common dural sheath and gives off the following branches:
- **Dorsal ramus:** provides sensation to the medial two-thirds of the back, the facet joint capsules, and the posterior ligaments. The dorsal ramus also innervates the deep spinal musculature.
- **Ventral ramus:** supplies all other skin and muscles of the body. In the cervical and lumbar regions, the ventral rami form plexuses (cervical plexus, brachial plexus, lumbar plexus, and lumbosacral plexus). In the thoracic levels, ventral rami form the intercostal nerve.
- **Recurrent meningeal branch (sinuvertebral nerve):** innervates the periosteum of the posterior aspect of the vertebral body, basivertebral and epidural veins, epidural adipose tissue, posterior annulus and posterior longitudinal ligament, and anterior aspect of the dural sac.

20. Describe the relationship of the exiting spinal nerve to the numbered vertebral segment for each spinal region.
In the cervical region, there are eight cervical nerve roots and only seven cervical vertebra. The **first seven cervical nerve roots** exit the spinal canal above their numbered vertebra. For example, the C1 root exits the spinal column between the occiput and the atlas (C1). The C5 nerve root passes above the pedicle of the C5 vertebra and occupies the intervertebral foramen between C4 and C5. The **C8 nerve root** is atypical because it does not have a corresponding vertebral element, and exits below the C7 pedicle and occupies the intervertebral foramen between

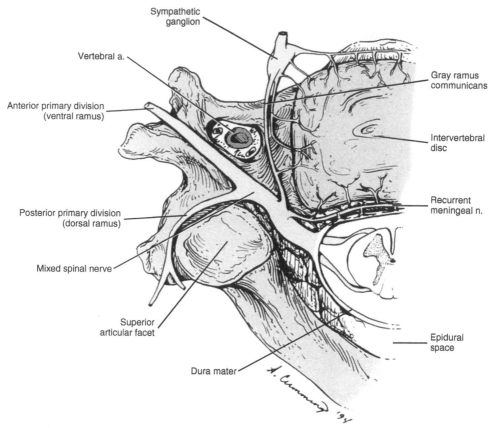

Fig. 1.9 Components of a spinal nerve: dorsal and ventral rami, mixed spinal nerve, recurrent meningeal branch (sinuvertebral nerve), and sympathetic ganglion. (From The Cervical Region. In: Cramer GD, Darby SA, editors. Basic and Clinical Anatomy of the Spine, Spinal Cord, and ANS. 3rd ed. St. Louis, MO: Mosby Year-Book; 2014, pp. 191, Fig. 5.31.)

C7 and T1. In the thoracic and lumbar spine, the relationship between the nerve root and vertebra changes as the nerve roots exit the spinal canal by passing below the pedicle of their named vertebra. The **T1 nerve root** passes below the T1 pedicle and exits the neural foramen between T1 and T2. The **T12 nerve root** passes below the T12 pedicle and exits the neural foramen between T12 and L1. The **L4 nerve root** passes beneath the L4 pedicle and exits the neural foramen between L4 and L5.

21. **How does the course of the recurrent laryngeal nerve differ from left to right?**
The recurrent laryngeal nerve originates from the vagus nerve and enters the tracheoesophageal groove. On the right side, it passes around the subclavian artery; on the left side, it passes under the aortic arch. Anterior surgical exposure of the lower cervical spine must be carefully performed in the interval between the tracheoesophageal sheath and carotid sheath to avoid injury to this nerve.

VASCULAR STRUCTURES

22. **Describe the blood supply to the spinal cord.**
The **anterior median spinal artery** and the **two posterior spinal arteries** supply the spinal cord (Fig. 1.10). The anterior spinal artery supplies 85% of the blood supply to the cord throughout its length. Radicular or segmental arteries feed these arteries. In the cervical spine, the majority of radicular arteries arise from the vertebral artery. These arteries enter the spinal canal through the intervertebral foramina and divide into anterior and posterior radicular arteries. The most consistent radicular artery in the cervical spine is located at the C5–C6 level. On average, there are 8 radicular feeders to the anterior spinal artery and 12 to the posterior spinal arteries throughout the length of the spinal cord. The basilar artery also anastomoses with the anterior spinal artery, variably supplying the cord to the fourth cervical level.

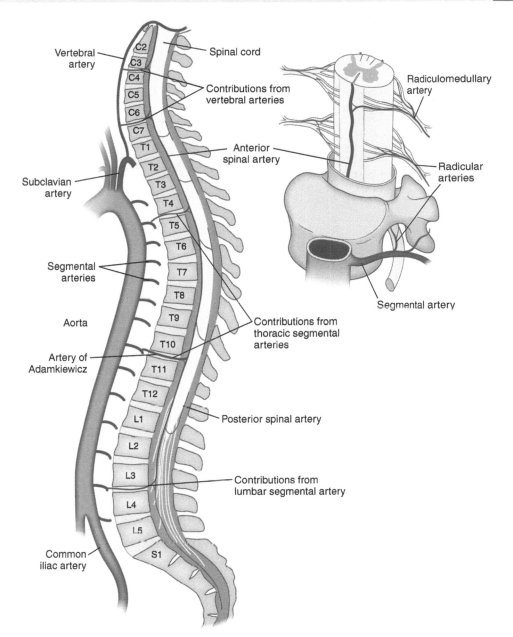

Fig. 1.10 The vasculature of the vertebral column. (From Shen FH. Chapter 5: Spine. In: Miller MD, Chhabra AB, Hurwitz S, et al., editors. Orthopaedic Surgical Approaches. Philadelphia, PA: Saunders; 2008, pp. 161–266, Fig. 5.18.)

23. **Describe the course of vertebral artery.**

The vertebral artery (Fig. 1.11) is the first branch of the subclavian artery and provides the major blood supply to the cervical spinal cord, nerve roots, and vertebrae. It can be divided into **four segments**. During its first segment, the vertebral artery passes from the subclavian artery anterior to C7 to enter the C6 transverse foramen. In the second segment, it continues from the C6 transverse foramina along its course through the cephalad transverse foramina to the level of the atlas. During its course, it lies lateral to the vertebral body and in front of the lateral mass. During its upward course, between C6 and C2, the vertebral artery gradually shifts to an anterior and

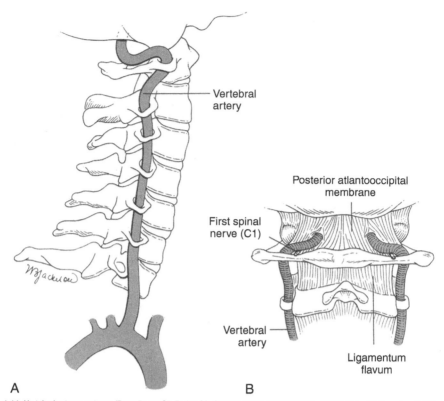

Fig. 1.11 Vertebral artery anatomy. (From Emery SE, Boden SD. Surgery of the Cervical Spine. Philadelphia, PA: Saunders; 2003, p. 6.)

medial position, thereby placing the artery at greater risk of injury during anterior decompressive procedures at the upper cervical levels. In its third segment, the artery exits C1 and curves around the C1 lateral mass, running medially along the cranial surface of the posterior arch of C1 in its sulcus, before passing through the atlanto-occipital membrane and entering the foramen magnum. The artery stays at least 12 mm lateral from midline of C1, making this a safe zone for dissection. In its fourth segment, the vertebral artery joins the contralateral vertebral artery to form the basilar artery.

FASCIA AND MUSCULATURE OF THE CERVICAL SPINE

24. What are the fascial layers of the anterior neck?
    The fascial layers of the neck consist of a superficial and deep layer. The superficial layer of the cervical fascia surrounds the platysma muscle. The deep cervical fascia consists of three layers:
    1. **Superficial layer:** surrounds the sternocleidomastoid and trapezius muscles.
    2. **Middle layer:** consists of the pretracheal fascia, which surrounds the strap muscles, trachea, esophagus, and thyroid gland. This layer is continuous with the lateral margin of the carotid sheath.
    3. **Deep layer:** consists of the prevertebral fascia, which surrounds the posterior paracervical and anterior prevertebral musculature.

25. Describe the muscular triangles of the neck.
    The anterior aspect of the neck is divided by the sternocleidomastoid into an anterior and posterior triangle. The **posterior triangle** borders are the trapezius, sternocleidomastoid, and middle third of the clavicle. The inferior belly of the omohyoid further divides this space into subclavian (lower) and occipital (upper) triangles. The **anterior triangle** is bounded by the sternocleidomastoid, the anterior median line of the neck, and lower border of the mandible. It is further subdivided into the submandibular, carotid, and muscular triangles. The posterior belly of the digastric separates the carotid from the submandibular triangles. The superior belly of the omohyoid separates the carotid from the muscular triangles (Fig. 1.12). The standard anterior approach to the midcervical spine is done through the muscular triangle.

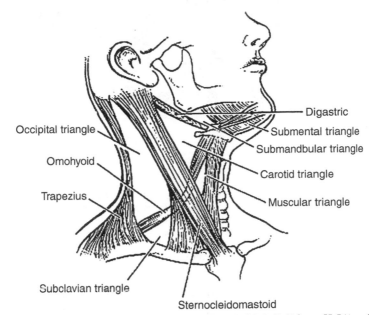

Fig. 1.12 Muscular triangles of the neck. (From Raiszadeh K, Spivak JM. Spine. In: Spivak JM, Di-Cesare PE, Feldman DS, et al., editors. Orthopaedics: A Study Guide. New York: McGraw-Hill; 1999, pp. 63–72, with permission.)

26. Name the muscles most commonly encountered during anterior and posterior cervical spine procedures.
    - **Anterior muscles:** platysma, sternocleidomastoid, strap muscles of the larynx, omohyoid, longus colli.
    - **Posterior muscles:** superficial layer—trapezius; middle layer—splenius capitis, splenius cervicis; deep layer—semispinalis capitis, longissimus capitis; muscles of the suboccipital triangle—rectus capitis posterior major and minor, obliquus capitis superior and inferior.

KEY POINTS

1. Appreciation of the distinguishing features of typical (C3–C6) and atypical (C1, C2, C7) vertebrae is important for understanding cervical spinal anatomy.
2. There are eight pairs of cervical nerve roots but only seven cervical vertebra.

Websites
1. Spinal cord, topographical, and functional anatomy: http://emedicine.medscape.com/article/1148570-overview
2. See cervical spine anatomy: http://www.orthogate.org/patient-education/cervical-spine/cervical-spine-anatomy.html
3. See spine anatomy index section: http://www.spineuniverse.com/displayarticle.php/article1297.html

BIBLIOGRAPHY

1. Aebi, M., Arlet, V., & Webb, J. K. (2007). *AO Spine Manual*. New York: Thieme.
2. An, H. S., & Simpson, J. M. (1994). *Surgery of the Cervical Spine*. Baltimore: William & Wilkins.
3. Benzel, E. C. (2012). *The Cervical Spine* (5th ed.). Philadelphia, PA: Lippincott.
4. Emery, S. E., & Boden, S. D. (2003). *Surgery of the Cervical Spine*. Philadelphia, PA: Saunders.
5. Kim, D. H., Vaccaro, A. R., Dickman, C. A., Cho, D., Lee, S., & Kim, I. (Eds.). (2013). *Surgical Anatomy and Techniques to the Spine* (2nd ed.). Philadelphia, PA: Saunders.
6. Shen, F. H., Samartzis, D., & Fessler, R. G. (Eds.). (2015). *Textbook of the Cervical Spine*. Maryland Heights, MO: Saunders.

CHAPTER 2

CLINICALLY RELEVANT ANATOMY OF THE THORACIC REGION

Vincent J. Devlin, MD and Darren L. Bergey, MD

OSTEOLOGY

1. Describe a typical thoracic vertebra.

   T1 and T10 through T12 possess unique anatomic features due to their transitional location between the cervico-thoracic and thoracolumbar spinal regions, respectively. Thoracic vertebra two through nine are termed **typical thoracic vertebra** because they share common structural features (Fig. 2.1):

   - **Vertebral body:** Heart shaped in cross-section. Posterior vertebral height exceeds anterior vertebral height, resulting in a wedged shape of the vertebral body when viewed in the lateral plane. This wedge shape contributes to the kyphotic alignment in the thoracic region.
   - **Costovertebral articulations:** The lateral surface of the vertebral body has both superior and inferior facets for articulation with adjacent ribs.
   - **Costotransverse articulation:** Rib articulation with the transverse process of vertebra.
   - **Vertebral arch**: Formed by laminae and two pedicles, which support seven processes:
   Spinous process (1)
   Transverse processes (2)
   Superior articular processes (2)
   Inferior articular processes (2)

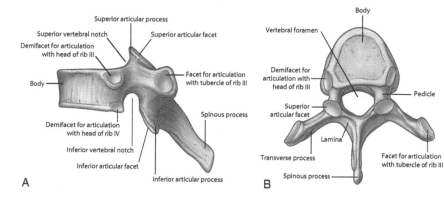

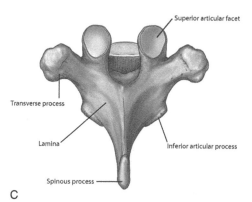

Fig. 2.1 Typical thoracic vertebra. (A) Lateral. (B) Superior. (C) Posterior. (From Drake RL, Vogl AW, Mitchell AWM. Gray's Atlas of Anatomy. Philadelphia, PA: Churchill Livingstone; 2015.)

2. What are the unique anatomic features of the first thoracic vertebra?

T1 vertebral body dimensions resemble a cervical vertebra more closely than a typical thoracic vertebra. The T1 vertebral body possesses a well-developed superior vertebral notch. The T1 spinous process is very prominent and may be larger than the C7 spinous process. The first rib articulates with the T1 vertebral body via a costal facet.

3. What are the unique anatomic features of T10, T11, and T12?

- Lack of costotransverse articulations (T11 and T12)
- Ribs articulate with vertebral bodies and do not overlie the disc space
- Vertebral body dimensions increase and approximate lumbar vertebral dimensions
- Facet morphology transitions from thoracic to lumbar in function and appearance
- T12 transverse process consists of three separate projections

4. What anatomic relationships are useful in determining the level of a thoracic lesion on a thoracic spine radiograph?

The first rib attaches to the T1 vertebral body. The second rib attaches to the T2 vertebral body. The third rib articulates with both the second and third vertebral bodies and overlies the T2–T3 disc space. This latter pattern continues until the tenth vertebral body. The tenth, eleventh, and twelfth ribs articulate only with the vertebral body of the same number and do not overlie a disc space.

5. Describe the anatomy of the thoracic pedicles.

The paired pedicles arise from the posterior-superior aspect of the vertebral bodies. The superior-inferior pedicle diameter is consistently larger than the medial-lateral pedicle diameter. Pedicle widths are narrowest at the T4–T6 levels, with medial-lateral pedicle diameter increasing both above (T1–T3) and below this region. The medial pedicle wall is two to three times thicker than the lateral pedicle wall across all levels of the thoracic spine. The medial angulation of the pedicle axis decreases from T1 to T12. The site for entry into the thoracic pedicle from a posterior spinal approach is located in the region where the facet joint and transverse process intersect and varies slightly, depending on the specific thoracic level.

ARTICULATIONS, LIGAMENTS, AND DISCS

6. What anatomic structures provide articulations between the thoracic vertebral bodies? Between the vertebral arches?

The structures that provide **articulations between the thoracic vertebral bodies** are:
1. Anterior longitudinal ligament
2. Posterior longitudinal ligament
3. Intervertebral disc

Five anatomic elements provide **articulations between the adjacent vertebral arches**:
1. **Articular capsules:** Thin capsules attach to the margins of the articular processes of adjacent vertebrae.
2. **Ligamentum flavum:** Yellow elastic tissue that connects laminae of adjacent vertebrae and attaches to the ventral surface of the lamina above and to the dorsal surface and superior margin of the lamina below.
3. **Supraspinous ligaments:** Strong fibrous cord that connects the tips of the spinous processes from C7 to sacrum.
4. **Interspinous ligaments:** Interconnect adjoining spinous processes. Attachment extends from base of each spinous process to the tip of the adjacent spinous process.
5. **Intertransverse ligaments:** Interconnect the transverse processes.

The pattern described above continues in the lumbar region as well.

7. What are the two types of articulations between the ribs and the thoracic vertebra?

The two types of articulations between the thoracic vertebra and ribs are costovertebral and costotransverse articulations. The **costovertebral articulation** is the articulation between the head of the rib *(costa)* and the vertebral body. The articular capsule, radiate ligaments, and intraarticular ligaments stabilize this articulation.

The **costotransverse articulation** occurs between the neck and tubercle of the rib and the transverse process. The ligaments that stabilize this articulation include the superior and lateral costotransverse ligaments (Fig. 2.2). The T11 and T12 transverse processes do not articulate with their corresponding ribs.

8. Describe the anatomy of the facet joints in the thoracic region.

The facet joints are located at the junction of the vertebral arch and the pedicle. The paired superior articular processes face posterolaterally, and the paired inferior articular processes face anteromedially. The thoracic facets are oriented 60° in the sagittal plane and approximate the coronal plane with a slight medial inclination (20°). Flexion-extension is minimal at T1–T2 and maximal at T12–L1, where facet joint orientation transitions to a lumbar pattern. Axial rotation is maximal at T1–T2 and minimal at the thoracolumbar junction. Lateral bending is more equally distributed across the thoracic region. Motion of the thoracic vertebrae is limited by anatomic

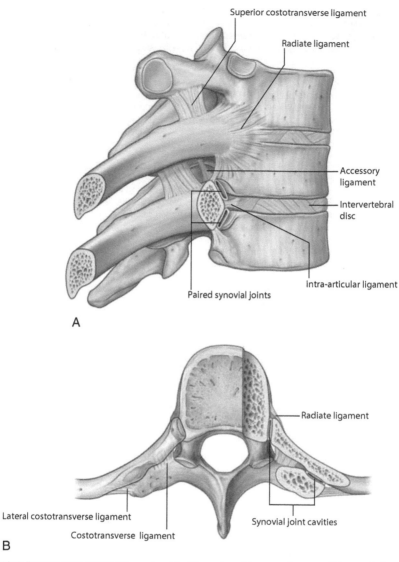

Fig. 2.2 Extrinsic ligaments of the thoracic spine: costovertebral ligaments, costotransverse ligaments. (A) Lateral. (B) Superior. (From Drake RL, Vogl AW, Mitchell AWM. Gray's Atlas of Anatomy. Philadelphia, PA: Churchill Livingstone; 2015.)

constraints, including the rib cage and its attachment to the sternum, ligamentous attachments at the costovertebral and costotransverse joints, narrow intervertebral discs, and overlap of the adjacent laminae and spinous processes.

NEURAL ANATOMY

9. Describe the contents of the spinal canal in relation to the vertebral segments in the thoracic and thoracolumbar spinal regions.
   In the fetus, the spinal cord extends the full length of the vertebral column. During childhood, the distal end of the spinal cord migrates proximally due to more rapid longitudinal growth of the osseous spinal elements and

generally reaches the lower border of L1 by 8 years of age. In the adult, the spinal cord occupies the upper four-fifths of the vertebral canal. It extends from the foramen magnum and ends distally at the level of the L1–L2 disc space (Fig. 2.3). The inferior region of the spinal cord, the **conus medullaris**, is characterized by the presence of both spinal cord and spinal nerve elements within the dural sac. Distal to the termination of the spinal cord *(conus)*, the lumbar, sacral, and coccygeal roots continue as a leash of nerves termed the **cauda equina**.

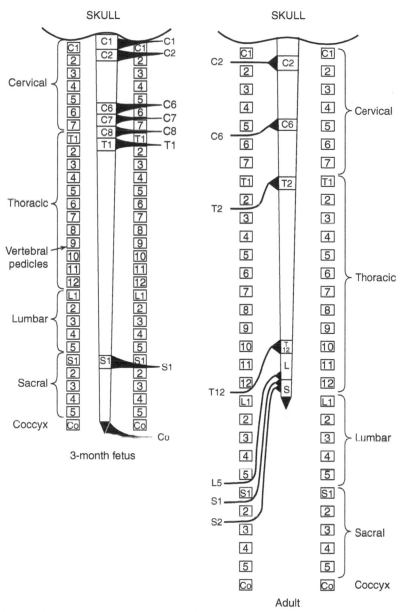

Fig. 2.3 Relationships between vertebral levels, spinal nerves, and spinal cord segments in the 3-month-gestation fetus and the adult *(dorsal view)*. In the fetus, the spinal cord extends the full length of the vertebral column, the spinal cord segments and vertebral levels correspond, and the spinal nerves course horizontally to exit from their intervertebral foramina. However, in adults the spinal cord ends at the L1–L2 vertebral level, only upper cervical cord segments correspond to their vertebral levels, with lower cord segments at progressively higher vertebral levels, and lower spinal nerves pursue increasingly more vertical courses. (From Shenk C. Functional and clinical anatomy of the spine. Phys Med Rehabil State Art Rev 1995;9[3]:577.)

10. Describe the anatomy of thoracic spinal nerves.

   Dorsal (sensory) and ventral (motor) roots originate from the spinal cord and join to form a spinal nerve in the region of the intervertebral foramen. The spinal nerve divides in the region of the foramen into a posterior (dorsal) primary ramus (innervates the posterior aspect of the associated dermatome and myotome) and an anterior (ventral) primary ramus, which continues as the intercostal nerve. The thoracic spinal nerves are numbered according to the pedicle of the vertebral body that the nerve contacts. For example, the T6 nerve root passes beneath the pedicle of the T6 vertebra.

11. Describe the contents of a thoracic neurovascular bundle.

   Each neurovascular bundle is composed of a posterior intercostal vein, posterior intercostal artery, and anterior primary ramus of a spinal nerve (mnemonic: **VAN** superior to inferior). The neurovascular bundle lies immediately below the inferior edge of each rib in the neurovascular groove.

12. Where is the thoracic portion of the sympathetic trunk located?

   The thoracic portion of the sympathetic trunk is located along the anterior surface of the rib head. The sympathetic chain or trunk consists of a series of **ganglia** that extend from the skull to the coccyx. There are two sympathetic chains, located on each of the anterolateral surfaces of the vertebral column. Each consists of approximately 22 ganglia. Each ganglia gives off a **gray ramus communicans** that joins the adjacent spinal nerve just distal to the junction of the anterior and posterior roots.

13. What is the innervation of the diaphragm?

   Innervation of the diaphragm is provided by the phrenic nerve, which originates from the C2 to C4 segments. Because the diaphragm receives its innervation and blood supply centrally, it can be incised and retracted from its insertion along the thoracic wall to permit surgical exposure of the thoracolumbar vertebral bodies without compromising its neurovascular supply.

VASCULAR STRUCTURES

14. Describe the vascular supply of the thoracic spinal cord.

   As in the cervical region, single anterior and paired posterior spinal arteries supply the spinal cord. Radicular (segmental) arteries enter the vertebral canal through the intervertebral foramina and divide into anterior and posterior radicular arteries, which supply the anterior and posterior spinal arteries, respectively. The majority of the vascular supply of the spinal cord is supplied by the anterior spinal artery. In the thoracic spine, the radicular arteries originate from intercostal arteries. The intercostal arteries arise segmentally from the aorta and course along the undersurface of each rib. Segmental arteries supplying the spine branch off from the intercostal arteries at the level of the costotransverse joint and enter the spinal canal via the intervertebral foramen. The number of radicular arteries is variable throughout the thoracic spine. The **radicular artery of Adamkiewicz** is the largest of these segmental arteries and is a major blood supply to the lower spinal cord. It originates from the left side in 80% of people and usually accompanies the ventral root of thoracic nerves 9, 10, or 11. However, it may originate anywhere from T5 to L5. Careful dissection near the intervertebral foramen and costotransverse joints is necessary to prevent injury to this vascular supply.

   The venous supply of the thoracic region parallels the arterial supply. It consists of an anterior and posterior ladder-like configuration of valveless veins that communicate with the inferior vena cava.

15. Explain the *watershed region* and *critical supply zone* of the thoracic spinal cord.

   The blood supply of the spinal cord is not entirely longitudinal. It is partly transverse and dependent on a series of radicular arteries that feed into the anterior and posterior spinal arteries at various levels. The limited number of radicular arteries supplying the thoracic spinal cord results in a less abundant blood supply in this region compared with the cervical and lumbar regions. Branches of the anterior median spinal artery supply the ventral two-thirds of the spinal cord, whereas branches of the posterior spinal arteries supply the dorsal third of the cord. The region where these two zones meet is relatively poorly vascularized and is termed the **watershed region**. The zone located between the fourth and ninth thoracic vertebrae has the least profuse blood supply and is termed the **critical vascular zone of the spinal cord**. This region corresponds to the narrowest region of the spinal canal. Interference with circulation in this zone during surgery is most likely to result in paraplegia. Surgical dissection in this region of the spine requires added care. Segmental vertebral arteries should be divided as far anteriorly as possible. Dissection in the region of the intervertebral foramen and costotransverse joint should be limited, and electrocautery should not be used in this area.

FASCIA, MUSCULATURE, AND RELATED STRUCTURES

16. Describe the anatomy of the posterior muscles of the thoracic and lumbar spinal regions.

   The anatomy of the posterior muscles of the back is confusing because of multiple overlapping muscle layers and because distinct muscle layers are not seen during posterior surgical dissection. It is helpful to divide the back muscles into three main layers:

   - **Superficial layer:** consists of muscles that attach the upper extremity to the spine and may be conceptualized as the appendicular muscle group. The trapezius (innervated by spinal accessory nerve), latissimus dorsi (thoracodorsal nerve), and levator scapulae muscles (dorsal scapular nerve) overlie the deeper rhomboid major and minor muscles (dorsal scapular nerve) (Fig. 2.4).

- **Intermediate layer:** consists of the serratus posterior superior and inferior and may be conceptualized as the respiratory group. These muscles of accessory respiration are innervated by the anterior primary rami of segmental nerves (Fig. 2.5).
- **Deep layer:** consists of the intrinsic back muscles, which function in movement of the head and spinal column. These muscles are innervated by the posterior rami of segmental thoracic and lumbar spinal nerves (Fig. 2.6).

The muscles comprising this deep layer can be subdivided into three layers:

1. Splenius capitis and splenius cervicis, which function as extensors and rotators of the head and neck.
2. Sacrospinalis (erector spinae), subdivided into spinalis, longissimus, and iliocostalis portions, and the transversospinales muscle group (semispinalis, multifidi, and rotatores), which function as extensors and rotators of the vertebral column.
3. Intertransversarii and interspinales, which are segmental muscles that stabilize adjacent vertebrae.

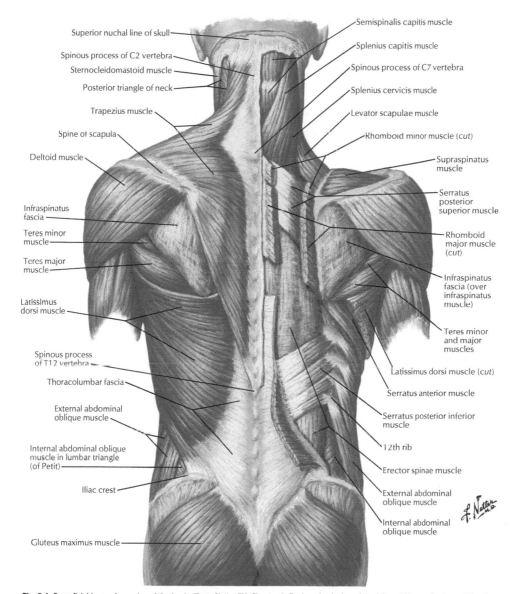

Fig. 2.4 Superficial layer of muscles of the back. (From Netter FH. Chapter 3. Back and spinal cord. In: Atlas of Human Anatomy. 7th ed. Philadelphia, PA: Saunders; 2019, Plates 180, 181, and 182.)

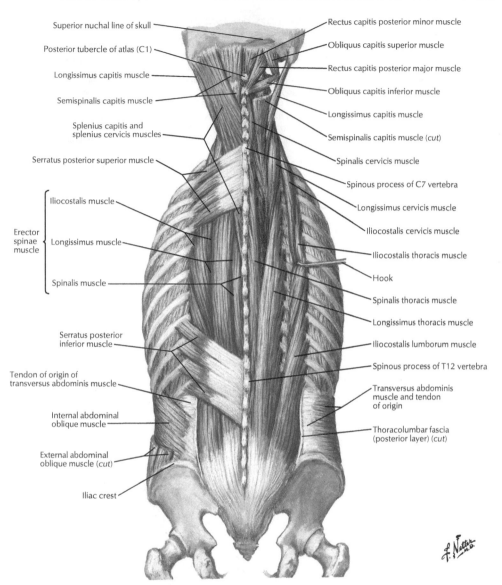

Fig. 2.5 Intermediate layer of muscles of the back. (From Netter FH. Chapter 3. Back and spinal cord. In: Atlas of Human Anatomy. 7th ed. Philadelphia, PA: Saunders; 2019, Plates 180, 181, and 182.)

17. Why should a spine specialist understand the anatomy of the thoracic cavity?

There are two important reasons why a spine specialist must possess a working knowledge of anatomy and pathology relating to the thoracic cavity. First, extraspinal pathologic processes within the thoracic cavity (e.g., aneurysm, malignancy) may mimic the symptoms of thoracic spinal disorders. Second, surgical treatment of many types of spinal problems involves exposure of the anterior aspect of the thoracic spine.

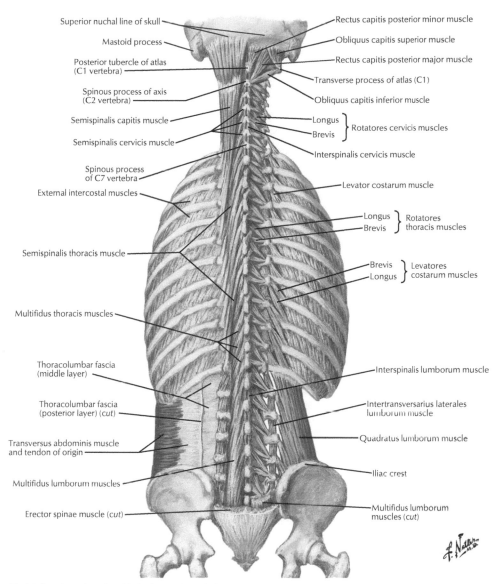

Superior nuchal line of skull

Mastoid process

Posterior tubercle of atlas (C1 vertebra)

Spinous process of axis (C2 vertebra)

Semispinalis capitis muscle

Semispinalis cervicis muscle

Spinous process of C7 vertebra

External intercostal muscles

Semispinalis thoracis muscle

Multifidus thoracis muscles

Thoracolumbar fascia (middle layer)

Thoracolumbar fascia (posterior layer) (*cut*)

Transversus abdominis muscle and tendon of origin

Multifidus lumborum muscles

Erector spinae muscle (*cut*)

Rectus capitis posterior minor muscle

Obliquus capitis superior muscle

Rectus capitis posterior major muscle

Transverse process of atlas (C1)

Obliquus capitis inferior muscle

Longus
Brevis } Rotatores cervicis muscles

Interspinalis cervicis muscle

Levator costarum muscle

Longus
Brevis } Rotatores thoracis muscles

Brevis
Longus } Levatores costarum muscles

Interspinalis lumborum muscle

Intertransversarius laterales lumborum muscle

Quadratus lumborum muscle

Iliac crest

Multifidus lumborum muscles (*cut*)

Fig. 2.6 Deep layer of muscles of the back. (From Netter FH. Chapter 3. Back and spinal cord. In: Atlas of Human Anatomy. 7th ed. Philadelphia, PA: Saunders; 2019, Plates 180, 181, and 182.)

The thoracic cavity contains the pleural cavities and the mediastinum. The pleural cavities contain the lungs. The **mediastinum** is the intrapleural region that separates the pleural cavities (Fig. 2.7) and is subdivided into four regions that contain the following structures:
1. Superior mediastinum (thymus gland, aortic arch and great vessels, trachea, bronchi, esophagus)
2. Anterior mediastinum (thymus gland, sternopericardial ligaments)
3. Middle mediastinum (pericardial cavity and related structures)
4. Posterior mediastinum (esophagus, thoracic aorta, inferior vena cava, azygos system, sympathetic chain)

Anterior mediastinum
Thymus (children),
connective tissue

Superior mediastinum
Trachea, aorta,
esophagus

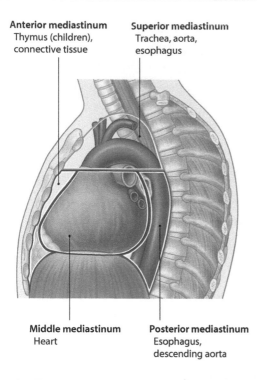

Middle mediastinum
Heart

Posterior mediastinum
Esophagus,
descending aorta

Fig. 2.7 Chest wall and mediastinum. (From Prakash K, Banks JC, Nava PB, et al. Chest wall and mediastinum. In: Atlas of Clinical Gross Anatomy. Philadelphia, PA: Elsevier Saunders; 2013, pp. 346–357, Fig. 29.1.)

KEY POINTS

1. Thoracic spinal motion is limited by multiple anatomic constraints.
2. The blood supply to the thoracic spinal cord is less abundant than in the cervical or lumbar region.
3. The third through ninth ribs overlap the posterolateral aspect of the adjacent disc space.
4. The intercostal artery and vein are located along the inferior surface of the rib.
5. The thoracic pedicle widths are most narrow at the T4–T6 levels and increase in width above (T1–T3) and below (T7–T12).

Websites
1. See spine anatomy index section, thoracic spine: http://www.spineuniverse.com/displayarticle.php/article 1397.html
2. See thoracic spine anatomy: http://www.orthogate.org/patient-education/thoracic-spine/thoracic-spine-anatomy.html

BIBLIOGRAPHY

1. An, H. S. (1998). *Principles and Techniques of Spine Surgery*. Baltimore: Williams & Wilkins.
2. Herkowitz, H. N., Garfin, S. R., Eismont, F. J., et al. (2018). *Rothman-Simeone: The Spine* (7th ed.). Philadelphia, PA: Saunders.
3. Hoppenfeld, S., & deBoer, P. (2003). *Surgical Exposure of the Spine and Extremities* (3rd ed.). Philadelphia, PA: Lippincott.
4. Schneck, C. (1995). Functional and clinical anatomy of the spine. *Physical Medicine and Rehabilitation State of the Art Reviews, 9*(3), 571–604.
5. Vaccaro, A. R. (1997). Spine anatomy. In S. R. Garfin & A. R. Vaccaro (Eds.), *Orthopaedic Knowledge Update—Spine* (Vol. 1, pp. 3–18). Rosemont, IL: American Academy of Orthopaedic Surgeons.

CHAPTER 3

CLINICALLY RELEVANT ANATOMY OF THE LUMBAR AND SACRAL REGION

Vincent J. Devlin, MD and Darren L. Bergey, MD

OSTEOLOGY

1. Describe a typical lumbar vertebra.

   The vertebral bodies are kidney shaped with the transverse diameter exceeding the anteroposterior diameter (Fig. 3.1). The vertebral body may be divided by an imaginary line passing beneath the pedicles into an upper and lower half. Six posterior elements attach to each lumbar vertebral body. Three structures lie above this imaginary line (superior articular process, transverse process, pedicle) and three structures lie below (lamina, inferior articular process, spinous process). The pars interarticularis is located along this imaginary dividing line. The transverse processes are long and thin except at L5, where they are thick and broad and possess ligamentous attachments to the pelvis. The five lumbar vertebral bodies increase in size from L1 to L5.

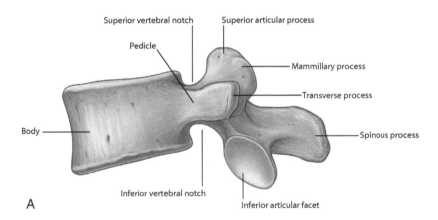

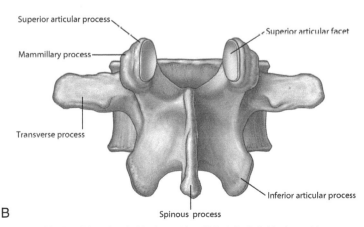

Fig. 3.1 (A) Lateral, typical lumbar vertebra. (B) Posterior, typical lumbar vertebra.

Continued

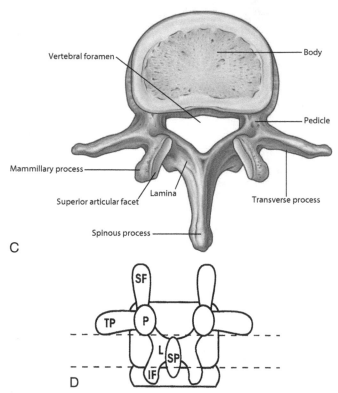

Fig. 3.1, cont'd (C) Superior, typical lumbar vertebra. (D) The six named posterior elements. *IF,* Inferior facet; *L,* lamina; *P,* pedicle; *SF,* superior facet; *SP,* spinous process; *TP,* transverse process. (A, B, & C: From Drake RL, Vogl AW, Mitchell AWM. Back. In: Gray's Atlas of Anatomy. Churchill Livingstone, Philadelphia, PA; 2015, pp. 19–55. D: From McCulloch JA, Young PH. Musculoskeletal and neuroanatomy of the lumbar spine. In: McCulloch JA, Young PH, editors. Essentials of Spinal Microsurgery. Philadelphia, PA: Lippincott-Raven; 1998, pp. 249–327, http://www.lww.com.)

2. **What region of the posterior elements of the spine is prone to failure when subjected to repetitive stress?**
   The **pars interarticularis** is an area of force concentration and is subject to failure with repetitive stress. A defect in the bony arch in this location is termed **spondylolysis.** The pars interarticularis is the concave lateral part of the lamina that connects the superior and inferior articular processes. The medial border of the pedicle is in line with the lateral border of the pars between L1 and L4. At L5, the lateral border of the pars marks the middle of the pedicle.

3. **Describe the anatomy of the lumbar pedicles.**
   The pedicle connects the posterior spinal elements (lamina, transverse processes, superior articular processes or facets) to the vertebral body. Lumbar pedicle widths are largest at L5 (18 mm) and smallest in the upper lumbar region at L1 (6 mm). The pedicles in the lumbar spine possess a slight medial inclination, which decreases from distal to proximal levels. The pedicles angle medially 30° at L5 and 12° at L1.

4. **What are the key anatomic features of the sacrum?**
   The sacrum is a triangular structure formed from five fused sacral vertebrae (Fig. 3.2). The S1 pedicle is the largest pedicle in the body. The **sacral promontory** is the upper anterior border of the first sacral body. The **sacral ala** (lateral sacral masses) are bilateral structures formed by the union of vestigial costal elements and the transverse processes of the first sacral vertebra. Four intervertebral foramina give rise to ventral and dorsal sacral foramina. Landmarks on the dorsal surface of the sacrum include **median, intermediate, and lateral sacral crests** which represent fused spinous, articular, and transverse processes respectively. The **sacral cornua (horns),** formed by remnants of the inferior articular processes, are the most caudal part of the intermediate sacral crest and articulate with the coccygeal cornua. The sacral cornua serve as a landmark for locating the **sacral hiatus,** an opening in the dorsal aspect of the sacrum due to absence of the fourth and fifth sacral lamina.

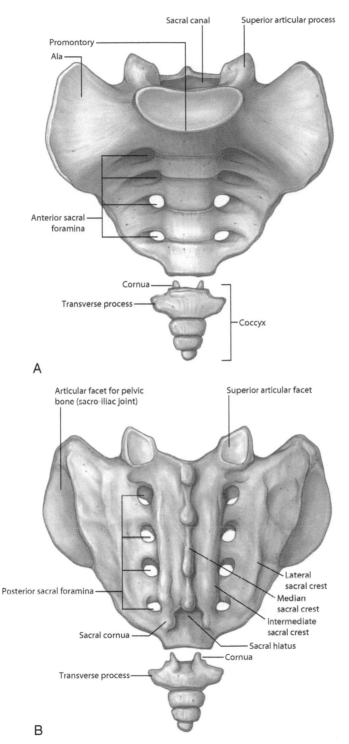

Fig. 3.2 (A) Sacrum, anterior. (B) Sacrum, posterior. (From Drake RL, Vogl AW, Mitchell AWM. Gray's Atlas of Anatomy. Philadelphia, PA: Churchill Livingstone; 2015.)

5. What are the key anatomic features of the coccyx?

The coccyx is a triangular structure that consists of three, four, or five fused coccygeal vertebrae. The coccyx articulates with the inferior aspect of the sacrum.

ARTICULATIONS, LIGAMENTS, AND DISCS

6. Describe the anatomy of the facet joints of the lumbar spine.

The inferior articular process of the cephalad vertebra is located posterior and medial to the superior articular process of the caudad vertebrae. The upper- and mid-lumbar facet joints are oriented in the sagittal plane. This orientation allows significant flexion-extension motion in this region but restricts rotation and lateral bending. The facet joints at L5–S1 are oriented in the coronal plane, thereby permitting rotation and resisting anterior-posterior translation.

7. What anatomic structures provide articulations between the lumbar vertebral bodies? Between the vertebral arches? Between L5 and the sacrum?

The structures that provide articulations between the lumbar vertebral bodies are the same as in the thoracic region: (1) anterior longitudinal ligament, (2) posterior longitudinal ligament, and (3) intervertebral disc.

The anatomic elements that provide articulations between the adjacent lumbar vertebral arches are the same as in the thoracic region: (1) articular capsules, (2) ligamentum flavum, (3) supraspinous ligaments, (4) interspinous ligaments, and (5) intertransverse ligaments.

Specialized ligaments connect L5 and the sacrum:
1. Iliolumbar ligament, which arises from the anteroinferior part of the transverse process of the fifth lumbar vertebra and passes inferiorly and laterally to blend with the anterior sacroiliac ligament at the base of the sacrum as well as the inner surface of the ilium.
2. Lumbosacral ligament, which spans from the transverse processes of L5 to the anterosuperior region of the sacral ala and body of S1.

8. Describe the alignment of the normal lumbar spine in reference to the sagittal plane.

The normal lumbar spine is lordotic (sagittal curve with its convexity located anteriorly). Normal lumbar lordosis (L1–S1) ranges from 30° to 80°, with a mean lordosis of 50°. Normal lumbar lordosis generally begins at L1–L2 and gradually increases at each distal level toward the sacrum. The apex of lumbar lordosis is normally located at the L3–L4 disc space. Normally, two-thirds of lumbar lordosis is located between L4 and S1 and one-third between L1 and L3 (Fig. 3.3).

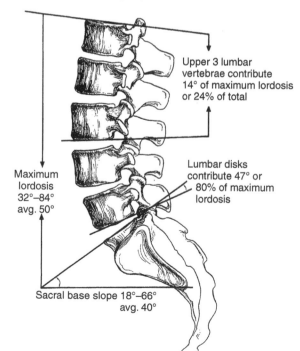

Upper 3 lumbar vertebrae contribute 14° of maximum lordosis or 24% of total

Lumbar disks contribute 47° or 80% of maximum lordosis

Maximum lordosis 32°–84° avg. 50°

Sacral base slope 18°–66° avg. 40°

Fig. 3.3 Sagittal alignment of the lumbar spine. Average maximum lordosis as measured from superior L1 to superior S1. (Reproduced with permission from DeWald RL. Revision surgery for spinal deformity. In: Eilert RE, editor. Instructional Course Lectures, Vol. 41. Rosemont: American Academy of Orthopaedic Surgeons; 1992.)

9. Which contributes more significantly to the normal sagittal alignment of the lumbar region—the shape of the intervertebral discs or the shape of the vertebral bodies?
   Eighty percent of lumbar lordosis occurs through wedging of the intervertebral discs, and 20% is due to the lordotic shape of the vertebral bodies. The wedge shape of the lowest three discs is responsible for one-half of total lumbar lordosis.

10. Describe the anatomy of the sacroiliac joint.
    The sacroiliac joint is a small, auricular-shaped synovial articulation located between the sacrum and ilium (Fig. 3.4). The complex curvature and strong supporting ligaments of the sacroiliac joint minimizes motion. Ligamentous support is provided by anterior sacroiliac ligaments, interosseous ligaments, and, most importantly, posterior sacroiliac ligaments. Other supporting ligaments in this region include the sacrospinous ligaments (ischial spine to sacrum) and sacrotuberous ligaments (ischial tuberosity to sacrum). The sacrum and pelvis can be considered as one vertebra (pelvic vertebra), which functions as an intercalary bone between the trunk and lower extremities.

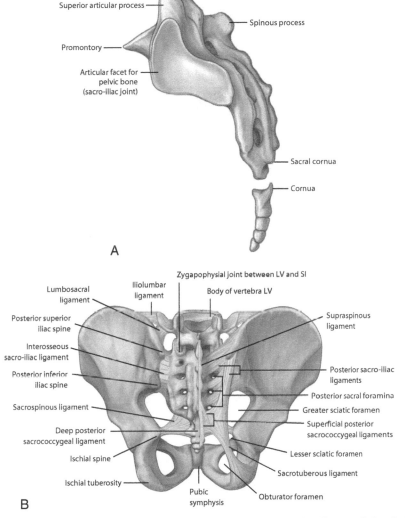

Fig. 3.4 (A) Sacrum and coccyx (lateral view). (B) Posterior view of sacrum and coccyx with associated ligaments. (A: From Drake RL, Vogl AW, Mitchell AWM. Back. In: Gray's Atlas of Anatomy. Philadelphia, PA: Churchill Livingstone; 2015, pp. 19–55. B: From Drake RL, Vogl AW, Mitchell AWM. Pelvis and perineum. In: Gray's Atlas of Anatomy. Philadelphia, PA: Churchill Livingstone; 2015, pp. 211–289.)

NEURAL ANATOMY

11. Describe the contents of the spinal canal in the lumbar region.
    The spinal cord terminates as the conus medullaris at the L1–L2 level in adults. Below this level, the **cauda equina,** composed of all lumbar, sacral, and coccygeal nerve roots, occupies the thecal sac. The lumbar nerves exit the intervertebral foramen under the pedicle of the same numbered vertebral body.

12. What structures comprise a lumbar anatomic segment? A lumbar motion segment?
    The vertebral body, its associated posterior elements, and the disc below, comprise an **anatomic segment.** In contrast, a **motion segment** is the smallest functional spinal unit and consists of two adjacent vertebrae, facet joints, an intervertebral disc, and adjoining ligaments.

13. What is the difference between an exiting nerve root and a traversing nerve root?
    Each lumbar anatomic segment possesses an exiting nerve root and a traversing nerve root. The **exiting nerve root** passes medial to the pedicle of the anatomic segment. The **traversing nerve root** passes through the anatomic segment to exit beneath the pedicle of the next caudal anatomic segment. For example, the exiting nerve root of the fifth anatomic segment is L5. This nerve passes beneath the L5 pedicle and exits the anatomic segment through the neural foramen of the L5 anatomic segment. The S1 nerve is the traversing nerve root and passes over the L5–S1 disc to exit beneath the pedicle of S1, which is located in the next caudad anatomic segment (Fig. 3.5).

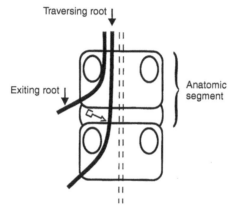

Fig. 3.5 The exiting nerve root and traversing root(s) of an unnumbered spinal segment. At the open *arrow,* the traversing nerve root becomes the exiting root of the anatomic segment below. (From McCulloch JA, Young PH. Musculoskeletal and neuroanatomy of the lumbar spine. In: McCulloch JA, Young PH, editors. Essentials of Spinal Microsurgery. Philadelphia, PA: Lippincott-Raven; 1998, pp. 249–327, http://www.lww.com.)

14. What analogy is commonly used to localize spinal pathology from caudad to cephalad within a lumbar anatomic segment?
    The analogy of a house with three floors is most commonly used to localize spinal pathology (Fig. 3.6A). The first story of the anatomic house is the level of the disc space. The second story is the level of the neural foramen and lower vertebral body. The third story is the level of the pedicle and includes the upper vertebral body and transverse process.

15. How is spinal pathology localized from medial to lateral within a lumbar anatomic segment?
    Neural compression may affect the thecal sac, nerve roots, or both structures. **Central canal spinal stenosis** refers to neural compression in the region of the spinal canal occupied by the thecal sac. **Lateral stenosis** involves the nerve root canal and its location is described in terms of three zones (see Fig. 3.6B,C) using the pedicle as a reference point. **Zone 1** (also called the subarticular zone, entrance zone, or lateral recess) includes the area of the spinal canal medial to the pedicle and under the superior articular process. **Zone 2** (also called the foraminal or midzone) includes the portion of the nerve root canal located below the pedicle. **Zone 3** (also called the extraforaminal or exit zone) refers to the nerve root in the area lateral to the pedicle.

16. An L4–L5 posterolateral disc protrusion located entirely within zone 1 of the nerve root canal results in compression of which nerve root?
    The most common location for a disc protrusion is *posterolateral*. This type of disc herniation impinges on the traversing nerve root of the L4 anatomic segment. This nerve is the L5 nerve root.

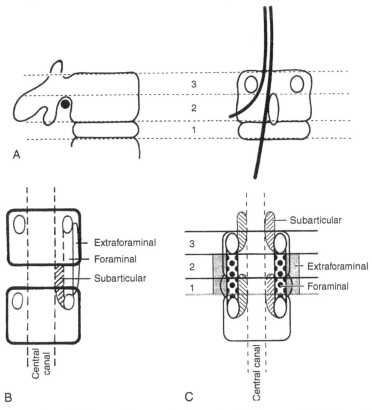

Fig. 3.6 (A) Conceptualization of the lumbar anatomic segment as a house. (B and C) Zone concept of the lumbar spinal canal. (From McCulloch JA. Microdiscectomy: The gold standard for minimally invasive disc surgery. Spine State Art Rev 1997;11[2]:382.)

17. An L4–L5 lateral disc protrusion located entirely within zone 3 of the nerve root canal results in compression of which nerve root?
    This describes the so-called *far-lateral* (extraforaminal) disc protrusion. This type of disc protrusion impinges on the exiting nerve of the L4 anatomic segment. This nerve is the L4 nerve root.

18. Compare the relationship of the nerve root to the pedicle and intervertebral disc in the cervical and lumbar spinal regions. Explain how anatomical differences affect the pattern of nerve root compression by a disc herniation in each region.
    Recall that the first seven cervical nerve roots exit the spinal canal above their numbered vertebra. As there are eight cervical nerve roots and seven cervical vertebrae, the C8 nerve root exits the spinal canal between C7 and T1. Due to the horizontal exit and course of the cervical nerve roots in relation to the dural sac, a C5–C6 disc herniation will impinge upon the C6 nerve root whether the herniation is located in a posterolateral or far-lateral location. In contrast, the lumbar nerve roots exit the spinal canal by passing below the pedicle of their named vertebra. For example, the L5 nerve root passes below the L5 pedicle. Due to the more vertically oriented course of the lumbar nerve root in contrast to a cervical nerve root, a lumbar nerve root may be impinged upon by disc material at two adjacent levels. For example, the L5 nerve root may be compressed by a posterolateral (zone 1) L4–L5 disc herniation or a far-lateral (zone 3) L5–S1 disc herniation.

19. Describe the location and significance of the superior hypogastric plexus. What can happen if it is injured during exposure of the anterior aspect of the spine?
    The superior hypogastric plexus is the sympathetic plexus located along the anterior prevertebral tissues in the region of the L5 vertebral body and anterior L5–S1 disc. This sympathetic plexus is at risk during anterior exposure of the L5–S1 disc space. Disruption of this plexus in men may cause retrograde ejaculation and sterility. Erection would not be affected because it is a parasympathetically mediated function (Fig. 3.7).

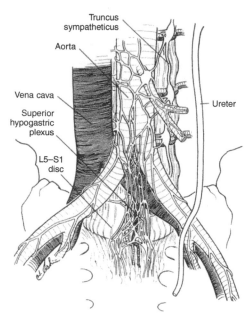

Fig. 3.7 Bifurcation of aorta and vena cava in relation to the spine. The superior hypogastric plexus. (From Hanley EN, Delmarter RB, McCulloch JA. Surgical indications and techniques. In: Wiesel SW, Weinstein JN, Herkowitz H. The Lumbar Spine. 2nd ed. Philadelphia, PA: Saunders; 1996, pp. 492–524.)

VASCULAR STRUCTURES

20. Describe the blood supply to the lumbar vertebral bodies.

Each lumbar vertebra is supplied by paired lumbar segmental arteries. The segmental arteries for L1 to L4 arise from the aorta. The origin of the segmental arteries for L5 is variable and may arise from the iliolumbar artery, fourth lumbar segmental artery, middle sacral artery, or aorta. As the segmental artery courses toward the inter-vertebral foramen, it divides into three branches.

1. The anterior branch (supplies the abdominal wall)
2. The posterior branch (supplies paraspinous muscles and facets)
3. The foraminal branch (supplies the spinal canal and its contents)

   The venous supply of the lumbar region parallels the arterial supply. It consists of an anterior and posterior ladderlike configuration of valveless veins that communicate with the inferior vena cava.

21. What is Batson's plexus?

Batson's plexus is a system of valveless veins located within the spinal canal and around the vertebral body. It is an alternate route for venous drainage to the inferior vena cava system. Because it is a valveless system, any in-crease in abdominal pressure (e.g., secondary to positioning during spine surgery) can cause blood to flow prefer-entially toward the spinal canal and surrounding bony structures. Batson's plexus also serves as a preferential pathway for metastatic tumor and infection spreading to the lumbar spine.

22. Where is the bifurcation of the aorta and vena cava located?

Most commonly, the bifurcation is over the L4–L5 disc or L5 vertebral body (see Fig. 3.7).

23. What is the significance of the iliolumbar vein?

The iliolumbar vein is a branch of the iliac vein that limits mobilization of the iliac vessels off the anterior aspect of the spine (Fig. 3.8). This vein should be carefully isolated and securely ligated before attempting mobilization of the vascular structures to expose the anterior aspect of the spine at the L4–L5 disc level.

FASCIA, MUSCULATURE, AND RELATED STRUCTURES

24. Why should a spine specialist be knowledgeable about the anatomy of the abdominal and pelvic cavities?

There are many important reasons why a spine specialist must possess a working knowledge of anatomy and pathology relating to the abdominal and pelvic cavities. Extraspinal pathologic processes within the abdominal and pelvic cavities (e.g., aneurysm, infection, and tumor) may mimic the symptoms of lumbosacral spinal disorders. Surgical treatment of many spinal problems involves exposure of the anterior lumbar spine and/or sacrum through a variety of surgical

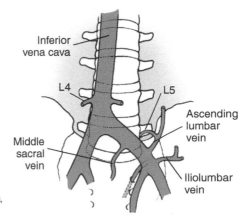

Fig. 3.8 Anatomy of the iliolumbar vein and environs. (From Canale ST, Beaty J. Campbell's Operative Orthopedics. 11th ed. Philadelphia, PA: Mosby; 2007.)

approaches. Evaluation of complications after spinal procedures requires assessment not only of the vertebral and neural structures, but also of vascular and visceral structures (e.g., bladder, intestines, spleen, kidney, and ureter).

25. What muscles of the posterior abdominal wall cover the anterolateral aspect of the lumbar spine?
    The psoas major and minor muscles originate from the lumbar transverse processes, intervertebral discs, and vertebral bodies, and insert distally at the lesser trochanter and iliopectineal region, respectively. They must be mobilized during exposure of the anterior lumbar spine, taking care to avoid nerves that cross the psoas muscles (genitofemoral nerve, sympathetic trunk), and the lumbar plexus, which passes within the substance of these muscles.

KEY POINTS

1. Lumbar lordosis begins at L1–L2 and gradually increases at each distal level toward the sacrum.
2. Six named posterior osseous elements attach to each lumbar vertebral body.
3. The spinal cord normally terminates as the conus medullaris at the L1–L2 level in adults.
4. The cauda equina occupies the thecal sac distal to the L1–L2 level in adults.

Websites
1. See lumbar spine anatomy: http://www.orthogate.org/patient-education/lumbar-spine/lumbar-spine-anatomy.html
2. See spine anatomy section, lumbar spine: http://www.spineuniverse.com/displayarticle.php/article1286.html

---

BIBLIOGRAPHY

1. Borenstein DG, Wiesel SW, Boden SD. Anatomy and biomechanics of the lumbosacral spine. In: *Low Back Pain: Medical Diagnosis and Comprehensive Management.* 2nd ed. Philadelphia, PA: Saunders; 1995, pp. 1–16.
2. Daubs MD. Anterior lumbar interbody fusion. In: Vaccaro AR, Baron EM, editors. *Spine Surgery.* Philadelphia, PA: Saunders; 2008, pp. 391–400.
3. Herkowitz HN, Dvorak J, Bell G, editors. *The Lumbar Spine.* 3rd ed. Philadelphia, PA: Lippincott; 2004.
4. Herkowitz HN, Garfin SR, Eismont FJ, editors. *The Spine.* 7th ed. Philadelphia, PA: Saunders; 2008.
5. McCulloch JA, Young PH. Musculoskeletal and neuroanatomy of the lumbar spine. In: McCulloch JA, Young PH, editors. *Essentials of Spinal Microsurgery.* Philadelphia, PA: Lippincott-Raven; 1998, pp. 249–327.
6. Wong DA. Open lumbar microscopic discectomy. In: Vaccaro AR, Albert TJ, editors. *Spine Surgery, Tricks of the Trade.* 2nd ed. New York, NY: Thieme; 2009, pp. 119–121.

CLINICAL EVALUATION OF THE SPINE PATIENT

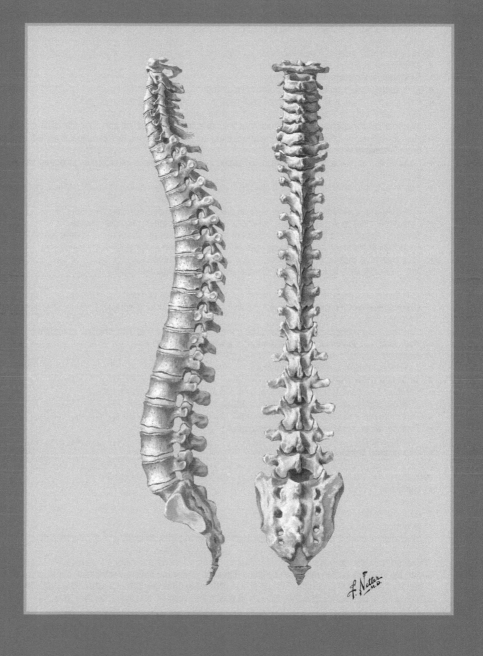

CHAPTER 4

EVALUATION OF CERVICAL SPINE DISORDERS

Jeffrey C. Wang, MD

1. **How does the evaluation of a patient with a spine complaint begin?**
   A complete history and physical examination are performed. The purpose of the history and physical examination is to make a provisional diagnosis that is confirmed by subsequent testing as medically indicated.

2. **What are some of the key elements to assess in the history of any spine problem?**
   - *Chief complaint:* pain, numbness, weakness, gait difficulty, deformity
   - *Symptom onset:* acute versus insidious
   - *Symptom duration:* acute, subacute, chronic, recurrent
   - *Pain location:* Is the pain primarily axial neck pain, arm pain, or a combination of both?
   - *Pain quality and character:* sharp versus dull; radiating versus stabbing versus aching
   - *Temporal relationship of pain:* Night pain, rest pain, or constant unremitting pain suggests systemic problems such as a tumor or infection. Morning stiffness that improves throughout the day suggests an arthritic problem or an inflammatory arthropathy.
   - *Relation of symptoms to neck position:* increased arm pain with neck extension suggests nerve root impingement
   - *Aggravating and alleviating factors:* Is the pain mechanical (activity-related) or nonmechanical (not influenced by activity) in nature?
   - *Family history:* inquire about diseases such as ankylosing spondylitis or rheumatoid arthritis.
   - *Concurrent medical illness:* diabetes, peripheral neuropathy, peripheral vascular disease
   - *Systemic symptoms:* a history of weight loss or fever suggests possibility of tumor or infection
   - *Functional impairment:* loss of balance, gait difficulty, loss of fine motor skills in the hands
   - *Prior treatment:* include both nonoperative and operative measures
   - *Negative prognostic factors:* pending litigation, Workers' Compensation claim

3. **What disorders should be considered in the differential diagnosis of neck/arm pain?**
   - *Degenerative spinal disorders:* discogenic pain, radiculopathy, myeloradiculopathy, myelopathy, facet joint-mediated pain
   - *Soft tissue disorders:* sprains, myofascial pain syndromes, fibromyalgia, and whiplash syndrome
   - *Rheumatologic disorders:* rheumatoid arthritis, ankylosing spondylitis
   - *Infections:* discitis, osteomyelitis
   - *Tumors:* metastatic versus primary tumors
   - *Intraspinal disorders:* tumors, syrinx
   - *Systemic disorders with referred pain:* angina, apical lung tumors (Pancoast tumor)
   - *Shoulder and elbow pathology:* rotator cuff disorders, medial epicondylitis
   - *Peripheral nerve entrapment syndromes:* radial, ulnar, or median nerve entrapment, suprascapular neuropathy
   - *Thoracic outlet syndrome or brachial plexus injury*
   - *Psychogenic pain*
   - *Cervicogenic headache*

4. **What are the basic elements of an examination of any spinal region?**
   - Inspection
   - Palpation
   - Range of motion (ROM)
   - Neurologic examination
   - Evaluation of related areas (e.g., shoulder, elbow, and wrist joints; scapula; supraclavicular area)

5. **What should the examiner look for during inspection of the cervical region?**
   During the initial encounter, much can be learned from observing the patient. Assessment of gait and posture of the head and neck is important. Patients should undress to allow inspection of anatomically related areas, including the neck muscles, shoulder, elbow and wrist joints, scapula, and supraclavicular area.

6. What is the purpose of palpation during assessment of the cervical region?
To examine for tenderness and locate bone and soft tissue pathology. Specific areas of palpation correspond to specific levels of the spine:
- Hyoid bone C3
- Thyroid cartilage C4–C5
- Cricoid membrane C5–C6
- First cricoid ring C6
- Carotid tubercle C6

Spinous processes should be palpated and checked for alignment. If tenderness is detected, it should be noted whether the tenderness is focal or diffuse, and the area of maximum tenderness should be localized.

7. In which three planes is range of motion assessed in the cervical spine?
- Flexion/extension
- Right/left bending
- Right/left rotation

8. What is a normal range of motion of the cervical spine?
- Flexion 45°
- Extension 55°
- Right/left bending 40°
- Right/left rotation 70°

Clinical estimates of motion are more commonly used in office practice. Flexion may be reproducibly measured using the distance from the chin to the sternum. For extension, the distance from the occiput to the dorsal spine may be helpful. Distances can be described in terms of fingerbreadths or measured with a ruler. The normal patient, for example, can nearly touch chin to chest in flexion and bring the occiput to within three or four fingerbreadths of the posterior aspect of the cervical spine in extension. Normal rotation permits the chin to align with the shoulder.

9. Describe an overview of the approach to the neurologic examination for cervical disorders.
The goal of examination is to determine the presence or absence of a neurologic deficit. If present, the level of a neurologic deficit is determined through testing of sensory, motor, and reflex function. The neurologic deficit may arise from pathology at the level of the spinal cord, nerve root, brachial plexus, or peripheral nerve. Examination of the cervical region is focused on the C5–T1 nerve roots because they supply the upper extremities. For each nerve root, the examiner tests sensation, strength, and if one exists, the appropriate reflex (Table 4.1).

Table 4.1 Testing Sensory, Motor, and Reflex Function.

LEVEL	SENSATION	MOTOR	REFLEX
C5	Lateral arm (axillary patch)	Deltoid	Biceps
C6	Lateral forearm	Wrist extension, biceps	Brachioradialis
C7	Middle finger	Triceps, wrist flexion, finger extension	Triceps
C8	Small finger	Finger flexion	None
T1	Medial arm	Interossei (finger abduction)	None

10. How is sensation examined?
Sensation can be examined using light touch, pin prick, vibration, position, temperature, and two-point discrimination. In assessing sensation, it is helpful to assess both sides of the body simultaneously. In this manner, sensation that is intact but subjectively decreased compared with the contralateral side can be easily documented. Light touch and pinprick sensation are graded as 0 = absent, 1 = impaired (partial or altered appreciation including hyperesthesia), or 2 = intact.

11. What neural pathways are tested during sensory examination?
- Spinothalamic tracts: transmit pain and temperature sensation
- Posterior columns: transmit two-point discrimination, position sense and vibratory sensation

12. How is motor strength graded? How are reflexes graded?
    See Table 4.2.

Table 4.2 Grading Motor Strength and Reflexes.	
MOTOR GRADE	**FINDINGS**
5	Full range of motion against full resistance
4	Full range of motion against reduced resistance
3	Full range of motion against gravity alone
2	Full range of motion with gravity eliminated
1	Evidence of contractility
0	No contractility
REFLEX GRADE	**FINDINGS**
4+	Hyperactive
3+	Brisk
2+	Normal
1+	Diminished
0	Absent

13. What is the significance of hyperreflexia? An absent reflex?
    Hyperreflexia signifies an upper motor neuron lesion (interruption in the neural pathway above the anterior horn cell). An **absent reflex** implies pathology at the nerve root level(s) that transmits the reflex (in the lower motor neuron, between the anterior horn cells of the spinal cord and the target muscle).

14. What is radiculopathy?
    Radiculopathy is a lesion that causes irritation of a nerve root (lower motor neuron). It involves a specific spinal level with sparing of levels immediately above and below. The patient may report pain, a burning sensation, or numbness that radiates along the anatomic distribution of the affected nerve root. Other signs may include severe atrophy of muscles and loss of the reflex supplied by the nerve. Severe radiculopathy may result in the flaccid paralysis of muscles supplied by the nerve.

15. What symptoms are associated with a C5–C6 disc herniation? Explain.
    A disc herniation at the C5–C6 level causes compression of the C6 nerve root. Thus weakness of biceps and wrist extensors, loss of the brachioradialis reflex, and diminished sensation of the radial forearm into the thumb and index finger, are expected. The nerve root of the inferior vertebra of a given motion segment (e.g., C3 for C2–C3 disc, C7 for C6–C7 disc) is the one typically affected by a herniated disc. Note that in the cervical region there are eight nerve roots and seven cervical vertebrae. The first seven cervical nerve roots exit the spinal canal above their numbered vertebra. The C8 nerve root is atypical because it does not have a corresponding vertebral element; it exits below the C7 pedicle, and occupies the intervertebral foramen between C7 and T1.

16. Describe testing of the cervical nerve roots.
    See Table 4.3.

Table 4.3 Testing the Cervical Nerve Roots.				
ROOT	**DISC LEVEL**	**SENSATION**	**REFLEX**	**MOTOR LEVEL**
C3	C2–C3	Posterior neck to mastoid	None	Nonspecific
C4	C3–C4	Posterior neck to scapula ± anterior chest	None	Nonspecific
C5	C4–C5	Lateral arm (axillary patch) to elbow	± Biceps	Deltoid ± biceps
C6	C5–C6	Radial forearm to thumb	Biceps, brachioradialis	Biceps, wrist extensors
C7	C6–C7	Midradial forearm to middle finger ± index/ring fingers	Triceps	Triceps, wrist flexors, finger extensors
C8	C7–T1	Ulnar forearm to little and ring fingers	None	Finger flexors ± intrinsics
T1	T1–T2	Medial upper arm	None	Hand intrinsics

17. What provocative maneuvers are useful in examining a patient with a suspected radiculopathy? Explain how each is carried out.

- **The Spurling test** (Fig. 4.1) is used to assess cervical nerve roots for stenosis as they exit the foramen. The patient's neck is extended and rotated toward the side of the pathology. Once the patient is in this position, a firm axial load is applied. If radicular symptoms are worsened by this maneuver, the test is said to be positive. The extended and rotated position of the neck decreases the size of the foramen through which the nerve roots exit, thereby exacerbating symptoms when an axial load is applied.
- **Axial cervical compression test:** Arm pain that is elicited by axial compressive force on the skull and relieved by distractive force suggests that radicular symptoms are due to neuroforaminal narrowing.
- **Valsalva maneuver:** This maneuver (moderately forceful attempted exhalation against a closed airway or holding the breath and "pushing downwards" with the diaphragm) may increase radicular symptoms. Increased intraabdominal pressure simultaneously increases cerebrospinal pressure, which in turn increases pressure on the cervical roots.
- **Shoulder abduction test:** Patients with cervical radiculopathy may obtain relief of symptoms by holding the shoulder in an abducted position, which decreases tension in the nerve root (Fig. 4.2)

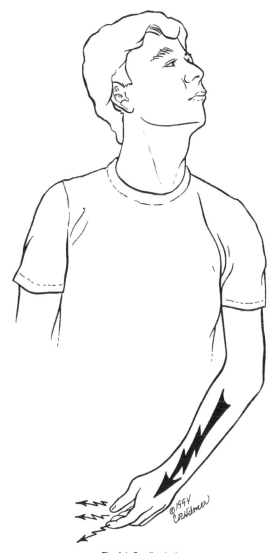

Fig. 4.1 Spurling test.

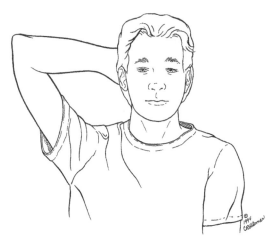

Fig. 4.2 Shoulder abduction test.

18. What is the Adson test?

    The Adson test helps to distinguish thoracic outlet syndrome from cervical radiculopathy. The affected arm is abducted, extended, and externally rotated at the shoulder while the examiner palpates the radial pulse. The patient turns the head toward the affected side and takes a deep breath. In a positive Adson test, the radial pulse on the affected side is diminished or lost during the maneuver, suggesting thoracic outlet syndrome (compression of the subclavian artery by a cervical rib, scalenus anticus muscle, or another cause).

19. What is cervical myelopathy? How does it present?

    Myelopathy is the manifestation of cervical spinal cord compression. **Cervical myelopathy** arising from spinal cord compression due to cervical degenerative changes is the most common cause of spinal cord dysfunction in patients older than 55 years. Vague sensory and motor symptoms involving the upper and/or lower extremities are common. **Lower motor neuron findings** occur at the level of the lesion, with atrophy of upper extremity muscles, especially the intrinsic muscles of the hands. **Upper motor neuron findings** are noted below the level of the lesion and may involve both the upper and lower extremities. Lower extremity spasticity and hyperreflexia are common. There may be relative hyperreflexia in the legs compared with the arms. Hoffmann sign and Babinski sign may be present. Additional findings may include neck pain and stiffness, spastic gait, loss of manual dexterity, or problems with sphincter control.

20. What reflexes or signs should be assessed when evaluating a patient with suspected cervical myelopathy? How are they evaluated?

    • **The Babinski test** is performed by stroking the lateral plantar surface of the foot from the heel to the ball of the foot, and curving medially across the heads of the metatarsals. A positive test (Babinski sign) occurs if there is dorsiflexion of the big toe and fanning of the other toes (Fig. 4.3).

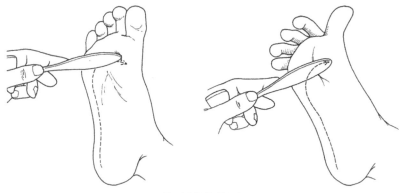

Fig. 4.3 Babinski test.

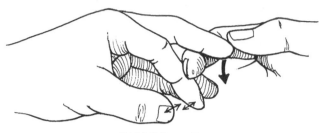

Fig. 4.4 Hoffmann sign.

- **The Hoffmann test** is performed on the patient's pronated hand while the examiner grasps the patient's middle finger (Fig. 4.4). The distal phalanx is forcefully and quickly flexed (almost a flicking motion) while the examiner observes the other fingers and thumb. The test is positive if flexion is seen in the thumb and/ or index finger. Hoffmann sign implies an upper motor lesion in the cervical spinal region as it is an upper extremity reflex. In contrast, pathology anywhere along the spinal cord can lead to a positive Babinski sign.
- **Finger escape sign (finger adduction test)** is performed by asking the patient to hold all digits of the hand in an extended and adducted position. With myelopathy, the two ulnar digits will fall into flexion and abduction, usually within 30 seconds.
- **Inverted radial reflex** is elicited by tapping the distal brachioradialis tendon. The reflex is present if spastic contraction of the finger flexors occurs, suggesting spinal cord compression at the C5–C6 level.
- The **scapulohumeral reflex** is performed by tapping the tip of the spine of the scapula. If the scapula elevates or the humerus abducts, it is termed a hyperactive reflex suggesting upper motor neuron dysfunction above the C4 spinal cord level.
- **Lhermitte sign** is a generalized electric shock sensation that involves the upper and lower extremities, as well as the trunk, and it is elicited by extreme flexion or extension of the head and neck.
- **Clonus.** Upward thrusting of the ankle joint leads to rhythmic, repetitive motion of the ankle joint due to reflex contraction of the gastrocnemius-soleus complex, caused by lack of central nervous system inhibition.

KEY POINTS

1. A comprehensive patient history and physical examination is the first step in diagnosing a spine complaint.
2. A major goal of the initial patient evaluation is to differentiate common nonemergent spinal conditions such as acute nonspecific neck pain and cervical spondylosis, from serious disorders such as spinal infections, spinal tumors, or cervical myelopathy.
3. Nonspinal pathology may mimic the symptoms of spinal disorders and must be considered in the differential diagnosis.

Websites
1. Cervical spine examination for neck and shoulder conditions (video): https://www.hss.edu/conditions_neck-and-shoulder-conditions-for-the-primary-care-physician-shoulder-exam.asp
2. Cervical examination: https://www.physio-pedia.com/Cervical_Examination

---

BIBLIOGRAPHY

1. Albert T, J. (2004). *Physical Examination of the Spine.* London, UK: Thieme.
2. Hoppenfeld, S. (1976). *Physical Exam of the Spine and Extremities* (1st ed.). New York, NY: Appleton & Lange.
3. Macnab, I., & McCulloch, J. A. (1994). *Neck Ache and Shoulder Pain* (1st ed.). Baltimore, MD: Lippincott Williams & Wilkins.
4. Rainville, J., Noto, D. J., Jouve, C., & Jenis, L. (2007). Assessment of forearm pronation strength in C6 and C7 radiculopathies. *Spine, 32,* 72–75.
5. Scherping, S. C. (2004). History and physical examination. In J. W. Frymoyer & S. W. Wiesel (Eds.), *The Adult Spine: Principles and Practice* (3rd ed., pp. 49–68.). Philadelphia, PA: Lippincott Williams & Wilkins.
6. Standaert, C. J., Herring, S. A., & Sinclair, J. D. (2018). Patient history and physical examina-tion—cervical, thoracic and lumbar. In H. N. Herkowitz, S. R. Garfin, & F. J. Eismont (Eds.), *Rothman-Simeone the Spine* (7th ed., pp. 183–200). Philadelphia, PA: Saunders.
7. Zeidman, S. M., Benzel, E. C., & Matheus, V. (2012). Neurologic and functional evaluation. In E. C. Benzel (Ed.), *The Cervical Spine* (5th ed., pp. 139–155). Philadelphia, PA: Lippincott Williams & Wilkins.

CHAPTER 5

EVALUATION OF THORACIC AND LUMBAR SPINE DISORDERS

Jeffrey C. Wang, MD

THORACIC SPINE EXAMINATION

1. **What are the most common reasons for referral to evaluate the thoracic spinal region?**
   Pain and spinal deformity. The differential diagnosis of thoracic pain is extensive and includes both spinal and nonspinal etiologies. Spinal deformities (e.g., scoliosis, kyphosis) are generally painless in children but may become symptomatic in adult life.

2. **What are some common causes of thoracic pain which are intrinsic to the spinal column?**
   - *Degenerative disorders:* spondylosis, spinal stenosis, disc herniation
   - *Fracture:* traumatic, pathologic
   - *Neoplasm*
   - *Infection:* disc space infection, vertebral osteomyelitis, epidural abscess
   - *Deformity:* kyphosis, scoliosis, trauma
   - *Vascular:* arteriovenous malformation
   - *Referred pain from a cervical spinal condition*

3. **What are some common nonspinal causes of thoracic pain?**
   - **Intrathoracic**
     - Cardiovascular (angina, aortic aneurysm)
     - Pulmonary (pneumonia, carcinoma)
     - Mediastinal (mediastinal tumor)
   - **Intraabdominal**
     - Hepatobiliary (hepatitis, cholecystitis)
     - Gastrointestinal (peptic ulcer, pancreatitis)
     - Retroperitoneal (pyelonephritis, aneurysm)
   - **Musculoskeletal/other**
     - Post-thoracotomy syndrome
     - Polymyalgia rheumatica
     - Fibromyalgia
     - Rib fractures
     - Intercostal neuralgia
     - Soft tissue disorders (sprains, myofascial pain syndromes)

4. **What should an examiner assess during inspection of the thoracic spinal region?**
   The patient should be undressed, and posture should be evaluated in both frontal and sagittal planes. Shoulder or rib asymmetry suggests the presence of scoliosis. A forward-bending test should be performed to permit assessment of rib cage and paravertebral muscle symmetry. If increased thoracic kyphosis is noted, it should be determined whether the kyphotic deformity is flexible or rigid. Leg lengths should be assessed. Look for any differences in height of the iliac crests. Note any skin markings such as café au lait spots, hairy patches, or birthmarks, which may suggest occult neurologic or bony pathology.

5. **What is the usefulness of palpation during examination of the thoracic spine?**
   Palpation allows the examiner to locate specific areas of tenderness, which aids in localization of pathology. Tenderness over the paraspinal muscles should be differentiated from tenderness over the spinous processes.

6. **How precisely is range of motion assessed in the thoracic region?**
   Range of motion (ROM) is limited in the thoracic region, and precise assessment is not an emphasized component of the thoracic spine examination. Nevertheless, thoracic ROM is tested in all planes. Flexion-extension is limited by facet joint orientation, rib cage stability, and narrow intervertebral discs. Thoracic rotation is typically greater than lumbar rotation due to facet orientation. Testing of lateral bending is relevant in assessing the flexibility of thoracic scoliosis. Asymmetric ROM, especially in forward-bending, suggests the presence of a lesion that irritates neural structures, such as a tumor or disc herniation.

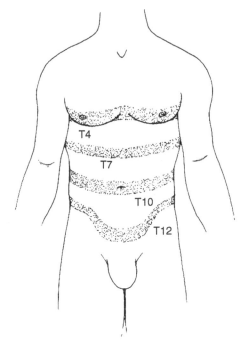

Fig. 5.1 Dermatomes of the trunk.

7. How is the neurologic examination of the thoracic spinal region performed?

Sensory levels are assessed by testing for light touch and pin-prick sensation. The exiting spinal nerves create band-like dermatomes (T4, nipple line; T7, xiphoid process; T10, umbilicus; T12, inguinal crease) (Fig. 5.1). **Motor function** is assessed by having the patient perform a partial sit-up and checking for asymmetry in the segmentally innervated rectus abdominis muscle. Upward movement of the umbilicus is consistent with isolated weakness in the lower portion of the rectus abdominis muscle (i.e., due to a spinal lesion between T10 and T12) and is termed **Beevor sign.** Reflex testing consists of evaluation of the **superficial abdominal reflex.**

8. What is the superficial abdominal reflex? What does it signify?

The superficial abdominal reflex is an upper motor neuron reflex. It is performed by stroking one of the four abdominal quadrants. The umbilicus should move toward the quadrant that was stroked. The reflex should be symmetric from side to side. Asymmetry suggests intraspinal pathology (upper motor neuron lesion) and is assessed with magnetic resonance imaging (MRI) of the spine.

9. What findings in the history and physical examination suggest the presence of a thoracic disc herniation?

Clinically significant thoracic disc herniation is rare. It is difficult to reach an accurate diagnosis from history and physical examination alone. Thoracic disc herniations may cause thoracic axial pain, thoracic radicular pain, myelopathy, or a combination of these symptoms. Neurologic findings may include nonspecific lower extremity weakness, ataxia, spasticity, numbness, hyperreflexia, clonus, and bowel or bladder dysfunction.

LUMBAR SPINE EXAMINATION

10. What pathologies should be considered in the differential diagnosis of low back pain?
- *Soft tissue disorders:* sprains, myofascial pain syndromes, fibromyalgia
- *Degenerative spinal disorders:* disc herniation, spinal stenosis, facet joint arthritis
- *Spinal instabilities:* for example, spondylolisthesis
- *Rheumatologic disorders:* rheumatoid arthritis, Reiter syndrome, psoriatic arthritis, ankylosing spondylitis
- *Infection:* bacterial, tuberculosis, fungal, HIV
- *Tumor:* primary spine tumors, metastatic tumors
- *Trauma:* fractures

- *Metabolic disorders:* osteoporosis, osteomalacia, Paget disease
- *Hematologic disorders:* sickle-cell disease
- *Systemic disorders with referred pain:* peptic ulcers, cholecystitis, pancreatitis, retrocecal appendicitis, dissecting abdominal aortic aneurysm, pelvic inflammatory disease, endometriosis, prostatitis
- *Psychogenic pain*

11. **What are some common causes of low back pain with or without lower extremity symptoms based on patient age at presentation?**
    Although no diagnosis is unique to a single age group, some generalizations apply:
    - **Less than 10 years:** consider spinal infection or tumor
    - **10–25 years:** disorders involving repetitive loading and trauma: spondylolysis, isthmic spondylolisthesis, Scheuermann disease, fractures, apophyseal ring injury
    - **25–50 years:** annular tear, disc herniation, isthmic spondylolisthesis
    - **Over 50 years:** spinal stenosis, degenerative spondylolisthesis, metastatic disease, osteoporotic compression fracture

12. **What factors in the patient history should prompt the examiner to consider further diagnostic testing, such as laboratory tests or imaging studies, during evaluation of symptoms of acute low back pain?**
    Factors that may indicate serious underlying pathology are termed **red flags** and include: fever, unexplained weight loss, bowel or bladder dysfunction, cancer history, significant trauma, osteoporosis, age older than 50 years, failure to improve with standard treatment, and history of alcohol or drug abuse.

13. **What is a simple method for helping patients to localize and describe spinal symptoms during a clinic visit?**
    Important clinical information can be obtained by having the patient complete a **pain diagram.** Pain diagrams can aid in differentiating various conditions such as mechanical low back pain, disc herniation, and spinal stenosis. Pain diagrams that contain markings of multiple body regions, nonanatomic pain distributions (i.e., pain outside of the body), or demonstrate inconsistency with physical examination findings, suggest the need to consider additional patient factors including psychological distress, magnified or inappropriate illness behavior, or somatoform-functional disorders.

14. **What are the basic elements of a physical examination of the lumbar spine?**
    Examination should address the lumbar region, pelvis, hip joints, lower limbs, gait, and peripheral vascular system. A complete examination should include:
    1. Inspection
    2. Palpation
    3. ROM (lumbar spine, hips, knees)
    4. Neurologic examination (sensation, muscle testing, reflexes)
    5. Assessment of nerve root tension signs
    6. Vascular examination
    7. Examination of the sacroiliac joint

15. **What is looked for during inspection?**
    During the initial encounter, much can be learned from observing the patient. Abnormalities of gait such as a *drop foot, Trendelenburg gait* (due to weakness of the hip abductor muscles), and abnormal posturing of the trunk, are important clues for the examiner. It is also helpful to observe patients undress, noting how freely and easily they can move the trunk and extremities. In addition, the base of the spine should be inspected for a hairy patch or any skin markings that may be associated with occult intraspinal anomalies. Waistline symmetry should be noted, as asymmetry suggests lumbar scoliosis. The overall alignment and balance of the spine should be assessed by dropping a plumb line from the C7 spinous process to see that it is centered on the sacrum. If it is not, the lateral distance from the gluteal cleft should be noted.

16. **What is the purpose of palpation?**
    To examine for tenderness and localize pathology. Palpation must include the spinous processes, as well as the adjacent soft tissues. The area of the sciatic notch should be deeply palpated to look for sciatic irritability. Specific areas of palpation correspond to specific levels of the spine (e.g., iliac crest, L4–L5; posterior superior iliac spine, S2).

17. **How is range of motion assessed in the lumbar spine?**
    Motion is assessed in three planes: flexion/extension, right/left bending, and right/left rotation. ROM can be estimated in degrees or measured with an inclinometer. It is important to note that a significant portion of lumbar flexion is achieved through the hip joints. The normal ROM for forward flexion is 40°–60°; for extension, 20°–35°; for lateral bending, 15°–20°; and for rotation, 3°–18°.

Table 5.1 Neurologic Examination of the Lumbar Region.

LEVEL	SENSATION	MOTOR	REFLEX
L1	Anterior thigh	Psoas (T12, L1, L2, L3)	None
L2	Anterior thigh, groin	Quadriceps (L2, L3, L4)	None
L3	Anterior and lateral thigh	Quadriceps (L2, L3, L4)	None
L4	Medial leg and foot	Tibialis anterior	Patellar
L5	Lateral leg and dorsal foot	Extensor hallucis longus	None
S1	Lateral and plantar foot	Gastrocnemius, peroneals	Achilles
S2–S4	Perianal	Bladder and foot intrinsics	None

18. What is the Schober test?

The Schober test is a simple and useful clinical test to evaluate spinal mobility. This test is based on the principle that the skin over the lumbar spine stretches as a person flexes forward to touch the toes. While the patient is standing, a tape measure is used to mark the skin at the midpoint between the posterior superior iliac crests, and at points 10 cm proximal and 5 cm distal to this mark. The patient is then asked to bend forward as far as possible, and the distance between the proximal and distal marked points is measured with the patient in the flexed position. In 90% of asymptomatic patients, there is an increase in length of at least 5 cm. This maneuver eliminates hip flexion and is a true indication of lumbar spine movement.

19. How is neurologic examination of the lumbar region performed?

Neurologic examination of the lumbar region focuses primarily on sequential examination of nerve roots. For each nerve root, the examiner tests sensation, motor strength, and, if one exists, the appropriate reflex (Table 5.1).

20. What provocative maneuvers are used to assess a patient with a suspected lumbar radiculopathy?

The **standard straight-leg raise test** and its variants increase tension along the sciatic nerve, and are used to assess the L5 and S1 nerve roots. The **reverse straight-leg raise test** increases tension along the femoral nerve and is used to assess the L2, L3, and L4 nerve roots.

21. Describe how the straight-leg raise test and the femoral nerve stretch test are performed.

The straight-leg raise test is a tension sign that may be performed with the patient supine (Lasègue test; Fig. 5.2) or seated (Fig. 5.3). The leg is elevated with the knee straight to increase tension along the sciatic nerve, specifically the L5 and S1 nerve roots. If the nerve root is compressed, nerve stretch provokes radicular pain.

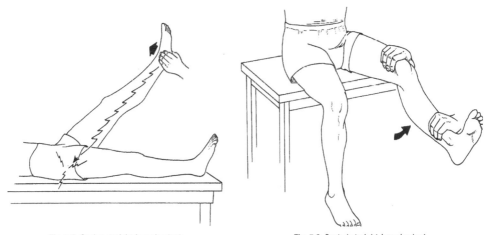

Fig. 5.2 Supine straight-leg raise test.   **Fig. 5.3** Seated straight-leg raise test.

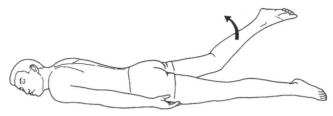

Fig. 5.4 Femoral nerve stretch test.

Back pain alone does not constitute a positive test. The most tension is placed on the L5 and S1 nerve roots during a supine straight-leg raise test between 35° and 70° of leg elevation. A variant of this test is the bowstring test, in which the knee is flexed during the standard supine straight-leg raise test to reduce leg pain secondary to sciatic nerve stretch. Finger pressure is then applied over the popliteal space at the terminal aspect of the sciatic nerve in an attempt to reestablish radicular symptoms.

The reverse straight-leg raise test, or femoral nerve stretch test, increases tension along the femoral nerve, specifically the L2, L3, and L4 nerve roots (Fig. 5.4). It may be performed with the patient in the prone or lateral position, with the affected side upward. The test is performed by extending the hip and flexing the knee. This is exactly opposite to the standard straight-leg raise test. The test is considered positive if radicular pain in the anterior thigh region occurs.

22. What is the contralateral straight-leg raise test? Why is it a significant test?
    This test is performed in the same fashion as the standard straight-leg raise test, except that the asymptomatic leg is elevated. If this test reproduces sciatic symptoms in the opposite extremity, it is considered positive. A positive test is strongly suggestive of a disc herniation medial to the nerve root (in the axilla of the nerve root). The combination of a positive straight-leg raise test on the symptomatic side, and a positive contralateral straight-leg raise test, is the most specific clinical test for a disc herniation, with accuracy approaching 97%.

23. What nerve root is affected by a posterolateral disc herniation?
    The nerve roots of the lumbar spine exit the spinal canal beneath the pedicle of the corresponding numbered vertebra and above the caudad intervertebral disc. The most common location for a lumbar disc herniation is posterolateral. This type of disc herniation compresses the *traversing nerve root* of the motion segment. For example, a posterolateral disc herniation at the L4–L5 level would compress the traversing nerve root (L5).

24. What nerve root is affected by a disc herniation lateral to or within the neural foramen?
    A disc herniation lateral to or within the neural foramen compresses the *exiting nerve root* of the motion segment. For example, a disc herniation at the L4–L5 level located in the region of the neural foramen, compresses the exiting nerve root (L4) and spares the traversing nerve root (L5).

25. What nerve roots are affected by a central disc herniation?
    A central disc herniation can compress one or more of the caudal nerve roots. A large central disc herniation is a common cause of a cauda equina syndrome.

26. What is cauda equina syndrome?
    Cauda equina syndrome is a symptom complex that includes low back pain, unilateral or bilateral sciatica, lower extremity motor weakness, sensory abnormalities, bowel or bladder dysfunction, and saddle anesthesia. It may result from acute or chronic compression of the nerve roots of the cauda equina caused by massive central lumbar disc protrusion, spinal stenosis, epidural hematoma, spinal tumor, and fracture. The syndrome can result in permanent motor deficit and bowel and bladder incontinence. Once identified, cauda equina syndrome generally requires urgent surgical intervention to prevent permanent neurologic deficits or incontinence.

27. What are Waddell signs?
    Waddell described five categories of tests that are useful in evaluating patients with low back pain. These signs do not prove malingering but are useful to highlight the potential contribution of psychologic and/or socioeconomic factors to spinal symptoms. Presence of three or more signs is considered significant. Isolated positive signs are not considered significant. Waddell tests include:
    1. **Superficial tenderness:** Nonorganic tenderness with light touch over a wide lumbar area, or deeper tenderness in a nonanatomic distribution.

2. **Simulation:** Maneuvers that should not be uncomfortable are performed. If pain is reported, nonorganic pathology is suggested. Examples of such tests include production of low back pain with axial loading of the head, or when the shoulders and pelvis are passively rotated in the same plane.
3. **Distraction:** The examiner performs a provocative test in the usual manner and rechecks the test when the patient is distracted. For example, a patient with a positive straight-leg raise test in the supine position, can be assessed with a straight-leg raise test in the seated position, under the guise of examining the foot or another part of the lower extremity. If the distraction test is negative but a formal straight-leg raise test in the supine position is positive, this finding is considered a positive sign.
4. **Regionalization:** Presence of findings that diverge from accepted neuroanatomy. For example, entire muscle groups, which do not have common innervation, may demonstrate *giving way* on strength testing, or sensory abnormalities may not follow a dermatomal distribution.
5. **Overreaction:** Disproportionate response to examination may take many forms such as collapsing, inappropriate facial expression, excessive verbalization, or any other type of overreaction to any aspect of the examination.

28. During assessment of a patient with lumbar pain involving the lower extremities, what nonspinal pathologies should be evaluated during the physical examination?
Pathology of the hip joints and vascular disease involving the lower extremities should be ruled out. The presentation of these pathologies and common spinal problems can overlap. Anterior thigh pain may be due to either nerve impingement involving the upper lumbar nerve roots (L2, L3, L4), or hip arthritis. ROM testing of the hip joints can rule out pathology. Lower extremity claudication may be due to either vascular disease or lumbar spinal stenosis (neurogenic claudication). Assessment for clinical signs of peripheral arterial disease (i.e., reduced or absent pulses in the lower extremity, thickened toenails, hair loss on the legs/feet, reduced temperature of one or both legs/feet, pallor or cyanosis of the legs/feet), and assessment of the ankle-brachial index, are helpful in diagnosing this problem.

29. How is the sacroiliac joint assessed?
Sacroiliac pain is difficult to confirm on clinical assessment alone and generally requires a diagnostic joint injection under radiographic control for confirmation. Clinical tests that have been described to assess this joint include:
- **Distraction test:** With the patient supine, a vertically oriented pressure is applied bilaterally to the anterior superior iliac spinous processes to distract the sacroiliac joints.
- **Patrick test:** With the patient supine, the knee on the affected side is flexed and the foot placed on the opposite patella. The flexed knee is then pushed laterally to stress the sacroiliac joint. This is also called the FABER (flexion-abduction-external rotation) test.
- **Gaenslen test:** With the patient supine, the hip and knee of the unaffected leg are flexed toward the chest, and the examiner hyperextends the affected leg at the hip joint.
- **Thigh thrust:** With the patient supine, the hip flexed to 90°, and the knee bent, the examiner applies a posteriorly directed force through the femur at varying angles of abduction/adduction.
- **Pelvic compression test:** With the patient either supine or in the lateral position, the iliac crests are pushed toward the midline in an attempt to elicit pain in the sacroiliac joint. Three or more positive tests in a patient whose symptoms cannot be made to centralize on physical examination support the diagnosis of sacroiliac joint pain.

KEY POINTS

1. A comprehensive patient history and physical examination is the first step in diagnosis of a spine complaint.
2. A major goal of the initial patient evaluation is to differentiate common nonemergent spinal conditions such as acute nonspecific thoracic or lumbar pain and degenerative spinal disorders, from serious and urgent problems such as spinal infections, spinal tumors, or cauda equina syndrome.
3. Nonspinal pathology (e.g., osteoarthritis of the hip joint, peripheral vascular disease) may mimic the symptoms of lumbar spinal disorders and must be considered in the differential diagnosis.

Websites
1. Low back examination (video): https://www.hss.edu/conditions_musculoskeletal-medicine-for-the-primary-care-physician-low-back-exam.asp
2. Musculoskeletal examination-low back pain: https://meded.ucsd.edu/clinicalmed/joints6.htm
3. Key points related to physical examination of the lumbar spine: http://www.wheelessonline.com/ortho/exam_of_the_lumbar_spine
4. United States Disability Examination Worksheets: https://www.vba.va.gov/pubs/forms/VBA-21-0960M-14-ARE.pdf
5. Sacroiliac Joint Tests: https://www.physio-pedia.com/Sacroiliac_Joint_Special_Test_Cluster

BIBLIOGRAPHY

1. Albert TJ. (2004). *Physical Examination of the Spine*. London, UK: Thieme; 2004.
2. Apeldoorn AT, Bosselaar H, Blom-Luberti T, Twisk JW, Lankhorst GJ. The reliability of nonorganic sign-testing and the Waddell score in patients with chronic low back pain. *Spine* 2008;33:821–826.
3. Hoppenfeld, S. Physical Examination of the Spine and Extremities. 1st ed. New York, NY: Appleton & Lange; 1976.
4. Laslett M. Evidence-based diagnosis and treatment of the painful sacroiliac joint. *J Man Manip Ther* 2008;16(3):142–152.
5. Rainville J, Jouve C, Finno M, Limke J. Comparison of four tests of quadriceps strength in L3 or L4 radiculopathies. *Spine* 2003; 28:2466–2471.
6. Scherping SC. (2004). History and physical examination. In: Frymoyer JW, Wiesel SW, editors. The Adult Spine: Principles and Practice. 3rd ed. Philadelphia, PA: Lippincott Williams & Wilkins; 2004, pp. 49–68.
7. Standaert CJ, Herring SA, Sinclair JD. Patient History and Physical Examination—Cervical, Thoracic and Lumbar. In: Herkowitz HN, Garfin SR, Eismont FJ, Bell GR, Fischgrund JS, Bono CM, editors. Rothman-Simeone and Herkowitz's The Spine. 7th ed. Philadelphia, PA: Saunders; 2018, pp. 183–200.

CHAPTER 6

EVALUATION OF SPINAL DEFORMITIES

Vincent J. Devlin, MD

1. **What is a spinal deformity?**

   A spinal deformity is an abnormality of the alignment, formation, or shape of the spinal column. Traditionally, spinal deformities have been classified into those that predominantly affect the coronal plane (e.g., idiopathic scoliosis) and the sagittal plane (e.g., Scheuermann kyphosis). In reality, spinal deformities are complex and simultaneously affect the sagittal, coronal, and axial plane alignment of the spinal column, and its relationship to the pelvis and thoracic cage. A spinal deformity may result from a pathologic process at a single vertebra level (e.g., spondylolisthesis), or multiple spinal levels (e.g., Scheuermann kyphosis), or it may involve the entire spinal column and pelvis due to compromised postural support mechanisms (e.g., neuromuscular scoliosis).

2. **Why does the assessment of spinal deformities require a comprehensive assessment of the patient's health status?**

   Multiple facets of human disease may be associated with a spinal deformity depending on its etiology. A spinal deformity may be only one manifestation of an underlying systemic disorder that may affect multiple organ systems. The etiology of spinal deformities is wide ranging and includes congenital, developmental, degenerative, neuromuscular and metabolic disorders, trauma, infection, tumors, and conditions whose precise etiology remains incompletely defined (e.g., idiopathic scoliosis). Radiographs are required to document the presence, severity, and extent of a specific spinal deformity. Higher-level imaging studies (computed tomography, magnetic resonance imaging [MRI]) are used to evaluate neural compression, anatomic detail, and to rule out the presence of coexisting intraspinal anomalies, and anomalies involving other body systems.

3. **What are the potential consequences of untreated spinal deformities?**

   The consequences of an untreated spinal deformity for a specific patient depend on many factors, including age, underlying health status, etiology, deformity magnitude and pattern, and the potential for future progression of the spinal deformity. Potential consequences of untreated spinal deformity may include cosmetic issues, pain, neurologic deficit, sagittal and/or coronal plane imbalance, and impairment in activities of daily living. Severe thoracic deformity may impair respiratory mechanics with resultant hypoxemia, pulmonary hypertension, cor pulmonale, or even death.

4. **Describe the basic components involved in the clinical assessment of a patient with spinal deformity.**

   A. **Detailed history:**
   - What is the presenting or chief complaint (e.g., deformity, pain, neurologic symptoms, impaired function in activities of daily living, cardiorespiratory symptoms)?
   - If pain is present, describe its location, severity, duration, frequency, and whether it is present during activity or at rest.
   - When was the spinal deformity first noticed?
   - Is the spinal deformity progressing in severity?
   - For pediatric patients: What is the patient's maturity and growth potential?

   B. **Past medical history:** Have prior spine treatments or diagnostic studies been performed? Are there any associated or general medical problems? Were there any abnormalities noted at birth or during development?

   C. **Medications:** include dose, route and frequency for each medication

   D. **Allergies:** include allergies to medication and nonmedication substances, such as iodine or shellfish

   E. **Review of Systems**

   F. **Family history:** Is there a family history of spinal deformity?

   G. **Social history:** occupation, history of tobacco and alcohol use, or drug abuse

   H. **Comprehensive physical examination:**

   Inspection. The patient must undress and change into a gown so the examiner can fully assess the trunk and extremities. Assess for asymmetry of the neckline, shoulder height, rib cage, waistline, flank, pelvis, and lower extremities. The patient is initially assessed in the standing position and next is bent forward to 90°. The patient should be inspected from both anterior and posterior aspects, and from the side. Note any skin lesions (e.g., midline hair patch, sinus tract, hemangiomas, café au lait pigmentation). Observe the patient's gait. Observe body proportions and height.

Palpation. Palpate the spinous processes and paraspinous region for tenderness, deviation in spinous process alignment, or a palpable step-off deformity.

Spinal range of motion. Test flexion-extension, side-bending, and rotation. Any restriction or asymmetry with range of motion (ROM) is noted.

Neurologic examination. Assess sensory, motor, and reflex function of the upper and lower extremities, including abdominal reflexes.

Spinal alignment and balance assessment in the coronal plane. Normally, the head should be centered over the sacrum and pelvis. A plumb line dropped from C7 should fall through the gluteal crease.

Spinal alignment and balance assessment in the sagittal plane. When the patient is observed from the side, assess the four physiologic sagittal curves (cervical and lumbar lordosis, thoracic and sacral kyphosis). When the patient stands with the hips and knees fully extended, the head should be aligned over the sacrum. The ear, shoulder, and greater trochanter of the hip should lie on the same vertical line.

Extremity assessment. Measurement of leg lengths, assessment of joint ROM and flexibility in the upper and lower extremities, are performed. Note any contractures or deformities involving the extremities (e.g., cavus feet).

Examination of related body systems. A detailed medical assessment should be performed. Certain spinal deformities are associated with abnormalities in other organ systems, especially the neurologic, renal, and cardiac systems. In specific situations, screening for vision problems, hearing loss, and learning disorders may be required.

EVALUATION OF PATIENTS WITH CORONAL PLANE SPINAL DEFORMITIES

5. What are some of the common types of scoliosis?
   - **Idiopathic scoliosis:** no apparent cause or related underlying etiology
   - **Neuromuscular scoliosis:** due to neuromuscular disorders such as cerebral palsy, muscular dystrophy, myelomeningocele, Friedreich ataxia, spina bifida, and spinal cord injury
   - **Congenital scoliosis:** due to failure of vertebrae to develop normally in utero including failure of formation (e.g., hemivertebra), or failure of segmentation (e.g., congenital bar)
   - **Thoracogenic scoliosis:** due to congenital rib fusions or chest wall tethering following thoracic surgery
   - **Syndromic scoliosis:** scoliosis in conjunction with a constellation of signs, symptoms or characteristics that are clinically recognizable (e.g., Marfan syndrome, Ehlers-Danlos syndrome, Prader-Willi syndrome, neurofibromatosis, and bone dysplasias)
   - **Posttraumatic scoliosis:** e.g., acute, chronic, and post-surgical causes
   - **Postinfectious scoliosis:** pyogenic, granulomatous
   - **Scoliosis related to metabolic bone diseases:** e.g., osteoporotic compression fractures
   - **Tumor-related scoliosis:** spinal cord or vertebral column tumors
   - **Adult degenerative or adult scoliosis:** develops in previously straight spines
   - **Scoliosis secondary to anomalies of the lumbosacral joint:** e.g., spondylolisthesis

6. How is scoliosis stratified according to patient age?
   - **Early onset scoliosis:** onset before age 10, regardless of etiology
   - **Adolescent idiopathic scoliosis:** onset from age 10 through adulthood
   - **Adult scoliosis:** two major types: *adult idiopathic scoliosis* (idiopathic scoliosis in an adult which began during childhood) and *adult de novo or degenerative scoliosis* (onset of new scoliosis in adulthood due to degenerative changes occurring in the spinal column). Additional causes of scoliosis in adults include all types of scoliosis that develop earlier in life and continue into adulthood, as well as scoliosis that develops in adulthood from miscellaneous etiologies, including trauma and osteoporosis.

   Traditionally, idiopathic scoliosis in pediatric patients was stratified into three groups based on age of onset: *infantile* (from birth through age 3), *juvenile* (age 4 through 10), and *adolescent* (age 10 through adulthood). As the natural history and treatment goals differ for patients less than age 10 compared to adolescent scoliosis patients, the term "early onset scoliosis" has been adopted by specialists worldwide to describe scoliosis with onset before age 10, regardless of etiology.

7. What are some important considerations in the evaluation of patients with early-onset scoliosis?
   Early onset scoliosis represents a heterogenous population consisting of patients with congenital, neuromuscular, syndromic, and idiopathic deformities. Unlike adolescent and adult scoliosis, early onset scoliosis occurs in patients with significant remaining growth potential and high likelihood for progressive deformity, and may adversely impact lung development and reduce life expectancy. Evaluation begins with a general medical history (birth, developmental, and family history) including details regarding the patient's spinal deformity (age at onset or diagnosis, progression, presence or absence of pain, prior treatment). Additional elements to assess include height, weight, nutritional status, achievement of age-appropriate developmental milestones, pulmonary status,

and investigation for comorbidities. Depending on deformity etiology, coexisting disorders may involve the neural axis, cardiac, urogenital, musculoskeletal, gastrointestinal, pulmonary, and integumentary systems.

8. Describe the assessment of an adolescent with possible scoliosis.
   The patient should be examined with the back exposed (Fig. 6.1). First, the patient is examined in the standing position. Second, the patient is examined as he or she bends forward at the waist, with arms hanging freely, knees straight, and feet together. Findings that suggest the presence of scoliosis include:
   - Shoulder height asymmetry
   - Scapula or rib prominence
   - Chest cage asymmetry
   - Unequal space between the arm and the lateral trunk on side to side comparison

Clinical Evaluation of Scoliosis

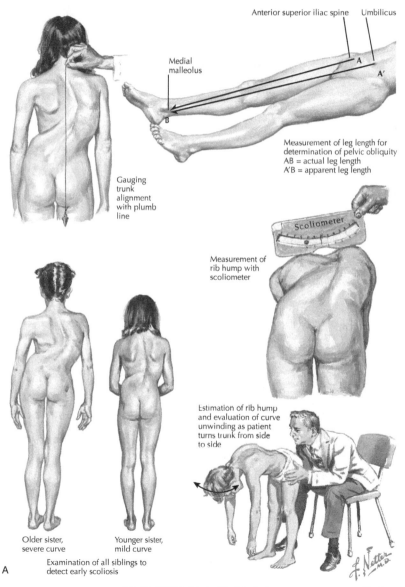

Anterior superior iliac spine   Umbilicus

Medial malleolus

Measurement of leg length for determination of pelvic obliquity
AB = actual leg length
A'B = apparent leg length

Gauging trunk alignment with plumb line

Scoliometer

Measurement of rib hump with scoliometer

Estimation of rib hump and evaluation of curve unwinding as patient turns trunk from side to side

Older sister, severe curve

Younger sister, mild curve

Examination of all siblings to detect early scoliosis

A

Fig. 6.1 (A) Clinical evaluation of scoliosis.   *Continued*

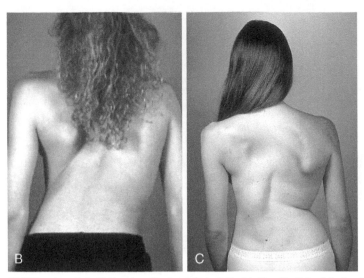

Fig. 6.1, cont'd (B) Thoracic scoliosis. (C) Thoracic and lumbar scoliosis. (A, Reprinted from The Netter Collection of Medical Illustrations – Musculoskeletal System, Part II, Developmental Disorders, Tumors, Rheumatic Diseases and Joint Replacements, p. 34. © Elsevier Inc. All Rights Reserved.)

- Waistline asymmetry
- Asymmetry of the paraspinous musculature

9. **What is a scoliometer? How is it used?**
   In North America, it is common for children in the 10- to 14-year age group to undergo a screening assessment at school for scoliosis. The *Adams test* (assessment for spinal asymmetry with the patient in the forward-bending position) is typically used to assess for possible scoliosis. The use of an *inclinometer (scoliometer)* has been popularized to quantitate trunk asymmetry and help decide whether radiographs should be obtained to further evaluate a specific patient. The scoliometer is used to determine the *angle of trunk rotation (ATR)*, the angle formed between the horizontal plane, and the plane across the posterior aspect of the trunk at the point of maximal deformity, with the patient in the forward-bending position. An ATR of 5° is correlated with an 11° curve, and an ATR of 7° is correlated with a 20° curve.

10. **How is scoliosis due to leg-length discrepancy distinguished from other types of scoliosis?**
    By performing the forward-bend test with the patient seated, the effect of leg-length discrepancy on the spine is eliminated. Alternatively, evaluating the patient after placing wood blocks beneath the shortened extremity eliminates the contribution of leg-length discrepancy to pelvic obliquity and scoliosis. True leg lengths should be determined by measuring the distances from the anterior-superior iliac spines to the medial malleoli and compared to apparent leg lengths measured from the umbilicus to the medial malleoli. Discrepancies should be confirmed using imaging techniques.

11. **What is the significance of painful scoliosis in a pediatric patient?**
    The presentation of painful scoliosis is atypical in the pediatric patient. If pain is present in a pediatric patient with idiopathic scoliosis, it is typically mild, nonspecific, intermittent, and nonradiating. Normally, the pain is mechanical (improves with rest), does not awaken the patient from sleep, and does not limit activity. Persistent severe back pain, or back pain with atypical features, should prompt the physician to further investigate the cause of the patient's symptoms. Workup (e.g., lateral spinal radiograph, MRI) is needed to rule out etiologies, such as a spinal tumor, spinal infection, spondylolisthesis, or Scheuermann disease.

12. **What conditions should be considered in the differential diagnosis of neckline asymmetry or shoulder height asymmetry?**
    In addition to an upper thoracic curvature secondary to idiopathic scoliosis, other conditions may be responsible for these clinical findings including torticollis, Klippel-Feil syndrome, and congenital vertebral anomalies.

13. **What is Klippel-Feil syndrome?**
    Klippel-Feil syndrome is a congenital fusion of the cervical spine associated with the clinical triad of a short neck, low posterior hairline, and limited neck motion.

14. **What should an examiner assess during evaluation of an adult patient with scoliosis?**
In contrast to pediatric patients, adult patients with scoliosis often present with back pain. However, the incidence of back pain in the adult population is significant regardless of the presence of a spinal deformity. Thus it cannot be assumed that symptoms of back pain are related to the presence of a spinal deformity. Examination of the adult patient should be directed at localizing painful areas of the spine. Is pain localized to an area of deformity, or to the lumbosacral junction? Does the patient have symptoms consistent with spinal stenosis or radiculopathy that warrant further workup with spinal canal imaging studies (i.e., MRI)? Is there evidence of deformity progression or cardiopulmonary dysfunction? There are no short cuts in the evaluation of spinal deformity, and a complete history and physical examination are mandatory.

15. **What is sciatic scoliosis?**
Pain due to lumbar nerve root irritation may lead to a postural abnormality that mimics a structural spinal curvature. This condition is termed *sciatic scoliosis*. This curvature is a nonstructural reaction to pain, therefore treatment should be directed toward the pain source, and not the curvature. In adolescents and young adults, this postural deformity may develop following a fall or trauma. Other causes of sciatic scoliosis include disc herniation and spinal stenosis. Sciatic scoliosis is characterized by the presence of a lateral curvature with an absence of vertebral rotation on an anterior-posterior radiograph. In contrast, idiopathic scoliosis is characterized by the presence of both lateral curvature and vertebral rotation.

EVALUATION OF PATIENTS WITH SAGITTAL PLANE SPINAL DEFORMITIES

16. **How are kyphotic spinal deformities classified based on etiology?**
A wide range of etiologies may lead to sagittal plane spinal deformities including:
- Postural kyphosis
- Scheuermann kyphosis
- Congenital kyphosis (i.e., defect of formation, defect of segmentation, mixed types)
- Neuromuscular kyphosis
- Myelodysplastic kyphosis
- Posttraumatic kyphosis
- Postsurgical kyphosis (i.e., postlaminectomy, proximal and distal junctional kyphosis)
- Ankylosing spondylitis
- Tumor-related kyphotic deformities
- Postinfectious kyphotic deformities (pyogenic, granulomatous)
- Postirradiation kyphosis
- Metabolic disorders (osteoporosis, osteomalacia, osteogenesis imperfecta)
- Skeletal dysplasias (achondroplasia, mucopolysaccharidoses, neurofibromatosis)
- Kyphosis due to degenerative spinal disorders

17. **What are some common causes of increased thoracic kyphosis?**
Thoracic kyphosis is one of the four physiologic sagittal curves in normal people. Many different spinal pathologies can lead to an abnormal increase in thoracic kyphosis. In the pediatric population, increased thoracic kyphosis is commonly associated with Scheuermann disease, poor posture, or congenital spinal anomalies. In the adult population, a wide range of spinal pathologies can manifest as increased thoracic kyphosis. Common causes include osteoporotic compression fractures (may lead to a deformity termed a *dowager hump*), degenerative spinal disorders, and postsurgical kyphosis.

18. **How are postural kyphosis and kyphosis due to Scheuermann disease distinguished clinically?**
Postural kyphosis (postural roundback) and Scheuermann kyphosis are common causes of abnormal sagittal plane alignment in teenagers (Fig. 6.2). These conditions can be distinguished on clinical assessment by performing a forward-bend test and observing the patient from the side. With postural kyphosis, the sagittal contour normalizes because the deformity is flexible. In kyphosis due to Scheuermann disease, the deformity is rigid (structural) and does not normalize on forward bending.

19. **Define gibbus.**
The term *gibbus* is derived from the Latin word for hump. It refers to a spinal deformity in the sagittal plane characterized by a sharply angulated spinal segment, with an apex that points posteriorly (Fig. 6.3).

20. **What condition should be considered in a child with limited lumbar flexion and a fixed lumbar lordosis?**
Lumbar lordosis that is rigid and does not correct when the patient performs a forward-bend test suggests the possibility of an intrathecal mass (tumor). A workup, including an MRI of the spine, should be initiated to rule out this possibility.

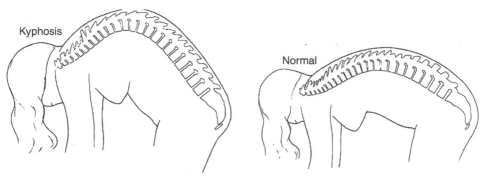

Fig. 6.2 Structural versus postural kyphosis. With structural kyphosis (i.e., Scheuermann kyphosis), the deformity does not normalize on forward bending. Postural kyphosis normalizes on forward bending because the deformity is flexible.

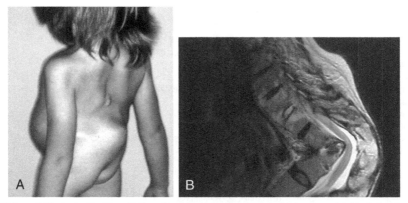

Fig. 6.3 (A) Congenital kyphosis with gibbus. (B) Magnetic resonance imaging demonstrates sharply angulated kyphotic deformity secondary to congenital kyphosis.

21. **What is meant by sagittal imbalance? What are some common causes?**
    A sagittally balanced spine is able to align with the gravity line and maintain a horizontal gaze with minimal muscular effort. *Sagittal imbalance* is a disabling postural disorder characterized by spinal pain, forward inclination of the trunk, and difficulty in maintaining an erect posture. The patient may attempt to maintain spinal balance through various compensatory mechanisms, including hyperextension of the hip joints, retroversion of the pelvis, hip and knee flexion, and compensation through mobile spinal segments outside the zone of any prior spinal surgery. The disorder was initially termed *flatback syndrome*. It was described in association with surgically treated cases of scoliosis in which a fusion extended distally into the lower lumbar spine in association with the use of distraction instrumentation, and resulted in loss of normal lumbar lordosis. When a patient with a sagittal imbalance syndrome due to loss of lumbar lordosis attempts to stand with the hips and knees fully extended, the head is no longer aligned over the sacrum (Fig. 6.4). Additional causes of sagittal imbalance include lumbar fusions performed in hypolordotic alignment, spinal degeneration, or vertebral fracture proximal or distal to a previous fusion mass, pseudarthrosis, posttraumatic kyphosis, multilevel laminectomies, and ankylosing spondylitis.

22. **Why is it helpful to examine a patient with sagittal imbalance in different positions?**
    Examination in different positions can provide information about the magnitude, flexibility, and location of the primary spinal deformity. To assess the true magnitude of the spinal deformity, the patient should be examined *standing* with the knees and hips as fully extended as possible. To assess flexibility of the spinal deformity in the sagittal plane, the patient should be examined in the *supine and prone* positions, and assessed for spontaneous correction with positioning. Examination in the *seated* position is helpful to eliminate the contribution of hip flexion contracture to the sagittal deformity. Differentiation between cervicothoracic deformity and lumbosacral deformity is aided by evaluation with the patient in the supine position. The patient's shoulders will remain elevated from the examination table in the presence of a primary cervicothoracic deformity. In contrast, a patient with a primary

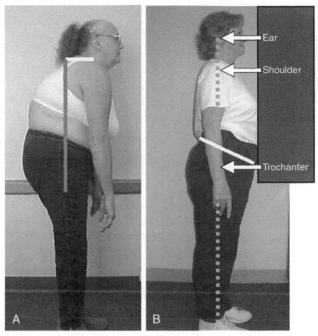

Fig. 6.4 (A) Sagittal imbalance (flatback) syndrome. (B) Normal sagittal plane alignment.

lumbosacral deformity may be able to lie flat on the examination table due to compensatory retroversion of the pelvis.

23. **What additional evaluation is indicated for a patient who presents with a congenital spinal deformity?**

    Assessment for associated anomalies in other organ systems is part of the workup of a patient with congenital scoliosis. The acronym VACTERL identifies the commonly involved organ systems: *v*ertebral, *a*nal, *c*ardiac, *t*racheal, *e*sophageal, *r*enal, and *l*imb. Associated anomalies of the neural axis (spinal dysraphism) are evaluated with an MRI of the spine. Nonspinal anomalies frequently involve the renal system, and may be evaluated with renal ultrasound or intravenous pyelography.

24. **Describe the key points to assess during examination of a patient with spinal deformity secondary to neuromuscular disease (Fig. 6.5).**

    • Assessment of level of function. Can the patient sit independently? Is the patient ambulatory? What is the Gross Motor Functional Classification System (GMFCS) level?

    • Assessment of general health status. Is there a history of seizures, frequent pneumonia, or poor nutrition?

    • Evaluation of head control, trunk control, and motor strength. Does the underlying neuromuscular problem result in a spastic, flaccid, or athetoid picture?

    • Assessment of curve flexibility. Curve flexibility can be assessed by grasping the head in the area of the mastoid process and lifting the patient from the sitting or standing position.

    • Is pelvic obliquity present? Is it correctable with traction and positioning?

    • Evaluation of the hip joints for coexistent pathology, including contractures.

    • Is the patient's underlying neuromuscular disorder associated with any other organ system problems? For example, Duchenne muscular dystrophy is associated with cardiomyopathy.

    • Documentation of pressure sores and areas of skin breakdown.

25. **What findings may be noted in a pediatric patient with spondylolisthesis?**

    Spondylolisthesis in children may present with a variety of symptoms and physical findings, depending on the degree of slippage, and the degree of kyphosis at the level of the slip. Low back pain and buttock pain are the most common presenting symptoms. A physical examination typically reveals localized tenderness with palpation at the level of slippage. Hamstring tightness is a commonly associated finding. In the most severe cases, the patient is unable to stand erect because of sagittal plane decompensation associated with compensatory lumbar hyperlordosis, and occasionally neurologic deficit (Fig. 6.6).

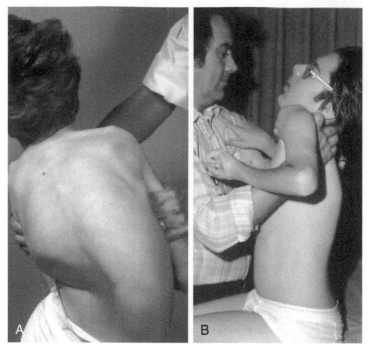

Fig. 6.5 Neuromuscular scoliosis. (A) Long sweeping curve with associated pelvic obliquity and loss of sitting balance. (B) Assessment of curve flexibility.

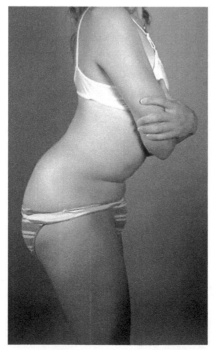

Fig. 6.6 Severe spondylolisthesis associated with sagittal plane decompensation.

KEY POINTS

1. The key components of the evaluation of a spinal deformity patient are a detailed patient history, comprehensive physical examination, appropriate diagnostic imaging studies, and assessment for potential abnormalities in other organ systems (e.g., renal, cardiac, gastrointestinal, pulmonary, integumentary, and central nervous system).
2. Consequences of untreated spinal deformity include cosmetic problems, pain, neurologic deficit, postural difficulty, pulmonary compromise, and impairment in daily living activities.

Websites
1. Scoliosis Research Society E-Text: http://www.srs.org/professionals/online-education-and-resources/srs-e-text
2. Scoliosis resources: http://www.nlm.nih.gov/medlineplus/scoliosis.html
3. Spondylolisthesis resources: http://www.nlm.nih.gov/medlineplus/ency/article/001260.htm
4. Overview of resources for spinal diseases: http://www.nlm.nih.gov/medlineplus/spinaldiseases.html

---

BIBLIOGRAPHY

1. Elsebaie, H. B., & Pawelek, J. (2016). Clinical examination and associated comorbidities of early onset scoliosis. In B. A. Akbarnia, M. Yazici, & G. A. Thompson (Eds.), *The Growing Spine: Management of Spinal Disorders in Young Children* (pp. 123–138). New York, NY: Springer.
2. Gaines, R. W. (2003). Clinical evaluation of the patient with spine deformity. In R. L. DeWald (Ed.), *Spinal Deformities: The Comprehensive Text* (pp. 267–271). New York, NY: Thieme.
3. Lamartina, C., & Berjano, P. (2014). Classification of sagittal imbalance based on spinal alignment and compensatory mechanisms. European Spine Journal, 23, 1177–1189.
4. Lonner, B. S. (2008). Spinal deformity in the clinical setting. In T. J. Errico, B. S. Lonner, & A. W Moulton (Eds.), *Surgical Management of Spinal Deformities* (pp. 61–70). Philadelphia, PA: Saunders.
5. Lonstein, J. E. (1995). Patient evaluation. In J. E. Lonstein, R. B. Winter, & D. S. Bradford, (Eds.), *Moe's Textbook of Scoliosis and Other Spinal Deformities* (3rd ed., pp. 45–56). Philadelphia, PA: Saunders.
6. McCarthy, R. E. (2001). Evaluation of the patient with deformity. In S. L. Weinstein (Ed.), *The Pediatric Spine – Principles and Practice* (2nd ed., pp. 133–160). Philadelphia, PA: Lippincott Williams & Wilkins.
7. Tolo, V. T. (2003). Clinical evaluation for neuromuscular scoliosis and kyphosis. In R. L. DeWald (Ed.), *Spinal Deformities: The Comprehensive Text* (pp. 272–283). New York, NY: Thieme.
8. Winter, R. B. (2006). Evaluation of the patient with congenital spine deformity. In R. L. DeWald (Ed.), *Spinal Deformities: The Comprehensive Text* (pp. 258–266). New York, NY: Thieme.

CHAPTER 7

EVALUATION OF IMPAIRMENT, DISABILTY, AND WORKERS' COMPENSATION

Stephen L. Demeter, MD, MPH, Christopher R. Brigham, MD, MMS, and Vincent J. Devlin, MD

1. **Distinguish between impairment, disability, and handicap.**

   An **impairment** is the "deviation of an anatomic structure, physiologic function, intellectual capability, or emotional status from that which the individual possessed prior to an alteration in those structures or functions or from that expected from population norms." (1)

   A **disability** is the "inability to complete a specific task successfully that the individual was previously capable of completing or that most members of a society are capable of completing owing to a medical or psychological deviation from prior health status or from the status expected of most members of a society." (1) In other words, a disability is the inability to perform a specified task because of an impairment.

   An impaired individual is considered to have a **handicap** if there are obstacles to accomplishing life's basic activities that can be overcome only by compensating in some way for the effects of the impairment. In this context, a *handicap* represents an impairment that is mitigated by the use of an assistive device or a task modification that allows an individual with an impairment to complete a task.

   An example contrasting impairment and disability serves well. Consider a person who sustains a cervical fracture with spinal cord compromise. There is loss of motor and sensory function in the upper and lower extremities with bowel/bladder dysfunction. That person has an impairment, or a deviation from normal anatomy and function. If the person were an accountant, this medical impairment may not translate into disability, and therefore not impact normal travel and work duties. On the other hand, if the person were a professional basketball player, the same medical impairment creates total disability. Thus, disability is task specific, whereas impairment merely reflects an alteration from normal body functions. Furthermore, the accountant may be considered to have a handicap, because they use a wheelchair, assistive equipment, and a specialized van to travel to work.

2. **What is an impairment evaluation?**

   An impairment evaluation is a medical evaluation that aims to define, describe, and measure the differences in a particular person compared with either the average person (e.g., an IQ of 86 compared with the expected average of 100), or that person's prior capability (e.g., a preinjury IQ of 134 compared with the current level of 100). Such differences may take the form of anatomic deviations (e.g., amputations), physical abnormalities (e.g., decreased ROM of a joint, decreased strength surrounding that joint, or abnormal neurologic input), physiologic abnormalities (e.g., diminished ability to breathe, electrical conduction disturbances in the heart), or psychological (e.g., diminished ability to think, reason, or remember).

3. **Who performs an impairment evaluation?**

   Impairment evaluations should be performed only by professionals with a medical background. Doctors of medicine and osteopathy are the logical choices. Other professionals, including chiropractic doctors, dentists, optometrists, psychologists, and physical therapists, also possess such training and background and often perform impairment evaluations. Further, an impairment evaluation should be performed only by professionals qualified by training or experience to assess the organ system that needs evaluation. Ideally, a neurologist should evaluate neurologic impairment, not cardiac impairment. However, many specialties cross boundaries so that an occupational medicine specialist or physiatrist can also evaluate orthopedic impairment, not just orthopedic surgeons.

4. **How does an impairment evaluation differ from a standard history and physical examination?**

   Several important differences are seen when these types of examinations are contrasted: the *goal* of the evaluation is different, the *patient* may be defined differently, and the *opportunity for reevaluation* is limited in impairment examinations.

   The goal of an impairment evaluation is to define deviations from normalcy. Having or arriving at a specific diagnosis or diagnoses is helpful. However, a specific diagnosis is not the end result in an impairment evaluation, unlike in the standard history and physical examination. Both evaluations require an appropriate educational background, skill, thoroughness, and dedication. In a standard history and physical examination, there is a doctor-patient relationship and the physician attempts to diagnose and determine any required treatment. In an impairment examination, the evaluator determines and quantifies deviations in the examinee's health status and does not enter into an active doctor-patient relationship.

The results of the standard history and physical belong to the person being evaluated (although not always, as in the case of a child). The results of an impairment evaluation are usually provided to the requesting source, such as an attorney, insurance company, or governmental agency (e.g., workers' compensation boards or the Social Security Department). This point raises an interesting legal concept. Physicians are not allowed to disclose medical information to anyone but the patient. To whom does such confidentiality apply in an impairment evaluation? Usually it exists between the physician and the referring agency or party, as opposed to the person evaluated.

Another basic difference is that the impairment evaluation report focuses on and addresses the questions asked by the referring party. For example, if the physician is asked to evaluate a person for a specific injury, such as an amputation or dysfunction of an arm, the entire evaluation focuses on the arm. The end result is a report that describes the injury, the differences in the function of the injured arm from a normal person's arm (or the individual's arm function prior to the injury), and provides a prognosis for future recovery. This information is then used by other parties to determine appropriate compensation. Other diagnoses discovered during the evaluation may be irrelevant. Other issues, such as causation, apportionment, and diagnostic or therapeutic recommendations, may or may not be desired. If these issues are not requested, they are not included in the report.

Lastly, impairment evaluations are generally limited to a single encounter with the examinee.

5. How does a disability evaluation differ from an impairment evaluation?
A disability results from a medical impairment that precludes a specific task. Generally, during a disability evaluation, that task will be the examinee's job. A disability evaluation is comprehensive and based on various factors. One of these factors is the medical impairment. Other factors may include a person's age, educational background, intellectual capabilities, and social factors. Such elements are used by the system to which the worker has applied for relief. For example, a person whose right arm has been amputated may be capable of entering the work force in some other capacity. If the person is young enough, smart enough, and sufficiently motivated, he or she may be capable of performing remunerative activities in some other job market. The referring agency uses such factors when determining whether a person is totally or partially disabled and which benefits are applicable. Thus in a disability evaluation, the physician must not only identify and quantify the impairment but address additional issues such as:
• What tasks is the examinee capable of performing?
• Can the examinee attend work?
• Are job modifications an option?
• When will the examinee reach maximum medical improvement (MMI)?

6. Define what is meant by causation and identify criteria used to determine causality in relation to the evaluation of impairment.
Causation refers to the legal or administrative system determination of the cause or causes of the injury or illness that has resulted in a temporary or permanent impairment. (2) According to the American Medical Association Guides to the Evaluation of Permanent Impairment, Sixth Edition (3), causality requires determination that each of the following has occurred to a reasonable degree of medical certainty:
• A causal event
• The patient experiencing the event has the condition (e.g., impairment)
• The event could cause the condition
• The event caused or materially contributed to the condition within medical probability
    Reasonable degree of medical certainty is generally interpreted in the setting of an impairment evaluation to mean that 50% or more of the evidence supports the determination of causality (i.e., "more probable than not" or "more likely than not" standard). If evidence is less than 50%, the degree of probability of an event's occurrence is merely a possibility, and does not establish causality.

7. What is the definition of apportionment?
Apportionment means that something is divided based on a specific issue. Causation can be apportioned. For example, if a person has arthritis in his knee, how much of the arthritic changes were caused by occupation, age, and prior meniscectomy? An impairment rating can be apportioned. If a person has a rating of 12% impairment because of a herniated disc with radiculopathy and low back pain, and also had three separate injuries to the same body area, how much of that impairment was caused by the first, second, or third injury? Treatment costs can be apportioned to both the old and the new injuries, and different employers. Most jurisdictions have their own rules as to whether apportionment is used and in which circumstances. A great deal of skill and expertise is needed for an examiner to apportion an individual's current condition to all the causative factors, including the normal aging process.

8. Distinguish between exacerbation and aggravation of a prior condition.
An *exacerbation* is a temporary worsening of a prior condition by an injury or illness, with an expectation that the condition will eventually return to baseline. An example of an exacerbation is a temporary increase in symptoms based on increased activity. This contrasts with an *aggravation,* which describes a permanent worsening of a prior

condition by a specific event or exposure. This distinction may have important legal consequences. For example, if a work injury aggravates a preexisting condition, the employer may become responsible for both the second injury and the preexisting condition.

9. **What is meant by maximum medical improvement, and permanent and stationary status?**
The concept of MMI, when used in impairment evaluations, means that a person's condition has achieved a state where no further substantial improvement is anticipated with time and/or additional treatment. Treatment may include medications, surgery, physical therapy, or other types of rehabilitation. Most impairment systems require that the person achieve MMI before a final impairment rating can be given. This rating is used as a basis for the final disability settlement. Note that this concept does not consider whether the individual will worsen with time. Further, the concept of MMI usually allows for an individual to accept further treatment (with MMI determined after an appropriate recovery time following that treatment) or to decline further treatment (in which case they have attained MMI). In other words, an individual may decline treatment that might mitigate the current level of impairment (as well as the impairment rating).

The concept of permanent and stationary (P&S) is generally synonymous with the concept of MMI. Legally, the terms are the same in the state of California. Other similar terms vary by state and statute, and include "medical stability," "medically stationary," "medical stabilization," "fixed and stable," and "of healing."

10. **List some of the major compensation systems which provide economic and other benefits to claimants who experience work incapacity due to injury, illness, or aging in the United States.**
Major compensation systems in the United States include:
- Social Security Administration system
- Federal and state workers' compensation systems
- Veterans Benefits Administration
- Personal injury claims
- Private disability systems (e.g., long-term disability insurance purchased through employer)

11. **Who determines the *rules* for impairment and disability evaluation?**
Various institutions pay the costs associated with disability, such as state governments (workers' compensation), the federal government (e.g., for veterans or longshoremen), insurance companies, and self-insured employers, and have input into the rules. Many systems that pay for disability have their own rules and regulations, including rules about performing the impairment examination and rating the impairment. The most commonly used system is a formal set of rules developed by the American Medical Association (AMA), which is frequently updated *(The Guides to the Evaluation of Permanent Impairment)*. Another system is the Social Security Administration (SSA) whose rules are outlined in the *Blue Book*. Specific rules are applied to impairments in each set of guidelines; for example, the SSA only recognizes total impairment, whereas the AMA *Guides* fractionates impairment from 1% to 100%. The impairment evaluator must be thoroughly familiar with the required system.

12. **What is the Americans with Disabilities Act?**
In 1990 Congress passed the Americans with Disabilities Act (ADA). This law protects people with disabilities from discrimination and mandates accommodation for disabled employees, customers, clients, patients, and others. It prohibits discrimination in public or private employment, governmental services, public accommodation, public transportation, and telecommunication. The ADA defines a person with a disability in three ways:
(1) Any person who has a physical or mental impairment that substantially limits one or more of the individual's major life activities.
(2) Any person who has a *record of* a substantially limiting impairment.
(3) Any person who is *regarded as* having a substantially limiting impairment, regardless of whether the person is in fact disabled.

According to the ADA, an employer may not inquire about a job applicant's impairment or medical history. In addition, preemployment inquiries about past injuries and/or workers' compensation claims are expressly prohibited. An employer may offer a position conditionally, based on completion of a medical examination or medical inquiry—but only if such examinations or inquiries are made of all applicants for the same job category and the results are kept confidential. A post-offer medical evaluation is also permissible and may be more comprehensive. The job offer may be withdrawn only if the findings of the medical examination show that a person is unable to perform the essential job functions, or if the person poses a direct threat to his or her own health or safety or to that of others, even with reasonable accommodation. It is important to have a list of essential job functions for comparison.

Over the years, the intent of the ADA became diluted based on a variety of judicial rulings. On July 26, 2008, President Bush signed the ADA Amendments Act into law that clarified and extended the original law:
- It added "major life activities" including "caring for oneself, performing manual tasks, seeing, hearing, eating, sleeping, walking, standing, lifting."
- It specified the operation of several "major bodily functions."

- It overturned two U.S. Supreme Court decisions that held that (1) an employee was not disabled if the impairment could be corrected by some device, and (2) an impairment that limits one major life activity must also limit other life activities to be considered a disability.

13. What is Social Security Disability (SSD)?

The SSA defines disability as "the inability to engage in any substantial gainful activity (SGA) by reason of any medically determinable physical or mental impairment(s) which can be expected to result in death or which has lasted or can be expected to last for a continuous period of not less than 12 months" (http://www.ssa.gov/disability/professionals/bluebook). In addition, for a person under age 18, disability can exist "if he or she has a medically determinable physical or mental impairment, or combination of impairments, that causes marked and severe functional limitations, and that can be expected to cause death, or that has lasted or can be expected to last for a continuous period of not less than 12 months." To comply with these definitions, a person may have a single medical impairment or multiple impairments that, when combined, are of such severity that the person can no longer perform his or her occupation or sustain any remunerative activity after age, education, and work experience are considered.

Two groups of people are eligible for SSD:

- Under Title II, Social Security Disability Insurance (SSDI) provides cash benefits for disabled workers and their dependents who have contributed to the Social Security Trust Fund through taxes.
- Title XVI (Supplemental Security Income [SSI]) provides a minimum income level for the needy, aged, blind, and disabled.

People qualify for SSI because of financial need. Under SSI, financial need exists when a person's income and resources are equal to or below an amount specified by law. In 2019, the limit for "countable" resources was $2000 for an individual or $3000 for a couple. The income limit (or SGA) for a blind person was $2040 per month and $1220 per month for non-blind persons (http://www.ssa.gov/ssi/spotlights/spot-resources.htm).

14. How do I fill out the forms from the SSA?

Social Security forms frequently cross a physician's desk. They are often multipaged documents asking many questions, which can be daunting for those who do not understand how the SSA determines disability. The completed forms are intended to provide background information to the impairment and disability evaluator in the Social Security system (in other words, the attending physician is not the final person responsible for his or her patient's approval for Social Security disability). An independent impairment examination may also be performed on such patients. Thus, the attending physician's report is used to provide background information so that a decision can be made whether or not a person qualifies for Social Security disability. If the information provided does not allow the decision makers to answer the questions regarding qualifications, then a separate examination, paid for and scheduled by the SSA, may be performed. The attending physician does not perform the evaluation, obtain consultation with other physicians, or perform additional diagnostic testing. Occasionally, the SSA will ask the attending physician to provide an opinion regarding a patient's ability to perform remunerative employment, but these opinions are not to be provided unless asked for.

15. What is workers' compensation?

Workers' compensation is a disability program that provides medical economic support to workers who have been injured or made ill from an incident arising out of employment. It is a complex program in the U.S. with separate systems for each state, the District of Columbia, and the U.S. territories. Several federal programs also cover civilian employees, longshore and harbor workers, military veterans, and certain high-risk workers (e.g., energy workers exposed to materials such as beryllium and radiation, and coal miners). This program originated as a social experiment by Otto von Bismarck in Germany in the 1880s. It is a *no-fault* compensation system designed to replace the traditional *tort system,* under which an injured worker had to sue his employer to get benefits. In a tort system, the employee was at a disadvantage for various reasons. To rectify this, states developed workers' compensation systems, beginning with Wisconsin in 1911. The federal government developed similar systems, which are often industry specific, and have their own rules regarding impairment, disability, and compensation.

16. What parties are involved in the workers' compensation system?

Parties involved in the workers' compensation system include physicians (i.e., primary treating, consulting, and medical-legal evaluating physicians), employers, insurers and/or claims administrators, case managers, and attorneys.

17. List the types of benefits available to the injured worker through the workers' compensation system?

A workers' compensation system generally provides the following benefits:

- Current and future medical treatment for the work-related injury
- Income benefits to cover lost wages (i.e., temporary total disability, temporary partial disability)
- Disability benefits (i.e., permanent total disability, permanent partial disability)
- Vocational rehabilitation services
- Death benefits paid to surviving dependents

18. **What are the basic eligibility requirements to receive workers' compensation benefits?**

There are three basic eligibility requirements for workers' compensation benefits. First, the worker must be an employee. Second, the employer must carry Workers' Compensation insurance. Third, the employee must have sustained a work-related injury or illness (i.e., the injury "arose out of employment" or "occurred in the course of employment").

In general, an injury or illness is considered work related if an event or exposure in the work environment either caused or contributed to the resulting condition, or significantly aggravated a preexisting condition. A claim is paid if the employer or insurance carrier agrees that the injury or illness was work related or occurred during the course of work. For example, an individual who sustained a finger amputation while working on a press clearly represents a work-related incident. However, if a person was driving a company car for personal business during work hours and sustained an injury as a result of a motor vehicle accident, this is also likely to be a compensable situation. Claims that are often denied by the insurance carrier include those for stress-related, self-inflicted and other psychiatric injuries, injuries occurring while under the influence of drugs or alcohol, or as a result of fighting, horseplay, or crime.

Workers' compensation benefits are available for workers in each state and for federal workers. Each state has slightly different rules, which are different from federal rules. Lastly, there are statutes of limitations on filing for these injuries, and certain categories of workers may not qualify for workers' compensation benefits as they are considered exempt in certain jurisdictions (e.g., seasonal workers, domestic workers).

19. **Outline the potential course of an injured worker from initial injury through determination of maximal medical improvement under a workers' compensation system.**

A worker who is injured on the job should obtain expeditious and appropriate medical treatment, and report the accident to their employer, who is responsible for filing a claim with the employer's workers' compensation insurance carrier and authorizing initial necessary medical treatment. Depending on the regulations of the system under which the injured worker is treated, there may be limitations regarding the worker's choice of treating physician. Coordination of subsequent medical care may be handled by a claims adjuster and subject to utilization review to assess medical necessity. If the injured worker remains off work after a specific waiting period, temporary total disability payments are paid to the worker while their injury is being treated. As treatment and recovery progress, the worker's status may improve to the point where they can return to modified duty (if such a position is available) with specific work restrictions, and receive temporary partial disability payments if they work less than their full work schedule and receive less pay than their usual salary. For workers who do not improve with initial treatment, additional specialized therapy termed *work rehabilitation,* is an option, and may include work conditioning or work hardening. *Work conditioning programs* address physical issues related to flexibility, strength, endurance, coordination, and work-related function with a goal of returning to work. *Work hardening programs* are interdisciplinary, addressing behavioral and vocational dysfunction, physical and functional needs, and may involve psychomedical counseling, ergonomic evaluation, and transitional work services. If the treating physician is unsure about the injured worker's capacity to perform activities related to employment, the injured worker can be referred for a *functional capacity evaluation.* This evaluation consists of advanced testing to determine safe matches for return to work and the level of reasonable accommodations necessary, and may be used to guide the development of *work limitations.* Treatment and disability payments continue until the injured worker can return to work at their full schedule or their condition stabilizes to the point where no further substantial improvement is anticipated with time and/or additional treatment (i.e., MMI or P&S status) (Fig. 7.1).

20. **How do I fill out back-to-work forms?**

For orthopedic problems, functional capacity assessment(s) may be used to determine if an individual can return to his or her normal occupation. Some of the basic principles from the ADA are also applicable. One starts with a description of the job, especially its essential functions, although peripheral functions may sometimes be important to include. For an assembly-line worker, the job description may include where the worker has to stand, how many times the worker has to bend over, whether the worker has to pick up a part and how heavy the part is, how often the worker does this activity, and other ergonomic issues. Ideally, one then matches the worker's capability with the requirements of the job. For example, if we can measure how long workers can stand, how often they bend over, how much bending they are capable of doing, and what strength they have while performing various tasks, we should be able to say whether they are capable of returning to their job or whether they need to be assigned to modified and/or restricted duties.

In most circumstances, we do not achieve this perfect state of knowledge and blending of the worker with the job and we do not need this level of evaluation. When physicians approach the issue of whether a patient can return to their normal job, they have two choices: either refer the person for appropriate testing, or make an *educated guess* based on their experience, knowledge, and background. The more educated the examiner and the better his or her understanding of the job requirements and the person being evaluated, the more valid his or her determination will be.

21. **What is a functional capacity assessment?**

A functional capacity assessment or evaluation (FCE) assesses how well a particular organ system is working. Thus any stress test (cardiac, pulmonary, heat tolerance) is a FCE, as are hearing tests and visual field examinations. On

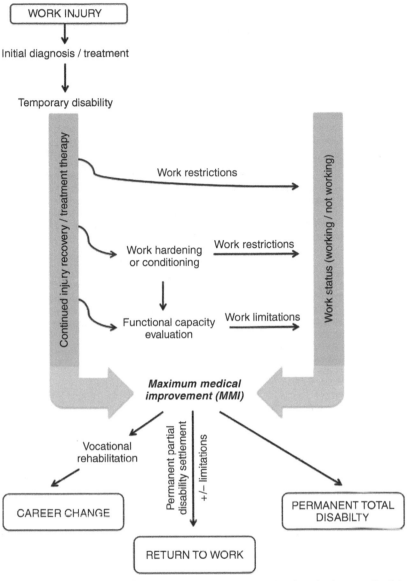

Fig. 7.1 Outline of progression following a work injury. Bible JE, Spengler DM, Mir HR. A primer for workers' compensation. Spine J 2014; 14:1325–1331.

a global level, FCE measures the body as a whole and determines how much and what kind of activity a person is capable of doing or will perform. The concept of testing how much activity (work) a person is able to perform was derived from studies performed by ergonomists and physical therapists.

When used as a descriptive phrase, FCE is a test of work capacity. Testing for a person's ability to work assesses many organ systems at one time. Generally, it is assumed that organ systems such as the cardiac, pulmonary, and neurologic systems are functioning normally. However, dysfunction in any organ system is a sufficient cause for an abnormal FCE.

Most FCEs assess the ability to work. There are many components, and it is common for an FCE to take 4 to 6 hours. Tests taking 2 or 3 days to perform are not unusual. The result is a list of body regions and both the maximum and sustainable levels of physical exertion that the examinee can perform in each body region. For example, the test will describe how much weight can be lifted, how many times it can be lifted, or for how long the examinee can perform the activities. The results can be linked to the specifics of a job. For example, if the job entails lifting 40–60 pounds on a frequent basis, and a person is capable of lifting only 20 pounds on a sustained basis (on a rare basis up to 50 pounds), one might conclude the person is not fit or qualified for the job. While this type of evaluation might seem ideal when determining if a person is able to do a job (for a new hire) or return to his or her normal job (for a recently injured individual who is deemed to have attained MMI), it must always be remembered these tests only measure how much the examinee is willing to do, not necessarily how much he or she can do.

22. **Outline some of the potential outcomes for an injured worker after maximum medical improvement status has been determined.**
Once MMI status has been determined, the injured worker is evaluated for impairment, return to work, and employability. A range of outcomes are possible at this stage (see Fig. 7.1). In some cases, the worker is able to return to a job with the same employer, with or without work limitations. If the injured worker is determined to have permanent limitations that can be accommodated by their employer, the alternate job with the same employer can be pursued, and a permanent partial disability settlement may be awarded. If the injured worker is determined to have limitations that cannot be accommodated by their employer, a new job may be pursued, and vocational rehabilitation may be considered. In other cases, the worker is unable to return to any gainful employment in any capacity, and is determined to have a permanent total disability. In some cases, the determination of impairment rating and disability may become contentious and require the involvement of independent medical evaluators and the legal system.

23. **What is an independent medical evaluation?**
An independent medical evaluation (IME) is a one-time evaluation performed by an independent medical examiner not involved in the treatment of the injured worker for the purpose of answering questions identified by the party requesting the evaluation. IMEs are requested by insurers, employers, claims administrators, and attorneys in the course of management and/or litigation related to workers' compensation, personal injury, medical malpractice, automobile injury, and disability claims. The content of an IME and report varies depending on the specific requirements of each case, and may include the following elements:
- Background information and descriptive data
- Review of medical records
- Current and preexisting status
- Occupational history
- Past medical history
- Family history
- Review of systems
- Physical examination
- Pain, behavioral, and psychological inventories
- Review of diagnostic tests (e.g., radiographs, magnetic resonance imaging [MRI], electrodiagnostic studies)
- Impressions
- Diagnoses
- Causation and apportionment
- Prognosis
- Work status
- Maximum medical improvement
- Functional abilities and work capacity
- Impairment rating
- Recommendations and answers to specific questions

24. **What are the American Medical Association's *Guides to the Evaluation of Permanent Impairment* (AMA *Guides*)?**
The AMA *Guides* evolved from a series of articles on impairment rating published in the *Journal of the American Medical Association* between 1958 and 1970, which were compiled into the First Edition of the AMA *Guides* in 1971. Subsequent updates and revisions have occurred and the most current version, the Sixth Edition, was published in 2008. The AMA *Guides* provide standardized medical criteria for determining medical impairment ratings. The evaluator is required to outline diagnostic criteria (based on the history, including prior clinical course), physical examination findings, diagnostic test results, and functional status, that place the patient in a specific impairment class, and requires assignment of a specific number within the options for that class. According to the AMA *Guides*, provision of an impairment rating does not directly equate to a work participation restriction or permanent disability rating. Although the AMA *Guides* are recognized as a reference in most states and outside the U.S., various editions are used in different jurisdictions. If the evaluator is unclear regarding the reference source to use for an impairment examination, they should contact the referral source to determine the appropriate version of the AMA *Guides* to use or if a different reference source is required.

25. Define the concept whole person impairment.

According to the AMA *Guides*, a normal individual is rated as 0% impaired, an individual who is totally dependent on others for care is considered >90% impaired, with 100% impairment reserved for those who are approaching death. Using the AMA *Guides*, a person whose right arm was amputated at the shoulder has a 60% impairment of the whole person; a leg amputation at the hip is equivalent to a 40% impairment of the whole person. A person with coronary disease may have whole person impairment (WPI) ranging from 0% to 65%. The precise amount of WPI depends on the degree of deviation from normalcy that can be found by performing a physical examination and reviewing medical records. Tables are provided in the AMA *Guides* that correlate the degree of dysfunction in a specific body part or organ system with the amount of WPI. Note that when impairment is rated for two or more body parts or organ systems, the total WPI is not calculated by adding the separate impairment ratings, but instead calculated using a Combined Values Chart to ensure that the total WPI does not exceed 100%.

26. Briefly explain the principles that are followed for evaluation of spine impairment according to the Fifth Edition of the AMA *Guides*.

Spinal impairment is rated only after MMI has been reached. Evaluation begins with a medical history, physical examination, and review of diagnostic and imaging studies. According to the Fifth Edition of the AMA *Guides*, there are two methods for spinal impairment rating: diagnosis-related estimate (DRE) and range of motion (ROM).

DRE is the principal method used to evaluate an individual who experiences a distinct injury. When the cause of the impairment is not easily determined and if the impairment can be characterized using the DRE method, the evaluator should use the DRE method. The evaluator starts by choosing the appropriate spinal region (cervical, thoracic, lumbar, and pelvic) and corresponding regional table. Each regional table has five categories, and the evaluator selects the category that best describes the examinee's spine condition, based on clinical criteria identified in the AMA *Guides*, and identifies the corresponding WPI within a 3% range. The exact percentage within the selected category is determined based on the degree of activity of daily living (ADL) deficits (if any). If the evaluator identifies WPI for more than one spinal region, the WPI values should be combined to identify the WPI for the spine. If the examinee has corticospinal (spinal cord) involvement with objective findings, this is rated according to specific criteria to determine the WPI percentage for corticospinal tract involvement, and the resultant percentage is combined with the spine DRE impairment.

The ROM method is required in certain circumstances. First, when an impairment is not caused by an injury, if the cause of the condition is uncertain and the DRE method does not apply, or an individual cannot be easily categorized in a DRE class. Second, when there is multilevel involvement in the same spinal region (e.g., fractures at multiple levels, disc herniations, or stenosis with radiculopathy at multiple levels or bilaterally). Third, where there is alteration of motion segment integrity (AOMSI), for example, fusions at multiple levels in the same spinal region, unless there is involvement of the corticospinal tract (DRE method is used for corticospinal tract involvement). Fourth, where there is recurrent radiculopathy caused by either a subsequent disc herniation or a recurrent injury in the same spinal region. Fifth, where there are multiple episodes of other pathology producing AOMSI and/or radiculopathy. The ROM method requires assessment of three elements that provide WPI percentages that are combined: (1) the ROM of the impaired spine region using an inclinometer, (2) diagnosis-based WPI according to the appropriate table, and (3) any sensory or motor spinal nerve deficit based on the appropriate tables in the AMA *Guides*.

27. Briefly explain the principles that are followed for evaluation of spine impairment, according to the Sixth Edition of the AMA *Guides*.

The Sixth Edition of the AMA *Guides* uses a diagnosis-based approach for rating of impairment of the spine and does not use ROM as a basis for defining impairment. A medical history and physical examination are performed to confirm that the examinee has reached MMI, and a diagnosis is provided for each spinal region requiring impairment rating. Diagnostic categories in the spine chapter include: non-specific spinal pain (soft tissues or strain/sprain), motion segment lesions (including intervertebral disc herniation, AOMSIs, pseudarthrosis, spinal stenosis, and spondylolisthesis [lumbar spine only]), fractures and dislocations, postoperative complications (non-neurologic), and fractures of the pelvis and acetabulum.

Diagnosis-Based Impairment (DBI) grids are provided for each anatomic spinal area and contain five potential impairment classes (Class 0: no objective findings, Class 1: mild, Class 2: moderate, Class 3: severe, Class 4: very severe, approaching total functional loss). The impairment ratings within each class are divided into 5 grades (A–E), and an impairment is provisionally assigned to the middle grade (C) by default. The final impairment grade within the class is determined using grade modifiers, which include Functional History (FH), Physical Examination (PE), and Clinical Studies (CS), and require use of a Net Adjustment Formula to determine the numerical rating for the impairment class and grade. Similar to the Fifth Edition of the AMA *Guides*, WPIs for multiple spinal regions are combined using a Combined Values Chart.

28. Can you provide an example of rating a cervical spine injury using the Fifth and Sixth editions of the AMA *Guides*?

A 64-year-old worker was involved in a motor vehicle accident when he was stopped at a red light. A car, traveling at 40 mph, struck the rear of his car. The worker was diagnosed with a "whiplash" injury. The worker was evaluated and treated on multiple occasions by his primary care physician. A computed tomography examination disclosed moderate-to-severe degenerative changes throughout the cervical spine. He complained of numbness and tingling in his right upper extremity but this remitted within a period of 2 months. He was treated with physical therapy and analgesics. One year later, when at MMI, he complained of neck pain radiating into both trapezii and shoulder regions. The pain was present with normal activities.

On examination, his cervical flexion was 28° with extension of 20°. Right lateral bending was 30° and left lateral bending was 32°. Right rotation was 18° and left rotation was 20°. There was discomfort at the extremes of all six ranges of motion. There was discomfort with palpation of the neck and trapezii. The neurologic examination was normal except for slightly diminished motor strength on shoulder shrugging. The Spurling Foraminal Compression Test caused only posterior neck pain.

Fifth Edition Rating

The Fifth Edition of the AMA *Guides* allows for rating spinal impairment in two distinctly different ways. The DRE method is principally used to evaluate an individual with a distinct injury and should be used here. This worker did not meet the criteria that required use of the range-of-motion (ROM) method for impairment analysis. As there were "no significant clinical findings, no observed muscle guarding or spasm, no documentable neurologic impairment, no documented alteration in structural integrity, no fractures, and no other indication of impairment related to injury or illness" (1), this individual qualified for a DRE Cervical Category I, reflecting 0% impairment of the whole person.

Sixth Edition Rating

When using the Sixth Edition, the steps in performing a spinal impairment rating are:
1. Perform history and physical examination, and determine if the individual is at MMI.
2. Establish the reliable diagnosis for each region of the spine to be rated.
3. Use the appropriate regional grid to determine the impairment class.
4. Use the adjustment grids to identify the grade modifiers for Functional History, Physical Examination, and Clinical Studies, as applicable. Then apply the Net Adjustment Calculation to determine the net adjustment and modification of the default value 'C' within the class.
5. Use the regional grid to identify the appropriate numerical impairment rating for the impairment class in grade.
6. Combine WPIs for multiple spinal regions when appropriate, using the Combined Values Chart.

When determining the impairment, the "key factor" for spinal disorders is the diagnosis (note: the key factor may differ according to the body system[s] involved). Each regional spinal grid has five classes (0–4) for the Class of Diagnosis (CDX). Each class has five ratings (A–E). There are three grade modifiers that may change the rating: Grade Modifier for Functional History (GMFH), Grade Modifier for Physical Examination (GMPE), and Grade Modifier for Clinical Studies (GMCS). These modifiers are used in a "Net Adjustment Formula" to modify the default rating, which is the middle value in the diagnosis grid. The default value (C) is adjusted up and down based upon grade modifiers. The formula is: $(GMFH - CDX) + (GMPE - CDX) + (GMCS - CDX)$.

In this case, the injured worker had a whiplash injury with continued axial symptoms. Therefore, he was assigned to the diagnostic category of "soft tissue and nonspecific conditions" for "nonspecific chronic, or chronic recurrent neck pain (also known as chronic sprain/strain, symptomatic degenerative disc disease, facet joint pain, chronic whiplash, etc.)" and was placed in Class 1 with a default rating of 2% impairment of the whole person. As described above, the default rating is typically "adjusted" based on grade modifiers. However, GMPEs or GMCSs are not applicable with a diagnosis of nonspecific chronic spinal pain. Therefore, the evaluator will rely exclusively on his or her professional judgement to determine the reliability of any FH formulated using the recommended Pain Disability Questionnaire (PDQ) or other valid functional assessment scale.

29. Can you provide an example of rating a thoracic spine injury using the Fifth and Sixth editions of the AMA *Guides*?

A 28-year-old worker fell off scaffolding at work. He struck a small wooden fence prior to coming to the ground. He complained of pain in the mid-back region. He was seen in the emergency room and diagnosed with a fracture in the thoracic spine. He received appropriate care and now, 6 months after the injury, he presents for an impairment rating. He has a nagging pain after a hard day of work, but is otherwise without problems. His physical examination was normal. On radiography, there was a 50% compression fracture of T10.

Fifth Edition Rating

According to the Fifth Edition, this worker qualifies for a DRE Thoracic Category III with an impairment rating of 15%–18% of the whole person. Based on the lack of significant symptoms and the normal physical examination, 15% impairment of the whole person is considered appropriate. If he reported more significant pain, his rating might have been adjusted to 16%, 17%, or 18% of the whole person. If the worker had sustained a 51% compression fracture, he would have qualified for a DRE Thoracic Category IV impairment with a minimum rating of 20%. Note that if the worker had sustained multiple thoracic fractures, he would have been rated using the ROM method.

Sixth Edition Rating

Using the Sixth Edition, this worker is rated as Class 2 impairment using the DBI grid.

The next step is to apply grade modifiers. Using the Functional History Adjustment Table, he qualifies for Grade Modifier 1 based on the level of his symptoms. Using the Physical Examination Adjustment Table, he qualifies for Grade Modifier 0 based upon the normal physical examination. The Clinical Studies Adjustment Table cannot be used as this refers to radiographic abnormalities used as the basis of his impairment rating.

In this case, the CDX is the radiographic diagnosis of compression fractures with a default value of 9% WPI. The GMFH result was -1. The GMPE result was 0. The Clinical Studies Adjustment could not be used (as noted above). The two adjustments diminished the default rating to an "A" $[(1 - 2) = -1; (0 - 2) = -2; (-1) + (-2) = (-3); (GMFH - CDX) + (GMPE - CDX)]$. The default value for Class 2 impairment is 9%. This is decreased to the lowest level in this class with the final impairment rating being 7% of the whole person.

30. **Can you provide an example of rating a lumbar spine injury using the Fifth and Sixth editions of the AMA *Guides*?**
During work hours, a worker slips on ice while delivering packages. He has the sudden onset of pain and discomfort in his lower back. An MRI disclosed a herniated disc at the L5–S1 interspace. He underwent a micro-discectomy because of persistent, severe symptoms. He had a successful outcome and returned to the workforce. He continues to have mild, low back pain radiating into the right lower extremity, except at the end of the workday when the lower back pain is worse. He rates his resting pain at 4 out of 10, and 7 out of 10 at the end of a long day, but this reverts to baseline by the next morning. His physical examination was normal with the following exceptions: diminished ROM, a diminished right ankle deep tendon reflex, slight weakness in the ankle plantar flexors, and hypesthesia of the lateral right foot.

Fifth Edition Rating
This worker has an impairment based on an anatomic deviation from normalcy. According to the Fifth Edition, this worker qualifies for a DRE Lumbar Category III with an impairment rating of 10%–13% of the whole person. Based on his symptoms, the 10% WPI baseline may be increased by 1%–3%, depending on the evaluator's recommendation. Using the Fifth Edition, the worker is rated as having a 12% impairment of the whole person because of the herniated disc, neurologic abnormalities, and current pain levels, despite the fact that he had a successful operation. Note that separate ratings are found in the Fifth Edition for the neurologic deficits (motor and sensory) but are only applicable when using the ROM method of rating spinal disorders.

Sixth Edition Rating
Using the Sixth Edition, the worker would be rated using the Lumbar Spine Regional Grid for "Motion Segment Lesions" with the diagnosis of intervertebral disc herniation and/or alteration of motion segment integrity (AOMSI). Based on an "intervertebral disc herniation or AOMSI **at a single level** with medically documented findings with or without surgery **and** with documented **residual radiculopathy at the clinically appropriate level** present at the time of examination," this worker qualifies for Class 2 with a default rating of 12% impairment of the whole person (CDX). Using the Functional History Adjustment Grid, he qualifies for a Grade 2 Modifier because of his symptoms of pain and symptoms with normal activity (GMFH). Using the Physical Examination Adjustment Grid, he qualifies for a Grade 1 Modifier based on the diminished light touch sensation that did not interfere with "some activities" (GMPE). Using the Clinical Studies Adjustment Grid (GMCS), he qualifies for Grade 2 Modifier based on the MRI, which showed the herniated disc consistent with the clinical presentation.

Recall that the net adjustment formula is $(GMFH - CDX) + (GMPE - CDX) + (GMCS - CDX)$. Inserting the numerical values, the result is $(2 - 2) + (1 - 2) + (2 - 2)$ or $(0) + (-1) + (0) = -1$. This modifies the default value of a grade "C" to one less, or a grade "B". According to the Lumbar Spine Regional Grid, this man qualified for a Motion Segment Lesion Class 3 with a 11% impairment of the whole person.

KEY POINTS

1. Impairment reflects an alteration from normal bodily functions, can be assessed using traditional medical means, and can be objectively determined using preselected reference guides.
2. Disability results from impairment, is task-specific, and is measured in the context of the system to which the worker has applied for relief. Disability determination is an administrative determination that uses both medical and nonmedical information.
3. One individual can be impaired significantly and have no disability, while another person can be severely disabled with only a limited impairment.
4. Workers' Compensation is a no-fault insurance program that provides medical economic support to workers who have been injured or made ill from an incident arising out of and in the course of employment.

Websites

1. Help for health professionals to understand the Social Security Disability determination process: http://www. ssa.gov/disability/professionals/index.htm
2. Impairment rating and disability determination: http://emedicine.medscape.com/article/314195-overview
3. Information and technical assistance relating to The Americans with Disabilities Act: http://www.ada.gov/
4. Musculoskeletal disorders and workplace factors: http://www.cdc.gov/niosh/docs/97-141/
5. Social Security Administration, U.S. Department of Health and Human Services: Disability Evaluation under Social Security. Available only online: http://www.ssa.gov/disability/professionals/bluebook

REFERENCES

1. Demeter SL. Introduction to disability and impairment. In: Demeter SL, Andersson GBJ, Smith GM, editors. *Disability Evaluation.* 2nd ed. St. Louis, MO: Mosby; 2003, pp. 3–7.
2. Grace TG. Causation and apportionment. In: Grace TG, editor, Independent Medical Evaluations. Chicago, IL: *American Academy of Orthopaedic Surgeons;* 2001; pp. 65–70.
3. Rondinelli RD, editors. *American Medical Association Guides to the Evaluation of Permanent Impairment.* 6th ed. Chicago, IL: American Medical Association; 2008.

BIBLIOGRAPHY

1. Bible JE, Spengler DM, Mir HR. A primer for workers' compensation. *Spine J* 2014;14:1325–1331.
2. Cocchiarella L, Andersson GBJ, editors. *American Medical Association Guides to the Evaluation of Permanent Impairment.* 5th ed. Chicago, IL: American Medical Association; 2001.
3. Demeter SL. Introduction to disability and impairment. In: Demeter SL, Andersson GBJ, Smith GM, editors. *Disability Evaluation.* 2nd ed. St. Louis, MO: Mosby; 2003, pp. 3–7.
4. Demeter SL. Contrasting the standard, impairment, and disability evaluation. In: Demeter SL, Andersson GBJ, Smith GM, editors. *Disability Evaluation.* 2nd ed. St. Louis, MO: Mosby; 2003, pp. 101–110.
5. Demeter SL. Appendix B. In: Demeter SL, Andersson GBJ, Smith GM, editors. *Disability Evaluation.* 2nd ed. St. Louis, MO: Mosby; 2003, pp. 871–891.
6. Grace TG. Causation and apportionment. In: Grace TG, editor. *Independent Medical Evaluations.* Chicago, IL: American Academy of Orthopaedic Surgeons; 2001, pp. 65–70.
7. Rondinelli RD, editor. *American Medical Association Guides to the Evaluation of Permanent Impairment.* 6th ed. Chicago, IL: American Medical Association; 2008.
8. Rondinelli RD, Ranavaya M. Disability assessment. In: Benzon HT, Rathmell JP, editors. *Practical Management of Pain.* 5th ed. Philadelphia, PA: Mosby; 2014, pp. 257–268.

SPINAL IMAGING

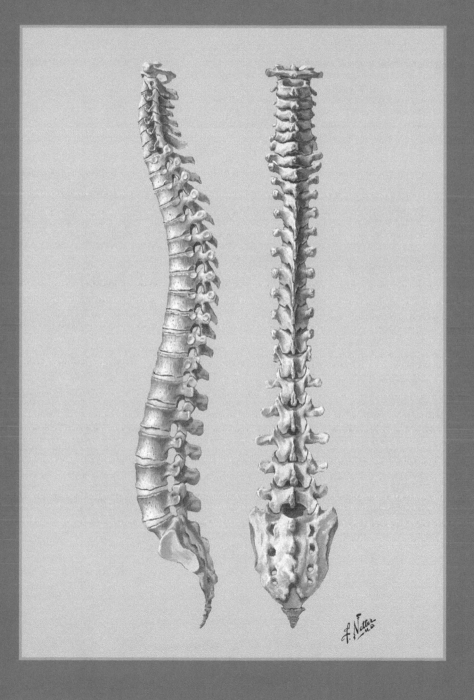

CHAPTER 8

STRATEGIES FOR IMAGING AND DIAGNOSIS IN SPINAL DISORDERS

Vincent J. Devlin, MD

1. **What are the major objectives of spinal imaging tests?**
   Common reasons to order spinal imaging studies are to:
   1. Rule out serious spinal pathology, such as tumor or infection.
   2. Screen the spinal column for injuries following trauma.
   3. Identify and assess spinal cord and/or nerve root compression.
   4. Identify and evaluate spinal instabilities and deformities.
   5. Create a topographic map to guide surgical intervention.
   6. Identify spinal levels intraoperatively.
   7. Evaluate the results of operative and nonoperative treatment.

2. **What steps can the clinician take to minimize inappropriate use of diagnostic imaging tests?**
   1. Perform a detailed history and physical examination before ordering any imaging tests.
   2. Formulate a working diagnosis to explain symptoms and guide testing.
   3. Order the imaging study best suited to evaluate the suspected pathologic process based on the working diagnosis, as well as the sensitivity, specificity, and accuracy of each imaging modality.
   4. Order imaging tests only when the information obtained from the test will affect medical decision making.
   5. Consider ways to limit radiation exposure when ordering imaging tests.

3. **What imaging modalities are used in the evaluation of spinal disorders?**
   - Plain radiographs
   - Magnetic resonance imaging (MRI)
   - Computed tomography (CT)
   - CT-myelography
   - Nuclear medicine studies
   - Angiography
   - Ultrasound
   - Fluoroscopy

4. **What is one of the greatest challenges facing patients and physicians regarding the use of spinal imaging tests for evaluation of spinal pain?**
   Both patients and physicians tend to overestimate the ability of modern imaging tests to detect symptomatic spinal pathology and guide treatment. Each imaging modality—radiograph, CT, MRI, bone scan—is extremely sensitive but relatively nonspecific. Studies have documented that spinal imaging reveals abnormalities in at least one-third of asymptomatic patients. One of the major challenges in utilization of imaging tests is to determine the clinical relevance of abnormal spinal morphology. This determination is especially challenging when one attempts to distinguish imaging abnormalities likely to have clinical relevance from those that are part of the normal aging process or part of a normal sequence of postoperative healing. In the absence of clinical assessment, imaging tests cannot determine whether a specific spinal structure is responsible for symptoms. Excessive emphasis on imaging tests without clinical correlation is hazardous to both the patient and physician, and may lead to inappropriate treatment.

5. **When should I order a spine radiograph?**
   Plain radiographs are the most commonly ordered initial imaging study for evaluation of the spinal column. Indications to order spinal radiographs include:
   - For diagnosis of spinal conditions, such as spinal degeneration, instability, fracture, spinal deformity, tumors and infection.
   - To provide follow-up regarding progression of a spinal disease process.
   - To evaluate progression of a spinal deformity.
   - As part of preoperative planning prior to spinal procedures.
   - For intraoperative localization of spinal levels (i.e., spinal enumeration).

- To provide postoperative assessment following spinal surgery.
- To identify postoperative adverse events, such as postsurgical instabilities, pseudarthroses, transition syndromes, and spinal implant failures.

6. What are the major advantages of using plain radiographs to assess spinal disorders?
   - Inexpensive and readily available
   - Provide rapid assessment of a specific spinal region or the entire spinal axis (occiput to sacrum) in orthogonal planes
   - Weight-bearing (standing) and dynamic studies (flexion-extension views, side-bending views) may be obtained
   - Plain radiographs are useful to assess osseous structure, vertebral alignment, spinal deformity, and implant position following spinal surgery

7. What are the major disadvantages of using plain radiographs to assess spinal disorders?
   - Radiographs have a low sensitivity and specificity for identification of symptomatic spinal pathology. It must be appreciated that age-related degenerative changes are present equally in symptomatic and asymptomatic populations.
   - Radiographs cannot visualize the spinal cord, nerve roots, and other soft tissue structures, such as intervertebral discs and spinal ligaments.
   - Radiographs cannot diagnose early-stage tumor or infection as significant bone destruction (at least 30%–40% of bone mass) must occur before a radiographic abnormality is detectable.

8. When should I order a spine MRI?
   An MRI is indicated if the clinical history and physical examination suggest a serious spinal condition (i.e., tumor, infection, or traumatic injury), if severe or progressive neurologic deficits are present, or when evaluation of the spinal canal and/or nerve root canals is required prior to spinal injections or surgical procedures. Caution is necessary when considering a spine MRI in patients with nonspecific axial pain, as positive findings of spinal degeneration may be unrelated to a specific patient's pain syndrome, as such findings are commonly observed in asymptomatic patients.

9. What are the major advantages of using MRI to assess spinal disorders?
   - Avoids ionizing radiation
   - Provides imaging in orthogonal planes
   - Visualizes an entire spinal region and detects pathology at transition zones between adjacent spinal regions
   - Provides excellent visualization of pathologic processes involving the disc, thecal sac, epidural space, neural elements, paraspinal soft tissues, and bone marrow

10. What are the major disadvantages of using MRI to assess spinal disorders?
    - Less definition of osseous anatomy compared with CT
    - Longer image acquisition time compared with CT
    - Some implanted devices are contraindications (e.g., pacemakers, drug pumps, and spine stimulators)
    - Claustrophobic or obese patients may have difficulty with the test
    - May be challenging to interpret in patients with major spinal deformities
    - Metal artifact due to spinal implants may adversely affect interpretation of MRI studies in postoperative patients. This may be mitigated in some situations by using metal artifact reduction sequences (MARS).

11. When should I order a CT scan?
    CT is most helpful in the evaluation of osseous anatomy. Clinical scenarios where CT is invaluable for assessment of spinal anatomy include: spinal fractures, facet arthrosis, spondylolysis, spondylolisthesis, ossification of the posterior longitudinal ligament, and evaluation of implant position and fusion status following surgery.

12. What are the major advantages of using CT to assess spinal disorders?
    - CT is the optimal test for assessment of bone detail.
    - Short image acquisition time.
    - Multiplanar two- and three-dimensional reconstructed images can be obtained to provide visualization of spinal anatomy with excellent resolution.
    - CT is useful when MRI is contraindicated (e.g., cardiac pacemaker).

13. What are the major disadvantages of using CT to assess spinal disorders?
    - Exposure to ionizing radiation.
    - CT provides poor delineation of neural elements, intervertebral discs, ligaments, and bone marrow changes.
    - Artifacts due to spinal implants may lead to image distortion and data loss.
    - Significant pathology can be missed if the physician is misled by a negative report and does not pursue additional workup and more definitive testing.

14. **When should I order a myelogram?**
    Myelography is infrequently used as a stand-alone test to evaluate spinal pathology. However, it continues to play a role in spinal imaging when combined with a CT scan.

15. **What are some disadvantages of myelography as an isolated test to assess spinal disorders?**
    - Myelography is an invasive test that requires introduction of nonionic, water-soluble contrast material into the subarachnoid space, and is associated with risks, including adverse reaction to contrast, spinal fluid leak, and spinal headache.
    - Myelography only provides indirect evidence of neural compression by demonstrating changes in contour of contrast-filled neural structures.
    - Myelography lacks diagnostic specificity as it is unable to differentiate whether extradural compression is due to disc, osteophyte, tumor, or infection.
    - Myelography is unable to visualize pathology in the lateral zone of the spinal canal because the contrast-filled nerve root sleeves end in the region of the pedicle.
    - Myelography cannot detect pathology below the level of a complete block to contrast.
    - Myelography is less accurate than CT or MRI in evaluating disc pathology and may fail to detect pathology at the L5–S1 level, where the spinal canal is very wide, and a large disc protrusion or osteophyte may not deform the dye column.
    - Upright myelographic studies have been supplanted by positional MRI which enables acquisition of images in multiple positions, including weight bearing and during movement.

16. **When should I consider ordering a CT-myelogram?**
    For complex spinal problems, high-quality MRI and noncontrast CT scans may be used as complementary studies to define a specific clinical problem. Nevertheless, a CT-myelogram remains the test of choice in certain situations including:
    - When MRI is contraindicated and detailed assessment of the spinal and nerve root canals is necessary.
    - Evaluation of the neural elements in a postoperative patient with stainless steel spinal implants.
    - Patients with significant clinical symptoms and equivocal MRI findings, in whom specific spinal pathology is suspected and requires additional investigation.
    - Preoperative planning for revision of spinal stenosis surgery, especially if symptoms suggest a relationship with postural change.
    - Preoperative planning for surgical treatment of complex spinal deformities such as symptomatic spinal stenosis in combination with severe lumbar scoliosis.
    - Evaluation of suspected cerebrospinal fluid leaks following spinal surgery.

17. **What are the major advantages of CT-myelography to assess spinal disorders?**
    The use of CT and myelography together exceeds the value of either test performed alone. The addition of contrast to the CT scan improves delineation of neural structures and permits distinction between the disc margins, thecal sac, and ligamentum flavum. As a result, the accuracy of CT-myelography is comparable to MRI for many spinal disorders, and can provide useful diagnostic information when MRI is contraindicated.

18. **What are the major disadvantages of using CT-myelography to assess spinal disorders?**
    The disadvantages of CT-myelography include its invasive nature, need for contrast administration, and use of ionizing radiation.

19. **When should I consider ordering a nuclear medicine study?**
    Imaging studies that use a variety of radionuclides, including technetium 99m (^{99m}Tc), gallium citrate (^{67}Ga), indium-labeled white blood cells (^{111}In), and 18F-fluorodeoxyglucose (^{18F}FDG) positron emission tomography (PET) imaging, have been described for a range of spinal indications:
    1. To screen the skeletal system for metastatic disease
    2. To screen the spinal column for primary bone tumors, disc space infection, or vertebral osteomyelitis
    3. To assess the relative biologic activity of bone lesions, such as pars interarticularis defects, or facet joint degenerative changes
    4. To aid in diagnosis of sacroiliac joint pathology, such as infection, arthritis, or insufficiency fractures

20. **What are the major advantages of using a ^{99m}Tc bone scan to assess spinal disorders?**
    - ^{99m}Tc bone scans provide an excellent method for rapidly screening the entire skeleton for osseous abnormalities; they are especially useful for detecting tumors and infections.
    - ^{99m}Tc bone scans are an effective method for determining the relative biologic activity of a bone lesion. For example, differentiation is possible between acute versus chronic vertebral fractures, or acute versus chronic pars defects.
    - Axial, sagittal, and coronal plane images may be obtained, for example, single-photon emission computed tomography (SPECT) and SPECT/CT.

21. **What are the major disadvantages of using a ^{99m}Tc bone scan to assess spinal disorders?**
    - ^{99m}Tc bone scans are highly sensitive but not highly specific.
    - ^{99m}Tc bone scans do not provide sufficient resolution for surgical planning.
    - Certain tumors, such as multiple myeloma or some purely lytic metastases, may not demonstrate increased activity on a bone scan, as they do not stimulate a significant osteoblastic response.

22. **What are some indications for use of spinal angiography?**
    A variety of angiographic techniques, including conventional, CT, or magnetic resonance angiography, play a role in select clinical scenarios. Examples include evaluation and localization of the vertebral artery following trauma or prior to craniocervical procedures, evaluation and treatment of spinal vascular malformations, and preoperative embolization of spinal tumors.

23. **What are some indications for use of ultrasonography for evaluation of spinal disorders?**
    Indications for use of ultrasonography include identification of spinal dysraphism in pediatric patients, intraoperative localization of spinal cord pathology, intraoperative assessment of spinal decompression, localization of postoperative fluid collections, guidance of catheter and needle placement, and monitoring distraction of pediatric magnetically controlled expandable rod systems.

24. **What are some indications for use of fluoroscopy for evaluation of spinal disorders?**
    Fluoroscopy is used when real-time visualization of anatomic structures is required. Fluoroscopy is integral to a range of diagnostic and therapeutic spinal procedures, including discography, spinal injections, and also plays an important role in intraoperative imaging.

25. **What are the adverse effects of radiation exposure and how are they classified?**
    Radiation exposure may cause indirect and/or direct damage to biological tissues at the cellular level. Adverse effects from radiation exposure may be classified as stochastic or nonstochastic. **Stochastic effects,** also referred to as probabilistic effects, occur randomly, have no threshold dose, and their severity is not dose related, although stochastic effects are more likely to occur after exposure to higher radiation doses. Stochastic effects include cancer in exposed individuals and heritable disease in offspring due to mutation of reproductive cells.

    In contrast, **deterministic effects**, also referred to as harmful tissue reactions, are directly related to a threshold radiation dose, and the severity of the reaction increases as dose is increased. Deterministic effects may occur early (days to weeks) or late (months to years) following a single high-dose exposure or multiple low-dose exposures. Examples of deterministic effects include cataracts, cutaneous burns, hair loss, and infertility. Radiation exposure during pregnancy poses risks to both the mother and unborn child; therefore ionizing radiation should be used only when the benefits outweigh the risks.

26. **What units are used to measure radioactivity and its effects?**
    There are various units for quantifying radioactivity and radiation effects:
    Exposure: Describes the amount of ionized radiation traveling through air. Units used to quantify the absorbed dose are the **roentgen** (R) and **coulomb/kilogram** (C/kg).
    Absorbed dose: Describes the amount of radiation absorbed by a specific mass of tissue. Units used to quantify the absorbed dose are the **rad** and **Gray** (Gy). One gray is equal to one joule of radiation energy absorbed per kilogram of matter, and is equivalent to 100 rads. Note that the absorbed dose does not take into account the location or radiosensitivity of the tissue exposed to radiation.
    Equivalent dose: Describes the amount of radiation absorbed by an individual organ or tissue. The units for equivalent dose are the sievert (Sv) or roentgen equivalent man (rem). Radiation doses from medical imaging are most commonly measured in millisieverts (mSv). Effective dose is calculated as the absorbed dose multiplied by the appropriate weighting factor to reflect the type of radiation. The weighting factor for radiation from medical imaging is equal to 1.0. Thus, the absorbed dose in Gy is equal to the equivalent dose in Sv. Note that 1 mSv equals 0.1 rem.
    Effective dose: This is the most common dose measurement used to estimate harm from radiological imaging. It is calculated for the whole body by addition of the equivalent doses to all organs exposed in the imaging examination after adjustment for the sensitivity of each organ to radiation. Effective dose is expressed in mSv and allows for comparison between different exposures and types of imaging modalities such as radiographs and CT.

27. **How does radiation exposure differ among various types of diagnostic imaging studies?**
    Many factors can cause the actual dose to vary significantly from the estimated effective radiation dose, including an individual's size, body region examined, and factors related to performance of the specific imaging procedure, including use of dose optimization techniques. The radiation exposure from medical imaging studies is often compared with natural background radiation to which humans are exposed, which is estimated as 3 mSv/year (Table 8.1). As MRI and ultrasonography do not emit radiation, their effective dose is zero. The effective dose from standard radiographic studies varies widely by a factor of 1000 (0.1–10 mSv). CT examinations have relatively high effective doses but these doses fall within a narrower range (2–10 mSv). Interventional procedures are associated with higher effective doses (5–70 mSv). Nuclear medicine studies are associated with effective doses ranging from 0.3 to 20 mSv.

Table 8.1 Radiation Dose to Adults Resulting From Common Imaging Studies and Procedures.

IMAGING STUDY/ PROCEDURE	ESTIMATED AVERAGE EFFECTIVE RADIATION DOSE (mSv)	COMPARES TO NATURAL BACKGROUND RADIATION EXPOSURE[a] FOR:
MRI or ultrasound	0	0 days
Chest radiograph (PA)	0.02	2.5 days
Chest radiograph (PA and Lateral)	0.1	10 days
Cervical spine radiograph	0.2	25 days
Thoracic spine radiograph	1.0	4 months
Lumbar spine radiograph	1.5	6 months
Pelvis radiograph	0.6	2 months
Dual x-ray absorptiometry (without CT)	0.001	3 hours
Dual x-ray absorptiometry (with CT)	0.04	5 days
CT spine	1.5–10	0.5–3 years
Head and/or neck angiography	5	1.7 years
Tecnetium[99] bone scan	6.3	2.1 years
PET scan	14.1	4.7 years
PET-CT scan	25	8 years
Gallium[67] citrate scan	15	5 years
Indium[111]I-labeled white blood cell scan	6.7	2.2 years

[a]Annual natural background radiation exposure reference value is 3 mSv/year.
CT, Computed tomography; *PA,* posteroanterior.
Data from Mettler FA, Huda W, Yoshizumi TT, et al. Effective doses in radiology and diagnostic nuclear medicine: A catalog. Radiology 2008;1: 254–263; Radiation dose in x-ray and CT exams <https://www.radiologyinfo.org/en/info.cfm?pg=safety-xray>.

To conceptualize the relative effective radiation doses from various medical imaging studies, comparison to a chest radiograph is sometimes used (estimated effective radiation dose of posteroanterior [PA] chest radiograph, 0.02 mSv). For example, a lumbar CT scan with an approximate effective radiation dose of 6 mSv is equivalent to 300 PA chest radiographs.

28. What steps can be taken to minimize radiation exposure to patients due to medical imaging studies?

The principle which guides radiation safety for medical imaging is **ALARA** (as low as reasonably achievable). It is recommended that health care providers consider the relative radiation exposures for various imaging studies, balance the medical benefit to the patient against any potential radiation risk associated with each examination, and optimize radiological protection. Radiation dose techniques specific to each imaging modality should be utilized. Radiation dose, and the age at which radiation is received, are related to radiation risk. Children are at increased risk due to greater sensitivity to radiation and a longer lifetime to manifest related changes. Education in radiological safety is available through professional societies, as well as the Image Gently Alliance (Alliance for Radiation Safety in Pediatric Imaging) and Image Wisely Alliance (joint initiative of the American College of Radiology, Radiological Society of North America, American Society of Radiological Technologists, and American Association of Physicists in Medicine).

29. What data is available regarding estimated radiation exposure experienced by pediatric patients who undergo treatment for spinal deformities?

Patients with early-onset scoliosis (EOS) and adolescent idiopathic scoliosis (AIS) undergo multiple imaging studies that involve ionizing radiation. For example, EOS patients with thoracic insufficiency syndrome (TIS) undergo CT scans of the chest and spine, plain radiography, ventilation and lung perfusion scans (V/Q), and intraoperative imaging with fluoroscopy, or surgical navigation systems. One analysis of TIS patients who completed treatment and underwent spinal fusion estimated the average cumulative total effective radiation dose as 60 mSV over 5.4 years (approximately 20 years of background radiation), with CT scans responsible for 74% of total radiation exposure. (1) In another study of skeletally immature patients with AIS, (2) the mean number of radiographs obtained per patient was 20.9 (range, 8–43) and the number of radiographs was higher in surgically treated patients compared with brace-treated patients (27.3 vs. 14.5 radiographs). For scoliosis radiographs obtained using a computed radiography (CR) system, the mean cumulative estimated effective dose over the course of treatment was 5.38 mSv, compared with 2.64 mSv with use of a filter.

KEY POINTS

1. One of the major challenges in utilization of spinal imaging tests is to determine the clinical relevance of abnormal spinal morphology.
2. Plain radiographs are inexpensive, widely available, involve relatively low radiation exposure, and provide valuable information about spinal alignment and bone structure, but are unable to define soft tissue and neural structures.
3. MRI is the best initial advanced spinal imaging modality for evaluation of most spinal disorders because it provides the greatest amount of diagnostic information regarding a specific spinal region and does not involve ionizing radiation.
4. CT is the best imaging modality for evaluation of bone detail but is associated with significant radiation exposure.
5. It is important that health care providers consider the relative radiation exposures for imaging studies which use ionizing radiation, and balance the medical benefit to the patient versus potential radiation risks associated with each examination.

Websites
1. MRI of the spine: http://www.radiologyinfo.org/en/pdf/spinemr.pdf
2. Radiological Safety: https://www.acr.org/Clinical-Resources/Radiology-Safety
3. Image Gently Alliance: https://www.imagegently.org/
4. Image Wisely Alliance: https://www.imagewisely.org/
5. Radiation-Emitting Products: https://www.fda.gov/Radiation-EmittingProducts/default.htm

REFERENCES

1. Luo TD, Stans AA, Schueler BA, Larson AN. Cumulative radiation exposure with EOS imaging compared with standard spine radiographs. *Spine Deform* 2015;3:144–150.
2. Mettler FA, Huda W, Yoshizumi TT, Mahesh M. Effective doses in radiology and diagnostic nuclear medicine: A catalog. *Radiology* 2008;248(1):254–263.

BIBLIOGRAPHY

1. Boden SD, McCowin PR, Davis DO, et al. Abnormal cervical spine magnetic-resonance scans in asymptomatic individuals: A prospective investigation. *J Bone Joint Surg* 1990;72:1178–1184.
2. Carragee EJ, Hannibal M. Diagnostic evaluation of low back pain. *Orthop Clin North Am* 2004;35:7–16.
3. Emch TM, Ross JS, Bell GR. Spine imaging. In: Garfin SR, Eismont FJ, Bell GR, editors. *Rothman-Simeone the Spine.* 7th ed. Philadelphia, PA: Saunders; 2018, pp. 201–240.
4. France JC. Radiographic imaging of the traumatically injured spine: plain radiographs, computed tomography, magnetic resonance imaging, angiography, clearing the cervical spine in trauma patients. In: Kim DH, Ludwig SC, Vaccaro AR, editors. *Atlas of Spine Trauma.* Philadelphia, PA: Saunders; 2008, pp. 37–67.
5. Gopinathan NR, Viswanathan VK, Crawford AH. Cervical spine evaluation in pediatric trauma: A review and an update of current concepts. *Indian J Orthop* 2018;52:489–500.
6. Hayda RA, Hsu RY, DePasse JM, Gil JA. Radiation exposure and health risks for orthopedic surgeons. *J Am Acad Orthop Surg* 2018;26:268–277.
7. Khorsand D, Song KM, Swanson J, Alessio A, Redding G, Waldhausen J. Iatrogenic radiation exposure to patients with early-onset spine and chest wall deformities. *Spine* 2018;38:E1108–E1114.
8. Luo TD, Stans AA, Schueler BA, Larson AN. Cumulative radiation exposure with EOS imaging compared with standard spine radiographs. *Spine Deform* 2015;3:144–150.
9. Mettler FA, Huda W, Yoshizumi TT, Mahesh M. Effective doses in radiology and diagnostic nuclear medicine: A catalog. *Radiology* 2008;248(1):254–263.

CHAPTER 9

RADIOGRAPHIC ASSESSMENT OF THE SPINE

Vincent J. Devlin, MD

GENERAL

1. What features distinguish screen-film radiography (SFR) versus computed radiography (CR) versus digital radiography (DR)?

   Screen-film radiography (SFR), also known as conventional or film-based radiography, utilizes a light-sensitive silver halide–coated film placed within a cassette containing two intensifying screens, which is placed behind the patient to be imaged and exposed to an x-ray beam. Radiographic contrast is dependent on differential attenuation of x-rays as they pass through different body tissues. The exposed film is removed from the cassette and passed through a developer to produce a hardcopy radiograph.

   Computed radiography (CR) involves the digital replacement of conventional x-ray film with a reusable cassette-based phosphor imaging plate, which temporarily stores an image within the phosphor layer following x-ray exposure. The CR cassette is placed into a scanner that reads the latent image from the plate by stimulating the plate with a laser beam and converting the image to a digital signal that is displayed on a computer monitor. Specialized software allows for image magnification, optimization of image contrast and brightness, and digital archiving.

   Digital radiography (DR) utilizes a digital detector panel that automatically generates a digital image upon exposure to x-ray and transfers the image in real time to a computer system without the use of an intermediate cassette as used in CR.

CERVICAL SPINE

2. What radiographic views are commonly used to assess the cervical spinal region?

   Standard cervical spine views include: lateral (Fig. 9.1), anteroposterior (AP) and open-mouth AP odontoid (Fig. 9.2), and right and left oblique (Fig. 9.3).

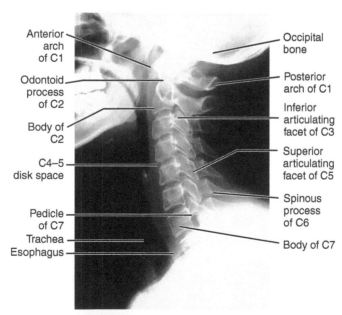

Anterior arch of C1

Odontoid process of C2

Body of C2

C4–5 disk space

Pedicle of C7

Trachea

Esophagus

Occipital bone

Posterior arch of C1

Inferior articulating facet of C3

Superior articulating facet of C5

Spinous process of C6

Body of C7

Fig. 9.1 Normal lateral cervical radiograph. (From Mettler FA. Essentials of Radiology. 3rd ed. Philadelphia, PA; Saunders; 2013.)

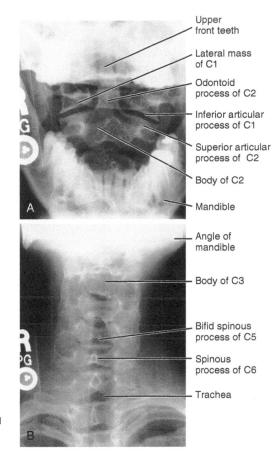

Upper
front teeth

Lateral mass
of C1

Odontoid
process of C2

Inferior articular
process of C1

Superior articular
process of C2

Body of C2

Mandible

Angle of
mandible

Body of C3

Bifid spinous
process of C5

Spinous
process of C6

Trachea

Fig. 9.2 (A) Normal anteroposterior (AP) odontoid view and (B) standard AP cervical view. (From Mettler FA. Essentials of Radiology. 3rd ed. Philadelphia, PA; Saunders; 2013.)

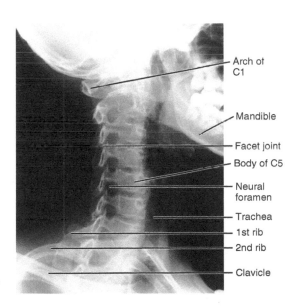

Arch ot
C1

Mandible

Facet joint

Body of C5

Neural
foramen

Trachea

1st rib

2nd rib

Clavicle

Fig. 9.3 Normal anatomy of the cervical spine on the oblique view. (From Mettler FA. Essentials of Radiology. 3rd ed. Philadelphia, PA; Saunders; 2014.)

3. **What important parameters require assessment on each cervical radiographic view?**

Lateral View
- Assess prevertebral and retropharyngeal soft tissue shadows
- Assess alignment via anatomic lines along anterior and posterior vertebral margins, spino-laminar junctions, and spinous processes
- Measure the distance from the posterior margin of the anterior C1 arch to the anterior aspect of the odontoid (atlantodens interval)
- Assess intervertebral disc space heights
- Confirm that the superior aspect of T1 is well visualized

Open-Mouth AP Odontoid View
- Check symmetry of the odontoid in relation to the lateral masses
- Assess the atlantoaxial joints for symmetry

AP View
- Confirm that spinous processes align with each other
- Assess distance between adjacent spinous processes and vertebral endplates
- Assess facet joint margins and uncinate processes

Oblique View
- Assess facet joint alignment
- Assess neural foramina and their bony boundaries

4. **What are the imaging options if the C7–T1 level cannot be visualized?**

A swimmer's view may be obtained when the C7–T1 level cannot be visualized on a lateral cervical spine radiograph. This view is obtained by raising the patient's arm overhead and directing the x-ray beam obliquely cephalad through the axilla. An alternative is to obtain a cross-table radiograph with traction applied to the patient's arms. Another option is to obtain bilateral oblique views of the C7–T1 level. Alternatively, a computed tomography (CT) scan of the cervical spine with sagittal reconstructions through the C7–T1 spinal level can be obtained.

5. **When are flexion-extension views of the cervical spine indicated?**

Lateral flexion-extension cervical views should be obtained only in neurologically intact, cooperative, and alert patients. Neck motion must be voluntary and there is no role for passive or assisted range of motion during these views. Outside of the acute trauma setting, lateral flexion-extension radiographs may be used to:
- Assess potential spinal instability due to soft tissue disruption when static radiographs show no significant bony injury or malalignment but clinical findings suggest a potential soft tissue injury.
- Assess healing of a cervical fusion
- Assess integrity of the C1–C2 articulation in patients at high risk for C1–C2 instability (e.g., rheumatoid arthritis, Down syndrome)

Lateral flexion-extension cervical radiographs are not indicated in the setting of acute trauma as they are difficult to obtain and have been shown not to provide additional clinically useful information. Because of protective muscle spasm, flexion-extension views are rarely of value in the acute postinjury period.

6. **What is the significance of the prevertebral soft tissue shadow distance?**

Increased thickness of the prevertebral soft tissue space may be a tip-off to the presence of a significant soft tissue injury involving the bony or ligamentous structures of the anterior cervical spine. This finding is less reliable in infants and children because of the wide, normal variation in the pediatric population. The normal prevertebral soft tissue shadow distance in adults is 7 mm at C2 and 22 mm at the C6 vertebral level. In general, prevertebral soft tissue thickness should not exceed 50% of the sagittal diameter of the vertebral body at the same level.

7. **What is the significance of an abnormal atlantoaxial interval?**

Abnormal widening of the space between the posterior aspect of the anterior arch of C1 and the anterior aspect of the odontoid (dens) defines an atlantoaxial subluxation and implies laxity of the transverse ligament. This space should not be greater than 3 mm in adults or 5 mm in children. Common causes of atlantoaxial subluxation include trauma, rheumatoid arthritis, and Down syndrome.

8. **What radiographic criteria are used to define instability of the spine in the region from C2 to T1?**

Commonly accepted radiographic criteria for diagnosing clinical instability in the middle and lower cervical spine (C2–T1) include sagittal plane translation greater than 3.5 mm or sagittal plane angulation greater than 11° in relation to an adjacent vertebra.

THORACIC SPINE

9. **What radiographic views are used to assess the thoracic spinal region?**

Standard thoracic spine views include an AP view and lateral view (Fig. 9.4).

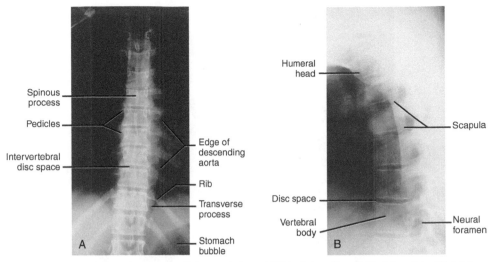

Fig. 9.4 Normal anatomy of the thoracic spine. (A) Anteroposterior, and (B) lateral views. (From Mettler F. Essentials of Radiology. 2nd ed. Philadelphia, PA: Saunders; 2005.)

10. What important structures are examined on AP and lateral thoracic radiographs?
    AP View
    - Soft tissue shadow
    - Spinous process alignment
    - Pedicle: check presence bilaterally
    - Vertebral body, ribs, transverse processes, costotransverse articulations, laminae
    Lateral View
    - Soft tissue shadow
    - Vertebral body contour and alignment
    - Intervertebral disc space height
    - Pedicles, spinous processes, superior and inferior articular processes, intervertebral foramina

LUMBAR SPINE

11. What radiographic views are commonly used to assess the lumbar spinal region?
    Standard lumbar spine views include upright (standing) AP (Fig. 9.5) and lateral views (Fig. 9.6). Oblique views, lateral flexion-extension views, spot lateral views, and Ferguson views are supplementary views that are valuable in specific situations but should not be ordered routinely to avoid unnecessary radiation exposure.

12. Why should lumbar spine radiographs be obtained with the patient in the standing position whenever possible?
    Lumbar spine pathology (e.g., spondylolisthesis) tends to be exacerbated in the upright position and relieved with recumbency. Most other spinal imaging procedures are performed in the supine position (e.g., CT, magnetic resonance imaging). Standing radiographs provide the opportunity to obtain valuable information about spinal alignment in the erect weight-bearing position.

13. What important structures may be assessed on lumbar radiographs?
    AP View
    - Psoas soft tissue shadow
    - Spinous process alignment
    - Pedicle; check presence bilaterally
    - Vertebral body and disc
    - Facet joints
    - Sacrum, sacral ala, sacroiliac joints
    Lateral View
    - Vertebral body contour and alignment
    - Intervertebral disc space height
    - Pedicles, spinous processes, superior and inferior articular processes, intervertebral foramina

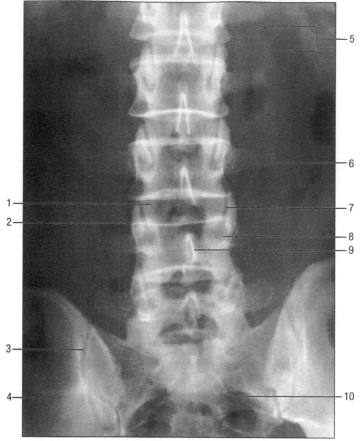

Fig. 9.5 Anteroposterior radiograph of the lumbar spine. *1,* L3 inferior articular process; *2,* L4 superior articular process; *3,* right sacroiliac joint; *4,* ilium, *5,* psoas lateral border; *6,* L3 transverse process; *7,* facet joint; *8,* L4 pedicle; *9,* L4 spinous process; *10,* anterior sacral foramen. (From Standring S. Gray's Anatomy. The Anatomical Basis of Clinical Practice. 41st ed. Philadelphia, PA: Elsevier; 2016, Fig. 43.45.)

- Sacrum
Oblique View
- Pars interarticularis
- Facet joints
- Neural foramina

14. What is the significance of an absent pedicle shadow?

An absent pedicle shadow on the AP view (Fig. 9.7) is an important radiographic finding because metastatic spinal disease may initially obscure a single pedicle. Pedicle absence may also result from destruction by primary tumors, histiocytosis, infection, or due to congenital absence/hypoplasia. Unilateral absence of a pedicle is termed the "winking owl sign." The visible pedicle represents the open eye, the absent pedicle represents the closed eye, and the spinous process represents the beak of the imaginary owl.

15. When are oblique views of the lumbar spine helpful?

- To diagnose spondylolysis
- To assess healing of lumbar posterolateral fusion

16. What anatomic structures comprise the "Scotty dog" on an oblique lumbar radiograph?

On the oblique lumbar radiograph, the vertebra and its processes can be imagined to outline the shape of a dog (Fig. 9.8): ear = superior articular process; head = pedicle; collar/neck = pars interarticularis; front leg/foot = inferior articular process; body = lamina; hind leg/foot = contralateral inferior articular process; tail = spinous process. **Spondylolysis** refers to a defect in the region of the pars interarticularis. It appears as a radiolucent defect in the region of the neck or collar of the *Scotty dog.*

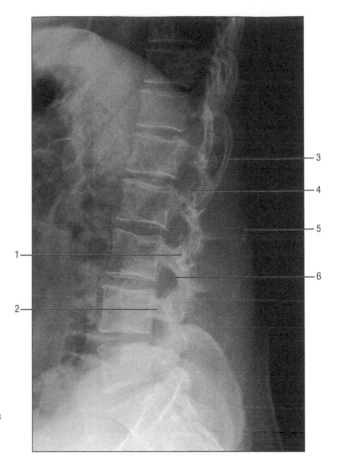

Fig. 9.6 Lateral radiograph of the lumbar spine. *1*, L3 transverse process; *2*, L4 pedicle; *3*, 12th rib; *4*, L2 superior articular process; *5*, L2 spinous process; *6*, L3-L4 intervertebral foramen. (From Standring S. Gray's Anatomy. The Anatomical Basis of Clinical Practice. 41st ed. Philadelphia, PA: Elsevier; 2016, Fig. 43.44.)

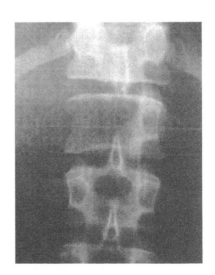

Fig. 9.7 Absent pedicle shadow due to vertebral tumor. (From Schajowicz F. Classification of tumors and tumor-like lesions of the spine. Spine State Art Rev 1988;169–181. with permission.)

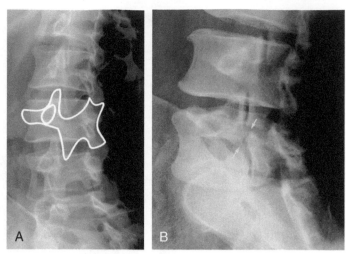

Fig. 9.8 Oblique radiographic view of the lumbar spine. (A) Outline on oblique radiograph resembles a *Scotty dog*. (B) Spondylolysis is a fracture in the pars interarticularis region *(arrows)*, which appears as a radiolucent band in the neck or collar of the dog. (From Pretorius ES, Solomon JA, editors. Radiology Secrets. 2nd ed. Philadelphia, PA: Elsevier; 2006.)

17. What is a Ferguson view and when should it be ordered?
A Ferguson view is an AP view of the lumbosacral junction taken with the x-ray tube angled 30°–35° cephalad. The x-ray beam goes through the plane of the L5–S1 disc, permitting the anatomy of the lumbosacral junction to be well visualized. This view is ordered when it is difficult to visualize the L5–S1 level in patients with severe spondylolisthesis and to assess an intertransverse fusion at the L5–S1 level.

18. What are coned-down views? When should they be ordered?
Coned-down views or spot views limit scatter of the x-ray beam and are useful to define bone detail for a limited area of the spine. For example, a spot lateral view of the lumbosacral junction is helpful to assess the L5–S1 level in cases of severe spondylolisthesis.

19. Explain the major pitfall involved in interpreting flexion-extension lumbar spine radiographs.
No universally accepted definition of radiographic instability of the lumbar spine exists. In asymptomatic subjects, up to 3 mm of translation and 7°–14° of angular motion may be present.

20. What is a lumbosacral transitional vertebra?
In the normal spine, the 24th vertebra below the occiput is the last presacral vertebra (L5), and the 25th vertebral segment is the body of S1. In the normal spine, there are five non–rib-bearing lumbar vertebrae above the sacrum. People who possess four non–rib-bearing lumbar vertebrae are considered to have sacralization of the L5 vertebra. People who possess six non–rib-bearing lumbar vertebrae are considered to have lumbarization of the S1 vertebral body. The term lumbosacral transitional vertebra has been adopted because it is difficult to determine whether the transitional vertebra is the 24th or 25th vertebra below the occiput without obtaining additional spinal radiographs. There are a variety of types of lumbosacral transitional vertebra. Vertebral anomalies ranging from hyperplasia of the transverse processes to large transverse processes that articulate with the sacrum or fusion of the transverse process and vertebral body with the sacrum may occur. These abnormalities may be partial or complete, unilateral or bilateral. Proper identification of lumbar spine segments in relation to the sacrum on plain radiographs is essential in planning lumbar spine procedures to ensure that surgery is carried out at the correct spinal level(s).

21. Define the following terms commonly used to describe abnormal vertebral alignment: spondylolisthesis, retrolisthesis, lateral listhesis, and rotatory subluxation.
Spondylolisthesis is defined as the forward displacement of the superior vertebra in relation to the vertebra below. The degree of spondylolisthesis is determined by measuring the percentage of vertebral body translation: 0%–25% (grade 1); 26%–50% (grade 2); 51%–75% (grade 3); and 76%–100% (grade 4). Other terms used to describe abnormal alignment between adjacent vertebra include **retrolisthesis** (posterior translation of the superior vertebra in relation to the vertebra below), **lateral listhesis** (lateral subluxation), and **rotatory subluxation** (abnormal rotation between adjacent vertebrae).

SPINAL DEFORMITY ASSESSMENT

22. What standard radiographs are used to evaluate spinal deformities?
Biplanar spinal deformity radiographs (posteroanterior [PA] and lateral radiographs with a field of view extending from the craniocervical junction to the proximal femurs) are the basic imaging studies used to assess spinal deformities (Fig. 9.9). The techniques for positioning, shielding, and performing this radiographic examination have been standardized. Radiographs are taken with the patient standing whenever possible. Sitting or supine radiographs may be required for patients who are unable to stand without support, including very young patients, tetraplegic/paraplegic patients, and patients with severe neuromuscular disorders.

23. When should I order a radiograph of a specific spinal region? When should I order a spinal deformity radiograph that images the entire spine?
Radiographs of a specific spinal region (cervical, thoracic, lumbar) are obtained for diagnosis and initial assessment of spinal pathology involving a specific vertebral or disc level within a spinal region (e.g., spondylolisthesis, fracture, infection, tumor). Spinal deformity radiographs are required for assessment of spinal pathology that involves multiple spinal segments (e.g., scoliosis, kyphosis). Spinal deformity radiographs are also necessary for planning spinal fusion procedures and for assessment of postoperative spinal alignment.

24. What specialized radiographs are commonly used to assess flexibility of spinal deformities?
- Supine AP side-bending radiographs (Fig. 9.10)
- Supine AP traction radiograph
- Lateral hyperextension radiograph
- Lateral hyperflexion radiograph
- Push-prone PA radiograph

Specialized radiographs are frequently obtained to assist in surgical planning before surgical correction of spinal deformities. *Side-bending films* are used to aid in selection of spinal levels that should be included in a scoliosis fusion. Supine AP side-bending films have been shown to be superior to standing side-bending films for

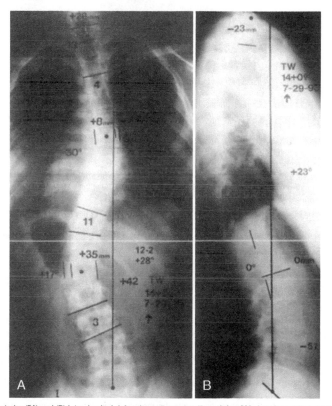

Fig. 9.9 (A) Posteroanterior (PA) and (B) lateral spinal deformity radiographs. (From Asher MA. Anterior surgery for thoracolumbar and lumbar idiopathic scoliosis. Spine State Art Rev 1998;12:701–711, with permission.)

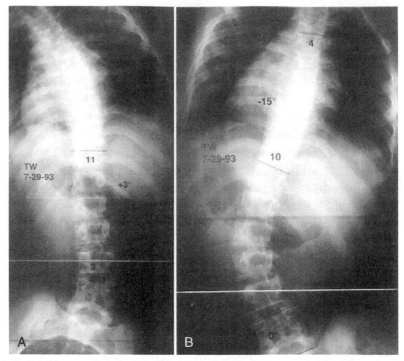

Fig. 9.10 Supine 36-inch long cassette side-bending radiographs. (From Asher MA. Anterior surgery for thoracolumbar and lumbar idiopathic scoliosis. Spine State Art Rev 1998;12:701–711, with permission.)

assessing coronal curve flexibility. *Supine AP traction radiographs* are helpful in patients with neuromuscular scoliosis to assess curve flexibility and correction of pelvic obliquity. A *hyperextension lateral radiograph* performed with a bolster placed at the apex of kyphosis may be useful for assessing the flexibility of a kyphotic deformity. A *hyperflexion lateral view* may be helpful to assess the flexibility of a lordotic spinal deformity.

25. What is the method used to quantify sagittal and coronal plane curvatures?
     The **Cobb method** is most commonly used to quantify curvature in the coronal and sagittal planes (Fig. 9.11). The following steps are involved in this measurement:
     1. Identify the end vertebra of the curvature whose measurement is desired.
     2. Construct lines along the superior endplate of the upper end vertebra and along the inferior endplate of the lower end vertebra.
     3. Next, construct lines perpendicular to the lines previously drawn along the end vertebra. Measure the angle between these two lines with a protractor or digital software to determine the Cobb angle.
     4. In large curves it is possible to measure the Cobb angle directly from the lines along the end vertebra without the need to construct perpendicular lines.

26. What is spinal balance?
     Balance has been defined as the ability to maintain the center of gravity of a body within its base of support with minimal postural sway. From the point of view of the spine, it implies that, in both the frontal and sagittal planes, the head is positioned correctly over the sacrum and pelvis in both a translational and angular sense. **Coronal plane balance** is present in a healthy young patient when a plumb line dropped from the center of the C7 vertebral body lies within 1 cm of the middle of the sacrum. **Sagittal plane balance** is present in a healthy young patient when a plumb line dropped from the center of C7 lies within 2.5 cm of the posterosuperior corner of S1. The plumb line measurement is also referred to as the **sagittal vertical axis (SVA)**. By convention, when the SVA falls behind the L5–S1 disc space, the SVA is considered **negative**. When the SVA falls through the L5–S1 disc, the SVA is considered **neutral**. When the SVA falls in front of the L5–S1 disc, the SVA is considered **positive**. In a normal young patient, the SVA is usually neutral or negative. With increasing age, the SVA becomes more positive. In the normal young patient, the SVA passes anterior to the thoracic spine, through the center of the L1 vertebral body, posterior to the lumbar spine, and through the posterior corner of S1.

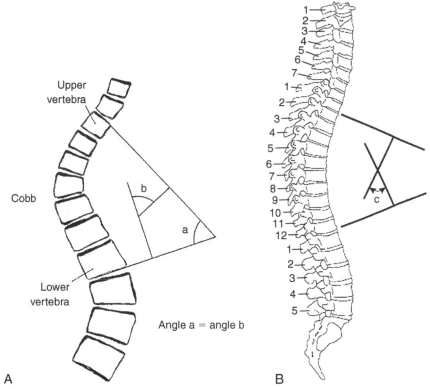

Fig. 9.11 (A) Measurement of scoliosis. (B) Measurement of kyphosis. (A: From Katz DS, Math KR, Groskin SA, editors. Radiology Secrets. Philadelphia, PA: Hanley & Belfus; 1998. B: From Devlin VJ, Narvaez JC. Imaging strategies for spinal deformities. Spine State Art Rev 1998;12:147–164

27. What are normal values for the sagittal curves of the different spinal regions?
    - **Cervical region:** Cervical lordosis (occiput–C7) averages 40°, with the majority of cervical lordosis occurring at the C1–C2 motion segment.
    - **Thoracic region:** Normal kyphosis (T1–T12) in young adults ranges from 20° to 50° with a tendency to increase slightly with age. The kyphosis in the thoracic region usually starts at T1–T2 and gradually increases at each level toward the apex (T6–T7 disc). Below the thoracic apex, segmental kyphosis gradually decreases until the thoracolumbar junction is reached.
    - **Thoracolumbar region:** The thoracolumbar junction (T12–L1) is essentially straight with respect to the sagittal plane. It serves as the transition area between the relatively stiff kyphotic thoracic region and the relatively mobile lordotic lumbar region.
    - **Lumbar region:** Normal lumbar lordosis (L1–S1) ranges from 30° to 80° with a mean lordosis of 60°. Lumbar lordosis generally begins at L1–L2 and gradually increases at each distal level toward the sacrum. The apex of lumbar lordosis is normally located at the L3–L4 disc space (Fig. 9.12).

28. Describe the relationship between thoracic kyphosis and lumbar lordosis in normal patients.
    The relationship between these two sagittal curves is such that lumbar lordosis generally exceeds thoracic kyphosis by 20°–30° in a normal patient. This relationship allows the body to maintain normal sagittal balance and maintain the SVA in a physiologic position. The body attempts to maintain the SVA in its physiologic position through a variety of compensatory mechanisms. Functionally, the sacrum and pelvis can be considered as one vertebra (pelvic vertebra), which functions as an intercalary bone between the trunk and the lower extremities. Alignment changes in the hip joints and lumbar spine can influence pelvic orientation and, in this manner, alter the sagittal orientation of the base of the spine. The body has an interrelated system of compensatory mechanisms to maintain sagittal balance involving the lumbar spine and pelvis, as well as the hip, knee, and ankle joints.

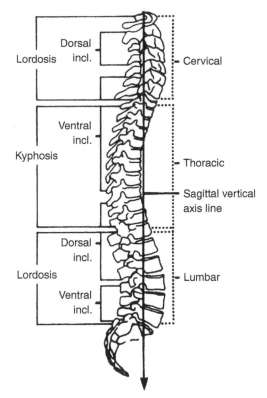

Dorsal
incl.

Lordosis

Cervical

Ventral
incl.

Kyphosis

Thoracic

Sagittal vertical
axis line

Dorsal
incl.

Lordosis

Lumbar

Ventral
incl.

Fig. 9.12 The sagittal curves of the spine. (From DeWald RL. Revision surgery for spinal deformity. In: Eilert RE, editor. Instructional Course Lectures, Vol. 41, Rosemont, IL: American Academy of Orthopaedic Surgeons; 1992, p. 241, with permission.)

29. What are the pelvic parameters that influence sagittal alignment of the spine?

Three pelvic parameters (Fig. 9.13) are measured: pelvic incidence (PI), sacral slope (SS), and pelvic tilt (PT). Pelvic incidence (PI) is a fixed anatomic parameter unique to the individual. Sacral slope (SS) and pelvic tilt (PT) are variable parameters. The relationship among the parameters determines the overall alignment of the sacropelvic unit according to the formula **PI = PT + SS.**
- **Pelvic incidence (PI)** is the angle defined by a line perpendicular to the sacral endplate line at its midpoint and a line connecting this point to the femoral rotational axis.
- **Pelvic tilt (PT)** is defined by a vertical reference line and a line from the midpoint of the sacral endplate to the femoral rotational axis.
- **Sacral slope (SS)** is the angle defined by a line along the sacral endplate line and a horizontal reference line.

30. What radiographic hallmarks indicate a *flatback syndrome*?

Flatback syndrome is a sagittal malalignment syndrome. Radiographically the hallmarks of flatback syndrome include a markedly positive sagittal vertical axis and decreased lumbar lordosis after a spinal fusion procedure. Classically, this condition was reported following use of a straight Harrington distraction rod to correct a lumbar or thoracolumbar curvature. When the thoracic and lumbar spine are fused in a nonphysiologic alignment with loss of lumbar lordosis, the patient is unable to assume a normal erect posture and instead assumes a stooped forward posture. The patient attempts to compensate for this abnormal posture by hyperextension of the hip joints, flexion of the knee joints, dorsiflexion of the ankle joints, and increased cervical lordosis. These compensatory mechanisms are ultimately ineffective in maintaining the SVA in a physiologic position and result in symptoms of back pain, knee pain, and inability to maintain an upright posture. There are many causes of sagittal plane malalignment in pediatric and adult spine patients. The development of imaging technology, which allow the capture of images that visualize from the head to the toes, has led to a deeper understanding of the interrelationship between alignment of the spine, pelvis, and lower extremities across all types of spinal disorders (Fig. 9.14).

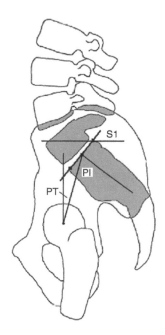

Fig. 9.13 Pelvic parameters: pelvic incidence (PI), pelvic tilt (PT), and sacral slope (SS). (From Staheli LT, Song KM, editors. Pediatric Orthopaedic Secrets. 3rd ed. Philadelphia, PA: Elsevier; 2007.)

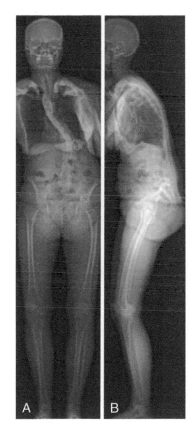

Fig. 9.14 Standing posteroanterior (A) and lateral radiographs (B) of a patient with sagittal imbalance taken with an EOS System. (From Celestre PC, Dimar JR, Glassman SD. Spinopelvic parameters: Lumbar lordosis, pelvic incidence, pelvic tilt, and sacral slope. What does a spine surgeon need to know to plan a lumbar deformity correction? Neurosurg Clin N Am 2018;29:323–329.)

31. What is EOS?

The EOS System (EOS Imaging SA, Paris, France) is a new imaging technology based on the invention of the multi-wire proportional chamber by Georges Charpak, recipient of the Nobel Prize in Physics in 1992. This system utilizes two pairs of orthogonally linked x-ray tubes and distal detectors. The chambers are positioned between the x-rays, which pass through the radiographed subject and toward the detectors, simultaneously capturing spatially calibrated AP and lateral images of the skeleton from the head to the feet as the system moves vertically along the patient. Due to the acquisition of calibrated images, these two-dimensional images can be precisely reconstructed in three dimensions. This technology enables capture of standing AP and lateral radiographs with substantially less radiation dose compared with conventional techniques and has enabled detailed evaluation of sagittal alignment and compensatory mechanisms involving the pelvis and lower extremities across a wide range of spinal conditions. Some of the relevant parameters (Fig. 9.15) that are evaluated include:

- **Sagittal vertical axis (SVA):** horizontal distance from the C7 plumb line and the posterosuperior corner of S1
- **T1 spinal pelvic inclination (T1SPi):** angle formed between a vertical line and a line from the center of the T1 vertebral body to the midpoint of a line connecting the center of the femoral heads (bicoxofemoral axis)
- **T1 pelvic angle (T1PA):** angle formed by a line from the center of the T1 vertebral body to the bicoxofemoral axis, and a line from the bicoxofemoral axis and the midpoint of the S1 endplate
- **Sacrofemoral angle (SFA):** angle formed by a line from the center of the S1 endplate and the bicoxofemoral axis, and a line between the bicoxofemoral axis and the femoral axis

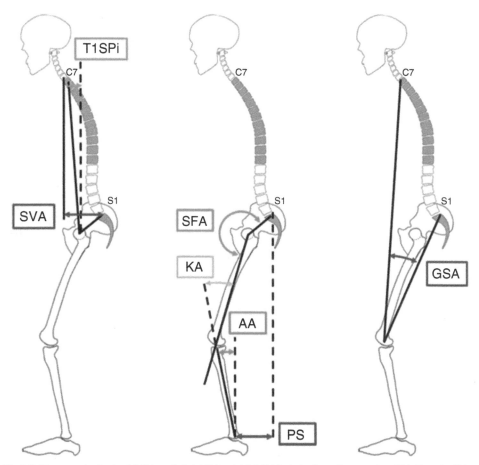

Fig. 9.15 Measurements of regional *(left)*, lower-limb *(middle)*, and global *(right)* spinal radiographic parameters. *AA,* Ankle angle; *GSA,* global sagittal angle; *KA,* knee angle; *PS,* posterior pelvic shift; *SFA,* sacrofemoral angle; *SVA,* sagittal vertical axis; *T1SPi,* T1 spinopelvic inclination. (From Jalai CM, Diebo BG, Cruz DL, et al., The impact of obesity on compensatory mechanisms in response to progressive sagittal malalignment. Spine J 2017;17:681–688.)

- **Knee flexion angle (KA):** angle between the mechanical axis of the femur and the mechanical axis of the tibia
- **Ankle angle (AA):** angle between a vertical line and the mechanical axis of the tibia
- **Posterior pelvic shift (PS):** distance between a vertical line extending from the posterosuperior corner of the sacrum and the anterior cortex of the distal tibia
- **Global sagittal angle (GSA):** angle between a line from the center of the C7 vertebral body to the femoral condyle, and a line from the femoral condyle to the posterosuperior corner of S1

KEY POINTS

1. Systematic review of spine radiographs provides important information regarding spinal alignment, degenerative changes, fractures, and spinal instability.
2. Cervical flexion-extension views should be obtained only in neurologically intact, cooperative, and alert patients and are not advised in the immediate postinjury period.
3. Important radiographic measurements for assessment of spinal deformities include coronal plane curvatures, coronal and sagittal plane balance, thoracic kyphosis, lumbar lordosis, and pelvic parameters.
4. Recent advances in whole body imaging technology permit analysis of sagittal alignment in conjunction with compensatory mechanisms involving the pelvis and lower extremities leading to a more comprehensive understanding of spinal deformities.

Websites
1. Standing balance and sagittal plane deformity: analysis of spinopelvic and gravity line parameters: http://www.medscape.com/viewarticle/578313
2. Three-dimensional terminology of spinal deformity: www.srs.org/professionals/online-education-and-resources/glossary/three-dimensional-terminology-of-spinal-deformity
3. Society of Skeletal Radiology Web Resources: https://skeletalrad.org/web-resources#tutorials

---

BIBLIOGRAPHY

1. Bernhardt, M., & Bridwell, K. H. (1989). Segmental analysis of the sagittal plane alignment of the normal thoracic and lumbar spine and lumbosacral junction. *Spine, 14,* 717–721.
2. Celestre, P. C., Dimar, J. R., & Glassman, S. D. (2018). Spinopelvic parameters: Lumbar lordosis, pelvic incidence, pelvic tilt, and sacral slope. What does a spine surgeon need to know to plan a lumbar deformity correction? *Neurosurgery Clinics of North America, 29,* 323–329.
3. Diebo, B. G., Varghese, J. J., Lafage, R., Schwab, F. J., & Lafage, V. (2015). Sagittal alignment of the spine: What do you need to know? *Clinical Neurology and Neurosurgery, 139,* 295–301.
4. Jalai, C. M., Diebo, B. G., Cruz, D. L., Poorman, G. W., Vira, S., Buckland, A. J., et al. (2017). The impact of obesity on compensatory mechanisms in response to progressive sagittal malalignment. *Spine Journal, 17,* 681–688
5. Lafage, R., Liabaud, B., Diebo, B. G., Oren, J. H., Vira, S., Pesenti, S., et al. (2017). Defining the role of the lower limbs in compensating for sagittal malalignment. *Spine, 42,* 1282–1288.
6. O'Brien, M. F., Kuklo, T. R., Blanke, K. M., & Lenke, L. G. (Eds.). (2005). *Spinal Deformity Study Group Radiographic Measurement Manual.* Memphis, TN: Medtronic Sofamor Danek USA, Inc.
7. Thawait, G. K., Chhabra, A., & Carrino, J. A. (2012). Spine segmentation and enumeration and normal variants. *Radiologic Clinics of North America, 50,* 587–598.
8. Wybier, M., & Bossard, P. (2013). Musculoskeletal imaging in progress: The EOS imaging system. *Joint, Bone, Spine, 80,* 238–243.

CHAPTER 10

MAGNETIC RESONANCE IMAGING OF THE SPINE

Vincent J. Devlin, MD

1. **What is magnetic resonance imaging (MRI)?**

   Magnetic resonance imaging (MRI) is a noninvasive imaging technology that uses magnetic fields and radiofrequency (RF) current to generate three-dimensional anatomical images without the use of ionizing radiation. The components of an MRI system include the main magnet, gradient coils, a RF coil, a computer system, and a patient table that passes through a horizontal tube (bore) running through the main magnet. The magnet is the most important component of the MRI system; it is comprised of multiple coils through which electric current is passed to create a magnetic field. The coils are cooled to superconducting temperatures (−269 degrees C, −452 degrees F) by bathing the wires in liquid helium, to decrease resistance to flow of electricity to near zero. Electric current passed through a superconducting magnet will flow continuously and create a permanent magnetic field whose strength is quantified in units called tesla (T). MRI systems used in clinical practice range between 0.5 and 3 Tesla (T) which is equivalent to 10,000–60,000 times the strength of the Earth's magnetic field (50 µT).

2. **How are MRI images generated?**

   MRI works by exciting and detecting changes in the rotational axis of protons that comprise living tissue. The hydrogen atoms (protons) in the human body are single charged atoms spinning on random axes such that the body's total magnetic field is zero. During an MRI scan, the patient is placed in a magnetic field, which causes the hydrogen nuclei to align parallel with the magnetic field. Application of **RF pulses** cause the hydrogen nuclei to realign and enter a higher energy state. Gradient coils within the main magnet alter the static field at a local level, which allows spatial encoding of the MRI signal. When the RF pulses are terminated, the excited **hydrogen nuclei** release energy as they realign in the direction of the main magnetic field at differential rates in different tissues, and return to a lower energy state in a process termed **relaxation**. The energy released during this transition is detected by the MRI receiver coil. Signal data are processed in terms of origin within the imaging plane and subsequently displayed on a monitor. The time between RF pulses is termed the **repetition time (TR).** The time between the application of RF pulses and the recording of the MRI signal is termed the **echo time (TE).** The process of relaxation is described in terms of two independent time constants, **T1** and **T2.**

3. **What is signal intensity?**

   Signal intensity describes the relative *brightness* of tissues on an MRI image. Tissues may be described as high (bright), intermediate (gray), or low (dark) intensity. Tissue intensity of a pathologic process relative to the intensity of surrounding normal tissue may be described as **hyperintense, isointense,** or **hypointense.** MRI signal intensity depends on the T1, T2, and proton density (number of mobile hydrogen ions) of the tissue under evaluation.

4. **Explain the differences between T1-weighted, T2-weighted, and proton density–weighted MRI images.**

   T1 (longitudinal plane relaxation time) and T2 (transverse plane relaxation time) are intrinsic physical properties of tissues. Different tissues have different T1 and T2 properties based on how their hydrogen nuclei respond to RF pulses during the MRI scan. MRI **contrast** is determined by varying the scanning parameters (TE and TR) to emphasize differences in tissue-specific properties and is referred to as *weighting* the image.
   - **T1-weighted images** are produced with a short TR (≤1000 msec) and a short TE (≤30 msec). T1 images are weighted toward fat. Fat typically appears bright on T1 images and less bright on T2 images. T1-weighted images are excellent for evaluating structures containing fat, hemorrhage, or proteinaceous fluid, all of which have a short T1 and demonstrate a high signal on T1-weighted images. Note that water will be dark on T1-weighted images. *T1 images demonstrate anatomic structures well because of their high signal-to-noise ratio.*
   - **T2-weighted images** are produced with a long TR (≥2000 msec) and a long TE (≥60 msec). T2 images are weighted toward water. Water appears bright on T2 images and dark on T1 images *(mnemonic: water [H_2O] is bright on T2)*. Signal intensity on T2 images is related to the state of tissue hydration. Tissues with high water content (cerebrospinal fluid, cysts, normal intervertebral discs) show an increased signal on T2 images. *T2 images are most useful for contrasting normal and abnormal anatomy.* In general, pathologic processes (e.g., neoplasm, infection, acute fractures) are associated with increased water content and appear hyperintense on T2 and hypointense on T1 images.

- **Proton density–weighted images** are produced with an intermediate TR (≥1000 msec) and a short TE (≤30 msec). Tissue contrast on proton density–weighted images is related to the number of protons within tissues. Water has intermediate signal intensity on proton density–weighted images.

5. Describe the signal intensity of common tissue types on T1- and T2-weighted and proton density–weighted MRI sequences.

On **T1-weighted sequences,** water has low-intermediate signal intensity, muscle has intermediate signal intensity, and fat has high signal intensity. T1-weighted sequences provide a good depiction of anatomic detail but are less sensitive to pathologic changes. T1-weighted sequences are useful to evaluate tissue enhancement after intravenous gadolinium contrast.

On **T2-weighted sequences,** water has high signal intensity while muscle and fat have intermediate signal intensity. T2-weighted sequences are useful in identification of pathologic processes (e.g., neoplasm, infection, acute fractures) as these entities are associated with increased water content.

On **proton density–weighted sequences,** fat has high signal intensity while muscle and water demonstrate intermediate signal intensity.

Note that cortical bone, tendons, and fibrous tissues demonstrate low signal intensity on both T1- and T2-weighted and proton density–weighted sequences, because these tissues contain few mobile hydrogen ions. Gas contains no mobile hydrogen ions and does not generate an MRI signal. Fat signal intensity may vary between each type of sequence depending on whether or not fat suppression is utilized. Fat signal may be suppressed using a variety of techniques for different purposes depending on the specific clinical scenario. The relative signal intensities of different tissue types on T1- and T2-weighted and proton density–weighted images are summarized in Table 10.1.

Table 10.1 Relative Intensity of Different Tissue Types on Various MRI Sequences.

TISSUE	T1	T2	PROTON DENSITY
Normal fluid (e.g., CSF)	Low-intermediate	High	Intermediate
Cortical bone	Low	Low	Low
Tendon/ligament	Low	Low	Low
Muscle	Intermediate	Intermediate	Intermediate
Fat	High	Intermediate	Intermediate
Red marrow	Intermediate	Intermediate	Intermediate
Yellow marrow	High	High	Intermediate
Intervertebral disc (central)	Intermediate	High	High
Intervertebral disc (peripheral)	Low	Intermediate	Intermediate

CSF, Cerebrospinal fluid; *MRI,* magnetic resonance imaging.

6. How do I know whether I am looking at a T1-weighted, T2-weighted, or proton density–weighted image?

One method is to look at the TE and TR numbers on the scan. T1 images are produced with a short TR (≤1000 msec) and a short TE (≤30 msec). T2 images are produced with a long TR (≥2000 msec) and a long TE (≥60 msec). Proton density–weighted images are produced with an intermediate TR (≥1000 msec) and short TE (≤30 msec).

An alternate method is to recall the signal characteristics of water. Locate a fluid-containing structure (e.g., CSF surrounding the spinal cord). If the **fluid is bright,** the image is probably a **T2-weighted image.** If the fluid is **dark,** the image is probably a **T1-weighted image.** Water has **intermediate** signal intensity on **proton density–weighted images.**

The above criteria refer to the most basic pulse sequence, spin echo (SE). In other pulse sequences, contrast phenomenology is more complex (Table 10.2).

7. What are pulse sequences?

The term **pulse sequence** refers to specific imaging parameters (i.e., timing, strength, and duration of RF pulses and magnetic gradients) used by an MRI scanner to collect imaging data. Various pulse sequences have been developed to optimize scan time, reduce artifact, and improve visualization of specific tissues and pathologic processes.

The **spin echo (SE) pulse sequence** is the most basic type of pulse sequence used for spinal imaging. It is obtained by applying an RF pulse that flips hydrogen nuclei by 90° (90° RF pulse), followed by a 180° RF

Table 10.2 T1-Weighted, T2-Weighted, and Proton Density–Weighted Image Parameters.

IMAGE TYPE	TE	TR
T1	≤30 msec	≤1000 msec
T2	≥60 msec	≥2000 msec
Proton density	≤30 msec	≥1000 msec

TE, Echo time; *TR,* repetition time.

refocusing pulse that manipulates the transverse vector of the relaxing protons to form an MRI signal called a spin echo, which is detected by the MRI coil. SE pulse sequences may be T1- or T2-weighted or proton density–weighted.

A **fast spin echo (FSE) pulse sequence** allows for faster image acquisition compared with an SE pulse sequence. A series of 180° RF refocusing pulses are utilized following the initial 90° RF pulse, which allows multiple SEs to be acquired in the time a single SE is obtained with a standard SE pulse sequence.

A **gradient echo pulse sequence** utilizes an excitation RF pulse with a flip angle less than 90°. Instead of using a 180° refocusing pulse, a magnetic gradient is used to manipulate the relaxing protons and form an echo.

As one becomes familiar with the basic science underlying MRI through formal study, and acquires experience interpreting spine MRI studies in daily practice, the advantages and disadvantages of specific pulse sequences in relation to various spine pathologies will be appreciated.

8. What is meant by fat suppression in relation to MRI?

MRI can selectively suppress or cancel out the signal from specific body tissues. Reduction of signal from fat tissue is useful in a variety of situations. For example, fat suppression can allow visualization of lesions that would otherwise be obscured by the fat signal, facilitate identification of fat-containing lesions, and aid in mitigating artifacts. Fat suppression is also useful for evaluation of tissues following administration of gadolinium contrast. A variety of techniques can be used to achieve fat suppression including *frequency-selective fat saturation* and *short tau inversion recovery (STIR) imaging.* STIR imaging is a nonselective technique as it suppresses signal from any tissue with a short T1 relaxation rate. STIR images are a sensitive tool for detection of pathology as the increased fluid and edema associated with pathological entities becomes conspicuous against the dark background signal from suppressed tissues. Frequency-selective techniques will suppress signal from fat without affecting signal from other water-containing tissues or gadolinium-based contrast agents.

9. What are indications for administration of an intravenous contrast agent in conjunction with a spine MRI study?

Intravenous gadolinium-based contrast agents (GBCAs) are used in conjunction with a spine MRI. GBCAs play a role in the MRI workup of suspected spinal infections, intradural tumors (e.g., diagnosis of *drop metastases,*) and evaluation of the spinal canal and its contents following laminectomy or discectomy. Vascularized structures such as tumors and inflammatory tissue are enhanced following administration of GBCAs and become more evident. As gadolinium acts primarily by shortening T1 relaxation times, T1-weighted images are typically obtained before and after contrast administration. A STIR sequence should not be used after GBCAs as this contrast agent has similar relaxation properties as fat protons, and the signal from GBCAs would be saturated on the STIR images.

Following administration, GBCAs are eliminated from the body via the kidneys. Renal function should be screened prior to GBCA administration, due to the risk of nephrogenic systemic sclerosis in patients with renal insufficiency and hepatorenal syndrome. According to an FDA Safety Announcement, small amounts of gadolinium may remain in the brain, bones, skin, and other parts of the body, for months to years following administration, but harmful effects have not been observed in patients with normal kidneys. Based on chemical structure, GBCAs are classified as linear or macrocyclic. Use of linear GBCAs has been shown to result in greater retention, and for longer than macrocyclic GBCAs. Use of GBCAs is contraindicated in pregnancy as these agents are assumed to cross the blood-placental barrier.

10. What are some contraindications to obtaining an MRI scan?

MRI scans are contraindicated in patients with metallic ocular foreign bodies, active implanted devices that are subject to magnetically induced malfunction, and certain passive implants (i.e., function without the supply of power) that are subject to potentially harmful movement or RF device heating with potential for tissue injury. Examples of contraindicated devices include insulin pumps, temporary transvenous pacing leads, as well as some types of cochlear and ocular implants, cardiac pacemakers, prosthetic heart valves and stents, implanted pain pumps, neurostimulators, brain aneurysm clips, carotid clips, and penile prostheses. Various online resources are available that provide detailed descriptions regarding the degree of MRI safety of medical devices. In 2005 ASTM (American Society for Testing and Materials) International developed a standard terminology regarding medical devices in patients for whom MRI examination is considered:

- **MRI Safe** refers to a device that has no known hazards in all MRI environments as they are nonconductive, nonmetallic, and nonmagnetic.

- **MRI Conditional** refers to a device that has been demonstrated to pose no known hazard in a particular MRI environment under specific conditions of use. Examples of conditions used to define the MRI environment include the strength of the main magnet, the gradient magnetic fields and the RF fields, and the specified absorption rate (SAR).
- **MRI Unsafe** refers to any device known to pose hazards in all MRI environments.

  The manufacturer and model of any implanted device should be identified, and the MRI safety information in the device manufacturer's labeling should be reviewed prior to imaging. Many passive spinal devices are comprised of nonferromagnetic materials and are considered "MRI Safe" or "MRI Conditional" based on specified conditions for MRI procedures. However, if devices are located near the intended site of imaging, significant **image artifact** may result and render the scan nondiagnostic over the instrumented levels. It may still be possible to obtain useful imaging data at spinal segments above and below the instrumented spinal segments. Stainless steel implants generally create excessive artifact compared to nonferromagnetic materials, such as titanium or polyetheretherketone (PEEK) implants; a computed tomography (CT) or CT-myelogram study may be necessary to evaluate spinal patients with stainless steel spinal implants.

  Claustrophobia is a relative contraindication to MRI but can be mitigated by use of patient sedation or an open-field scanner. Pregnancy is not a contraindication to MRI but it is a contraindication for use of GBCAs.

11. Describe the normal appearance of critical bone and soft tissue structures on MRI scans of the cervical spine.
    See Fig. 10.1.

12. Describe the important anatomic structures of the thoracic spine on MRI scans.
    See Fig. 10.2.

13. What anatomic structures should be routinely assessed on an MRI study of the lumbar spine?
    See Fig. 10.3.

14. When is MRI indicated for a specific spinal region versus a screening MRI study of the entire spine?
    The protocol should be designed to image the spinal area of clinical interest. When a regional spinal condition is suspected, such as radiculopathy or spinal stenosis, an MRI of the specific spinal region of clinical interest is appropriate. However, in some clinical situations, it is appropriate to screen the entire spinal cord and vertebral column from foramen magnum to distal sacrum. A screening MRI is indicated to evaluate patients with spinal deformities known to be associated with abnormalities of the neural axis such as syrinx, Arnold-Chiari malformation, diastematomyelia, spinal cord tumors, tethered spinal cord, and congenital spinal stenosis. A screening MRI is also important for the assessment of patients with spinal conditions that may involve multiple spinal regions, such as metastatic tumors, infections, and certain traumatic injuries.

15. Define the terms used to describe abnormal disc morphology on MRI studies.
    - **Annular tear:** A disruption of the ligament surrounding the periphery of the disc.
    - **Bulge:** Extension of disc tissue beyond the disc space with a diffuse, circumferential, nonfocal contour.
    - **Protrusion:** Displaced disc material extending focally and asymmetrically beyond the disc space. The displaced disc material is in continuity with the disc of origin. The diameter of the base of the displaced portion, where it is continuous with the disc material within the disc space of origin, has a greater diameter than the largest diameter of the disc tissue extending beyond the disc space.
    - **Extrusion:** Displaced disc material extending focally and asymmetrically beyond the disc space. The displaced disc material has a greater diameter than the disc material maintaining continuity (if any) with the disc of origin.
    - **Sequestration:** A fragment of disc that has no continuity with the disc of origin. Another commonly used term is *free disc fragment*. By definition, all sequestered discs are extruded; however, not all extruded discs are sequestered (Fig. 10.4).

16. Match each MRI image of a disc abnormality in Fig. 10.5A–E with the appropriate description: (1) annular tear, (2) disc bulge, (3) disc protrusion, (4) disc extrusion, and (5) disc sequestration.
    Answers: (1) annular tear, B; (2) disc bulge, E; (3) disc protrusion, C; (4) disc extrusion, A; (5) disc sequestration, D.

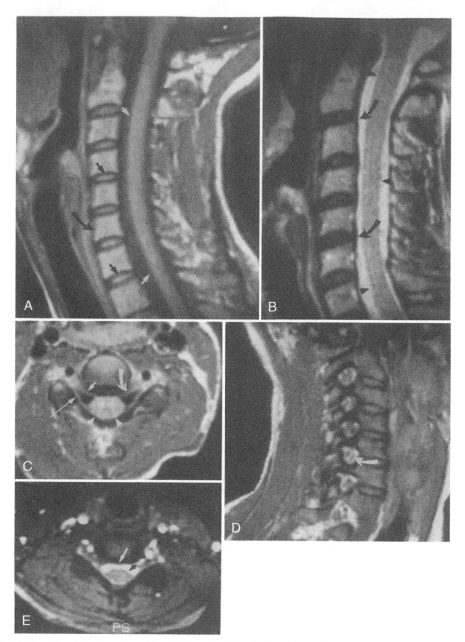

Fig. 10.1 Normal cervical spine anatomy. The sagittal T1-weighted image (A) provides excellent anatomic delineation of the vertebral bodies *(curved black arrows)*, intervertebral discs *(straight black arrows)*, and spinal cord *(white arrows)*. On the sagittal T2-weighted image (B), a myelographic effect is created by the increased signal intensity in the cerebrospinal fluid (CSF). There is an excellent interface between the posterior margin of the discovertebral joints *(curved black arrows)* and the CSF, as well as excellent delineation of the spinal cord *(black arrowheads)*. The axial T1-weighted image (C) provides excellent delineation of the spinal cord *(white arrowheads)*, ventral *(short white arrow)* and dorsal *(long white arrow)* nerve roots, and the intervertebral canals *(curved white arrow)*. On the oblique T1-weighted image (D), the fat in the intervertebral canals outlines the neural *(curved arrow)* and vascular structures. On the axial gradient echo image (E), the high signal intensity of the CSF produces excellent contrast for the delineation of the spinal cord *(black arrow)* and the posterior margin of the intervertebral disc *(white arrow)*. (With permission from Herzog RJ. State of the art imaging of spinal disorders. Phys Med Rehabil State Art Rev 1990;4:230.)

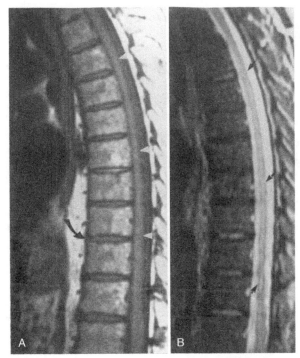

Fig. 10.2 Normal thoracic spine anatomy. The sagittal T1-weighted image (A) provides excellent anatomic delineation of the vertebral bodies, intervertebral discs *(curved black arrow),* and spinal cord *(white arrowheads).* On the sagittal T2-weighted image (B), the myelographic effect results in an excellent cerebrospinal fluid–extradural interface along with delineation of the thoracic spinal cord *(black arrows).* (With permission from Herzog RJ. State of the art imaging of spinal disorders. Phys Med Rehabil State Art Rev 1990;4:231.)

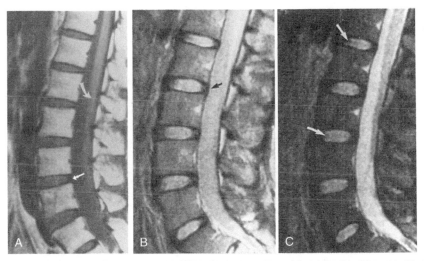

Fig. 10.3 Normal lumbar spine anatomy. The sagittal T1-weighted image (A) provides excellent delineation of the vertebral bodies, intervertebral discs, thecal sac, lower thoracic cord, and conus medullaris *(curved white arrow).* The high signal intensity of the vertebral bodies is secondary to the fat in the cancellous marrow. The interface between the posterior outer annular fibers *(straight white arrow)* and the cerebrospinal fluid (CSF) is not well defined. On the sagittal proton density–weighted image (B), increased signal intensity in the disc is identified, along with increased signal intensity of the CSF. This results in improved delineation of the posterior annular–posterior longitudinal ligament complex *(arrow).* On the sagittal T2-weighted image (C), increased signal intensity in the disc is identified, along with a linear horizontal area of decreased signal intensity in the center of the disc representing the intranuclear cleft *(arrows).* Increased signal intensity in the CSF creates a myelographic effect and provides an excellent CSF-extradural interface.

Continued

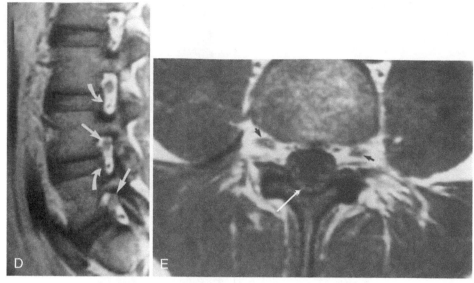

Fig. 10.3, cont'd The sagittal T1-weighted image (D) through the intervertebral canals provides excellent delineation of the dorsal root ganglia *(straight white arrows)* positioned subjacent to the vertebral pedicles. The posterolateral margin of the discs *(curved white arrows)* is well delineated. The axial T1-weighted image (E) provides excellent delineation of the individual nerve roots *(long white arrow)* in the thecal sac. The presence of fat in the epidural space and intervertebral canals provides an excellent soft-tissue interface to evaluate nerve roots *(short black arrows)*, ligaments, and osseous elements. (With permission from Herzog RJ. State of the art imaging of spinal disorders. Phys Med Rehabil State Art Rev 1990;4:232–233.)

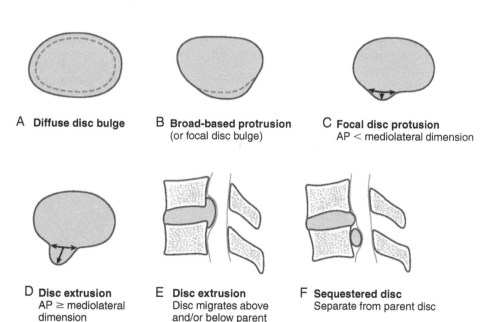

A **Diffuse disc bulge**

B **Broad-based protrusion** (or focal disc bulge)

C **Focal disc protusion** AP < mediolateral dimension

D **Disc extrusion** AP ≥ mediolateral dimension

E **Disc extrusion** Disc migrates above and/or below parent disc, maintaining continuity with it

F **Sequestered disc** Separate from parent disc

Fig. 10.4 Abnormalities of disc morphology. (A) Bulge, (B and C) protrusion, (D and E) extrusion, (F) sequestration. The *dashed lines* in (A) and (B) indicate the vertebral bodies, whereas the *solid lines* represent the disc material. *AP,* anteroposterior. (With permission from Helms CA, Major NM, Anderson, M, et al., editors. Helms: Musculoskeletal MRI. 2nd ed. Philadelphia, PA: Saunders; 2008.)

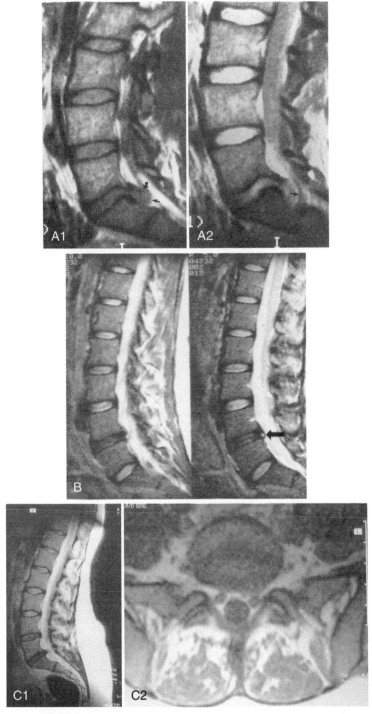

Fig. 10.5 Lumbar disc abnormalities. (A: With permission from Herzog RJ. State of the art imaging of spinal disorders. Phys Med Rehabil State Art Rev 1990;4:239. B: With permission from Gundry CR, Heithoff KB, Pollei SR. Lumbar degenerative disk disease. Spine State Art Rev 1995;9:151. *Continued*

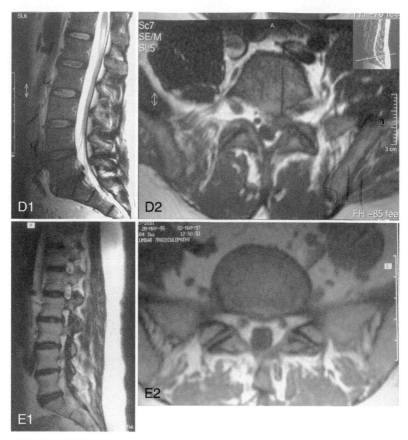

Fig. 10.5, cont'd C, D, and E: With permission from Russo RB. Diagnosis of low back pain: role of imaging studies. Phys Med Rehabil State Art Rev 1999;13:437–439.)

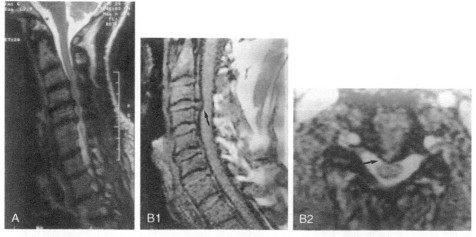

Fig. 10.6 Cervical degenerative conditions. (A: From Oishi M, Onesti ST, Dorfman HD. Pathogenesis of degenerative disc disease of the cervical spine. Spine State Art Rev 2000;14:538. B: From Schwartz AJ. Imaging of degenerative cervical disease. Spine State Art Rev 2000;14:558.

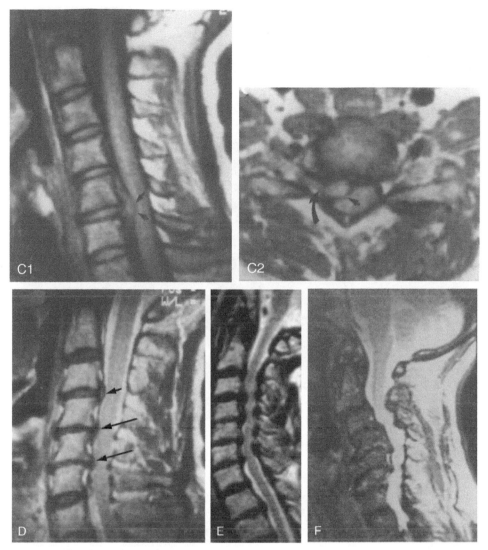

Fig. 10.6, cont'd C and D: From Herzog RJ. State of the art imaging of spinal disorders. Phys Med Rehabil State Art Rev 1990;4:236.
E: From Floman Y, Ashkenazi E. Expansive open-door laminoplasty in the management of multilevel cervical myelopathy. Spine State Art Rev 2000;14:639. F: From Ducker TB. Complex cervical myeloradiculopathy (S-shaped spinal deformity): Case report. Spine State Art Rev 1991;5:317.)

17. Match each cervical MRI image in Fig. 10.6A–F with the appropriate description. Each image depicts a patient who presents with symptoms consistent with cervical radiculopathy and/or cervical myelopathy.
    1. Complex cervical spinal deformity. Cervical kyphosis is associated with C3–C4 anterolisthesis and C4–C5 retrolisthesis. Posterior spinal cord compression from C2 to C4 and anterior spinal cord compression from C4 to C6 are noted.
    2. Severe multilevel cervical spinal stenosis (C2–C3 through C6–C7) with anterior and posterior cord compression.
    3. Single-level cervical disc extrusion associated with severe spinal cord compression.
    4. Multilevel cervical spondylosis superimposed on developmental stenosis. The anteroposterior diameter of the central spinal canal is narrowed on a developmental basis from the C3–C4 level and distally to this. Cervical disc protrusions and spondylotic ridges cause cord impingement at C3–C4, C4–C5, and C5–C6.
    5. Single-level cervical disc protrusion associated with mild spinal cord impingement.
    6. Congenital stenosis of the cervical spinal canal associated with multilevel disc protrusions and severe multilevel spinal cord compression. Congenital fusion of the C6 and C7 vertebral bodies is noted.
       Answers: (1), F; (2), E; (3), C; (4), D; (5), B; (6), A.

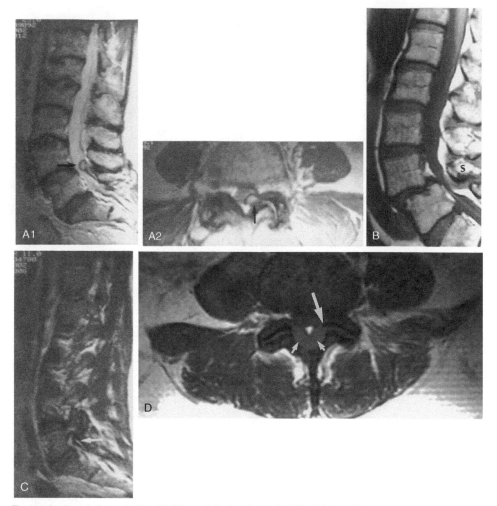

Fig. 10.7 Lumbar spinal stenosis. (A and C: With permission from Gundry CR, Heithoff KB, Pollei SR. Lumbar degenerative disk disease. Spine State Art Rev 1995;9:169. B: With permission from Barckhausen RR, Math KR. Lumbar spine diseases. In: Katz DS, Math KR, Groskin SA, editors. Radiology Secrets. Philadelphia, PA: Hanley & Belfus; 1998. D: With permission from Figueroa RE, Stone JA. MRI imaging of degenerative spine disease: MRI myelography and imaging of the posterior spinal elements. In: Castillo M, editor. Spinal Imaging: State of the Art. Philadelphia, PA: Hanley & Belfus; 2001.)

18. Match each lumbar MRI image in Fig. 10.7A–D with the appropriate description. Each image depicts a patient who presents with symptoms consistent with lumbar spinal stenosis.
    1. Ligamentum flavum hypertrophy causes stenosis of the central spinal canal and lateral recess.
    2. Hypertrophy of the superior articular process at L5–S1 associated with thickened ligamentum flavum results in front-to-back narrowing of the L5–S1 intervertebral nerve root canal with compression of the L5 ganglion.
    3. A synovial cyst arises from the L4–L5 facet joint, resulting in compression of the left side of the thecal sac, and the left L5 nerve root.
    4. Degenerative spondylolisthesis associated with L4–L5 central spinal stenosis.
       Answers: (1), D; (2), C; (3), A; (4), B.

19. A 50-year-old diabetic man presents with a 2-month history of low back pain refractory to bedrest and analgesics. An MRI (Fig. 10.8) is obtained by the patient's primary physician, and the patient is referred for consultation. What is the diagnosis?
    The imaging findings are classic for a *disc space infection.* Pyogenic infection typically begins at the vertebral endplates, then involves the disc, and finally spreads to involve the adjacent vertebral bodies. T1-weighted images show decreased signal intensity in the disc and vertebral bodies. T2-weighted images show increased signal

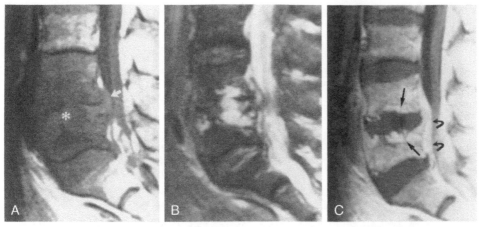

Fig. 10.8 Magnetic resonance of *Streptococcus pneumoniae* discitis/osteomyelitis. (A) Sagittal T1-weighted conventional spine-echo (CSE) image reveals an extensive hypointensity involving the L4–L5 disc space *(asterisk)* and the adjacent vertebral bodies. An extradural soft tissue mass compresses the thecal sac *(arrow)*. (B) Sagittal T2-weighted CSE image shows mixed hyperintensity and isointensity in the involved L4–L5 intervertebral disc and adjacent vertebrae. (C) Sagittal T1-weighted CSE image following gadolinium administration reveals peripheral enhancement of the disc *(straight arrows)* and uniform enhancement of the epidural mass *(curved arrows)*, representing discitis and epidural phlegmon. (With permission from Reddy S, Leite CC, Jinkins JRZ. Imaging of infectious disease of the spine. Spine State Art Rev 1995;9:135.)

intensity in the disc and vertebral bodies. Additional findings may include inflammatory changes in the paravertebral soft tissues and abscess formation in either the epidural space or anterior paravertebral tissues.

20. A 70-year-old woman presents with back pain and a thoracic fracture. She has a history of breast cancer and a documented history of osteoporosis. How can MRI help determine whether the fracture is the result of osteoporosis or metastatic breast cancer?
Findings on MRI that support a diagnosis of *metastatic tumor* include: a convex posterior margin of the vertebral body (i.e., an expanded appearance); abnormal signal intensity extending into the pedicle or posterior osseous elements; compression of the entire vertebral body, including its posterior third; presence of an epidural or extraosseous soft tissue mass; and diffuse marrow replacement throughout the vertebral body without focal fat preservation (Fig. 10.9).

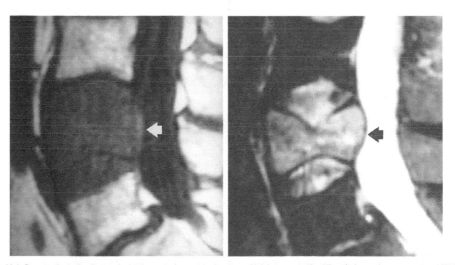

Fig. 10.9 Bone metastasis. *Arrows* depict the posterior vertebral cortex, which has a smooth, diffuse bulge and convex contour. (With permission from Palmer WE, Suri R. MR. Differentiation of benign versus malignant collapse. In: Castillo M, editor. Spinal Imaging: State of the Art. Philadelphia, PA: Hanley & Belfus; 2001.)

Findings on MRI that support a diagnosis of a *benign osteoporotic compression fracture* include: a horizontally oriented low signal line paralleling the vertebral body endplate, normal or mildly abnormal signal in the fractured vertebral body, a region of spared normal bone marrow signal intensity, a wedge-shaped vertebral body without compression of the posterior third, and the presence of multiple vertebral body fractures (Fig. 10.10).

MRI can be useful in determining the *age of an osteoporotic vertebral fracture*. The presence of marrow edema indicates that the fracture is relatively acute. The STIR pulse sequence is extremely sensitive to marrow edema. Gadolinium contrast will also show enhancement in acute fractures. The absence of marrow edema indicates a more chronic fracture.

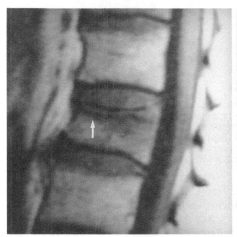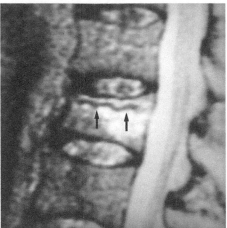

Fig. 10.10 Benign osteoporotic compression fracture. *Arrows* depict a linear fracture plane. The line does not extend all the way to the posterior vertebral cortex and posterior cortical height is maintained. (With permission from Palmer WE, Suri R. MR. Differentiation of benign versus malignant collapse. In: Castillo M, editor. Spinal Imaging: State of the Art. Philadelphia, PA: Hanley & Belfus; 2001.)

The MRI findings in acute osteoporotic compression fractures and fractures due to malignancies may overlap. Fracture edema and hemorrhage can surround a vertebral body and give the appearance of a soft tissue mass. Fracture-related edema in acute osteoporotic fractures may cause diffuse vertebral body enhancement similar to the findings in metastatic disease. However, after osteoporotic fractures heal, signal intensities in the collapsed and adjacent normal vertebral bodies are identical. In equivocal cases, a follow-up MRI scan can be performed to reassess the bone marrow for resolution of signal abnormalities and reversion to normal fat signal. A CT-guided biopsy is indicated when questions about the cause of a spine fracture remain after imaging studies have been performed.

KEY POINTS

1. MRI is a noninvasive imaging technology that utilizes magnetic fields and radiofrequency (RF) current to generate three-dimensional anatomical images without the use of ionizing radiation.
2. MRI provides excellent visualization of pathologic processes involving the disc, thecal sac, epidural space, neural elements, paraspinal soft tissues, and bone marrow.
3. Gadolinium contrast-enhanced MRI of the spine is valuable for evaluating patients with infection, tumor, or history of prior decompressive surgery.

Websites
1. MRI sequences: http://www.mr-tip.com/serv1.php?type=seq
2. MRI Pulse Sequences: https://pubs.rsna.org/doi/full/10.1148/rg.262055063
3. Gadolinium-based contrast agents: https://www.fda.gov/Drugs/DrugSafety/ucm589213.htm
4. MRI Safety: www.mrisafety.com
5. Patient Safety: https://radiology.ucsf.edu/patient-care/patient-safety

BIBLIOGRAPHY

1. Czervionke, L. F., Fenton, D. S. (Eds.). (2011). *Imaging Painful Spine Disorders.* Philadelphia, PA: Saunders.
2. Helms, C. A., Major, N. M., Kaplan, P. A., Anderson, M., Dussault, R. (Eds.). (2008). *Helms: Musculoskeletal MRI.* (2nd ed.). Philadelphia, PA: Saunders.
3. Khanna, A. J. (Ed.). (2014). *MRI Essentials for the Spine Specialist.* New York, NY: Thieme.
4. Ly, J. Q. (2007). Systematic approach to interpretation of the lumbar spine MR imaging examination. *Magnetic Resonance Imaging Clinics of North America, 15,* 155–166.
5. Maus, T. P., Miller, F. H. (Eds.). (2012). Spinal imaging. *Radiologic Clinics of North America, 50,* 569–860.
6. Naidich, T. P., Castillo, M., Cha, S. et al., (Eds.). (2003). *Imaging of the Spine.* Philadelphia, PA: Saunders.
7. Woods, T. O. (2007). Standards for medical devices in MRI: present and future. *Journal of Magnetic Resonance Imaging, 26,* 1186–1189.

CHAPTER 11

COMPUTED TOMOGRAPHY AND CT-MYELOGRAPHY

Vincent J. Devlin, MD

1. **What is computed tomography?**

   Computed tomography (CT) is a noninvasive imaging technology that generates detailed cross-sectional images using a computer and rotating x-ray emitter. The CT scanner is a circular, rotating frame with an x-ray emitter mounted on one side and x-ray detectors mounted on the opposite side. As the patient lies on a mechanical table, which moves through the CT gantry, the scanner rotates and emits an x-ray beam that passes through the body and interacts with a series of rotating detectors. Cross-sectional images are generated based on mathematical reconstruction of tissue beam attenuation. Images are represented on a gray scale in which the shade of gray is determined by the density of the imaged structure. Dense structures such as bone appear white, less dense structures appear as various shades of gray, and the least dense structures (containing gas) appear black. With early-generation CT scanners, termed *sequential* CT scanners, one cross-sectional image was obtained for each complete rotation of the CT frame, before the table moved the patient into position for the next image. Contemporary CT scanners, termed *helical* or *spiral* CT scanners, move continuously around the patient as the patient moves through the scanner, and use multiple rows of x-ray detectors (multidetector row CT [MDCT]). When indicated, contrast agents may be injected into the thecal sac to enhance visualization of the spinal cord and nerve roots, or intravenously to permit visualization of vascular structures.

2. **What are Hounsfield units?**

   Hounsfield units (HU) measure the relative attenuation or density of a structure imaged on CT. By convention, the attenuation is −1000 for air, 0 for water, and +1000 for dense cortical bone. The operator adjusts the level and width of the displayed range of HU (window) to study different tissues optimally (e.g., bone window, soft tissue window).

3. **What is multiplanar reconstruction?**

   CT data are recorded in the axial plane as image slices composed of small boxes of tissue called *voxels*. These volume elements can be made equivalent in size in three orthogonal axes (isotropic voxels) permitting the axial data to be reconstructed in multiple planes by computer software (e.g., sagittal and coronal reformatted images). Advances in modern software permit reconstruction in nonorthogonal (oblique) and curved planes. Three-dimensional rendering techniques allow models of the spine to be created to facilitate understanding of complex three-dimensional anatomy (Fig. 11.1).

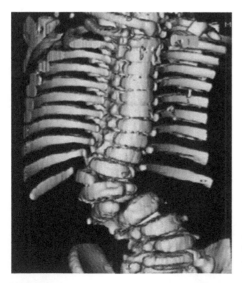

Fig. 11.1 Three-dimensional computed tomography of a patient with scoliosis due to multiple hemivertebra. (With permission from Hedequist DJ. Surgical treatment of scoliosis. Ortho Clin North Am 2007;38:497–509.)

4. **What is the role of CT in assessment of spinal trauma?**
   Multiplanar CT is the imaging study of choice for evaluation of adult spine trauma. In many situations, the complex osseous anatomy of the spine is not visualized in sufficient detail on plain radiographs and CT scan is required to accurately diagnose and classify spinal fractures (Fig. 11.2). Magnetic resonance imaging (MRI) plays a complementary role to CT for assessment of ligamentous injury, spinal cord injury, and neurologic compression syndromes in the spine trauma patient. However, routine use of CT in pediatric patients is not indicated due to concerns regarding radiation exposure, and plain radiographs are recommended for initial evaluation in most circumstances.

5. **Compare the use of CT and MRI for assessment of spinal tumors and infections.**
   MRI is the optimal test for initial evaluation of spinal tumors and infections after plain radiographs have been obtained. MRI provides information about the spinal canal, disc, bone, and surrounding soft tissues that may not be evident on CT. CT plays a role in determining the extent of bone destruction due to an infection or tumor. This determination is important for assessment of spinal stability, risk of pathologic vertebral fracture, and planning surgical treatment.

6. **What questions should be considered before ordering a CT-myelogram study of the spine?**
   CT-myelography is used infrequently due to its invasive nature, requirement for contrast administration, and use of ionizing radiation. Some questions to consider prior to ordering a CT-myelogram include:
   1. Can the pertinent clinical question be answered with noninvasive diagnostic imaging, such as MRI or a combination of MRI and CT?
   2. Will the information obtained from the study have an important impact on clinical management of the patient?
   3. Does the patient have any history of adverse reaction to iodinated contrast media or any conditions that increase the risk of an adverse reaction?

7. **What are some factors that increase the risk of an adverse reaction to iodinated contrast media?**
   Some factors considered to increase the risk include a previous reaction to radiologic contrast media, renal insufficiency, diabetic nephropathy, significant cardiac or pulmonary disease, asthma, multiple allergies, and patients at the extremes of age. Although there is no premedication regimen that can eliminate the risk of a severe reaction, recommended strategies combine pretreatment with corticosteroids (e.g., oral prednisone) and antihistamines (e.g., oral diphenhydramine), with or without addition of a H-2 antagonist (e.g., oral ranitidine).

8. **What types of adverse reactions can occur during a CT-myelogram procedure?**
   Initially, patients may experience discomfort during intrathecal injection of the nonionic water-soluble contrast agent. After injection, patients may experience an anaphylactoid (idiosyncratic) reaction (urticaria, facial and

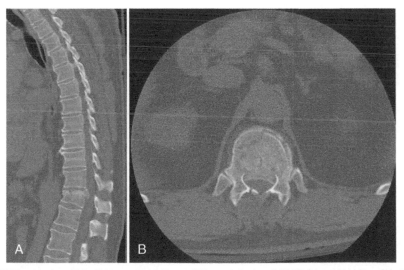

Fig. 11.2 T12 burst fracture. (A) Sagittal image. (B) Axial image. (With permission from Sethi MK, Schoenfeld AJ, Bono CM, et al. The evolution of thoracolumbar injury classification systems. Spine J 2009;9:780–788.)

laryngeal edema, bronchospasm, hypotension), or a nonidiosyncratic reaction due to the adverse effect of contrast on a specific organ system (nephrotoxicity, cardiac arrhythmia, myocardial ischemia, vasovagal reaction). Specific treatment depends on the exact clinical circumstance.

9. Compare the utility of CT and MRI for assessment of cervical radiculopathy.
Cervical radiculopathy typically results from nerve root impingement in the neural foramen by disc material, bone spurs, or a combination of osseous and disc pathology. MRI is the best test for visualizing disc material, as well as adjacent neural structures, and is generally the first test obtained in the evaluation of cervical radiculopathy. CT is the best test for visualizing osseous pathology responsible for radiculopathy but does not optimally visualize the spinal cord or nerve roots and requires use of ionizing radiation. Use of intrathecal contrast can enhance the ability of CT to visualize adjacent soft tissue and neural structures but requires an invasive procedure and is not necessary for routine cases.

10. Compare the utility of MRI, CT, and CT-myelography for assessment of cervical stenosis presenting with myelopathy.
MRI is usually the next test obtained in the imaging workup for cervical myelopathy after plain radiographs are obtained. MRI provides a noninvasive method of visualizing the entire cervical spine, including the discs, vertebra, spinal cord, and nerve roots, in multiple planes.
   CT plays a role when assessment of bone detail is required or when MRI is contraindicated. Clinical scenarios where CT has utility include preoperative planning prior to complex spinal instrumentation procedures (e.g., assessment of potential screw fixation sites, templating for spinal implants) and postoperative assessment of healing of spinal fusions.
   CT-myelography may play a role when MRI is contraindicated or when osseous pathology contributes to spinal canal encroachment. In the presence of complex cervical stenosis, CT-myelography continues to play a role, particularly in patients with ossification of the posterior longitudinal ligament (OPLL) in whom progressive mineralization of this ligament narrows the diameter of the cervical spinal canal (Fig. 11.3A, B).

11. Contrast the utility of CT and MRI for assessment of lumbar disc pathology.
Both CT and MRI can be used to define disc contour abnormalities (bulge, protrusion, extrusion, and sequestration) and guide treatment. Advantages of MRI include lack of ionizing radiation, superior contrast resolution, ability to detect intrathecal pathology, and the capacity to depict changes in disc pathoanatomy and chemistry (e.g., disc desiccation, annular tears) prior to changes in disc contour. For these reasons, MRI is the imaging modality of choice for assessment of lumbar disc pathology.

12. How is the location of neural compressive pathology such as lumbar disc material or lumbar spinal stenosis defined and described on CT and MRI studies?
The location of spinal pathology is described in relation to specific anatomic landmarks:
   • thecal sac
   • medial edge of facet joints

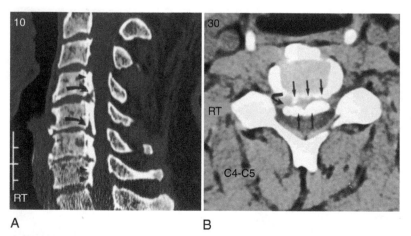

Fig. 11.3 Ossification of the posterior longitudinal ligament (OPLL), cervical stenosis, and cervical myelopathy. Sagittal image (A) depicts continuous OPLL *(arrowheads, straight arrows)*. Axial image (B) shows double layer sign characterized by ventral and dorsal OPLL *(straight arrows)* surrounding a central hypodense dural remnant *(curved arrow)*. Double layer sign is pathognomonic for an absent dural plane and risk of cerebrospinal fluid fistula. (From Epstein NE. From the imaging department. Spine J 2001;1:77, with permission.)

- pedicles (medial, lateral, upper and lower borders)
- intervertebral disc
  In the **axial plane**, these landmarks define the following **zones**:
- *Central zone:* central region of the spinal canal occupied by the thecal sac
- *Subarticular zone:* region between the medial edge of the superior articular process and the medial aspect of the ipsilateral pedicle.
- *Foraminal zone:* region bounded by the medial and lateral aspects of the pedicle
- *Extraforaminal zone:* region lateral to the lateral border of the pedicle
  In the **sagittal plane**, these anatomic landmarks are used to describe the location of spinal pathology in terms of **levels**. In the cephalocaudal direction, spinal pathology is described as located at the *disc, infrapedicular, pedicular,* or *suprapedicular levels.*
  The location of displaced disc material is described in terms of *levels* and *zones.* When describing lumbar spinal stenosis, a distinction is made between central spinal stenosis and lateral spinal stenosis. *Central spinal stenosis* refers to compression in the region of the spinal canal occupied by the thecal sac. *Lateral spinal stenosis* involves the nerve root canal and is described in terms of the three zones that use the pedicle as a reference point: zone 1 (subarticular zone), zone 2 (foraminal zone), and zone 3 (extraforaminal zone) (Fig. 11.4).

13. A 65-year-old woman presents with symptoms of back pain and neurogenic claudication. Available imaging studies include a lateral myelogram image (Fig. 11.5A) and an axial CT image (Fig. 11.5B). What is the patient's diagnosis? Explain what neural structures are compressed.
    The clinical and radiographic findings are classic for L4–L5 degenerative spondylolisthesis (grade 1). The lateral myelogram image shows an intact neural arch at the level of spondylolisthesis, leading to the diagnosis of degenerative spondylolisthesis. Disc degeneration, facet joint and ligamentum flavum hypertrophy, and spondylolisthesis, result in central spinal stenosis *(open arrow and opposing arrows)* and zone 1 (subarticular) lateral canal stenosis *(small arrows).* L4–L5 degenerative spondylolisthesis typically results in central spinal stenosis at the L4–L5 level associated with compression of the traversing L5 nerve roots bilaterally. The exiting L4 nerve roots are not typically involved unless there is advanced loss of disc space height, at which time the L4 nerve roots become compressed in the region of the neural foramen. Degenerative spondylolisthesis does not progress beyond a grade 2 (50%) slip unless prior surgery has been performed at the level of listhesis.

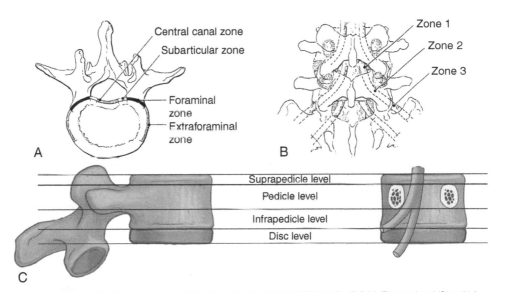

Fig. 11.4 Localization of lumbar neural compression due to disc material or spinal stenosis. (A) Axial, (B) coronal, and (C) sagittal views demonstrate anatomic relationships of the thecal sac and nerve roots to relevant adjacent lumbar anatomical structures. The thecal sac may be compressed in the central zone of the spinal canal. A nerve root may be compressed along its course through the subarticular zone (zone 1), the foraminal zone (zone 2), or the extraforaminal zone (zone 3). In the sagittal plane, these landmarks are used to describe the location of spinal pathology in the cephalocaudal direction as located at the disc level, the infrapedicular level, the pedicular level, or the suprapedicular level. (A and B: From Devlin VJ. Degenerative lumbar spinal stenosis and decompression. Spine State Art Rev 1997;11:107–128. C: From Lee IS. Imaging diagnosis of the degenerative spine. In: Kim DH, Kim YC, Kim KH, editors. Minimally Invasive Percutaneous Spinal Techniques. Philadelphia, PA: Saunders; 2011, pp. 58–110.)

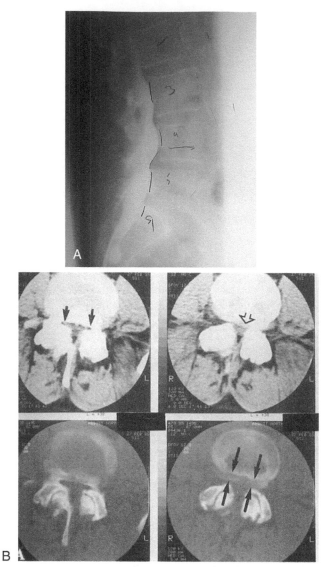

Fig. 11.5 (A) Lateral myelographic view shows L4–L5 spondylolisthesis and spinal stenosis. (B) Axial computed tomography (CT) scans at the L4–L5 level show central spinal stenosis *(open arrow and opposing arrows)* and zone 1 *(subarticular)* lateral canal stenosis *(small arrows)*. (With permission from Cole AJ, Herring SA. The Low Back Pain Handbook. Philadelphia, PA: Hanley & Belfus; 1997.)

14. What is the role of CT in evaluation of a patient following spinal decompression and spinal fusion with instrumentation? When should a myelogram be added?

A CT scan can provide critical information following spinal decompression and fusion procedures. A myelogram should be performed in conjunction with the CT scan if it is necessary to assess the spinal canal and nerve root canals at the operative site, and MRI is either contraindicated or unable to adequately image the target spinal levels (e.g., due to metal artifact). Problems that can be diagnosed with CT with or without myelography include:

- Persistent neural compression
- Adjacent level spinal stenosis or instability
- Nonunion following attempted spinal fusion (pseudarthrosis) (Fig. 11.6A,B)
- Incorrect placement of spinal implants, including pedicle screws, interbody grafts, or fusion cages (Fig. 11.6C).

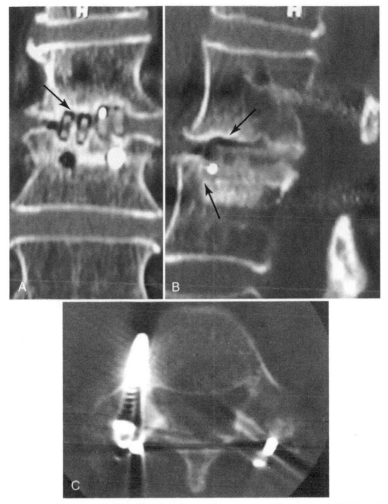

Fig. 11.6 (A) Coronal computed tomography (CT). (B) Sagittal CT image shows nonunion following attempted L1–L2 posterior interbody fusion. Note the lucencies around the interbody cages *(superior arrows)* and subsidence of cages into the L2 vertebral body *(inferior arrows)*. (C) Right-sided pedicle screw is improperly placed because it is not contained within bone and impinges on the adjacent nerve root. (A and B: With permission from Fogel GR, Toohey JS, Neidre A, Brantigan JW. Spine J 2006;6:421–427. C: With permission from. Devlin VJ. Spine Secrets. Philadelphia, PA: Hanley & Belfus; 2003.)

MRI may adequately image the spine in the presence of titanium or polyetheretherketone (PEEK) spinal implants. However, in some situations, significant artifact may persist and CT with or without myelography remains the next best imaging test. MRI in the presence of stainless steel spinal implants generally will not provide adequate visualization of the instrumented spinal segments due to artifact, and CT with or without myelography is indicated in this situation.

KEY POINTS

1. Multiplanar CT is the imaging study of choice for evaluating the complex osseous anatomy of the spine.
2. Contrast agents may be injected into the thecal sac or intravenously to enhance CT visualization of the spinal cord, nerve roots, and vascular structures.
3. The radiation dosage associated with CT is an important concern and may be minimized by following appropriate protocols.

Websites
1. Principles of CT and CT Technology: http://tech.snmjournals.org/cgi/content/full/35/3/115
2. Parameters for CT of the Spine: https://www.acr.org/-/media/ACR/Files/Practice-Parameters/CT-Spine.pdf

BIBLIOGRAPHY

1. Haaga, J. R., & Boll, D. T. (Eds.). (2017). *CT and MRI of the Whole Body* (6th ed.). Philadelphia, PA: Elsevier.
2. Resnick, D., & Kransdorf, M. J. (Eds.). (2005). *Resnick: Bone and Joint Imaging* (3rd ed.). Philadelphia, PA: Saunders.
3. Lee, I. S. (2011). Imaging diagnosis of the degenerative spine. In: D. H. Kim, Y. C. Kim, & K. H. Kim (Eds.), *Minimally Invasive Percutaneous Spinal Techniques* (pp. 58–110). Philadelphia, PA: Saunders.
4. Maus, T. P. (2014). Radiologic assessment of the patient with spine pain. In: H. T. Benzon, J. P. Rathmell, C. L. Wu, et al. (Eds.), *Practical Management of Pain* (5th ed., pp. 185–242). Philadelphia, PA: Mosby.

CHAPTER 12

NUCLEAR IMAGING AND SPINAL DISORDERS

Vincent J. Devlin, MD

1. **What nuclear medicine studies play a role in the evaluation of spinal pathology?**

   The technetium-99m (^{99m}Tc) bone scan has demonstrated utility in the evaluation of osseous lesions. Positron emission tomography (PET) with ^{18}F-fluoro-2-deoxy-2D-glucose (FDG) has shown utility in diagnosis of spinal metastatic disease, infection, and bone marrow abnormalities, while ^{18}F-sodium fluoride (NaF) PET has shown utility in the assessment of skeletal metabolism and osseous lesions. Hybrid studies that combine nuclear studies with structural imaging techniques, such as computed tomography (CT) and magnetic resonance imaging (MRI), provide improved image quality and higher spatial resolution.

2. **What principles are important for basic understanding of diagnostic nuclear medicine imaging tests related to the spine?**

   Nuclear medicine imaging tests produce images that reflect the biodistribution of an administered radioactive tracer, which may emit either gamma rays (i.e., ^{99m}Tc) or positrons (i.e., ^{18}F-FDG).

   In planar scintigraphy and single-photon emission computed tomography (SPECT), the gamma rays emitted by ^{99m}Tc exit from the body, pass through a collimator, and are detected by a gamma camera. Sodium iodide crystals in the camera convert the gamma energy to photons, which are detected by photomultiplier tubes, converted to voltage, digitized, and used by computers to generate an image.

   In PET, positrons are emitted by the radioactive tracer and travel several millimeters in tissue before colliding with negatively charged electrons, which results in *annihilation* and production of two high-energy gamma rays traveling in opposite directions. These annihilation photons are detected by crystals within the rings of scintillation detectors in the PET scanner, to localize the sites of radiotracer uptake in the body without the need for a collimator, a process termed *coincidence detection*. With the patient in the same position, data from the PET scan are co-registered with data from a CT (PET/CT) or MR (PET/MR). See Table 12.1.

3. **How is a ^{99m}Tc bone scan performed?**

   The radiopharmaceutical ^{99m}Tc, typically attached to a diphosphonate derivative, is administered intravenously and rapidly distributed throughout the body. Before excretion through the renal system, the technetium is adsorbed into the hydroxyapatite matrix of bone. A gamma camera is used to record the distribution of radioactivity throughout the body. Areas of increased blood flow and osteoblastic activity are detected by an increased concentration of radionuclide tracer. A decrease or absence of radionuclide tracer reflects either an interruption of blood flow or decreased osteoblastic activity.

4. **What is the difference between a planar bone scan, a SPECT scan, and a SPECT-CT scan?**

   A **planar bone scan** displays imaging data on a single planar image similar to a radiograph. As three-dimensional imaging data is superimposed on a single planar image, relevant pathology may not be appreciated due to overlap of anatomic structures (Fig. 12.1).

Table 12.1 Radionuclides for Use in Diagnostic Nuclear Medicine Imaging Studies.

Photon-Emitting Radionuclides
Technetium-99m (^{99m}Tc)
Indium-111 (^{111}In)
Gallium-67 (^{67}Ga)
Positron Emission Tomography (PET) Radionuclides
^{18}F-fluoro-2-deoxy-2D-glucose (^{18}FDG)
^{18}F-sodium fluoride (^{18}NaF)
Gallium-68 (^{68}Ga)

SPECT uses a computer-aided gamma camera and the radionuclides of standard nuclear imaging to provide cross-sectional images by 360° rotation of the camera around the patient. The images can be reconstructed in the sagittal, transverse, and coronal planes similar to a CT scan (Fig. 12.2). A SPECT study is more sensitive than planar scintigraphy in detecting lesions in the spine and allows for localization of spinal lesions to the vertebral body, disc space, or vertebral arch.

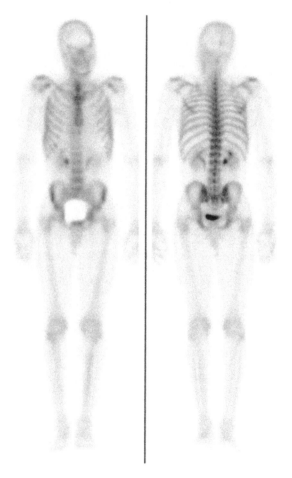

Fig. 12.1 Normal 99mTc–MDP distribution on whole-body bone scan in anterior *(left)* and posterior *(right)* projections. Note uniform radiotracer uptake throughout bones with some uptake in kidneys and bladder. (From Torigan DA, Ramchandani P. Radiology Secrets Plus. 4th ed. Philadelphia, PA: Elsevier; 2017, p. 759.)

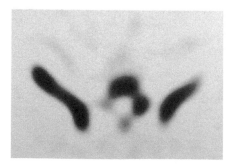

Fig. 12.2 Cross-sectional single-photon emission computed tomography image at the L5 level showing increased uptake in the left posterior neural arch consistent with spondylolysis.

SPECT-CT is a hybrid technology that combines SPECT and CT in an integrated system, which permits sequential scanning in the same position to facilitate fusion of nuclear and CT images. This technology provides increased diagnostic capabilities depending on the quality of the CT scanner but exposes patients to increased radiation dose.

5. What is a three-phase bone scan?
A three-phase bone scan is most commonly ordered during a workup for infection. It consists of three parts:
1. **Flow phase study:** Assesses vascular spread of the injected radionuclide immediately after injection. Detects perfusion abnormalities in suspect tissue
2. **Blood pool phase study:** Detects hyperemia in bone and soft tissue due to abnormal pooling of the radionuclide shortly following contrast injection (5 minutes)
3. **Delayed static phase study:** Usually obtained 2–4 hours after injection. Can detect abnormal increased uptake in areas of active bone remodeling

6. For which common spinal disorders does a ^{99m}Tc bone scan provide potentially useful diagnostic information?
^{99m}Tc bone scanning may provide potentially useful diagnostic information regarding osseous pathology including spine fractures, primary and metastatic spine tumors, spinal infections, and lumbar spondylolysis. Although ^{99m}Tc bone scans are very sensitive for detection of osseous pathology, these studies lack specificity, provide a significant radiation dose, and often require use of additional imaging modalities. As a result, ^{99m}Tc bone scans have been replaced in many clinical scenarios by MRI or CT. However, ^{99m}Tc bone scans continue to play a role in select patients, including patients unable to undergo MRI.

7. What is the typical appearance on a ^{99m}Tc bone scan in a patient with acute vertebral compression fractures secondary to osteoporosis?
The typical appearance of osteoporotic compression fractures on a ^{99m}Tc bone scan (Fig. 12.3) consists of multiple transverse bands of increased uptake on a posteroanterior image. However, the etiology of the fracture (trauma, tumor, metabolic bone disease) cannot be definitively diagnosed based solely on a bone scan. Increased activity can be noted within 72 hours of fracture, and the average time for a bone scan to revert to normal following an osteoporotic vertebral compression fracture is 7 months.

8. A 70-year-old woman complains of increasing low back and upper sacral pain. A ^{99m}Tc bone scan was obtained (Fig. 12.4). What is the most likely diagnosis?
The scan shows increased radionuclide activity above the bladder in the sacral area in a H-shaped pattern (Honda sign). Bilateral increased radionuclide uptake in the sacral ala in association with a transverse region of increased radionuclide activity is typical of a sacral insufficiency fracture, most commonly due to osteoporosis.

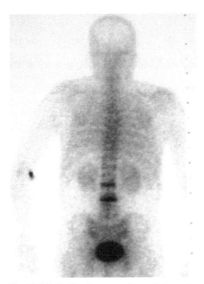

Fig. 12.3 Technetium bone scan demonstrates acute two-level osteoporotic compression fractures.

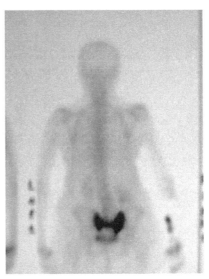

Fig. 12.4 Increased radionuclide uptake in a H-shaped pattern (Honda sign) in the sacrum is consistent with an insufficiency fracture.

9. Discuss the advantages and disadvantages of a ^{99m}Tc bone scan as part of the workup for spine infections.

Advantages of a ^{99m}Tc bone scan include the ability to detect a pyogenic infectious process before plain radiographs demonstrate an abnormality. A ^{99m}Tc bone scan is a highly sensitive study for diagnosis of spinal osteomyelitis in the absence of prior spine surgery or medical comorbidities.

Disadvantages of a ^{99m}Tc bone scan are related to its lack of specificity, especially in patients with a history of recent spine surgery, spinal implants, Paget disease, fracture, or pseudarthrosis. In addition, ^{99m}Tc bone scans are flow-dependent studies and may be falsely negative in situations associated with decreased perfusion to target tissues. A high false-negative rate is associated with their use in the diagnosis of granulomatous infections (e.g., tuberculosis). Gadolinium-enhanced MRI is the imaging test of choice for diagnosis of spinal infection. If MRI is contraindicated, ^{18}FDG PET scanning is an option. Gallium citrate (^{67}Ga) scans and indium-labeled (^{111}In) white blood cell scans are additional diagnostic options, although not widely used in clinical practice.

10. What is the role of a ^{99m}Tc bone scan in the evaluation of pediatric patients with back-pain symptoms?

Back pain may be difficult to localize in pediatric patients. A bone scan may be considered to evaluate the axial skeleton in patients with normal spinal radiographs and back pain persisting for longer than 4 weeks in the absence of constant pain, night pain, positive neurologic findings, or constitutional symptoms, in which case a spinal MRI should be ordered. A bone scan can diagnose osseous pathology such as fractures, spinal osteomyelitis, and some spinal tumors, but is unable to assess intraspinal and paraspinal soft tissue structures or neurologic structures. Addition of SPECT images can increase the ability to detect a stress reaction (impending spondylolysis) or pars interarticularis fracture. MRI is the study of choice in the presence of neurologic signs or symptoms, or if there is suspicion of infection, inflammation, or neoplasm.

11. What information can a ^{99m}Tc bone scan provide about lumbar spondylolysis?

A bone scan with SPECT images can provide useful information about lumbar spondylolysis. It can determine whether a spondylolysis detectable by radiography is acute or chronic. When radiographs are negative, a bone scan can diagnose an impending spondylolysis (stress reaction). In some cases, the bone scan may be positive on the side opposite to a radiographically detectable pars defect which aids in diagnosis of an impending spondylolysis. Bone scans can also be used to assess healing of an acute spondylolysis. However, bone scans are unable to identify nonosseous spinal pathology such as disc pathology or Scheuermann disease, which may be associated with or mimic spondylolysis. MRI is also an effective imaging modality for detecting spondylolysis and can visualize both osseous and nonosseous pathology without the use of ionizing radiation or need for a radiotracer injection.

12. What is the role of a ^{99m}Tc bone scan in the assessment of adults with back pain?

A ^{99m}Tc bone scan is a sensitive test for identifying osseous abnormalities such as fracture, infection, and metastatic disease, but is not very specific as it cannot distinguish spinal degenerative changes from other types of spinal pathology. ^{99m}Tc bone scans play a role in the evaluation of patients unable to undergo MRI, but their role is limited by the inability to visualize intraspinal and paraspinal soft tissue abnormalities and neurologic structures.

13. What are the advantages and pitfalls regarding use of a ^{99m}Tc bone scan in the evaluation of primary osseous tumors involving the spinal column?

^{99m}Tc bone scans have a limited role in the evaluation of primary osseous tumors. Tracer uptake is variable across different types of benign osseous lesions. ^{99m}Tc bone scans play a role in detection of osteoid osteoma, osteochondroma, and chondroblastoma, which typically demonstrate intense tracer uptake. However, there is a limited role for bone scintigraphy in the evaluation of other benign lesions, such as aneurysmal bone cysts and bone infarcts. Primary bone malignancies such as osteosarcoma and Ewing sarcoma demonstrate intense uptake on bone scintigraphy. However, bone scintigraphy is not helpful in delineating the extent of tumor involvement or identifying skip lesions, which are more clearly depicted on MRI. Bone scintigraphy may play a role in detecting metastatic disease after the primary tumor has been identified.

14. What are the advantages and pitfalls regarding use of a ^{99m}Tc bone scan in the evaluation of metastatic osseous tumors involving the spinal column?

^{99m}Tc bone scans play a role in the evaluation of metastatic tumors which involve the spinal column, particularly osteoblastic or osteosclerotic metastases arising from prostate, breast, and lung primary tumors (Fig. 12.5). Findings that support a diagnosis of metastatic disease include solitary or multiple focal areas of increased radiotracer uptake in the axial skeleton. However, ^{99m}Tc bone scans are not reliable for diagnosis of osteolytic (myeloma) or marrow-infiltrating tumors (renal-cell carcinoma, lymphoma) as these lesions do not typically stimulate increased osteoblastic activity. PET scanning using ^{18}FDG is useful for detection of symptomatic spinal metastases not

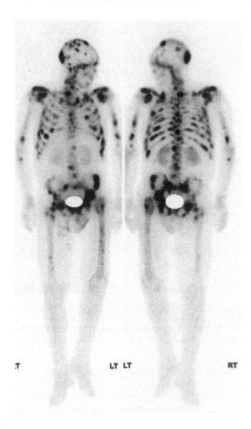

Fig. 12.5 Anterior and posterior views of a ^{99m}Tc bone scans show a patient with multiple foci of intense activity involving the ribs, spine, skull, scapula, pelvis, and extremities due to widespread bone metastases from metastatic prostate cancer. (From Waller ML, Chowdhury FU. The basic science of nuclear medicine. Ortho Trauma 2015;30:201–222, p. 208.)

identified on radiographs, CT, or technetium bone scans, due to its ability to detect tumor in the bone marrow directly. Other pitfalls to be aware of with respect to use of ^{99m}Tc bone scans for assessment of metastatic disease include the "superscan" phenomenon, the "flare" phenomenon, and the potential for multifocal tracer uptake to occur due to other pathologies such as osteoarthritis, Paget disease, or ankylosing spondylitis rather than metastatic disease.

15. What is the superscan phenomenon?

The superscan phenomenon occurs when the distribution of metastatic disease is so widespread and uniformly distributed that the ^{99m}Tc bone scan is incorrectly interpreted as negative. Increased radionuclide uptake is noted throughout the skeleton in the presence of diminished or absent uptake in the kidneys and bladder. This phenomenon can occur with metastatic prostate and breast cancer, renal osteodystrophy, and Paget disease.

16. How is a PET scan performed?

Hybrid PET imaging consisting of PET/CT or PET/MRI is performed sequentially. First, a positron-emitting radionuclide tracer is injected into the body. Next, a scout CT or MRI is performed, which images from the skull base to the proximal thighs. Following injection of the radionuclide tracer, positrons are emitted that travel through tissue and collide with electrons, resulting in production of gamma rays. A PET scanner records and analyzes these data and creates an image. CT or MRI are combined with PET data to maximize image quality, aid in localization of radionuclide uptake, and enhance diagnostic accuracy.

^{18F}FDG is the most commonly used radiotracer. ^{18F}FDG accumulates at sites of neoplasia and inflammation, as cells in these regions have an increased metabolic rate. ^{18F}FDG is transported and becomes trapped intracellularly as a result of phosphorylation by hexokinase. Because ^{18F}FDG competes with nonradioactive glucose, recent food consumption or elevation of blood glucose greater than 150 mL/dL in diabetic patients will decrease scan sensitivity. An alternative to ^{18F}FDG is ^{18F}NaF, a bone-specific tracer that has application in PET imaging of the musculoskeletal system (Fig. 12.6).

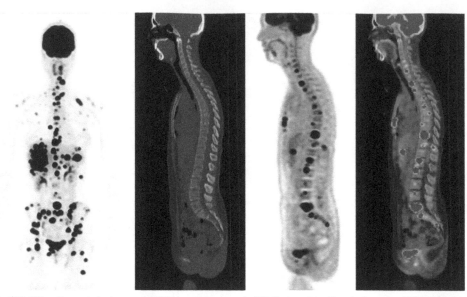

Fig. 12.6 FDG positron emission tomography (PET)/computed tomography (CT). Maximum intensity projection and sagittal CT, PET, and fused PET/CT images (from left to right) in a patient with metastatic melanoma. There are disseminated liver and bone metastases. Note that many of the vertebral metastases cannot be detected on the CT. (From Waller ML, Chowdhury FU. The basic science of nuclear medicine. Ortho Trauma 2015;30:201–222, p. 218.)

17. For which common pathologies can a PET scan provide useful diagnostic information?

    PET scans are most commonly used in the evaluation of cancer for diagnosis, staging, and assessment of treatment effectiveness. Utility in head and neck tumors, colorectal tumors, melanoma, lymphoma, multiple myeloma, lung cancer, and metastatic breast cancer have been reported. [18]FDG PET is very accurate for diagnosis of metastatic bone lesions, including osteolytic metastases and marrow infiltrative tumors, but is less reliable for diagnosis of osteoblastic metastases. The PET tracer [18]FNaF may be used as a complementary agent as it targets locations where osteogenesis is ongoing and images the osteogenic reaction to the tumor, rather than the tumor itself, and provides excellent visualization of osteoblastic metastases. The role of PET scans in the diagnosis of spinal infections is evolving. [18]FDG PET has been used in the evaluation of the postsurgical spine, for monitoring response to infection treatment, and for evaluation of nonspecific clinical presentations, such as fever of unknown origin.

KEY POINTS

1. A technetium-99m bone scan can detect regions of increased blood flow or osteoblastic activity.
2. FDG-PET scans have utility in diagnosis of spinal neoplasia and spinal infection.

Websites

Nuclear medicine: https://www.nibib.nih.gov/science-education/science-topics/nuclear-medicine#1001

Society of Nuclear Medicine and Molecular Imaging: http://www.snmmi.org/AboutSNMMI/Content.aspx?ItemNumber=15627

BIBLIOGRAPHY

1. Georgakopoulos, A., Pneumaticos, S. G., Sipsas, N., & Chatziioannou, S. (2015). Positron emission tomography in spinal infections. *Clinical Imaging, 39,* 553–558.
2. Gnanasegaran, G., Paycha, F., Strobel, K., van der Bruggenm, W., Kampen, W. U., Kuwert, T., et al. (2018). Bone SPECT/CT in postoperative spine. *Seminars in Nuclear Medicine, 48,* 410–424.
3. Mettler, F. A., & Guiberteau, M. J. (2019). *Essentials of Nuclear Medicine and Molecular Imaging* (7th ed.). Philadelphia, PA: Elsevier.
4. Parghane, R. V., & Basu, S. (2018). PET/Computed tomography and PET/MR imaging: Basic principles, methodology, and imaging protocol for musculoskeletal applications. *PET Clinics, 13,* 459–476.
5. Torigan, D. A., & Ramchandani, P. (2017). *Radiology Secrets Plus* (4th ed.). Philadelphia, PA: Elsevier.
6. Waller, M. L., & Chowdhury, F. U. (2015). The basic science of nuclear medicine. *Orthopaedic and Trauma, 30,* 201–222.
7. Ziessman, H. A., O'Malley, J. P., Thrall, J. H., & Fahey, F. H. (2014). *Nuclear Medicine—The Requisites* (4th ed.). Philadelphia, PA: Saunders.

NONSURGICAL MANAGEMENT OF SPINAL DISORDERS

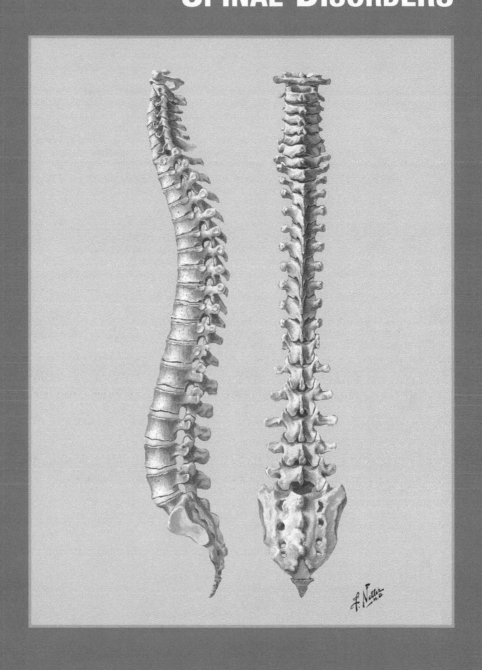

CHAPTER 13

CERVICAL SPINAL DISORDERS: NONSURGICAL MANAGEMENT STRATEGIES

Vincent J. Devlin, MD

1. **What etiologies are included in the differential diagnosis of patients who present for initial assessment and management of symptoms attributed to the cervical spine in an outpatient setting?**
   The most common cervical diagnoses in patients who present for initial evaluation for nonsurgical management in an outpatient clinic or office setting include axial neck pain, radiculopathy, and myelopathy. These conditions may present singly or in combination. Axial neck pain is most often mechanical in nature as it is provoked or relieved by specific activities or postures. **Mechanical neck pain** is attributed to stimulation of nociceptors located in intervertebral discs, zygapophyseal (facet) joints, ligaments, muscles, and tendons, and arises as a consequence of spinal degeneration or an injury. **Radiculopathy** and **myelopathy** occur as a consequence of impingement of neurologic structures from narrowing of the nerve root canals or central spinal canal by pathologies including disc herniation, spondylosis, and congenital stenosis or as a consequence of ischemic injury to neural structures. Specific pathologies that may lead to neck and/or arm pain symptoms include:
   - Cervical fractures/dislocations not previously diagnosed
   - Cervical spine infections: discitis, osteomyelitis
   - Cervical spine tumors: metastatic, primary
   - Rheumatologic disorders: rheumatoid arthritis, ankylosing spondylitis, fibromyalgia
   - Visceral disorders presenting with referred pain: angina, apical lung tumors (Pancoast tumor)
   - Shoulder and elbow pathology: rotator cuff disorders, medial epicondylitis
   - Peripheral nerve entrapment syndromes: thoracic outlet syndrome, suprascapular neuropathy; radial, ulnar, or median nerve entrapment

   Patients with a cervical spine problem sometimes report neck or upper extremity symptoms in combination with **headaches** secondary to a source in the cervical spine (cervicogenic headaches). Familiarity with the presentation of primary and secondary headaches is important to avoid misdiagnosis or delayed diagnosis of serious conditions that may manifest with headache symptoms, including vascular disorders (i.e., vertebral artery or aortic aneurysm dissection), intracranial tumors, and meningitis.

2. **What are the most important initial steps in the assessment of a patient with a cervical pain syndrome?**
   The medical history and physical examination remain the most important part of the initial assessment of a patient with cervical pain.

3. **For patients who present with a cervical complaint, what are some important areas to investigate in relation to the patient's history?**
   A comprehensive medical history should include the following elements:
   - Is this the first episode or a recurrent problem?
   - Was there a specific injury (i.e., motor vehicle, work-related, or sport-related injury; a fall)?
   - What factors increase and decrease symptoms?
   - What is the pattern of pain over a 24-hour period? Is the pain intermittent or constant?
   - Is the most intense pain localized to the neck and surrounding areas or to one or both arms?
   - Is there focal weakness or numbness in the upper extremities?
   - Are there changes in gait including clumsiness and imbalance?
   - Are there difficulties with fine-motor tasks such as buttoning a shirt or manipulating small objects?
   - Are there new bowel or bladder symptoms?
   - Is morning stiffness present?
   - Are headaches a major reason for seeking evaluation?
   - Is neck pain associated with dizziness, chest pain, or shortness of breath?
   - Are any red flag-symptoms present?

- Are any yellow-flag symptoms present?
- Consider use of a validated tool to assess pain and function (Visual Analog Pain Scale, Neck Disability Index).

4. **What are red flags in the evaluation of cervical pain syndromes?**
   Red flags are risk factors that suggest significant and/or potentially life-threatening pathologies associated with neck pain. Red flag conditions are rare and are estimated to occur in less than 5% of patients who present for cervical spine evaluation (Table 13.1).

5. **What are yellow flags in the evaluation of cervical pain syndromes?**
   Yellow flags are factors used to identify patients at risk of developing chronicity, disability, and poor treatment outcomes. These high-risk patients can potentially benefit from more intensive nonsurgical management with greater emphasis on a return to activity and focus on functional recovery. Some examples of yellow flags include:
   - Fear avoidance (avoid activity due to fear of worsening neck pain)
   - Catastrophizing (excessively negative thoughts and beliefs about the future)
   - Depression
   - Lack of motivation to return to work
   - High baseline functional impairment
   - Medicolegal issues
   - Work-related injury
   - Presence of nonorganic signs (suggests psychological component to pain)

6. **What are the key elements to include in the physical examination of a patient referred for initial evaluation of cervical pain with or without arm pain?**
   - Observation: assess gait, balance, neck posture
   - Palpation: assess for cervical tender points, lymphadenopathy
   - Range of motion: cervical flexion, extension, rotation, side bending
   - Neurologic examination
     - Assess sensory, motor, and reflex function

Table 13.1 Red Flags in Patients Presenting for Cervical Spine Evaluation.

SUSPECTED CONDITIONS	RED FLAGS
Fracture, dislocation, or ligament disruption	Neck pain with recent significant trauma: • Fall >3 feet • High speed motor vehicle accident • Axial loading head injury • Bicycle collision with stationary object
Malignancy	• History of cancer • Unexplained weight loss • Age >50
Infection	• Intravenous drug abuse • Urinary tract infection • Skin infection • Recent spinal procedure • Immunocompromise
Myelopathy/spinal cord compression	• Upper extremity weakness • Increased reflexes • Long tract signs • Difficulty with gait • Loss of manual dexterity • Incontinence
Inflammatory arthritis	• Morning stiffness • Swelling in multiple joints • Pain improved with activity but not rest
Atlantoaxial instability	• Rheumatoid arthritis • Down syndrome • Ankylosing spondylitis

- Screen for radiculopathy: Spurling test, shoulder abduction test, cervical compression, and cervical distraction tests
- Screen for myelopathy: plantar reflex (Babinski sign), Hoffman sign, tandem gait assessment
- Evaluation of related areas as indicated (e.g., shoulder joints)

7. **When are imaging studies important for evaluation of the cervical spine?**
Caution is necessary when deciding to order spinal imaging studies in patients with cervical pain syndromes. Degenerative changes involving the discs and facet joints are commonly observed in asymptomatic patients and may be unrelated to a specific patient's pain syndrome. In general, imaging studies are used to exclude serious conditions. An initial screening evaluation generally consists of plain radiographs. Patients who present with risk factors for cervical spine fracture or dislocation based on valid screening protocols (i.e., National Emergency X-Radiography Utilization Study [NEXUS] criteria, Canadian C-Spine Rule) should be evaluated with cervical computed tomography (CT). For other patients, magnetic resonance imaging (MRI) is the preferred initial imaging modality because it provides the most diagnostic information regarding a specific spinal region and does not involve ionizing radiation. Reasons to order an MRI include a clinical history and physical examination that suggest a serious spinal condition (i.e., tumors, infection, traumatic injury), positive neurologic signs or symptoms, or if evaluation of the spinal canal and/or nerve root canals is required prior to spinal injections or surgical procedures.

8. **How are common cervical disorders classified in patients who present for evaluation and treatment?**
Various criteria are helpful for stratifying patients and guiding treatment for common cervical spine conditions:
- Duration of symptoms: acute (<6 weeks); subacute (6 weeks to 3 months); chronic (>3 months)
- Pain pathophysiology: nociceptive pain, neuropathic pain, mixed nociceptive-neuropathic pain
- Presumed pain generator: soft tissue structures, zygapophyseal (facet) joint, cervical disc
- Clinical syndrome: neck pain, radiculopathy, degenerative cervical myelopathy (DCM)
- Location of dominant pain: neck (axial), arm (radicular), pain referred from nonspinal structures (e.g., shoulder joint)
- Neck Pain Task Force *Classification for Neck Pain and Associated Disorders*

9. **What is the Neck Pain Task Force** *Classification for Neck Pain and Associated Disorders?* **How does it guide evaluation and treatment for patients with cervical spine disorders?**
The Task Force on Neck Pain and Associated Disorders was designated by the Steering Committee of the Bone and Joint Decade 2000–2010 to systematically review literature on neck pain and associated disorders and to conduct original research projects as part of an initiative of the United Nations and the World Health Organization. The Neck Pain Task Force (NPTF) developed a four-grade severity classification system for use in the interpretation of scientific evidence and clinical decision making for cervical disorders (Table 13.2). Grade 1 and 2 patients present with neck dominant pain. Grade 3 patients present with arm dominant pain (radiculopathy). Grade 4 patients present with signs and symptoms due to major structural pathology which may manifest as neck pain, radiculopathy, or myelopathy.

Table 13.2 Classification of Neck Pain and Its Associated Disorders (NPTF Grades 1–4).

SEVERITY	CRITERIA	IMAGING	INTERVENTION
Grade 1	No signs or symptoms that suggest major structural pathology and no or minor interference with ADLs (cervical axial pain)	Not needed	Likely to respond to minimal interventions such as reassurance and self-care. Ongoing care likely not needed.
Grade 2	No signs or symptoms which suggest major structural pathology but major interference with ADLs is present (cervical axial pain)	Not needed initially	Provide pain relief and early activation/intervention directed toward preventing long-term disability.
Grade 3	No signs or symptoms of major structural pathology, but neurologic signs are present (i.e., radiculopathy)	May require imaging and further investigation	Monitor neurologic status and consider benefits versus risks of more invasive treatments.
Grade 4	Signs and symptoms of major structural pathology (i.e., fracture, myelopathy, neoplasm, infection, or systemic disease)	Prompt imaging and investigation	Prompt treatment is directed toward specific condition which is present.

ADLs, Activities of daily living.
Data from Guzman J, Haldeman S, Carroll LJ, et al. Clinical practice implications of the Bone and Joint Decade 2000–2010 Task Force on Neck Pain and Its Associated Disorders. Spine 2008;33(S4):S199–S213.

10. Compare and contrast the clinical presentation of patients with axial neck pain and cervical radicular pain.

Cervical axial pain is experienced in the region bound by the inferior occiput, the lateral margins of the neck, and the scapula. Cervical axial pain generally localizes to the posterior midline or paramidline, but may also be referred into the proximal upper extremities or anterior upper chest area. Axial neck pain may also be associated with headaches that involve the retro-orbital, suboccipital, and jawline regions. Referred pain arises from stimulation of nonneural structures of the neck, such as muscles, ligaments, intervertebral discs, and facet joints, and is termed *somatic pain*. Studies have outlined recognizable and specific pain patterns which are produced by stimulation of zygapophyseal joints and dorsal rami (Fig. 13.1A,B). Cervical axial pain tends to increase with activity and reduce with recumbency. Patients may complain of neck stiffness and decreased neck mobility.

Cervical radiculopathy presents with pain that is most intense in the upper arm below the deltoid insertion, and most commonly extends below the elbow to involve the thumbs or fingers of the hand according to the specific pattern of dorsal root ganglion and cervical nerve root involvement. Arm pain may be constant and aggravated by neck movement, coughing, or sneezing. Some combination of sensory loss, motor weakness, or impaired reflexes occurs in a segmental distribution (Fig. 13.2).

11. What are some recommendations for initial management of acute nonradiating cervical pain?

The clinician should first evaluate the patient to rule out major structural pathology. If there are no red flags suggesting serious pathology, the patient should be reassured that recovery is likely within 2–3 months. The patient should be encouraged to stay active and return to normal activities. A home exercise program, with stretching and strengthening and aerobic exercise, is initially recommended. Referral to physical therapy is considered based on patient preference, for patients with yellow flag symptoms or if symptoms persist despite initial self-treatment. Structured patient education combined with exercise, as well as multimodal care consisting of ROM exercise in combination with manipulation or mobilization, are additional nonoperative treatment options. It is recommended that nonoperative treatment of acute neck pain emphasizes patient education and active treatments over passive modalities. Nonnarcotic medications such as nonsteroidal antiinflammatory medications (NSAIDs) or short-term use of a nonbenzodiazepine muscle relaxant may be considered.

12. Describe the epidemiology, risk factors, and natural history of cervical pain in adults.

Self-reported neck pain is very common and is experienced by 30%–50% of the adult population annually. The source of neck pain is often unidentified. According to the NPTF, 50%–75% of patients with neck pain report neck pain 1–5 years later. The prevalence of neck pain peaks during middle age and is higher among women, who are more likely to experience persistent neck pain and less likely to experience pain resolution, compared with men.

Neck pain has a multifactorial etiology, including genetic factors, older age, female gender, physical activity participation, poor psychological health, tobacco use, prior history of neck or low back pain, and rear-end automobile accidents. The presence of cervical spinal degeneration on imaging studies is not considered a risk factor for neck pain.

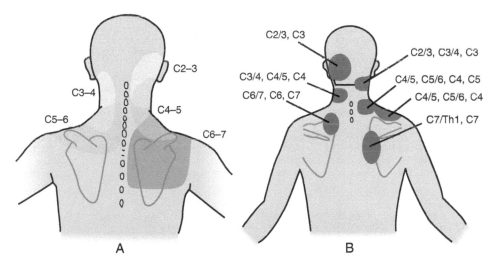

Fig. 13.1 Distribution of cervical pain (A) following cervical zygapophyseal joint injections, (B) following zygapophyseal joint injections from C2/3 through C7/Th1 which is blocked by denervation of the dorsal rami from C3 through C7. (From Sial KA, Simpouloa TT, Bajwa ZH, et al. Cervical facet syndrome. In: Walman SD, editor. Pain Management. 2nd ed. Philadelphia, PA: Saunders; 2011, pp. 516–521, Figs. 57.1 and 57.2.)

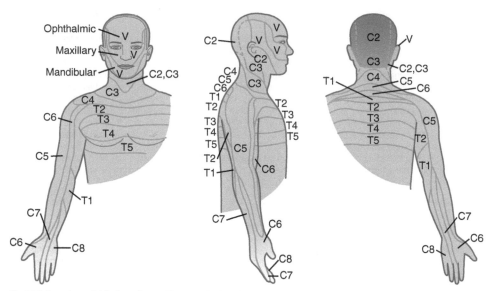

Fig. 13.2 Dermatome distributions of nerve fibers from C1 through T5 which transmit sensation to the head, neck, arm, forearm, hand, and thoracic areas. (From Cheng JS, Vasquez-Castellanos R, Wong C. Neck pain. In: Firestein GS, Budd R, Gabriel SE, et al., editors. Kelley and Firestein's Textbook of Rheumatology. 10th ed. Philadelphia, PA: Elsevier; 2017, pp. 654–668, Fig. 45.5.)

The natural history of neck pain in adults is favorable overall. However, there are notable rates of recurrent pain and chronicity. For patients with acute neck pain, recovery is rapid in the first 6–12 weeks and gradually slows with little recovery noted after 1 year. Up to 30% of patients with acute neck pain will develop chronic symptoms. Patients with chronic neck pain may experience a stable or fluctuating course with episodes of remission and exacerbation over time.

13. **Outline some recommended approaches for nonoperative treatment of chronic cervical pain.**
A clinician should reassess the patient for red flags (serious underlying conditions) and yellow flags (barriers to recovery). Treatment of chronic neck pain should address both the biomechanical issues and the psychosocial factors that contribute to pain and disability. Evidence-based treatment for chronic neck pain includes active rehabilitation therapy with supervised exercise. This may include stretching, strengthening with isometric and/or dynamic exercises, cervicothoracic stabilization, and aerobic conditioning. Multimodal care, which includes exercise in conjunction with manipulation or mobilization, is an additional treatment option. The potential benefits of cervical manipulation should be weighed against the risk of uncommon serious adverse events including nerve root injury, spinal cord injury, vascular injury (cervical artery dissection and stroke), or even death. Pharmacologic treatment options include NSAIDs or serotonin-norepinephrine reuptake inhibitors (SNRIs), such as duloxetine. Alternatively, a short course of a nonbenzodiazepine muscle relaxant may be considered. Opioid medications are not indicated for treatment of chronic musculoskeletal cervical pain. Alternative therapies supported by randomized controlled evidence include qigong (a holistic system of coordinated body posture and movement), and Iyengar yoga (emphasizes precision and alignment in all postures). Selected patients may benefit from cognitive behavioral therapy or a functional restoration program. For patients in whom zygapophyseal joint pain is considered, diagnosis is confirmed with nerve blocks performed by anesthetizing the medial branch nerves innervating the target facet joint(s). Anesthetic agents of varying duration of effect are used during two separate injection sessions. If the diagnosis is confirmed, percutaneous radiofrequency neurotomy to ablate the medial branch nerves innervating the target facet joint(s) is a treatment option. Although cervical disc degeneration is a cause of neck pain in some patients, distinguishing painful from nonpainful cervical discs remains challenging.

14. **Describe the epidemiology, risk factors, and natural history of cervical radiculopathy in adults.**
Cervical radiculopathy commonly results from dorsal root ganglion and nerve root compression due to cervical spondylosis (most common etiology) or from a herniated disc. The association of preceding trauma with cervical radiculopathy is low. In order of frequency, the C7 nerve root (2° to C6-C7 disc herniation) is most commonly involved, followed by the C6 nerve root (2° to C5-C6 disc herniation), and C8 nerve root (2° to C7-T1 disc herniation). A population-based study from Minnesota showed an annual incidence of cervical radiculopathy of 83.2 per 100,000 population (107.3 per 100,000 in men and 63.5 per 100,000 in women).

Some risk factors associated with cervical radiculopathy include manual jobs, lifting heavy objects, operation of vibrating equipment, frequent automobile travel, tobacco use, and coughing.

Studies have described a favorable history for patients with cervical radiculopathy. The majority of patients with cervical radiculopathy improve within several weeks. Longer term follow-up (2–19 years) has shown the majority of patients experience no, mild, or intermittent symptoms. Patients who experience progressive or persistent neurologic weakness, myelopathy, or intractable pain should be referred for surgical evaluation.

15. **Outline a nonoperative treatment plan for patients with cervical radiculopathy.**
    - Supervised active physical therapy
    - Use of ergonomic modifications and postural relieving positions
    - Medication: NSAIDs, SNRIs, anticonvulsants (conflicting evidence regarding efficacy), oral corticosteroids (often prescribed as a short-term agent despite lack of evidence regarding efficacy), opioids (not recommended as a first-line treatment, prescribe only for short period after failure of other pharmacologic and nonpharmacologic interventions)
    - Cervical epidural injections or selective nerve root blocks
    - Intermittent cervical traction
    - Soft cervical collar (short-term use only, <1–2 weeks; little evidence to support this practice)

16. **Describe the clinical presentation of patients with degenerative cervical myelopathy.**
    DCM is the most common cause of spinal cord dysfunction in adult patients. Age-related spinal column tissue degeneration leads to static spinal cord compression and, in some cases, repetitive dynamic injury secondary to spinal column hypermobility due to concomitant spinal instability. The first symptoms of DCM are often poor balance and lower extremity weakness with resultant gait dysfunction. Patients may also present with gradual weakness and numbness of the hands, and fine motor coordination deficits ("clumsy hands"). Some patients may complain of neck pain, although the condition is often painless. Neck flexion may produce a shock-like sensation involving the trunk and upper extremities (Lhermitte phenomenon). Bowel and bladder function may be affected in later stages of the disease. Progressive DCM may eventually result in cord ischemia and paralysis as a consequence of cervical cord compression.

17. **What is the natural history of degenerative cervical myelopathy?**
    DCM is a disease with an often unpredictable course. The natural history of DCM is characterized by stepwise deterioration in neurologic function with variable intervals of clinical stability. Current literature shows that more than half of patients with DCM will deteriorate over a follow-up period of 3 to 6 years based on assessment of modified Japanese Orthopedic Association (mJOA) scores. The severity of DCM is graded objectively using the mJOA assessment scale, an investigator administered tool that provides scores for upper extremity motor function (0–5), lower extremity motor function (0–7), sensation (0–3), and bladder function (0–3), which are combined in a composite score. Severity of myelopathy is graded as mild ($\geq$15 points), moderate (12–14 points) or severe (<12 points).

18. **Outline the treatment plan for patients with degenerative cervical myelopathy.**
    Nonsurgical management does not alter the natural history of the disease. Surgical intervention is the only treatment that can arrest the progression of DCM and is recommended for patients with moderate or severe DCM. Nonsurgical management may be considered for patients with mild myelopathy. However, it is unclear which types of nonoperative treatment provide benefit when compared with the natural history of DCM. Operative treatment is indicated for mild DCM with neurologic deterioration or mild DCM that fails to improve.
    Nonsurgical management for mild DCM may include:
    - Immobilization in a cervical collar
    - Isometric neck exercises
    - Strengthening exercises of upper and lower extremities
    - Analgesic medications
    - Passive modalities
    - Balance exercises
    - Assistive devices (cane, walker) to minimize risk of falls
    - Education and instructions to avoid hyperextension of the cervical spine, for example, in high-risk environments and activities:
        - Adjust computer screen and TV height.
        - Avoid using high shelves.
        - Avoid sports activities with prolonged neck hyperextension, such as breaststroke swimming.
        - During dental work, the dentist should be informed about neck ROM restrictions and the need to avoid hyperextension postures.

19. **Outline some of the benefits and risks of commonly recommended nonoperative treatments for degenerative spinal disorders involving the cervical spine.**
    See Table 13.3.

Table 13.3 Nonoperative Treatments for Cervical Degenerative Disorders.

TREATMENT	BENEFITS	RISKS
Education and reassurance	Effective when included as a component of an active management program	Not effective as an isolated treatment
Home exercise program	Specific isometric and range-of-motion exercises may provide similar benefits as a supervised program	Potential for poor patient compliance
Supervised exercise and physical therapy	Combined programs including strengthening, range of motion, flexibility, aerobic conditioning, and ergonomic counseling are effective for treatment for axial neck pain	Poor patient participation and noncompliance may limit potential benefits
Cervical manipulation and mobilization	Positive benefit for acute and subacute neck pain	Limited evidence to support long-term improvement versus other treatments; potential for rare complications including myelopathy, spinal cord injury, and vascular injury.
Cognitive behavioral therapy	Benefit shown in treatment of chronic whiplash disorder and subacute neck pain	Chronic neck pain improvement may be statistically significant but not always clinically meaningful
Acupuncture	Recommended by various clinical practice guidelines	Data does not clearly demonstrate effectiveness, potential for adverse events
Massage therapy	Provides immediate and short-term relief of pain and tenderness	Long-term effects of treatment remain undefined
Active CAM therapies	Supervised yoga (Iyengar) and qigong shown to provide clinically important improvement chronic neck pain	Risk of injury if not correctly practiced
TENS	Noninvasive and nonpharmacologic treatment based on gate control theory of pain	Limited data to support positive benefit compared to placebo
Passive modalities	Appropriate as an adjunct to an active therapy program; cooling may relieve pain and spasm; heat may provide benefit when attempting to regain motion; ultrasound may increase tissue blood flow and healing	Limited evidence of long-term clinically important benefits; may harm patients by exacerbating fear and anxiety about being physically active when in pain
Neck collar	Immobilization may decrease acute inflammation and muscle spasm	Unproven benefit; muscle atrophy and dependence may result from prolonged use
Cervical traction	Benefit in treatment of radiculopathy when used in combination with exercise program; positioning neck in flexion, may relieve foraminal narrowing	Positioning neck in extension may worsen foraminal narrowing; avoid in patients with myelopathy
NSAIDs	Effective for decreasing inflammation and acute neck pain	Gastrointestinal side effects, acute kidney injury, cardiovascular risks with COX-2 inhibitors

Table 13.3 Nonoperative Treatments for Cervical Degenerative Disorders. *(Continued)*

TREATMENT	BENEFITS	RISKS
Antidepressants (SNRI)	Duloxetine provides an analgesic effect independent of its effect on depression, effective for neuropathic pain	Adverse effects include nausea, insomnia, fatigue, dry mouth, hepatotoxicity
Anticonvulsants (gabapentinoids)	Conflicting low level evidence to support use in axial radiating pain	Adverse effects include fatigue, dizziness, somnolence, ataxia, and concentration difficulty
Muscle relaxants (nonbenzodiazepine)	Benefit for acute or exacerbation of acute, nonradiating pain	Not recommended for chronic pain; adverse effects include sedation, fatigue, abuse potential
Opioids	Rapid and reliable relief of acute pain but not indicated for chronic musculoskeletal cervical pain	Constipation, sedation, depression, potential for misuse, overdose, opioid use disorder; lack of evidence for sustained pain relief or functional improvement with long-term use for noncancer pain
Oral corticosteroids	Low level evidence is available to support use for acute radicular pain	Avascular necrosis, elevated blood glucose, insomnia, unproven long-term benefit
Cervical steroid injections	Benefit for acute radiating pain due to antiinflammatory effect and interruption of nociceptive input	Rare complications include dural puncture, meningitis, epidural abscess, epidural hematoma, adrenal suppression, paralysis
Radiofrequency rhizotomy	Provides short-term relief of facet-mediated cervical pain	Repeat procedures may be required; risks include temporary numbness, pain, bruising hematoma, or infection at procedure site

CAM, Complementary and alternative medicine; *NSAID,* nonsteroidal antiinflammatory medication; *SNRI,* serotonin-norepinephrine reuptake inhibitor; *TENS,* transcutaneous electrical nerve stimulation.

20. What is a *whiplash injury*? How is this condition treated?

Whiplash injury is a term used to describe an acute cervical sprain or strain caused by an acceleration and deceleration motion without direct application of force to the head or neck. Rear-end automobile collisions are the most common injury mechanism, although whiplash injury may result due to head-on or side-impact collisions.

Whiplash may result in injury to the cervical facet joints, cervical musculature (trapezius, levator scapulae, scalene, sternocleidomastoid, and paraspinal muscles), and cervical disc. Common symptoms include neck pain and headaches. Patients may variably report upper limb paresthesias, shoulder girdle pain, and weakness. Less common symptoms may include dizziness, fatigue, malaise, dizziness, and tinnitus. Although the symptoms of nonradicular neck and shoulder pain are often self-limiting (2–4 months), some patients continue to experience chronic symptoms.

Nonoperative treatment options include cervical traction, isometric neck exercises, a soft cervical collar, analgesic medications, passive modalities (heat, ice, ultrasound), and massage. Neurologic symptoms or intractable pain symptoms that are not responsive to treatment indicate the need for further evaluation. Patients with persistent pain may have annular tears, coexisting degenerative joint and disc pathology, nerve root entrapment, spinal stenosis, or myelopathy. In patients with chronic symptoms, diagnostic medial branch blocks may be used to identify facet joint-mediated pain, which may benefit from percutaneous radiofrequency neurotomy. Clinicians must be aware of the role of psychosocial factors, including litigation, when evaluating and treating patients with chronic whiplash symptoms.

21. What are cervicogenic headaches?

The *International Classification of Headache Disorders* divides headaches into two main categories: primary headaches (e.g., migraine, cluster and tension headaches, and other types) and secondary headaches (multiple etiologies). Cervicogenic headaches are defined as pain referred to the head from a source in the cervical spine and are classified as secondary headaches. Cervicogenic headaches are usually, but not invariably, accompanied by neck pain. The prevalence of cervicogenic headaches ranges from 0.4% to 2.5% in the general population, up to 17.5% in patients with severe headaches, and exceeds 50% in patients with headaches associated with whiplash injuries. Women are more commonly affected than men. The underlying mechanism responsible for cervicogenic headaches is attributed to the convergence of nociceptive afferents from the upper three cervical spinal nerves and the trigeminal nerve (CN V) in the trigeminocervical nucleus. This convergence provides an explanation for how pain from the upper cervical region is simultaneously referred to regions of the head innervated by cervical nerves (occipital and auricular regions), as well as regions innervated by the trigeminal nerve (parietal, frontal, and orbital). The C2–C3 zygapophyseal joints are considered the most common source of cervicogenic headaches, but cervicogenic headaches may also originate from facet joints or intervertebral discs at other spinal levels.

Clinical criteria used to diagnose cervicogenic headaches include:
- Unilateral dominant headaches (zygapophyseal source) or bilateral headache (discogenic source)
- Symptoms exacerbated by neck movement or posture
- Pain episodes of varying duration or continuous pain with fluctuating intensity
- Moderate, nonexcruciating pain, usually nonthrobbing in nature
- Pain starts in the neck and spreads to the oculo-frontotemporal area
- Related events during a headache attack may include autonomic symptoms, nausea, dizziness, photophobia, and blurred vision in the ipsilateral eye

Cervicogenic headaches arising from a zygapophyseal source may be diagnosed with nerve blocks or intraarticular blocks. The C1–C2 joint is anesthetized with intraarticular blocks. The C2–C3 zygapophyseal joint is blocked by anesthetizing the third occipital nerve where it crosses the joint and provides articular branches. The C3–C4 joint is blocked by anesthetizing the medial branches of the C3 and C4 dorsal rami or with intraarticular blocks. A discogenic source may be evaluated with cervical discography, but use of this test is controversial.

Treatment is directed toward the identified painful structure. Treatment options include medication, exercise, spinal manipulation, mobilization, and steroid injections. Radiofrequency neurotomy may be considered if a zygapophyseal source has been identified with injections. In patients with cervical radiculopathy or myelopathy (C3–C7) and concomitant headaches, evidence supports the role of both anterior cervical fusion and cervical total disc arthroplasty in providing relief of symptoms.

It is important to recognize the differential diagnosis of cervicogenic headaches includes several serious disorders. Cervical artery dissection involving the carotid or vertebral arteries may initially present with headache, with or without neck pain, and may have a gradual or sudden onset. Failure to recognize this condition may be fatal if the patient is misdiagnosed with a cervicogenic headache and treated with cervical manipulation. Posterior cranial fossa tumors may present as headaches associated with imbalance, nausea, ataxia, and occasionally, neck pain. Meningitis may present as neck stiffness, fever, headache, and/or nausea.

22. How can patients be screened in the outpatient setting to assess the need for cervical spine radiographs if they report a history of recent blunt cervical trauma?
In patients who present for outpatient evaluation for acute neck pain, initial assessment may reveal a history of recent blunt cervical trauma. Screening with the Canadian C-Spine Rules, initially developed for use in the Emergency Room (ER), may be used for screening in the outpatient setting to assess the need for radiographs to rule out a clinically important cervical injury (fracture, dislocation, or ligamentous instability). Assessment is performed using three questions:
- *Question 1: Are there any high-risk factors that mandate diagnostic imaging such as age ≥65 years, a dangerous injury mechanism, or paresthesias in the extremities?*
  If yes, diagnostic imaging is required. If no, then go to question 2.
- *Question 2: Are there any low-risk factors which allow safe assessment of ROM?*
  Examples of low-risk factors include: simple rear-end motor vehicle collision, sitting position in the ER, ambulatory at any time after injury, delayed onset of neck pain, absence of midline cervical spine tenderness.
  If no, diagnostic imaging is required. If yes, go to question 3.
- *Question 3: Is the patient able to actively rotate their neck 45° to the right and left?*
  If no, diagnostic imaging is required. If yes, diagnostic imaging is not needed.

The above rules have been found to be highly sensitive and reliable, and may be used to reassure the patient that their acute neck pain is not due to a serious injury. The Canadian C-Spine Rules are not applicable in specific circumstances including in patients with a known vertebral disease (prior cervical spine surgery, rheumatoid arthritis, ankylosing spondylitis, cervical spinal stenosis), nontraumatic injuries, acute paralysis, and age <16 years.

23. Can fibromyalgia present as neck and/or upper extremity pain?
Yes. In its early stages, fibromyalgia may present as pain limited to the cervical region or upper extremities. However, fibromyalgia may be distinguished from axial neck pain or radiculopathy by the diffuse nature of its clinical presentation as the condition evolves and progresses. Fibromyalgia is a chronic, widespread musculoskeletal pain syndrome of uncertain etiology. It is a noninflammatory, nonautoimmune central afferent processing disorder, which leads to a diffuse pain syndrome. Core symptoms include multifocal pain, fatigue, stiffness, sleep disturbance, cognitive difficulties, paresthesias, and psychologic distress. Physical examination of patients with

fibromyalgia shows widely distributed tender points above and below the waist and on both sides of the body. Treatment options include physical therapy, medication (duloxetine, milnacipran, pregabalin), cognitive behavioral therapy, and multidisciplinary care.

KEY POINTS

- Medical history and physical examination provide important information that guides nonoperative treatment based on whether the diagnosis is axial cervical pain, radiculopathy, degenerative cervical myelopathy, or a serious structural disorder involving the cervical spine.
- Although the natural history of acute axial cervical pain in adults is favorable, there is a notable rate of recurrent pain and chronicity.
- Treatment of chronic neck pain should address both the biomechanical issues and the psychosocial factors that contribute to the patient's pain and disability.
- The natural history of cervical radiculopathy is favorable and the majority of patients experience improvement over time regardless of the specific type of treatment provided.
- Surgical intervention is the only treatment that can arrest the progression of degenerative cervical myelopathy. Nonsurgical management is an option for patients with mild myelopathy but surgery is recommended for patients with moderate or severe myelopathy.

Websites
1. Clinically Organized Relevant Exam (CORE) Neck Tool and Headache Navigator:
   https://cep.health/clinical-products/core-neck-tool-and-headache-navigator/
2. Neck Pain Care Process Model, Intermountain Healthcare:
   https://intermountainhealthcare.org/ext/Dcmnt?ncid=526837557
3. Spine Health: A pain in the neck:
   https://www.cbi.ca/documents/12741/633624/JCCC_neck_pain.pdf/83aeb449-3abd-4952-b7bd-b138f21a1c3a
4. Quality-based pathway clinical handbook for nonemergent integrated spine care:
   http://www.health.gov.on.ca/en/pro/programs/ecfa/docs/hb_spine.pdf

BIBLIOGRAPHY

1. Badhiwala, J. H., & Wilson, J. R. (2018). The natural history of degenerative cervical myelopathy. *Neurosurgery Clinics of North America, 29,* 21–32.
2. Bogduk, N., & Govind, J. (2009). Cervicogenic headache: An assessment of the evidence on clinical diagnosis, invasive tests, and treatment. *Lancet Neurology, 10,* 959–968.
3. Blanpied, P. R., Gross, A. R., Elliott, J. M., Devaney, L. L., Clewley, D., Walton, D. M., et al. (2017). Neck pain: Revision 2017. Clinical practice guidelines linked to the International Classification of Functioning, Disability and Health. Orthopaedic Section of the American Physical Therapy Association. *Journal of Orthopaedic and Sports Physical Therapy, 47,* 1–83.
4. Guzman, J., Haldeman, S., Carroll, L. J., Carragee, E. J., Hurwitz, E. L., Peloso, P., et al. Clinical practice implications of the Bone and Joint Decade 2000–2010. Task Force on Neck Pain and Its Associated Disorders. *Spine, 33*(Suppl. 4), S199–S213.
5. Hurwitz, E. L., Carragee, E. J., van der Velde, G., Carroll, L. J., Nordin, M., Guzman, J., et al. (2008). Treatment of neck pain: Noninvasive interventions. Results of the Bone and Joint Decade 2000–2010 Task Force on Neck Pain and Its Associated Disorders. *Spine, 33,* S123–S52.
6. Iyer, S., & Kim, H. J. (2016). Cervical radiculopathy. *Current Reviews in Musculoskeletal Medicine, 9,* 272–280.
7. Southerst, D., Nordin, M. C., Côté, P., Shearer, H. M., Varatharajan, S., Yu, H., et al. (2016). Is exercise effective for the management of neck pain and associated disorders or whiplash-associated disorders? A systematic review by the Ontario Protocol for Traffic Injury Management (OPTIMa) Collaboration. *The Spine Journal, 16,* 1503–1523.
8. Stiell, I. G., Wells, G. A., Vandemheen, K. L., Clement, C. M., Lesiuk, H., De Maio, V. J., et al. (2001). The Canadian C-spine rule for radiography in alert and stable trauma patients. *JAMA, 285,* 1841–1845.

CHAPTER 14

THORACIC AND LUMBAR SPINAL DISORDERS: NONSURGICAL MANAGEMENT STRATEGIES

Vincent J. Devlin, MD

THORACIC SPINE

1. What etiologies are included in the differential diagnosis of patients who present for initial assessment and management of symptoms attributed to the thoracic spine in an outpatient setting?

Diagnosis of patients referred for evaluation of thoracic spine conditions is not always straightforward. Thoracic spine pain may arise from a variety of sources including thoracic and cervical spinal structures, chest wall structures, as well as referral from cardiopulmonary, gastrointestinal, and miscellaneous causes. Although musculoskeletal thoracic and chest wall pain are the most common etiologies presented at outpatient spine consultations, less common etiologies must also be considered to avoid delayed diagnosis of serious or life-threatening conditions. Etiologies to consider in the differential diagnosis of patients referred for evaluation include:

Thoracic pain of spinal origin
- Musculoskeletal thoracic spine pain (sprain, strain)
- Thoracic spine degeneration and (disc degeneration, disc herniation, stenosis, facet joint degeneration)
- Scheuermann disease
- Ankylosing spondylitis
- Diffuse idiopathic skeletal hyperostosis (DISH)
- Spinal deformities
- Spinal neoplasm
- Spinal infection
- Spinal fractures (osteoporotic, pathologic, traumatic)
- Referred pain from the cervical spinal region
- Postural disorders

Thoracic pain of chest wall origin
- Referred pain from costovertebral, sternocostal, or costochondral joints or thoracic cage musculature

Thoracic pain referred from nonspinal structures
- Cardiovascular-related pain: myocardial ischemia, myocardial infarction, aortic aneurysm, valvular disease
- Pulmonary-related pain: bronchitis, lung diseases, pneumothorax, pulmonary embolism, Pancoast tumor
- Gastrointestinal-related pain: esophageal disorders, peptic ulcer disease, reflux, pancreatitis
- Breast-related pain: macromastia

Postsurgical or iatrogenic thoracic pain
- Postthoracotomy pain
- Poststernotomy pain
- Miscellaneous postprocedural pain (i.e., thoracostomy tube placement)

Miscellaneous causes of thoracic pain
- Fibromyalgia
- Diabetic thoracic radiculopathy
- Postherpetic neuralgia
- Thoracic outlet syndrome
- Thoracic pain in association with motor vehicle accidents

2. What nonoperative treatments are recommended for musculoskeletal thoracic pain?

Musculoskeletal thoracic *pain* occurs in the absence of significant pathologies such as infection, neoplasm, metastatic disease, osteoporosis, inflammatory arthropathies, fracture, or pain referred from abdominal or pelvic viscera. Thoracic strain or sprain refers to acute or subacute pain caused by injury to soft tissue structures including muscles, ligaments, tendons, and fascia, in an otherwise normal spine. *Sprain* is defined as an injury to ligament fibers without total rupture. *Strain* is defined as an injury that affects muscles or tendons. Evidence guiding nonoperative treatment of musculoskeletal thoracic pain is limited. Active interventions, including stretching, postural, strengthening, and stabilization exercises, are the most commonly recommended treatments.

Passive interventions, including mobilization, soft tissue massage, acupuncture, and electrotherapy, are commonly prescribed, but supporting evidence is limited. A multimodal program of care with manual therapy, soft tissue therapy, exercises, heat/ice, and education is recommended by many providers. A limited course of nonsteroidal antiinflammatory medication (NSAIDs) or acetaminophen may provide benefit.

3. **What are some important considerations in the evaluation and treatment of thoracic pain in patients with radicular symptoms?**
Thoracic radiculopathy is an uncommon spinal disorder. The most common etiologies of thoracic radiculopathy are diabetes and thoracic disc pathology. Other less common causes include primary spine tumors, metastatic spine tumors, scoliosis, and herpes zoster. Patients typically present with band-like chest or abdominal wall pain. A T1 radiculopathy is challenging to distinguish from a C8 radiculopathy, and characteristics include diminished axillary sensation, motor deficits of the intrinsic muscles of the hand, and Horner syndrome. Electrodiagnostic testing can aid in the diagnosis of radiculopathy.

Thoracic disc herniation are documented on MRI in up to 40% of asymptomatic individuals. The number of patients with objective neurologic findings due to thoracic disc herniation is estimated as 1 per million annually. Thoracic disc herniations occur most commonly in the lower third of the thoracic spine (T9–T10 through T12–L1), less commonly in the middle third (T5–T6 through T8–T9), and least commonly in the upper thoracic region (T1–T2 through T4–T5).

Thoracic disc herniations may present with axial spine pain, thoracic radiculopathy, thoracic myelopathy, or with a mixed presentation. Patients with thoracic axial pain, radiculopathy, or mild myelopathy are appropriate for initial nonoperative treatment. Nonsurgical treatment options include postural, strengthening, and stabilization exercises, medication (NSAIDs, gabapentinoids), transcutaneous electrical nerve stimulation (TENS) and other modalities, and transforaminal injections. Recognition of patients with myelopathy is important; severe or progressive myelopathy requires prompt evaluation for surgical treatment.

LUMBAR SPINE

4. **What etiologies are included in the differential diagnosis of patients who present for initial assessment and management of symptoms attributed to the lumbar spine in an outpatient setting?**
The most common reason for referral for outpatient evaluation of the lumbar spine is axial low back pain. Conditions to consider in the differential diagnosis include:
- Lumbar strain or lumbar sprain
- Discogenic low back pain
- Zygapophyseal joint pain
- Radiculopathy due to a herniated lumbar disc
- Lumbar spinal stenosis
- Lumbar spondylolysis
- Lumbar spondylolisthesis
- Osteoporotic compression fracture
- Scoliosis
- Spine infections: discitis, osteomyelitis
- Spine tumors: metastatic, primary
- Disorders involving the hip joint
- Sacroiliac joint pain
- Rheumatologic disorders: rheumatoid arthritis, ankylosing spondylitis, fibromyalgia
- Visceral disorders presenting with referred pain: pyelonephritis, pancreatitis, renal stones
- Vascular disorders: peripheral vascular disease, aortic aneurysm

5. **For patients who present with a complaint attributed to the lumbar spine, what are some important areas to investigate in relation to the patient's history?**
- Is this the first episode or a recurrent problem?
- Was there a specific injury (i.e., motor vehicle injury, work-related injury, sport-related injury, or fall from a height)?
- What factors increase and decrease symptoms?
- What is the pattern of pain over a 24-hour period? Is pain intermittent or constant?
- Is the most intense and bothersome pain localized to the low back and surrounding areas or to one or both legs?
- Is there focal weakness or numbness in the lower extremities?
- Are there new bowel or bladder symptoms?
- Is morning stiffness present?
- Are any red-flag symptoms present?
- Are any yellow-flag symptoms present?
- Consider use of a self-assessment questionnaire to evaluate pain (i.e., Visual Analog Pain Scale [VAS], Numerical Rating Scale [NRS])

- Consider use of a validated scale to measure level of disability and function (Oswestry Disability Index [ODI], Roland-Morris Disability Questionnaire [RMDQ], or Patient Reported Outcomes Measurement Information System [PROMIS])
- Consider use of a screening tool to identify patients with acute low back pain at risk of poor outcomes and to stratify patients for appropriate level and intensity of future treatment (i.e., Keele Subgrouping for Targeted Treatment [STarT] Screening Tool)

6. **What is the difference between red flags and yellow flags in the context of evaluation of low back pain symptoms?**
   Red flags are risk factors that suggest significant or potentially life-threatening pathologies associated with low back pain. Examples of red flag conditions are spine fractures, neurologic emergencies such as cauda equina syndrome (CES), spinal infections, and spinal tumors. Red flag conditions are rare and are estimated to occur in less than 5% of patients. **Yellow flags** are factors that are used to identify psychosocial barriers, which place patients at risk of developing chronicity, disability, and poor outcomes. Examples include fear and avoidance of activity or movement, a belief that lumbar pain is harmful or disabling, depression, and an expectation that passive treatment without active participation in treatment will resolve back pain. Patients who are identified as high risk can potentially benefit from more intensive nonsurgical management, with a greater emphasis on return to activity and focus on functional recovery.

7. **What are the key elements to include in the physical examination of a patient referred for initial evaluation for lumbar pain with or without leg pain?**
   - Observation: assess gait, balance, lumbar posture, waistline or trunk asymmetry
   - Palpation: assess for lumbar tender points
   - Range of motion: lumbar flexion, extension, rotation, side bending
   - Neurologic examination
     - Sensory, motor, reflex function
     - Provocative maneuvers to assess for radiculopathy when pain involves the lower extremities (straight-leg raise tests, femoral nerve stretch test)
     - Screen for myelopathy: plantar reflex (Babinski sign), tandem gait
   - Evaluation of related areas (e.g., hip joints, sacroiliac joints)
   - Peripheral vascular exam (assess dorsalis pedis and posterior tibial pulses)
   - Waddell signs (superficial tenderness, simulation, distraction, regionalization, and overreaction)

8. **What are some indications for obtaining imaging studies and laboratory tests in the evaluation of a lumbar spine complaint?**
   Caution is necessary when considering spinal imaging studies in patients with lumbar pain syndromes as positive imaging findings of spinal degeneration are commonly observed in asymptomatic patients and may be unrelated to a specific patient's pain syndrome. An initial screening evaluation generally consists of plain radiographs. Magnetic resonance imaging (MRI) is the preferred initial advanced imaging modality because it provides the greatest amount of diagnostic information regarding a specific spinal region and does not involve ionizing radiation. Some reasons to order an MRI include a clinical history and physical examination that suggest a serious spinal condition (i.e., tumor, infection, traumatic injury), if positive neurologic findings are detected, or when preprocedural evaluation of the spinal canal and/or nerve root canals is required prior to spinal injections or surgical procedures. Laboratory tests including complete blood count (CBC), erythrocyte sedimentation rate (ESR), and C-reactive protein (CRP) are appropriate when spinal infection or tumors are suspected.

9. **What are some ways to classify common lumbar disorders which present for evaluation and treatment?**
   No universally accepted classification exists for lumbar disorders. Some factors which are used to stratify patients and guide treatment include:
   - Duration of symptoms: acute (<6 weeks); subacute (6 weeks to 3 months); chronic (>3 months)
   - Level of disability and function (ODI, RMDQ)
   - Location of dominant symptoms (low back pain vs. leg pain)
   - Etiology: lumbar strain or sprain, discogenic pain, facet joint pain, radiculopathy secondary to lumbar disc herniation, spinal stenosis, pain secondary to nonspinal conditions

10. **Describe how a patient referred for initial evaluation of an acute lumbar spine condition may be classified into one of four clinical syndromes as a guide to future stratified treatment.**
    A patient may be classified into one of four clinical syndromes (1) based on pattern recognition without the need for imaging studies or identification of a specific pain generator. The **medical history** guides classification:
    - **Is the pain worse in the back or leg?**
      Note: Many patients will report that they experience both back and leg pain. Back-dominant pain may be experienced in the back, greater trochanteric region, or groin region, and is worsened with activity and

certain positions. Leg-dominant pain is located below the gluteal fold, and may involve the thigh, leg, or foot.

- **Is the pain constant or intermittent?**
- **What movements or postures aggravate and relieve the pain (i.e., flexion vs. extension)?**
  Physical examination is used to confirm the medical history and evaluate neurologic status.
  Four clinical syndromes are identified:
  Pattern 1: Back-dominant pain and always aggravated with flexion.
  Note: Pain may be constant or intermittent. Two subtypes are identified: fast responders and slow responders. **Fast responders** have a clear directional preference with relief in extension, while **slow responders** have pain with movement in both directions. Pain origin in pattern 1 is most likely discogenic.
  Pattern 2: Back-dominant pain. Aggravated by extension and never increases with flexion.
  Pain is always intermittent. Pain origin in pattern 2 is most likely related to the posterior spinal elements.
  Pattern 3: Constant leg-dominant pain. Pattern 3 corresponds to sciatica.
  Pattern 4: Intermittent leg-dominant pain. Pattern 4 corresponds to neurogenic claudication.
  Patients who do not fit into one of the four patterns or who do not respond to initial treatment are considered for additional evaluation to rule out an alternate condition responsible for persistent symptoms.

11. What are some recommendations for initial management of acute back-dominant pain?
   Patients are provided with education and reassurance. In the days following pain onset, cold packs may provide relief of acute pain, and may be followed by use of alternate heat and/or cold depending on patient preference. NSAIDs or a short-term course of a muscle relaxant may be prescribed. Patients should be advised to stay active and continue usual activities as pain permits, including work. For pattern 1 patients with a clear directional prefer-ence, prone-lying passive extension exercises are advised. For pattern 1 patients without a directional preference, treatment begins with short rest periods in the position that provides maximal pain control and progresses to movements in the least painful direction. For pattern 2 patients, recommendations include sitting in a chair and slumping forward to lower the torso between the knees, followed by use of the arms to raise the upper body, which unloads the trunk muscles.

12. How is the Keele STarT Screening Tool used to stratify patients with acute low-back pain into low-, medium-, and high-risk groups regarding risk for ongoing disability?
   The Keele STarT Screening Tool (https://www.keele.ac.uk/sbst/startbacktool/) is a nine-item tool used to identify patients at low, moderate, or high risk for development of chronic, disabling, low back pain. Items focus on radiating leg pain, pain elsewhere (neck, shoulder), walking ability, dressing ability, fear of activity, anxiety, catastrophizing, depressed mood, and bothersomeness of pain. The total score (questions 1–9) identifies low risk versus moderate/high risk, and a distress subscale score (questions 5–9) discriminates between moderate and high risk.
   Low-risk patients are likely to improve with reassurance, education, self-management, and a prescription for NSAIDs. Some low-risk patients may benefit from referral for a one-time visit with a physical therapist.
   Medium-risk patients receive the same treatments as low-risk patients, and a course of physical therapy, which includes manual therapy and specific exercises.
   High-risk patients receive all of the treatments recommended for low- and medium-risk patients, including phys-ical therapy, using a combined physical and cognitive-behavioral approach. Mental health screening may iden-tify psychosocial barriers to recovery such as depression, anxiety/stress disorders, mood disorders, sleep dis-turbance, personal or family history of abuse or trauma, substance abuse, or general impairment.

13. What is the natural history of acute low back pain?
   Many patients with a new episode of low back pain recover by 6–12 weeks. However, pain recurrences are com-mon and some patients fail to improve, developing chronic disabling pain. Up to two-thirds of patients will report some pain at 3 months. Up to one-third of patients will experience a recurrence of low back pain within 1 year of recovering from previous low back pain. Factors considered to increase the risk of development of persistent, disabling, low back pain include initial high pain intensity, psychological distress, and concomitant pain at multiple body sites.

14. What are some recommendations for initial management of constant leg-dominant pain consistent with a diagnosis of sciatica?
   Management of an acute episode of sciatica focuses on identifying positions of comfort that result in decreased leg pain. Lying supine with the lower legs on a chair (Z-position) or side-lying are suggested, but alternative po-sitions may be effective. First-line medications prescribed to decrease pain intensity are NSAIDs. The acute pain phase resolves in many patients over period of 4–6 weeks as patients are able to become more mobile and gradually return to daily activities. Referral to physical therapy for instruction in a home exercise program or supervised exercise program is an option. Patients who continue to experience severe radicular pain after initial nonoperative treatment may benefit from epidural steroid injections. Patients who present with or develop symp-toms and physical examination findings consistent with CES or a progressive neurologic deficit require urgent evaluation with MRI and surgical consultation.

15. **What is the natural history of an acute lumbar disc herniation?**
    The natural history of an acute lumbar disc herniation is quite favorable. Gradual improvement in symptoms over several weeks is noted in the majority of patients. Comparison of nonsurgical and surgical treatment has shown that surgically treated patients recover more quickly from sciatic pain symptoms, report better long-term functional status, and higher satisfaction. Both nonsurgical and surgical treatments are associated with clinically significant improvement over time and the differences between treatment groups narrows over time.

16. **What is cauda equina syndrome?**
    CES develops when the nerve roots in the central lumbar spinal canal area compress leading to disruption of sensory and motor function to the lower extremities and bladder. One of the most common causes of CES is a massive lumbar disc herniation. Clinical features that may indicate CES include severe low back pain, motor weakness, sensory loss or pain in one or, more commonly, both legs, bilateral lower extremity pain with single leg straight-leg raising, recent onset of bowel or bladder dysfunction, and sensory abnormalities involving the bladder or rectum. Once the diagnosis is confirmed with imaging studies, prompt surgical decompression is indicated.

17. **What are some recommendations for initial management of neurogenic claudication?**
    Symptoms of neurogenic claudication are generally relieved with sitting in a forward-flexed posture. It is important to distinguish neurogenic claudication from vascular claudication, which is unrelieved with positional change. Nonoperative treatments for neurogenic claudication secondary to lumbar spinal stenosis include education, active physical therapy, transfer and gait training, manual therapy, and NSAIDs. Epidural injections are frequently performed but there is limited evidence to support this practice. For patients with symptoms of neurogenic claudication which limit function, surgical treatment has been demonstrated to provide substantially greater improvement in pain and function compared with continued nonoperative treatment.

18. **What is the natural history of symptomatic lumbar spinal stenosis?**
    The natural history of symptomatic lumbar spinal stenosis is favorable in approximately 50% of patients, regardless of initial or subsequent treatment. Significant deterioration in symptoms with nonsurgical treatment is uncommon. Surgery has been shown to be more effective than nonoperative management in patients with symptomatic lumbar spinal stenosis, as well as degenerative spondylolisthesis associated with spinal stenosis in short- to medium-term follow-up (2–4 years). At long-term follow-up (8–10 years), certain outcome parameters converged between operative and nonoperative treatment groups, but the overall benefit of surgical treatment appeared to be maintained.

19. **Compare and contrast current guidelines for treatment of acute and subacute low back pain with guidelines for treatment of chronic low back pain.**
    Patients with chronic low back pain are more challenging to treat than those with acute or subacute low back pain and require different treatment approaches (Table 14.1). Multiple factors may contribute to development of chronic low back pain including biophysical, psychological, social, and genetic factors. Generalized treatment recommendations (2) for chronic low back pain include:
    • A graded activity or exercise program directed toward improvement in function
    • Psychologic therapies such as cognitive behavioral therapy and mindfulness-based stress reduction
    • Adjunctive interventions including tai chi, yoga, acupuncture, and manipulation as second-line treatment options
    • Pharmacologic treatment is recommended only following inadequate response to nonpharmacologic therapy (avoid use of paracetamol and routine use of opioids)
    • Recommended interventional therapies are limited to epidural steroid injections for severe radicular pain (epidural or facet injections are not recommended for low back pain)
    • Surgical spinal decompression is recommended for radicular pain due to disc herniation or spinal stenosis refractory to nonsurgical management
    • Spinal fusion surgery or disc replacement outcomes are marginally greater than results of multidisciplinary rehabilitation and surgery is associated with a greater risk of adverse events

20. **What is the McKenzie exercise approach? How and when is it applied?**
    The McKenzie method includes an assessment and intervention component and is commonly referred to as a mechanical diagnosis and therapy (MDT). The McKenzie exercise philosophy is based on the finding that certain spinal movements may aggravate pain, whereas other movements relieve pain. McKenzie believed that accumulation of flexion forces caused dysfunction of posterior aspect of the disc. Most McKenzie exercises are extension biased. The positions and movement patterns that relieve pain are individually determined for each patient. McKenzie classified lumbar disorders into three syndromes based on posture and response to movement: *postural*, *dysfunctional*, and *derangement syndrome*. Each syndrome has a specific treatment and postural correction. Treatment objectives include identifying the directional preference of lumbosacral movement for a patient that induces **centralization of the pain** (change in pain location from a distal location in the lower extremity to a proximal or central location). Examples of McKenzie exercises include:
    • Repeat end-range movements while standing: back extension, side gliding (lateral bending with rotation)
    • Recumbent end-range movement: passive extension while prone, prone lateral shifting of hips off midline
    McKenzie exercises (Fig. 14.1) are most commonly prescribed for disc herniation and lumbar radicular pain.

Table 14.1 Overview of Interventions Endorsed for Nonspecific Low Back Pain in Evidence-Based Clinical Practice Guidelines (Danish,[4] US,[5] and UK[6] guidelines).

	ACUTE LOW BACK PAIN (<6 WEEKS)	PERSISTENT LOW BACK PAIN (>12 WEEKS)
Education and Self-care		
Advice to remain active	First-line treatment, consider for routine use	First-line treatment, consider for routine use
Education	First-line treatment, consider for routine use	First-line treatment, consider for routine use
Superficial heat	Second-line or adjunctive treatment option	Insufficient evidence
Nonpharmacologic Therapy		
Exercise therapy	Limited use in selected patients	First-line treatment, consider for routine use
Cognitive behavioral therapy	Limited use in selected patients	First-line treatment, consider for routine use
Spinal manipulation	Second-line or adjunctive treatment option	Second-line or adjunctive treatment option
Massage	Second-line or adjunctive treatment option	Second-line or adjunctive treatment option
Acupuncture	Second-line or adjunctive treatment option	Second-line or adjunctive treatment option
Yoga	Insufficient evidence	Second-line or adjunctive treatment option
Mindfulness-based stress reduction	Insufficient evidence	Second-line or adjunctive treatment option
Interdisciplinary rehabilitation	Insufficient evidence	Second-line or adjunctive treatment option
Pharmacologic Therapy		
Paracetamol	Not recommended	Not recommended
Nonsteroidal antiinflammatory drugs	Second-line or adjunctive treatment option	Second-line or adjunctive treatment option
Skeletal muscle relaxants	Limited use in selected patients	Insufficient evidence
Selective norepinephrine reuptake inhibitors	Insufficient evidence	Second-line or adjunctive treatment option
Antiseizure medications	Insufficient evidence	Role uncertain
Opioids	Limited use in selected patients, use with caution	Limited use in selected patients, use with caution
Systemic glucocorticoids	Not recommended	Not recommended
Interventional Therapies		
Epidural glucocorticoid injection (for herniated disc with radiculopathy)	Not recommended	Limited use in selected patients
Surgery		
Discectomy (for herniated disc with radiculopathy)	Insufficient evidence	Second-line or adjunctive treatment option
Laminectomy (for symptomatic spinal stenosis)	Insufficient evidence	Second-line or adjunctive treatment option

(Continued on following page)

Table 14.1 Overview of Interventions Endorsed for Nonspecific Low Back Pain in Evidence-Based Clinical Practice Guidelines (Danish,[4] US,[5] and UK[6] guidelines). *(Continued)*

	ACUTE LOW BACK PAIN (<6 WEEKS)	PERSISTENT LOW BACK PAIN (>12 WEEKS)
	Surgery	
Spinal fusion (for nonradicular low back pain with degenerative disc findings)	Insufficient evidence	Role uncertain
Subacute low back pain is a transition period between acute and chronic low back pain; evidence on optimal therapies for subacute low back pain is scarce but a reasonable approach is to shift towards therapies recommended for chronic low back pain.		

From Foster NE, Anema JR, Cherkin D, et al. Low back pain 2: Prevention and treatment of low back pain: Evidence, challenges, and promising directions. Lancet 2018; 391(10137):2368–2383. http://dx.doi.org/10.1016/S0140-6736(18)30489-6.

21. **What are spinal stabilization exercises? When are they used?**

Strengthening exercises for a dynamic *corset* of muscle control to maintain a neutral position are known as spinal stabilization exercises. Recently, there has been a focus on the role of the transversus abdominis and lumbar multifidi muscles in enhancing spinal stability. The goal of stabilization exercises is to reduce mechanical stress on the spine. Spinal stabilization exercises can be prescribed for most causes of low back pain. Key concepts of a spinal stabilization exercise program include:

• Determination of the functional range (the most stable and asymptomatic position) for all movements
• Strengthening of transversus abdominis, abdominal obliques (oblique crunches), rectus abdominis (sagittal plane crunches, supine pelvic bracing with alternating arm and leg raises), gluteus maximus (prone gluteal squeezes, supine pelvic bridging, bridging and marching), and gluteus medius (sidestepping)
• Neuromuscular reeducation, mobility, and endurance exercises
• Progression of therapy from gross and simple movements to smaller, isolated, and complex movements
• Progression to dynamic stabilization exercises (quadruped opposite upper and lower extremity extension, quadruped hip extension and contralateral arm flexion, prone hip extension and contralateral arm flexion, balancing on a gymnastic ball, wall slides, squatting, and lifting) (Fig. 14.2)

22. **Explain what is meant by a functional restoration program and how it differs from other types of nonsurgical spine care.**

Nonsurgical spine care may be conceptualized in terms of three levels of care:

• **Primary care** is applied to patients with acute back and neck pain problems. Symptoms are controlled with medical or surgical management, exercise therapy, medications, modalities, and manual techniques.

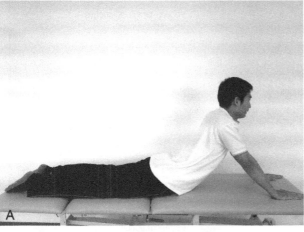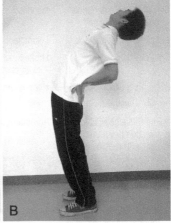

Fig. 14.1 McKenzie exercises with trunk extension. (A) Extension in lying. (B) Standing extension. (From Purepong N, Jitvimonrat A, Boonyoung S, et al. Effect of flexibility exercise on lumbar angle: A study among nonspecific low back pain patients. J Bodyw Mov Ther 2012;16:236–243.)

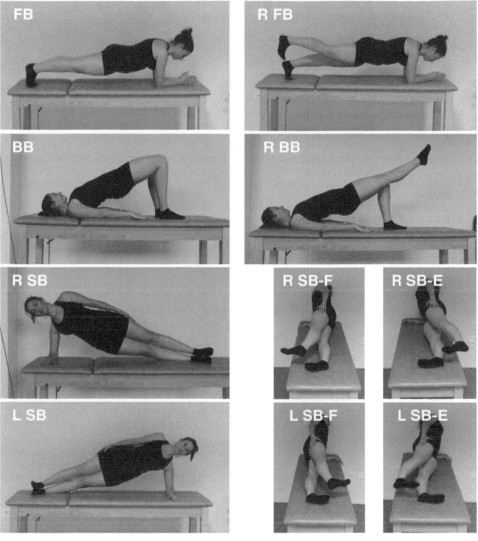

Fig. 14.2 Lumbar stabilization bridge exercises. *BB*, back bridge; *FB*, front bridge; *L SB*, left side bridge; *L SB-E*, left side bridge with hip extension; *L SB-F*, left side bridge with hip flexion; *R BB*, back bridge with elevated right leg; *R FB*, front bridge with elevated right leg; *R SB*, right side bridge; *R SB-E*, right side bridge with hip extension; *R SB–F*, right side bridge with hip flexion. (From García-Vaquero MP, Moreside JM, Brontons-Gil E, et al. Trunk muscle activation during stabilization exercises with single and double leg support. J Electromyogr Kinesiol 2012;22:398–406.)

- **Secondary care** is applied to patients who did not respond to the initial primary care level of treatment. Such patients require more comprehensive management involving interdisciplinary care of medical specialists, physical therapists, occupational therapists, psychologists, social workers, and disability managers. During this phase, restorative exercise and education are applied to prevent deconditioning and chronic disability. Work-conditioning and work-hardening approaches are included in secondary care.
- **Tertiary care** is indicated for patients who did not respond to primary and secondary conservative care or surgical treatment. Tertiary care or functional restoration involves interdisciplinary team care with all disciplines on site. Functional restoration programs can be provided by pain clinics. Functional restoration programs include:
  - Quantification of physical deconditioning (strength, endurance, aerobic capacity)
  - Addressing psychosocial problems (psychopathology, use of narcotics)

- Identification of socioeconomic factors in disability (compensation, psychogenic pain)
- Cognitive behavioral training (relaxation techniques, improve self-esteem)
- Restoration of fitness
- Work simulation activities
- Individual, family, and group counseling
- Disability and vocational management
- Outcome monitoring

23. What is "complementary and alternative medicine"?

Various terms (3) have been used to distinguish conventional medicine (CM) from complementary health approaches:

- *Alternative medicine:* treatment used in place of CM
- *Complementary medicine:* treatment used in combination with CM
- *Integrative medicine:* practiced by traditionally trained physicians and uses a combination of CM and complementary and/or alternative therapies
- *Integrated medicine:* care is by teams of CM providers and clinicians versed in complementary and alternative therapies
- *Holistic medicine:* treatments consider body, mind, and spirit in health and healing
- The National Center for Complementary and Integrative Health (NCCIH), a unit of the US National Institute of Health (NIH) identified the 10 most common complementary health approaches used by U.S. adults as:
  - Natural products
  - Deep breathing
  - Yoga, tai chi, or qigong
  - Chiropractic or osteopathic manipulation
  - Meditation
  - Massage
  - Special diets
  - Homeopathy
  - Progressive relaxation
  - Guided imagery

Information on specific complementary health treatments and related research may be found at: https://nccih.nih.gov/health.

KEY POINTS

1. The natural history of acute low back pain is variable. Although low back pain is short lasting in many patients, recurrent pain is common, and some patients end up with persistent disabling pain.
2. Based on patient history and physical examination, patients presenting with "nonspecific" mechanical low back pain symptoms may be classified into one of four patterns as a guide to initial treatment: back-dominant pain aggravated by flexion, back-dominant pain aggravated by extension, constant leg-dominant pain, and intermittent leg-dominant pain.
3. Patients with chronic low back pain are more challenging to treat than those with acute or subacute low back pain and require different treatment approaches.
4. Identification and resolution of psychosocial barriers to recovery is critical for successful treatment of chronic spinal pain syndromes.

Websites

1. Clinically Organized Relevant Exam (CORE) Back Tool
   http://www.effectivepractice.org/lowbackpain
2. Low Back Pain Care Process Model, Intermountain Healthcare:
   https://intermountainhealthcare.org/ext/Dcmnt?ncid=522579081
3. Management of Chronic Noncancer Pain Care Process Model, Intermountain Healthcare:
   https://intermountainhealthcare.org/ext/Dcmnt?ncid=521023323
4. Pain Assessment Tools and Clinical Guidelines, Pain BC™:
   https://www.painbc.ca/health-professionals/assessment-tools

REFERENCES

1. Hall, H., McIntosh, G., & Boyle, C. (2009). Effectiveness of a low back pain classification system. *Spine Journal, 9*, 648–657.
2. Foster, N. E., Anema, J. R., Cherkin, D., Chou, R., Cohen, S. P., Gross, D. P., et al. (2018). Low back pain 2: Prevention and treatment of low back pain: Evidence, challenges, and promising directions. *The Lancet, 391*(10137), 2368–2383. Retrieved from http://dx.doi.org/10.1016/S0140-6736(18)30489-6.

3. Simpson, C. A. (2015). Complementary medicine in chronic pain treatment. *Physical Medicine and Rehabilitation Clinics of North America, 26*, 321–347.
4. Stochkendahl, M. J, Kjaer, P., Hartvigsen, J., Kongsted, A., Aaboe, J., Andersen, M., et al. (2018). National clinical guidelines for nonsurgical treatment of patients with recent onset low back pain or lumbar radiculopathy. *European Spine Journal, 27*, 60–75.
5. Qaseem, A., Wilt, T. J., McLean, R. M., & Forciea, M. A. (2017). Noninvasive treatments for acute, subacute and chronic back pain: A clinical practice guideline from the American College of Physicians. *Annals of Internal Medicine, 166*(7), 514–530.
6. National Institute for Health and Care Excellence, UK. *Low Back Pain and Sciatica in Over 16s: Assessment and Management.* 2016. Retrieved from https://www.nice.org.uk/guidance/ng59.

BIBLIOGRAPHY

Thoracic Spine

1. Briggs, A. M., Smith, A. J., Straker, L. M., & Bragge, P. (2009). Thoracic spine pain in the general population: Prevalence, incidence and associated factors in children, adolescents and adults: A systematic review. *BMC Musculoskeletal Disorders, 10*, 77–89.
2. Heneghan, N. R., Gormley, S., Hallam, C., & Rushton, A. (2009). Management of thoracic spine pain and dysfunction: A survey of clinical practice in the UK. *Musculoskeletal Science & Practice, 29*, 58–66.
3. Southerst, D., Marchand, A. A., Côté, P., Shearer, H. M., Wong, J. J., Varatharajan, S., et al. (2015). The effectiveness of noninvasive interventions for musculoskeletal thoracic spine and chest wall pain: A systematic review. The Ontario Protocol for Traffic Injury Management (OPTIMa) Collaboration. *Journal of Manipulative and Physiological Therapeutics, 38*, 521–531.

Lumbar Spine

1. Alleyne, J., Hall, H., & Rampersaud, R. *Clinically Organized Relevant Exam (CORE) Tool for the Low Back Pain Toolkit for Primary Care Providers. Centre for Effective Practice. Funded by the Government of Ontario.* 2013. ontario.ca/lowbackpain and http://www. effectivepractice.org/lowbackpain.
2. Della Mora, L. S., Perruccio, A. V., Badley, E. M., & Rampersaud, Y. R. (2016). Differences among primary care patients with different mechanical patterns of low back pain: A cross-sectional investigation. *BMJ Open, 6*, e013060. doi:10.1136/bmjopen-2016-013060.
3. Deyo, R. A., Dworkin, S. F., Amtmann, D., Andersson, G., Borenstein, D., Carragee, E., et al. (2014). Report of the NIH task force on research standards for chronic low back pain. *Spine Journal, 14*, 1375–1391.
4. Foster, N. E., Anema, J. R., Cherkin, D., Chou, R., Cohen, S. P., Gross, D. P., et al. (2018). Low back pain 2: Prevention and treatment of low back pain: Evidence, challenges, and promising directions. *The Lancet, 391*(10137), 2368–2383. Retrieved from http://dx. doi.org/10.1016/S0140-6736(18)30489-6.
5. Hall, H., McIntosh, G., & Boyle, C. (2009). Effectiveness of a low back pain classification system. *Spine Journal, 9*, 648–657.
6. Hartvigsen, J., Hancock, M. J., Kongsted, A., Louw, Q., Ferreira, M. L., Genevay, S., et al. (2018). Low back pain 1: What is low back pain and why we need to pay attention. *The Lancet, 391*, 2356–2367. Retrieved from http://dx.doi.org/10.1016/S0140-6736(18)30480-X.
7. Hill, J. C., Whitehurst, D. G., Lewis, M., Bryan, S., Dunn, K. M., Foster, N. E., et al. (2011). Comparison of stratified primary care management for low back pain with current best practice (STarT Back): A randomized controlled trial. *Lancet, 378*, 1560–1571.
8. Qaseem, A., Wilt, T. J., McLean, R. M., & Forciea, M. A. (2017). Noninvasive treatments for acute, subacute and chronic back pain: A clinical practice guideline from the American College of Physicians. *Annals of Internal Medicine, 166*(7), 514–530.
9. Rampersaud, Y. R., Bidos, A., Fanti, C., & Perruccio, A. V. (2017). The need for multidimensional stratification of chronic low back pain. *Spine, 42*, 1318–1325.
10. Simpson, C. A. (2015). Complementary medicine in chronic pain treatment. *Physical Medicine and Rehabilitation Clinics of North America, 26*, 321–347.
11. Stochkendahl, M. J., Kjaer, P., Hartvigsen, J., Kongsted, A., Aaboe, J., Andersen, M., et al. (2018). National clinical guidelines for nonsurgical treatment of patients with recent onset low back pain or lumbar radiculopathy. *European Spine Journal, 27*, 60–75.
12. National Institute for Health and Care Excellence, UK. Low Back Pain and Sciatica in Over 16s: *Assessment and Management.* 2016. Retrieved from https://www.nice.org.uk/guidance/ng59.

CHAPTER 15

PHARMACOLOGIC MANAGEMENT OF PAIN IN SPINE DISORDERS

Vincent Huang, MD, Jonathan Ramin, DO, and Thomas N. Bryce, MD

1. **What is the definition of pain?**
   Pain is an unpleasant sensory and emotional experience associated with actual or potential tissue damage.

2. **What are some common criteria used to classify spinal pain?**
   Various criteria may be used to classify pain. For example:
   Time course: acute (<1 month), subacute (1–3 months), or chronic (>3 months)
   Intensity: mild, moderate, or severe (e.g., based on visual or numerical rating scale)
   Pathophysiology: nociceptive, neuropathic, or nociplastic
   Location: axial, radicular, or referred pain
   Presence/absence of radiation: axial non-radiating, axial radiating pain

3. **Distinguish between acute and chronic pain.**
   Acute pain is pain of recent onset, and usually has a well-defined cause, such as peripheral nerve or tissue injury. It is expected to diminish with time or following appropriate treatment, as tissue heals and inflammation resolves. **Chronic pain** is pain that persists beyond its expected duration and does not respond to usual treatments. It may be the result of an initial injury or may have no clear cause. Chronic pain is often accompanied by other problems such as fatigue, sleep disturbance, changes in appetite and weight, decreased libido, and depressed mood.

4. **Describe how pain is classified based on pathophysiological mechanism.**
   Nociceptive pain arises from actual or threatened damage to non-neural tissue due to activation of sensory neurons referred to as nociceptors by mechanical, thermal or chemical stimuli. Nociceptive pain occurs in the presence of a normally functioning somatosensory nervous system and is categorized as somatic or visceral. Somatic nociceptive pain may arise from skin, muscles, tendons, ligaments, or bone, while visceral nociceptive pain arises from thoracic, pelvic, or abdominal organs. Somatic nociceptive pain is described as localized, sharp, or dull, aching and is typically worsened by activity and decreased with rest. Examples of somatic nociceptive pain include back pain due to a lumbar strain or immediately following posterior lumbar surgery. Visceral nociceptive pain is poorly localized, described as deep, squeezing or cramping and is often associated with involvement of the autonomic nervous system leading to symptoms such as nausea, vomiting, sweating, and changes in vital signs. Examples of visceral pain include symptoms associated with myocardial infarction or appendicitis.
   Neuropathic pain is caused by a lesion or disease of the somatosensory nervous system. Patient descriptors for neuropathic pain include burning, shooting, stabbing, electric shock-like, tingling, or numbness. Patients with neuropathic pain may exhibit pain with stimuli which are normally not painful (allodynia) or show a marked or prolonged response to painful stimuli (hyperalgesia). Neuropathic pain may be categorized by location as central (e.g., spinal cord injury related pain) or peripheral (e.g., cervical or lumbar radiculopathy).
   Nociplastic pain arises from altered nociception despite lack of clear evidence of actual or threatened tissue damage causing the activation of peripheral nociceptors or evidence for a disease or lesion of the somatosensory nervous system. Pain is considered to arise due to persistent dysfunction of neurons throughout the central nervous system which lowers pain thresholds and amplifies sensory signaling. Examples of conditions in this category include fibromyalgia, tension headaches and cervical and lumbar pain without a structural cause.
   More than one type of pain may be responsible for a patient's pain symptoms and result in a **mixed pain syndrome.**

5. **What pharmacologic agents are frequently used to treat spinal pain?**
   The most commonly prescribed medications for spinal pain include acetaminophen, nonsteroidal antiinflammatory medications (NSAIDs), antidepressants, anticonvulsants, muscle relaxants, opioids, and topical agents.
   Recognition of the different types of pain is clinically important because some medications are more effective for certain types of pain. The medications of choice for nociceptive pain are analgesics. Acetaminophen and NSAIDs are recommended as first-line analgesics. While opioids are also effective, they are considered as second-line analgesics due to the risk of drug-related adverse events associated with opioid use. The medications of choice for neuropathic and nociplastic pain are anticonvulsants and antidepressants. While opioids are also effective for treatment of neuropathic pain, they are generally avoided in nociplastic pain. For treatment of patients with mixed pain syndromes, a combination of different medications may be used (Table 15.1).

Table 15.1 Common Pharmacological Agents for Treatment of Spinal Pain.

DRUG CLASS	MODE OF ACTION	COMMENTS
Acetaminophen	Mechanism of action is not completely understood. Inhibits COX-mediated production of prostaglandins	• Effective against fever • Adverse effects include liver toxicity
NSAID	Nonselective (COX-1 and COX-2) and selective (COX-2) inhibitors of cyclooxygenase	• Adverse effects include dyspepsia, peptic ulcers, bleeding, cardiovascular risk, and renal toxicity
TCA	Inhibit presynaptic reuptake of serotonin and norepinephrine	• Effective against comorbid depression • Risk of anticholinergic adverse effects • Risk of serotonin syndrome
SNRI (duloxetine)	Serotonin/norepinephrine reuptake inhibition	• Effective against comorbid depression and anxiety • Adverse effects include nausea, sleep disturbances, and sexual dysfunction
Anticonvulsants (gabapentin and pregabalin)	Alpha-2-delta calcium channel modulators	• Adverse effects include sedation, dizziness, and peripheral edema
Opioids	μ-Opioid receptor agonist	• Not recommended for first-line and long-term treatment • Risk of gastrointestinal adverse effects, tolerance, and abuse
Tramadol	Weak μ-Opioid receptor agonist and serotonin/norepinephrine reuptake inhibitor	• Lower potential for abuse compared to other opioids • Risk of seizure or serotonin syndrome when used with various antidepressant medications
Nonbenzodiazepines Muscle relaxant	• Varies according to specific medication	• May be used short term for acute spinal pain • Long-term use is not recommended
Topical agents: Capsaicin Lidocaine	• Selective agonist of transient receptor potential vanilloid 1 • Sodium channel blocker	• Limited risk of systemic adverse effects and drug interactions • May be combined with oral therapies

COX, Cyclooxygenase; *NSAID*, nonsteroidal antiinflammatory drug; *SNRI*, serotonin norepinephrine reuptake inhibitor; *TCA*, tricyclic antidepressant.

6. Discuss the advantages and disadvantages of the use of acetaminophen and NSAIDs.

Acetaminophen (paracetamol) and NSAIDs are first-line pharmacologic treatment options commonly prescribed for patients with spinal conditions. Acetaminophen has antipyretic and analgesic properties, but lacks antiinflammatory properties. The exact mechanism of action of acetaminophen remains incompletely understood. Although acetaminophen is less effective in providing analgesia than NSAIDs, acetaminophen has a more favorable overall safety profile. Acetaminophen has minimal effects on platelet inhibition. However, as this medication is metabolized in the liver, it is associated with the risk of hepatotoxicity and intake should not exceed the recommended maximum daily dose of 3000 mg/day.

NSAIDs provide antipyretic, antiinflammatory, and analgesic effects, mediated by inhibition of the proinflammatory enzyme cyclooxygenase (COX). NSAIDs provide more effective pain relief compared with acetaminophen, but are associated with potentially serious gastrointestinal, renal, and cardiovascular risks. As such, the lowest effective dose of NSAIDs given for the shortest duration needed for pain relief should be used. NSAIDs have variable effects depending on their chemical structure and may be classified as:

- Salicylic acids: acetylsalicylic acid (aspirin), salsalate, diflunisal
- Acetic acids: diclofenac, indomethacin, sulindac, ketorolac, etodolac, tolmetin
- Propionic acids: ibuprofen, naproxen (Naprosyn), fenoprofen, ketoprofen, oxaprozin, flurbiprofen
- Fenamic acids: sodium meclofenamate (Meclomen)
- Enolic acids (oxicams): piroxicam, meloxicam
- Nonacidic compounds: nabumetone
- COX-2 selective inhibitors: celecoxib

7. **What is the difference between a selective and a nonselective NSAID?**

NSAIDs may be classified as nonselective or traditional NSAIDs (e.g., aspirin, ibuprofen, naproxen) and selective NSAIDs or cyclooxygenase-2 (COX-2) inhibitors (e.g., celecoxib). Traditional NSAIDs act as nonselective inhibitors of the COX enzyme and inhibit both cyclooxygenase-1 (COX-1) and COX-2 enzymes. Selective NSAIDs were developed in an attempt to provide antiinflammatory action without the gastrointestinal adverse drug reactions attributed to inhibition of the COX-1 enzyme. Although clinical studies have shown COX-2 selective inhibitors reduce the risk of NSAID-related ulcers and complications by half when compared with traditional NSAIDs, other clinical studies have also revealed an increased incidence of adverse cardiac effects (e.g., myocardial infarction and cardiovascular death) with the use of COX-2 inhibitors when compared with non-selective NSAIDs. Given the increased incidence of adverse cardiovascular effects, and the finding that use of a proton pump inhibitor (e.g., omeprazole, 20 mg daily) with a traditional NSAID achieves a similar gastrointestinal risk profile without increasing the risk of cardiac events, the use of COX-2 inhibitors has declined.

All NSAIDs also increase the risk of hemodynamically mediated acute kidney injury. NSAIDs are not recommended for use in high-risk patients, such as those with a history of chronic kidney disease, electrolyte abnormalities (i.e., hypercalcemia), and nephrotic syndrome. Monitoring of hemoglobin, electrolytes, renal function, liver function, and blood pressure is recommended for patients maintained on NSAIDs, especially for elderly patients. Aspirin and traditional NSAIDs inhibit platelet aggregation through a COX-1-mediated effect. Concomitant use of aspirin for secondary prevention of cardiovascular disease and traditional NSAIDs is associated with increased gastrointestinal adverse events and aspirin resistance (failure to prevent thrombotic events). In patients taking aspirin for prevention of cardiovascular disease who are prescribed another NSAID, it is recommended to take aspirin at least 2 hours prior to ingestion of other NSAIDs (Table 15.2).

8. **When are antidepressants useful for patients with chronic spinal pain?**

Antidepressant medications are commonly prescribed to treat chronic spinal pain, particularly neuropathic pain. These medications are prescribed as they have an analgesic effect, independent of their effect on depression. Options include serotonin-norepinephrine reuptake inhibitors (SNRIs; e.g., duloxetine), tricyclic antidepressants (TCAs; e.g., amitriptyline, nortriptyline, desipramine), and selective serotonin reuptake inhibitors (SSRIs;

Table 15.2 Characteristics of Common Oral Nonsteroidal Antiinflammatory Drugs.

NSAID (DOSE)	HALF-LIFE (HOURS)	CV RISK	GI RISK	COX-2 SELECTIVITY	NNT[a]	SELECTED CHARACTERISTICS
Aspirin (1200 mg)	4–6	L	M	L	2.4	Unlike other NSAIDs, irreversibly inhibits platelet functioning for the life of the platelet (7–10 days)
Celecoxib (400 mg)	11	M to H	L	H	2.1	• Relative reduction in GI toxicity compared with nonselective NSAIDs • No effect on platelet function
Diclofenac (100 mg)	2	H	M	H	1.8	• Also available in topical, solution, and gel • Incidence of elevated transaminase levels higher than with other NSAIDs
Etodolac	6–7	M	L	H	NA	• Relatively COX-2 selective at lower total daily dose of 600–800 mg
Ibuprofen (600 mg)	2	M to H	L	M	1.7	• Short duration of effect • Useful alternative to naproxen in patients without CV risks
Indomethacin	4.5	L	M to H	L	NA	• Useful for treatment of acute gout • Potent inhibitory effects on renal prostaglandin synthesis
Ketorolac (20 mg)	4–6	NA	H	L	1.8	• Available in injectable form • Indicated for short-term use (up to 5 days) • Risk of serious GI complications, concurrent GI protection is suggested

NSAID (DOSE)	HALF-LIFE (HOURS)	CV RISK	GI RISK	COX-2 SELECTIVITY	NNTª	SELECTED CHARACTERISTICS
Table 15.2 Characteristics of Common Oral Nonsteroidal Antiinflammatory Drugs. *(Continued)*						
Meloxicam	15–20	M	L	H	NA	• Long duration of effect; slow onset • Relatively COX-2 selective and minimal effect on platelet function at lower total daily dose of 7.5 mg
Naproxen (400 mg)	12–15	L to M	M	L	2.7	• Useful for treatment of acute or chronic pain
Piroxicam (40 mg)	50	L	H	M	1.9	• Long-acting option for treatment of chronic pain • Daily doses ≥20 mg increase risk of serious GI complications

ªNNT are calculated for the proportion of patients with at least 50% pain relief over 4–6 hours compared with placebo according to the milligram in parentheses in Table 15.2.
CV, Cardiovascular; *COX-2*, cyclooxygenase-2; *GI*, gastrointestinal; *H*, high; *L*, low; *M*, moderate; *NA*, not available; *NNT*, numbers needed to treat; *NSAID*, nonsteroidal antiinflammatory drug.

e.g., paroxetine, citalopram, fluoxetine, sertraline). Duloxetine, a prototypical SNRI, has shown effectiveness in treating pain and improving function in people with chronic axial nonradiating pain. TCAs may be considered for use in certain patients with axial nonradiating spinal pain, especially in those who have difficulty sleeping. However, duloxetine seems to be a more effective and safer alternative than TCAs if there are no contraindications to SNRI use. Although SSRIs are not as effective for pain control compared to other classes of antidepressants, they play a role in treatment due to their favorable safety profile and the overlap of symptoms due to chronic pain and depression.

9. What are some adverse effects associated with use of antidepressants for spinal pain?
   SNRIs: Nausea, insomnia, dry mouth, constipation, sexual dysfunction, somnolence, and fatigue are reported adverse effects for duloxetine. Duloxetine should not be used in individuals with significant liver disease due to risk of hepatotoxicity.
   TCAs: Anticholinergic adverse effects are prominent with TCA use. These effects include dry mouth, urinary retention, constipation, weight gain, blurry vision, and orthostatic hypotension. In addition, caution should be taken when prescribing TCAs to individuals with cardiac disease. TCA use in combination with other serotonergic medications increases the risk of serotonin syndrome and therefore this combination should be used with caution.
   SSRIs: Adverse effects reported with SSRIs include weight gain, sexual dysfunction, sleep disturbance, headaches, dry mouth, gastrointestinal problems, and a slightly increased risk of bleeding due to platelet dysfunction (Table 15.3).

10. When should anticonvulsants be used in the management of spinal pain?
    Gabapentinoids (i.e., gabapentin and pregabalin) are the most commonly used anticonvulsant class of medications used for the treatment of neuropathic pain. These gamma-aminobutyric acid analogs are alpha-2-delta ligands that act on voltage-gated calcium channels. Gabapentinoids are first-line agents for the treatment of neuropathic pain due to spinal cord injury. However, there is only low-level evidence supporting the use of gabapentinoids for

DRUG	TYPE	INITIAL DOSE (mg/day)	TARGET DOSE RANGE (mg/day)
Table 15.3 Commonly Prescribed Oral Antidepressant Medications.			
Duloxetine	SNRI	30	60
Venlafaxine	SNRI	25	225
Amitriptyline	TCA	10–25	75–100
Nortriptyline	TCA	10–25	75–100
Desipramine	TCA	10–25	75–100
Paroxetine	SSRI	20	20–50
Citalopram	SSRI	20	40

SNRI, Serotonin-norepinephrine inhibitor; *SSRI*, selective serotonin reuptake inhibitors; *TCA*, tricyclic antidepressants.

axial radiating spinal pain. Side effects of gabapentinoids include fatigue, dizziness, somnolence, ataxia, difficulty with mental concentration, headaches, peripheral edema, and loss of balance. Additional anticonvulsants indicated for neuropathic pain include oxcarbazepine, carbamazepine, and valproic acid (Table 15.4).

11. Name two categories of muscle relaxants and describe the role of each category in the treatment of spinal pain.

Muscle relaxants can be divided into two categories: *benzodiazepines* and *nonbenzodiazepines*. There is a lack of evidence to support the use of benzodiazepines (i.e., diazepam, alprazolam) for treatment of spinal pain. Moderate evidence supports the use of nonbenzodiazepines (i.e., baclofen, tizanidine, cyclobenzaprine, metaxalone, and methocarbamol) for muscle spasm related to acute axial nonradiating spinal pain or an acute exacerbation of chronic pain, although the evidence indicates benefit is limited to short-term use (7–14 days). There is no evidence to suggest benefit for chronic spinal pain. In addition, the potential for abuse and overdose resulting in respiratory depression and death do not justify their long-term use. These associated risks are further compounded when combined with opioids. There is no clear evidence that one muscle relaxant is superior to another; however, it is important to recognize that the agents differ significantly in their adverse effect profiles. The adverse effects of muscle relaxants include primarily central nervous system–mediated effects including sedation, dizziness, and headache. Agents such as cyclobenzaprine that have anticholinergic adverse effects may be of concern in the geriatric population. This agent, in combination with other serotonergic medication, may also increase risk of serotonin syndrome (Table 15.5).

12. Are oral corticosteroids useful in the treatment of spinal pain?

Oral corticosteroids are frequently prescribed for treatment of spinal pain. However, randomized control trials (RCTs) have not shown that oral corticosteroids are effective for the treatment of axial radiating or nonradiating spinal pain. A single large RCT involving patients with sciatica showed modestly improved function compared to placebo but no significant improvement in radicular pain. Use of oral corticosteroids has not been shown to decrease the likelihood of undergoing surgery for relief of radiculopathy. Oral corticosteroid use has been associated with increased rates of adverse events including insomnia and nervousness.

13. What is the role of topical analgesics?

Topical analgesics are applied directly over a painful site and are available as aerosols, creams, gels, lotions, lozenges, ointments, patches, and solutions. Analgesic activity is limited to the peripheral soft tissues. For the treatment of low back pain, there is limited evidence to recommend for or against the use of topical preparations. However, since topical agents exhibit minimal absorption and have few systemic adverse reactions or drug

Table 15.4 Commonly Prescribed Oral Anticonvulsant Medications.

DRUG	STARTING DOSE	TARGET DOSE RANGE
Gabapentin	100–300 mg daily	300–800 mg tid
Pregabalin	25–75 mg bid	50–300 mg bid
Oxcarbazepine	150 mg bid	150–600 mg bid
Carbamazepine	100 mg bid	200–400 mg bid
Valproic acid	250 mg bid	500–1000 mg bid

bid, Twice a day; *tid,* three times per day.

Table 15.5 Commonly Prescribed Oral Muscle Relaxant Medications.

DRUG	STARTING DOSE	DOSE RANGE	MECHANISM OF ACTION
Baclofen	5–10 mg tid	10–30 mg tid	Acts as a GABA-B receptor agonist to inhibit gamma motor neuron activity at spinal cord level
Tizanidine	2 mg bid or tid	4–8 mg tid	Acts as a central alpha-2-adrenergic agonist to increase presynaptic inhibition of motor neurons
Cyclobenzaprine	5 mg tid	5–10 mg tid	Acts on locus coeruleus with increase NE release via gamma fibers, which innervate and inhibit the alpha motor neurons in the ventral horn
Methocarbamol	500 mg qid	1000 mg qid	Mechanism of action has not been established
Metaxalone	400 mg tid	800 mg tid or qid	Mechanism of action has not been established

bid, Twice a day; *tid,* three times a day; *qid,* four times a day; *NE, norepinephrine.*

interactions, they are often prescribed in axial nonradiating spinal pain. Many of the agents are available as over-the-counter products for the treatment of spinal pain.

Common analgesics include:

- **Capsaicin,** the active component of chili peppers, is a topical analgesic cream that depletes substance P in small nociceptors. It may provide pain relief in patients with peripheral neuropathy, arthritis of small joints, and, occasionally, complex regional pain syndrome.
- **Lidoderm patch** (5% prescription or 4% over-the-counter strength) is a topical treatment initially approved for treatment of neuropathic pain. It works by blocking voltage-gated sodium channels to stabilize neuronal membranes. The patch is applied over small areas of neuropathic and/or nociceptive pain. The patches are worn for 12 hours and then taken off for 12 hours, but the analgesia is sustained.

Other topical agents that have shown benefit as adjunct treatment for spinal pain include: lidocaine 5% cream, diclofenac gel, and menthol salicylate cream. These agents are generally safe to use and are not associated with the same systematic adverse effect profiles as oral analgesics.

14. What is the role of opioid analgesics in acute and chronic spinal pain?

Opioids play a role in management of spinal pain related to cancer, as well as acute spinal pain following trauma and surgery. In other clinical situations requiring medication for treatment of spinal pain, opioids should only be used for the relief of severe acute axial nonradiating spinal pain during short-lived painful events if other nonopioid interventions are not effective. Opioids are never first-line treatment options for either nociceptive or neuropathic chronic spinal pain in a primary care setting. Opioids should always be prescribed with caution to avoid their associated risks (e.g., misuse, overdose, and opioid-use disorder). There is no evidence that pain relief is sustained or that function improves when opioids are prescribed long-term for chronic noncancer pain.

Although, opioids continue to play a role in the acute management of severe pain immediately following spine surgery, there has been a shift toward use of multimodal pain management protocols that minimize or do not involve opioids. These protocols target different mechanisms of action in the peripheral and/or central nervous system, combined with nonpharmacologic interventions, during the preoperative, intraoperative, and postoperative periods.

15. Briefly explain how opioid medications exert their effect and describe some common opioid medications used for treatment of spinal pain.

Opioids work by binding to receptors found in the brain, spinal cord, and other nervous tissue. These receptors are G-protein-coupled-receptors comprised of various subtypes (i.e., mu [μ], kappa [κ], delta [δ], and orphan-like receptor). Opioids may be described as pure agonists, partial agonists, or agonist/antagonists. Most of the opioids used for treatment of spinal pain are *agonists* and rely primarily on binding to μ receptors to achieve their analgesic effect. *Partial agonists* bind with great affinity to μ receptors but excite these receptors less than the pure agonists. *Mixed agonists/antagonists* show varying activity depending on the opioid receptor type and medication dose.

Opioids used for treatment of spinal pain may be classified as short- or long-acting based on duration of action. Short-acting opioids have a more rapid increase and decrease in serum levels compared to long-acting opioids. Short-acting opioids commonly prescribed for spinal pain include immediate-release morphine, oxycodone, hydromorphone, oxymorphone, hydrocodone, and codeine. Long-acting opioids either have an inherently long action or are formulated to release more gradually into the bloodstream. Long-acting opioids commonly prescribed for spinal pain are extended-release (ER), controlled-release (CR), or sustained-release (SR) versions of morphine, oxycodone, oxymorphone, and fentanyl and are commonly referred to as extended-release and long-acting (ER/LA) opioid formulations (Table 15.6).

A more recently developed class of analgesics acts through a dual mode of action. Tramadol is a weak agonist at the μ receptor that provides additional analgesia through inhibition of norepinephrine and serotonin reuptake. Tapentadol is a dual action opioid that is a weak agonist at the μ receptor but only inhibits norepinephrine uptake.

Opioid antagonists are medications that bind to opioid receptors and reverse and block the effect of opioids. Spine care providers should be knowledgeable regarding use of the opioid antagonist naloxone, available in a nasal spray or prefilled autoinjection device for treatment of opioid overdose.

16. What are some of the major health-related risks associated with opioid analgesics?

Some of the health-related risks include:

- Physical dependence
- Tolerance
- Opioid use disorder
- Respiratory depression*
- Fatal and nonfatal overdose*
- Falls and injury, especially in older adults
- Chronic use during pregnancy can lead to neonatal opioid withdrawal syndrome.

---

*Risk of respiratory depression and overdose increase when opioids are combined with other central nervous system depressants (e.g., benzodiazepines)

Table 15.6 Commonly Prescribed Opioid Medications.

| | Equivalent Doses (mg) | | DURATION OF |
	IV	PO	ACTION (HOURS)
Opioid Agonists			
Morphine	10	30	SA: 3–6; LA: 8–12
Oxycodone	N/A	20	SA: 3–6; LA: 8–12
Hydrocodone	N/A	30	SA: 4–6; LA: 8–12
Hydromorphone	1.5	7.5	SA: 3–6; LA: 18–24
Oxymorphone	1	10	SA: 4–8; LA: 12
Fentanyl	0.1	N/A	TD: 72
Codeine	75–120	130–200	4–6
Meperidine	100	300	2–4
Methadone	3.75	7.5	6–12 (for analgesia)
Dual-Action Opioid Agonists			
Tramadol	N/A	50	3–7
Tapentadol	N/A	100	4–6

IV, Intravenous; *LA*, long-acting; *N/A*, not applicable; *PO*, oral; *SA*, short-acting; *TD*, transdermal.

17. **What are some additional adverse effects and toxicities associated with opioid analgesics?**
    - Sedation
    - Constipation
    - Nausea and vomiting
    - Chronic dry mouth
    - Dry skin and pruritus
    - Increased pain sensitivity (hyperalgesia)
    - Neuroendocrine effects
    - Urinary retention
    - Thermoregulatory dysfunction

18. **What are early, late, and prolonged opioid withdrawal symptoms?**
    See Table 15.7.

19. **What is opioid-use disorder?**
    Opioid-use disorder is a problematic pattern of opioid use leading to clinically significant impairment or distress, defined by Diagnostic and Statistical Manual of Mental Disorders (DSM)-V if two or more of the following criteria are met:
    - Taking the opioid in larger amounts and for longer than intended
    - Wanting to cut down or quit but not being able to do it

Table 15.7 Early, Late, and Prolonged Opioid Withdrawal Symptoms.

EARLY (HOURS TO DAYS)	LATE (DAYS TO WEEKS)	PROLONGED (WEEKS TO MONTHS)
• Anxiety/restlessness • Rapid short respirations • Runny nose, tearing eyes, sweating • Insomnia • Dilated reactive pupils	• Runny nose, tearing eyes • Rapid breathing, yawning • Tremor, diffuse muscle spasms/aches • Piloerection • Nausea, vomiting, or diarrhea • Abdominal pain • Fever, chills • Increase in white blood cells if sudden withdrawal	• Irritability, fatigue • Bradycardia • Decreased body temperature • Craving • Insomnia

- Spending a lot of time obtaining the opioid
- Craving or a strong desire to use opioids
- Repeatedly unable to carry out major obligations at work or home from opioid use
- Continued use despite persistent or recurring social or interpersonal problems caused or made worse by opioid use
- Stopping or reducing important social, occupational, or recreational activities due to opioid use
- Recurrent use of opioids in physically hazardous situations
- Consistent use of opioids despite acknowledgement of persistent or recurrent physical or psychological difficulties from using opioids
- Tolerance
- Withdrawal

20. What factors increase the risk of developing an opioid use disorder?
- Family history of opioid-use disorder
- Age 18–25
- History of drug overdose
- Significant underlying psychiatric disorder such as major depression
- Magnitude of daily opioid dose (the greater the dose, the greater the risk)
- Duration of opioid prescription (the greater the duration, the greater the risk)

21. What are Morphine Milligram Equivalents?
To compare opioid doses, tools have been developed to equate different opioids into one standard value. This standard value is based on morphine and its potency, referred to as Morphine Milligram Equivalents (MME). MME measurement allows for direct comparison of different opioids by accounting for different potencies. Caution must be exercised when using these calculators to guide switching from one medication to another as equianalgesic doses are affected by a range of factors such as interpatient variability, drug tolerance, drug-drug interactions, genetics, renal or hepatic insufficiency, and patient age. It is recommended to begin with a 50% lower dose than the equianalgesic dose when changing drugs and then titrate to a safe/effective response (Table 15.8).

22. What is the magnitude of risk of opioid overdose or death based on MME?
As the daily dose of opioids increases, the risk of overdose increases. Relative to taking <19 MME/day, the adjusted hazard ratio for any overdose event (consisting of mostly nonfatal overdose) is:
- one and one-half times the risk for taking 20–49 MME/day
- over three times the risk for taking 50–99 MME/day
- nearly nine times the risk for taking ≥100 MME/day

Table 15.8 Morphine Milligram Equivalent Doses for Commonly Prescribed Opioids.

OPIOID	CONVERSION FACTOR
Codeine	0.15
Fentanyl transdermal (in mcg/hr)	2.4
Hydrocodone	1
Hydromorphone	4
Methadone	
• 1–20 mg/day	4
• 21–40 mg/day	8
• 41–60 mg/day	10
• ≥61–80 mg/day	12
Morphine	1
Oxycodone	1.5
Oxymorphone	3
Tramadol	0.1

A similar pattern is found for serious overdose with a dose-dependent association with risk of overdose death. Relative to taking 1–19 MME/day, the adjusted odds ratio of dying from an opioid overdose is:
- nearly one and one-half times the risk for taking 20–49 MME/day
- nearly twice the risk for taking 50–99 MME/day
- over twice the risk for taking 100–199 MME/day
- nearly three times the risk for taking ≥200 MME/day

23. **What information should be disclosed to the patient prior to prescribing opioids?**
    - Receive controlled medications from only one prescriber and fill prescriptions at only one pharmacy.
    - Keep the medication in a secure location, preferably locked.
    - Your body may become used to the drug (physical dependence) and stopping the drug may make you miss it or feel sick.
    - Opioids can cause your body to develop an enhanced pain response to noxious stimuli (hyperalgesia) and pain elicited by innocuous stimuli (allodynia) called opioid-induced pain sensitivity.
    - You will likely develop tolerance and need more medication to get the same effect.
    - There is a risk of opioid dependence when taking this medication.
    - Take the medication exactly as shown on the label and not more frequently or less frequently.
    - An overdose of this medicine can slow or stop your breathing and even lead to death. You may experience adverse effects such as confusion, drowsiness, slowed breathing, nausea, vomiting, constipation, and dry mouth.
    - Avoid alcohol and other drugs that are not part of the treatment plan (e.g., benzodiazepines) because they may worsen adverse effects and increase risk of overdose. Be careful when driving or operating heavy machinery. Opioids may slow your reaction time.
    - Do not share medication with anyone.
    - Return or properly dispose of unused medication.

24. **What are some recommendations to clinicians who are treating adult patients with chronic pain and opioid use in an outpatient setting?**
    See Box 15.1.

Box 15.1 CDC Recommendations for Prescribing Opioids for Chronic Pain Outside of Active Cancer, Palliative, and End-of-Life Care.

Determining When to Initiate or Continue Opioids for Chronic Pain

1. Consider opioid therapy only if expected benefits for both pain and function are considered to outweigh risks to the patient, as nonpharmacologic therapy and nonopioid therapy are preferable.
2. Prior to starting opioid therapy for chronic pain, establish treatment goals, and continue opioid therapy only if there is clinically meaningful improvement in pain and function that outweighs risks to patient safety.
3. Clinicians should discuss with patients the known risks and realistic benefits as well as patient and clinician responsibilities regarding opioid therapy.

Opioid Selection, Dosage, Duration, Follow-Up, and Discontinuation

4. Prescribe immediate-release opioids instead of extended-release/long-acting (ER/LA) opioids when initiating therapy.
5. When initiating opioid therapy, prescribe the lowest effective dose. Use caution when prescribing opioids at any dosage, and carefully reassess the benefits and risks when increasing dosage to ≥50 morphine milligram equivalents (MME)/day and avoid increasing the dose to 90 MME/day unless this decision is carefully justified.
6. For treatment of acute pain, prescribe the lowest effective dose of immediate-release opioids and limit the quantity to cover the expected duration of severe pain (3 days or less will often be sufficient; more than 7 days will rarely be needed).
7. Evaluate the benefits and harms within 1–4 weeks of starting opioid therapy for chronic pain or after dose escalation. Evaluate the benefits and harms of continued therapy with patients every 3 months or more frequently. If benefits do not outweigh harms of continued opioid therapy, the clinician should optimize other therapies and work with patients to taper opioids to lower dosages or to taper and discontinue opioids.

Assessing Risk and Addressing Harms of Opioid Use

8. Prior to initiating and periodically during opioid therapy, clinicians should evaluate for factors that increase risk for opioid overdose, such as history of overdose or substance abuse disorder, opioid dosages ≥50 MME/day, or concurrent benzodiazepine use, and consider offering naloxone when such factors are present.
9. Clinicians should review the patient's history of controlled substance prescriptions using state prescription drug monitoring program (PDMP) data to determine whether the patient is receiving opioid dosages or dangerous combinations that put the patient at high risk for overdose.

Box 15.1 CDC Recommendations for Prescribing Opioids for Chronic Pain Outside of Active Cancer, Palliative, and End-of Life Care. *(Continued)*

10. Clinicians should use urine drug testing prior to starting opioid therapy and consider urine drug testing at least annually to assess for prescribed medications as well as other controlled prescription drugs and illicit drugs.
11. Clinicians should avoid prescribing opioid pain medication and benzodiazepines concurrently whenever possible.
12. Clinicians should offer or arrange evidence-based treatment (usually medication-assisted treatment with buprenorphine or methadone in combination with behavioral therapies) for patients with opioid use disorder.

Adapted from Dowell D, Haegerich TM, Chou R. CDC guideline for prescribing opioids for chronic pain—United States, 2016. MMWR Recomm Rep 2016;65:1.

Table 15.9 Pharmacologic Management for Acute, Subacute, and Chronic Axial Nonradiating Spinal Pain.

PHARMACOLOGIC MANAGEMENT	Duration of Axial Nonradiating Spinal Pain		
	ACUTE	SUBACUTE OR CHRONIC	ACUTE EXACERBATION OF CHRONIC
Acetaminophen	R	DNR	IE
NSAIDs	R	R	R
Nonbenzodiazepine skeletal muscle relaxant	R	DNR	R
Benzodiazepine	DNR	DNR	DNR
Antidepressant	IE	R	IE
Systemic steroids	DNR	DNR	DNR
Gabapentinoids	IE	IE	IE
Opioids	R[a]	DNR	DNR
Topical agents	IE	IE	IE

[a]Opioids should not be considered first-line medication for any spinal pain. Use lowest effective dose, immediate-release instead of extended-release/long-acting opioids, and dosing should not exceed ≥50 MME/day.
DNR, Do not recommend; *IE*, insufficient evidence; *NSAID*, nonsteroidal antiinflammatory drug; *R*, recommend.

25. **Summarize current recommendations regarding pharmacological treatment options for nonradiating axial spine pain, according to recent evidence-based guidelines.**
According to recent evidence-based guidelines, recommended pharmacologic treatment options for patients with acute or subacute low back pain include NSAIDs and skeletal muscle relaxants. For patients with chronic low back pain who do not respond to nonpharmacologic treatments, use of NSAIDs as first-line therapy, or tramadol or duloxetine as second-line therapy, is recommended. Opioids should only be considered for patients who do not respond to first- and second-line treatments and only if the potential benefits outweigh the risks for a specific patient, following a discussion of the risks and benefits of treatment (Table 15.9).

26. **Summarize the pharmacologic treatment recommendations for radiating axial spine pain according to recent systematic reviews.**
There is insufficient evidence to support a strong recommendation for the use of a particular medication for treatment of radiating axial pain. There is low level evidence supporting the use of gabapentinoids, and a lack of evidence supporting the effects of NSAIDs, systemic steroids, antidepressants, anticonvulsants, muscle relaxants, and opioid analgesics on pain intensity. In view of this uncertainty, factors which may be considered when selecting medication for radiating spine pain include duration of use, pain severity, patient age, concomitant medications, comorbidities, medication safety profile and side effects, as well as patient preference.

KEY POINTS

1. Acetaminophen and NSAIDs are first-line treatment for acute axial nonradiating spinal pain.
2. There is moderate evidence to support the use of nonbenzodiazepines muscle relaxants for acute or acute exacerbation of chronic axial nonradiating spinal pain, although the evidence indicates benefit is limited to short-term use of 7–14 days. There is no evidence to suggest benefit for chronic spinal pain.
3. Duloxetine or tramadol are recommended for treatment of chronic axial nonradiating spinal pain. TCAs may also be considered for use in certain patients with axial nonradiating spinal pain.

KEY POINTS—cont'd

4. There is insufficient evidence to support a specific recommendation regarding pharmacologic management of patients with axial radiating spinal pain.
5. There is insufficient evidence to recommend for or against the use of gabapentinoids for acute or chronic axial nonradiating or radiating spinal pain.
6. Systemic steroids should not be prescribed for patients with acute or subacute low back pain, even with radicular symptoms.
7. Opioids are not first-line treatments for acute spinal pain. Opioids should be prescribed for a short period only after failure of other pharmacologic and nonpharmacologic interventions for acute severe pain. There is no literature supporting the long-term use of opioids for treatment of chronic spinal pain.
8. CDC recommends caution when prescribing opioids at any dosage; carefully reassess risks and benefits when increasing dosage to ≥50 MME/day; and avoid increasing dosage to ≥90 MME/day.

Websites

1. AAOS Opioid Tool kit: https://www.aaos.org/Quality/PainReliefToolkit/?ssopc=1
2. American Pain Society Clinical Practical Guidelines: http://americanpainsociety.org/education/guidelines/overview
3. Calculator opioid dose: https://www.cdc.gov/drugoverdose/pdf/calculating_total_daily_dose-a.pdf
4. CDC guidelines for prescribing opioids: https://www.cdc.gov/drugoverdose/prescribing/guideline.html
5. DEA schedule changes: https://www.deadiversion.usdoj.gov/schedules/#define
6. International Association for the Study of Pain: https://www.iasp-pain.org/
7. New York City Health Department—opioid prescribing: https://www.nyc.gov/site/doh/providers/health-topics/opioid-prescribing.page
8. Oxford League Table of Analgesics in Acute Pain. Bandolier website at: http://www.bandolier.org.uk/booth/painpag/Acutrev/Analgesics/Leagtab.html
9. Prescription Drug Monitoring Program by State: https://www.deadiversion.usdoj.gov/faq/rx_monitor.htm
10. VA/DoD Clinical practice guideline for diagnosis and treatment of low back pain. 2017: https://www.healthquality.va.gov/guidelines/Pain/lbp/VADoDLBPCPG092917.pdf

---

BIBLIOGRAPHY

1. Chou, R., Deyo, R., Friedly, J., Skelly, A., Weimer, M., Fu, R., et al. (2017). Systemic pharmacologic therapies for low back pain: A systematic review for an American College of Physicians clinical practice guideline. *Annals of Internal Medicine, 166*(7), 480–493.
2. Dowell, D., Haegerich, T. M., & Chou, R. (2016). CDC guideline for prescribing opioids for chronic pain—United States. *MMWR Recommendations and Reports, 65*(1), 1–49.
3. Frieden, T. R., & Houry, D. (2016). Reducing the risks of relief—the CDC opioid-prescribing guideline. *New England Journal of Medicine, (16)*, 1501–1504.
4. Lewis, R. A., Williams, N., Sutton, A. J., Burton, K., Din, N. U., Matar, H. E., et al. (2015). Comparative clinical effectiveness of management strategies for sciatica: Systematic review and network meta-analyses. *Spine Journal, 15*(6), 1461–1477.
5. Ong, C. K. S., Lirk, P., Tan, C. H., & Seymour, R. A. (2007). An evidence-based update on nonsteroidal antiinflammatory drugs. *Clinical Medicine & Research, 5*(1), 19–34.
6. Pinto, R., Maher, C., Ferreira, M., Ferreira, P. H., Hancock, M., Oliveira, V. C., et al. (2012). Drugs for relief of pain in patients with sciatica: Systematic review and meta-analysis. *BMJ, 344,* 497.
7. Pinto, R. Z., Verwoerd, A. J. H., & Koes, B. W. (2017). Which pain medications are effective for sciatica (radicular leg pain)? *BMJ, 359,* 4248.
8. Qaseem, A., Wilt, T. J., McLean, R. M., & Forciea, M. A. (2017). Noninvasive treatments for acute, subacute, and chronic low back pain: A clinical practice guideline from the American College of Physicians. *Annals of Internal Medicine, 166*(7), 514–530.
9. Rasmussen-Barr, E., Held, U., Grooten, W. J., Roelofs, P. D., Koes, B. W., van Tulder, M. W., et al. (2017). Nonsteroidal anti-inflammatory drugs for sciatica: *An updated Cochrane review. Spine, 42*(8), 586–594.

CHAPTER 16

DIAGNOSTIC AND THERAPEUTIC SPINAL INJECTIONS

Vincent J. Devlin, MD

GENERAL CONSIDERATIONS

1. **What specialists perform diagnostic and therapeutic spinal injections?**
   A diverse community of physicians from many specialties perform spinal injections including anesthesiologists, physiatrists, interventional radiologists, neurologists, and spine surgeons.

2. **What is the preferred setting for performing spinal injections?**
   The preferred setting for both diagnostic and therapeutic spinal injections is the sterile environment of an outpatient/ambulatory surgery suite or hospital operating room. Fluoroscopy is used to improve accuracy, safety, and efficacy of injections. Monitoring, including pulse oximetry, blood pressure, and pulse rate, should be performed during the procedure and during the recovery period in case of an adverse reaction to the injected local anesthetic or intravenous sedation. Emergency resuscitating equipment, including crash carts, should be available.

3. **What are the pain generators of the spine?**
   Symptoms of axial and radicular pain may be attributed to pathology involving bone, spinal soft tissues (muscles, ligaments, and tendons), intervertebral discs, facet joints, sacroiliac joints, and neurologic structures (spinal cord and nerve roots). The interventional pain physician uses injection techniques in an attempt to identify a specific pain generator responsible for a patient's symptoms and guide subsequent treatment. It may be challenging or impossible to identify a specific pain generator in the setting of diffuse age-related degenerative spinal pathology. Consensus regarding the scientific basis for a single pain generator to explain the morbidity of chronic axial pain does not exist. The major pain generators of the spine include:
   Soft tissue spinal structures: Pain from injury to spinal soft tissue structures including muscles, tendons, and ligaments are the most common disorders responsible for neck and low back pain. This diagnosis is generally based on clinical assessment without the need for interventional procedures. Soft tissue injuries may be classified as strains or sprains, but are more commonly referred to as nonspecific neck or low back pain.
   Intervertebral discs: Displaced disc material can impinge on the spinal cord or nerve roots and cause axial and/or radiating pain involving the extremities. Evidence also suggests that the disc itself can cause pain in the absence of neural compression, which is termed **discogenic pain**. Histologic studies demonstrate the presence of nerve endings throughout the outer third of the annulus fibrosus. These nerve endings are branches of the sinuvertebral nerves, the gray rami communicantes, and the lumbar ventral rami. Annular tears may result from injury or degeneration. These fissures in the outer margins of the annulus may lead to pain due to mechanical or chemical irritation of these small nerve endings.
   Facet joints (zygapophyseal joints or *z-joints*) are paired synovial joints in the posterior column of the spine, which are innervated by medial branches of primary dorsal rami. Lumbar facet pathology may result in referred pain involving the buttock, groin, hip, or thigh. Cervical facet joint pathology can manifest as neck pain, referred pain involving the scapular area, or headaches.
   Sacroiliac joints are a potential pain generator due to the presence of nociceptors within and adjacent to these joints. However, clinical diagnosis and appropriate treatment remains controversial.

4. **List the basic interventional spine procedures.**
   Epidural injections, medial branch nerve blocks, intraarticular facet joint injections, discography, and sacroiliac joint injections.

EPIDURAL INJECTIONS

5. **What are the indications for epidural injections?**
   Treatment of radicular symptoms secondary to disc herniation is the most common and well-supported indication for epidural steroid injections. Epidural steroid injections are also a treatment option for patients with radicular symptoms due to neuroforaminal stenosis or central canal stenosis. Limited evidence supports the role of epidural injections for treatment of axial pain. Epidural injections are also used to aid in localization of symptomatic spinal levels and for treatment of ongoing radicular and/or axial pain following spine surgery.

6. **What are some contraindications to epidural injections?**
   Absolute contraindications for epidural steroid injections include: a bleeding disorder or requirement for maintenance on a therapeutic dose of an anticoagulant; systemic or local infection at the injection site; history of significant allergic or hypersensitivity reaction to injected medications or contrast agents; tumor at the injection site;
   and lack of informed consent. Relative contraindications include uncontrolled diabetes mellitus, congestive heart
   failure, hypertension, pregnancy, and patients with unrealistic expectations and goals regarding treatment.

7. **What is the composition of the injectate delivered into the epidural space?**
   The composition of the injectate varies and may include a corticosteroid, local anesthetic, or normal saline, either
   singly or in combination. Corticosteroids are used in epidural injections because of their inhibitory effects on
   cytokines and chemokines generated at sites of inflammation, as well as their suppressive effects on leukocyte
   distribution, aggregation, and function, but are not approved by the US Food and Drug Administration (FDA) for this
   indication. Corticosteroids used for epidural injections differ with respect to microscopic particle size, solubility,
   and duration of effect, and are classified as particulate (methylprednisolone, triamcinolone and betamethasone) or
   nonparticulate (dexamethasone). As particulate steroids are insoluble in water, these medications may bind and
   form sizeable aggregates, increasing the risk of blood vessel occlusion. The potential for particulate steroids to
   embolize following inadvertent intravascular injection and occlude terminal blood vessels in the brain or spinal
   cord has been linked to catastrophic neurologic injuries, particularly following transforaminal epidural injections.

8. **Describe the different approaches for injections into the epidural space.**
   After the skin at the needle entry point is infiltrated with a local anesthetic, a spinal needle is advanced towards
   the epidural space under fluoroscopic guidance via an interlaminar, transforaminal, or caudal approach.
   The **interlaminar approach** is an option for cervical, thoracic, and lumbar epidural injections (Fig. 16.1A,B).
   Epidural needles are directed between the lamina via a midline or paramedian approach. As the needle penetrates
   the ligamentum flavum, the epidural space is identified by the loss-of-resistance method and fluoroscopy is used
   to check depth of needle insertion. A small amount of contrast is used to assess epidural distribution and confirm
   the absence of intrathecal, subdural, or intravascular injection. Typically 5–10 mL of corticosteroid and local
   anesthetic solution is injected in the lumbar spine. In the cervical and thoracic spine, 2–5 mL is injected. The
   injectate is delivered to the posterior epidural space, and indirect spread to the anterior epidural space is anticipated. It is recommended that cervical interlaminar epidural injections be performed at C7–T1 and not higher than
   C6–7 as the epidural space narrows proximally. An interlaminar injection is not recommended at the site of prior
   posterior spine surgery or in patients with severe central stenosis.
   The **transforaminal approach** is an option for all spinal regions. It uses an oblique needle trajectory to
   inject medication into the epidural space within the lateral aspect neuroforamen. This approach delivers the
   injectate to the anterior epidural space and targets the region where the disc contacts the nerve root (Fig. 16.2).
   Transforaminal injections should be performed only under real-time fluoroscopic guidance for accuracy and
   safety reasons. A small amount of contrast is used to confirm spread of contrast medially and adjacent to the
   pedicle, as well as laterally and distally along the exiting spinal nerve, and to confirm the absence of intravascular injection. When available, use of digital subtraction imaging can increase the ability to detect vascular uptake
   of contrast medium. Because the medication is placed directly at the target nerve root, less volume is required
   to achieve pain relief. In the lumbar spine, 3–5 mL of corticosteroid and local anesthetic solution is injected.

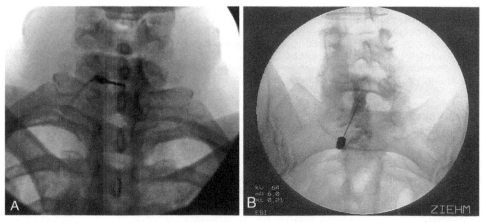

Fig. 16.1 (A) Cervical epidural-interlaminar approach, C7–T1. (B) Lumbar epidural-interlaminar approach. (A: From House L, Barette K, Ryan M, et al. Cervical epidural steroid injection. Phys Med Rehabil Clin N Am 2018;29:1–17, Fig. 3.)

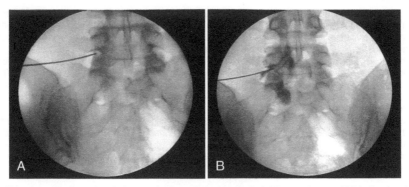

Fig. 16.2 (A) Lumbar epidural-transforaminal approach. The needle is placed in the left L5 neuroforamen. (B) Injection of contrast shows epidural dye flow.

In the cervical and thoracic spine, 1–1.5 mL is required to adequately block the target nerve root. Nonparticulate corticosteroids are recommended for all cervical transforaminal injections and for initial lumbar transforaminal injections.

The **caudal approach** is the safest approach for injection into the lumbar epidural space and has the lowest risk of dural puncture. The needle is inserted between the sacral cornu into the sacral hiatus, which leads to the caudal epidural space. The drawback of this approach is the large volume of injection required to reach the target area in the lumbar spine. Frequently, 10–15 mL of corticosteroid and local anesthetic solution is needed to achieve pain relief.

An epidural catheter may be used to deliver medication to the lumbar spine in patients with a history of spine surgery (Fig. 16.3). Various manufacturers offer epidural catheters specifically designed for pain procedures. An introducer needle is placed caudally, and the flexible epidural catheter is advanced cephalad to the target. These catheters can also be steered to the left or right to reach the target area. By using a catheter, less volume is necessary to achieve pain relief if the catheter tip is in close proximity to the target area.

9. What are some potential complications associated with epidural injections?
The most common adverse events encountered following epidural injections are side effects due to steroids, increased pain, and vasovagal reaction. However, serious and even catastrophic adverse events may occur including:
- **Allergic reaction** to injected medications, contrast material, or topical antiseptics.
- **Bleeding:** Hematoma may develop in superficial tissue sites or in the epidural space. This risk is elevated in patients with coagulopathy or liver disease, or in patients maintained on anticoagulant medications.
- **Infection:** Multiple factors may cause infection including translocation of skin organisms, violation of aseptic technique, or injection of contaminated medications. The risk of infection is elevated in diabetic and immunocompromised patients.

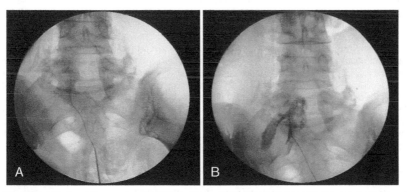

Fig. 16.3 (A) Lumbar epidural-caudal approach using epidural catheter. Note that the patient had previous decompression and fusion. The catheter tip is in the vicinity of the left L5 neuroforamen. (B) Injection of contrast showing epidural dye flow and left L5 and S1 radiculogram.

- **Dural puncture and subarachnoid injection:** Spinal headache may occur due to spinal fluid leak secondary to inadvertent dural puncture. In some cases, the dural puncture site seals by itself with bedrest. An epidural blood patch is the treatment for persistent spinal headache. Medication intended for the epidural space that is injected into the subarachnoid space may lead to respiratory depression, arachnoiditis, and pain.
- **Intravascular injection:** Inadvertent vascular injection of anesthetic agents may lead to serious complications including catastrophic neurologic injuries or toxicity, leading to seizures, cardiac arrest, or even death. The advantages of the transforaminal approach must be weighed against the risk of spinal cord or brain infarction due to unrecognized intravascular injection, which is less likely to occur with caudal or translaminar approaches.
- **Neurologic complications:** These may result from direct penetrating trauma to the spinal cord or nerves, infarction of the spinal cord, brainstem, cerebrum, or cerebellum due to intravascular injection into a radicular artery, ischemia resulting from neural compression by hematoma, or neurotoxicity secondary to injected medications.
- **Miscellaneous complications:** Pneumothorax (following lung injury during thoracic or lower cervical injections) or bladder dysfunction (due to blockade of sacral nerve roots).

10. Discuss the systemic side effects of epidural corticosteroids.
    Specific adverse effects are associated with use of corticosteroid medications and are not unique to spinal corticosteroid injections. Dose-dependent side effects of corticosteroids include nausea, facial flushing, insomnia, low-grade fever (usually <100°F), and nonpositional headache. Following an epidural injection, hypo-thalamic-pituitary-adrenal axis suppression may occur depending on the steroid dose and last for several weeks. Corticosteroid-related immune suppression is associated with increased infection risk following surgery. Increased rates of postoperative infection have been reported if spine surgery is performed within 3 months of an epidural injection. Additional adverse effects associated with epidural corticosteroids include changes in fluid and electrolyte balance, elevated blood pressure, exacerbation of peptic ulcer disease, menstrual flow abnormalities, and allergic reaction. It is not uncommon to see elevation in blood glucose for 48–72 hours after a steroid injection. Multiple corticosteroid injections have been associated with additional adverse effects including decreased bone mineral density and avascular necrosis.

11. How often can epidural injections be repeated for treatment of an acute radicular pain syndrome?
    Recommendations regarding the timing and number of epidural injections vary. As a general guide, one to three epidural injections can be performed with an interval of at least 1 month between injections. Reevaluation by a physician after each injection is indicated to determine the need for additional procedures. If a patient does not respond to an initial technically accurate injection, repeating the same injection is not indicated. Pursuing a series of three epidural injections regardless of clinical response is not warranted. Current recommendations are to per-form no more than three epidural injections in a 6-month period and no more than four epidural injections in a 1-year period.

MEDIAL BRANCH NERVE BLOCKS AND FACET JOINT INJECTIONS

12. Explain the difference between a facet joint injection and a medial branch block.
    A painful facet joint can be blocked by injecting into the joint itself or by blocking the nerves that innervate the joint. Most facet joints receive innervation from medial branches of the dorsal rami of the spinal nerves above and below the joint. Because each facet joint is dually innervated, it can be blocked by injecting the medial branch above and below the joint. For example, the L4–5 facet joint is innervated at its upper aspect by medial branches from L3 and at its lower aspect by medial branches from L4. Therefore, two injections are necessary to block the innervation of this single facet joint (Fig. 16.4).

13. How does the innervation of the facet joints vary by spinal region?
    Standard nomenclature describes facet joints using a hyphen (i.e., L3–4 facet joint) and medial branch nerves us-ing a comma (i.e., L3,4 medial branches). Facet joints are typically innervated by two medial branches on each side—the medial branch from the spinal nerve above the joint and the medial branch from the spinal nerve below the joint. In the cervical region from C3–4 to C6–7, the medial branches that innervate the facet joints are num-bered similarly (i.e., the C5,6 medial branches innervate the C5–6 facet joints). As there are eight cervical nerves and only seven cervical vertebrae, the C7–T1 facet joints are innervated by the C7,8 medial branches. From T1–2 distally, the medial branches that supply the facet joints at each spinal level are numbered one less than the in-nervated joint (i.e., T7–8 facet joints are innervated by the T6,7 medial branches; L4–5 facet joints are innervated by the L3,4 medial branches).
    In the upper cervical region there is a different pattern of innervation. The atlanto-occipital (O-C1) and atlan-toaxial (C1–2) joints are innervated by the ventral rami of the corresponding spinal nerves. Diagnostic blocks at these levels are performed using intraarticular blocks. Innervation of the C2–3 facet joint is by a single nerve, the medial branch of the dorsal ramus of the C3 spinal nerve (third occipital nerve), and is blocked with injections in the region dorsal to the C2–3 facet joint.

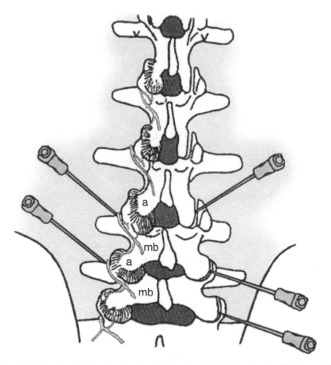

Fig. 16.4 Posterior view of lumbar spine showing location of medial branches *(mb)* of dorsal rami, which innervate lumbar facet joints *(a)*. Needle position for L3 and L4 medial branch blocks shown on left half of diagram would be used to anesthetize L4–5 facet joint. Right half of diagram shows L3–4, L4–5, and L5–S1 intraarticular facet joint injection positions. (From Canale S, Beaty J. Campbell's Operative Orthopedics. 11th ed. Philadelphia, PA: Mosby; 2007. Redrawn from Boduk N. Back pain: Zygapophyseal blocks and epidural steroids. In: Cousins MJ, Bridenbaugh PO, editors. Neural Blockade in Clinical Anesthesia and Management of Pain. 2nd ed. Philadelphia, PA: Lippincott; 1988.)

14. Briefly explain the role of diagnostic and therapeutic injections used to target pain attributed to the facet joint.

The spinal facet joints are recognized as a frequent source of axial pain and also play a role in cervicogenic headaches. It is not possible to reliably diagnose level specific–facet mediated pain solely on the basis of medical history, physical examination, or imaging tests, so physicians use anesthetic blocks. Based on studies that injected specific facet joints in normal and symptomatic subjects, pain maps have been created for the facet joints in all spinal regions, and serve as a diagnostic guide to depict the distribution of pain arising from specific spinal levels.

Intraarticular facet joint injections may be performed purely as a diagnostic block by injecting only local anesthetic or for therapeutic purposes by adding corticosteroid to the local anesthetic (Figs. 16.5 and 16.6). Although diagnostic intraarticular facet joint injections are commonly used for diagnostic purposes, this has not been validated. Similarly, therapeutic intraarticular facet joint injections are commonly used but their effectiveness has not been confirmed in rigorous clinical studies.

Medial branch nerve blocks are the most reliable way to diagnose facet-related pain for cervical levels below C3 and throughout the lumbar region. However, there is a notable false-positive rate (up to one-third of patients) with medial branch blocks, so controlled comparative blocks including placebo injections are necessary before diagnosis of facet joint pain can be confirmed. Two comparative medial branch blocks (performed on separate occasions using local anesthetics with different durations of actions) that are both positive and concordant with negative placebo control injections are necessary to confirm a specific facet joint as a pain generator. If the diagnosis of facet joint pain is confirmed, radiofrequency thermocoagulation of the medial branches of the identified facet joints can provide pain relief.

15. Explain what is involved in performance of a radiofrequency neurotomy.

Radiofrequency neurotomy is used to denervate a painful facet joint by thermocoagulation of the medial branches that supply sensation. To denervate a particular joint, the medial branch above and below the joint are treated. The insulated probe is inserted percutaneously to the target nerve tissue and connected to the generator, which supplies a radiofrequency current. This current generates heat in the surrounding tissues, creating a lesion that destroys the nerve tissue. Pain relief may last for 6–9 months following a single treatment (Fig. 16.7).

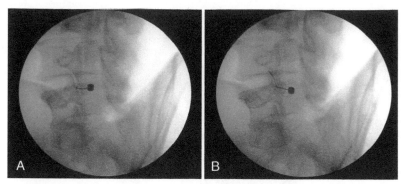

Fig. 16.5 (A) Lumbar facet injection. The needle is placed in the left L4–5 facet joint. (B) Injection of contrast shows dye flow into joint space, confirming the needle placement.

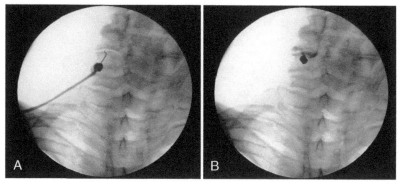

Fig. 16.6 (A) Cervical facet injection. The needle is placed in the cervical facet joint. (B) Injection of contrast confirms needle placement.

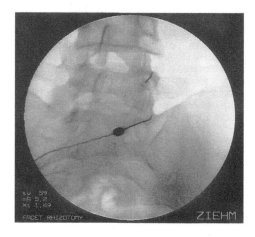

Fig. 16.7 Radiofrequency probe in position for L5 and S1 medial branch neurotomies.

INJECTIONS TARGETING THE INTERVERTEBRAL DISC

16. Describe pathophysiologic changes associated with discogenic pain.

Disc degeneration refers to abnormal disc morphology secondary to aging or injury. Discs that exhibit decreased signal intensity in their central region on a T2-weighted magnetic resonance imaging (MRI) are frequently termed *degenerative*. Not all degenerative discs are painful. In certain patients, it is thought that the disc becomes

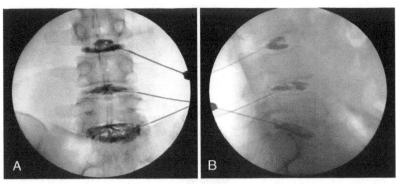

Fig. 16.8 (A) Lumbar discography, anteroposterior view. (B) Lateral view showing normal lobular nucleogram of the top disc and abnormal posterior fissures in the lower two discs.

sensitized and generates pain as a result of chemical or mechanical irritation. Histologic studies have demonstrated the presence of nerve endings throughout the outer third of the annulus fibrosus. These nerve endings are branches of the sinu-vertebral nerves, the gray rami communicantes, and the lumbar ventral rami. Phospholipase A_2, a known inflammatory mediator, is found in high levels in the intervertebral disc. Chemical irritation is most likely due to leaking of inflammatory mediators, such as phospholipase A_2, from the nucleus with subsequent irritation of nerve endings in the annulus.

17. **What is provocative discography?**
Provocative discography is a test used to identify a painful intervertebral disc. It is most commonly used in the lumbar spine, but its use has also been reported in the cervical and thoracic regions. Using a double needle technique, a thin needle is placed percutaneously into the center of the disc in an awake patient. Once appropriate needle placement is confirmed, a small amount of fluid (usually a water-soluble contrast dye) is injected into the center of the targeted discs. As the contrast is injected, the lateral fluoroscopic projection is used to monitor the contrast pattern. In theory, if the particular disc is a source of pain, the patient will experience the familiar type of axial or arm/leg pain as pressure increases within the disc upon injection of fluid. The patient is asked to rate the degree of pain on an analog scale for each injected disc level, and to report whether the pain experienced during injection is the typical pain for which he or she is seeking relief. The volume of fluid injected is recorded for each disc level. The resistance of each disc to injection and the quality of the endpoint with injection are recorded. A disc with an intact annulus will have a high resistance to injection and a firm endpoint. A severely degenerated disc is likely to have reduced resistance to injection and almost no endpoint as the contrast leaks out of the disc without pressurizing the disc. Manometry may be used to monitor pressure as dye is injected, to record the opening pressure, and the pressure at which pain is reproduced. In addition to the suspected disc(s), at least one adjacent disc is tested as a control. Injection of normal discs is not generally associated with pain.

Postdiscography images are recorded as plain x-rays (Fig. 16.8) or as a computed tomography (CT) scan to document the contrast dye pattern (nucleogram). Nucleograms can be described as cotton ball, lobular, irregular, fissured, or ruptured (Fig. 16.9). Cotton ball and lobular nucleogram patterns are considered normal. As the disc degenerates, nucleograms deteriorate from irregular to fissured, and finally to a ruptured pattern.

18. **What criteria are used to make the diagnosis of discogenic pain based on provocative discography?**
To diagnose discogenic pain, one must document evidence of disc degeneration on a nucleogram and concordant pain during injection of the target disc. The sole purpose of discography is to identify painful intervertebral discs. At least one normal-appearing adjacent disc is tested as a control. A valid test requires the absence of pain in the control disc. It has been observed that some discs can be made painful if sufficient pressure is applied. False-positive results can be reduced by using manometry to record pressure during discography. Some criteria suggested for diagnosis of lumbar discogenic pain using manometry include:
1. Stimulation of the suspected disc reproduces concordant or familiar pain.
2. The pain reproduced is registered as at least 7 on a 10-point visual analog scale.
3. The pain reproduced occurs at a pressure less than 50 psi or less than 15 psi above the opening pressure. (Opening pressure is defined as the amount of pressure that must be exerted to start the flow of contrast into the disc.)
4. Stimulation of adjacent discs provides controls such that when only one adjacent disc can be stimulated, that disc is painless or pain from that disc is not concordant, and is produced at a pressure greater than 15 psi above opening pressure.

Discogram type		Degeneration
1. Cottonball	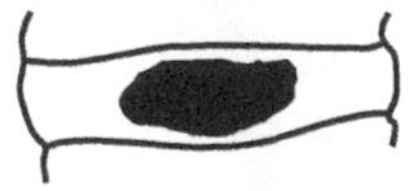	No signs of degeneration. Soft white amorphous nucleus
2. Lobular	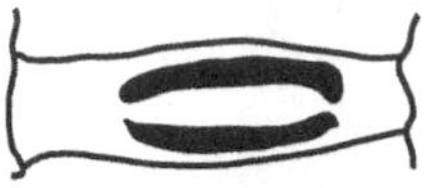	Mature disc with nucleus starting to coalesce into fibrous lumps
3. Irregular	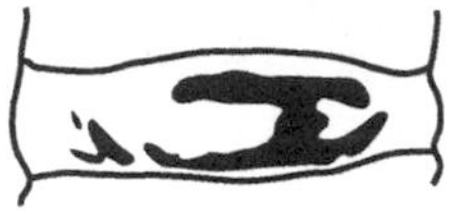	Degenerated disc with fissures and clefts in the nucleus and inner annulus
4. Fissured	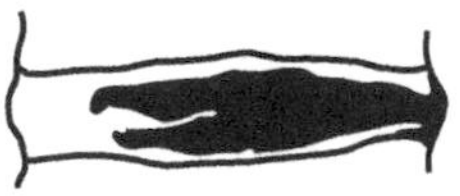	Degenerated disc with radial fissure leading to the outer edge of the annulus
5. Ruptured	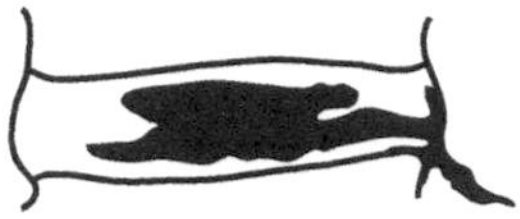	Disc has a complete radial fissure that allows injected fluid to escape. Can be in any state of degeneration.

Fig. 16.9 The five types of discogram and the stages of disc degeneration that they represent. (From Adams M, Dolan P, Hutton W. The stages of disc degeneration as revealed by discograms. J Bone Joint Surg 1986;68:36–41.)

19. Discuss the controversy surrounding provocative discography.

Discography remains a controversial test. Proponents of discography opine that disc morphology on MRI cannot be used to distinguish a painful disc from asymptomatic age-appropriate degenerative changes as justification for this test. Opponents of discography cite a high percentage of false-positive results with discography in patients with psychological distress, chronic pain syndromes, increased somatic awareness, annular disruption, and individuals involved in litigation or workers' compensation cases. In addition, provocative discography has not been shown to improve treatment outcomes for patients with axial pain syndromes and may lead to unnecessary and ineffective spinal surgery. Use of discography to identify candidates for surgical treatment, such as a lumbar fusion, remains controversial.

20. What are some possible complications of discography?

Nausea, headache, and increased pain may occur but are typically limited and readily treatable. Discitis is a serious common complication, with an incidence of less than 1%. False-positive discograms may lead to misdiagnosis and set off a cascade of inappropriate and/or ineffective invasive treatments. Other complications relate to misplacement of the needle, including nerve injury, dural puncture, and bowel perforation. Accelerated progression of disc degeneration following discography is also a concern.

21. What are some treatment options for discogenic pain?

There is no consensus concerning the optimal treatment of discogenic pain. Nonsurgical treatment options include therapeutic exercise, medications, injections, and use of a lumbar support. Surgical treatment options include spinal fusion and disc replacement surgery.

SACROILIAC INJECTIONS

22. When are sacroiliac (SI) joint injections indicated?

Patient history and physical examination have shown low reliability in diagnosing SI joint pain. In patients with low back, buttock, or groin pain not attributed to other causes, SI joint pain can be considered in the differential diagnosis. The clinical diagnosis of SI joint pain is supported when a patient demonstrates positive responses to at least three of the following examination maneuvers: FABER (flexion, abduction, and external hip rotation), thigh

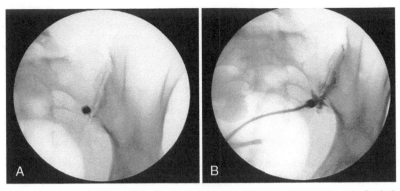

Fig. 16.10 (A) Sacroiliac joint injection. The needle is placed in the joint space. (B) Injection of contrast shows dye flow in the joint space, confirming needle placement.

trust, Gaenslen test, distraction, sacral thrust, and compression test. No radiographic or CT findings are diagnostic for SI joint pain.

An analgesic response to a fluoroscopically or CT-guided diagnostic SI joint block is considered the most reliable test to diagnose SI joint–mediated pain. Several injection techniques have been described. One common technique involves positioning the patient in the prone oblique position to facilitate visualization of the inferior portion of the joint. A 22-gauge spinal needle is placed in the inferior aspect of the joint, and a small amount of contrast is injected to confirm needle position. Then a small amount of corticosteroid, combined with a local anesthetic, is injected (Fig. 16.10). Extraarticular SI joint blocks that target the lateral branches of the sacral nerve roots have also been described. These extraarticular blocks are used to screen for candidates who could benefit from RF ablation of these nerves to provide relief of SI pain.

INJECTIONS TO ASSESS CONDITIONS WHICH MIMIC SPINAL PATHOLOGY

23. What injection techniques can help identify other pain generators that mimic cervical and lumbar pathology?
    Symptoms due to various types of shoulder pathology may overlap symptoms of a cervical spine disorder. Careful examination of the shoulder joint should always be performed in a patient presenting with neck pain. Diagnostic injections into the subacromial space, glenohumeral joint, and/or the acromioclavicular joint can help differentiate pain originating from the shoulder region from pain originating in the cervical spine.

    Degenerative arthritis of the hip joint may present with symptoms that mimic an upper lumbar disc herniation or spinal stenosis. Injection of the hip joint with a local anesthetic under fluoroscopic, CT, or ultrasound guidance can help differentiate hip and spine pathology.

KEY POINTS

1. Access options for epidural injections include translaminar, transforaminal, and caudal approaches.
2. Medial branch nerve blocks are the most reliable way to diagnose facet-related pain.
3. Use of provocative discography in the management of axial pain syndromes remains controversial.
4. An analgesic response to a properly performed diagnostic SI joint block is considered the most reliable test to diagnose SI join–mediated pain.

Websites
1. Discography: http://emedicine.medscape.com/article/1145703-overview
2. Epidural steroid injections: http://emedicine.medscape.com/article/325733-overview
3. Injection, sacroiliac: treatment and medication: http://emedicine.medscape.com/article/103399-treatment
4. Paraspinal injections—facet joint and nerve root blocks: http://emedicine.medscape.com/article/345382-overview
5. Safe Use Initiative: epidural steroid injections: https://www.fda.gov/Drugs/DrugSafety/SafeUseInitiative/ucm434387.htm#esi

BIBLIOGRAPHY

1. Adams, M. A., Dolan, P., & Hutton, W. (1986). The stages of disc degeneration as revealed by discograms. *Journal of Bone and Joint Surgery, 68,* 36–41.
2. Carragee, E. J., & Stauff, M. (2018). Discography. In S. R. Garfin, F. J. Eismont, & G. R. Bell, et al., (Eds.), *Rothman-Simeoone the Spine* (7th ed., pp. 301–314). Philadelphia, PA: Saunders.
3. El-Yahchouchi, C. A., Plastaras, C. T., Maus, T. P., Carr, C. M., McCormick, Z. L., Geske, J. R., et al. (2016). Adverse event rates associated with transforaminal and interlaminar epidural steroid injections: A multi-institutional study. *Pain Medicine, 17,* 239–247.
4. Kennedy, D. J., Engel, A., Kreiner, D. S., Nampiaparampil, D., Duszynski, B., & MacVicar, J. (2015). Fluoroscopically guided diagnostic and therapeutic intra-Articular sacroiliac joint injections: Systematic review. *Pain Medicine, 16,* 1500–1518.
5. King, W., & Borowczyk, J. M. (2011). Zygapophysial joint pain: Procedures for diagnosis and treatment. In T. A. Lennard, S. Walkowski, A. K. Singla, et al. (Eds.), *Pain Procedures in Clinical Practice* (3rd ed., pp. 357–389). Philadelphia, PA: Elsevier.
6. Radcliff, K., Kepler, C., Hilibrand, A., Rihn, J., Zhao, W., Lurie, J., et al. (2013). Epidural steroid injections are associated with less improvement in patients with lumbar spinal stenosis: A subgroup analysis of the Spine Patient Outcomes Research Trial. *Spine, 38,* 279–291.
7. Rathmell, J. P., Benzon, H. T., Dreyfuss, P., Huntoon, M., Wallace, M., Baker, R., et al. (2015). Safeguards to prevent neurologic complications after epidural steroid injections. *Anesthesiology, 122,* 974–984.
8. Soto, D. A., & Loperena, E. O. (2018). Sacroiliac joint interventions. *Physical Medicine and Rehabilitation Clinics of North America, 29,* 171–183.
9. Singla, A., Yang, S., Werner, B. C., Cancienne, J. M., Nourbakhsh, A., Shimer, A. L., et al. (2017). The impact of preoperative epidural injections on postoperative infection in lumbar fusion. *Journal of Neurosurgery Spine, 26,* 645–649.
10. Young, I. A., Hyman, G., Packia-Raj, L., & Cole, A. J. (2007). The use of lumbar epidural/transforaminal steroids for managing spinal disease. *Journal of the American Academy of Orthopaedic Surgeons, 15,* 228–238.

CHAPTER 17

ELECTRODIAGNOSIS IN SPINAL DISORDERS

Paul M. Kitei, MD, Sayed E. Wahezi, MD, and Mark A. Thomas, MD

1. List the common reasons for requesting electrodiagnostic tests for the evaluation of patients with spinal disorders.
   - *To establish and/or confirm a clinical diagnosis.* Electrodiagnostic tests (EDX) may help determine whether extremity symptoms are due to radiculopathy, peripheral entrapment neuropathy, or polyneuropathy.
   - *To localize nerve lesions.* EDX can assist in differentiation between root lesions (radiculopathy), brachial or lumbosacral plexus lesions (plexopathy), and peripheral nerve lesions (entrapment neuropathy). EDX can help distinguish central lesions (e.g., motor neuron disease) from peripheral neuropathy and spinal stenosis.
   - *To determine the severity and extent of nerve injury.* EDX can differentiate myelin injury (conduction block or neurapraxia) from either axonal degeneration alone (axonotmesis) or axonal degeneration along with damage to a nerve's supporting structures (neurotmesis). EDX can help to determine whether a lesion is acute or chronic, progressive or improving, and preganglionic or postganglionic. EDX can provide information regarding prognosis and a timeline for recovery after nerve injury. It is the only diagnostic test that assesses the *function* of a nerve.
   - *To correlate findings noted on spinal imaging studies.* EDX may help determine whether an abnormality noted on spinal magnetic resonance imaging (MRI) is contributing to a patient's neurologic complaints.
   - *To provide documentation in medicolegal settings.*

2. When should EDX be avoided in the assessment of patients with spinal disorders?
   - *During the first 2–4 weeks after symptom onset.* During this time many EDX findings are difficult to detect, and testing is not recommended, unless a baseline study for comparison would be useful.
   - *When the diagnosis of radiculopathy is unequivocal.* EDX adds little to the treatment plan.
   - *When findings will not change medical or surgical management.* For example, patients with extreme illness, patients who refuse treatment, or patients with isolated neck or back pain without radiculopathy.
   - *Patients with potential contraindications to EDX testing.* For example, anticoagulated patients whose needle electromyography (EMG) test would require studying muscles that are not easily compressible in the case of bleeding; patients with open skin lesions; or patients with pacemakers and defibrillators whose nerve conduction studies (NCS) would require studying nerves near the pacemaker and pacing leads.

3. What are the basic components of an electrodiagnostic examination?
   EDX is an extension of the history and physical examination. Its goal is to help differentiate the variety of causes for numbness, weakness, and pain. The standard EDX examination consists of two parts: EMG and NCS.
   EMG (needle electrode examination) uses a needle "antenna" to detect and record electrical activity directly from a muscle. The distribution of abnormalities is used to identify the site of nerve or muscle pathology. **EMG is the most useful electrodiagnostic test for the evaluation of radiculopathy**. Muscles are assessed at rest and during contraction to evaluate four characteristics:
   1. *Insertional activity:* EMG needle insertion into normal muscle generates brief electrical discharges by muscle fibers.
   2. *Spontaneous activity:* In a normal relaxed muscle there should be no electrical activity.
   3. *Motor-unit action potentials:* Slight contraction of the target muscle generates motor unit action potentials which are assessed for amplitude, duration, and configuration.
   4. *Recruitment:* With more forceful muscle contraction of a normal muscle, a larger number of motor units are recruited and their firing rate increases.
   NCS record and analyze biological electrical waveforms elicited in response to a nonbiological electrical stimulus over a nerve or nerves. NCS assess the ability of a specific nerve or nerves to transmit an impulse between two sites along the nerve following an electrical stimulus. When NCS are abnormal, they provide information that a specific nerve is not conducting impulses properly in the measured nerve segment. Both sensory and motor NCS can be performed, allowing for the evaluation of sensory, motor, and mixed nerves. **NCS are most useful for diagnosis of peripheral entrapment neuropathy and peripheral neuropathy**. NCS are generally expected to be normal in radiculopathy. Specialized NCS—H-reflex, F-wave, and somatosensory evoked potentials (SEPs)—have limited value in specific clinical settings for diagnosis of radiculopathy (see questions 8–11).

4. **What is the anatomic basis for EDX as it relates to the assessment of spinal disorders?**

The purpose of the EDX is to assess the function of the peripheral sensory and motor nervous system. Each spinal nerve contains both motor and sensory fibers which contribute to the formation of a peripheral nerve. The cell bodies of the motor axons that comprise the ventrally exiting motor roots are situated within the anterior horn of the spinal cord (primary motor neurons). The cell bodies of the sensory axons (primary sensory neurons) are located outside the spinal cord within the dorsal root ganglion (DRG). The DRG are bipolar cells with central projections that form the sensory roots, which enter the dorsal aspect of the spinal cord, and peripheral projections, which continue as sensory nerve fibers in peripheral nerves. After the dorsal and ventral roots join to form the mixed spinal nerve, usually in the region of the intervertebral foramina, the mixed spinal nerve divides into anterior (ventral) and posterior (dorsal) rami. The anterior rami supply the anterior trunk muscles and, after entering the brachial or lumbosacral plexus, the muscles of the extremities. The posterior rami supply the paraspinal muscles and skin over the neck and trunk (Fig. 17.1).

Lesions can be classified as either *preganglionic* (localized to spinal cord or sensory nerve root proximal to the DRG) or *postganglionic* (localized anywhere along the motor nerve root, sensory nerve root distal to the DRG, brachial or lumbosacral plexuses, or peripheral nerves). Myelin lesions within the spinal canal (myelopathy, most radiculopathies) are undetectable with standard NCS studies, as it is impossible to stimulate proximally to these lesions. Axonal lesions within this same region compromise sensory fibers proximal to their cell bodies in the DRG. Such lesions do not affect the sensory NCS, because the injured sensory fibers degenerate centrally between the cell body in the DRG and the nerve root. Cells in the DRG continue to supply nutrition to the peripheral sensory fibers, thereby preserving sensory nerve conduction in this region, even though physical examination findings of sensory loss can be present. With more peripheral lesions (e.g., those affecting the plexuses or peripheral nerves), sensory fibers degenerate distally, resulting in abnormal sensory NCS. In contrast, nerve root compression distal to the motor cell bodies in the anterior horn cell results in distal degeneration of motor fibers that can be detected with EMG studies and sometimes motor NCS. Note that the muscles most commonly recorded from during NCS are innervated by at least two nerve roots, and thus only severe single- or multi-level root compression will result in abnormal motor NCS waveforms (the waveform amplitude is maintained due to numerous unaffected nerve root fibers that contribute to the amplitude, while needle EMG may be able to detect even mild axonal lesions. For these reasons, needle EMG is the single most valuable electrodiagnostic test for diagnosis of radiculopathy affecting motor fibers.

It is possible for the DRG to be situated more proximally in the neural foramina, or even in an intraspinal location. In these instances, the DRG and/or more distal fibers can be affected by direct compression or indirectly by vascular insult and edema formation. While sensory NCS are typically normal in discogenic radiculopathies, they may be affected if the DRG is located more proximally, which is relatively common in the case of the L5 DRG (12%–21% of cases of L5 radiculopathy may have reduced superficial peroneal SNAP amplitudes). The DRG can

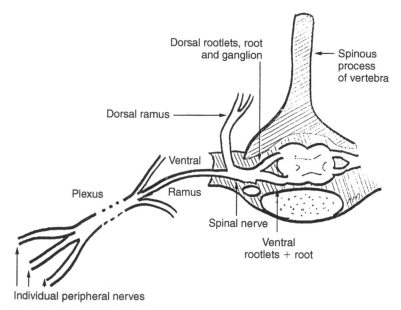

Fig. 17.1 General organization of the somatic peripheral system to show the formation of rootlets, spinal nerve rami and plexuses, and individual nerve trunks.

Table 17.1 Temporal Sequence of Electrophysiologic Abnormalities Possibly Seen in a Radiculopathy.

DAYS AFTER ONSET	ELECTROPHYSIOLOGIC ABNORMALITIES
0+	Reduced recruitment *(earliest abnormality observed on electromyography)* Reduced number of motor unit potentials Increased firing rates of motor potentials Fasciculations may appear H-reflex latency prolonged Reduced number of F-waves
4+	Compound motor action potential amplitude may be reduced, reaching its nadir at 7 days
7+	Positive sharp waves appear in paraspinal muscles
12+	Positive sharp waves appear in proximal limb muscles Fibrillations appear in paraspinal muscles
15+	Positive sharp waves appear in distal limb muscles Fibrillations occur in proximal limb
18+	Fibrillations potentials seen in most affected muscles

also be damaged in diseases such as diabetes mellitus, herpes zoster, and malignancy. In these conditions, the sensory NCS may be abnormal.

5. **Explain how EMG is used to assess radiculopathy in patients with spinal disorders.**
Specific muscles are selected for EMG assessment. Six upper limb muscles, including paraspinal muscles, consistently identify more than 98% of cervical radiculopathies *that are confirmable by electrodiagnosis*. For upper-limb EMG evaluation, a suggested screen includes deltoid, triceps, pronator teres, abductor pollicis brevis, extensor digitorum communis, and cervical paraspinal muscles. Six lower limb muscles, including paraspinal muscles, consistently identify more than 98% of lumbosacral radiculopathies *that are confirmable by electrodiagnosis*. A suggested lower-limb EMG screen for optimal identification includes the vastus medialis, anterior tibialis, posterior tibialis, short head of biceps femoris, medial gastrocnemius, and lumbar paraspinal muscles. For both lumbosacral and cervical disorders, when paraspinal muscles are unreliable to study, eight distal muscles are needed to achieve optimal identification. It is important to note, however, that a significant percentage of radiculopathies are not confirmable by electrodiagnosis, regardless of the number of muscles tested (see question 16).

Localization of a nerve injury to a specific root level is achieved by testing a variety of muscles in a multi-segmental distribution that are innervated by different peripheral nerves. If the abnormalities are confined to a single myotome and cannot be localized to the distribution of a single peripheral nerve, the diagnosis is consistent with radiculopathy. The paraspinous musculature is generally affected in radiculopathies. However, on occasion, especially in cervical radiculopathies and long-standing radiculopathies, the paraspinous muscles may be normal.

EDX findings must be interpreted in view of the time interval between the onset of the lesion and the performance of the electrical study, as the development of specific EMG abnormalities occur in a somewhat predictable time course (Table 17.1). Specific diseases are more likely to develop certain abnormalities than others. Table 17.2 identifies the EMG abnormalities commonly associated with various pathologies.

6. **What are fibrillation potentials? Why are they important in assessing radiculopathy?**
Fibrillation potentials are spontaneous, regularly firing action potentials of individual denervated muscle fibers. Fibrillation potentials are a sensitive indicator of motor axon loss. They can be observed in neuropathy, direct nerve and muscle trauma, myopathy, and some neuromuscular transmission disorders. Fibrillation potentials appear approximately 14 days after nerve fiber injury. However, they appear within 1 week in paraspinal muscles and within 3–6 weeks in the distal limb. Fibrillations can persist for 18–24 months or longer, until muscle fibers are reinnervated. Importantly, while the presence of fibrillations is indicative of motor axonal loss, it is not indicative of the degree of motor axonal loss (i.e., a muscle with countless fibrillations could have minimal axonal loss, while a muscle with few fibrillations could have significant axonal loss, and vice versa).

7. **How are NCS obtained? For what diagnoses are NCS most likely to be helpful?**
NCS are obtained by application of an electrical impulse at one point, resulting in an action potential (motor or sensory) that is recorded at a second point at a predetermined distance along the nerve. The NCS measures the time (latency) required to travel between the stimulating and recording site as well as the velocity (nerve conduction velocity [NCV]) and amount of potential conducted (amplitude). Sensory responses (sensory nerve action potential [SNAP]) are recorded over a sensory nerve, whereas motor responses (compound motor action

Table 17.2 Needle Electromyographic Findings.

EMG FINDING	PATHOPHYSIOLOGY	ASSOCIATED DISEASES
Increased insertional activity	Excessive irritability of muscle fibers to mechanical disturbances	• Acute/ongoing inflammatory myopathy • Neuropathy • Lower motor neuron disease, such as radiculopathy
Fibrillation potentials	Denervation of muscle fibers Membrane instability	• Acute/ongoing myopathy • Neuropathy • Anterior horn cell disease • Neuromuscular transmission disorders • Radiculopathy
Positive sharp waves	Denervation of muscle fibers Membrane instability	• Acute/ongoing myopathy • Neuropathy • Anterior horn cell disease • Neuromuscular transmission disorders • Radiculopathy (may be present with normal foot and paraspinal muscles)
Fasciculation	Motor unit spontaneous discharge	• Any lower motor neuron pathology of any chronicity • May also be a normal variant
Increased duration, amplitude, phase number ("neuropathic"/polyphasic potentials)	Reduced motor unit number Collateral sprouting Reinnervation	• Any ongoing/chronic neuropathic lesion • Late-stage muscle disease
Decreased duration, amplitude, phase number ("myopathic" potentials)	Pathologic muscle fibers Reinnervation	• Early myopathy • Late-stage chronic neuropathy
Increase in recruitment frequency	Reduced number of motor units available to produce desired contractile force	• Neuropathic processes
Decrease in recruitment frequency	Reduced number of healthy muscle fibers per motor unit	• Myopathic processes

potential [CMAP]) are recorded over a muscle. The SNAP amplitude represents the sum of the action potentials of the sensory fibers of individual sensory or mixed nerves. The CMAP amplitude represents the sum of the action potentials of individual muscle fibers innervated by a motor nerve. Special types of nerve conduction studies include F-wave, H-reflex, SEPs, and motor-evoked potentials (MEPs).

NCS are most likely to yield positive findings in conditions that may mimic the symptoms of radiculopathy, such as compression neuropathy or peripheral neuropathy. Sensory NCS are expected to be normal in radiculopathy because the pathologic lesion is often preganglionic. Motor NCS can be abnormal in severe radiculopathy (i.e., reduced CMAP amplitude).

8. What are H-reflexes and F-waves?
H-reflexes and F-waves are special types of conduction studies that provide information regarding nerve conduction in proximal sections of nerves that are difficult to assess using standard NCS techniques. These studies are of limited value in diagnosing radiculopathy (see questions 9 and 10), although they are excellent screening tests for polyneuropathy.

9. Describe the H-reflex and its clinical use.
The H-reflex is a monosynaptic spinal reflex first described by Hoffmann in 1918. It is the electrical equivalent of the triceps surae (ankle jerk) reflex when recorded from the gastrocnemius/soleus muscle. Submaximal stimulation of the proximal tibial nerve is transmitted toward the spinal cord and causes motor neuron cells in the anterior horn to transmit impulses via the spinal nerve to the gastrocnemius muscle. An abnormal H-reflex localizes the lesion to the S1 root or any points along this neural pathway. Prolonged latency and reduced amplitude may indicate an S1 radiculopathy; however, H-reflex studies are neither highly sensitive nor specific. H-reflexes demonstrate approximately 50% sensitivity for S1 root involvement and may be used to distinguish S1 from L5 radiculopathies. Unfortunately,

once abnormal, the H-reflex remains so indefinitely, independent of the patient's clinical status (a patient with a history of prior, resolved S1 radiculopathy who presents with a new, acute L5 radiculopathy may have an abnormal H-reflex), which may confuse the clinical picture. The H-reflex is often of limited utility in patients over 60 years of age and in those who have undergone lumbar laminectomy, as it is frequently absent bilaterally in these populations.

10. How is the F-wave elicited? What is the value of the F-wave in the assessment of radiculopathy?

The F-wave is a compound action potential evoked from a muscle by a *supramaximal* electrical stimulus to its related peripheral nerve. This procedure results in an antidromic activation of the motor neuron. As the electrical impulse travels backward along the nerve to the spinal cord, a small number of anterior horn cells are activated and nerve impulses are subsequently transmitted via the spinal nerve and result in small motor action potentials that can be recorded from the associated muscle. The F-wave has variable configuration, latency, and amplitude. F-waves are abnormal immediately after nerve root injury, even when the needle EMG is normal. However, an F-wave study has low utility for diagnosing a radiculopathy, because multiple roots innervate most muscles tested during EDX, and lesions along any of these multiple roots can render an F-wave abnormal. Abnormal F-waves are observed only in multiple and severe motor root compromise. Clinically, F-waves have been shown to be useful in the diagnosis of multiple root lesions, such as Guillain-Barré syndrome, and extensive proximal neuropathies, such as plexopathies.

11. What is SEP testing? What is its value in the investigation of radiculopathy?

SEPs are waveforms recorded over the scalp or spine following electrical stimulation of a mixed or sensory nerve in the periphery. SEPs are conducted in the posterior columns of the spinal cord, which represent nerve fibers carrying joint position and vibratory sensation. SEPs are used successfully in monitoring spinal cord function during spinal surgery, and prolonged SEPs latency can be the earliest sign in extensive multiple root lesions (see question 21). As previously discussed, patients with radiculopathy will typically have normal sensory NCS (due to the lesion usually being preganglionic). Further, without significant motor involvement, motor NCS, and sometimes EMG, will be unremarkable. Thus it would be ideal if another EDX tool existed that provided useful diagnostic information for radiculopathy. Some believe that dermatomal SEPs are useful in diagnosing radiculopathy or other spinal pathologies, in particular in patients who have NCS and EMG that are negative but clinical suspicion for radiculopathy is high. This notion is largely based on case reports and case series that have demonstrated the value of dermatomal SEPs. At the present time, however, the American Association of Neuromuscular and Electrodiagnostic Medicine (AANEM) recommends that dermatomal SEPs not be performed to evaluate lumbar or cervical radiculopathy, as they are unproven diagnostic procedures. SEPs have low sensitivity and specificity for radiculopathy, likely due to the fact that the nerve fibers assessed by SEPs are not typically affected in radiculopathy.

12. What are the EDX findings in a single-level radiculopathy?
- Abnormal EMG findings in a myotomal distribution
- Normal sensory NCS (unless the DRG is located more proximally, as is relatively common in L5 radiculopathy)
- Normal motor NCS (unless motor fiber compromise is severe, in which case reduced CMAP amplitude and normal or reduced conduction velocity may be observed)
- Normal F-waves
- Abnormal H-reflex in most acute or chronic S1 radiculopathies

13. What are the most common root levels involved in cervical and lumbar radiculopathies?

The C7 root is most commonly involved in cervical radiculopathy (31%–81%), followed by C6 (19%–25%), C8 (4%–10%), and C5 (2%–10%). Nerve roots C1–C4 have no extremity representation, and lesions affecting these roots cannot be diagnosed on EDX testing.

The L5 and S1 roots are most commonly involved in lumbar radiculopathy (70%–90%), followed by the L4 root. This is because the vast majority of lumbar disc herniations (95%) occur at the L4–L5 and L5–S1 spinal levels.

14. Which muscles are most frequently involved in common cervical and lumbosacral radiculopathies, and how are these radiculopathies differentiated from other pathologies that may present similarly?

See Table 17.3.

15. Can needle EMG detect thoracic radiculopathy?

EMG of the anterior abdominal wall muscles may be used to diagnose thoracic radiculopathy. Fibrillations may be noted in the paraspinal musculature in the thoracic region. Seventy-five percent of herniated thoracic discs occur between T8 and T12. EMG cannot differentiate between compressive thoracic radiculopathy and diabetic thoracic radiculopathy. If fibrillation potentials are observed in the thoracic region, it may be pertinent to consider other causes of these electrical findings (e.g., amyotrophic lateral sclerosis), as thoracic radiculopathy is relatively uncommon and accounts for <2% of all radiculopathies.

Table 17.3 Most Commonly Involved/Affected Muscles in Various Cervical and Lumbosacral Radiculopathies and Clinical Pearls Regarding the Differential Diagnosis of Common Radiculopathies.

ROOT INVOLVED	MOST COMMONLY INVOLVED/AFFECTED MUSCLES	CLINICAL PEARLS REGARDING DIFFERENTIAL DIAGNOSIS OF COMMON RADICULOPATHIES
C5	- rhomboids - supraspinatus - infraspinatus - levator scapulae - deltoid - biceps brachii - brachialis	• Distinguish from suprascapular/axillary neuropathy and upper trunk brachial plexopathy with EDX. • Distinguish from rotator cuff tear (EDX is typically normal)
C6	- biceps brachii - pronator teres - extensor carpi radialis	• Distinguish from upper trunk brachial plexopathy with EDX • May present similarly to carpal tunnel syndrome and may be differentiated on the basis of NCS • Median and radial nerve entrapment around the elbow/forearm can mimic C6 radiculopathy
C7	- anconeus - flexor carpi radialis - triceps - extensor digitorum communis	• May present similarly to carpal tunnel syndrome and may be differentiated on the basis of NCS
C8/T1	- flexor digitorum profundus - abductor digiti minimi - 1st dorsal interosseous - pronator quadratus - abductor pollicis brevis - opponens pollicis	• C8, and especially T1, radiculopathies are uncommon and difficult to distinguish • NCS should be performed to rule out other pathologies that may present similarly (ulnar neuropathy, brachial plexopathy, thoracic outlet syndrome) • If NCS is indicative of lower trunk plexopathy, it is essential to rule out Pancoast tumor
L4	- quadriceps - hip adductors	• May present similarly to lumbar plexopathy, femoral neuropathy, or diabetic amyotrophy • Evaluation of hip range of motion may be used to rule out hip joint arthropathy
L5	- gluteus medius and minimus - tensor fascia lata - medial hamstrings - tibialis anterior - extensor hallucis longus - extensor digitorum brevis - peronei - tibialis posterior - flexor digitorum longus	• May present similarly to peroneal neuropathy or lumbosacral plexopathy
S1	- gastrocnemius - soleus - lateral hamstrings - gluteus maximus - intrinsic foot muscles	• If EMG abnormalities are limited to the intrinsic foot muscles, further evaluation with NCS should be performed to confirm or exclude the diagnosis of tarsal tunnel syndrome

EDX, Electrodiagnostic tests; *EMG,* electromyography; *NCS,* nerve conduction studies.

16. **What are the sensitivity and specificity of EMG for evaluating radiculopathy?**
The sensitivity of needle EMG for lumbosacral radiculopathies varies depending on the diagnostic gold standard used and ranges from 29% to 90%. For cervical radiculopathy, the sensitivity has been reported to range from 50% to 71%. It is generally considered that the value of EMG in the diagnosis and localization of radiculopathy resides in its specificity (often >85%) rather than its sensitivity. This ability allows EMG to play a role as a complementary test to MRI. If an anatomic lesion, such as a disc herniation, is noted on MRI, EMG can help determine whether the lesion is associated with axonal damage. Alternatively, if MRI fails to identify an anatomic lesion but clinical suspicion remains high, needle EMG can occasionally be useful to confirm the diagnosis of radiculopathy. Needle EMG and diagnostic imaging findings correlate in 65%–85% of patients.

17. **What are some limitations of needle EMG for the diagnosis of radiculopathy?**
   1. Needle EMG detects motor axonal loss, motor axonal reinnervation, and decreased recruitment seen with motor conduction block or axonal loss. However, needle EMG cannot detect pure sensory radiculopathy (consisting of myelin and/or axonal damage), which is unfortunate as pure sensory radiculopathy is the most common form of radiculopathy.
   2. False-negative studies can occur in instances of focal demyelination secondary to root compression, when axon loss involves only sensory root fibers, when only a few motor fibers are injured by root compression, during the early postinjury period before denervation potentials appear, or several months after the onset of a radiculopathy (late postinjury period) when significant reinnervation has already occurred.
   3. False-positive studies are possible when signs of reinnervation are the only electrodiagnostic findings indicating radiculopathy.
   4. A normal EMG of the paraspinal muscles does not rule out the presence of root lesions.
   5. Abnormal spontaneous activity can be found in asymptomatic individuals and is only significant in the appropriate clinical context.

18. **Does electrodiagnostic confirmation of radiculopathy predict response to lumbar and/or cervical epidural steroid injections?**
Several studies in recent years have investigated this issue, and the answer is somewhat controversial. The topic is an important one, as epidural steroid injections (ESIs) are commonly used for the treatment of radicular pain, and having an effective tool to appropriately identify patients who are more likely to respond to these interventions would be useful from both patient-care and cost-savings perspectives.
   Data regarding EDX and ESIs for lumbar radiculopathy are mixed. A number of studies have reviewed patients who underwent transforaminal, interlaminar, or caudal ESIs for lumbar radiculopathy after undergoing EDX studies. There are some data indicating that patients with EMG-confirmed lumbar radiculopathy have more favorable outcomes based on pain and/or disability scores that is statistically significant compared with those who have EMG-negative lumbar radiculopathy. However, not all studies found the observed improvements to be clinically significant. Additionally, some patients had questionable clinical diagnoses and those with clear-cut lumbosacral radiculopathy were often excluded. It is possible that some patients with EMG-negative lumbar radiculopathy did not have pain that was due to lumbar radiculopathy, as there are many pain conditions that mimic radiculopathy (e.g., referred pain from the lumbosacral facets or sacroiliac joints). Accordingly, EMG may not provide added value in predicting response to ESIs in patients with clear-cut lumbosacral radiculopathy, but may be helpful when the diagnosis is more ambiguous.
   As for whether EDX provides any prognostic value regarding ESIs for cervical radiculopathy, data are more limited. Only a single study sought to address this question, and it failed to demonstrate any difference in pain reduction following ESI between EMG-confirmed and EMG-negative groups. However, as only 22 subjects were enrolled, it is difficult to draw significant conclusions from this limited data.

19. **What EDX findings are present in patients with spinal stenosis?**
EDX does not reveal abnormalities in mild or early-stage lumbar spinal stenosis. In patients with severe lumbar stenosis, multilevel and bilateral abnormalities are noted on needle EMG. Sensory and motor nerve conduction are usually normal. The F-wave may be abnormal, and an abnormal H-reflex may be elicited bilaterally.
   In mild or early-stage cervical spinal stenosis, similar to lumbar spinal stenosis, EDX is usually not informative. In patients with later stage cervical stenosis with cervical myelopathy, positive findings may be present and vary depending on whether involvement is limited to the descending corticospinal tracts or whether there is additional involvement of the anterior horn cells. Use of SEPs have been described for evaluation of cervical spinal stenosis. In cervical spinal stenosis, the median nerve SEP reveals a normal Erb's point potential and abnormal proximal latencies. The cortical potential may be either prolonged or absent, depending on the severity of neural compromise. Multiple absent or abnormally prolonged SEPs may be helpful in the diagnosis of multiple nerve root compromise that is not evident on needle examination.

20. **Is an EDX evaluation informative after a laminectomy?**
Postoperative EDX studies are of limited value after a laminectomy. Abnormalities in the paraspinal muscles are difficult to interpret because denervation potentials can originate from traumatic muscle injury secondary to

surgery. In the first 10–14 postoperative days, the EDX study can only reveal preexisting abnormalities, and thus the purpose of obtaining EDX studies during this time is usually to establish a baseline for future comparison. Between 3 weeks and 4 months after surgery, EDX results can reliably investigate a previously unsuspected lesion or be used to assess postoperative weakness. When the EDX examination is performed 4–6 months after cervical laminectomy or 6–12 months after lumbar laminectomy, it is difficult to interpret the clinical significance of the EDX findings. Abundant fibrillation potentials found in proximal and distal muscles of the myotome may suggest a recurrent or ongoing radiculopathy.

21. **What is intraoperative neurophysiologic monitoring, and what is its utility in spine surgery?**
Intraoperative neurophysiologic monitoring (IOM) is a system used to monitor neurologic function during surgery, and its goal is to prevent intraoperative neurologic damage. IOM uses several different technologies, including MEPs, SEPs, electroencephalography (EEG), electromyography (EMG), brainstem auditory evoked potentials (BAEPs), and/or visual evoked potentials (VEPs). IOM during spine surgery is somewhat controversial. Some experts recommend using IOM when spine surgery is performed as it is a sensitive and specific modality for intraoperative detection of neurologic injury. Other experts argue that using IOM is not warranted despite its proven diagnostic value due to the additional costs involved and insufficient evidence that IOM improves outcomes.

KEY POINTS

1. Electrodiagnostic evaluation, *in particular needle electromyography,* may be useful to establish and/or confirm a clinical diagnosis of radiculopathy. It is less useful when the diagnosis of radiculopathy is already certain.
2. NCS are most useful for diagnosis of peripheral entrapment neuropathy and peripheral neuropathy but are generally normal in patients with radiculopathy.
3. EMG has limited usefulness in the evaluation of spinal stenosis and postlaminectomy syndrome.
4. Electrodiagnostic testing should be deferred during the first 2–4 weeks following clinical onset of radiculopathy, because false-negative studies are common during this time period.

Websites
1. Electrodiagnostic Testing, American Academy of Orthopedic Surgeons: https://orthoinfo.aaos.org/en/treatment/electrodiagnostic-testing/
2. Practice Guidelines, American Association of Neuromuscular & Electrodiagnostic Medicine: http://www.aanem.org/Practice/Practice-Guidelines.aspx
3. American Association of Neuromuscular & Electrodiagnostic Medicine—Choosing Wisely: http://www.choosingwisely.org/wp-content/uploads/2015/02/AANEM-Choosing-Wisely-List.pdf

---

BIBLIOGRAPHY
1. Annaswamy, T. M., Bierner, S. M., Chouteau, W., & Elliott, A. C. (2012). Needle electromyography predicts outcome after lumbar epidural steroid injection. *Muscle & Nerve, 45,* 346–355.
2. Botez, S. A., Zynda-Weiss, A. M., Logigian, E. L. (2014). Diffuse age-related lumbar MRI changes confound diagnosis of single (L5) root lesions. *Muscle & Nerve, 50*(1), 135–137.
3. Cho, S. C., Ferrante, M. A., Levin, K. H., Harmon, R. L., & So, Y. T. (2010). Utility of electrodiagnostic testing in evaluating patients with lumbosacral radiculopathy: An evidence-based review. *Muscle & Nerve, 42,* 276–282.
4. Fish, D. E., Shirazi, E. P., & Pham, Q. (2008). The use of electromyography to predict functional outcome following transforaminal epidural spinal injections for lumbar radiculopathy. *Journal of Pain, 9*(1), 64–70.
5. Marchetti, J., Verma-Kurvari, S., Patel, N., & Ohnmeiss, D. D. (2010). Are electrodiagnostic study findings related to a patient's response to epidural steroid injection? *PM & R, 2*(11), 1016–1020.
6. McCormick, Z., Cushman, D., Caldwell, M., Marshall, B., Ghannad, L., Eng, C., et al. (2015). Does electrodiagnostic confirmation of radiculopathy predict pain reduction after transforaminal epidural steroid injection? A multicenter study. *Journal of Nature and Science, 1*(8), e140.
7. Mondelli, M., Aretini, A., Arrigucci, U., Ginanneschi, F., Greco, G., & Sicurelli, F. (2013). Sensory nerve action potential amplitude is rarely reduced in lumbosacral radiculopathy due to herniated disc. *Clinical Neurophysiology, 124*(2), 405–409.
8. Streib, E. W., Sun, S. F., Paustian, F. F., Gallagher, T. F., Shipp, J. C., & Ecklund, R. E. (1986). Diabetic thoracic radiculopathy: Electrodiagnostic study. *Muscle & Nerve, 9,* 548–553.
9. Tsao, B. (2007). The electrodiagnosis of cervical and lumbosacral radiculopathy. *Neurologic Clinics, 25*(2), 473–494.
10. Wilbourn, A. J., & Aminoff, M. J. (1998). AAEM Minimonograph 32: The electrodiagnostic examination in patients with radiculopathies. *Muscle & Nerve, 21,* 1612–1631.

CHAPTER 18

SPINAL ORTHOSES

Vincent J. Devlin, MD

1. **What is a spinal orthosis?**

    A spinal orthosis is a device that provides support or restricts motion of the spine. Spinal orthoses may also be prescribed to treat spinal deformities such as scoliosis. All orthoses are force systems that act on body segments. The forces that an orthosis generates are limited by the tolerance of the skin and subcutaneous tissue.

2. **List some common indications for prescribing a spinal orthosis.**
    - To immobilize a painful or unstable spinal segment (e.g., spinal fracture)
    - To prevent or correct a spinal deformity (e.g., scoliosis, kyphosis)
    - To protect spinal instrumentation from potentially dangerous externally applied mechanical loads (e.g., postoperative immobilization following instrumented spinal fusion).

3. **How are spinal orthoses classified?**

    Orthoses may be described according to method of production (prefabricated, custom fit, computer-aided design and computer-aided manufacture [CAD-CAM]), rigidity (i.e., rigid, semirigid, flexible), location of origin (e.g., Milwaukee brace, Charleston brace), inventor (e.g., Knight, Williams), or appearance (e.g., halo). The most universally accepted classification system describes spinal orthoses according to the region of the spine immobilized by the orthosis:
    - Cervical orthosis (CO): for example, Philadelphia collar
    - Cervicothoracic orthosis (CTO): for example, sternal occipital mandibular immobilizer (SOMI) brace
    - Cervicothoracolumbosacral orthosis (CTLSO): for example, Milwaukee brace
    - Thoracolumbosacral orthosis (TLSO): for example, Jewett brace
    - Lumbosacral orthosis (LSO): for example, Chairback brace
    - Sacroiliac orthosis (SIO): for example, Sacroiliac belt

4. **What factors require consideration in order to prescribe the most appropriate orthosis for a specific spinal problem?**
    - The patient's body habitus
    - Likelihood of patient compliance
    - The intended purpose of the orthosis (motion control, deformity correction, pain relief, postoperative immobilization)
    - The location of the spinal segment(s) that require immobilization
    - The degree of motion control required

5. **What orthoses are available for treating cervical disorders?**
    - CO
    - CTO
    - Halo skeletal fixator

6. **What motions do cervical orthoses attempt to control?**

    Cervical orthoses variably restrict flexion-extension, axial rotation, and lateral bending based on their design characteristics. In the normal cervical spine, axial rotation approaches 90°, lateral bending approaches 45°, flexion approaches 45°, and extension approaches 55°. Approximately 50% of cervical flexion-extension occurs at the occipital-C1 level and 50% of cervical axial rotation occurs at the C1–C2 level. Normal ranges of motion for each subaxial cervical spine segment are estimated as 8°–10° of flexion-extension, 3°–5° of axial rotation, and 2°–6° of lateral bending.

7. **What are COs? When are COs prescribed? How do they work? What are some examples of different types of COs?**

    COs are cylindrical in design and encircle the neck region. They may be anchored to the mandible and/or occiput to increase stiffness and motion control. COs are commonly prescribed for pain associated with cervical spondylosis, stabilization following cervical spinal surgery, and protection and immobilization of the cervical spine following trauma.

    COs may be soft or rigid. Soft collars provide no meaningful motion control. Rigid COs (e.g., Philadelphia, Miami-J) provide some restriction of flexion-extension, and to a lesser degree, restriction of rotation and lateral bending in the middle cervical region. However, motion restriction is less effective in the occiput to C2 region and lower cervical (C6–C7) region. COs are inadequate for immobilization of unstable spine fractures. Common types of COs include:

SOFT COLLAR (Fig. 18.1)
Design: Nonrigid; made of firm foam covered by cotton and fastened posteriorly with Velcro. Provides minimal restriction of cervical movement.

Indications: Cervical spondylosis, cervical strains. Allows soft tissues to rest, provides warmth to muscles, and reminds patients to avoid extremes of neck motion. Contraindicated in conditions in which cervical motion must be restricted (e.g., ligamentous injuries, fractures).

PHILADELPHIA COLLAR (Fig. 18.2)
Design: Two-piece polyethylene foam (Plastazote) collar with Velcro fasteners. Includes ventilation apertures, a molded chin support, and an occipital support. Tracheostomy style is available.

Indications: Stable cervical spine injuries, emergent mobilization of cervical injuries, and postsurgical immobilization. Contraindicated if the patient cannot tolerate pressure over the chin, occiput, or upper sternum.

MIAMI-J COLLAR (Fig. 18.3)
Design: Ventilated, two-piece polyethylene collar. Adjustable mandible and occipital components. Reported by patients to be more comfortable than Philadelphia collar. Provides greater limitation of cervical motion than Philadelphia collar.

Indications: Similar to Philadelphia collar. More appropriate for use in patients with altered mental status because collar-skin contact pressures generated by this brace are below maximal capillary skin pressure.

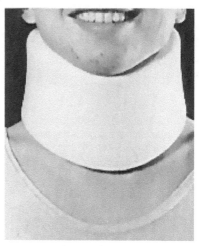

Fig. 18.1 Soft collar.

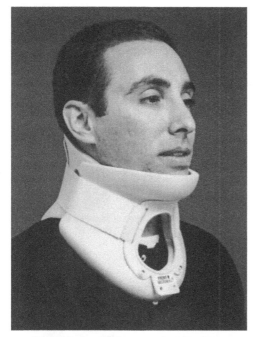

Fig. 18.2 Philadelphia collar. (From Fisher TJ, Williams SL, Levine AM. Spinal orthoses. In: Browner BD, Jupiter JB, Levine AM, et al., editors. Skeletal Trauma. 4th ed. Philadelphia, PA: Saunders; 2008, pp. 793–812.)

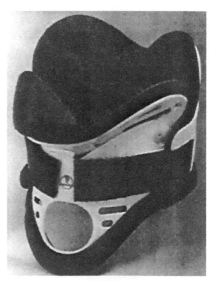

Fig. 18.3 Miami-J collar.

8. What are CTOs? When are CTOs prescribed? How do they work? What are some examples of different types of CTOs?

CTOs encircle the cervical region to a variable degree and use chin and occiput fixation attached to the trunk via straps or rigid circumferential supports. Two to four rigid uprights may be used to increase stiffness and improve motion control. CTOs are prescribed when greater motion restriction is desired in the middle and lower cervical spine compared with the motion restriction achieved with COs. These designs are generally reported to be more uncomfortable by patients. Common types of CTOs include:

TWO-POSTER CTO (Fig. 18.4)

Design: A metal orthosis consisting of single anterior and posterior uprights. Occipital, mandibular, sternal, and thoracic pads are attached. Difficult to use if the patient cannot sit erect.

Indications: Provision of support following cervical fusion procedures

FOUR-POSTER CTO (Fig. 18.5)

Design: Similar to two-poster CTO but with two anterior and two posterior uprights

Indications: Provision of support following cervical fusion procedures

SOMI CTO (Fig. 18.6)

Design: The *s*ternal *o*ccipital *m*andibular *i*mmobilizer (SOMI) derives its name from its points of attachment. It consists of a sternal plate with shoulder components, a waist belt, and occipital and mandibular pads

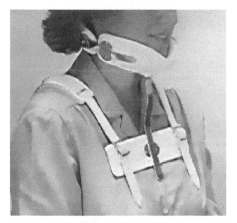

Fig. 18.4 Two-poster orthosis.

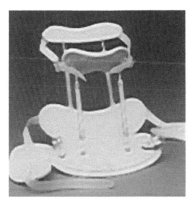

Fig. 18.5 Four-poster orthosis.

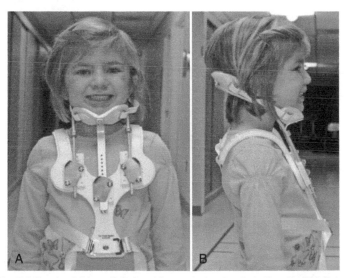

Fig. 18.6 Sternal occipital mandibular immobilizer cervicothoracic orthosis. (From Kim DH, Ludwig SC, Vaccaro AR, et al., editors. Atlas of Spine Trauma. Philadelphia, PA: Saunders; 2008, pp. 523.)

connected by uprights to create a three-post design. A head band may be added and is useful if the chin piece must be temporarily removed due to skin irritation. This orthosis can be more easily fitted to the supine patient than poster type CTOs because the uprights that maintain position of the occipital pad are attached anteriorly to the sternal plate. This brace is not compatible with magnetic resonance imaging (MRI).

Indications: Provision of additional support after cervical fusion procedures, immobilization of stable cervical fractures, and as a transition brace after treatment with a halo orthosis.

ASPEN CTO SYSTEM (Fig. 18.7)

Design: Consists of a CO attached to a thoracic vest via two or four posts

Indications: For maximum possible stabilization of the lower cervical and upper thoracic spinal regions. Indicated for minimally unstable fractures.

MINERVA CTO (Fig. 18.8)

Design: An occipitocervical support encircles the lower skull and supports the chin and subsequently attaches to an adjustable vest. This orthosis reduces axial load on the cervical spine and provides immobilization across the cervical region, as well as the cervicothoracic junction.

Indications: Similar to SOMI

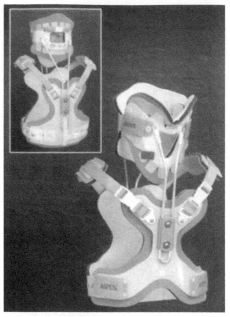

Fig. 18.7 Aspen cervicothoracic orthosis. (From Kim DH, Ludwig SC, Vaccaro AR, et al., editors. Atlas of Spine Trauma. Philadelphia, PA: Saunders; 2008, pp. 95.)

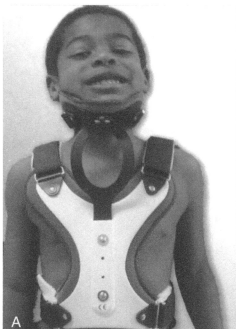 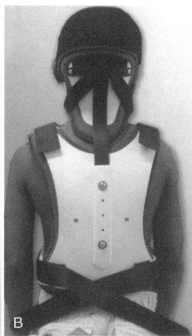

Fig. 18.8 Minerva cervicothoracic orthosis. (From Kim DH, Ludwig SC, Vaccaro AR, et al., editors. Atlas of Spine Trauma. Philadelphia, PA: Saunders; 2008, pp. 96.)

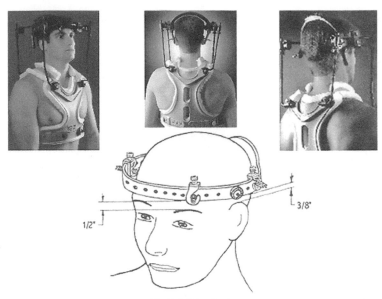

Fig. 18.9 Halo orthosis.

9. Describe the components of a halo skeletal fixator (halo vest orthosis).
The halo skeletal fixator (Fig. 18.9) stabilizes the cervical spine by fixing the skull in reference to the chest through an external mechanical apparatus. A rigid ring is fixed around the periphery of the skull. A snug-fitting fleece-lined plastic vest immobilizes the chest. Adjustable rods and bars stabilize the ring and vest with respect to each other. The halo vest orthosis provides the most effective restriction of cervical motion, especially for the upper cervical region. Traction may be applied to the cervical spine by use of turnbuckles.

10. When should a halo skeletal fixator be prescribed?
Indications for use of a halo skeletal fixator include:
    1. Treatment of select cervical fractures (especially C1 and C2 fractures)
    2. Postoperative immobilization (e.g., to supplement and protect nonrigid spinal fixation such as C1–C2 wiring)
    3. Maintenance of cervical spinal alignment when spinal stability is compromised by tumor or infection and surgical stabilization has not yet been performed or is contraindicated.

11. How is the halo skeletal fixator applied?
The patient is placed supine with the head position controlled by the physician in charge (Fig. 18.10). The correct ring size (should permit 1–2 cm of circumferential clearance around the skull) and vest size are determined. Critical measurements to determine correct vest size include:
    1. Waist circumference
    2. Chest circumference at level of xiphoid
    3. Distance from shoulder to iliac crest
Pin sites are identified. The skin is cleaned with povidone-iodine, and pin sites are injected with 1% lidocaine. The patient is instructed to keep the eyes closed during placement of the anterior pins to prevent skin tension in the eyebrow area, which could cause difficulty with eyelid closure. Anterior pins are placed 1 cm above the orbital rim, below the equator (greatest circumference) of the skull, and above the lateral two-thirds of the orbit. This pattern avoids the temporalis muscle laterally and the supraorbital and supratrochlear nerves and frontal sinus medially. Posterior pins are placed opposite the anterior pins at the 4 o'clock and 8 o'clock positions. The pins are tightened to 8 in-lb (0.9 Nm) in adults. The vest is applied, and the upright posts are used to connect the ring to the vest. Cervical radiographs are

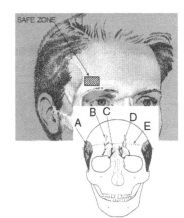

Fig. 18.10 Halo pin placement. *A,* Temporalis muscle. *B,* Supraorbital nerve. *C,* Supratrochlear nerve. *D,* Frontal sinus. *E,* Equator. (From Garfin SR, Bottle MJ, Waters RL, et al. Complications in the use of the halo fixation device. J Bone Joint Surg 1986;68:320–325.)

obtained to check spinal alignment. The pins are retightened with a torque wrench once at 24–48 hours after initial application. The pin sites are cleaned daily with hydrogen peroxide.

12. **What problems have been associated with the use of halo skeletal fixator?**
Complications associated with use of a halo skeletal fixator include pin-loosening, pin-site infection, discomfort secondary to pins, scars after pin removal, nerve injury, dysphagia, pin-site bleeding, dural puncture (following trauma to the halo ring), pressure sores secondary to vest irritation, reduced vital capacity, brain abscess, and psychological trauma.

    Although the halo skeletal fixator is the most restrictive of the various CTOs, significant motion may occur due in part to difficulty in fitting the vest securely to the chest. Both supine and upright radiographs should be assessed to ensure that cervical alignment and restriction of cervical motion are maintained with changes in posture. A phenomenon termed *snaking* may occur, in which there is movement between individual cervical vertebrae without significant motion between the occiput and C7. Use of the halo skeletal fixator is not well tolerated in older patients, patients with severe rheumatoid arthritis and coexistent hip and knee arthritis, or patients with severe kyphotic deformities (e.g., ankylosing spondylitis). Such patients experience difficulties with ambulation, balance, feeding, and self-care. Increased morbidity and mortality associated with halo-vest immobilization has been documented in patients over 65 years of age. Rigid internal fixation of the spine to avoid use of a halo skeletal fixator is the preferred treatment option whenever feasible.

13. **What special techniques are required to apply a halo skeletal fixator in pediatric patients?**
General anesthesia is frequently required. Various ring and vest sizes are required. A computed tomography (CT) scan of the skull is obtained to guide pin placement in very small children. This permits assessment of skull thickness and aids in avoiding suture lines and skull anomalies associated with congenital malformations. There is risk of perforation of the inner table of skull during pin placement in pediatric patients. In patients younger than 3 years, use of multiple pins (10–12) inserted with a maximum torque of 2 in-lb is recommended. In children 4–7 years of age, 8 pins are used and are tightened with 4 in-lb of torque. In children 8–11 years of age, 6–8 pins are used and are tightened with 6 in-lb of torque. For children 12 years or older, the adult guidelines for halo placement are used (4 pins, 8 in-lb of torque).

14. **What is a noninvasive halo system? (Fig. 18.11)**
A noninvasive halo system attempts to provide immobilization of the cervical spine approaching that of a conventional halo in a less invasive fashion. This orthosis avoids the use of skull pins, which eliminates many of the complications associated with the conventional halo system. It consists of a total contact orthosis made of Kydex (acrylic-polyvinyl chloride). Anterior and posterior bars connect the vest to an attachment, which encompasses the occiput, mandible, and forehead. This orthosis provides immobilization from C1 to T1, with similar intersegmental immobilization of the cervical spine as a halo except at the C1–C2 segment. It provides a less invasive alternative to the halo orthosis or an alternative for post-halo immobilization.

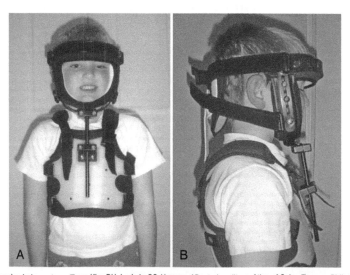

Fig. 18.11 Noninvasive halo system. (From Kim DH, Ludwig SC, Vaccaro AR, et al., editors. Atlas of Spine Trauma. Philadelphia, PA: Saunders; 2008, pp. 527.)

15. Describe three methods for classifying TLSOs.

TLSOs are prescribed for disorders involving the thoracic and lumbar regions. TLSOs may be classified according to:

1. **Method of fabrication:** TLSOs may be *prefabricated* (e.g., cruciform anterior spinal hyperextension [CASH] brace, Jewett brace), *custom-molded* to the body contours of the individual patient (custom TLSO, body cast), or *hybrid* (prefabricated module customized to a specific patient with a variety of modifications including Velcro straps, pulley systems, adjustable sternal pads, and pneumatic bladders). More recently, use of CAD-CAM technology has been popularized, and allows rapid fabrication of precise fit orthoses comparable to custom-molded orthoses.

2. **Intended function:** TLSOs may be further differentiated on the basis of intended function:
   - *Static support and immobilization* (e.g., treatment of stable thoracic and lumbar fractures, postoperative bracing after spine fusion)
   - *Deformity correction* (spinal deformities such as idiopathic scoliosis, Scheuermann kyphosis)
   - *Postural support* (e.g., to relieve axial pain)

3. **Degree of soft tissue contact**: TLSOs can be distinguished by the degree of contact with skin and soft tissues. *Limited-contact orthoses* (e.g., Jewett, CASH, Knight-Taylor) utilize discrete pads or straps to restrict motion. *Full-contact orthoses* (TLSO, body cast) distribute orthotic pressure over a wide surface area.

16. What motions do TLSOs attempt to restrict?

The thoracic region is the most stable and least mobile portion of the spinal column. Thoracic ranges of motion have been estimated as 34° combined flexion-extension, 15° unilateral lateral bending, and 35° unilateral axial rotation. The thorax provides stability to thoracic spine segments through rib attachments and the sternum. The coronal orientation of the thoracic facet joints is such that rotation is the major motion requiring restriction. This motion is difficult to control and requires a custom-molded orthosis if maximal motion control is required. The lower thoracic spinal segments are the most mobile segments of the thoracic spine due to the presence of free floating ribs and indirect attachment to the sternum. The thoracolumbar junction is a transition region between the stable upper and middle thoracic regions and the mobile lumbar region. Facet joint orientation transitions from a coronal to a sagittal orientation in this region. Lumbar ranges of motion have been estimated as 60° flexion, 20° extension, 25°–30° lateral bending, and 10°–15° axial rotation, with flexion-extension motion predominating due to the sagittal orientation of the lumbar facet joints.

Experimental studies have shown that full-contact TLSOs can effectively restrict motion between T8 and L4. If motion control is required above T8, a cervical extension should be added to the TLSO. Experimental studies have also shown that a TLSO paradoxically increases motion at the L4–L5 and L5–S1 levels. As a result, a thigh cuff must be added to the TLSO if motion control is desired at the L4–L5 and L5–S1 levels. Because limited-contact braces function by applying forces via sternal and pubic pads, these orthoses provide only mild restriction of sagittal plane motion (flexion-extension) and do not effectively limit coronal or transverse plane motion.

17. What are some examples of different types of limited contact TLSOs?

JEWETT (Fig. 18.12)

Design: Consists of a three-point fixation system with anterior pads located over the sternum and pubic symphysis and a posterior pad located over the thoracolumbar region. This orthosis restricts flexion but permits free extension. It is reported to be uncomfortable due to force concentration over a small area as a result of its three-point design.

Indications: For pain relief associated with minor, stable thoracic and upper lumbar fractures (e.g., fractures secondary to osteoporosis)

CASH (Fig. 18.13)

Design: The CASH orthosis is shaped like a cross with bars and pads anteriorly that are opposed by a posterior thoracolumbar strap.

Indications: Similar to Jewett

KNIGHT-TAYLOR (Fig. 18.14)

Design: Pelvic and thoracic bands are connected by a pair of posterior and lateral metal uprights. An interscapular band stabilizes the uprights and serves as an attachment for axillary straps. Over-the-shoulder straps attempt to limit lateral bending and flexion-extension. A cervical extension may be added. This orthosis provides poor rotational control.

Indications: Minor stable fractures and stable soft tissue injuries

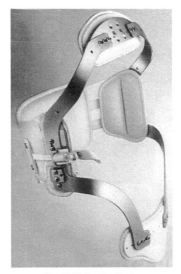

Fig. 18.12 Jewett orthosis.

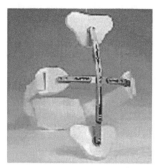

Fig. 18.13 Cruciform anterior spinal hyperextension orthosis.

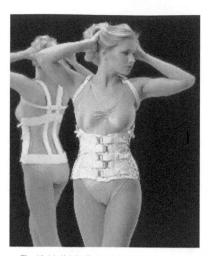

Fig. 18.14 Knight-Taylor thoracolumbosacral orthosis.

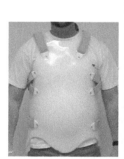

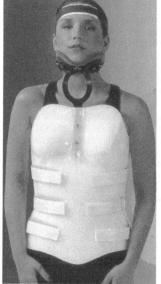

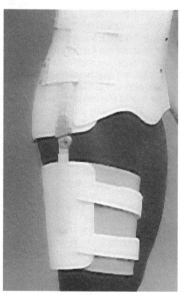

Fig. 18.15 Custom-molded thoracolumbosacral orthosis.

Fig. 18.16 Custom-molded thoracolumbosacral orthosis with cervical extension.

Fig. 18.17 Custom-molded thoracolumbosacral orthosis with thigh cuff.

18. **What are some examples of different types of full-contact TLSOs?**

   CUSTOM-MOLDED TLSO (Fig. 18.15)

   Design: Plastic jacket provides total body contact except over bony prominences. Available in one- or two-piece construction with anterior, posterior, or side-opening styles.

   Indications: Immobilization of the spine between T8 and L4. Provides adequate rotational control for treatment of stable spine fractures in this region.

   CUSTOM-MOLDED TLSO WITH CERVICAL EXTENSION (Fig. 18.16)

   Design: Custom-molded TLSO with attached chin and occiput support.

   Indications: Immobilization of the spine between T1 and T7. Provides adequate rotational control for treating stable spine fractures in this region.

   CUSTOM-MOLDED TLSO WITH THIGH CUFF (Fig. 18.17)

   Design: Custom-molded TLSO with attached thigh cuff. Thigh cuff may be fixed or attached via hinges with a drop lock.

   Indications: Immobilization of the spine between L4 and S1

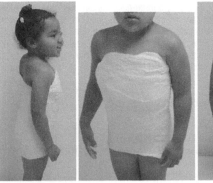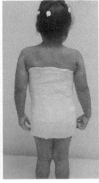

Fig. 18.18 Hyperextension cast.

HYPEREXTENSION CAST (Fig. 18.18)
Design: Custom-molded cast is placed with the patient positioned on a table or frame, which extends the injured spine segment.

Indications: Treatment of select thoracolumbar fractures (burst fractures without neurologic deficit, chance fractures limited to bone). A reasonable option in unreliable patients who are likely to be noncompliant with bracing.

19. **When an orthosis is indicated for immobilization of a stable thoracic or lumbar fracture, what are some factors to consider in selection of the appropriate type of orthosis?**
    The *level of injury* is a critical factor to consider in orthotic selection for a thoracic or lumbar fracture. For an orthosis to limit motion in a specific region of the spine, it must extend proximal and distal to the level of injury and immobilize the adjacent spinal segments. A TLSO is generally recommended if rigid immobilization is required from the T8 to L4 level. If the fracture involves L5, a thigh cuff should be added. If control is required proximal to T8, a cervical extension should be added. A halo or Minerva orthosis can effectively immobilize from the T1 level cephalad. The *type of spine fracture* (high-energy injury vs. low-energy osteoporotic compression fracture), *associated injuries* (e.g., pulmonary, abdominal), and the patient's *body habitus* are additional important factors to consider in decision-making. For example, orthotic treatment of thoracic and lumbar osteoporotic compression fractures is poorly tolerated in elderly populations and has not been shown to positively impact functional outcomes.

20. **What are some contraindications to orthotic treatment for thoracic and lumbar spine fractures?**
    - Unstable fracture types (fracture-dislocation, significant ligamentous injury, e.g., Chance fracture, flexion-distraction injury)
    - Incomplete neurologic deficit (surgery for decompression and stabilization indicated)
    - Morbid obesity
    - Polytrauma or associated injuries that prohibit brace wear (e.g., pulmonary or abdominal injury)
    - Impaired mental status
    - Impaired skin sensation
    - Noncompliant patient

21. **What are reasons to consider use of an orthosis following a spinal fusion procedure?**
    At present, spinal fusion procedures are most commonly performed in conjunction with the placement of segmental spinal instrumentation across the operated spinal levels. If the patient is reliable, possesses good bone quality, and multiple fixation points are used, postoperative bracing is not mandatory after a spinal instrumentation and fusion procedure. Potential reasons to consider using spinal orthosis following a spinal fusion procedure include:
    - To provide a splinting effect to relieve pain and limit trunk motion. Use of an orthosis can increase intraabdominal pressure, which has the potential to provide a splinting effect that may help relieve pain during the initial recovery period. An orthosis can also provide a postural reminder to limit extreme body motions.
    - To protect spinal implants from excessive forces. Young children tend to become active prematurely and may disrupt spinal fixation. Adults with osteopenia may also benefit from bracing to protect the implant-bone interface.
    - To provide immobilization after a lumbar fusion performed without use of spinal implants.

22. **What are the most commonly prescribed orthoses for treatment of lumbar and lumbosacral disorders?**
    Various types of LSOs exist ranging from custom-molded LSOs to elastic binders. LSOs stabilize the lumbar and sacral regions by encircling the upper abdomen, rib cage, and pelvis. Motion restriction provided by molded LSO does not approach the restriction provided by a molded TLSO. In contrast to a TLSO, an LSO does not

extend over the thorax and cannot limit motion by a three-point bending mechanism. Instead, LSOs function by fluid compression of the abdominal cavity and restriction of gross body motion. They provide only mild restriction of flexion and extension, and minimal restriction of side bending and rotation. LSOs are not sufficiently restrictive for immobilization of lumbar spine fractures. Nonrigid LSOs such as corsets, sports supports, and binders do not provide meaningful restriction of spinal motion but exert an effect by providing a reminder to maintain proper posture, supporting weak abdominal musculature, and reducing pain by limiting gross trunk motion.

CUSTOM-MOLDED LSO (Fig. 18.19)
Design: Custom made from patient mold
Indications: Chronic low back pain of musculoskeletal origin, post-surgical immobilization

CHAIRBACK LSO (Fig. 18.20)
Design: Composed of a posterior frame of Kydex with a fabric abdominal panel. Adjustable laces provide side closure and front straps provide front tightening.
Indications: Low back pain exacerbated by lumbar extension

CORSET (Fig. 18.21)
Design: Canvas garment with side-pull tightening straps and paraspinal steel stays
Indications: Mechanical low back pain

ELASTIC BINDER (Fig. 18.22)
Design: Broad elastic straps are fastened with Velcro closure
Indications: For postural support with minimal discomfort. Good choice for a patient with a pendulous abdomen or weak abdominal musculature.

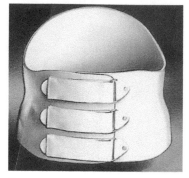
Fig. 18.19 Custom-molded lumbosacral orthosis.

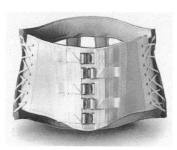
Fig. 18.20 Chairback lumbosacral orthosis.

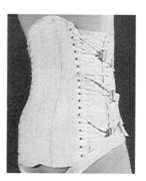
Fig. 18.21 Corset.

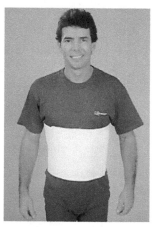
Fig. 18.22 Elastic binder.

SPORTS SUPPORT (Fig. 18.23)
Design: Consists of a heavy-duty elastic binder with a posterior neoprene pocket. The pocket holds a thermoplastic panel that is heated and contoured to the patient's lumbosacral region.
Indications: For patients whose shape or activity level precludes use of a more restrictive orthosis.

SACROILIAC ORTHOSIS (Fig. 18.24)
Design: A belt that wraps around the pelvis between the trochanters and iliac crests
Indications: During pregnancy, when laxity of the sacroiliac or anterior pelvic joints may cause pain, or for other conditions affecting the sacroiliac joints.

23. What are some examples of orthoses used for treatment of adolescent idiopathic scoliosis?
Orthoses are recommended for adolescent idiopathic scoliosis patients who have curves of 20°–40° and who are likely to have significant growth remaining. Patients with curves less than 20° are usually observed for progression, whereas those with curves approaching 50°

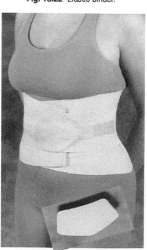
Fig. 18.23 Sports support.

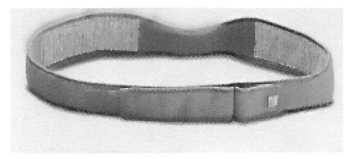

Fig. 18.24 Sacroiliac orthosis.

are generally considered for surgical treatment. There is a lower likelihood of successful orthotic treatment in male patients with scoliosis and for patients with significant curves detected prior to age 10. Options for orthotic treatment include:

- **Milwaukee brace** (Fig. 18.25): Basic components include a custom-molded pelvic girdle, one anterior and two posterior uprights extending from the pelvic girdle to a plastic neck ring, corrective pads, straps, and accessories. This brace can be used for all curve types and is the most effective orthosis for curves with an apex above T8. The cosmetic appearance of this brace is a concern to patients and limits brace compliance and the frequency of its prescription.
- **TLSO** (Fig. 18.26): The TLSO encompasses the pelvis and thorax. Curve correction is obtained through placement of corrective pads within the orthosis. This orthosis is effective for treatment of thoracic curves with an apex located below T8, as well as thoracolumbar and lumbar scoliosis. The best known orthosis in this category is the Boston brace.
- **Charleston brace** (Fig. 18.27): Designed to be worn only at night while the patient is lying down. This allows fabrication of a brace that overcorrects the curve and creates a mirror image of the curve. For

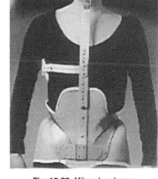

Fig. 18.25 Milwaukee brace.

example, a left lumbar curve is treated by designing a brace that creates a right lumbar curve. The relative success of this brace depends on the flexibility of the spine. It is most effective for single curves in the lumbar or thoracolumbar region. It provides a treatment option for patients who are noncompliant with daytime brace use. Another orthosis designed for night-time use, the **Providence Nocturnal Scoliosis System,** relies on application of controlled, direct-lateral, and derotational corrective forces to shift curves toward the midline as an alternative option to the Charleston brace.

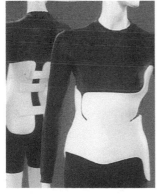

Fig. 18.26 Thoracolumbosacral orthosis (Boston).

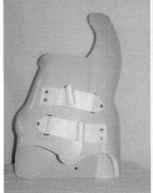

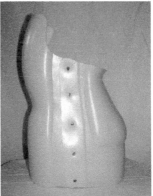

Fig. 18.27 Charleston brace.

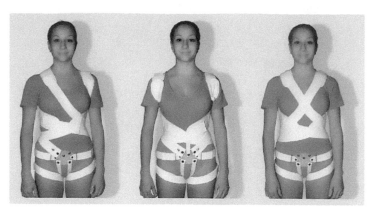

Fig. 18.28 SpineCor brace.

- **SpineCor brace** (Fig. 18.28): This novel design is a flexible brace that utilizes fabric pelvic and thoracic harnesses connected by elastic straps. The elastic straps are tightened to provide lateral and rotational corrective forces.

24. **What orthoses are used for treatment of adolescent patients with Scheuermann kyphosis?**
In adolescents, the CTLSO (Milwaukee brace) is the traditional method for orthotic management of sagittal plane (kyphotic) spinal deformities, but its appearance limits patient acceptance. A TLSO with an anterior sternal extension or padded, anterior shoulder outriggers may be considered as an alternative. A TLSO is most effective for treatment of low thoracic kyphotic deformities (apex below T9) or thoracolumbar-lumbar Scheuermann disease. In very severe deformities, cast treatment can be considered prior to use of an orthosis to gain greater deformity correction.

25. **What orthoses are used for treatment of an adolescent with low back pain and spondylolysis?**
Adolescent athletes may sustain injuries to the lumbar region that result in spondylolysis or stress reaction in the pars interarticularis. Various types of orthoses have been recommended for use in the treatment of this condition. Improvement in symptoms following bracing has been reported whether or not healing of the stress fracture occurs. Orthotic options for an adolescent with spondylolysis include a corset, Boston-type LSO, or custom TLSO.

KEY POINTS

1. A spinal orthosis may be prescribed to provide support to the spine, restrict spinal motion, or correct a spinal deformity.
2. Spinal orthoses are classified according to the region of the spine immobilized by the orthosis: cervical orthosis (CO), cervicothoracic orthosis (CTO), or thoracolumbosacral orthosis (TLSO).
3. The halo vest orthosis provides the most restrictive immobilization of the cervical spine, but is associated with a higher rate of complications than other cervical orthoses, and is not well tolerated in the older population.
4. The TLSO provides effective motion restriction between T8 and L4 but paradoxically increases motion at the L4–L5 and L5–S1 levels.

Websites
1. Spinal Orthoses for Idiopathic Scoliosis: http://www.spine-health.com/conditions/scoliosis/bracing-treatment-idiopathic-scoliosis
2. Cervical, Thoracic, and Lumbosacral Orthoses: https://now.aapmr.org/cervical-thoracic-and-lumbosacral-orthoses/

BIBLIOGRAPHY

1. Agabegi, S. S., Asghar, F. A., & Herkowitz, H. N. (2010). Spinal orthoses. *Journal of the American Academy of Orthopaedic Surgeons, 18,* 657–667.
2. Bible, J. E., Biswas, D., Whang, P. G., Simpson, A. K., Rechtine, G. R., & Grauer, J. N. (2009). Postoperative bracing after spine surgery for degenerative conditions: A questionnaire study. *Spine Journal, 9,* 309–316.
3. Carter, K. D., Roberto, R. F., & Kim, K. D. (2008). Nonoperative treatment of cervical fractures: Cervical orthoses and cranioskeletal traction in patients with cervical spine fractures. In D. H. Kim, S. C. Ludwig, A. R. Vaccaro, et al. (Eds.), *Atlas of Spine Trauma* (pp. 88–103). Philadelphia, PA: Saunders.

4. Perry, A., Newton, P. O., & Garfin, S. R. (2008). The use of cervical and thoracolumbar orthoses, halo devices, and traction in children. In D. H. Kim, S. C. Ludwig, A. R. Vaccaro, et al. (Eds.), *Atlas of Spine Trauma* (pp. 519–530). Philadelphia. PA: Saunders.
5. Sawers, A., DiPaola, C. P., & Rechtine, G. R. (2009). Suitability of the noninvasive halo for cervical spine injuries: A retrospective analysis of outcomes. *Spine Journal, 9,* 216–220.
6. Truumees, E. (2008). Bracing for thoracolumbar trauma. In D. H. Kim, S. C. Ludwig, A. R. Vaccaro, et al. (Eds.), *Atlas of Spine Trauma* (pp. 279–310). Philadelphia, PA: Saunders.
7. Vives, M. J. (2018). Chapter 81: Spinal orthoses for traumatic and degenerative disease. In S. R. Garfin, F. J. Eismont, G. R. Bell, et al. (Eds.), *Rothman-Simeone the Spine* (7th ed., pp. 1409–1429). Philadelphia, PA: Saunders.
8. Webster, J. B., & Murphy, D. P. (2019). *Atlas of Orthoses and Assistive Devices* (5th ed.). Philadelphia, PA: Elsevier.

SURGICAL INDICATIONS AND PERIOPERATIVE MANAGEMENT OF THE SPINE PATIENT

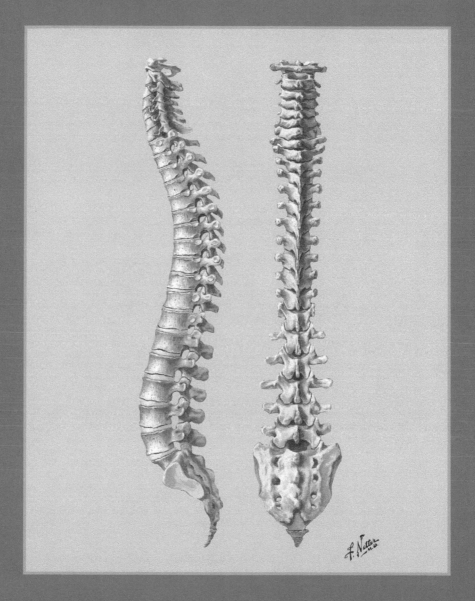

F. Netter
M.D.

CHAPTER 19

INDICATIONS FOR SURGICAL INTERVENTION IN SPINAL DISORDERS AND WHEN NOT TO OPERATE

Vincent J. Devlin, MD

1. **What are some critical factors that determine the outcome of a spinal procedure?**
Critical factors that determine whether a spinal procedure is a success or failure include:
   - Surgical indications
   - Surgical procedure (type and invasiveness)
   - Surgical technique
   - Timing of surgery
   - Patient psychosocial factors
   - Medical comorbidities
   - Biologic factors

   It is critical to perform the appropriate surgical procedure for the correct indications with technical proficiency at the appropriate time. However, patient psychosocial factors, medical comorbidities, and biologic factors that adversely impact spinal arthrodesis or neural recovery can all negatively influence the outcome of appropriate and well-executed surgery in powerful ways. The relationship among these factors may be summarized in a formula:

$$\text{Surgical Success} = \frac{\text{Indications} \times \text{Procedure} \times \text{Technique} \times \text{Timing}}{(\text{Psychosocial Factors})^4 \times \text{Comorbidities} \times \text{Biologic Factors}}$$

2. **What are the major indications for spinal procedures?**
   - Decompression of symptomatic neural compression
   - Stabilization of unstable spinal segments
   - Realignment of spinal deformities
   - Maintenance of intersegmental spinal motion following disc removal

3. **Describe some common indications for spinal decompression procedures.**
Spinal decompression procedures are indicated for symptomatic spinal cord or nerve root impingement. Common indications for decompression procedures include disc herniation, spinal stenosis, and spinal cord and/or nerve root impingement secondary to fracture, tumors, or infection.

4. **Describe some common indications for spinal stabilization procedures.**
Spinal stabilization procedures are indicated when the structural integrity of the spinal column is compromised to prevent initial or additional neurologic deficit, spinal deformity, or intractable pain. Common indications for spinal stabilization procedures include fractures, tumors, spondylolisthesis, and spinal instability after laminectomy.

5. **Describe some common indications for spinal realignment procedures.**
Spinal realignment procedures are performed to correct spinal deformities. Spinal deformities may result from single-level spinal pathology (e.g., spondylolisthesis, fracture, tumors) or pathology involving multiple spinal levels (e.g., kyphosis, scoliosis, complex multiplanar deformity).

6. **How do the indications for lumbar and cervical total disc arthroplasty differ?**
Lumbar total disc arthroplasty is most commonly indicated for reconstruction of the disc at one spinal level (L4–L5 or L5–S1) following single-level discectomy for treatment of patients with symptomatic degenerative disc disease. Cervical total disc arthroplasty is indicated for reconstruction of the disc (C3–C7) following discectomy at one or two contiguous levels for treatment of radiculopathy with or without neck pain, or myelopathy due to degenerative spinal pathology localized to the level of the disc space.

7. **How is the timing of spinal procedures prioritized?**
Indications for spinal surgery are prioritized based on the physician's responsibility to prevent irreversible harm to the patient as a result of spinal pathology, and must take into account the window of time within which surgical

intervention likely remains effective. Although there is no universally accepted classification or time frames, surgical indications may be broadly prioritized as:

1. **Emergent indications**. Patients in this category are at risk of permanent loss of function if surgery is not performed immediately. Delayed intervention for spinal emergencies may lead to irreversible harms including death, paralysis, or permanent sphincter dysfunction. Emergent surgical intervention is indicated for treatment of progressive neurologic deficits due to spinal cord or nerve root compression caused by conditions such as fractures, dislocations, tumors, abscesses, or massive disc herniations.

2. **Urgent indications**. Patients in this category have a serious spinal condition and require surgical intervention soon to prevent development of a significant permanent neurologic deficit or spinal deformity. Absence of a progressive or severe initial neurologic deficit or acute high-grade spinal instability permits limited time for additional spinal imaging studies, preoperative medical optimization, and formulation of a comprehensive surgical plan that enables the spinal procedure to be performed under more ideal conditions. Examples include patients with unstable spinal fractures without significant neurologic deficits and certain spinal tumors and infections.

3. **Elective indications**. Patients in this category have the opportunity to explore nonsurgical treatment alternatives and carefully evaluate the benefit-risk ratio of surgical versus nonsurgical treatment. Examples include patients with degenerative spinal disorders and spinal deformities.

8. In what situations is it unrealistic to perform surgery for a patient with a spinal disorder?
Decisions can only be made on a case-by-case basis after a complete medical history and physical examination, imaging workup, and medical risk assessment have been completed. Input from the surgeon, consulting physicians, patient, and family members play a role in decision-making. Some situations in which spinal surgery would not be advised include:

- When the general medical condition of the patient is a contraindication to an appropriate surgical procedure (i.e., the amount of surgery required to address the patient's spinal problem exceeds the patient's likely ability to tolerate the indicated surgical procedure).
- In the presence of global spinal pathology not amenable to focal surgical treatment (e.g., axial pain secondary to diffuse degenerative disc changes involving the cervical, thoracic, and lumbar spine may be beyond surgical remedy).
- Poor soft tissue coverage over the posterior aspect of the spine, which is not reconstructible with plastic surgery techniques.
- Severe infection that cannot be eradicated.
- Lack of correlation between imaging studies and the patient's symptoms.
- Patients with unrealistic expectations and goals with respect to surgical outcome.
- Patients with profound psychological disorders.

9. Is severe back pain ever an indication for spinal surgery?
Only in limited specific circumstances. Back pain is a symptom, not a diagnosis. The lifetime prevalence of back pain exceeds 70%. Surgery is not indicated for treatment of nonspecific low back pain. In specific clinical situations, spinal fusion is a reasonable option for treatment of axial spine pain following adequate nonsurgical treatment if a definite nociceptive focus is identified in a patient without negative psychosocial factors. However, caution is advised when the indication for surgery is spinal pain, as this complaint is subjective and personal, and surgical outcomes may be negatively influenced by a myriad of factors, including concomitant depression, tobacco use, and litigation. Back pain may be a prominent symptom in patients with neural impingement, spinal instability, or certain spinal deformities. In such situations, appropriate spinal decompression, stabilization, and/or realignment may improve back pain symptoms associated with these other spinal pathologies.

10. How is surgical decision-making for degenerative spinal disorders different from decision-making for spinal disorders secondary to trauma, tumor, or infection?
Patients who require operative treatment for spinal tumors, trauma, and infections often require surgical intervention on an emergent or urgent basis. Surgical decision-making for these types of spinal pathologies is often limited to determination of the optimal surgical approach and timing for performing a spinal decompression and spinal stabilization procedure. In contrast, patients with degenerative spinal problems usually undergo surgical treatment on an elective basis. In these situations, the patient has an opportunity to maximize available nonsurgical treatment before considering surgery. Decision-making for degenerative disorders not only involves selection of the optimal surgical approach for achieving spinal decompression and restoration of spinal biomechanics but, in many patients, also encompasses a myriad of psychologic and socioeconomic issues. It is important that patients considering elective spine surgery for treatment of degenerative spinal disorders are educated about the range of available nonsurgical and surgical options, as well as realistic expectations and goals regarding improvement in pain and physical function following surgery.

11. Is the presence of degenerative disc changes, disc herniation, or spinal stenosis on magnetic resonance imaging (MRI) a sufficient basis for determining the need for surgical intervention?
No. MRI of the spine is a highly sensitive but not highly specific imaging test. Many findings reported on MRI and other spinal imaging studies are common in asymptomatic individuals. Decisions about the need for surgical

intervention must consider whether or not the results of imaging studies correlate with a patient's medical history and physical examination findings prior to recommending treatment.

12. When is surgery indicated for treatment of a lumbar disc herniation?

Elective lumbar disc excision is an option for patients who meet the following criteria:
- Functionally incapacitating leg pain in a specific nerve root distribution
- Nerve root tensions signs with or without neurologic deficit
- Failure of nonoperative treatment for at least 4–8 weeks
- Imaging findings on MRI that demonstrate a lumbar disc herniation located at a level and side which correlate with the patient's physical findings and pain distribution.

Early surgical intervention is indicated for treatment of cauda equina syndrome associated with a lumbar disc herniation. If MRI confirms the presence of cauda equina compression due to a lumbar disc herniation when patients present with any combination of bladder or bowel dysfunction, saddle anesthesia, acute lower extremity sensory or motor loss, and positive sciatic tension signs, prompt surgical treatment is necessary.

13. When is surgery indicated for treatment of lumbar spinal stenosis?

Spinal stenosis is frequently detected on spinal imaging studies performed in an adult population. However, imaging findings must be correlated with clinical signs and symptoms prior to indicating surgical treatment, as more than 20% of asymptomatic patients over age 60 have spinal stenosis on lumbar MRI studies. Patients with symptomatic spinal stenosis generally present for evaluation due to neurogenic claudication and a variable combination of low back, buttock, thigh, and/or leg symptoms. Severe progressive neurologic deficits are not typically present, but may occasionally occur. Surgery is considered for patients who have failed nonsurgical management. Indications for surgery include: persistent functional incapacity due to neurogenic claudication; persistent or increased buttock, thigh, and/or leg symptoms; and neurologic deficits. The patient's general medical condition is factored into the decision whether to pursue surgical treatment. Patients should be educated regarding realistic expectations and goals following surgical treatment. Surgical goals include improved function, decreased pain, and improvement of neurologic symptoms.

14. What are the indications for surgical treatment of a cervical disc herniation in a patient who reports symptoms consistent with cervical radiculopathy?

The natural history of cervical radiculopathy secondary to a cervical disc herniation is favorable. Improvement is reported with nonoperative management in more than 70% of patients. Surgical treatment is an option for patients with:
- Persistent or recurrent arm pain unresponsive to nonoperative treatment
- Progressive functional neurologic deficits
- Static neurologic deficit associated with significant radicular pain
- Spinal imaging results that correlate with clinical history and physical examination findings

15. What are the indications for surgical treatment of cervical spinal stenosis?

Patients with symptomatic cervical spinal stenosis may present with radiculopathy, myelopathy, or a combination of radiculopathy and myelopathy.

Surgical indications for cervical spondylotic radiculopathy are similar to those for a cervical disc herniation.

Patients with degenerative cervical myelopathy are considered for surgical treatment as nonsurgical management has not been shown to alter the natural history of degenerative cervical myelopathy. Surgical intervention is the only treatment that can arrest the progression of degenerative cervical myelopathy. Initial nonsurgical management may be considered for patients with mild myelopathy. Surgical treatment is recommended for patients with mild myelopathic findings who experience pain refractory to nonsurgical measures, progressive neurologic deficit, or progressive impairment of function (e.g., ambulation, balance, upper extremity coordination difficulties). Surgery is recommended for patients with moderate or severe myelopathy to prevent decline in neurologic function.

16. Discuss some factors which play a role in decision-making regarding the choice between surgical versus nonsurgical management of traumatic spinal injuries.

Factors that play a role in treatment decision-making for spinal trauma include the injury pattern, spinal stability, neurologic status, and the presence of associated injuries. Various classification systems have been developed to guide treatment and identify the presence of posttraumatic mechanical instability at spinal levels between the occipitocervical junction and the sacropelvic region. Neurologic deficits following spinal trauma are classified as transient neurologic deficits that have resolved, nerve root injuries, incomplete spinal cord injuries, and complete spinal cord injuries.

Nonoperative treatment using a spinal orthosis is considered for fractures that are mechanically stable in neurologically intact patients without significant spinal deformity. Upright radiographs in the orthosis are recommended to assess the ability of the orthosis to provide relative stability of the spine under physiologic loads and limit worrisome patterns of displacement, such as increased segmental kyphosis or subluxation, which indicate the need for surgical stabilization.

Surgical treatment is indicated for mechanically unstable spine fractures and for spine fractures accompanied by progressive or significant neurologic deficits. The goals of operative treatment are to obtain and maintain anatomic spinal alignment, restore adequate stability to allow for early mobilization, and decompress neurologic structures as indicated.

17. **When are pyogenic vertebral infections most appropriately treated nonoperatively and when is surgical treatment a better option?**
The majority of pyogenic spinal infections can be managed effectively with appropriate antibiotic therapy and brace treatment. Biopsy and blood cultures are mandatory to guide appropriate antibiotic therapy. Parenteral antibiotics should be administered for a minimum of 6 weeks. Effectiveness of antibiotic therapy can be assessed with serial erythrocyte sedimentation rates (ESR) and C-reactive protein (CRP) levels. Indications for surgical intervention include:
    - To perform an open biopsy (when closed biopsy is negative or considered unsafe)
    - Following failure of appropriate nonsurgical management as documented by persistently elevated ESR or CRP, or refractory severe back pain
    - To drain a clinically significant abscess (e.g., associated with sepsis)
    - To treat neurologic deficit due to spinal cord, conus, cauda equina, or nerve root compression
    - To treat progressive spinal instability (e.g., secondary to extensive vertebral body or disc space destruction)
    - To correct a progressive or unacceptable spinal deformity

18. **Discuss some factors which play a role in decision-making regarding the selection of surgical versus nonsurgical management of primary spinal tumors.**
Decision-making regarding treatment of primary spinal tumors is dependent on a range of factors, including tumor type and location, presence or absence of metastases, and sensitivity of the tumor to radiation and/or chemotherapeutic agents. Diagnostic imaging, biopsy, metastatic workup, oncologic staging, and surgical staging play a role in the development of an appropriate multidisciplinary treatment strategy. For benign primary tumors, treatment options include observation, intralesional curettage, or marginal en bloc resection. For a localized malignant primary spine tumor that is poorly responsive to radiation and chemotherapy, en bloc resection is indicated in an attempt to achieve a surgical cure. When en bloc resection is not feasible or metastatic lesions are present, palliative surgery and/or adjuvant therapies are indicated.

19. **Discuss some of the critical factors which play a role in decision-making regarding the selection of surgical versus nonsurgical management of metastatic spinal tumors.**
In the majority of patients, the goal of treatment for metastatic spinal tumors is palliation rather than achievement of a cure. A wide range of treatments are available, including conventional external-beam radiation, stereotactic radiosurgery, conventional open surgical intervention, separation surgery, and percutaneous vertebral body augmentation procedures. Evidence-based decision-making regarding treatment selection is facilitated by use of the NOMS algorithm. *Neurologic* (N) considers the presence or absence of myelopathy and/or radiculopathy, as well as the degree of epidural cord compression. *Oncologic* (O) considers whether the primary tumor is radiosensitive or radioresistant or previously irradiated. *Mechanical* (M) factors assess whether the spine is stable or unstable. *Systemic* (S) factors consider the patient's ability to tolerate surgery.

20. **When is surgery indicated for treatment of metastatic spinal tumors?**
Indications for surgical intervention in patients with metastatic spinal disease include:
    - When biopsy is needed to obtain a definitive histologic diagnosis
    - Impending pathologic spine fracture
    - Spinal instability
    - Pathologic spine fracture with bone retropulsed into the spinal canal
    - Increasing neurologic deficit despite steroid administration or during the course of radiation therapy
    - Neurologic compromise at a previously irradiated level
    - Radioresistant tumors associated with high-grade epidural spinal cord compression

21. **What are some contraindications to surgical treatment of metastatic spinal tumors?**
Contraindications to surgical intervention for patients with metastatic spinal disease include:
    - Widespread visceral or brain metastases
    - Severe nutritional depletion
    - Immunosuppression
    - Significant metastases in all three spinal regions
    - Active infection
    - Expected survival less than 3 months
    - Inability to survive the proposed procedure

22. **What factors are considered in deciding whether surgical treatment is indicated for adolescent idiopathic scoliosis?**

Patients with adolescent idiopathic scoliosis do not typically present for evaluation due to major back pain symptoms and do not exhibit neurologic deficits. Surgery is most commonly considered to prevent future consequences of curve progression and for treatment of trunk asymmetry. Curve magnitude, clinical deformity, risk of curve progression, skeletal maturity, and curve pattern are factors considered when deciding whether to recommend surgery. Curves greater than 50° are generally recommended for surgical treatment because of the risk for continued curve progression in adulthood. Surgical treatment is also often recommended for patients whose curves are greater than 45° while still growing, or are continuing to progress greater than 45° when growth has stopped. In these cases, surgery is elective and should be decided by the patient and family after discussion of the benefits and risks that can be expected if surgery is elected.

23. **What are some common indications for surgical treatment of adult scoliosis?**

Unlike adolescent patients with idiopathic scoliosis, adult scoliosis patients commonly present for evaluation of back pain symptoms. Indications for surgical treatment of patients with adult idiopathic or degenerative scoliosis include pain, progressive deformity, functional disability cardiopulmonary symptoms, neurologic symptoms, and cosmesis. Studies suggest that operative treatment for younger patients (<50 years of age) is driven by increased coronal plane deformity, while operative treatment for older patients (>50 years of age) is driven by pain and disability, independent of radiographic measures.

24. **What psychosocial factors may negatively influence a patient's outcome following a spine procedure?**

Preoperative psychologic evaluation can identify the presence of psychosocial factors, which can influence the outcome of spine surgery, such as:
- Depression
- Anxiety
- Fear avoidance behavior
- Substance abuse (alcoholism, drug dependence)
- Psychologic disturbance (e.g., borderline personality)
- Passive coping strategies (e.g., catastrophizing behavior, neuroticism)
- Injury reinforcers (litigation, financial factors, social factors, job dissatisfaction)
- Childhood developmental risk factors (physical abuse, sexual abuse, abandonment, neglect, chemically dependent parents)

25. **What biologic factors can potentially be modified before a spinal fusion procedure to improve a patient's surgical outcome?**
- *Nutritional status:* Poor nutritional status adversely impacts infection risk, wound healing, and spinal fusion. Preoperative evaluation and nutritional counseling are indicated for patients with compromised nutritional status prior to spinal fusion surgery.
- *Smoking:* Nicotine increases the risk of postoperative pulmonary complications, wound healing complications, wound infections, and pseudarthrosis. Smoking cessation is recommended prior to spinal fusion procedures.
- *Medications:* Various medications negatively impact spinal fusion including corticosteroids, chemotherapeutic agents, and nonsteroidal antiinflammatory drugs (NSAIDs). Although a controversial area, some evidence suggests the association between decreased spinal fusion rates and use of NSAIDs is dose-dependent and duration-dependent, and that low-dose NSAID administration for the first several postoperative days is not associated with decreased fusion rates.
- *Osteoporosis:* Osteoporosis compromises spinal implant fixation and is associated with adjacent-level fractures following posterior instrumented spinal fusion. Assessment of bone density and treatment with calcium, vitamin D, and anabolic agents when indicated can help mitigate related adverse events.
- *Alcohol consumption:* Alcohol consumption has been identified as an independent risk factor for pseudarthrosis following spinal fusion. Patients with alcohol disorder can benefit from evaluation and treatment prior to elective surgery.

26. **When a patient reports that an initial spinal procedure has failed to improve their spinal condition, when is revision spine surgery indicated?**

A comprehensive clinical and imaging assessment is required to address this complex question. Pain severity or disability, in and of itself, is not an indication for additional spinal surgery. Patients with symptoms attributed to scar tissue (arachnoiditis, perineural fibrosis), systemic medical disease, or psychosocial instability are unlikely to have positive outcomes if additional surgery is undertaken. It is also important to recognize that a patient with unrealistic expectations and goals will not benefit from additional surgical intervention. Assuming the patient can medically tolerate an appropriate surgical procedure, additional intervention may potentially be indicated if surgically correctable pathology is present and the patient's symptoms can be explained on the basis of this pathology. Factors to consider during a patient's workup include whether the persistent symptoms are related to a prior spinal decompression (e.g., incomplete decompression, undecompressed adjacent level stenosis, recurrent disc herniation) or spinal fusion (e.g., pseudarthrosis, instrumentation-related issues, suboptimal spinal alignment). Previously undetected spinal infection must always be ruled out. Timing of symptom onset in relation to the initial procedure is an important clue to diagnosis. Commonly encountered problems for which revision spinal surgery may provide benefit in the appropriately selected patient include:

- Recurrent or persistent disc herniation
- Recurrent or persistent spinal stenosis
- Postlaminectomy instability
- Infection
- Symptomatic pseudarthrosis
- Sagittal imbalance syndrome (flatback deformity)
- Adjacent-level degenerative changes or stenosis (transition syndrome)
- Spinal implant misplacement, migration, or failure

27. Describe factors that may influence decision-making regarding spinal surgery in clinical scenarios where multiple treatment options exist or evidence to support the best treatment is unclear. How can patients and physicians work together in this situation?

Decision-making regarding treatment options for certain spinal disorders is challenging as the best available evidence regarding treatment may be conflicting. Factors that have been reported to influence surgeon decision-making include surgeon training, anecdotal experience, value judgments, and local standards, as well as external and/or market forces. In these scenarios where several choices for treatment exist, the use of *shared decision-making* is advocated. The surgeon's role is to:

1. Describe the patient's condition accurately.
2. Present the best available medical evidence regarding risks, benefits, and realistic outcomes of various treatment options.
3. Assist the patient in clarifying his or her preferences and values regarding treatment alternatives.
4. Guide the patient through this process while maintaining neutrality. Use of *decision aids* is an option to facilitate this process. However, the desire to be involved in the decision-making process varies from patient to patient. Although all patients want to be well informed, some prefer to delegate basic decisions and technical details to their surgeons.

28. What are some methods that can be used to inform patient decision-making regarding spinal surgery?

Informed decision-making regarding the benefits and risks of spine surgery for a specific patient may be enhanced through *risk stratification*. Quantification of patient risk can inform realistic expectations and goals regarding spine surgery outcomes, and guide strategies directed toward minimization of medical and surgical complications. Useful strategies include use of tools such as American Society of Anesthesiologist (ASA) physical status classification or frailty indexes, as well as predictive modeling techniques, which incorporate a broad range of patient and procedural factors to estimate patient risk.

KEY POINTS

1. General indications for surgical intervention for spinal disorders include decompression, stabilization, deformity correction, and motion preservation following intervertebral disc excision.
2. Inappropriate patient selection and failure to optimize the patient for the proposed surgery guarantees a poor surgical result despite how expertly a surgical procedure is performed.
3. Risk stratification strategies can inform decision-making regarding the benefits and risks of spine surgery and guide strategies directed toward minimization of medical and surgical complications.
4. By providing evidence-based information on surgical options and outcomes, surgeons can partner with patients through *shared decision-making* to determine the preferred treatment course for spine pathologies having multiple potential treatment options.

Websites
1. Dartmouth-Hitchcock Center for Shared Decision Making: http://www.dhmc.org/shared_decision_making.cfm
2. Which patients undergo presurgical psychological evaluation before spine surgery? https://www.spineuniverse.com/professional/news/which-patients-undergo-pre-surgical-psychological-evaluation-spine-surgery
3. Risk stratification approach to spinal surgical management: https://www.spineuniverse.com/professional/news/risk-stratification-approach-spinal-surgical-management

BIBLIOGRAPHY

1. Akbarnia, B., Ogilvie, J. W., & Hammerberg, K. W. (2006). Debate: Degenerative scoliosis: To operate or not operate. *Spine, 31,* 195–201.
2. Boden, S. D., & Sumner, D. R. (1995). Biologic factors affecting spinal fusion and bone regeneration. *Spine, 20,* 1025–1125.
3. Clark, M. J., Mendel, E., & Vrionis, F. D. (2014). Primary spine tumors: Diagnosis and treatment. *Cancer Control, 21,* 114–123.
4. Epstein, N. E. (2013). Are recommended spine operations either unnecessary or too complex? Evidence from second opinions. *Surgical Neurology International, 4,* 353–358.
5. Gaudin, D., Krafcik, B. M., Mansour, T. R., & Alnemari, A. (2017). Considerations in spinal fusion surgery for chronic lumbar pain: Psychosocial factors, rating scales, and perioperative patient education—a review of the literature. *World Neurosurgery, 98,* 21–27.
6. Joaquim, A. F., Powers, A., Laufer, I., & Bilsky, M. H. (2015). An update in the management of spinal metastases. *Arquivos de Neuro-psiquiatria, 73,* 795–802.
7. Laufer, I., Rubin, D. G., Lis, E., Cox, B. W., Stubblefield, M. D., Yamada, Y., et al. (2013). The NOMS framework: Approach to the treatment of spinal metastatic tumors. *Oncologist, 18,* 744–751.
8. Weinstein, J. N. (2000). The missing piece: Embracing shared decision-making to reform health care. *Spine, 25,* 1–4.
9. Weinstein, J. N., Lurie, J. D., Tosteson, T. D., Hanscom, B., Tosteson, A. N., Blood, E. A., et al. (2007). Surgical versus nonsurgical treatment for lumbar degenerative spondylolisthesis. *New England Journal of Medicine, 356,* 2257–2270.
10. Weinstein, J. N., Tosteson, T. D., Lurie, J. D., Tosteson, A. N., Hanscom, B., Skinner, J. S., et al. (2006). Surgical versus nonoperative treatment for lumbar disc herniation: The spine patient outcomes research trial (SPORT): A randomized trial. *JAMA, 296,* 2451–2459.
11. Weinstein, J. N., Tosteson, T. D., Lurie, J. D., Tosteson, A. N., Blood, E., Hanscom, B., et al. (2008). Surgical versus nonsurgical therapy for lumbar spinal stenosis. *New England Journal of Medicine, 358,* 794–810.
12. ter Wengel, P. V., Feller, R. E., Stadhouder, A., Verbaan, D., Oner, F. C., Goslings, J. C., et al. (2018). Timing of surgery in traumatic spinal cord injury: A national, multidisciplinary survey. *European Spine Journal, 27,* 1831–1838.

PREOPERATIVE ASSESSMENT AND PLANNING FOR PATIENTS UNDERGOING SPINE SURGERY

CHAPTER 20

Vincent J. Devlin, MD

1. **What are some factors which influence complication rates associated with spinal procedures?**
   - Type of procedure
   - Whether elective or emergency
   - Chronologic age of the patient
   - General health status of the patient and medical comorbidities
   - Institution where surgery is performed

2. **What are some examples of types of elective spinal procedures that are associated with a relatively low risk of complications and perioperative morbidity?**
   When performed in patients without significant medical comorbidities, elective spinal procedures associated with a relatively low-risk profile include:
   - Lumbar microdiscectomy
   - Lumbar laminectomy
   - Anterior cervical discectomy and fusion
   - Single-level lumbar spinal instrumentation and fusion (anterior or posterior)

3. **What are some examples of types of spinal procedures associated with a relatively high risk of complications and perioperative morbidity?**
   Spinal procedures associated with a relatively high-risk profile, often referred to as complex spinal procedures, include:
   - Surgery involving >6 spinal levels or lasting >6 hours
   - Revision spinal deformity procedures
   - Same-day or staged multilevel anterior-posterior spinal procedures or circumferential multilevel spinal procedures performed through a single posterior surgical approach.
   - Emergent spinal procedures for trauma, infections, and tumors, especially if associated with preoperative neurologic deficit.
   - Spine surgery in patients with significant medical comorbidities (coronary artery disease, congestive heart failure, cirrhosis, dementia, emphysema, renal insufficiency, pulmonary hypertension, stroke, age >80 years, chronic steroid use, pediatric spinal deformities due to neuromuscular or syndromic disorders).

4. **How is the surgical invasiveness of spinal procedures quantified?**
   Increased surgical invasiveness is correlated with higher intraoperative blood loss, longer surgical times, and increased risk of developing a surgical site infection requiring return to the operating room for treatment. Mirza et al. (5) developed an index to characterize the invasiveness of spine surgery and quantify spine surgery complexity. Points are assigned per vertebral unit (defined as one vertebra and the caudal intervertebral disc) based on each surgical component performed at each vertebral unit: anterior decompression (ad), anterior fusion (af), anterior instrumentation (ai), posterior decompression (pd), posterior fusion (pf), and posterior instrumentation (pi). For example:
   - L4–L5 posterior discectomy: invasiveness score is 1 (pd = 1)
   - C6–C7 anterior cervical discectomy, fusion, and plating: invasiveness score is 5 (ad = 1 [one disc] + af = 2 [two vertebra] + ai = 2 [two vertebra]).
   - L4–L5 laminectomy, posterolateral fusion, posterior pedicle instrumentation, and interbody fusion: invasiveness score is 10 (pd = 2 [two vertebra] + pi = 2 [two vertebra] + pf = 2 [two vertebra] + af = 2 [two vertebra] + ai = 2 [two vertebra]).

5. **What tools may assist surgeons in stratifying spine surgery risks as a guide to counseling patients regarding their procedure-specific risks for complications prior to deciding to have surgery?**
   Patients considering spinal surgery may be counseled regarding their specific risk for medical complications, infection, and dural tear, based on their personal comorbidity profile and the surgical invasiveness of the proposed

operative intervention using an online risk calculator (SpineSage™). Risk factors considered in this predictive model include chronic obstructive pulmonary disease (COPD), asthma, congestive heart failure, prior cardiac complications, body mass index (BMI), diabetes, renal conditions, age, gender, spinal diagnosis, prior spine surgery, and whether the surgery is a revision procedure. Surgical invasiveness is determined based on the number of spinal levels that are decompressed, fused, or instrumented, and whether the surgical approach is anterior or posterior. Additional surgical risk calculators are available online and include the Seattle Spine Score and the American College of Surgeons National Surgical Quality Improvement Program (ACS-NSQIP) Surgical Risk Calculator. Recently, frailty scores rather than chronologic age have been suggested for use in preoperative risk stratification prior to adult spinal deformity surgery, as frailty has been shown to be a better predictor of adverse events compared to chronologic age.

6. Once a patient and surgeon decide to pursue spine surgery, what are some important areas to address to optimize the patient for surgery?

The details and sequence for presurgical assessment varies based on multiple factors, including patient age, medical comorbidities, procedure type and magnitude, surgical acuity, and whether the surgical procedure is performed in an inpatient or outpatient facility. Patients undergoing major spine surgery are increasingly evaluated and managed using systems-based protocols, which comprehensively evaluate patients prior to surgery and guide intraoperative and postoperative management to optimize surgical outcomes. Such protocols often include:

(1) Comprehensive assessment by the spine surgeon who:
   - performs a detailed preoperative medical history and physical examination
   - obtains appropriate radiographs and spinal imaging studies
   - develops and finalizes a detailed surgical plan
   - coordinates equipment and personnel required for the surgical procedure
   - obtains informed consent for surgical procedure
   - orders appropriate preoperative testing according to when the specific test has a reasonable pretest probability of being abnormal, and when the abnormal test result would directly impact perioperative care. These tests may include:
     i. complete blood count (CBC)
     ii. comprehensive metabolic panel (CMP)
     iii. hemoglobin (hgb) A1c
     iv. albumin and prealbumin levels (baseline nutritional status)
     v. chest x-ray (CXR)
     vi. electrocardiogram (ECG)
     vii. bleeding profile (prothrombin time, partial thromboplastin time, bleeding time)
     viii. urine analysis
     ix. type and screen or type and cross-match if blood transfusion may be required
     x. pregnancy (as indicated)
     xi. urine screening for nicotine use and controlled substances (select patients)
(2) Multidisciplinary spine conference (for complex spine surgery cases) to confirm that the patient is a reasonable candidate for the proposed surgical procedure from medical, anesthesia, rehabilitation medicine, and surgical perspectives.
(3) Preoperative anesthesia consultation.
(4) Appropriate subspecialty medical consultations as indicated for specific medical comorbidities.
(5) Optimization of modifiable conditions such as nutritional status, diabetes control, tobacco use, alcohol abuse, osteoporosis, and opioid use to decrease risk of related complications.
(6) Patient education course with patient and caregivers to review surgery preparation and postoperative care details.
(7) Presurgical conference with surgeon, patient, and family members, which covers a range of topics, including presurgical education, diagnosis, available treatment options, informed consent, and expectations regarding recovery, including discharge planning.

7. List key areas to assess during the preoperative medical evaluation of a patient undergoing major spinal reconstructive surgery.

- **Cardiovascular**: Assess for risk factors such as coronary artery disease history, congestive heart failure, hypertension, carotid disease, history of transient ischemic attacks (TIAs), peripheral vascular disease and/or vascular claudication, history of thromboembolic disease, presence and types of stents or pacemaker, use of antiplatelet therapy or anticoagulants. Investigate for presence of cardiac disease in patients with congenital spinal deformities.
- **Pulmonary**: Recognize patients at risk for pulmonary complications, including patients with severe neuromuscular disorders, severe thoracic scoliosis, COPD, asthma, sleep apnea, emphysema, poor exercise tolerance, and tobacco use.
- **Neurologic**: Document preoperative neurologic status and baseline cognitive status. Check antiseizure medication levels when appropriate.
- **Hematologic**: Inquire regarding history of abnormal bruising or bleeding, or conditions associated with coagulopathy, including renal and hepatic disorders. Assess issues regarding blood donation and blood transfusion.

Determine plan for management of nonsteroidal antiinflammatory drugs (NSAIDs), aspirin, antiplatelet and other anticoagulant medications in the perioperative period.

- **Endocrine**: Assess risk factors for osteoporosis and order testing as indicated (DEXA scan, Vitamin D level), optimize control of blood glucose in diabetic patients, determine need for perioperative steroids in chronic steroid users or adrenal insufficiency.
- **Renal**: Document history of chronic renal insufficiency. Additional precautions and preoperative consultations required for patients potentially requiring or in need of dialysis.
- **Hepatic**: Document history of chronic or active liver disease due to association with thrombocytopenia, coagulopathy, encephalopathy, sepsis, renal failure, and increased perioperative morbidity.
- **Rheumatologic**: Assess for cervical instability, especially in rheumatoid arthritis patients. Consultation indicated for perioperative management of disease-modifying antirheumatic drugs as appropriate.
- **Immune status**: Caution is required if surgery is planned for immunocompromised patients (e.g., oncology, human immunodeficiency virus [HIV], rheumatology patients) due to associated comorbidities.
- **Nutritional status**: Assess nutritional status and correct any deficits prior to elective surgery due to association with impaired wound healing and increased risk of infection.
- **Orthopedic**: Assess for extremity contractures, presence of total joint replacements, cervical instability, or previously undiagnosed cervical myelopathy, which may influence safe patient positioning prior to and during spine surgery.
- **Medications**: Obtain a list of all medications and nutritional supplements, evaluate potential impact on spine surgery and hemostasis, and determine a plan for perioperative medication management in coordination with medical subspecialists.
- **Patient habits**: Inquire regarding history of smoking, alcohol use, narcotic use, and address these areas prior to surgery by referral to a smoking cessation program, psychosocial evaluation, or pain management specialist.
- **Psychological and social factors**: Assess barriers to recovery including depression, chronic pain, and lack of home/family support, and refer for psychosocial evaluation as appropriate.
- **Rehabilitation**: Refer patients with poor exercise tolerance to preoperative rehabilitation program (prehabilitation) to improve ambulation, strength, and facilitate postoperative recovery.
- **Weight-management**: Morbidly obese patients ($>$40 kg/m^2) are referred to a nutritionist for a weight-loss program consisting of diet and exercise, or to bariatric surgery.

8. What are the three leading causes of death after noncardiac surgery?
Cardiac events, major bleeding, and sepsis in the perioperative period are the three leading cause of death after noncardiac surgery.

9. How is cardiac risk stratified before surgery?
Risk for major adverse cardiac events (MACE) after noncardiac surgery are related to surgery-specific characteristics and patient-specific factors. Most spinal procedures are intermediate risk (1%–5% MACE risk). Functional capacity may be used as a predictor of cardiac risk and is expressed in metabolic equivalents (1 MET is the resting oxygen uptake in a sitting position, or 3.5 mL of oxygen uptake/kg per minute). Perioperative and long-term cardiac risks are increased in patients who are unable to perform 4 METS of work in daily activities (i.e., are not able to climb a flight of stairs, walk up a hill, or walk on level ground at 4 mph). Identification of risk factors such as angina, dyspnea, syncope, palpitations, or history of heart disease, hypertension, diabetes, chronic renal disease, cerebrovascular disease, or peripheral artery disease also impact cardiac risk. The Revised Cardiac Risk Index (RCRI), alternatively referred to as the Lee index, ACS-NSQIP risk prediction rule, or Gupta Cardiac Index, may be used to establish a patient's cardiac risk and are available online. An ECG is obtained in patients with cardiac disease to serve as a baseline. Additional testing may be indicated if it will influence perioperative care (echocardiography, stress testing, 24-hour ambulatory monitoring, and cardiology consult). Additionally, the biomarkers brain natriuretic peptide (BNP) and N-terminal pro-BNP (NT-proBNP), as well as C-reactive protein (CRP) may be used for prediction of perioperative major cardiovascular events in noncardiac surgery.

10. What are the risk factors for perioperative stroke in relation to spine surgery?
Major risk factors for stroke in the noncardiac and nonvascular surgical population include advanced age, history of TIAs, hypertension, cardiac abnormalities (e.g., atrial fibrillation), diabetes, female sex, renal disease, and prior stroke. Patients with a history of prior stroke or TIA should be referred for neurologic consultation and assessment for evaluation with brain and vascular imaging, especially if the events were not previously evaluated. The incidence of stroke in a broad postsurgical population is approximately 1 per 1000 cases based on the ACS-NSQIP database. However, early data from the NeuroVision trial in noncardiac surgery patients with cardiac risk factors suggest that the incidence of covert stroke (i.e., stroke without obvious neurologic deficit) in patients ≥65 years of age is 10% based on postoperative MRI.

11. When is a pulmonary consultation advisable before spinal surgery?
- Thoracic spinal deformities
- Neuromuscular spinal deformities
- Patients with known pulmonary problems (asthma, COPD, sleep apnea, emphysema) or smoking history.

12. **Which patients are likely to require ventilator support after spinal surgery?**
Patients are extubated following spine surgery according to accepted anesthesia protocols. Examples of situations where it may be wise to delay extubation include:
- Patients with significant preoperative impairment of pulmonary function
- Patients undergoing same-day multilevel anterior and posterior thoracolumbar fusion procedures, involving extensive blood loss, fluid shifts, and prolonged operative time.
- Patients undergoing extensive anterior or circumferential cervical surgery associated with prolonged operative times (>5 hours), extensive blood loss (>300 mL), extensive anterior exposures (>3 levels), exposures involving the C2–C4 spinal levels, or in the presence of high-risk patient factors (morbid obesity) or anesthetic factors (multiple intubation attempts) due to risk of postoperative neck edema and resultant airway obstruction.

13. **Why are smokers at increased risk of complications following spinal procedures compared with nonsmokers?**
Smoking increases the risk of cardiopulmonary complications after surgery (e.g., atelectasis, pneumonia). Cessation of smoking 2 months before surgery reduces the risk of pulmonary complications fourfold. Smoking also decreases the success rate of spinal fusion and increases the risks for postoperative wound complications and infection.

14. **List some key points relating to neurologic assessment prior to spinal procedures.**
- Document the presence of any preoperative neurologic deficits
- Routinely screen for myelopathic signs and symptoms, including gait abnormalities
- Determine the patient's ability to cooperate with a wake-up test (if need is anticipated)
- Consider a neurology consultation if a history of seizure disorder is present
- Obtain neurosurgery consultation if spinal deformity correction is planned in a patient with a CNS shunt.

15. **Why is nutritional assessment important? How is a patient's nutritional status quantified?**
Malnutrition increases the chance of postoperative infection and wound healing complications and is associated with increased length of hospital stay. Serum albumin less than 3.5 mg/dL, total lymphocyte count less than 1500–2000 cells/mm, transferrin less than 200 mg/dL, and prealbumin less than 20 mg/dL are considered to represent clinical malnutrition.

16. **What are the options for blood transfusion if significant blood loss is anticipated during a spinal procedure?**
1. Autologous blood transfusion (use of the patient's own blood)
   - Reinfusion of predonated autologous blood
   - Acute normovolemic hemodilution
   - Use of an intraoperative cell saver device
   - Postoperative cell salvage of blood collected from surgical drains
2. Transfusion of blood from a directed donor (e.g., family member)
3. Allogenic blood transfusion (i.e., community blood pool).

17. **Does the presence of diabetes increase the risk of complications associated with spine surgery?**
Yes. The presence of diabetes increases the rate of overall postoperative complications following spine surgery, including the risks of impaired wound healing and wound infection. In addition, insulin-dependent diabetic patients who undergo decompression for radiculopathy have less favorable outcomes, especially if peripheral neuropathy is present. Optimization of blood glucose levels preoperatively can result in improved wound healing and decreased infection rates. A preoperative HgbA1c of <7% is recommended prior to spine surgery in diabetic patients to decrease these risks.

18. **What problems may occur due to alcohol intake in patients who undergo spine surgery?**
Patients should be screened for alcohol use and the possibility of alcohol withdrawal during hospital admission to prevent related complications. The two most useful screening tools to identify those patients who may benefit from referral for evaluation and subsequent intervention are the CAGE (Cut down, Annoyed, Guilty, Eye-opener) questionnaire and AUDIT (Alcohol Use Disorders Identification Test) tool. Useful lab markers for excessive alcohol use include gamma-glutamyltransferase (GGT), carbohydrate-deficient transferrin (CDT), and red-cell mean corpuscular volume. Some problems associated with alcohol use in surgical patients include:
- Altered metabolism of medications including anesthetic agents
- Abnormal hemostasis due to decrease in vitamin K-dependent clotting factors and platelet abnormalities.
- Metabolic abnormalities: hypoglycemia, ketoacidosis, malnutrition, nutrient deficiencies (thiamine, folate, and magnesium).
- Alcohol withdrawal symptoms (autonomic dysfunction, seizures, hallucinations, delirium).
- Postoperative complications, including increased surgical bleeding time, increased hospital length of stay, intensive care unit admission, wound complications, postoperative infections, pseudarthrosis following spine fusion, pulmonary complications, and postoperative ileus.

19. **What problems are encountered following spinal procedures in patients who use opioids preoperatively?**
It has been estimated that over 50% of patients presenting for spine surgery use opioids. Opioid consumption prior to elective spine surgery is associated with worse postoperative patient-reported outcomes with respect to pain, function, and quality of life. In addition, patients treated with opioids are less likely to be satisfied following surgery and have an increased risk of postoperative complications. Use of a multidisciplinary approach, including psychologic and opioid screening, with weaning from opioids preoperatively and close opioid monitoring postoperatively, is recommended.

20. **List basic equipment/facility requirements for undertaking complex spinal procedures.**
Although not an all-inclusive list, some basic requirements include:
    - Range of spinal implants and ancillary instrumentation
    - Power equipment (e.g., surgical drills and burrs)
    - Imaging capability (radiographs, fluoroscopy, surgical navigation)
    - Radiolucent spine table
    - Anesthesiologists familiar with anesthetic requirements for complex spine surgery
    - Intraoperative neurophysiologic monitoring capability
    - Surgical microscope
    - Blood recovery system (cell saver)
    - Bone bank access
    - Appropriate perioperative medical and surgical support services including intensive care facilities when indicated.

21. **What is the best way to ensure that a patient has been adequately educated about their diagnosis, treatment, and recovery before an elective spinal procedure?**
The surgeon should arrange and attend a meeting with the patient and caregivers prior to surgery. Important points to cover during this meeting include:
    - Review patient's specific spinal problem and treatment alternatives
    - Review pertinent diagnostic studies
    - Explain specific surgical procedures using spine models (incisions, bone graft, implants, Food and Drug Administration status of spinal devices).
    - Discuss realistic expectations and goals of surgical treatment (pain relief, deformity correction, neurologic improvement, likely outcome of procedure).
    - Discuss possible surgical complications, obtain informed consent, and document this process in the medical record.
    - Confirm arrangements for blood donation, cessation of aspirin and antiinflammatory medication (as appropriate), cessation of smoking, spinal monitoring, review of wake-up test (if needed), and orthosis (if needed).
    - Order any additional imaging studies required for final preoperative planning
    - Review final recommendations and evaluations by consultants (anesthesiologist, internist, cardiologist, pulmonologist)
    - Remind patient of the importance of preoperative chlorhexidine skin wash at home prior to surgery to decrease infection risk.
    - Outline events on the day of surgery for the patient and family: check-in procedures and waiting area, duration of surgery, and patient's postoperative location and status (ICU vs. step down vs. standard floor vs. outpatient); discuss need for postoperative ventilatory support (when appropriate). Arrange for hospital tour (when appropriate).
    - Review anticipated hospital course/discharge arrangements: length of stay, discharge planning concerns, work-related issues, psychologic support during recovery period, and chemical dependency issues related to use of narcotic medication.

22. **What are some complications which should be explained to the patient as part of the informed consent process prior to performing a procedure for decompression of the spinal cord and/or nerve roots?**
    - Neurologic injury
    - Dural tear
    - Spinal instability
    - Persistent or increased back and/or extremity pain
    - Blood loss
    - Epidural hematoma
    - Wound infection
    - Complications related to the surgical approach or surgical positioning
    - Potential need for subsequent spinal surgery including stabilization procedures
    - Medical complications—urinary tract infection, myocardial infarction, deep vein thrombosis
    - Anesthetic complication
    - Postoperative visual loss or blindness
    - Arachnoiditis
    - Death

23. **What are some complications which should be explained to the patient as part of the informed consent process prior to surgical procedures that involve spinal instrumentation and fusion?**
    - Implant/bone graft failure, misplacement, or dislodgement
    - Neurologic injury, including paralysis and loss of bowel and bladder control
    - Pseudarthrosis (failure of fusion)
    - Bone graft donor site pain
    - Infection
    - Blood loss
    - Epidural hematoma
    - Diseases transmitted by blood transfusion or allograft bone
    - Dural tear
    - Persistent or increased back and/or extremity pain
    - Need for subsequent spinal surgery
    - Medical complications: urinary tract infection, myocardial infarction, pneumonia, deep vein thrombosis, pulmonary embolism, stroke.
    - Allergic reaction (to drugs, metallic devices)
    - Surgical approach-related complications (e.g., hernia, retrograde ejaculation in men, vascular injury, visceral injury, dysphagia)
    - Visual difficulty or blindness postoperatively
    - Injury due to surgical positioning including brachial plexus injury and pressure sores on chest, facial areas, pelvis, and lower extremities.
    - Anesthetic complication
    - Death

24. **What is an enhanced recovery after surgery program?**
    Enhanced recovery after surgery (ERAS) involves the systematic implementation of an evidence-based perioperative multimodal protocol to optimize patient outcomes in the preoperative, intraoperative, and postoperative periods, and is directed toward attenuation of the surgical stress response, optimization of pain management, and reduction in morbidity. ERAS emphasizes a multidisciplinary approach to perioperative care which emphasizes preoperative education, multimodal pain management, minimization of blood loss, minimally invasive surgical approaches, enhanced nutrition, and early rehabilitation so that patients are able to recover more quickly. Various components of ERAS have been applied to spinal surgery in recent years, and there is strong interest in implementing such approaches. For example, multimodal analgesia regimens that include preoperative, intraoperative, and postoperative components using medications with different mechanisms of action such as NSAIDs, gabapentin and pregabalin, acetaminophen, muscle relaxants, and extended-release local anesthesia provide improved pain control and reduced complications, compared with patients treated with traditional postoperative patient-controlled analgesia using opioids.

KEY POINTS

1. Comprehensive preoperative evaluation and planning decreases perioperative complications and optimizes patient outcomes following spine surgery.
2. Patient education regarding diagnosis, treatment alternatives, complications, and anticipated recovery is an integral component of the preoperative planning process.
3. Patients considering spinal surgery may be counseled regarding their specific risk for medical complications, infection, and dural tear based on their personal comorbidity profile and the surgical invasiveness of the proposed operative intervention using an online risk calculator.
4. Enhanced recovery after surgery (ERAS) involves the systematic implementation of an evidence-based perioperative multimodal protocol to optimize patient outcomes in the preoperative, intraoperative, and postoperative periods.

Websites
1. 2014 ACC/AHA guideline on perioperative cardiovascular evaluation and management of patients undergoing noncardiac surgery: https://www.ahajournals.org/doi/10.1161/CIR.0000000000000106
2. Alcohol Use Disorders Identification Test (AUDIT): http://whqlibdoc.who.int/hq/2001/WHO_MSD_MSB_01.6a.pdf
3. ACS-NSQUIP Surgical Risk Calculator: https://riskcalculator.facs.org/RiskCalculator/
4. ERAS Society: http://erassociety.org/guidelines/list-of-guidelines/
5. Perioperative pocket manual: http://enotes.tripod.com/periop-0.htm
6. The Safety in Spine Surgery Project: http://safetyinspinesurgery.com/about-us/
7. SpineSage™: http://depts.washington.edu/spinersk/about.php

BIBLIOGRAPHY

1. Ali, Z. S., Ma, T. S., Ozturk, A. K., Malhotra, N. R., Schuster, J. M., Marcotte, P. J., et al. (2018). Preoptimization of spinal surgery patients: Development of a neurosurgical enhanced recovery after surgery (ERAS) protocol. *Clinical Neurology and Neurosurgery, 164,* 142–153.
2. Buchlak, Q., Yanamadala, V., Leveque, J. C., & Sethi, R. (2016). Complication avoidance with preoperative screening: Insights from the Seattle spine team. *Current Reviews in Musculoskeletal Medicine, 9,* 316–326.
3. Lee, D., Armaghani, S., Archer, K. R., Bible, J., Shau, D., Kay, H., et al. (2014). Preoperative opioid use as a predictor of adverse postoperative selfreported outcomes in patients undergoing spine surgery. *Journal of Bone and Joint Surgery. American Volume, 96,* 89.
4. Lee, M. J., Cizik, A. M., Hamilton, D., & Chapman, J. R. (2014). Predicting medical complications after spine surgery: A validated model using prospective surgical registry data. *Spine Journal, 14,* 291–299.
5. Mirza, S. K., Deyo, R. A., Heagerty, P. J., Konodi, M. A., Lee, L. A., Turner, J. A., et al. (2008). Development of an index to characterize the "invasiveness" of spine surgery: Validation by comparison to blood loss and operative time. *Spine, 33,* 2651–2661.
6. Hu, S. S., & Berven, S. H. (2006). Preparing the adult deformity patient for spine surgery. *Spine, 31,* 126–131.
7. Sethi, R. K., Pong, R. P., Leveque, J. C., Dean, T. C., Olivar, S. J., & Rupp, S. M. (2014). The Seattle spine team approach to adult deformity surgery: A systems-based approach to perioperative care and subsequent reduction in perioperative complication rates. *Spine Deformity, 2,* 95–103.
8. Sugrue, P. A., Halpin, R. J., & Koski, T. R. (2014). Treatment algorithms and protocol practice in high-risk spine surgery. *Neurosurgery Clinics of North America, 24,* 219–230.
9. Wainright, T. W., Immins, T., & Middleton, R. G. (2016). Enhanced recovery after surgery (ERAS) and its applicability for major spine surgery. Best Practice & Research. *Clinical Anesthesiology, 30,* 91–102.

CHAPTER 21

ANESTHETIC CONSIDERATIONS AND INTRAOPERATIVE MANAGEMENT DURING SPINE SURGERY

Vincent J. Devlin, MD

1. **What are some key areas of focus in relation to perioperative anesthetic management of spinal surgery patients?**
   1. Preanesthetic patient risk assessment and optimization for surgery
   2. Assessment of procedure-specific risk factors
   3. Identification of a potentially difficult airway, cervical instability, or spinal cord compression
   4. Hemodynamic monitoring requirements
   5. Intraoperative neurophysiologic monitoring and anesthetic agent selection
   6. Intraoperative positioning
   7. Maintenance of normothermia
   8. Fluid and blood loss management
   9. Preparation for potential intraoperative crises
   10. Postoperative care coordination including tracheal extubation and pain management

2. **How do anesthesiologists assess anesthetic risk for a patient scheduled to undergo spinal surgery?**
   Anesthesiologists perform a preanesthetic evaluation and assign an American Society of Anesthesiologist (ASA) physical status classification (Table 21.1). Preanesthetic assessment includes a review of medical records, patient interview, and a focused history and physical examination, including assessment of any comorbid conditions. Preoperative testing and subspecialty medical consultations are obtained as indicated. Areas of particular interest include current medications, allergies, anesthetic history, history of surgical procedures, history of bleeding disorder or excessive bleeding, cardiovascular and respiratory risk factors, identification of patients who may pose challenges related to airway management, and assessment of functional capacity (metabolic equivalents of task score [METS]). An informed consent for anesthesia care is obtained. Factors that contribute to development of the anesthetic plan for a specific patient include the surgical site, number of operatively treated spinal levels, surgical approach, anticipated blood loss, surgical duration, and use of intraoperative neurophysiologic monitoring. Standardized high-risk spine protocols have been defined for patients, including those who undergo surgery lasting >6 hours, >6 surgical levels, staged procedures, adult and pediatric spinal deformity procedures, and patients with significant medical comorbidities. Online surgical risk calculators (e.g., ACS-NSQIP, SpineSage) may be used to provide a more detailed estimate of patient and procedural risk.

3. **What are some of the major categories of intraoperative adverse events associated with spinal surgery?**
   Various classification systems have been developed to categorize intraoperative adverse events associated with spine surgery. (1) Some general categories of potential intraoperative adverse events during spinal surgery are listed in Table 21.2.

4. **What types of cervical spine pathologies are at risk for neurologic injury with endotracheal intubation?**
   Patients with an unstable cervical spine (e.g., fracture, rheumatoid arthritis, odontoid hypoplasia) or severe cervical stenosis are at risk for neurologic injury with endotracheal intubation. Important factors for minimizing neurologic injury include recognizing cord compression and/or spinal instability, performing intubation with care, and avoiding neck movement, especially extension of the cervical spine. Many anesthesiologists prefer fiber-optic intubation in this setting. Monitoring of neurologic function can be performed directly if an awake intubation technique is utilized or indirectly with neurophysiologic monitoring if an unconscious fiber-optic–guided intubation is performed. A variety of alternative intubation methods have been described, including manual inline cervical immobilization and orotracheal intubation, nasal intubation, as well as use of specialized laryngoscope blades, video laryngoscopes, lighted stylets, and bronchoscopes. Intubation technique is guided by the ASA Difficult Airway Algorithm and the skills and preferences of the anesthesiologist.

Table 21.1 American Society of Anesthesiologists Physical Status Classification System.

CLASS	DESCRIPTION
1	Normal, healthy patient
2	Patient with mild systemic disease
3	Patient with severe systemic disease
4	Patient with severe systemic disease that is a constant threat to life
5	Moribund patient who is not expected to survive without the operation
6	A declared brain-dead patient whose organs are being removed for donor purposes
E	Patient undergoing an emergency procedure[a]

[a]Emergency exists when delay in treatment would lead to a significant increase in the threat to life or body part (https://www.asahq.org/standards-and-guidelines/asa-physical-status-classification-system).

Table 21.2 General Categories of Intraoperative Adverse Events During Spinal Surgery.

1. Airway or ventilation related	11. Ophthalmologic injury
2. Allergic reactions	12. Respiratory
3. Anesthesia related	13. Spinal implant–related
4. Cardiac	14. Sterile field contamination
5. Coagulopathy	15. Surgical instrument breakage or failure
6. Death	16. Surgical positioning injury
7. Dural tear	17. Unplanned change in surgical procedure
8. Hypotension	18. Vascular injury
9. Massive blood loss	19. Visceral injury
10. Neurologic injury	20. Wrong level/side surgery

5. **What are some strategies that can be used to avoid operating at the wrong site during spinal procedures?**
Wrong site spinal surgery can involve operating at the wrong spinal level, the wrong side of the spine, or even performing surgery on the wrong patient. Various guidelines and safety checklists exist to ensure that wrong site surgery does not occur. The North American Spine Society developed a Sign, Mark, and X-Ray Checklist for safety which includes:
   - Preprocedure verification of patient identity, procedure site, and imaging studies. It is important to confirm that level identification on preoperative MRI correlates with level identification based on preoperative radiographs.
   - Marking of the surgical site prior to surgery.
   - Time-out prior to start of procedure to confirm correct surgical site, surgical side, and patient identity.
   - Intraoperative imaging to locate and mark the appropriate vertebral level with a radiopaque marker, preferably at the level of the pedicle.
   - Time-out during surgery to confirm radiographic localization of the appropriate surgical level(s).

   Intraoperative localizing imaging studies require correlation with preoperative radiographs and MRI studies, as anatomic variations (i.e., Klippel-Feil anomaly, nonstandard number of ribs, transitional lumbosacral junction) may lead to incorrect level identification. Regional anatomic landmarks and visualization of radiologically evident pathology (e.g., vertebral fracture, spondylolisthesis) may be used as a secondary check to confirm appropriate level selection. Localization of thoracic levels during anterior approaches may be especially challenging, and preoperative placement of polymethyl methacrylate impregnated with barium sulfate or radiopaque coils have been described to facilitate identification of the correct thoracic spinal level.

6. **What types of spinal procedures benefit from use of single-lung ventilation?**
Thoracic spine procedures performed with the assistance of thoracoscopy require single-lung ventilation to maintain a safe working space within the thoracic cavity. Anterior thoracic spine procedures performed through an open thoracotomy approach for exposure of the spine above the level of T8 also benefit from single-lung

ventilation. In open anterior thoracic spine procedures, single-lung ventilation decreases the difficulty of retracting the lung from the operative field in the upper thoracic region. For open procedures below the T8 level, the lung can more easily be retracted out of the operative field without the need for single-lung ventilation. Options for single-lung ventilation include use of a double-lumen endotracheal tube or a bronchial blocker inserted into a single-lumen tube. Remember that a double-lumen tube will need to be changed to a single-lumen tube at the end of the procedure if extubation is not planned as it is not suitable for postoperative ventilation.

7. **What patient populations are at increased risk of latex allergy?**
Prior exposure to latex as a result of medical treatment (e.g., multiple bladder catheterizations, multiple surgical procedures at a young age) or occupational exposure may lead to an IgE-mediated anaphylactic reaction upon subsequent exposure to the latex antigen. In addition to health-care workers, patient populations with an increased risk of latex allergy include those with myelodysplasia, congenital genitourinary tract abnormalities, spinal cord injuries, cerebral palsy, and ventriculoperitoneal shunts. Anaphylaxis secondary to latex allergy may occur intraoperatively (usually 20–60 minutes following induction) and must be included in the differential diagnosis of intraoperative emergencies. A detailed history is the best means of detecting patients at risk. Patients with a history of latex allergy may be treated with pharmacologic prophylaxis (diphenhydramine, ranitidine, prednisone), but this may not prevent an anaphylactic reaction. A latex-safe environment must be provided in the operating room (OR).

8. **What types of anesthetic monitoring are recommended during spinal procedures?**
Basic intraoperative anesthetic monitoring for spine surgery includes continuous assessment of heart rate, electrocardiogram, blood pressure, oxygen saturation (SaO_2), end tidal carbon dioxide, temperature, fluid intake, and urine output. Additional monitoring modalities include intraoperative neurophysiologic monitoring, neuromuscular blockade monitoring, and depth of anesthesia monitoring. Vascular access for major spine procedures includes two large-bore peripheral intravenous lines, intraarterial blood pressure monitoring, and a central line. Use of minimally invasive cardiac output measurement techniques (e.g., FloTrac/Vigileo system) enables use of goal-directed fluid management to optimize intraoperative hemodynamic management.

9. **What are some important considerations regarding management of fluid administration, blood loss, and coagulopathy during major spinal reconstructive procedures?**
Detailed recording of fluid administration, hourly estimated blood loss, and laboratory values on a tracking sheet or display board is recommended. Crystalloid solutions are administered initially, followed by infusion of colloid solutions for losses in excess of maintenance fluid requirements. Traditional parameters for guiding adequacy of fluid replacement such as heart rate, blood pressure, and central venous pressure react slowly to changes in intravascular volume, and various goal-directed fluid therapy approaches based on variables such as stroke volume variation, pulse pressure variation, and cardiac filling pressures have been suggested to optimize fluid management. (2) For complex procedures at the spinal cord level, use of intraoperative neurophysiologic monitoring and maintenance of mean arterial pressure (MAP) in a range of 85–90 mm have been recommended to prevent ischemic injury to the spinal cord.

There is no universally accepted threshold at which to transfuse blood during spinal procedures, although a restrictive intraoperative transfusion trigger (hemoglobin [Hgb] <8 g/dL, hematocrit [HCT] <25%), has been associated with lower morbidity and shorter length of stay compared to use of a liberal trigger. An intraoperative Hgb level ranging from 8 to 10 g/dL is often targeted, depending on patient comorbidities and case-specific factors including procedure type, procedure duration, and the rate and volume of blood loss anticipated. Institution-specific transfusion protocols have been described for use in cases of massive, life-threatening intraoperative blood loss.

Options for treatment of coagulopathy include fresh frozen plasma, cryoprecipitate (fibrinogen level <150 mg/dL), platelet infusion (platelet count <100,000 U/µL),), desmopressin (for persistent oozing after correction of fibrinogen and platelet levels), and recombinant factor VIIa (for persistent oozing if international normalized ratio [INR] >2 and desmopressin has been administered). (3) In rare cases, disseminated intravascular coagulation (DIC) may develop due to widespread activation of the coagulation system with excessive consumption of coagulation factors, platelets, fibrinogen, and associated microvascular thrombi formation, and life-threatening bleeding.

10. **What are some methods that can be used to reduce allogeneic blood transfusion during spine surgery?**
   - Preoperative autologous blood donation
   - Preoperative marrow stimulation (erythropoietin)
   - Acute normovolemic hemodilution
   - Intraoperative salvage (use of cell saver)
   - Use of antifibrinolytic agents (epsilon aminocaproic acid [EACA], tranexamic acid [TXA])
   - Accepting a lower threshold Hgb level before transfusion (restrictive transfusion trigger)
   - Use of topical hemostatic agents as an adjunct to surgical hemostasis

11. **What complications have been reported in association with hypothermia during surgery?**
Complications reported in association with intraoperative hypothermia (core temperature <35.5 degrees C) include myocardial depression, cardiac arrhythmias, thrombocytopenia, decreased mobilization of calcium, prolongation of

drug half-lives, lactic acidosis, and surgical site infection. Steps that can be taken to prevent hypothermia during spine surgery include:
- Use of forced-air warming systems
- Use of fluid warmers
- Use of humidified, warmed (40 degrees C) inspired gases
- Use of warm lavage for wound irrigation
- Warming of the OR

12. What are the options for monitoring neurologic function during spinal procedures?
A variety of methods may be used to monitor neurologic function during spinal surgery including:
- Somatosensory-evoked potentials (SSEPs)
- Transcranial electric motor–evoked potentials (tceMEPs)
- Electromyography (EMG)
- Stagnara wake-up test
- Ankle clonus test

13. What difficulties have been reported in association with use of the Stagnara intraoperative wake-up test?
- Extubation secondary to patient movement
- Dislodgement of intravenous access
- Air embolus
- Dislodgement of spinal implants
- Difficulty using the test in patients with reduced capacity (e.g., deafness, language barrier)
- Contamination of the surgical field

14. How do anesthetic requirements differ for various spinal monitoring techniques?
For **surgery at the level of the spinal cord or conus medullaris**, multimodality monitoring with a combination of SSEPs and tceMEPs is indicated. The preferred anesthetic technique in this situation is total intravenous anesthesia (TIVA) using propofol and a short-acting opioid infusion. If TIVA is not used, anesthesia with a combined low-level volatile agent (e.g., 0.3 minimum alveolar concentration [MAC]) augmented by combination intravenous drugs may be used, although even this low concentration of volatile anesthetic is known to compromise cortical SSEP and tceMEP amplitudes, as well as increase signal variability. Hence, use of any inhalational anesthetics should be viewed only as a "last resort" measure. When propofol is either precluded or is not readily available, TIVA alternatives include ketamine, etomidate, and/or dexmedetomidine.

For **surgery in the lumbar region below the level of the conus medullaris**, monitoring typically is directed toward assessment of lumbar nerve root function with recording of spontaneous and stimulus-evoked EMG from lower extremity myotomes in conjunction with upper extremity SSEPs to identify impending positional brachial plexopathy. This permits a less restrictive anesthesia protocol and allows greater flexibility in the use of inhalational agents rather than TIVA. In such cases, it is critical to ensure that the neuromuscular junction is unblocked. Once decompression commences, there should be no muscle relaxants on-board as evidenced by a train-of-four ratio of at least 0.7, measured preferably from a foot versus a hand muscle. Recent studies have shown that absence or cessation of spontaneous neurotonic electromyographic activity provides limited information about the functional integrity of spinal nerve roots and appears to be insensitive to slow-onset traction injuries or vascular insult to the nerve root. Consequently, some centers have modified their neurophysiologic monitoring strategy during instrumented lumbosacral spine surgery to include tceMEPs in order to provide ongoing information regarding nerve root functional integrity. When tceMEPs are recorded, a TIVA protocol is preferred. In such cases, the anesthetic requirements for TIVA are the same as for cervical or thoracic spine surgery (propofol, opioid [preferably remifentanil], midazolam [low dose of 1–2 mg/h if needed], and no neuromuscular blockade).

15. In addition to use of intraoperative neurophysiologic monitoring, what are two additional practices that can help minimize the risk of intraoperative neurologic injury?
- *Careful patient positioning for surgery.* Neurologic injury related to positioning can be minimized with attention to detail and use of strategies to avoid compression and traction injuries, which most commonly involve the ulnar nerve and brachial plexus.
- *Maintain normal or slightly elevated MAP and avoid episodes of hypotension.* In high-risk patients (e.g., severe myelopathy, preexistent neurologic deficit), maintenance of MAP in the range of 85–90 mm maintains spinal cord perfusion and minimizes the risk of ischemic neurologic injury.

16. What are some important considerations when positioning patients for a spinal procedure in the supine position?
The supine position is used for procedures that involve anterior access to the cervical or lumbar spinal regions. For cervical procedures, the neck is maintained in a neutral position, the arms are tucked at the patient's side,

and the elbows are cushioned with foam padding to protect the ulnar nerves. The shoulders may be taped to enhance visualization of the lower cervical region with fluoroscopy. If intraoperative cervical traction is planned, cervical tongs are applied. For lumbar procedures, the arms may be tucked or abducted to less than 90° depending on the location of the required abdominal incision.

17. List some important considerations when positioning a patient for a spinal procedure in the lateral decubitus position.

The lateral decubitus position is used for surgical procedures involving the anterior spinal column in the thoracic and lumbar regions. Important considerations include:

- In the lateral decubitus position, pulmonary blood flow is greater to the dependent lung, while the nondependent lung receives preferential ventilation leading to ventilation and perfusion mismatch
- Neutral alignment of the head and cervical spine should be maintained
- Protection of the dependent eye and ear from pressure
- Placement of an axillary roll caudal to the axilla to relieve pressure on the dependent shoulder and prevent compression of the brachial plexus and vascular structures by the humeral head
- Protection of the peroneal nerve in the dependent leg by knee flexion and use of a pillow
- Placement of a pillow between the legs to prevent pressure from bony prominences
- Sequential compression stockings to prevent venous pooling in the lower extremities

18. What are some important concerns when the kneeling or tuck position is used for spinal procedures?

The extreme degree of hip and knee flexion required to achieve this position is not possible for many patients, especially those with total joint replacements or severe hip or knee arthritis. This position can significantly compromise perfusion to the lower extremities, resulting in ischemia, thrombosis, compartment syndrome, and neurologic deficits. Use of this position is restricted to brief spinal procedures such as lumbar discectomy.

19. What are some concerns with use of the sitting position for cervical spine procedures?

The sitting position is preferred by some surgeons for procedures involving the posterior cervical spine. A major advantage of this position is reduced blood pooling in the surgical field and potentially reduced blood loss because of improved venous drainage. The airway is easily accessible, and optimal ventilation of lungs is facilitated. The disadvantages include systemic hypotension and the creation of a negative pressure gradient that may result in air entrainment and venous air embolus (VAE). Careful management and monitoring are essential to prevent serious complications associated with this operative position. Prior hydration and gradual transfer to the sitting position help avoid undue systemic hypotension. Insertion of a central venous pressure catheter is recommended to monitor intravascular pressure, confirm the potential diagnosis of air embolism, and provide access to retrieve air in the event that a large embolus obstructs cardiac outflow. A precordial Doppler placed on the right chest is a sensitive marker for sounds of air embolus.

20. List some important considerations when positioning patients for a spinal procedure in the prone position.

Most patients readily tolerate spine surgery in the prone position (Fig. 21.1). Important considerations include:

- Transfer from the supine to the prone position requires coordination with all OR staff. Specific protocols are used for patients with unstable spine conditions. Use of a spine-specific turning frame has been shown to generate significantly less spine motion compared with a log-roll technique during supine to prone transfers onto the OR table in unstable spine conditions.
- The prone position is associated with a decrease in cardiac index and increase in abdominal pressure, which may be transmitted to the venous system and increase blood loss.
- The head should be kept at or slightly above the level of the heart to maintain brain perfusion. The head-down position should be avoided because it decreases intraocular perfusion pressure.
- The cervical spine should be kept in a neutral or slightly flexed position. Hyperextension, hyperflexion, and extreme rotation of the cervical spine should be avoided.
- Cushioning should be placed beneath the forehead and chin, to keep the eyes, chin, and face free of pressure. Soft foam with preconfigured cutouts, gel pads, and helmet systems are available for use in prone head positioning. Alternatively, cervical tongs or a halo ring with pin fixation may be used to suspend the head using traction or through use of table-specific attachments.
- The upper extremities should be positioned with the shoulders and elbows abducted and flexed below 90° (for thoracic and lumbar procedures) or tucked at the patient's sides (for cervical procedures).
- Compression of the thoracic region should be minimized to avoid adverse impact on ventilation and airway pressure.
- Padding should be placed beneath the elbow to protect the ulnar nerve from compression.
- The abdomen should be free of compression to reduce venous backflow through Batson's plexus with resultant vertebral venous plexus engorgement.

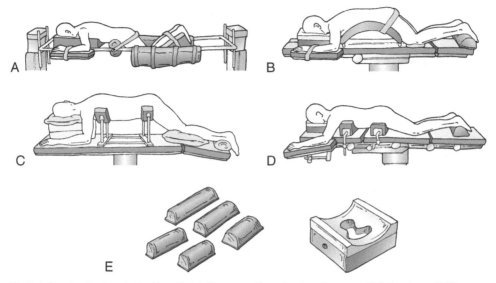

Fig. 21.1 Examples of equipment utilized for patients in the prone position undergoing spine surgery. (A) Jackson frame; (B) Wilson frame pad; (C) Relton-Hall accessory frame; (D) regular operating room table with bolster supports under sternum, iliac crest, and lower legs; (E) gel foam pads and prone head pillows. (From Stier GR, Asgarzadie F, Cole DJ. Neurosurgical diseases and trauma of the spine and spinal cord: anesthetic considerations. In: Cottrell JE, Patel P, editors. Cottrell and Patel's Neuroanesthesia. 6th ed. Philadelphia, PA: Elsevier; 2017, pp. 351–398, Fig. 21.34, p. 390.)

- The breast, chest, and iliac areas should be adequately padded to prevent compression injury.
- If the surgical procedure involves lumbar fusion, the hips should be extended to create a lordotic alignment of the lumbar spinal segments.
- Male genitalia should be checked to verify absence of compression.
- Sequential compression stockings should be placed to prevent venous pooling in the lower extremities.
- The Foley catheter should be secured to prevent dislodgement.

21. **What ophthalmologic complications are encountered in relation to spinal procedures?**
Ophthalmologic complications associated with spinal procedures include corneal abrasions, periorbital edema, and postoperative visual loss (POVL). Corneal abrasions are the most commonly reported ophthalmologic complication and are attributed to loss of the natural lid reflex and decreased tear production as a consequence of general anesthesia. Preventive measures include taping of the eyelids and use of ophthalmic ointments. POVL is a rare but disastrous complication associated with spine surgery in the prone position. POVL most commonly occurs due to ischemic optic neuropathy (ION) and less commonly due to central retinal artery occlusion (CRAO) or occipital infarct. According to the visual loss registry established by the ASA, patients at increased risk are those who undergo lengthy procedures in the prone position (>6 hours) or who experience substantial blood loss (>1 L), or both. Preoperative factors that may increase the risk for POVL include, but are not limited to, male gender, obesity, and the presence vascular disease risk factors (hypertension, peripheral vascular disease, diabetic retinopathy). Mitigating measures include positioning the head level with or higher than the heart, administration of colloids in addition to crystalloids to maintain intravascular volume in patients with substantial blood loss, and staging lengthy procedures in high-risk patients.

22. **What types of spinal procedures are associated with venous air embolus (VAE)?**
VAE is most commonly reported in association with posterior cervical surgery in the sitting position, but may also occur with posterior spine surgery in the prone position. VAE is due to air entering the venous system through multiple venous channels that remain open above the level of the heart. Monitoring for cervical procedures in the sitting position includes a central venous pressure catheter, precordial Doppler, and end tidal CO_2 monitoring. When signs of VAE are detected on Doppler, recommendations include filling the wound with saline irrigation fluid and obtaining hemostasis. Transient jugular venous compression has been suggested as a method to decrease air inflow through the exposed veins. Aspiration of air from the central venous catheter may be attempted. Nitrous oxide should be discontinued from the anesthetic gas mixture. If symptoms resolve, surgery can continue.

In severe cases, surgery is terminated and the head is lowered to allow the patient to be placed in a left lateral decubitus position to optimize the ability to aspirate air from the right atrium.

VAE may also occur during multilevel posterior thoracic and lumbar spinal instrumentation and fusion procedures in the prone position. Visible air bubbling at the operative site has been reported as the first sign of VAE. Treatment follows the principles outlined for posterior cervical procedures. If air continues to enter the venous system, hypotension, arrhythmias, hypoxemia, and cardiac arrest may occur. VAE has been associated with a patent foramen ovale, but this lesion is not present in all cases.

23. **What is malignant hyperthermia (MH)?**
MH is an uncommon autosomal-dominant inherited disorder of skeletal muscle characterized by a hypermetabolic response of skeletal muscle to specific anesthetic agents, primarily volatile, halogenated inhalation agents and the depolarizing muscle relaxant succinylcholine. An important pathophysiologic process in this disorder is intracellular hypercalcemia due to excessive calcium release from the sarcoplasmic reticulum attributed to a genetic anomaly involving the ryanodine or dihydropyridine receptor. Intracellular hypercalcemia activates metabolic pathways that, if left untreated, result in depletion of adenosine triphosphate, high temperature, acidosis, and cell death. No simple preoperative diagnostic test is available but MH susceptibility may be assessed with a muscle biopsy and caffeine-halothane contracture test or with genetic testing.

Early signs of MH include unexplained tachycardia or rise in end-tidal CO_2. Patients may exhibit muscle rigidity, metabolic derangements, elevated body temperature (may exceed 43 degrees C), acute renal failure, coagulation abnormalities, and cardiac arrhythmias leading to death in the absence rapid and appropriate treatment. The Malignant Hyperthermia Association of the United States (MHAUS) maintains a MH Hotline (1-800-644-9737) and website (https://www.mhaus.org/healthcare-professionals/) to assist in managing a crisis. Immediate treatment recommendations when MH is diagnosed include:
1. Call for additional assistance for management of the emergency.
2. Discontinue inhalation agents and succinylcholine.
3. Hyperventilate the patient with 100% oxygen and change the anesthesia circuit.
4. Conclude surgery if possible. If surgery must be continued, maintain anesthesia with intravenous (IV) nontriggering agents such as IV sedatives, narcotics, amnestics, and nondepolarizing muscle relaxants.
5. Administer dantrolene intravenously at 2.5 mg/kg and repeat as needed until the patient responds with a decrease in end-tidal carbon dioxide, decreased muscle rigidity, and/or decreased heart rate.
6. Obtain a blood gas to assess for significant metabolic acidosis and administer 1–2 mEq/kg of bicarbonate for pH <7.1.
7. Treat hyperkalemia with calcium chloride or calcium gluconate, sodium bicarbonate, and insulin.
8. Treat cardiac arrhythmias with standard agents but avoid calcium channel blockers because they may induce hyperkalemia in the presence of dantrolene.
9. Elevation of body temperature should be managed with measures such as iced fluids and cooling blankets.
10. Administer fluid and diuretics to maintain urine output.

24. **What risk factors have been associated with cardiac arrest in the prone position?**
Risk factors associated with intraoperative cardiac arrest in patients undergoing spine surgery in the prone position include hypovolemia, cardiac disease, electrolyte abnormalities, air or fat embolism, mechanical vessel obstruction (e.g., due to poor patient positioning), anaphylaxis, tension pneumothorax, and wound irrigation with hydrogen peroxide. When feasible, the patient is turned to the supine position for cardiopulmonary resuscitation (CPR), taking care to protect the wound from contamination. Prone resuscitation is an option and may be initiated using either a two-handed technique if the patient's sternum is supported, or by providing hand support to the sternum in combination with posterior thoracic compression. An additional option is to access the thorax directly through a left-sided posterior thoracotomy to access the heart and perform internal cardiac massage. (4)

25. **How often do unintentional dural tears complicate spinal decompression procedures and what principles guide treatment of incidental durotomies that occur intraoperatively?**
Dural tears with cerebrospinal fluid (CSF) leakage may occur intraoperatively with reported rates ranging from approximately 1%–17% depending on the location and type of spinal procedure. Risk factors for incidental durotomy include revision surgery for spinal stenosis, ossification of the posterior longitudinal ligament (OPLL) or ligamentum flavum, and advanced age. Optimal treatment for dural tears identified intraoperatively is a water-tight primary closure of the dura. Repair of even partial thickness dural tears has been recommended to avoid sequellae associated with delayed rupture and subsequent CSF leakage. General principles which facilitate successful dural repair include adequate exposure, meticulous hemostasis, use of magnification for optimal visualization, containment of neural tissue, and watertight closure of the incidental durotomy with either an interrupted or locked suture technique. The adequacy of a dural repair should be tested by increasing intrathecal pressure with a Valsalva maneuver and observing whether CSF leakage occurs. If persistent CSF leakage is observed or the dural tear is unable to be closed without tension, augmentation of the dural repair using autologous, allogenic, or synthetic

grafts, and/or use of a dural sealant as an adjunct to the dural repair is recommended. Incidental durotomies involving the cervical spinal region are uncommon. Dural tears occurring during anterior cervical surgery may not be reparable due to limited surgical exposure. In this situation, treatment options include use of a dural sealant and/or an onlay dural patch. Postoperative use of a closed lumbar subarachnoid drainage system to divert CSF drainage from the site of the dural tear is an option for primary treatment in cases where the dura tear is unable to be repaired primarily with suture, or as an adjunctive treatment following dural repair in any spinal region.

26. What major vascular structures are at risk during cervical, thoracic, and lumbar procedures and what are some pearls regarding prevention and management of these injuries?

In the cervical region, vertebral artery injury is the most feared type of vascular injury due to its association with massive blood loss, neurologic sequellae, and mortality. Posterior cervical surgery involving the upper cervical spine exposes the vertebral artery to injury from excessive lateral dissection of the C1 posterior arch (>15 mm from midline) or from placement of screws at the C1 and C2 levels. Strategies to prevent vertebral artery injury during upper posterior cervical surgery include preoperative mapping of the course of the vertebral artery on cross-sectional imaging studies, limiting lateral dissection of the C1 arch, and use of proper technique for place-ment of upper cervical screws. The vertebral artery is also at risk of injury during anterior procedures involving the subaxial cervical region. Preoperative cross-sectional images of the surgical levels should be routinely scruti-nized for an anomalous position of the vertebral artery. Vertebral artery injuries during anterior cervical procedures are most often due to excessive lateral vertebral body resection or failure to recognize the presence of an anoma-lous vertebral artery. Initial management of a vertebral artery injury involves controlling bleeding with direct pressure and activation of a massive transfusion protocol. Immediate evaluation of available management options include vascular surgery consultation, exploration and possible surgical repair or vessel ligation, bypass surgery, or angiography and endovascular treatment with stenting or vessel occlusion.

Iatrogenic intraoperative injury to the thoracic aorta and/or vena cava is uncommon but may occur due to surgical disruption or from misplaced thoracic screws. An acute iatrogenic tear of the thoracic aorta or vena cava is a life-threatening injury and requires immediate treatment upon recognition with direct surgical repair or emergent endovascular techniques. Perforation of the aorta by a thoracic pedicle screw may not be identified intraoperatively, and subsequent successful treatment with screw removal and endovascular repair has been reported.

Iatrogenic vascular injury during lumbar surgery may occur with anterior, lateral, and posterior procedures. During open anterior and lateral lumbar procedures, injuries involving the distal aorta, vena cava, and iliac vessels are treated with direct vascular repair. Injuries to the iliolumbar vein and middle sacral vessels are treated with vessel ligation. For injuries which occur during minimally invasive approaches, treatment is emergent conversion to open surgery and vascular repair or ligation. Vascular injuries during posterior lumbar surgery are most com-monly due to a direct vessel injury following penetration of the anterior longitudinal by a pituitary rongeur. Vascu-lar injury may not be evident initially as bleeding into the surgical field is uncommon. If hemodynamic instability is present, blood and fluid resuscitation and urgent abdominal exploration for vessel repair is carried out. If the patient is hemodynamically stable, consultation for endovascular intervention may be considered.

27. What types of visceral injuries have been reported in association with spine surgery and what are some clinical findings which suggest the presence of a previously unrecognized intraoperative visceral injury?

Visceral injuries reported in association with spinal surgery include injuries to the bowel, ureter, bladder, pancreas, spleen, lung, heart, and esophagus. Clinical manifestations of visceral injuries associated with spine surgery are extremely variable, and depend on the extent and site of injury. Clinical presentation of previously unrecognized visceral injury may include unexplained hypotension or decrease in Hgb, fever, persistent wound infection despite appropriate treatment, cardiac or pulmonary dysfunction, dysphagia, esophagocutaneous fistula, or abdominal pain.

28. What are some practical intraoperative strategies recommended by experts to reduce surgical site infection related to spinal procedures?

- Administration of prophylactic antibiotics within 30 minutes of surgery with redosing intraoperatively for proce-dures lasting longer than twice the half-life of the antibiotic or for cases with blood loss in excess of 1500 mL.
- Preoperative warming and avoidance of intraoperative hypothermia
- Skin preparation with chlorhexidine and alcohol solution
- Limiting unnecessary personnel traffic in the OR
- Initial double gloving by the surgical team with change of outer gloves prior to handling spinal instrumentation.
- Appropriate measures to avoid contamination by intraoperative fluoroscopy and surgical navigation equipment.
- Use of antimicrobial-impregnated sutures
- Copious wound irrigation at the end of the procedure
- Application of vancomycin powder to the wound prior to closure

29. **What are some recommendations regarding how to minimize intraoperative radiation exposure to surgeons and operating room staff?**
Recommendations related to intraoperative radiation safety during spine surgery include (1):
- Utilize appropriate protective equipment including lead aprons, thyroid shields, and leaded eyeglasses.
- Utilize fluoroscopic techniques and practices that minimize radiation exposure and enhance safety of OR personnel including:
  - Use of personal dosimeter
  - Minimize total fluoroscopy time
  - Use pulsed fluoroscopy instead of continuous fluoroscopy
  - Position the image intensifier as close to the patient as possible to limit scatter radiation
  - Use collimation and automatic exposure control when possible
  - Essential staff should stand opposite the x-ray source (near the image intensifier) during lateral fluoroscopy.
  - Nonessential staff should stand far away from fluoroscope, behind lead shield or leave the room when possible (inverse square law).
- Consider use of surgical navigation or intraoperative computed tomography

---

KEY POINTS

1. Spine surgery patients provide a wide range of challenges to the anesthesiologist in relation to airway management, positioning, blood loss, fluid management, and requirements for invasive monitoring.
2. Successful outcomes for complex spine procedures are dependent on implementation of standardized and coordinated team-based approaches to optimize care and minimize intraoperative and postoperative adverse events.

Websites
1. American Society of Anesthesiologists Standards and Guidelines: https://www.asahq.org/standards-and-guidelines
2. Sign, Mark & X-ray—North American Spine Society: https://www.spine.org/Documents/ResearchClinicalCare/SMAX2014Revision.pdf
3. Latex allergy: https://www.aana.com/docs/default-source/practice-aana-com-web-documents-(all)/latex-allergy-management.pdf?sfvrsn=9c0049b1_8
4. Malignant hyperthermia: http://www.mhaus.org/
5. World Health Organization Surgical Safety Checklist: https://www.who.int/patientsafety/safesurgery/checklist/en/

REFERENCES

1. Rampersaud, Y. R., Anderson, P. A., Dimar, J. R., & Fisher, C. G. (2016). Spinal Adverse Events Severity System, version 2 (SAVES-V2): inter- and intraobserver reliability assessment. *Journal of Neurosurgery: Spine, 25*, 256–263.
2. Tandon, M. S., & Saigal, D. (2017). Chapter 24: Spinal surgery. In H. Prabhakar (Ed.), *Essentials of Neuroanesthesia* (pp. 399–439). Philadelphia, PA: Elsevier.
3. Sugrue, P. A., Halpin, R. J., & Koski, T. R. (2013). Treatment algorithms and protocol practices in high-risk spine surgery. *Neurosurgery Clinics of North America, 24*, 219–230.
4. Ramayya, A. G., Abdullah, K. G., Tsai, E. C. (2017). Intraoperative crisis management in spine surgery: what to do when things go bad. In M. P. Steinmetz & E. C. Benzel (Eds.), *Benzel's spine surgery: techniques, complication avoidance, and management* (4th ed., pp. 1848–1858). Philadelphia, PA: Elsevier.

BIBLIOGRAPHY

1. Epstein, N. E. (2013). A review article on the diagnosis and treatment of cerebrospinal fluid fistulas and dural tears occurring during spinal surgery. *Surgical Neurology International, 4*, S301–S317.
2. Kamel, I., & Barnette, R. (2014). Positioning patients for spine surgery: avoiding uncommon position-related complications. *World Journal of Orthopedics. 5*, 425–443.
3. Rankin, D., Zuleta-Alarcon, A., Soghomonyan, S., Abdel-Rasoul, M., Castellon-Larios, K., & Bergese, S. D. (2017). Massive blood loss in elective and orthopedic surgery: Retrospective review of intraoperative transfusion strategy. *Journal of Clinical Anesthesia, 37*, 69–73.
4. Ramayya, A. G., Abdullah, K. G., Tsai, E. C. (2017). Intraoperative crisis management in spine surgery: what to do when things go bad. In M. P. Steinmetz & E. C. Benzel (Eds.), *Benzel's Spine Surgery: Techniques, Complication Avoidance, and Management* (4th ed., pp. 1848–1858). Philadelphia, PA: Elsevier.
5. Rampersaud, Y. R., Anderson, P. A., Dimar, J. R., & Fisher, C. G. (2016). Spinal Adverse Events Severity System, version 2 (SAVES-V2): inter- and intraobserver reliability assessment. *Journal of Neurosurgery: Spine, 25*, 256–263.
6. Sugrue, P. A., Halpin, R. J., & Koski, T. R. (2013). Treatment algorithms and protocol practices in high-risk spine surgery. *Neurosurgery Clinics of North America, 24*, 219–230.
7. Srinivasan, D., Than, K. D., Wang, A. C., La Marca, F., Wang, P. I., Schermerhorn, T. C., et al. (2014). Radiation safety and spine surgery: Systematic review of exposure limits and methods to minimize radiation exposure. *World Neurosurgery, 82*, 1337–1343.

8. Stier, G. R., Asgarzadie, F., & Cole, D. J. (2017). Neurosurgical diseases and trauma of the spine and spinal cord: Anesthetic considerations. In J. E. Cottrell & P. Patel (Eds.), *Cottrell and Patel's Neuroanesthesia* (6th ed., pp. 351–398). Philadelphia, PA: Elsevier.
9. Tandon, M. S., & Saigal, D. (2017). Chapter 24: Spinal surgery. In H. Prabhakar (Ed.), *Essentials of Neuroanesthesia* (pp. 399–439). Philadelphia, PA: Elsevier.
10. Wills, J., Schwend, R. M., & Paterson, A. (2005). Intraoperative visible bubbling of air may be the first sign of venous air embolism during posterior surgery for scoliosis. *Spine. 30*, 629–635.

INTRAOPERATIVE NEUROPHYSIOLOGIC MONITORING DURING SPINAL PROCEDURES

Vincent J. Devlin, MD

1. **What is intraoperative neurophysiologic monitoring?**
   Intraoperative neurophysiologic monitoring refers to the various neurophysiologic techniques used to assess functional integrity of the nervous system during surgical procedures that place these structures at risk.

2. **What neurologic structures are at risk during spinal surgery?**
   - Spinal cord and/or nerve roots at the surgical site
   - Spinal cord and/or peripheral nervous system structures remote from the surgical site, including spinal nerve roots, brachial plexus, lumbosacral plexus, and peripheral nerves (e.g., placed at risk of injury from positioning of extremities, head, or neck)
   - Optic nerve

3. **What criteria need to be met if intraoperative neurophysiologic monitoring is used during spinal surgery?**
   Three criteria need to be met if monitoring is used during spinal surgery:
   - Neurologic structures are at risk
   - Those structures can be monitored reliably and efficiently by qualified personnel
   - The surgeon is willing and able to alter surgical technique based on information provided

4. **List common types of spinal procedures during which intraoperative neurophysiologic monitoring is commonly utilized.**
   - Correction of spinal deformities (scoliosis, kyphosis, spondylolisthesis)
   - Insertion of spinal implants (e.g., pedicle screw systems, intervertebral body fusion devices, especially if inserted via a direct lateral surgical approach)
   - Decompression performed at the level of the spinal cord
   - Surgical treatment of spinal cord tumors

5. **Which intraoperative personnel may perform intraoperative neurophysiologic monitoring? Why is it important for surgeons to be knowledgeable regarding their qualifications?**
   Intraoperative neurophysiologic monitoring involves a technical component and an interpretive component. Technical aspects of monitoring include equipment set-up and execution of specific monitoring modalities. Interpretative aspects of monitoring include development of an intraoperative spinal monitoring plan and assessment of the clinical significance of waveform changes during the spinal procedures. The surgeon should be knowledgeable regarding the credentials of spinal monitoring service providers since the medicolegal burden of interpretation becomes the responsibility of the surgeon if the monitoring provider is not certified to interpret neurophysiologic potentials. Personnel who may be involved in provision of spinal monitoring services include:
   - **Physician:** Most often a neurologist who may work with or without technologists
   - **Neurophysiologist, D.ABNM (Diplomate of the American Board of Neurophysiologic Monitoring):** Neurophysiologist with a minimum of a master's and often a doctorate degree in audiology, neurophysiology, or neurosciences.
   - **Neurophysiologist:** Noncertified neurophysiologist with a minimum of a master's degree and often a doctorate in neurophysiology or neurosciences.
   - **Certified neurophysiologic intraoperative monitoring technologist (CNIM):** Usually a registered electroencephalography (EEG) technologist who has completed a course of study, demonstrated competence in acquiring intraoperative data over a number of cases, and passed a nationally recognized technologist examination.
   - **Audiologist (CCC-A, Certified Clinical Competence-Audiology):** Certified audiologist with a minimum of a master's degree in audiology and related neurophysiology.

6. **What mechanisms may be responsible for neurologic injury during spine procedures?**
   - **Direct injury** due to surgical trauma (e.g., during spinal canal decompression or placement of spinal implants)

- **Traction and/or compression** affecting neural structures. Injury may occur during spinal realignment and deformity correction using spinal instrumentation or as a result of epidural hematoma following corpectomy procedures. Traction or compression injury to neural structures remote from the surgical site may occur due to patient positioning (e.g., brachial plexus traction injury, ulnar nerve compression injury).
- **Ischemia** resulting in decreased perfusion of the spinal cord and/or nerve roots, resulting in ischemic injury to neurologic structures (e.g., following ligation of critical segmental vessels supplying the spinal cord or after an episode of sustained hypotension). Ischemia is the most common mechanism responsible for neurologic injury during scoliosis surgery.

7. What techniques are available for monitoring spinal cord function?
   - Stagnara wake-up test
   - Ankle clonus test
   - Somatosensory-evoked potentials (SSEPs)
   - Transcranial electric motor-evoked potentials (tceMEPs)

8. What techniques are available for monitoring nerve root function during spinal surgery?
   - Electromyographic (EMG) monitoring
   - tceMEP monitoring from multiple myotomes

CLINICALLY BASED SPINAL MONITORING TESTS

9. What is the Stagnara wake-up test?
   The Stagnara wake-up test is used to assess the gross integrity of spinal cord motor tract function during spinal surgery. Discussion of this test with the patient before surgery increases its success. During the procedure, anesthesia is temporarily reduced to a degree where the patient is able to follow simple commands (move both hands and then both feet). Most patients have no recollection of being awakened, and those who recall do not report the experience to be unpleasant. This test has significant limitations. It does not provide information about spinal cord sensory tract function or individual nerve root function. In addition, it cannot be administered in a continuous fashion during surgery. A spinal cord injury may not manifest immediately following a specific surgical maneuver and thus may not be detected with a wake-up test. In addition, impending spinal cord compromise due to ischemia cannot be detected using this test. Furthermore, during the wake-up test, patient movement may disrupt sterility of the operative field or displace the endotracheal tube. The limitations associated with clinically based tests, such as the wake-up and ankle clonus tests, stimulated the development of intraoperative neurophysiologic monitoring techniques.

10. What is the ankle clonus test?
    Ankle clonus is the rhythmic contraction of the calf muscles following sudden, passive dorsiflexion of the foot. Clonus is produced by elicitation of the stretch reflex. In the normal, awake person, clonus cannot be elicited because of central inhibition of this stretch reflex. The clonus test relies on the presence of central inhibition and clonus to confirm that the spinal cord and peripheral neurologic structures are functionally intact. Neurologically intact patients emerging from general anesthesia normally have temporary ankle clonus bilaterally since lower motor neuron function returns before the return of inhibitory upper motor neuron impulses. Absence of transient ankle clonus has been correlated with neurologic compromise, but is not sufficiently reliable for use as a primary test for monitoring spinal cord function.

NEUROPHYSIOLOGIC MONITORING MODALITIES

11. What are SSEPs?
    SSEPs are a modification of the basic EEG in which a cortical or subcortical response to repetitive stimulation of a peripheral mixed nerve is recorded at sites cephalad and caudad to the operative field (Fig. 22.1B). Data consists of a plot of voltages over time and appear as a series of peaks and valleys. Signal amplitude (height from a peak to an adjacent valley) and latency (time from stimulation to a response peak) are recorded continuously during surgery and compared with baseline data. SSEPs provide direct information about the status of the ascending spinal cord sensory tracts (located in the dorsal medial columns of the spinal cord). SSEPs provide only indirect information about the status of the spinal cord motor tracts (located in the anterolateral columns of the spinal cord). SSEPs do not provide real-time data regarding neurologic function because there is a slight delay (usually <1 minute) while the SSEP response is averaged for extraction from background noise.

12. Discuss important limitations of SSEPs.
    SSEPs directly assess spinal cord sensory tracts but provide only indirect information about motor tracts. Damage to the spinal cord motor tracts can occur without a concomitant change in SSEPs. SSEPs are better for detecting mechanical damage than ischemic damage to motor tracts because these cord regions have different blood supplies. The spinal cord motor tracts are supplied by the anterior spinal artery, whereas the spinal cord sensory

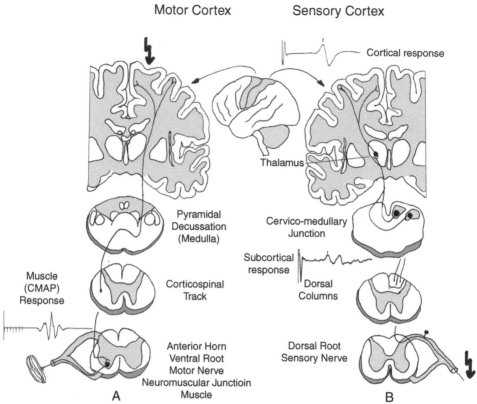

Fig. 22.1 Pathways of the motor evoked potential (MEP) and somatosensory-evoked potential (SSEP). (A) The muscle MEP *(left)* is produced by transcranial electric stimulation of the motor cortex *(arrow)*. The response travels down the corticospinal tract, crossing the midline in the medulla. It continues in the white matter tracts of the spinal cord and activates the motor nuclei in the anterior horn cell of the spinal cord. The response travels via the ventral root to the neuromuscular junction where the response is usually measured as a compound muscle action potential (CMAP). (B) The cortical SSEP *(right)* is produced by electric stimulation of a peripheral sensory nerve *(arrow)*. It enters the spinal cord via the dorsal root and ascends the spinal cord in the dorsal columns. It synapses in the cervicomedullary junction, crosses the midline, and synapses in the thalamus before producing a response in the sensory cortex. The response is typically recorded over the sensory cortex (the cortical SSEP) and the cervical spine (the subcortical response). (From Sloan TB, Edmonds HL, Koht A. Intraoperative electrophysiologic monitoring in aortic surgery. J Cardiothorac Vasc Anesth 2013;27[6]:1364–1373.)

tracts are perfused by radicular arteries. SSEPs may be unrecordable in patients with severe myelopathy, peripheral neuropathy, or obesity. In addition, recording SSEPs is not a sensitive technique for monitoring individual nerve root function as these potentials reflect electrophysiologic signals arising from multiple nerve roots.

13. **What factors other than neurologic injury can have an adverse effect on SSEP recordings?**
    Operating room power equipment (due to electrical interference), halogenated anesthetic agents, nitrous oxide, hypothermia, and hypotension.

14. **When should the surgeon be notified about changes in SSEPs?**
    The surgeon should be notified when SSEPs show a persistent unilateral or bilateral loss of amplitude of 50% or greater, relative to baseline amplitude. Although a 10% increase in latency is often identified as a criterion for surgeon notification, changes in latency are common and less significant, and spinal cord injury is unlikely if amplitude is unchanged.

15. **What are tceMEPs?**
    tceMEPs are neuroelectric impulses elicited by transcranial application of a high-voltage stimulus to electrodes placed over specific scalp regions to excite specific areas of the motor cortex. These descending impulses stimulate corticospinal tract axons and are typically recorded from electrodes placed over key upper and lower extremity peripheral muscles as a compound muscle action potential (CMAP). Motor-evoked potentials can also be recorded from the spinal cord (D- and I-waves) via electrodes placed percutaneously or through a laminotomy (Fig. 22.1A).

16. What is the advantage of using tceMEPs?

tceMEPs can provide information about the functional integrity of the spinal cord motor tracts and individual nerve roots that cannot be obtained using SSEPs. They are extremely sensitive to alterations in spinal cord blood flow resulting from intraoperative hypotension or evolving vascular injury. In addition, alterations in tceMEPs present earlier than changes in SSEPs in patients with evolving neurologic injury, which permits earlier initiation of corrective action to prevent permanent neurologic compromise. Although not a replacement for SSEPs, tceMEPs are used in combination with SSEPs to provide a direct measure of both spinal cord sensory and motor tract function, thereby increasing the efficacy of spinal monitoring.

17. When should the surgeon be notified about changes in tceMEPs?

The surgeon should be notified when the CMAP shows a persistent unilateral or bilateral loss of amplitude of 60% or greater relative to baseline amplitude.

18. Is the use of tceMEPs associated with any dangers or complications?

Only rare and minor complications have been reported in association with the use of tceMEPs in spine surgery. The most common complication is a tongue or lip laceration, which may be avoided by ensuring that a single or double bite block is placed following intubation. Transcranial stimulation has been utilized without untoward effects in patients with cardiac disease, pacemakers, and a history of seizures. Movement-related injury has not been a problem even with patients who are positioned in tongs or with a Mayfield positioner.

19. What is the role of EMG monitoring during spinal procedures?

Electromyography is used to assess the functional integrity of individual nerve roots. EMG techniques are classified into two categories based on method of elicitation: mechanical and electrical. **Mechanically elicited electromyograms (EMGs)** are used during the dynamic phases of surgery (pedicle screw preparation and insertion, nerve root manipulation, drilling, and intervertebral body fusion device insertion via a direct lateral approach) to detect nerve root irritation. Mechanically elicited EMGs are also termed *spontaneous* or *free-running* EMGs. **Electrically elicited EMGs** should be used during the static phases of surgery (immediately before or after pedicle screw placement). An electrically elicited EMG is also termed a *stimulus-evoked* EMG or *triggered* EMG.

20. How does a surgeon use electromyography to check that screws have been properly placed within the lumbar pedicles?

The surgeon places an EMG probe onto the pedicle screw and electrically stimulates the screw. If the pedicle wall is intact, the passage of electrical current will be restricted, and the adjacent nerve root will not be stimulated. If the pedicle wall has been fractured, current passes through the pedicle wall and stimulates the adjacent nerve root. This results in contraction of the associated peripheral muscle, which is recorded as an EMG. Electrical thresholds for EMG activity consistent with safe screw placement have been determined and provide a reference for use in clinical practice (e.g., absence of a stimulation-induced myogenic response up to 10 mA). It is important to place the EMG probe in contact with the hexagonal screw port or directly on the screw shank to avoid false-negative results that could occur when only the crown of the screw is stimulated.

21. What is the difference between *burst* EMG and *train* EMG?

Burst EMG activity is indicative of a nerve root being mechanically irritated, resulting in a brief burst of muscle activity of a few seconds duration. Multiple irritations or insults result in the muscle going into spasm, which is termed *train*. **Train EMG** activity is consistent with nerve root injury and must be dealt with immediately because it often predicts postoperative motor nerve deficit.

22. How is intraoperative spinal monitoring used to prevent neurologic injury secondary to patient positioning?

Tetraplegia or paraplegia may result from hyperextension positioning of the stenotic cervical or lumbar spine. Spinal monitoring of both upper and lower extremity neurologic function can permit prompt recognition and repositioning, thereby preventing permanent neurologic deficit. Monitoring of ulnar nerve SSEPs is performed to assess possible brachial plexopathy due to changes in arm positioning. During anterior spinal procedures, monitoring of peroneal and femoral nerve function is performed. Peroneal nerve monitoring can alert staff to the onset of an impending peroneal nerve palsy secondary to pressure of the leg against the operating room table. A permanent injury can be averted by moving the patient's leg or adjusting the leg padding. Monitoring of femoral nerve function can alert the surgeon to excessive traction on the iliopsoas muscle and adjacent lumbosacral plexus to avoid neurologic injury.

23. What are the effects of the anesthetic agents on neurophysiologic signals and how does the spinal monitoring plan affect anesthetic choice?

Inhalational agents cause a dose-related increase in latency and reduction in amplitude, thereby exerting a suppressive effect on tceMEPs and SSEPs. Cortical SSEPs are less sensitive than tceMEPs to suppression by

Inhalational agents, while EMG, D-waves, and subcortical SSEPS are not generally affected. Neuromuscular blocking agents suppress tceMEPs and EMG as these modalities require recording of muscle responses, but enhance SSEPs due to reduction in noise from muscle activity. When tceMEPs and SSEPs are recorded, a total intravenous anesthesia (TIVA) regimen comprised of infusion of a sedative agent (e.g., propofol) and an opioid (e.g., fentanyl, remifentanil) is optimal. Inhalational agents should be avoided after induction and intubation. All depolarizing and nondepolarizing paralytic agents should be avoided, except at the beginning of the procedure during spinal exposure, because these agents block neuromuscular junction transmission and preclude muscle contraction.

24. **What protocol should be followed if a neuromonitoring alert (significant decrease or loss of neurophysiologic potentials) occurs during surgery?**
    The surgeon and anesthesiologist should remain calm and communicate with the spinal monitoring personnel, anesthesia staff, and operating room staff as the following steps (1) are taken:
    1. Check that the electrodes have not become displaced
    2. Elevate and maintain the mean arterial blood pressure between 85 and 95 mm Hg
    3. Assess for change in anesthetic technique
    4. Elevate body temperature and irrigate the wound with warm saline
    5. Check arterial blood gas and laboratory tests and optimize hemoglobin, blood pH, and pCO_2 levels
    6. Assess the patient's neck and limb position on the operating room table
    7. Reverse any antecedent surgical events (e.g., strut graft/cage placement; surgical maneuvers including distraction, compression, translation, or osteotomy closure)
    8. Inspect for an obvious source of neural compression (e.g., bone fragment, hematoma)
    9. Perform intraoperative imaging of the surgical site
    10. If tceMEP and/or SSEP data fail to recover, a wake-up test and an awake clinical examination are considered.
    11. Depending on the specific spinal problem undergoing treatment, spinal instrumentation may require removal. The individual clinical scenario and stability of the spine must be considered in decision-making. Intraoperative consultation with a surgeon colleague is an additional consideration.
    12. Use of steroids (spinal injury protocol) is an option

CLINICAL APPLICATIONS OF NEUROPHYSIOLOGIC MONITORING

25. **What is meant by multimodal intraoperative neurophysiologic monitoring?**
    Multimodal intraoperative neurophysiologic monitoring refers to the use of multiple monitoring modalities (SSEPs, tceMEPs, EMG) to provide specific and complementary data regarding the functional integrity of the afferent dorsal sensory spinal cord tracts, efferent ventral spinal cord motor tracts, spinal nerve roots, and peripheral nerves. Multimodal intraoperative monitoring provides higher sensitivity and specificity for detection of neurologic deterioration compared with single modality monitoring and is the preferred approach.

26. **A 60-year-old man with cervical myelopathy is scheduled for C4–C6 corpectomies, anterior fibula grafting, and posterior spinal instrumentation and fusion (C2–T1). What neurophysiologic monitoring modalities are appropriate for this case?**
    Monitoring of spinal cord function is performed with tceMEPs and SSEPs recorded from both upper and lower extremities. Upper extremity SSEPs will also provide monitoring for brachial plexopathy due to positioning. Cervical nerve roots can be monitored with spontaneous electromyography and tceMEPs recorded from the deltoid and hand muscles. Brainstem auditory-evoked responses (BAERs) can be considered to monitor brainstem perfusion because the vertebral artery is at risk with this surgical exposure.

27. **A 50-year-old woman is undergoing surgical treatment for adult scoliosis, consisting of transforaminal lumbar interbody fusions (L3–S1) and posterior spinal instrumentation (pedicle screws) and fusion (T4-pelvis). What neurophysiologic monitoring modalities are indicated for this type of surgical procedure?**
    Multimodality, intraoperative neurophysiologic monitoring is indicated. A combination of SSEPs and tceMEPs is required to optimally assess spinal cord function. EMG and tceMEPs are used to assess nerve root function. Upper extremity SSEPs are indicated to monitor positional brachial plexopathy. A wake-up test can be performed if significant deterioration of SSEPs and/or tceMEPs occurs during surgery, but is rarely indicated.

28. **A 40-year-old man is scheduled for revision surgery which includes L2–L3 and L3–L4 posterior and transforaminal lumbar interbody fusion and pedicle screw instrumentation. What neurophysiologic monitoring modalities are indicated?**
    In lumbar procedures, monitoring modalities are determined by the level of surgery. The spinal cord extends distally to the L1–L2 region, and monitoring of both spinal cord (SSEPs, tceMEPs) and nerve root function (EMG, tceMEPs) is recommended. Ulnar nerve SSEP monitoring is performed to assess the brachial plexus during surgery.

29. **A 20-year-old man with grade 3 L5–S1 isthmic spondylolisthesis is scheduled for L4–S1 posterior spinal instrumentation and fusion, L5–S1 interbody fusion, and reduction of the spondylolisthesis. What neurophysiologic monitoring modalities are indicated?**
For procedures below L2, neurophysiologic monitoring is directed to assessment of nerve root function utilizing EMG and tceMEPs. Ulnar nerve SSEPs are indicated to permit identification of impending brachial plexus injury due to prolonged prone positioning. Addition of anal sphincter electromyography can be considered for intraoperative assessment of S2–S4 nerve root integrity. Loss of dorsiflexion strength is a known complication following spondylolisthesis reduction, and monitoring of tceMEPs from two myotomes (tibialis anterior, extensor hallucis longus) has been shown to be more accurate than EMG for predicting a new postoperative dorsiflexion injury. (2)

KEY POINTS

1. Multimodality, intraoperative neurophysiologic monitoring permits assessment of the functional integrity of the spinal cord, spinal nerve roots, brachial plexus, lumbosacral plexus, and peripheral nerves during spinal surgery.
2. Intraoperative assessment of spinal cord function is optimally achieved with a combination of transcranial electric motor-evoked potentials (tceMEPs) and somatosensory-evoked potentials (SSEPs).
3. Intraoperative assessment of nerve root function is achieved with electromyographic (EMG) monitoring techniques and monitoring of tceMEPs from specific myotomes.
4. The optimal anesthesia maintenance protocol for successful intraoperative neurophysiologic monitoring of spinal cord function is a total intravenous anesthesia (TIVA) regimen and avoidance of muscle relaxation, nitrous oxide, and inhalational agents.

Websites
1. American Board of Neurophysiologic Monitoring (ABNM): http://www.abnm.info/
2. American Board of Registration of Electroencephalographic and Evoked Potential Technologists: http://abret.org/
3. American Society of Neurophysiologic Monitoring: http://www.asnm.org/default.aspx
4. Scoliosis Research Society Neuromonitoring Information Statement, 2009: https://www.srs.org/about-srs/quality-and-safety/position-statements/neuromonitoring-information-statement

REFERENCE
1. Vitale, M. G., Skaggs, D. L., Pace, G. I., Wright, M. L., Matsumoto, H., Anderson, R. C., et al. (2014). Best practices in intraoperative neuromonitoring in spine deformity surgery: Development of an intraoperative checklist to optimize response. *Spine Deformity, 2*(5), 333–339.
2. Lieberman, J. A., Lyon, R., Jasiukaitis, P., Berven, S. H., Burch, S., & Feiner, J. (2019). The reliability of motor evoked potentials to predict dorsiflexion injuries during lumbosacral deformity surgery: Importance of multiple myotomal monitoring. *Spine Journal, 19*(3), 377–385.

BIBLIOGRAPHY
1. Devlin, V. J., Anderson, P. A., Schwartz, D. M., & Vaughan, R. (2006). Intraoperative neurophysiologic monitoring: Focus on cervical myelopathy and related issues. *Spine Journal, 6*(6), 212–224.
2. Devlin, V. J., & Schwartz, D. M. (2007). Intraoperative neurophysiologic monitoring during spinal surgery. *Journal of the American Academy of Orthopaedic Surgeons, 15*(9), 549–560.
3. Hilibrand, A. S., Schwartz, D. M., Sethuraman, V., Vaccaro, A. R., & Albert, T. J. (2004). Comparison of transcranial electric motor and somatosensory evoked potential monitoring during cervical spine surgery. *Journal of Bone and Joint Surgery, 86*(6), 1248–1253.
4. Hoppenfeld, S., Gross, A., Andrews, C., & Lonner, B. (1997). The ankle clonus test for assessment of the integrity of the spinal cord during operations for scoliosis. *Journal of Bone and Joint Surgery, 79*(2), 208–212.
5. Laratta, J. L., Ha, A., Shillingford, J. N., Makhni, M. C., Lombardi, J. M., Thuet, E., et al. (2018). Neuromonitoring in spinal deformity surgery: A multimodality approach. *Global Spine Journal, 8*(1), 68–77.
6. Lieberman, J. A., Lyon, R., Jasiukaitis, P., Berven, S. H., Burch, S., & Feiner, J. (2019). The reliability of motor evoked potentials to predict dorsiflexion injuries during lumbosacral deformity surgery: importance of multiple myotomal monitoring. *The Spine Journal, 19*(3), 377–385.
7. Schwartz, D. M., Auerbach, J. D., Dormans, J. P., Flynn, J., Drummond, D. S., Bowe, J. A., et al. (2007). Neurophysiological detection of impending spinal cord injury during scoliosis surgery. *Journal of Bone and Joint Surgery, 89*(11), 2440–2449.
8. Schwartz, D. M., Sestokas, A. K., Dormans, J. P., Vaccaro, A. R., Hilibrand, A. S., Flynn, J. M., et al. (2011). Transcranial electric motor evoked potential monitoring during spine surgery: Is it safe? *Spine, 36*(13), 1046–1049.
9. Stecker, M. M. (2012). A review of intraoperative monitoring for spinal surgery. *Surgical Neurology International, 3*(3), 174–187.
10. Vitale, M. G., Skaggs, D. L., Pace, G. I., Wright, M. L., Matsumoto, H., Anderson, R. C., et al. (2014). Best practices in intraoperative neuromonitoring in spine deformity surgery: Development of an intraoperative checklist to optimize response. *Spine Deformity, 2*(5), 333–339.

CHAPTER 23

POSTOPERATIVE MANAGEMENT AND ADVERSE EVENTS AFTER SPINE SURGERY

Vincent J. Devlin, MD

1. **What types of adverse events are encountered in the early postoperative period following spinal procedures?**

   In the postoperative period, adverse events (AEs) may involve the surgical site or arise due to systemic or medically related causes. Surgical site AEs include those related to the surgical approach, neural decompression, spinal instrumentation, bone graft site, wound healing, and wound infection. Systemic or medically related AEs include events that involve the cardiac, pulmonary, gastrointestinal, hematological, renal, and neurological systems, as well as AEs such as electrolyte abnormalities, medication-related side effects, and alcohol or narcotic withdrawal. A spine surgery focused AE classification system, the Spine Adverse Events Severity (SAVES) system, has been developed and validated to facilitate identification and recording of AEs related to spine surgery (Table 23.1).

2. **What is the rationale that supports a distinction between the terms "adverse event" and "complication"?**

   As noted by Rampersaud, (1), the terms "adverse event" and "complication" are often used interchangeably despite their different meanings. An AE is defined as "any event that is due to medical or surgical management, and not due to the underlying disease process or injury, which leads to harm of the patient or requires additional monitoring or treatment." In contrast, complications are defined as "a disease or disorder, which, as a direct or indirect consequence of a surgical procedure, will change the expected outcome of the patient." It has been documented that AEs occur frequently in association with spine surgery, but the majority of these events are not associated with clinical sequelae. To improve patient safety it is recommended to track all AEs regardless of clinical consequence to facilitate quality improvement, patient safety activities, and consistent AE reporting.

SURGICAL ADVERSE EVENTS

3. **What are some factors that increase the risk for airway compromise following anterior cervical surgery and how do these factors influence postoperative airway management?**

   Acute airway compromise following anterior cervical procedures is associated with the need for reintubation and/or prolonged intubation, as well as additional sequellae, including pneumonia, prolonged intensive care admission, tracheostomy, and death. Postoperative airway compromise may develop following anterior cervical surgery due to hematoma, laryngopharyngeal edema, prevertebral soft tissue swelling, displacement of anterior spinal implants, or bone grafts or retropharyngeal abscess. Surgical risk factors associated with postoperative airway compromise following anterior cervical procedures include exposure of more than three vertebral bodies, blood loss >300 mL, exposures involving C2–C4, operative time >5 hours, combined anterior-posterior cervical surgery, and use of bone morphogenetic protein (BMP). Patient risk factors for development of postoperative airway compromise include morbid obesity, obstructive sleep apnea, pulmonary disease, spinal cord injury, cervical myelopathy, and previous anterior cervical surgery.

   Various protocols are suggested for safe airway management following anterior cervical surgery based on surgical and patient-related risk factors. Lower risk patients are extubated following surgery. It is recommended that higher risk patients remain intubated overnight following surgery, with the head of the bed elevated 30°. Patients are evaluated for extubation based on weaning parameters obtained without sedation and following a cuff-leak test or fiber-optic bronchoscopy to verify airway patency. A cuff-leak test is performed in an awake patient by verifying air flow around the endotracheal tube after deflating the cuff and occluding the end of the endotracheal tube. The optimal time to extubate a high-risk patient following cervical surgery is controversial. Extubation should be attempted only when appropriate staff are available to manage a failed extubation. The peak time for development of airway compromise is 24–48 hours following surgery. Patients intubated beyond 1 week are considered for tracheostomy.

4. **Describe the management of a patient who develops acute respiratory compromise following anterior cervical surgery.**

   An acute postoperative respiratory crisis in a patient who has been extubated following anterior cervical surgery is most commonly due to hematoma or laryngopharyngeal edema. Some general management guidelines related to management of patients with postoperative respiratory compromise include:
   - The hospital's emergency response system should be activated and additional staff called for assistance, including members of the anesthesia and surgical teams.

Table 23.1 Categories of Postoperative Adverse Events Following Spine Surgery.

1. Cardiac arrest/failure/arrhythmia
2. Construct failure with loss of correction
3. Construct failure without loss of correction
4. Cerebrospinal fluid leak/meningocele
5. Deep vein thrombosis
6. Deep wound infection
7. Delirium
8. Dysphagia
9. Dysphonia
10. Gastrointestinal bleeding
11. Hematoma
12. Myocardial infarction
13. Neurologic deterioration ≥1 motor grade in American Spinal Injury Association (ASIA) motor scale
14. Nonunion
15. Pneumonia
16. Postop neuropathic pain
17. Pressure sores
18. Pulmonary embolism
19. Superficial wound infection
20. Systemic infection
21. Urinary tract infection
22. Wound dehiscence
23. Other (specify:_____)

From Street JT, Lenehan BJ, DiPaola CP, et al. Morbidity and mortality of major adult spinal surgery. A prospective cohort analysis of 942 consecutive patients. Spine J 2012;12(1):22–34.

- If the patient's status is noncritical and not life-threatening, the patient should be transported to an operating room as this is the optimal setting for securing an airway.
- For patients in respiratory arrest, ventilation is initiated with oxygen using a bag-valve mask system.
- If ventilation remains inadequate after 1 minute, oral intubation is attempted.
- If the initial intubation attempt is unsuccessful, the anterior surgical wound is opened and decompressed by removal of any hematoma if present.
- A second attempt at intubation is performed.
- If the second attempt at intubation is unsuccessful, the physician should perform a cricothyroidotomy.

5. **What are some causes of dysphagia and dysphonia following anterior cervical spine surgery?**
   Dysphagia is defined as difficulty swallowing solids and/or liquids. The etiology of dysphagia following anterior cervical surgery is multifactorial and includes denervation, soft tissue swelling, and scar tissue formation. Risk factors for postoperative dysphagia include multilevel anterior surgical exposures, extended operating times, advanced age, use of rhBMP-2, prominent anterior cervical plates, and use of postoperative cervical immobilization. Swallowing is a complex multiphase activity, involving oral, pharyngeal, and esophageal phases, each phase controlled by different neurologic mechanisms. Important neurologic structures involved in swallowing that are placed at risk during anterior cervical procedures include the hypoglossal nerve (C3 level or above), superior laryngeal nerve, and pharyngeal plexus (C2–C5 levels) and the recurrent laryngeal nerve (C5–C7 levels). Postoperative dysphagia occurs in over half of patients who undergo anterior cervical spine surgery but the majority of patients experience improvement by 6 months. Persistent dysphagia after 1 year is reported in 12%–14% of patients. Evaluation of patients with severe and/or persistent dysphagia should include imaging of the operative site, speech pathology evaluation, swallowing studies, and evaluation for placement of a feeding tube.
   Dysphonia is defined as hoarseness or alteration in the volume, pitch, or quality of the voice. Causes include nerve injury, vocal cord trauma, or postoperative edema, involving the larynx and vocal folds. Hoarseness is most

commonly associated with injury to the recurrent laryngeal nerve. Injury to the superior laryngeal nerve during anterior cervical surgery can also produce hoarseness, as well as adversely affecting vocal quality, pitch elevation control, and vocal range. Dysphonia following anterior cervical surgery is less common than dysphagia, and has been reported in up to 30% of patients. Patients with severe and/or chronic dysphonia should be referred for evaluation by a speech therapist and/or otolaryngologist.

6. List some potential causes of neurologic deficits that are diagnosed following spinal procedures.
   - Direct intraoperative neural trauma (e.g., during surgical exposure, related to decompression procedures, or as a result of neural impingement by spinal implants)
   - Spinal deformity correction (e.g., L5 root injury during L5–S1 spondylolisthesis reduction)
   - Acute vascular etiology (e.g., intraoperative hypotension, disruption of critical segmental blood vessels supplying the spinal cord during anterior surgical approaches)
   - Subacute vascular etiology (neurologic deterioration may develop as late as 96 hours after spinal reconstructive surgery due to poor perfusion of the spinal cord and/or nerve roots)
   - Patient positioning during surgery (e.g., brachial plexopathy, compressive neuropathy involving the ulnar or peroneal nerves, lower extremity compartment syndrome, cervical cord injury secondary to intraoperative neck positioning in a patient with cervical stenosis)
   - Postoperative bleeding resulting in epidural hematoma and neural compromise
   - Miscellaneous causes: cerebrovascular accident, transient ischemic attack, subarachnoid or intracerebral hemorrhage, and seizures

7. What basic elements comprise an adequate neurologic assessment of the postoperative spine patient?
   Initial neurologic assessment after spine surgery should, at a minimum, include assessment of upper and lower extremity neurologic function (motor strength, sensation). It is not adequate to simply record that a patient was able to move their fingers or wiggle their toes as documentation of intact upper or lower extremity neurologic status. Documentation of function of the major motor groups in both upper and lower extremities is required. Neurologic examination is performed at regular intervals following surgery (i.e., every 2 hours for the first 24 hours, every 4 hours for the next 48 hours, and once every shift until discharge following major surgical procedures). When clinically appropriate, results of evaluation of voluntary anal contraction, deep anal pressure, perineal sensation, and bladder function are recorded. New-onset neurologic deficits require prompt imaging to rule out acute spinal cord or nerve root compression.

8. Describe the clinical presentation of a postoperative epidural hematoma.
   Epidural hemorrhage involving the cervical or thoracic region may compress the spinal cord and classically produces an acute, painful myelopathy. Reports of pain unrelieved with narcotic analgesics, or atypical neurologic symptoms or findings (e.g., unexplained numbness, balance difficulty, mild weakness), require careful evaluation because such symptoms may represent early manifestations of an epidural hematoma. Epidural hematoma involving the lumbosacral region may manifest as a cauda equina syndrome. Risk factors include postoperative coagulopathy, multilevel laminectomies, intraoperative blood loss exceeding 1000 mL, spinal cord vascular malformations, previous spine surgery, advanced age, and preoperative use of nonsteroidal antiinflammatory medications (NSAIDs). Treatment of a symptomatic epidural hematoma is emergent spinal decompression.

9. What is cauda equina syndrome?
   Cauda equina syndrome is a complex of low back pain, bilateral lower extremity pain and/or weakness, saddle anesthesia, and varying degrees of bowel and/or bladder dysfunction. Treatment is prompt surgical decompression. Inadequate decompression of lumbar spinal stenosis is a risk factor for developing cauda equina syndrome in the postoperative period.

10. After an uneventful posterior spinal instrumentation procedure for idiopathic scoliosis in a teenage patient, unilateral anterolateral thigh numbness and discomfort are noted. What is the most common cause of this problem?
    Pressure injury to the lateral femoral cutaneous nerve (also known as meralgia paresthetica) secondary to intraoperative positioning. If there is no associated motor deficit and the sensory examination confirms a deficit limited to the distribution of the lateral femoral cutaneous nerve, the diagnosis is confirmed. The prognosis for recovery is good.

11. An adult patient with grade 1 L5–S1 isthmic spondylolisthesis undergoes L5–S1 posterior spinal instrumentation (pedicle fixation), decompression, and fusion. Before surgery, the patient experienced only right leg symptoms. After surgery, the patient reports relief of right leg pain but has a new left L5 radiculopathy, which was not present before surgery. What are the likely causes?
    A problem related to the left L5 pedicle screw resulting in neural impingement must be ruled out. Rates of pedicle screw malposition range from 0% to 2%. However, most of these screw misplacements do not result in any long-term sequelae. Radiographs can be helpful in ruling out gross screw misplacement. However, a computed tomography (CT) scan is preferred because it can provide an axial view and depict the exact screw location in relation to the

L5 nerve root. Other potential causes of new-onset left leg pain include intraoperative nerve root injury, inadequate L5 nerve root decompression, L5–S1 disc herniation, and postoperative hematoma.

12. **A nurse taking care of your patient calls you and reports that this patient has developed a small amount of wound drainage 5 days after a posterior lumbar decompression and fusion procedure for spondylolisthesis. The discharge planner has already made arrangements to transfer this patient to a skilled nursing facility today. What should you advise?**
The patient's transfer should be postponed, and the patient should remain hospitalized to permit evaluation by the surgical team. As a general principle, postoperative spine patients with wound drainage should not be discharged if drainage persists past the fourth or fifth postsurgical day as surgical exploration is frequently indicated. The differential diagnosis of postoperative wound drainage includes superficial or deep wound infection, seroma, hematoma, wound dehiscence, suture abscess, and cerebrospinal fluid (CSF) leak. Expectant management and oral antibiotic treatment are not appropriate when infection is suspected.

The most common symptom in a patient with a postoperative spinal wound infection is pain at the surgical site. Clinical signs may include tenderness with palpation along the incision, erythema, induration, and wound drainage. Additional findings may include general malaise, pain out of proportion to the expected typical postoperative course, and a low-grade fever. Cultures of drainage from the superficial wound are unreliable due to potential for contamination with skin flora, and cultures obtained via aspiration of deeper layers of the wound are preferable, but are associated with a low diagnostic yield. Laboratory tests including complete blood count (CBC) with differential, erythrocyte sedimentation rate (ESR), C-reactive protein (CRP) levels, and blood cultures are obtained. CRP levels peak within 2–3 days postoperatively and generally decrease towards normal within 14 days, and are superior compared to monitoring of ESR or white blood cell counts for detection of early infection. If infection is suspected on a clinical basis, surgical exploration should be undertaken to allow for debridement, intraoperative wound cultures and gram stain, and initiation of broad-spectrum antibiotic therapy.

13. **How is a surgical site infection defined?**
The United States Center for Disease Control classifies a surgical site infection (SSI) as superficial, deep, or organ space. A superficial infection occurs within 30 days of surgery, involves only skin and subcutaneous tissues, and is associated with one of the following: purulent drainage; positive culture obtained aseptically; wound opened by surgeon or designee, and presence of signs or symptoms such as localized pain, swelling, erythema, or heat; or diagnosis as such by a surgeon or designee. A deep infection occurs within 30 or 90 days depending on procedure (laminectomy, 30 days; fusion, 90 days), and involves the fascia and muscles along with one of the following: purulent drainage from deep tissues; a dehiscence or opening or aspiration by the surgeon with positive identification of microorganisms; abscess or other histologic signs of infection; and the presence of at least one sign or symptom, including fever (>38 degrees C), localized pain, or tenderness. An organ space infection occurs deep to the muscles and fascia and has similar criteria as deep infection.

14. **Describe the initial steps involved in surgical treatment of a patient with an acute wound infection 2 weeks after a posterior lumbar spinal instrumentation and fusion procedure.**
In the operating room, the wound is opened sequentially to allow irrigation and debridement. Following evaluation of the superficial wound layer, the deep fascial layer is most commonly opened and explored for a deep infection, since communication generally occurs between the superficial and deep aspects of the wound. It is recommended that at least three to five samples from both the superficial and deep levels of the wound are sent for aerobic and anaerobic cultures, and Gram stain. Spinal implants are left in place if they are intact and appropriately placed. Loose bone graft is removed. All nonviable tissue is debrided. All layers of the wound are irrigated with multiple liters of saline. Broad-spectrum intravenous (IV) antibiotics that cover both gram-positive organisms (including methicillin-resistant *Staphylococcus aureus* [MRSA]) and gram-negative organisms (including *Pseudomonas*) are administered and subsequently modified based on culture results. Following debridement, the wound may be closed primarily or left open in anticipation of future wound exploration and debridement procedures.

15. **What are the options for management of spinal wounds that require multiple debridements?**
In patients who develop infection following instrumented spine surgery, it is common to re-explore the wound in 24–72 hours to reassess the need for additional debridement versus wound closure. Some factors associated with the need for repeat debridement include diabetes, infection with MRSA, polymicrobial infections, infection secondary to bacteremia from distant infection sites (i.e., urinary tract infection [UTI], pneumonia), presence of spinal instrumentation, use of allograft, BMP or synthetic graft material, lumbosacral location, immunocompromised status, compromised nutritional status, and cigarette smoking.

Options for management of spinal wounds following debridement include wound closure over drains, use of a suction-irrigation system, open wound packing with healing by secondary intention, and vacuum-assisted wound closure. The use of vacuum-assisted wound closure devices has been popularized for management wounds treated with serial debridement. A reticulated polyurethane ether foam dressing is inserted, and the open wound is converted into a closed wound by placement of an adhesive barrier. Subatmospheric pressure is maintained by the therapy device and provides a favored environment to promote wound healing. Wound drainage is directed into a specially designed canister and simplifies care. Complications associated with use of vacuum-assisted closure devices include bleeding, retention of sponge fragments, and CSF leaks, which may be associated with severe neurologic AEs. Complex wound closure scenarios may require plastic surgery consultation for local, rotational, or free flap coverage.

16. **What are some recommendations regarding postoperative management of patients who undergo surgical repair of an incidental durotomy?**
The postoperative management protocol for a patient who undergoes operative repair of an incidental durotomy commonly includes a variable period of bedrest. It is recommended that bedrest be prescribed in the position that minimizes CSF pressure at the durotomy site. Patients with lumbar durotomies are maintained in the supine position, while patients with cervical durotomies are maintained in the upright position. Oral or IV administration of caffeine or theophylline is recommended for treatment of headache symptoms. Options for treatment of persistent CSF leakage include an epidural blood patch, insertion of a subarachnoid drain, or surgical exploration and direct dural repair.

17. **What is the incidence of late-presenting dural tears following spine surgery and what treatment is recommended in this clinical scenario?**
The incidence of late-presenting dural tears (LPDTs) following spine surgery is 2 per 1000 surgeries. (2) LPDTs may result from a dural tear that was not recognized at the time of initial surgery or delayed presentation of an inadequately repaired dural tear. The majority of readmissions and reoperations for this condition occur within 2 weeks of surgery. Lumbar procedures, surgeries involving both cervical and lumbar levels, decompression procedures, and procedures lasting ≥250 minutes have been associated with LPDTs. LPDTs are associated with an increased likelihood of SSI, sepsis, pneumonia, UTI, wound dehiscence, thromboembolism, acute kidney injury (AKI), and liability risk.
    The clinical presentation of an LPDT generally includes headache, which most often increases with standing. Additional symptoms may include nausea, vomiting, dizziness, vertigo, fever, and infection. As a CSF fistula develops, CSF passes through the wound or a drain tract and presents as clear wound drainage. Laboratory testing for beta-2-transferrin can be used to confirm the presence of CSF in wound drainage fluid. Magnetic resonance imaging (MRI) or CT-myelography may be used to identify the extent and location of CSF fluid collections. Nonsurgical management options include bedrest, oversewing the wound margins, aspiration of CSF followed by application of an epidural blood patch, or placement of a subarachnoid drainage catheter. Surgical management consists of primary dural repair and may require augmentation of the repair with tissue grafts, dural sealants, collagen matrices, or dural allografts. A subarachnoid catheter may be placed through the durotomy repair site at the time of surgery. In some cases a CSF fluid collection or a pseudomeningocele may develop, and is often asymptomatic. However, occasionally a large compressive pseudomeningocele may lead to major neurologic deficits and require urgent treatment.

18. **You are called to assess a 49-year-old man in the recovery room immediately after an anterior L4–S1 fusion performed via a left retroperitoneal approach. The nurse reports that the left leg is cooler than the right leg. The patient reports severe left leg pain. What test should be ordered?**
An emergent arteriogram and a vascular surgery consultation are indicated. The scenario is consistent with a vascular injury. The temperature change should not be attributed to the sympathectomy effect that is routinely noted following anterior lumbar surgery (in which case increased temperature is noted on the side of the exposure).

19. **List some causes of spinal implant construct failure in the early postoperative period**
    - Improper initial implant placement
    - Rod fracture due to rod strength compromise resulting from excessive bending or notching
    - Loosening of rod-bone anchor connections due to inadequate intraoperative tightening
    - Bone anchor fracture, loosening, or displacement
    - Subsidence of anterior column grafts or devices in osteoporotic vertebral bodies
    - Anterior column device or graft migration
    - Fracture at the proximal or distal extent of an implant construct or adjacent level fracture
    - An inadequate length implant construct
    - Inadequate anterior column load sharing within a spinal construct
    - Facet joint impingement or soft tissue disruption at the ends of posterior instrumentation construct leading to a transition syndrome

MEDICAL ADVERSE EVENTS

20. **What types of pulmonary AEs are encountered after spinal procedures?**
Atelectasis, bronchospasm, pneumonia, pleural effusion, pneumothorax, prolonged intubation, acute respiratory distress syndrome (ARDS), transfusion-related acute lung injury (TRALI), pulmonary thromboembolism, hypoxemia, respiratory failure, prolonged ventilation, and reintubation.

21. **What is the most common pulmonary AE following spinal surgery?**
Atelectasis. Clinical signs include tachypnea, tachycardia, and fever secondary to collapse of peripheral lung alveoli. Treatment includes adequate pain control, lung expansion therapy (deep breathing exercises, incentive

spirometry, coughing, chest physiotherapy, continuous positive airway pressure [CPAP]), suctioning, frequent turning in bed, and early mobilization. For patients with extensive atelectasis despite these measures, bronchoscopy is considered.

22. **What factors are associated with an increased risk of pulmonary AEs after spine surgery?**
Some factors associated with an increased risk of pulmonary AEs following spine surgery include spinal cord injury, nonidiopathic scoliosis, cognitive disability, age over 60 years, chronic obstructive pulmonary disease, obstructive sleep apnea, smoking, and the American Society of Anesthesiologists (ASA) physical status class $\geq$2. Patients undergoing anterior thoracic spine procedures and combined anterior and posterior spinal procedures associated with large blood loss and fluid shifts also have an increased risk of postoperative pulmonary AEs.

23. **What prophylaxis is recommended for venous thromboembolic events including deep vein thrombosis and pulmonary embolism following spinal procedures?**
Current estimates of baseline risk of developing symptomatic venous thromboembolic events (VTE) range between 0.05% and 1.5% and exceed 2% in high-risk patients. Decision-making regarding appropriate VTE prophylaxis for patients undergoing spine surgery is based on individual patient risk factors including spinal diagnosis, procedure type, patient age, and comorbid conditions. Specific factors associated with elevated VTE risk include a history of previous VTE, known thrombophilia, advanced age, spinal cord injury, malignancy, extended operative times, and procedure type. Procedures with an elevated risk of VTE include posterior cervical procedures, anterior or posterior thoracic procedures, anterior lumbar procedures, procedures involving combined anterior-posterior approaches, and multilevel fusions ($\geq$4 levels).

Options for prophylaxis for VTE include mechanical and pharmacologic treatments. Use of lower extremity intermittent pneumatic compression or sequential compression devices prior to, during, and after surgery, in addition to early postoperative mobilization, are recommended for patients undergoing spine surgery. The use of pharmacologic agents for anticoagulation in patients undergoing low-risk procedures such as posterior lumbar decompressions, or 1 or 2 level anterior cervical fusion, is not recommended in the absence of additional risk factors, as the risk of a clinically significant VTE is balanced by the potential for development of an epidural hematoma. For patients with elevated risk factors, the most common options for pharmacologic prophylaxis include low-molecular-weight heparin or low-dose unfractionated heparin initiated when primary hemostasis is evident, generally within 24–48 hours following surgery. Use of warfarin is not recommended due to associated bleeding risk. Limited data exist to support the use of aspirin for prophylaxis. Insertion of an inferior vena cava filter as primary prophylaxis against pulmonary embolism (PE) or routine use of an inferior vena cava filter in addition to anticoagulation is not recommended.

24. **How does deep vein thrombosis most commonly present after spine surgery? What is the preferred diagnostic test and treatment for deep vein thrombosis in this setting?**
Fewer than half of patients with deep vein thrombosis (DVT) present with positive clinical findings. Signs and symptoms suggestive of DVT include calf or thigh pain, foot or ankle edema, calf tenderness with or without a palpable cord, elevated skin temperature, and a positive Homan's sign (calf pain with ankle dorsiflexion). Duplex ultrasound examination, using both B-mode and color flow analysis, is the diagnostic test of choice. Other diagnostic modalities include impedance plethysmography, magnetic resonance venography, and contrast venography, but are less commonly utilized. The main treatment of DVT is anticoagulation to prevent clot propagation, PE, and development of postphlebitic syndrome. Various anticoagulation regimens have been described for treatment of postoperative DVT, including use of heparin infusion in combination with an oral agent, low-molecular-weight heparin, selective factor Xa inhibitors, and selective thrombin inhibitors, but limited data are available to guide treatment of DVT following spine surgery. In a postoperative spine trauma population, therapeutic anticoagulation led to an unplanned reoperation rate of 18% compared with 10% in nonanticoagulated control patients, and an epidural hematoma rate of 3% compared with 1% in controls. Initiation of anticoagulation with a heparin infusion increased the rate of reoperation compared with use of low-molecular-weight heparin, and led to a recommendation against use of an initial heparin bolus if an initial heparin infusion is administered. (3) For patients who are not candidates for systemic anticoagulation, placement of an inferior vena cava filter is considered.

25. **How does PE present following spine surgery? What is the preferred diagnostic test and treatment for PE in this setting?**
The most common presenting symptom in a patient with PE is dyspnea. Additional clinical features associated with PE include tachypnea, cough, chest pain, wheezing, and syncope. Most PEs following spine surgery are attributed to propagation of vein thrombi proximally from the calf to the popliteal, femoral, and/or iliac veins. However, it has been reported that PE may arise in the absence of DVT (*de novo* pulmonary emboli) in the trauma setting, and are attributed to a local response to injury or inflammation. Multidetector CT pulmonary angiography is the preferred test for diagnosis of PE and has replaced ventilation-perfusion lung scanning. The main treatment of PE is anticoagulation. In patients with severe hemodynamic compromise, systemic or catheter-based thrombolytic therapy,

catheter-based thrombus removal, or surgical embolectomy are potential options. PE patients who have contraindications to anticoagulant therapy are evaluated for insertion of an inferior vena cava filter.

26. **What is acute respiratory distress syndrome?**

ARDS results from diffuse, multilobar capillary transudation of fluid into the pulmonary interstitium, which dissociates the normal relationship of alveolar ventilation with lung perfusion. Persistent perfusion of poorly ventilated lung regions creates a shunt that results in hypoxia. ARDS has many causes including sepsis, aspiration, pulmonary contusion, and fluid overload or massive transfusions. Typically ARDS presents several days after surgery with fever, respiratory distress, reduced arterial oxygen, diffuse bilateral infiltrates on chest radiographs, pulmonary capillary wedge pressure <18 mmHg and a PaO_2 to FiO_2 ratio of 200 or less. Treatment includes ventilator support with positive end-expiratory pressure (PEEP) to promote ventilation of previously trapped alveoli and minimize shunting.

27. **What is transfusion-related acute lung injury?**

TRALI is defined as a new acute lung injury or ARDS occurring during or within 6 hours after blood product administration in the absence of another temporally associated cause. Management is similar to ARDS and consists of respiratory and circulatory support. Differential diagnosis includes transfusion-associated circulatory overload (TACO), anaphylaxis, and sepsis.

28. **After an anterior thoracic fusion performed through an open thoracotomy approach, a patient has persistent high chest tube outputs after the fourth postoperative day. The fluid has a milky color. What diagnosis should be suspected?**

Chylothorax. Injury to the thoracic duct or its tributaries may not be recognized intraoperatively and lead to leakage from the lymphatic system into the thoracic cavity. Treatment consists of continued chest tube drainage and decreasing the patient's fat intake. Hyperalimentation is of benefit during this period. Failure of these measures may require surgical exploration and repair of the lymphatic ductal injury.

29. **Explain how a hemothorax or pneumothorax may occur in association with posterior spinal procedures.**

There are several mechanisms that may be responsible for development of a hemothorax or pneumothorax in association with posterior spinal procedures. During posterior surgical procedures, the chest cavity may be entered inadvertently if dissection is carried too deeply between the transverse processes. Hemothorax or pneumothorax may also occur when thoracoplasty is performed to decrease rib prominence as part of a posterior procedure for scoliosis. A tension pneumothorax may result from respirator malfunction or rupture of a pulmonary bleb. Insertion of a central venous pressure (CVP) line in the operating room may result in a pneumothorax that is not diagnosed before beginning the surgical procedure. Prompt diagnosis and chest tube insertion are required for treatment of hemothorax or pneumothorax.

30. **What is the rate of cardiac AEs following inpatient spinal surgery and what percentage of cardiac AEs are diagnosed after hospital discharge?**

The rate of cardiac AEs following spine surgery is estimated between 0.67%–1.6% and 30% of cardiac events are diagnosed after hospital discharge. Cardiovascular AEs occurring in the postoperative period include myocardial infarction (MI), cardiac arrhythmias, and cardiac arrest and are referred to as major cardiac adverse events (MACEs). Perioperative cardiac events are the leading cause of death following noncardiac surgery. Risk factors associated with perioperative cardiac complications such as cardiac arrest or myocardial infarction include advanced age, insulin-dependent diabetes mellitus, preoperative anemia, and history of cardiac disorders or prior cardiac treatment. MI is diagnosed in 1%–2% of patients following spine surgery. The reported median time for a perioperative MI following spinal fusion surgery is 2 days. Preoperative risk assessment, medical optimization, and close postoperative monitoring of high-risk patients are critically important components of perioperative management of patients undergoing spine surgery.

31. **What is the most common gastrointestinal problem after spinal surgery?**

Ileus. Common causes include general anesthesia, prolonged use of narcotics, immobility after surgery, and significant manipulation of intestinal contents during anterior spinal exposures. Clinical findings include abdominal distention and the inability to pass stool or flatus. Absent bowel sounds, abdominal cramping or discomfort, pain, nausea, and vomiting may be present. Diet restriction is the initial treatment. Nasogastric suction may be placed to provide relief of symptoms. Preventative strategies include preoperative carbohydrate loading, use of chewing gum, early enteral feeding, minimization of opioids, and early patient mobilization.

32. **What is Ogilvie syndrome?**

Acute massive dilation of the cecum and ascending and transverse colon in the absence of mechanical obstruction is termed Ogilvie syndrome. Patients present with normal small bowel sounds and a colonic ileus. It is a potentially dangerous entity that can result in cecal dilation, colonic rupture, and mortality. The incidence appears to be increasing and may be related to use of opioids for postoperative analgesia. Diagnosis is made with an upright abdominal radiograph and may require a water-soluble enema or CT to rule out mechanical obstruction. Initial treatment consists of stopping oral intake, insertion of nasogastric and rectal tubes, IV hydration, electrolyte monitoring and discontinuation of opioids. Pharmacologic treatment has been described using neostigmine, which acts by increasing parasympathetic stimulation. If pharmacologic treatment is contraindicated or unsuccessful, endoscopic decompression or surgical treatment with cecostomy or subtotal colectomy may be necessary.

33. **Define superior mesenteric artery syndrome.**
    Superior mesenteric artery (SMA) syndrome refers to proximal intestinal obstruction due to narrowing of the space between the SMA and aorta in the region where the SMA crosses over the third portion of the duodenum. This condition has been reported in thin patients who undergo significant correction of a spinal deformity or who are immobilized in hip spica or body casts. Patients present with persistent postoperative emesis. Physical examination reveals hyperactive, high-pitched bowel sounds. Diagnosis is confirmed with an upper gastrointestinal contrast study or CT with IV and oral contrast. Initial treatment includes complete restriction of oral intake, gastric decompression with a nasogastric tube, adequate IV hydration, and initiation of hyperalimentation if symptoms persist. Patients should be encouraged to lie in the prone or left lateral position. If symptoms persist, surgical intervention is indicated.

34. **What are the most common genitourinary AEs reported following spine surgery?**
    Postoperative urinary retention (POUR) is the most frequently reported genitourinary AE reported after spinal procedures with an incidence ranging from 5% to 38%. Factors associated with POUR include advanced age, previous AKI or UTI, male sex, benign prostatic hypertrophy, history of joint replacement surgery, hypertension, preoperative beta-blocker use, and diabetes mellitus. POUR has been identified as a significant risk factor for development of a UTI, sepsis, increased length of stay, discharge to a skilled facility, and readmission within 90 days. Management involves decompression of the bladder based on clinical assessment, ultrasonic assessment of bladder volume, and/or hospital protocols.

    Hospital-acquired UTIs occur in association with 1.3% of spinal surgeries, and have been associated with an increased risk for systemic sepsis and SSIs. Three-quarters of hospital acquired UTIs are associated with a urinary catheter. Most UTIs are due to *Escherichia coli* and other gram-negative rods. Initial treatment of UTIs is with broad spectrum antibiotic coverage with subsequent adjustment based on urinary culture results.

35. **What are some factors responsible for the development of acute kidney injury in patients undergoing spinal surgery?**
    AKI is a syndrome attributed to multiple etiologies (prerenal, intrinsic renal, postrenal) and causes an abrupt decrease in kidney function that results in failure to manage fluid, electrolyte, and acid-base homeostasis. Reported rates of AKI following multilevel spine surgery in pediatric and adult patients range from 3.9% to 17%. Etiology is multifactorial and includes renal hypoperfusion, intravascular hypovolemia, and administration of nephrotoxic medications. Postoperative AKI has been associated with increased postoperative morbidity and mortality. The increase in the reported rates of AKI reflects the use of more sensitive diagnostic criteria, as well as surgical treatment of spine patients with multiple medical comorbidities. In 2004, the term "acute renal failure" was replaced by AKI, and a consensus definition for AKI, the Risk, Injury, Failure, Loss, and End-stage Kidney (RIFLE) criteria, was proposed. Subsequently, the Acute Kidney Injury Network (AKIN) proposed modified criteria, which were followed by criteria from the Kidney Disease: Improving Global Outcomes (KDIGO) Foundation that defined AKI as any of the following:
    - Increase in serum creatinine level by $\geq$0.3 mg/dL ($\geq$26.5 µmol/L) within 48 hours
    - Increase in serum creatinine level to $\geq$1.5 times baseline within 7 days, or
    - Decrease in urine output <0.5 mL/kg/hour for 6 hours

36. **What is the most common electrolyte disorder encountered in hospitalized patients?**
    Hyponatremia. Hyponatremia is reported in up to 30% of patients who undergo spinal surgery and is associated with increased perioperative morbidity, increased length of hospital stay, and mortality. Hyponatremia is commonly defined as a serum sodium concentration <135 mEq/L, and further subdivided as mild (130–135 mEq/L), moderate (120–130 mEq/L), or severe (<120 mEq/L). Hyponatremia may also be classified by plasma osmolality (hypotonic, isotonic, hypertonic), volume status (hypervolemic, euvolemic, hypovolemic), and duration and rate of onset. While severe hyponatremia may lead to cerebral edema resulting in seizures or coma, mild postoperative hyponatremia may be asymptomatic or associated with unrecognized symptoms, including gait disturbances, falls, headaches, cognitive deficits, and nausea. Hyponatremia has been associated with multiple factors, including use of thiazide diuretics, NSAIDs, hypotonic IV fluids during surgery, the syndrome of inappropriate secretion of antidiuretic hormone (SIADH), and increasing age. When hyponatremia is diagnosed postoperatively, it is important to distinguish between patients with SIADH and patients with hypovolemia, as the treatment for SIADH is free-water

restriction and high dietary salt intake while the treatment of hypovolemia is fluid replacement with isotonic normal saline.

37. **What is the most common postoperative AE in patients undergoing spine surgery after the age of 65 years?**

Postoperative delirium is recognized as the most common postoperative AE in seniors, occurring in 5%–50% of patients postoperatively. Delirium is characterized by an acute, fluctuating alteration in mental function and disturbance in attention. Delirium is associated with an increased number of AEs during hospitalization, prolonged hospitalization, an increased need for discharge to a skilled facility, and mortality. Risk factors for development of delirium include:
- Preoperative factors: age ≥65 years, cognitive impairment, functional impairment, depression, psychotropic drug use, visual or hearing impairment, alcohol use, prior episodes of delirium, and hypoalbuminemia
- Intraoperative factors: intraoperative hypotension, multiple blood transfusion, and prolonged anesthesia time
- Postoperative factors: infection, hypoxia, substance withdrawal, narcotic use, medication side effects, anemia, electrolyte disturbances, inadequate pain control, and interrupted sleep

    Management is directed toward preventive measures because once delirium symptoms develop, treatment is challenging. Preventative measures include early mobilization, reorientation, uninterrupted sleep, family presence, availability of sensory aids including personal items such as hearing aids and glasses, avoidance of anticholinergic medications, minimization or discontinuation of narcotic medications, treatment of constipation, and evaluation of the necessity for urinary catheters, IV lines, and restraints. Pharmacologic treatment with haloperidol and second-generation antipsychotics is reserved only for patients with severe agitation at risk for harm to self or others.

38. **What is the incidence of ophthalmic complications after spinal surgery? What are the risk factors?**

The overall incidence of ophthalmic complications after spine surgery is estimated at 1 in 1000 procedures. The most common perioperative eye injury is a corneal abrasion. Postoperative visual loss may also occur and is due to a variety of mechanisms that have been classified as anterior and posterior ischemic optic neuropathy, central retinal artery or vein occlusion, decreased visual acuity, and visual field deficits. Spinal procedures performed in the prone position (i.e., scoliosis surgery, extensive lumbar spinal fusions) have the highest rates, but this complication may develop following procedures performed in the supine position. An eye check should be included in the postoperative patient assessment. Symptoms or abnormal examination findings should prompt an urgent ophthalmology consult.

39. **What are some current trends regarding pain management for patients undergoing major spinal reconstructive procedures?**

IV opioid medications have traditionally been the most widely used method for postoperative pain management after spine surgery. In alert and cooperative patients, these medications have most commonly been administered via a patient-controlled anesthesia (PCA) pump. However, short-term AEs of opioids associated with this regimen include nausea, vomiting, ileus, pruritus, urinary retention, somnolence, and respiratory depression. Following recognition of the "opioid epidemic" and realization that the risk for chronic opioid use is highest after orthopedic and neurosurgical procedures, there has been a trend away from reliance solely on IV opioids and toward use of multimodality strategies for perioperative pain management. Preoperative patients are educated regarding the negative effects of chronic opioid use and encouraged to wean from opioids prior to surgery, with the assistance of an addiction specialist if necessary. Preemptive analgesia is implemented prior to surgery with use of an NSAID, acetaminophen, gabapentinoid, or sustained release opioid as prophylaxis against central autonomic hyperactivity, which accompanies painful stimuli resulting from spine surgery. Intraoperatively, infiltration with extended-release local anesthetics such as lidocaine and bupivacaine are used to decrease postoperative analgesic requirements. Postoperatively, as a substitute for opioid infusion via PCA, a combination of medications with different mechanisms of action (e.g., NSAID, acetaminophen, gabapentinoids) in combination with judicious use of an oral opioid are utilized, resulting in decreased total opioid consumption and decreased opioid-related side effects.

KEY POINTS

1. Adverse events (AEs) following spine surgery are unavoidable, but their negative effects can be lessened by prompt diagnosis followed by appropriate and expedient treatment.
2. Procedure-specific AEs following spine surgery may be related to the surgical approach, neural decompression, or spinal instrumentation.
3. Systemic AEs after spine surgery may involve the entire spectrum of body organ systems.

Websites
1. Acute Kidney Injury (AKI): https://kdigo.org/guidelines/acute-kidney-injury/
2. CDC Surgical Site Infection Event: https://www.cdc.gov/nhsn/pdfs/pscmanual/9pscssicurrent.pdf
3. Cricothyroidotomy: https://emedicine.medscape.com/article/1830008-overview#a3
4. Dysphagia after anterior cervical spine surgery: http://www.csrs.org/wp-content/uploads/2014/06/dysphagia-outcome-study.pdf
5. Hyponatremia: https://www.hyponatremiaupdates.com/what-is-hyponatremia
6. Perioperative visual loss (POVL): https://www.apsf.org/videos/perioperative-visual-loss-povl-video/

REFERENCES

1. Rampersaud, Y. R., Anderson, P. A., Dimar, J. R., & Fisher, C. G. (2016). Spinal Adverse Events Severity System, version 2 (SAVES-V2): inter- and intraobserver reliability assessment. *Journal of Neurosurgery: Spine, 25*(2), 256–263.
2. Durand, W. M., DePasse, J. M., Kuris, E. O., Yang, J., & Daniels, A. H. (2018). Late-presenting dural tear: Incidence, risk factors, and associated complications. *The Spine Journal, 18*(11), 2043–2050.
3. Shiu, B., Le, E., Jazini, E., Weir, T. B., Costales, T., Caffes, N., et al. (2018). Postoperative deep vein thrombosis, pulmonary embolism, and myocardial infarction: Complications after therapeutic anticoagulation in the patient with spine trauma. *Spine, 43*(13), 766–772.

BIBLIOGRAPHY

1. Bovonratwet, P., Bohl, D. D., Malpani, R., Haynes, M. S., Rubio, D. R., Ondeck, N. T., et al. (2019). Cardiac complications related to spine surgery: Timing, risk factors and clinical effect. *Journal of the American Academy of Orthopaedic Surgeons, 27*(7), 256–263.
2. Debkowska, M. P., Butterworth, J. F., Moore, J. E., Kang, S., Appelbaum, E. N., & Zuelzer, W. A. (2019). Acute postoperative airway complications following anterior cervical spine surgery and the role for cricothyrotomy. *Journal of Spine Surgery, 5*(1), 142–154.
3. Durand, W. M., DePasse, J. M., Kuris, E. O., Yang, J., & Daniels, A. H. (2018). Late-presenting dural tear: incidence, risk factors, and associated complications. *The Spine Journal 18*(11), 2043–2050.
4. Golubovsky, J. L., Ilyas, H., Chen, J., Tanenbaum, J. E., Mroz, T. E., & Steinmetz, M. P. (2018). Risk factors and associated complications for postoperative urinary retention after lumbar surgery for lumbar spinal stenosis. *The Spine Journal 18*(9), 1533–1539.
5. Hennrikus, E., Ou, G., Kinney, B., Lehman, E., Grunfeld, R., Wieler, J., et al. (2015). Prevalence, timing, causes, and outcomes of hyponatremia in hospitalized orthopaedic surgery patients. *Journal of Bone and Joint Surgery 97*(22), 1824–1832.
6. Joaquim, A. F., Murar, J., Savage, J., & Patel, A. A. (2014). Dysphagia after anterior cervical spine surgery: a systematic review of potential preventative measures. *The Spine Journal, 14*(9), 2246–2260.
7. Rampersaud, Y. R., Anderson, P. A., Dimar, J. R., & Fisher, C. G. (2016). Spinal Adverse Events Severity System, version 2 (SAVES-V2): inter- and intraobserver reliability assessment. *Journal of Neurosurgery: Spine, 25*(2), 256–263.
8. Raudenbush, B. L., Molinari, A., & Molinari, R. W. (2017). Large compressive pseudomeningocele causing early major neurologic deficit after spinal surgery. *Global Spine Journal 7*(3), 206–212.
9. Schairer, W. W., Pedtke, A. C., & Hu, S. S. (2014). Venous thromboembolism after spine surgery. *Spine 39*(11), 911–918.
10. Shiu, B., Le, E., Jazini, E., Weir, T. B., Costales, T., Caffes, N., et al. (2018). Postoperative deep vein thrombosis, pulmonary embolism, and myocardial infarction: Complications after therapeutic anticoagulation in the patient with spine trauma. *Spine, 43*(13), 766–772.
11. Street, J. T., Lenehan, B. J., DiPaola, C. P., Boyd, M. D., Kwon, B. K., Paquette, S. J., et al. (2012). Morbidity and mortality of major adult spinal surgery. A prospective cohort analysis of 942 consecutive patients. *The Spine Journal, 12*(1), 22–34.
12. Swann, M. C., Hoes, K. S., Aoun, S. G., & McDonagh, D. L. (2016). Postoperative complications of spine surgery. Best Practice & Research. *Clinical Anaesthesiology, 30*(1), 103–120.

VI

BASIC SPINAL PROCEDURES, SURGICAL APPROACHES, AND SPINAL INSTRUMENTATION

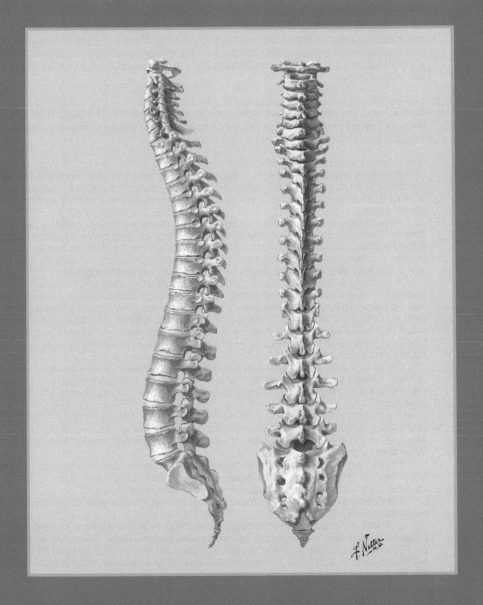

CHAPTER 24

PROCEDURES FOR DECOMPRESSION OF THE SPINAL CORD AND NERVE ROOTS

Vincent J. Devlin, MD

GENERAL PRINCIPLES

1. **What is spinal decompression surgery?**

   Spinal decompression is a general term that refers to a range of surgical procedures that are performed to relieve symptoms due to compression of the spinal cord and/or nerve roots. Spinal decompression may be accomplished using direct and/or indirect methods and is often performed in conjunction with spinal implants and/or spinal fusion.

2. **Explain what is meant by direct spinal decompression.**

   Direct spinal decompression accomplishes neural decompression by resection of the causes of neural compression, which can include bone, ligaments, and disc material. Examples of procedures that involve direct spinal decompression include discectomy, laminectomy, and corpectomy.

3. **Explain what is meant by indirect spinal decompression.**

   Indirect spinal decompression achieves decompression of neural elements without resection of the structures responsible for neural compression. (1) Indirect decompression may be accomplished by distraction between adjacent vertebrae, by spinal realignment using implants, or by excision or realignment of posterior compressive structures.

   Indirect decompression by distraction between adjacent vertebrae is commonly used in the treatment of lumbar spinal stenosis. For example, in patients with single-level central spinal canal and neuroforaminal stenosis, restoration of disc space height through placement of an interbody device or posterior element distraction by insertion of an interspinous process device can provide indirect decompression by increasing the cross-sectional area of the central spinal canal and increasing the height and volume of the neural foramina.

   An example of indirect decompression using spinal instrumentation across multiple spinal segments is the treatment of a lumbar burst fracture with kyphotic deformity and spinal canal compromise due to retropulsed bone fragments from the posterior vertebral body. Insertion of a pedicle screw-rod system spanning the fractured level permits application of distractive forces to correct the kyphotic deformity and restore spinal canal patency by reduction of fracture fragments that are attached to the posterior longitudinal ligament (PLL). Indirect reduction of fracture fragments attached to the PLL is termed "ligamentotaxis" and is only possible for fractures in which the PLL is not completely disrupted.

   Cervical laminoplasty is an example of an indirect decompression procedure that realigns posterior compressive structures to expand spinal canal area and allow posterior spinal cord migration away from anterior compression. However, for posterior migration of the cervical spinal cord to occur, neutral or lordotic alignment of the cervical spine is necessary.

4. **Distinguish between laminotomy, laminectomy, and laminoplasty.**

   All procedures are performed through a posterior approach and are intended to provide posterior decompression of neural structures (Fig. 24.1A).

   A **laminotomy** consists of partial lamina removal to access the spinal canal and permit direct decompression of the nerve root and/or dural sac. Partial removal of laminar bone and facet joints to expose and decompress the nerve root is referred to as a foraminotomy or laminoforaminotomy (see Fig. 24.1B).

   A **laminectomy** consists of removal of the spinous process and the entire lamina to directly relieve neural compression (see Fig. 24.1C).

   A **laminoplasty** provides decompression of the neural elements by enlarging the spinal canal with a surgical technique that avoids removal of the posterior spinal elements. Various laminoplasty techniques permit preservation and reconstruction of the posterior osseous and ligamentous structures of the spinal column without the need for fusion. Laminoplasty techniques are most commonly utilized in the cervical spine (Fig. 24.2).

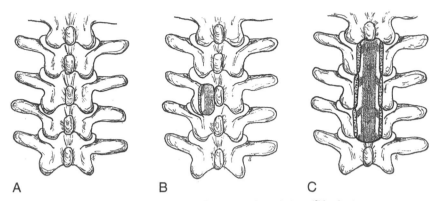

A   B   C

Fig. 24.1 Lumbar decompression. (A) Preoperative. (B) Laminotomy. (C) Laminectomy.

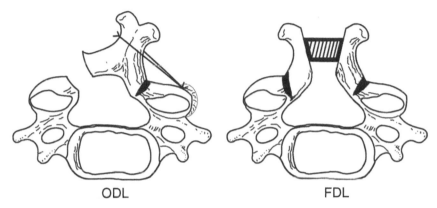

ODL   FDL

Fig. 24.2 Cervical laminoplasty methods. *ODL*, Open door laminoplasty; *FDL*, French door laminoplasty. (From Wang L, Wang Y, Yu B et al. Open-door versus French-door laminoplasty for the treatment of cervical multilevel compressive myelopathy. J Clin Neurosci 2015; 22[3]:450–455.)

5. Distinguish between anterior discectomy, corpectomy, and vertebrectomy.
   - An **anterior discectomy** procedure is indicated to relieve anterior neural compression localized to the level of the disc space. It involves removal of the intervertebral disc and any osteophytes that compress the neural elements. The space formerly occupied by the disc is filled with bone graft or an intervertebral body fusion device (Fig. 24.3).
   - A **corpectomy** (*corpus* meaning "body") entails removal of the vertebral body combined with removal of the superior and inferior adjoining discs (Fig. 24.4). The resultant anterior spinal column defect is reconstructed

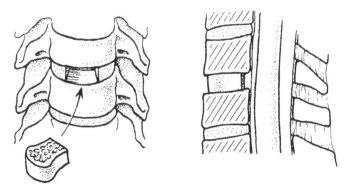

Fig. 24.3 Anterior cervical decompression: discectomy. (From Muller EJ, Aebi M. Anterior fusion of the cervical spine. Spine State Art Rev 1992;6:459–474.)

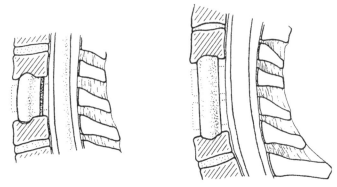

Fig. 24.4 Anterior cervical decompression: single-level and multilevel corpectomy. (From Muller EJ, Aebi M. Anterior fusion of the cervical spine. Spine State Art Rev 1992;6:459–474.)

with an anterior bone graft or vertebral body replacement device (also called a fusion cage) and usually stabilized with anterior and/or posterior spinal instrumentation. A corpectomy is indicated to relieve anterior neural compression that extends behind a vertebral body or to remove a vertebral body whose structural integrity is compromised (e.g., tumors, infection, fracture).

- A **vertebrectomy** is a more radical procedure consisting of removal of the posterior spinal elements (spinous process, lamina, pedicles) in addition to the vertebral body. This procedure creates severe spinal instability and is performed in conjunction with anterior and posterior spinal instrumentation and fusion. Spinal pathologies treated with vertebrectomy include primary spine tumors and spondyloptosis.

6. Describe the three basic steps involved in performing a corpectomy after the anterior aspect of the vertebral bodies have been exposed.
   1. Remove the discs above and below the target vertebral body. This facilitates subsequent removal of the vertebral body by providing reference landmarks for the depth and position of the spinal canal.
   2. Remove the vertebral body. The anterior two-thirds of the vertebral body is rapidly removed with a rongeur, osteotome, or burr. The remaining posterior wall of the vertebral body is thinned with a burr. This technique facilitates the more delicate removal of the posterior vertebral cortex with a curette or Kerrison rongeur to expose the spinal canal, PLL, and dural sac.
   3. Fill the space created after corpectomy with a structural bone graft or a vertebral body replacement device to restore anterior spinal column support. Anterior and/or posterior spinal implants are used to provide additional stability.

7. What steps can spinal surgeons follow to maximize the likelihood of a successful outcome following spinal decompression procedures?
   - Operate only when the clinical history and physical examination correlate with spinal imaging studies.
   - Rely on high-quality imaging studies (full length spinal deformity radiographs, computed tomography [CT], magnetic resonance imaging [MRI], CT-myelography) for preoperative planning.
   - Administer prophylactic intravenous antibiotics immediately prior to surgery
   - Minimize exposure-related damage to spinal structures (muscles, ligaments, facet joints, bone, and nerve tissue).
   - Operate with adequate lighting, exposure, and use of loupe magnification or a microscope.
   - Confirm that the proper surgical level(s) have been exposed by taking an intraoperative radiograph or fluoroscopic image.
   - Assess spinal stability before wound closure. Perform a spinal fusion if spinal instability has been created as a result of the decompression procedure or if spinal instability was present before surgery.
   - When spinal fusion is performed, use of spinal instrumentation is indicated to maintain or restore age-appropriate sagittal plane alignment parameters.

CERVICAL SPINAL REGION

8. Describe treatment of spinal cord compression with myelopathy due to cranial settling and instability at the occipitocervical junction in a patient with rheumatoid arthritis using a posterior surgical approach.
   Posterior laminectomy of C1 and occipitocervical fusion is a treatment option. The rheumatoid pannus usually decreases in size after stability is provided by posterior instrumentation and fusion. In select cases, an anterior transoral resection of the odontoid process is performed as a subsequent procedure.

9. **What is a transoral decompression? Describe two indications for this procedure.**
Transoral decompression is performed through the mouth. Surgical dissection through the posterior pharynx permits exposure of the odontoid process, C1 arch, and the base of the skull. Anterior surgical access to the occipitocervical junction is indicated for treatment of tumors (e.g., chordoma in the region of the clivus) and for resection of the odontoid process in rheumatoid arthritis patients with irreducible C1–C2 subluxations.

10. **What are the options for surgical decompression of a C5–C6 disc herniation?**
    - An **anterior surgical approach** is commonly used to excise a cervical disc herniation, especially when the disc herniation is large and centrally located. Following removal of disc material from within the disc space, the posterior annulus and the PLL are partially excised, and any loose disc fragments are removed from the epidural space. Options for reconstruction of the disc space following anterior discectomy include **anterior cervical fusion** or **artificial disc replacement**. Anterior cervical fusion involves placement of a structural bone graft or intervertebral body fusion device into the disc space and stabilization with spinal instrumentation such as an anterior cervical plate. Alternatively, an artificial disc replacement device may be placed into the disc space to provide stabilization while preserving segmental spinal motion.
    - An alternative surgical option is to perform a **posterior laminoforaminotomy**. The lamina and facets are partially removed to provide posterior exposure and decompression of the nerve root and subjacent disc. A posterior laminoforaminotomy approach is appropriate for removal of disc fragments located lateral to the spinal cord or for decompression of foraminal stenosis due to facet hypertrophy, but does not provide adequate exposure for safe removal of central disc herniations.

11. **When is a posterior surgical approach considered for decompression of cervical spinal stenosis with myelopathy?**
Posterior surgical approaches for cervical spinal stenosis are most commonly recommended when three or more levels require decompression. Posterior cervical decompression procedures involve direct removal of posterior compressive structures but rely on indirect decompression of anterior neural compression due to posterior migration of the spinal cord. An important prerequisite for achievement of adequate decompression from a posterior approach is the presence of a neutral or lordotic sagittal alignment, which permits posterior migration of the spinal cord away from anterior compressive pathology (Fig. 24.5).

12. **What are some tips regarding selection of patients for treatment of cervical spinal stenosis with myelopathy using a laminoplasty procedure?**
It is recommended to avoid laminoplasty in patients with severe neck pain, spinal instability, marked kyphotic cervical alignment, and single level anterior cervical stenosis amenable to treatment with an anterior-based cervical decompression procedure. In patients with mild cervical kyphosis, favorable outcomes have been reported with local kyphosis measuring ≤13°. In patients with ossification of the posterior longitudinal ligament (OPLL), measurement of the kyphosis line (K-line) is recommended. The K-line is a straight line connecting the midpoints of

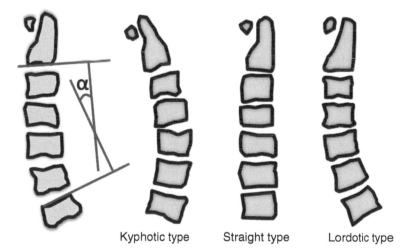

Kyphotic type   Straight type   Lordotic type

Fig. 24.5 Cervical alignment is identified as kyphotic, straight (neutral), or lordotic by measurement of the angle between the endplates of the C2 and C7 vertebra. (From Sun JC, Zhang B, Shi J, et al. Can K-line predict the clinical outcome of anterior controllable antedisplacement and fusion surgery for cervical myelopathy caused by multisegmental ossification of the posterior longitudinal ligament? World Neurosurg 2018;116:118–127.)

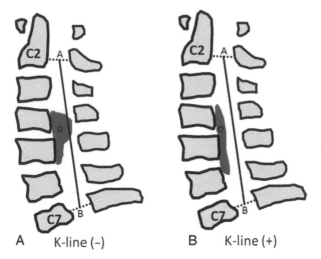

A   K-line (−)   **B   K-line (+)**

Fig. 24.6 The K-line is a straight line connecting the midpoints of the spinal canal at C2 and C7 on a neutral lateral radiograph. (A) Ossification of the posterior longitudinal ligament (OPLL) that does not extend past the K-line is identified as K-line positive. (B) OPLL extending past the K-line is identified as K-line negative. (From Sun JC, Zhang B, Shi J, et al. Can K-line predict the clinical outcome of anterior controllable antedisplacement and fusion surgery for cervical myelopathy caused by multisegmental ossification of the posterior longitudinal ligament? World Neurosurg 2018;116:118–127.)

the spinal canal at C2 and C7 on a neutral lateral radiograph. OPLL that does not extend past the K-line (K-line positive) will respond favorably to posterior decompression, while OPLL extending past the K-line (K-line negative) will not experience adequate posterior cord shift and neural decompression. Preoperative measurement of a modified K-line (mK-line) connecting the midpoints of the spinal cord at C2 and C7 on a T1-weighted sagittal MRI identified that patients with ≤4 mm clearance between an anterior cord compression-causing structure and the mK-line will experience unsatisfactory indirect decompression with laminoplasty (Fig. 24.6).

13. When is the anterior surgical approach considered for decompression of cervical spinal stenosis?
Anterior surgical approaches for treatment of cervical spinal stenosis are widely used for treatment of cervical spinal stenosis in patients with three or fewer levels of involvement. Successful decompression can be achieved regardless of whether the patient has lordotic, neutral, or kyphotic sagittal plane alignment. Multilevel discectomy and interbody fusion are appropriate when neural compression is localized to the level of the disc space. Anterior corpectomy and reconstruction with a strut graft or vertebral body replacement device are appropriate when cord compression extends beyond the level of the disc space or when a significant kyphotic deformity is present.

14. When is a combined anterior and posterior approach considered for treatment of cervical spinal stenosis?
- Multilevel cervical stenosis requiring three or more levels of anterior decompression
- Multilevel cervical stenosis requiring two or more levels of corpectomy
- Multilevel cervical stenosis associated with a rigid cervical kyphotic deformity
- Rigid posttraumatic or postlaminectomy kyphotic deformities

15. Compare the advantages and disadvantages of cervical laminectomy, cervical laminoplasty, and cervical laminectomy with fusion for treatment of multilevel cervical spinal stenosis.
- **Cervical laminectomy** has been widely used for decompression of cervical stenosis with satisfactory results in a many patients. Its advantage is its simplicity. Disadvantages include the tendency to produce segmental instability, postoperative kyphotic deformity, and late neurologic deterioration in certain patients. However, modifications of cervical laminectomy, including skip laminectomy and muscle-preserving selective laminectomy have been developed to minimize adverse events associated with traditional laminectomy.
- **Cervical laminoplasty** has been popularized to address some of the problems associated with cervical laminectomy. Retention of the posterior spinal elements decreases the likelihood of postoperative spinal instability and extensive postoperative epidural scar formation. Because the procedure is performed without fusion, cervical motion is preserved. However, postoperative neck pain may be problematic after laminoplasty procedures.
- **Cervical laminectomy combined with facet fusion and screw-rod fixation** plays a major role in the treatment of multilevel cervical spinal stenosis. It is an effective means of decompressing the spinal canal in patients with neutral or lordotic cervical alignment. Fusion prevents the development of postoperative kyphosis and can improve neck pain symptoms. Spinal implants provide the ability to restore and maintain cervical lordosis. Disadvantages include loss of cervical motion and the complexity of the procedure.

16. What nerve root injury is most common after cervical laminectomy or laminoplasty?
Nerve root dysfunction at the C5 level is the most common nerve root problem after cervical laminectomy or laminoplasty. Nerve root dysfunction may be noted immediately, or it may develop 1–5 days after surgery. The exact cause of C5 dysfunction is incompletely understood, but has been attributed to several factors: (1) the C5 root is the shortest cervical root and is susceptible to traction injury due to posterior cord shift, (2) C5 foraminal stenosis, (3) local spinal cord ischemia, (4) excessive width of laminar decompression, and (5) a segmental disorder of the spinal cord. C5 root deficits are readily detectable on clinical examination because the C5 root provides sole innervation to the deltoid muscle.

17. Provide three examples of clinical situations in which a cervical corpectomy is indicated.
A corpectomy is indicated for treatment of anterior spinal cord compression due to:
1. Vertebral body tumor extending into the spinal canal
2. Vertebral body fracture with retropulsion of bone fragments into the spinal canal
3. OPLL in a patient with a severe and rigid kyphotic deformity

THORACIC AND LUMBAR SPINAL REGIONS

18. What factors are involved in determining the appropriate surgical approach for treatment of a thoracic disc herniation?
Factors to consider in determining the appropriate surgical approach include:
- Location of the disc herniation relative to the spinal cord (central, centrolateral, lateral)
- Level of the disc herniation (upper thoracic, midthoracic, thoracolumbar junction)
- Whether the disc herniation is calcified
- Neurologic signs and symptoms (none, radiculopathy, myelopathy)

19. What are the surgical approach options for decompression to treat a symptomatic thoracic disc herniation?
Current surgical approach options include:
- **Anterior transthoracic surgical approaches** including transpleural thoracotomy, retropleural mini-open thoracotomy, and video-assisted thoracoscopic approaches
- **Posterolateral surgical approaches** including transfacet, transpedicular, transforaminal, and costotransversectomy approaches, and
- **Lateral surgical approaches** including the lateral extracavitary approach and laterally-based minimally invasive approaches using tubular or dual-blade retractors
  The midline posterior laminectomy approach has been abandoned due to poor outcomes and associated high rate of neurologic injury.

20. List three indications for performing a corpectomy in the thoracic and/or lumbar spine.
1. Burst fracture with retropulsion of bone into the spinal canal causing anterior cord compression
2. Tumor extending from the posterior part of the vertebral body into the spinal canal
3. Vertebral osteomyelitis with vertebral body collapse and retropulsion of bone and disc material into the spinal canal, resulting in anterior spinal cord compression

21. In treatment of spinal infections associated with neural compression, how does the surgeon determine the optimal surgical approach for spinal decompression?
Spinal discitis/osteomyelitis is a disease process that predominantly affects the anterior spinal column. Adequate surgical treatment includes debridement of nonviable and infected tissue, direct decompression of neural elements, and reconstruction of the anterior column with bone graft or a fusion cage, often in combination with spinal instrumentation. Surgical approach options include anterior approaches, combined anterior and posterior approaches, and circumferential surgical approaches through a single posterior incision. Various minimally invasive surgical approaches, including anterior column debridement in combination with percutaneous stabilization have also been described. The optimal surgical approach is one which allows adequate access for debridement, decompression, and surgical reconstruction.
  The surgical approach for treatment of a **spinal epidural abscess** is determined by its location. An abscess located posteriorly and extending over multiple levels is best treated by multiple-level laminotomies or laminectomy, taking care to preserve the facet joints. An abscess located anteriorly and associated with vertebral osteomyelitis is most directly treated with an anterior surgical approach. If an abscess involves both the anterior and posterior epidural space, an anterior and posterior approach combined with spinal stabilization is indicated.

22. Describe three techniques for decompression of a thoracolumbar burst fracture associated with a retropulsed bone fragment that causes neurologic deficit.
1. Indirect decompression achieved by use of posterior spinal instrumentation, fusion, *ligamentotaxis*, and realignment of the spinal deformity

2. Direct posterolateral decompression via a laminectomy or transpedicular approach, in combination with use of posterior spinal instrumentation and fusion
3. Direct anterior decompression with corpectomy and reconstruction, combined with anterior and/or posterior spinal instrumentation

23. **What is the primary factor that determines the surgical approach for treatment of a lumbar disc herniation?**
The primary factor guiding selection of the operative approach is the **location of the disc fragment**. Disc herniations located in the central or posterolateral region of the spinal canal are excised through a **laminotomy approach**. Disc herniations located in the foraminal and extraforaminal zone are most directly decompressed through a **paraspinal or intertransverse approach**.

24. **Describe a lumbar laminotomy procedure for removal of a disc herniation.**
A laminotomy is performed on the side of the disc herniation. An intraoperative radiograph or fluoroscopic image is taken to confirm the proper level of exposure. Sufficient bone and ligamentum flavum are removed to permit visualization of the lateral edge of the nerve root. Retraction of the nerve root and removal of the disc fragment are performed under magnification (loupes or microscope).

25. **Describe a paraspinal approach for removal of a foraminal lumbar disc herniation.**
The muscles attached to the midline bony structures are left intact. An incision is made in the fascia lateral to the midline. Blunt dissection is carried down to the transverse processes. The transverse processes are identified, and the intertransverse membrane is exposed. A radiograph is obtained to confirm that the correct spinal level has been exposed. The intertransverse membrane is then released, the nerve root is identified and retracted medially, and the disc herniation is removed.

26. **What are the surgical options for decompression of lumbar spinal stenosis?**
- **Single-level or multilevel laminectomy**. This technique may be used for any type of spinal stenosis problem and is required for treatment of congenital lumbar spinal stenosis. The disadvantage of this technique is its tendency to destabilize the spinal column (see Fig. 24.1C).
- **Single or multilevel laminotomy**. This technique can be used for single-level or multilevel stenosis when the neural compression is localized to the level of the disc space. Bilateral stenosis can be decompressed with separate bilateral approaches or through a unilateral approach for bilateral decompression. Use of a laminotomy technique has the advantage of preserving the stability provided by midline bony and ligamentous structures. It is somewhat more difficult and more time-consuming than a laminectomy when performed for multilevel stenosis (see Fig. 24.1B).
- **Interlaminar decompression.** Various techniques have been described which utilize temporary distraction between adjacent spinous processes to increase the interlaminar working space and facilitate undercutting of the cephalad and caudad lamina and facet joints to decompress the dural sac and nerve roots.
- **Microendoscopic decompressive laminotomy using tubular retractor systems**. Bilateral decompression of spinal stenosis may be performed through a unilateral approach or separate bilateral surgical approaches using tubular retractors and specialized instruments.
- **Implantation of an interspinous device.** An example of this device class is the Superion Indirect Decompression System (Vertiflex, Inc., Carlsbad, CA). This device is implanted by percutaneous means through a cannula inserted between adjacent spinous processes to provide distraction and restrict extension for treatment of moderate degenerative lumbar spinal stenosis.

27. **When should the surgeon perform a spinal arthrodesis after decompression for lumbar spinal stenosis?**
- Following intraoperative destabilization (removal of more than 50% of both facet joints, complete removal of a single facet joint, or disruption of the pars interarticularis)
- For patients with significant lumbar scoliosis
- For patients with spondylolisthesis or lateral listhesis at the level of decompression

KEY POINTS

1. The selection of the appropriate procedure for spinal decompression depends on a variety of factors including clinical symptoms, spinal level, location of compression, number of involved levels, and the presence/absence of spinal instability or spinal deformity.
2. Spinal arthrodesis and spinal instrumentation are indicated in conjunction with decompression in the presence of spinal deformity or spinal instability or when decompression results in destabilization at the surgical site.

Websites
1. Cervical spine: https://www.aans.org/Patients/Neurosurgical-Conditions-and-Treatments/Cervical-Spine;
2. Laminoplasty: https://emedicine.medscape.com/article/1890493-overview#showall
3. Spinal decompression and fusion: https://reference.medscape.com/features/slideshow/spinal-decompression#page51
4. Thoracic disc herniation: https://www.ncbi.nlm.nih.gov/pmc/articles/PMC3609007/;
5. Herniated disc: https://www.hss.edu/condition-list_herniated-disc.asp; Laminotomy versus laminectomy: http://www.spineuniverse.com/treatments/surgery/laminotomy-versus-laminectomy

REFERENCE
1. Yoshihara, H. (2017). Indirect decompression in spinal surgery. *Journal of Clinical Neuroscience, 44*, 63–68.

BIBLIOGRAPHY
1. Baron, E. M., & Vaccaro, A. R. (2018). *Operative Techniques: Spine Surgery*. Philadelphia: Elsevier.
2. Carr, D. A., Volkov, A. A., Rhoiney, D. L., Setty, P., Barrett, R. J., Claybrooks, R., et al. (2017). Management of thoracic disc herniations via posterior unilateral modified transfacet pedicle-sparing decompression with segmental instrumentation and interbody fusion. *Global Spine Journal, 7*(6), 506–513.
3. Fujiyoshi, T., Yamazaki, M., Kawabe, J., Endo, T., Furuya, T., Koda, M., et al. (2008). A new concept for making decisions regarding the surgical approach for cervical ossification of the posterior longitudinal ligament: The K-line. *Spine, 33*(26), 990–993.
4. Kim, D. H., Vaccaro, A. R., Dickman, C. A., Cho, D., Lee, S., & Kim, I. (2013). *Surgical Anatomy and Techniques to the Spine* (2nd ed.). Philadelphia, PA: Saunders.
5. McCulloch, J. A., & Young, P. H. (1998). *Essentials of Spinal Microsurgery*. Philadelphia, PA: Lippincott-Raven.
6. Nori, A., Shiraishi, T., Aoyama, R., Ninomiya, K., Yamane, J., Kitamura, K., et al. (2018). Muscle-preserving selective laminectomy maintained the compensatory mechanism of cervical lordosis after surgery. *Spine, 43*(8), 542–549.
7. Taniyama, T., Hirai, T., Yoshii, T., Yamada, T., Yasuda, H., Saito, M., et al. (2014). Modified K-line in magnetic resonance imaging predicts clinical outcome in patients with nonlordotic alignment after laminoplasty for cervical spondylotic myelopathy. *Spine, 39*(21), 1261–1268.
8. Wang, L., Wang, Y., Yu, B., Li, Z., & Liu, X. (2015). Open-door versus French-door laminoplasty for the treatment of cervical multilevel compressive myelopathy. *Journal of Clinical Neuroscience, 22*(3), 450–455.
9. Yoshihara, H. (2017). Indirect decompression in spinal surgery. *Journal of Clinical Neuroscience, 44*, 63–68.

CHAPTER 25

SPINAL ARTHRODESIS, GRAFT MATERIALS, AND GRAFT TECHNIQUES

Vincent J. Devlin, MD

1. **What is spinal arthrodesis?**

   Spinal arthrodesis is defined as osseous union (fusion) between adjacent vertebrae due to surgical intervention. During surgery, adjacent bone surfaces are decorticated and graft material is applied to promote bone growth between adjacent vertebrae. Spinal instrumentation or external immobilization may be utilized to limit motion at the surgical site and enhance fusion. Spinal arthrodesis procedures are broadly categorized by location as anterior spinal column fusions, posterior spinal column fusions, or circumferential spinal fusions (also called 360° fusions, global fusions, or combined anterior and posterior column fusions).

2. **Describe some of the functions of spinal instrumentation in relation to spinal arthrodesis procedures.**

   Spinal instrumentation is used to limit intersegmental motion and create a favorable mechanical environment that promotes spinal fusion. Other functions of spinal instrumentation include correction of spinal deformities and restoration of immediate mechanical stability to spinal segments whose structural integrity has been compromised by spinal pathologies such as fracture, tumor, infection, and degenerative disorders.

3. **What factors influence successful healing of a spinal fusion?**

   (1) **Type of graft material** (e.g., autograft, allograft, synthetic biomaterials)
   (2) **Local factors:**
      - Quality of the soft tissue bed into which bone graft is placed
      - Method of preparation of the graft recipient site
      - Mechanical stability of the spine segment(s) to be fused
      - Graft location (anterior vs. posterior spinal column)
      - Spinal region (the cervical region is considered a more favorable environment for fusion versus the thoracic or lumbar regions)
   (3) **Systemic host factors**:
      - Patient age
      - Presence of metabolic bone disease
      - Nutritional status
      - Perioperative medications
      - Tobacco use

4. **How does patient age and medical history influence healing of a spinal fusion and selection of an appropriate graft material?**

   The bones of skeletally immature patients have an inherent osteogenic potential, and high rates of arthrodesis are reported regardless of whether autograft, allograft, composite grafts, or ceramics are utilized as graft material. Lower fusion rates are encountered in the adult population and union rates have been shown to decline with increasing age. Additional factors that negatively impact fusion rates in adults include endocrine disorders (e.g., diabetes), medications, and tobacco use.

   Certain medications have the potential to impair fusion if used in the perioperative period because they inhibit or delay bone formation. Examples include nonsteroidal antiinflammatory drugs (NSAIDs, e.g., ibuprofen, ketorolac tromethamine), cytotoxic drugs (e.g., methotrexate, doxorubicin), certain antibiotics (e.g., ciprofloxacin), corticosteroids, and anticoagulants (e.g., warfarin [Coumadin]). Recent evidence suggests that the adverse effects of NSAIDs on spinal fusion healing are related to dose and duration of use, and that incorporation of normal-dose NSAIDs into postoperative pain management protocols for spine fusion patients is reasonable and is associated with improved pain control and reduction in adverse events associated with use of opioids. In contrast, other medications such as teriparatide have been reported to enhance healing of spinal fusions and are under investigation for this purpose.

5. **How does tobacco use interfere with spinal fusion?**

   The rate of successful spinal arthrodesis in smokers is lower than in nonsmokers. Cigarette smoking has been shown to interfere with bone metabolism and inhibit bone formation. Nicotine is considered the agent responsible for these adverse effects. The precise mechanisms responsible remain under investigation and include inhibition of graft revascularization and neovascularization, as well as osteoblast suppression. These effects are mediated by inhibition of cytokines.

6. **What are some of the common types of graft materials used in spinal arthrodesis procedures?**
   Common graft material options for use in spinal fusion include:
   - **Autograft**: Autograft bone is obtained from the patient undergoing surgery. Sources include the patient's ilium, fibula, or ribs. Autograft bone may also be obtained from the operative site and is termed *local bone graft*. Vascularized autografts (e.g., rib, fibula) are an option for use in complex reconstruction scenarios. Bone marrow aspirate (BMA) is an autologous source of stem cells, osteoblasts, and growth factors and may be used in conjunction with other graft materials.
   - **Allograft**: Allograft bone is human cadaveric bone, which is available in a variety of shapes and compositions.
   - **Demineralized Bone Matrix (DBM)**: Allograft bone may undergo processing by acid extraction to remove bone mineral while retaining collagen and noncollagenous proteins. The end product is DBM, an allograft form with osteoinductive activity.
   - **Bone Morphogenetic Proteins (BMPs)**: BMPs are osteoinductive proteins that are members of the transforming growth factor beta (TGF-β) superfamily of growth factors. As BMPs are soluble proteins, use of a carrier is required to maintain an effective local concentration and prevent diffusion away from the operative site.
   - **Ceramics**: Various ceramics are available for use as bone graft material, including beta-tricalcium phosphate (β-TCP), hydroxyapatite (HA), calcium sulfate, silicate-substituted calcium phosphate (Si-CaP), and beta-calcium pyrophosphate (β-CPP).
   - **Composite grafts**: Various types of scaffolds may be combined with biologic elements (e.g., BMA, growth factors) to promote fusion.

7. **Which three properties are desirable in an ideal graft material for use in spinal fusion?**
   1. **Osteoinduction:** The graft should contain growth factors (noncollagenous bone matrix proteins) that can induce osteoblast precursors to differentiate into mature bone-forming cells.
   2. **Osteoconduction:** The graft should provide a framework or scaffold (bone mineral and collagen) onto which new bone can form.
   3. **Osteogenesis:** The graft should contain viable progenitor stem cells that can form new bone matrix and remodel bone as needed.
      Autograft bone has been considered the gold standard for spinal fusion bone graft materials. Autograft bone possesses all of the properties required to achieve spinal fusion as it is osteoinductive, osteoconductive, and osteogenic.

8. **Compare the properties of current graft materials in relation to an ideal graft material for use in spinal fusion.**
   See Table 25.1.

9. **How are graft materials classified according to their intended use?**
   Graft materials may be compared to autograft bone and classified according to their intended use:
   - **Extender:** This type of graft material is indicated for use in combination with autograft bone. Such graft material permits use of a lesser volume of autograft without compromising fusion rates. A bone graft extender can also permit a finite amount of autograft to be utilized over a greater number of spinal levels without compromising the fusion rate when compared with fusion using autograft alone.

Table 25.1 Properties of Graft Materials for Spinal Fusion.

GRAFT MATERIAL	OSTEOGENESIS	OSTEOINDUCTION	OSTEOCONDUCTION
Autograft	+	+	+
Allograft	−	±	+
Demineralized bone matrix	−	+	+
Bone morphogenetic proteins	−	+	−
Ceramics	−	−	+
Composite grafts	−	+	+
Bone marrow aspirate	+	±	−

+, Present; −, absent; ±, weak or variable property.

- **Enhancer:** This type of graft material is used in conjunction with autograft bone to increase the rate of successful arthrodesis above the rate of fusion achieved with use of autograft alone.
- **Substitute:** This type of graft material is used as an alternative to autograft bone and is intended to provide equivalent or superior fusion success compared with autograft bone.

10. What are some differences between cortical and cancellous bone graft in relation to use of each type of graft in spinal fusion procedures?

Cortical bone comprises the outer portion of skeletal structures. It is compact and exhibits high resistance to bending and torsional forces. These properties allow cortical bone to provide structural support when used as a graft material. Cortical bone is incorporated by creeping substitution, which occurs slowly over years. *Cancellous bone* is less dense than cortical bone and provides a porous matrix essential for osteogenesis in areas not requiring immediate structural support. Cancellous bone is incorporated more rapidly than cortical bone because of direct bone apposition onto the scaffold provided by its bony trabeculae. Bone graft used in spinal fusion procedures may be comprised entirely of cancellous or cortical bone, or a combination of both. The ratio of cancellous to cortical bone varies depending on the bone graft donor site and technique used for graft procurement and graft preparation.

11. Explain the difference between nonstructural and structural graft material.

Nonstructural grafts (also termed *morselized* grafts) consist of particles of bone (e.g., cancellous bone from the iliac crest). This graft type does not provide structural stability when used by itself. Adjunctive spinal instrumentation is generally used to facilitate bony union. **Structural grafts** provide mechanical support during the process of fusion consolidation.

12. Compare and contrast the healing potential of the anterior spinal column and posterior spinal column with respect to spinal fusion.

Biologic factors and *biomechanical factors* are different in the anterior and posterior spinal columns. Graft materials placed in the anterior column are subject to compressive loading, which promotes fusion. Structural grafts are commonly used to restore the load bearing capacity of the anterior spinal column. In the anterior spinal column, the wide bony surface area combined with excellent vascularity of the fusion bed, which is composed primarily of cancellous bone, creates a superior biologic milieu for fusion. High fusion success rates in the anterior column may be achieved using autograft bone, allograft bone, as well as specific bone graft substitutes. In contrast, the posterior spinal column is composed primarily of cortical bone and subject to tensile forces, which provide a less favorable healing environment for spinal fusion. Posterior column graft materials are generally not required to provide structural support. Posterior column fusion is highly dependent on biologic factors, including the presence of osteogenic cells, osteoinductive factors, as well as the quality of the soft tissue and osseous bed into which the graft material is placed. In view of this more challenging healing environment, autogenous iliac bone graft has traditionally been the gold standard for achieving posterior spinal fusion. Fusion rates also vary by spinal region, with the highest fusion rates associated with cervical and thoracic fusions and the lowest rates with lumbar fusions, especially posterolateral lumbar fusions.

13. What anatomic structures provide potential sites for posterior spinal arthrodesis?

In the *cervical region*, posterior spinal fusions are achieved by applying bone graft to the lamina, facet joints, and spinous processes. In the *thoracic and lumbar regions*, the lamina, facet joints, spinous processes, and transverse processes are available sites for arthrodesis. These bone surfaces require meticulous preparation including removal of all overlying soft tissue prior to graft application. In addition, it is critical to remove the outer cortical bone surface (decortication) to expose underlying cancellous bone and provide access to the pluripotent stem cells within the patient's bone marrow to achieve a consistent and high likelihood of successful fusion (Fig. 25.1).

14. Discuss some considerations involved in selection of graft materials for use in posterior spinal fusion procedures.

Autogenous cancellous iliac crest bone graft has been considered the traditional gold standard for graft material for posterior spinal fusion procedures, as it possesses osteogenic, osteoconductive, and osteoinductive properties, and provides a consistently high rate of successful arthrodesis. Local bone graft obtained from the operative site is an alternate source of autogenous bone graft, and avoids concerns regarding potential morbidity associated with harvest of iliac autograft. A graft extender (e.g., nonstructural allograft, DBM, BMA) may be added to iliac autograft or local bone graft to increase the total amount of graft material available for a specific procedure.

Allograft bone in the form of cancellous chips or DBM has been evaluated as a graft substitute and graft extender in posterior fusion procedures. In adult patients, when used as the sole source of graft material for posterior fusion, nonstructural allograft bone in the form of cancellous chips or DBM does not achieve a sufficiently high fusion rate to warrant use as a substitute for autograft bone. However, acceptable fusion rates have been reported with use of allograft cancellous bone chips or DBM when used as a graft extender in combination with autograft bone or BMA in adults. In contrast, in the pediatric population, success has been reported using nonstructural allograft bone or DBM as a graft substitute in posterior fusion procedures, including scoliosis surgery.

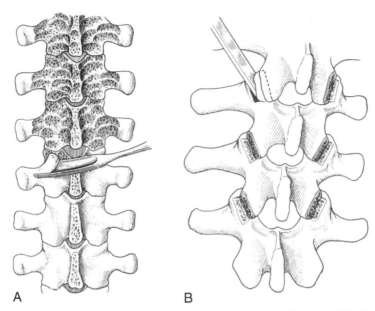

A **B**

Fig. 25.1 Posterior spinal arthrodesis technique. (A) Posterior fusion. Posterior osseous structures (lamina, facet joints, transverse processes) are cleaned of soft tissue, and the outer cortical bone is removed (decortication) to expose underlying cancellous bone. (B) Facet joint fusion. The facet joint cartilage is excised, and the joint surfaces are prepared for bone graft application. (From Laurin CA, Riley LH. Atlas of Orthopaedic Surgery: General principles. Spine. Chicago: Year Book Medical Publishers; 1989.)

This success is attributed to the greater potential for osseous union inherent in pediatric patients and the creation of local bone graft by meticulous decortication of the posterior bony structures during surgery.

Multiple studies report success with use of bone morphogenetic protein (rhBMP-2) in combination with synthetic carriers, with or without the addition of local autograft, in posterior fusion procedures. However, at the current time posterior use of rhBMP-2 remains an off-label use in the United States. Additional graft material options for use in posterior spinal fusion include ceramics, polymers, and composite materials, which may be combined with BMA or synthetic osteoinductive factors. However, available evidence to support these alternatives is more limited.

15. Describe some of the factors to consider in selection of graft materials for use in anterior spinal fusion procedures.

Both autograft and allograft bone grafts (structural and nonstructural) have been reported to provide acceptable fusion rates when used in the anterior spinal column as graft materials. When a structural graft is required, the high rate of fusion obtained with autograft must be weighed against the morbidity of harvesting large sections of autogenous bone graft from the pelvis or other graft donor sites. Additional graft options include synthetic cages used in combination with a variety of graft materials including, nonstructural autograft, nonstructural allograft, BMPs used with a carrier, and synthetic osteoconductive materials.

16. How are structural grafts used to reconstruct the anterior spinal column classified by their location?

Anterior column structural graft constructs are classified according to location as *strut grafts, interbody grafts,* or *transvertebral grafts*. **Strut grafts** reconstruct the anterior spinal column following removal of a vertebral body (i.e., corpectomy). **Interbody grafts** reconstruct the anterior spinal column following discectomy. **Transvertebral grafts** are used to stabilize adjacent vertebrae and achieve fusion across an intervening disc space (Fig. 25.2).

17. What are fusion cages?

Fusion cages are intended to provide structural support to the anterior spinal column and promote fusion following removal of an intervertebral disc (i.e., **intervertebral body fusion device**) or vertebral body (i.e., **vertebral body replacement device**). These devices are filled with a variety of graft material and are generally used in conjunction with some type of supplemental fixation. The cage is intended to restore immediate mechanical stability to the anterior spinal column and provide a favorable environment for fusion. Cages are available in a variety of shapes and materials (e.g., titanium, carbon fiber, polyetheretherketone [PEEK], cortical bone). Cages may be implanted through a variety of surgical approaches (e.g., anterior, lateral, posterolateral, transforaminal) depending on the specific spinal region, spinal level, and type of pathology requiring surgical treatment (Fig. 25.3).

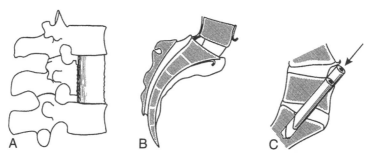

Fig. 25.2 (A) Anterior graft constructs may be described as strut grafts, (B) interbody grafts, or (C) transvertebral grafts. (From Devlin VJ, Pitt DD. The evolution of surgery of the anterior spinal column. Spine State Art Rev 1998;12:493–528.)

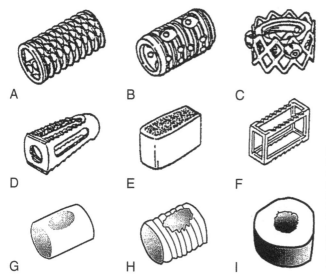

Fig. 25.3 Options for lumbar interbody fusion. (A) Ray cylindrical threaded fusion cage. (B) BAK cylindrical threaded fusion cage. (C) Surgical titanium mesh. (D) Tapered (lordotic) fusion cage. (E) Iliac crest autograft or allograft bone. (F) Carbon fiber fusion cage. (G) Nonthreaded femoral cortical bone dowel. (H) Threaded femoral cortical bone dowel. (I) Femoral ring allograft. (From Devlin VJ, Pitt DD. The evolution of surgery of the anterior spinal column. Spine State Art Rev 1998;12:493–528.)

18. What graft material options are available for use in interbody fusion in the cervical, thoracic, and lumbar spinal regions?
    - In the **cervical region,** structural allograft bone grafts or intervertebral body fusion devices comprised of metals or polymers and filled with a variety of graft materials, are most commonly used. Iliac autograft bone graft remains an excellent graft option but has become less popular due to concerns regarding donor site morbidity, additional surgical time required to obtain iliac graft, and the widespread availability of allografts and cages.
    - In the **thoracic region,** interbody graft options include structural allograft and intervertebral body fusion devices. Local rib graft may be harvested for use as graft material during surgical procedures that involve rib exposure or resection (e.g., costotransversectomy or transthoracic spinal exposures).
    - In the **lumbar spine,** both nonstructural and structural grafts may be used. Structural graft options for interbody fusion include autograft (iliac crest); allograft (femur, ilium, tibia); and a variety of interbody fusion cage devices that are generally used in combination with nonstructural bone graft, BMPs on a carrier, or synthetic osteoconductive materials (Figs. 25.4 and 25.5).

19. What graft options are available after corpectomy in the cervical, thoracic, and lumbar spinal regions?
    - In the **cervical region,** one- or two-level corpectomies are most commonly reconstructed using tricortical iliac autograft, fibula allograft, or a fusion cage used in combination with spinal instrumentation. For reconstruction of two or more vertebral levels, a fibular allograft or fusion cage is most commonly used in combination with posterior spinal instrumentation.
    - In the **thoracic and lumbar regions,** a variety of structural graft options are available including autograft, allograft, and fusion cages. Adjunctive spinal instrumentation is used in combination with strut grafts (Fig. 25.6).

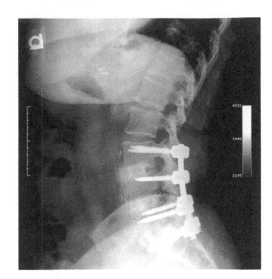

Fig. 25.4 Allograft femoral rings packed with various graft materials are used with a high rate of success for anterior lumbar interbody fusion.

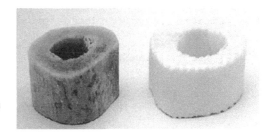

Fig. 25.5 Examples of femoral allograft rings. (Kim DH, Chang UK, Kim SH, et al. Tumors of the Spine. Philadelphia, PA: Saunders; 2008.)

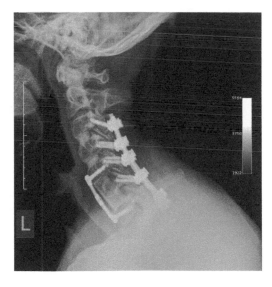

Fig. 25.6 Fibula strut graft and anterior plate *(lower levels)*; machine-prepared structural interbody allografts *(upper levels)*.

20. What is the most common indication for placement of a transvertebral graft?

A transvertebral graft is most commonly used in the surgical treatment of high-grade L5–S1 spondylolisthesis when a reduction or resection procedure is undesirable. Typically a fibular autograft, fibular allograft, or a cylindrical fusion cage is placed from either a posterior or anterior approach to bridge L5 and the sacrum. The graft is typically combined with posterolateral spinal fusion and instrumentation.

21. Discuss some sources and uses of local autograft bone in spinal fusion procedures.

Local graft material may be recovered whenever a high-speed burr is used for spinal decompression or decortication through use of an inline suction trap to collect bone dust from the surgical field. Local bone graft may also be recovered in spinal decompression procedures during which pieces of bone from the spinous processes, lamina, facet joints, and resected osteophytes may be collected and saved for use as graft material, following removal of any soft tissue or cartilage. If a surgical procedure involves rib resection or spinal osteotomy, local bone graft from these procedures may be collected and used as graft material.

Local bone graft may be used to augment the volume of available graft material in all types of spinal fusion procedures. Use of local bone graft with or without a bone graft extender has been extensively reported for use in short-segment (i.e., one- or two-level) lumbar spinal fusion procedures with achievement of acceptable fusion rates.

22. When does a surgeon use the anterior iliac crest or the posterior iliac crest as the site for harvesting bone graft?

Factors to consider in selecting the graft site include the volume of bone graft required and the patient's position during surgery. The posterior iliac crest can supply a greater volume of bone than the anterior iliac crest. Patient position during surgery is also a factor. When the patient is in the prone position, the posterior third of the ilium is more easily accessible, whereas in the supine position, the anterior third of the ilium is easier to access (Fig. 25.7).

23. What are some limitations regarding use of iliac autograft bone for spinal fusions?

- The supply of autograft is limited and graft quality may be less than optimal.
- Increased operative time and a second incision are required for graft harvest.
- Complications reported following iliac crest bone graft procedures include:
  - Wound infection, hematoma, or seroma
  - Acute and/or chronic donor site pain
  - Superior gluteal artery injury
  - Pelvic fracture
  - Sacroiliac joint violation
  - Injury to the sciatic nerve
  - Meralgia paresthetica (lateral femoral cutaneous nerve injury)
  - Superior cluneal nerve injury or transection
  - Lumbar hernia

24. What are two available methods for preserving allograft bone grafts?

Allograft bone is harvested under sterile conditions and preserved by freezing or freeze-drying. These methods reduce immunogenicity and permit extended storage. Allograft bone is available either as a nonstructural graft

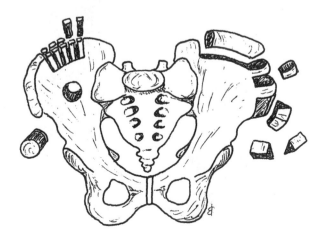

Fig. 25.7 Types of anterior and posterior iliac grafts.

(e.g., corticocancellous or cancellous chips) or as a structural graft (e.g., femoral rings, tricortical wedges, fibular shaft, tibial or femoral shaft, machine-contoured ramps, or threaded dowels).

25. **What is the risk of disease transmission with allograft bone graft?**
The risk of disease transmission with allograft bone is extremely low. Donors are screened for a history of medical problems, and serologic tests are performed to identify HIV, hepatitis B, and hepatitis C. The incidence of HIV transmission from allograft bone is estimated as 1 in 1.6 million. Bone allografts have a much lower incidence of disease transmission than blood transfusions.

26. **Compare some advantages and disadvantages of freeze-dried and fresh-frozen allograft bone.**
    • Freeze-dried allograft bone can be stored at room temperature, whereas fresh-frozen grafts require storage in a −70 degrees C freezer.
    • As a result of processing, fresh-frozen allograft bone contains more viable osteoinductive factors than freeze-dried allograft.
    • Freeze-dried bone is brittle if not hydrated adequately. Fresh-frozen bone must be thawed to body temperature and consequently requires more preparation time but has better mechanical properties and higher fusion rates than freeze-dried bone.

27. **How does allograft incorporate into a spinal fusion mass?**
The method of incorporation into a fusion mass depends on the type of allograft bone graft. Allograft cortical bone can take years to incorporate fully because it is remodeled by creeping substitution. Osteoclasts resorb the allograft, and osteoblasts form new bone as the graft is revascularized. Corticocancellous allograft bone is incorporated more rapidly because bone apposition on existing bony trabeculae is the primary mode of incorporation.

28. **What are the advantages of allograft bone in spinal fusion procedures?**
Nonstructural allograft can be used as a graft extender in posterior fusion procedures when the volume of autograft available is insufficient. Structural allograft (e.g., fibula, femoral cortical shaft) can be used to fill anterior column defects following discectomies and corpectomies. Structural allograft provides superior mechanical strength compared with autograft iliac crest wedges or rib grafts and avoids the morbidity and increased operative time associated with graft harvest.

29. **What are the disadvantages of allograft bone in spinal fusion procedures?**
Allograft bone weakens as it undergoes remodeling. In rare instances, allograft can transmit infections. In some countries allograft bone is not allowed to be used based on cultural, religious, or ethical grounds. Lastly, the expense involved in processing, preserving, and storing allograft can make this graft type difficult to obtain.

30. **What is demineralized bone matrix?**
DBM is an osteoconductive scaffold produced by acid extraction of allograft bone. It lacks structural and mechanical properties. Its constituents include noncollagenous proteins, osteoinductive growth factors, and type 1 collagen. During manufacture, DBM powder is combined with a variety of carrier substances to improve handling characteristics. DBM is available in a variety of formulations including powders, fibers, gels, granules, putties, and strips. DBM is more osteoinductive than allograft bone because the demineralization process makes growth factors (BMPs) more accessible. Clinical data support the use of DBM as a bone graft extender or enhancer in posterior spinal fusion procedures performed with autograft bone. It is not intended to be used in isolation as a bone graft substitute. Fewer studies address its efficacy in anterior spinal fusion procedures. Significant variation in the biologic activity of DBM preparations has been documented, and may occur within production lots from the same manufacturer. Bioassays are available to assess osteoinductivity, although no universally accepted standards exist.

31. **What is the role of ceramics in spinal fusion procedures?**
Ceramic materials (β-TCP, HA, calcium sulfate, natural coral ceramics, bioactive glass) have been evaluated for use in spinal fusion. Data support the role of ceramic material as a scaffold for bone growth. Ceramics are recommended for use as bone graft extenders in combination with osteoinductive materials, but not for use as bone graft substitutes. Ceramics also play a role as a component of a composite graft composed of a ceramic delivery vehicle and osteoinductive bone growth factors or osteoprogenitor cells.
Ceramic materials possess a wide range of properties depending on porosity, mechanical properties, and resorption rates. As ceramics are brittle and possess low shear strength, these materials are not suited to provide a structural support function.

32. **Explain what is meant by a composite graft and provide an example of this class of graft material.**
A composite graft consists of a synthetic scaffold that is combined with biologic elements to stimulate fusion. An ideal composite graft material provides an osteoconductive matrix, osteoinductive proteins, and osteogenic cells. Various matrices have been investigated for use in combination with a range of biologic elements, including bone

marrow aspirate, autograft, BMPs, growth factors, and synthetic peptides for use as composite graft materials for spinal fusion.

33. What are bone morphogenetic proteins?

BMPs are part of a larger TGF-β superfamily that contains multiple related proteins. These proteins are cytokines that function as signaling molecules. BMPs were first identified as the active osteoinductive fraction of DBM. Molecular cloning techniques permitted subsequent identification and characterization of specific proteins. Although over 20 different BMPs have been identified, only BMP-2, -4, -6, -7, and -9 have significant osteogenic properties. Using genetically modified cell lines, recombinant BMP can be produced in large quantities using a bioreactor. The most extensively studied BMP for use in spinal fusion surgery is recombinant human bone morphogenetic protein-2 (rhBMP-2). Subsequent research discovered that BMPs function as body morphogenetic proteins and affect a wide range of structures and processes across different organ systems, ranging from embryogenesis and organogenesis to adult tissue hemostasis. Dysregulated BMP signaling has been associated with a range of human diseases including skeletal diseases, vascular diseases, and cancer.

34. How do BMPs signal for bone formation on a cellular level?

BMPs bind to two types of receptors (type I and type II) on the cell surface. Both type I and type II receptors are required for signal transduction. These receptors are serine/threonine protein kinases that phosphorylate and activate proteins called Smads. Smads are intracellular proteins that bind BMP ligands and transduce signals from the cell surface to the nucleus where they regulate gene expression. Different types of Smads are present and include receptor-regulated Smads (R-Smads), common mediator Smads (C-Smads), and antagonistic-inhibitory Smads (I-Smads). In addition, Smad-independent pathways also play a role in the transduction of BMP signals.

35. Discuss the use of rhBMP-2 in anterior lumbar fusion procedures.

Recombinant human bone morphogenetic protein-2 (rhBMP-2) is approved in the United States for use in the anterior lumbar spinal region as the INFUSE Bone Graft/Medtronic Interbody Fusion Device. The components of this device include INFUSE Bone Graft (rhBMP-2 placed on an absorbable collagen sponge carrier made from bovine type 1 collagen) and specific titanium or PEEK interbody fusion cages. This device is indicated for use in single level anterior/oblique fusion procedures (L2–S1) in skeletally mature patients for treatment of degenerative disc disease and up to grade 1 spondylolisthesis at the involved spinal level. The compressible collagen sponge is protected by the structural support of the cage and maintains an effective local concentration of rhBMP-2 while it serves as a scaffold for new bone formation. It slowly degrades as mesenchymal stem cells surround the implant and differentiate into osteoblasts, and form trabecular bone at the surgical site.

36. Describe some concerns with use of rhBMP-2 for spinal fusions.

Initial clinical studies using INFUSE reported high fusion rates and low adverse event rates, and led to FDA approval of its use in specific anterior lumbar interbody fusion procedures. Based on these initial favorable results, the use of rhBMP-2 was expanded through physician-directed or "off-label" use to other types of spinal procedures, including cervical fusions, thoracic fusions, posterolateral lumbar fusions, as well as posterior lumbar interbody and transforaminal lumbar interbody fusions. Subsequently, an increasing number of adverse events associated with use of rhBMP-2 were reported. In 2008 an FDA Public Health Notification was issued regarding risks associated with use of INFUSE in the anterior cervical spine due to potentially life-threatening complications. Marked soft tissue inflammation and delayed swelling occurred in some patients and led to airway-related complications (i.e., dyspnea, respiratory failure, airway obstruction, dysphagia, reintubation, hospital readmission).

In 2011, a *Special Issue on The Evolving Safety Profile of rhBMP-2 Use in the Spine* was published in *The Spine Journal* and identified specific areas of concern including:

1. Bone overgrowth and uncontrolled bone formation
2. Adverse events related to stimulation of osteoclasts such as implant subsidence, loosening, and migration.
3. Wound related issues including inflammation, edema, seroma, and hematoma
4. Potential negative effects on neurologic structures leading to retrograde ejaculation, urinary retention, back pain, leg pain, radiculitis, and functional loss.
5. Concerns regarding carcinogenicity related to rhBMP-2 use

In response to these concerns, Medtronic Sofamor Danek engaged the Yale University Open Data Access (YODA) Project to independently analyze data from all known prior clinical trials involving rhBMP-2. This led to two publications (1,2) in the *Annals of Internal Medicine* in 2013, and a summary (3) of the important findings of YODA in the *Yale Journal of Biology and Medicine* in 2014 as:

"1. No difference in fusion rates between rhBMP-2 and autograft iliac crest bone graft
2. Both rhBMP-2 and iliac crest bone graft are associated with similar rates of retrograde ejaculation and neurological complications when used in anterior interbody lumbar fusion or posterolateral fusion
3. There is clear evidence that rhBMP-2 usage leads to high rates of complication in anterior cervical procedures and high rates of ectopic bone formation in posterior lumbar interbody procedures
4. Although there is a slight increased relative risk of cancer with the use of rhBMP-2, the absolute risk remains very small and therefore most likely clinically insignificant."

37. Define nonunion following a spinal fusion procedure.

Nonunion or pseudarthrosis is defined as the failure of an attempted fusion to heal within 1 year after surgery.

38. What are the major risk factors for nonunion following a spinal fusion procedure?
- **Biologic factors:** Tobacco use, medications (steroids, high doses of NSAIDs), deep wound infection, metabolic disorders
- **Mechanical factors:** Inadequate spinal fixation
- **Inadequate surgical technique:** Inadequate preparation of the fusion site
- **Graft-related factors:** Inadequate volume of bone graft, inappropriate selection of graft material (e.g., use of allograft as the sole graft material in an adult posterior fusion).

39. How is a failed spine fusion diagnosed?

Clinical symptoms such as localized pain over the fusion site should prompt suspicion of a nonunion. Confirmatory tests include plain radiographs (include flexion-extension radiographs to assess for an abnormal degree of motion) and computed tomography with multiplanar reconstructions (to assess for bridging bone). Radiographic findings that suggest pseudarthrosis include broken or loose spinal implants, progressive spinal deformity after surgery, and discontinuity in the fusion mass on imaging studies. Surgical exploration is the most reliable method of determining whether a fusion has successfully healed.

40. Does the presence of a nonunion after an attempted spinal fusion always cause symptoms?

No. Although many patients who develop a nonunion report pain symptoms, this is not always the case. Fusion success does not always correlate with favorable patient outcomes. However, many studies support a strong positive correlation between successful arthrodesis and positive patient outcomes.

KEY POINTS

1. Graft material options for use in spinal arthrodesis include autograft bone, allograft bone, demineralized bone matrix, ceramics, bone marrow aspirate, and osteoinductive proteins.
2. An ideal graft material for use in spinal fusion possesses osteoinductive, osteoconductive, and osteogenic properties.
3. Graft materials may function as bone graft extenders, bone graft enhancers, or bone graft substitutes.
4. Spinal fusion cages are devices that contain graft material and provide structural support to the anterior spinal column following removal of an intervertebral disc or vertebral body.

Websites
1. Bone grafting: http://www.medscape.com/viewarticle/449880
2. Bone graft substitutes: https://www.ncbi.nlm.nih.gov/pmc/articles/PMC6314336/pdf/i2211-4599-12-6-757.pdf
3. Bone graft options for spine fusion: https://www.spine-health.com/treatment/spinal-fusion/bone-graft-options-spine-fusion
4. Lumbar pseudarthrosis: http://www.medscape.com/viewarticle/462180
5. The YODA project: http://yoda.yale.edu/modtronic-systematic-reviews

REFERENCES
1. Fu, R., Selph, S., McDonagh, M., Peterson, K., Tiwari, A., Chou, R., et al. (2013). Effectiveness and harms of recombinant human bone morphogenetic protein-2 in spine fusion: A systematic review and meta-analysis. *Annals of Internal Medicine,* 158(12), 890–902.
2. Simmonds, M. C., Brown, J. V., Heirs, M. K., Higgins, J. P., Mannion, R. J., Rodgers, M. A., et al. (2013). Safety and effectiveness of recombinant human bone morphogenetic protein-2 for spinal fusion: A meta-analysis of individual-participant data. *Annals of Internal Medicine,* 158(12), 877–889.
3. Hustedt, J. W., & Blizzard, D. J. (2014). The controversy surrounding bone morphogenetic proteins in the spine: A review of current research. *Yale Journal of Biology and Medicine,* 87(4), 549–561.

BIBLIOGRAPHY
1. Carragee, E. J., Hurwitz, E. L., & Weiner, B. K. (2011). A critical review of recombinant human bone morphogenetic protein-2 trials in spine surgery: Emerging safety concerns and lessons learned. *The Spine Journal, 11*(6), 471–491.
2. Carragee, E. J., Comer, G. C., & Smith, M. W. (2011). Local bone graft harvesting and volumes in posterolateral lumbar fusion: A technical report. *The Spine Journal, 11*(6), 540–544.
3. Fisher, C. R., Cassilly, R., Cantor, W., Edusei, E., Hammouri, Q., & Errico, T. (2013). A systematic review of comparative studies on bone graft alternatives for common spine fusion procedures. *European Spine Journal, 22*(6), 1423–1435.

4. Fu, R., Selph, S., McDonagh, M., Peterson, K., Tiwari, A., Chou, R., et al. (2013). Effectiveness and harms of recombinant human bone morphogenetic protein-2 in spine fusion: A systematic review and meta-analysis. *Annals of Internal Medicine, 158*(12), 890–902.
5. Gao, R., Street, M., Tay, M. L., Callon, K. E., Naot, D., Lock, A., et al. (2018). Human spinal bone dust as a potential local autograft. *Spine, 43*(4), 193–199.
6. Hustedt, J. W., & Blizzard, D. J. (2014). The controversy surrounding bone morphogenetic proteins in the spine: A review of current research. *Yale Journal of Biology and Medicine, 87*(4), 549–561.
7. Kadam, A., Millhouse, P. W., Kepler, C. K., Radcliff, K. E., Fehlings, M. G., Janssen, M. E., et al. (2016). Bone substitutes and expanders in spine surgery: A review of their fusion efficacies. *International Journal of Spine Surgery, 10,* 33.
8. Simmonds, M. C., Brown, J. V., Heirs, M. K., Higgins, J. P., Mannion, R. J., Rodgers, M. A., et al. (2013). Safety and effectiveness of recombinant human bone morphogenetic protein-2 for spinal fusion: A meta-analysis of individual-participant data. *Annals of Internal Medicine, 158*(12), 877–889.
9. Tuchman, A., Brodke, D. S., Youssef, J. A., Meisel, H. J., Dettori, J. R., Park, J. B., et al. (2016). Iliac crest bone graft versus local autograft or allograft for lumbar spinal fusion: Systematic review. *Global Spine Journal, 6*(6), 592–606.
10. Winter, H. A., Kraak, J., Oosterhuis, J. W., & de Kleuver, M. (2013). Spinal reconstruction with free vascularized bone grafts; Approaches and selection of acceptor vessels. *Scandinavian Journal of Surgery, 102*(1), 42–48.
11. Zachos, T. A., Piuzzi, N. S., Mroz, T., et al. (2018). Principles of bone fusion. In S. R. Garfin, F. J. Eismont, & G. R. Bell (Eds.), *Rothman-Simeone the Spine* (7th ed., pp. 1085–1122). Philadelphia, PA: Elsevier.

CHAPTER 26

SURGICAL APPROACHES TO THE OCCIPUT AND CERVICAL SPINE

Kern Singh, BS, MD, Justin Munns, MD, Daniel K. Park, MD, and Alexander R. Vaccaro, MD, PhD

1. **What are the most common surgical approaches to the occiput and cervical spine?**
   A. **Posterior**
      * Midline
   B. **Anterior**
      * Transoral approach
      * Extra/lateral/retropharyngeal approaches
      * Anterolateral (Smith-Robinson) approach

POSTERIOR SURGICAL APPROACHES

2. **What are the major palpable posterior anatomic landmarks and their corresponding anatomic levels?**
   * *Posterior occipital prominence:* Inion (external occipital protuberance)
   * *First palpable spinous process:* C2 spinous process
   * *Most prominent spinous process at cervicothoracic junction:* Vertebra prominens (C7)

3. **Describe the posterior exposure of the occiput and upper cervical spine.**
   The patient is placed into a reverse Trendelenburg position with a midline incision made from the external occipital protuberance to the spinous process of C2. The C2 vertebra (axis) has a large lamina and bifid spinous process that provides attachments for the rectus major and inferior oblique muscles. The bony topography between the lamina and the lateral mass of the axis is indistinct. Surgical dissection on the occiput and the ring of the atlas should be done in a careful manner. It is advisable to use gentle muscle retraction and Bovie (monopolar and bipolar) cauterization rather than any forceful subperiosteal stripping.

4. **What is the significance of the ligamentum nuchae?**
   The ligamentum nuchae (Fig. 26.1) represents the midline fascial confluence. Dissection should be carried through this ligament to decrease blood loss and to maintain a stout tissue layer for closure.

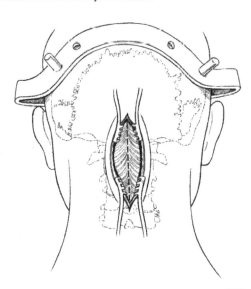

Fig. 26.1 Ligamentum nuchae. (From Winter RB, Lonstein JE, Denis F, Smith MD. Posterior upper cervical procedures. In: Atlas of Spinal Surgery. Philadelphia, PA: Saunders; 1995, p. 21.)

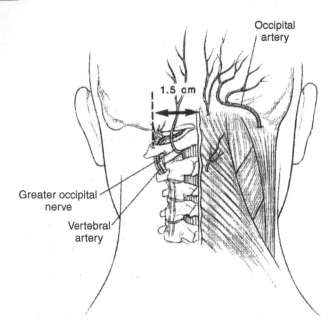

Fig. 26.2 Vertebral artery. (From Winter RB, Lonstein JE, Denis F, Smith MD. Posterior upper cervical procedures. In: Atlas of Spinal Surgery. Philadelphia, PA: Saunders; 1995, p. 23.)

5. **What structure is at risk with lateral dissection of the atlas?**
   The vertebral artery lies lateral to the ring of the atlas (Fig. 26.2); therefore, the dissection should not be carried more than 1.5 cm lateral to the posterior midline and 8–10 mm laterally along the superior C1 border to avoid injury to the vertebral artery. Once the greater occipital nerve is encountered and the fragile venae comitantes of the paravertebral venous plexus are exposed, further lateral dissection endangers the vertebral artery. If bleeding is encountered from disruption of the venous plexus between C1 and C2, packing and hemostatic agents are usually adequate to control bleeding. If vertebral artery injury occurs, direct repair, manual pressure, endovascular treatment, and ligation are options for control of hemorrhage.

6. **Describe the course of the vertebral artery in the cervical spine.**
   The vertebral artery arises from the subclavian artery. It enters the transverse foramen at C6 in 95% of people and courses upward through the foramina above. At C1, the vertebral artery exits from the foramen, courses medially on the superior groove of the posterior ring of the atlas, and enters the foramen magnum to unite with the opposite vertebral artery to form the basilar artery.

7. **Where is the vertebral artery injured most frequently in upper cervical spine exposures?**
   The vertebral artery is injured most frequently just lateral to the C1–C2 facet articulation and at the superior lateral aspect of the arch of C1.

8. **Why is the patient placed in a reverse Trendelenburg position?**
   The reverse Trendelenburg position allows venous drainage away from the surgical field and toward the heart, which decreases bleeding during the procedure.

9. **Describe the posterior exposure of the lower cervical spine.**
   The midline posterior exposure is the most common approach used in the cervical spine. Care is taken to carry dissection through the ligamentum nuchae to minimize blood loss. Once the tips of the spinous processes are identified at the appropriate levels through radiographic confirmation, subperiosteal dissection of the posterior elements is then carried out. The posterior approach is extensile and is easily extended proximally to the occiput and distally to the thoracic spinal region.

10. **What functional consequences may arise from lateral dissection of the paraspinal muscles?**
    Lateral dissection carries the potential risk of denervation of the paraspinal musculature. Inadequate approximation of the posterior cervical musculature may lead to a fish gill appearance of the posterior paraspinal muscles and possible loss of the normal cervical lordosis.

11. Why is it important to expose only the levels to be fused, especially in children?

A process termed *creeping fusion extension* may occur when unwanted spinal levels are exposed during the fusion procedure. This is especially common in children and may lead to unintended fusion at these spinal levels.

12. What complications are associated with the posterior approach to the cervical spine?

Complications include postlaminectomy kyphosis due to muscular denervation or following decompression, radiculopathy, epidural hematoma, and loss of neck range of motion. Postoperative paralysis and paresis, particularly of the C5 nerve root, are also associated with a posterior cervical laminectomy or laminoplasty.

ANTERIOR SURGICAL APPROACHES

13. What are the indications for a transoral approach to the upper cervical spine and craniocervical junction?

Pathology at the craniocervical junction (CCJ) with an anterior midline component (e.g., tumor), which is not amenable to decompression by a posterior approach. A transoral approach allows direct access to CCJ from mid-clivus to the superior aspect of C3.

14. During the transoral approach to the odontoid, what is the key palpable landmark used to determine exposure location?

The anterior tubercle of the atlas. The vertebral artery lies a minimum of 2 cm from this anatomic landmark within the foramen transversarium.

15. Describe the transoral exposure to the upper cervical spine.

Transoral retractors are inserted to expose the posterior oropharynx (Fig. 26.3). A soft rubber catheter is placed through the nostril and looped about the uvula to facilitate its cephalad retraction. The area of the incision is infiltrated with 1:200,000 epinephrine. A midline 3-cm vertical incision centered on the anterior tubercle of the atlas is made through the pharyngeal mucosa and muscle. The anterior longitudinal ligament and tubercle of the atlas are exposed subperiosteally, and the longus colli muscles are mobilized laterally. A high-speed burr may be used to remove the anterior arch of the atlas to expose the odontoid process (Fig. 26.4).

16. What preoperative patient care factors must be addressed before undergoing a transoral decompression?

All oropharyngeal or dental infections must be treated before elective surgery because wound infection rates are high with this approach. The oral cavity is cleansed with chlorhexidine before surgery, and perioperative antibiotics are given for 48–72 hours after surgery (often cephalosporin and metronidazole).

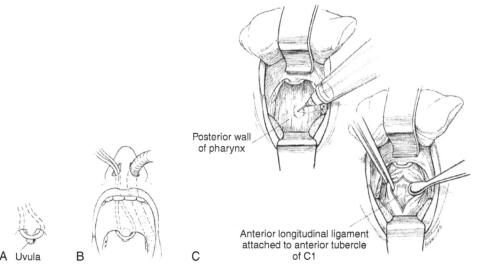

Posterior wall of pharynx

Anterior longitudinal ligament attached to anterior tubercle of C1

A   Uvula   B   C

Fig. 26.3 Transoral exposure. (A) A soft rubber catheter is used to retract the uvula. (B) Nasotracheal intubation is performed. (C) A specialized self-retaining retractor system is assembled to facilitate a midline vertical incision in the posterior wall of the pharynx centered on the anterior tubercle of the atlas. (From Winter RB, Lonstein JE, Denis F, Smith MD. Anterior upper cervical procedures. In: Atlas of Spinal Surgery. Philadelphia, PA: Saunders; 1995, p. 3.)

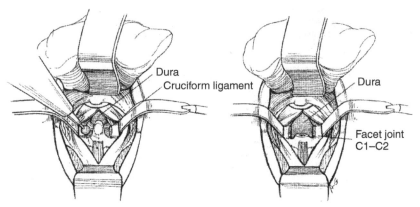

Fig. 26.4 Removal of C1 arch. (From Winter RB, Lonstein JE, Denis F, Smith MD. Anterior upper cervical procedures. In: Atlas of Spinal Surgery. Philadelphia, PA: Saunders; 1995, p. 5.)

17. **Describe the incision and superficial dissection for the retropharyngeal approach to the upper cervical spine.**
A skin incision is made along the anterior aspect of the sternocleidomastoid muscle and is curved toward the mastoid process. The platysma and the superficial layer of the deep cervical fascia are divided in the line of the incision to expose the anterior border of the sternocleidomastoid. The submandibular gland and the posterior belly of the digastric muscle are identified. The posterior belly of the digastric muscle runs obliquely across the surgical field towards the hyoid bone and separates the submandibular triangle from the carotid triangle (Figs. 26.5 and 26.6).

18. **What two vessels are ligated once the sternocleidomastoid is retracted?**
The superior thyroid artery and the lingual vessels.

19. **What nerve may be potentially injured in this approach, resulting in a painful neuroma?**
The marginal branch of the facial nerve.

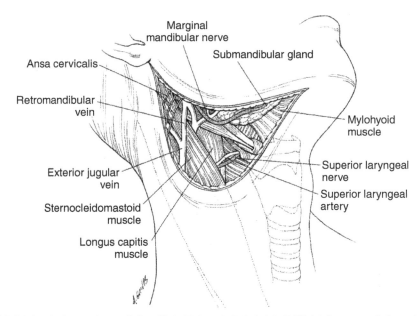

Fig. 26.5 Anterior retropharyngeal approach. (From Winter RB, Lonstein JE, Denis F, Smith MD. Anterior upper cervical procedures. In: Atlas of Spinal Surgery. Philadelphia, PA: Saunders; 1995, p. 10.)

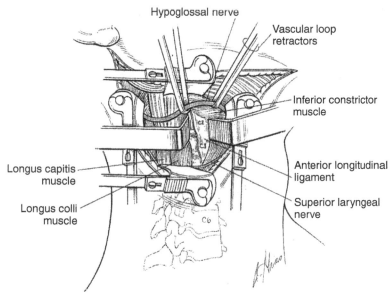

Fig. 26.6 Anterior retropharyngeal approach–deep dissection. (From Winter RB, Lonstein JE, Denis F, Smith MD. Anterior upper cervical procedures. In: Atlas of Spinal Surgery. Philadelphia, PA: Saunders; 1995, p. 11.)

20. What is the importance of the facial artery as an anatomic landmark?
   The facial artery helps to identify the location of the hypoglossal nerve, which lies adjacent to the digastric muscle.

21. Stripping of what muscle helps to identify the anterior aspect of the upper cervical spine and basiocciput?
   The longus colli.

22. Describe the functional consequence of excessive retraction on the superior laryngeal nerve.
   Excessive retraction may lead to hoarseness, inability to sing high notes, and aspiration.

23. Name the palpable anatomic landmarks used to identify the level of exposure of the lower cervical spine.
   The angle of the mandible (C2–C3), the hyoid bone (C3), upper aspect of thyroid cartilage (C4–C5), cricoid membrane (C5–C6), carotid tubercle (C6), and the cricoid cartilage (C6).

24. Describe the anterior lateral or Smith-Robinson approach to the lower or subaxial cervical spine.
   A transverse incision is made over the interspace of interest in Langer's lines to improve the cosmetic appearance of the surgical scar. The incision is carried slightly laterally beyond the anterior border of the sternocleidomastoid muscle and almost to the midline of the neck. The subcutaneous tissue is divided in line with the skin incision. The platysma may be divided along the line of the incision, or its fibers may be bluntly dissected and its medial-lateral divisions retracted (Fig. 26.7). The anterior border of the sternocleidomastoid is identified, and the fascia anterior to this muscle is incised. The sternocleidomastoid is retracted laterally and the strap muscles are retracted medially to permit incision of the pretracheal fascia medial to the carotid sheath. The sternocleidomastoid and carotid sheath are retracted laterally, and the strap muscles and visceral structures (trachea, larynx, esophagus, and thyroid) are retracted medially. The anterior aspect of the spine, including the paired longus colli muscles, are now visualized.

25. What is the function of the platysma muscle and its corresponding innervation?
   The platysma is an embryologic remnant serving no functional importance. It receives its innervation from the seventh cranial nerve.

26. Once the platysma and the superficial cervical fascia are divided, what neurovascular structure is at risk for injury?
   The carotid sheath. It contains three neurovascular structures: internal jugular vein, carotid artery, and vagus nerve.

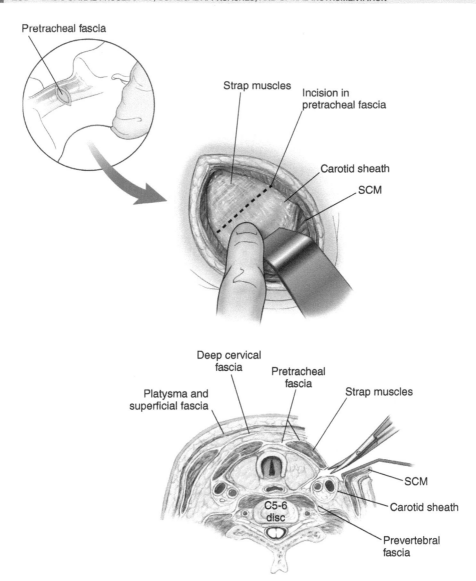

Fig. 26.7 Exposure of the lower anterior cervical spine. Incise the skin, subcutaneous tissue and platysma muscle. Identify the sterno-cleidomastoid *(SCM)* muscle and develop the interval between the SCM and strap muscles. Palpate the pulse of the carotid artery within the carotid sheath and divide the pretracheal fascia medial to the carotid sheath. Blunt dissection and retraction will permit visualization of the anterior aspect of the cervical spine. (From Shen FH. Spine. In: Miller MD, Chhabra BA, Brown JA, et al., editors. Orthopedic Surgical Approaches. 2nd ed. Philadelphia, PA: Saunders; 2015, pp. 161–266, Fig. 5.26.)

27. **What structures are at risk when dissecting through the pretracheal fascia of the neck?**
    The superior and inferior thyroid arteries may be injured during dissection through the pretracheal fascial layer.
    Dissection is normally done in a longitudinal manner, using digital dissection.

28. **What fascial layer is encountered after dissection through the pretracheal fascia?**
    After dissection through the pretracheal fascia, the prevertebral fascia or retropharyngeal space is encountered.
    The prevertebral fascia is split longitudinally, exposing the anterior longitudinal ligament. The longus colli muscle
    is elevated bilaterally and retracted laterally until the anterior surface of the vertebral body is exposed.

29. **What structures are at risk when the dissection is carried too far laterally on the vertebral body in the subaxial spine?**
Dissection carried too far laterally may risk injury to the vertebral artery traversing through the foramen transversarium or damage the sympathetic plexus.

30. **What are the advantages and disadvantages of approaching the cervical spine anteriorly from the right or left side?**
Smith and Robinson advocated using the left-sided approach to decrease the risk of damaging the recurrent laryngeal nerve. On the right side, this nerve loops beneath the right subclavian artery and then travels in a relatively horizontal course in the neck, increasing its chances of damage with exposure in this region. However, most right-handed surgeons find the right-sided approach more facile because the mandible is not an obstruction. A right-sided exposure avoids damage to the thoracic duct. Also, the cervical esophagus is retracted less due to its normal anterior position on the left side of the neck. Overall, either side can be used for the anterior approach because evidence does not suggest one side to be safer than the other.

31. **Name the potential causes of dysphagia after anterior cervical surgery.**
Dysphagia may be secondary to postoperative edema, hemorrhage, denervation (recurrent laryngeal nerve), or infection. If persistent dysphagia is present, a barium swallow or endoscopy should be considered.

32. **Damage to the sympathetic chain may result in what clinical condition?**
Horner syndrome, which is manifested by a lack of sympathetic response resulting in anhydrosis, ptosis, miosis, and enophthalmos. The cervical sympathetic chain lies on the anterior surface of the longus colli muscles posterior to the carotid sheath. Subperiosteal dissection is important to prevent damage to these nerves. Horner syndrome is usually temporary; permanent sequelae occur in less than 1% of cases.

33. **Describe the rare but serious complication of esophageal perforation.**
Patients usually manifest symptoms in the postoperative period related to development of an abscess, tracheoesophageal fistula, or mediastinitis. The usual treatment consists of intravenous antibiotics, nasogastric feeding, drainage, debridement, and repair.

KEY POINTS

1. The transoral approach to the craniocervical junction is indicated for fixed deformity causing anterior midline neural compression.
2. The posterior midline cervical approach is extensile and provides access from the occiput to the thoracic region.
3. A key to the anterior approach to the subaxial cervical spine is understanding the anatomy of the fascial layers of the neck.

Websites
1. Approaches to the spinal column: http://medind.nic.in/jae/t02/i1/jaet02i1p76.pdf
2. Endoscopic endonasal approach for craniovertebral junction pathology: https://consultqd.clevelandclinic.org/endoscopic-endonasal-surgery-for-craniovertebral-junction-pathology/

BIBLIOGRAPHY
1. An, H. (1998). Surgical exposures and fusion techniques of the spine. In H. An (Ed.), *Principles and Techniques of Spine Surgery* (pp. 31–62). Baltimore: Williams & Wilkins.
2. Ghobrial, G. M., Mukherjee, D., Baron, E. M., Choi, D., Harrop, J. S., Johnson, J. P., et al. (2018). Anterior odontoid resection: The transoral approach. In E. Baron & C. Vaccaro (Eds.), *Operative Techniques: Spine Surgery* (3rd ed., pp. 16–26). Philadelphia, PA: Elsevier.
3. Liu, J. K., Apfelbaum, R. I., & Schmidt, M. H. (2005). Anterior surgical anatomy and approaches to the cervical spine. In D. Kim, A. Vaccaro, & R, Fessler (Eds.), *Spinal Instrumentation: Surgical Techniques* (pp. 59–69). New York, NY: Thieme.
4. McAfee, P. C., Bohlman, H. H., Riley, L. H., Robinson, R. A., Southwick, W. O., & Nachlas, N. E. (1987). The anterior retropharyngeal approach to the upper part of the cervical spine. *Journal of Bone and Joint Surgery, 69*(9), 1371–1383.
5. Misra, S. (2005). Posterior cervical anatomy and surgical approaches. In D. Kim, A. Vaccaro, R. Fessler (Eds.), *Spinal Instrumentation: Surgical Techniques* (pp. 267–274). New York: Thieme.
6. Winter, R. B., Lonstein, J. W., Denis, F., & Smith, M. D. (1995). *Atlas of Spinal Surgery* (pp. 1–104). Philadelphia, PA: Saunders.

CHAPTER 27

SURGICAL APPROACHES TO THE THORACIC, LUMBAR, AND LUMBOSACRAL SPINE

Vincent J. Devlin, MD and Mohammad E. Majd, MD

1. **What are the various posterior surgical approaches to the thoracic and lumbar spine?**
   A. Thoracic
      - Midline posterior thoracic approach
      - Posterolateral thoracic approaches
         - Transpedicular
         - Costotransversectomy
         - Lateral extracavitary
   B. Lumbar
      - Midline posterior lumbar approach
      - Paraspinal lumbar approach
   C. Specific surgical approaches for lumbar interbody fusion
      - Posterior lumbar interbody approach
      - Transforaminal lumbar interbody approach

2. **What are some advantages and disadvantages of posterior approaches to access the thoracic and lumbar spine?**
   Posterior surgical approaches are the most common surgical approaches used by spine surgeons due to their extensile nature, which enables surgical exposure from T1 to the sacrum and ilium. Advantages of posterior surgical approaches include direct visualization of posterior spinal structures including spinous processes, laminae, pars interarticularis, facet joints, and transverse processes, as well as the ability to simultaneously access anterior spinal column structures through a single surgical incision. Disadvantages of a posterior approach include muscle injury, blood loss, and surgical site pain.

3. **Describe the options for patient positioning when posterior surgical approaches to the thoracic and lumbar spinal regions are performed.**
   Patients are positioned prone on a radiolucent operative frame or spine-specific surgery table for posterior approaches to the thoracic and lumbar spine. An exception is the use of a lateral decubitus position during simultaneous anterior and posterior surgical procedures. When surgery includes spinal instrumentation and fusion of the lumbar region, patients are positioned with the hips and thighs in an extended position to preserve and enhance lumbar lordosis. During posterior lumbar spinal decompression procedures, reduction of lumbar lordosis by positioning the hips in a flexed position may be used to facilitate access to the lumbar spinal canal by increasing the distance between the spinous processes and lamina. However, as patients with lumbar spinal stenosis are most symptomatic in an extended posture, the patient's position on the operating table is a factor to consider when determining the extent of lumbar neural decompression.

4. **Outline the key steps involved in a midline posterior exposure of the thoracic and/or lumbar spine.**
   - Incise the skin and subcutaneous tissues with a scalpel
   - Place Weitlander and cerebellar retractors to tamponade superficial bleeding by exerting tension on surrounding tissues.
   - Electrocautery dissection is carried out down to the level of the spinous processes.
   - Cobb elevators and electrocautery are used to elevate the paraspinous muscles from the lamina at the level(s) requiring exposure.
   - Dissection is continued laterally to expose the pars interarticularis and medial aspect of the facet joints without disrupting the facet joint capsules. This provides sufficient exposure for discectomy and laminectomy procedures.
   - If an intertransverse fusion is planned, Cobb elevators and electrocautery are used to elevate the paraspinous muscles lateral to the facet joints to expose the transverse processes on each side for decortication

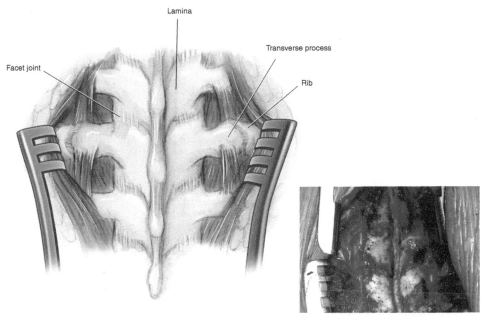

Fig. 27.1 Subperiosteal exposure of the posterior thoracic spine. (From Shen FH. Spine. In: Miller M, Chhabra BA, Browne B, et al., editors. Orthopaedic Surgical Exposures. 2nd ed. Philadelphia, PA: Saunders; 2015, Fig. 5-91, p. 238.)

and grafting. The facet joints are excised and prepared for fusion. Care is taken to preserve the soft tissue structures (interspinous ligaments, supraspinous ligaments, and facet capsules) at the transition between fused and nonfused levels.
- Hemostasis is maintained by coagulating bleeding points with electrocautery and packing with surgical sponges (Figs. 27.1 and 27.2).

5. **Where are blood vessels encountered during a posterior surgical exposure of the thoracic and lumbar spinal regions?**
   The arterial blood supply of the posterior thoracic and lumbar spine is consistent at each spinal level (Fig. 27.3). Arteries are encountered at the lateral border of the pars Interarticularis, upper medial border of the transverse process, and intertransverse region. Sacral arteries exit from the dorsal sacral foramen. The superior gluteal artery enters the gluteal musculature and may be encountered during iliac crest bone grafting.

6. **What methods are used by the surgeon as a guide to exposure of the correct anatomic levels during a posterior approach to the thoracic or lumbar spine?**
   A combination of methods is used to guide exposure of correct anatomic levels:
   - **Preoperative radiographs** are reviewed to determine bony landmarks and presence of anatomic variants that may affect numbering of spinal levels (i.e., altered number of rib-bearing thoracic vertebrae, lumbarized or sacralized vertebrae) to plan for surgery.
   - **Intraoperative osseous landmarks** are referenced: C7 (vertebra prominens), T8 (inferomedial angle of the scapula), T12 (most distal palpable rib), L4–L5 (superior lateral edge of ilium).
   - An **intraoperative radiograph** with a metallic marker at the level of exposure is obtained to confirm exposure of the appropriate spinal level. A permanent copy should be made to document the correct level of exposure for every procedure.

7. **What are some examples of spinal pathologies that are appropriately treated using a thoracic laminectomy approach?**
   Spinal pathologies that involve the posterior osseous structures or the posterior aspect of the spinal cord are appropriate for treatment using a laminectomy approach. Examples include thoracic spinal stenosis secondary to ligamentum flavum hypertrophy or tumors involving the dorsal aspect of the spinal cord. An isolated laminectomy approach is not indicated for treatment of spinal pathologies anterior or lateral to the thoracic spinal cord due to risks of neurologic injury and spinal destabilization (Fig. 27.4).

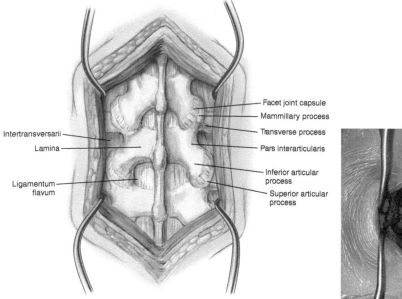

Fig. 27.2 Posterior midline approach to the lumbar spine. (From Shen FH. Spine. In: Miller M, Chhabra BA, Browne B, et al., editors. Orthopaedic Surgical Exposures. 2nd ed. Philadelphia, PA: Saunders; 2015, Fig. 5.106A, p. 251.)

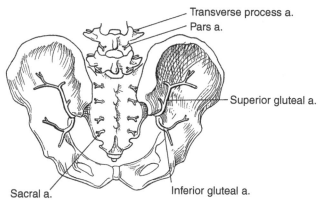

Fig. 27.3 Blood vessels encountered during posterior midline approach. (From Wiesel SW, Weinstein JN, Herkowitz H, et al., editors. The Lumbar Spine. 2nd ed. Philadelphia, PA: Saunders; 1996.)

8. **What is a thoracic transpedicular approach and when is this surgical approach used?**
   After the spine is exposed by a posterior midline approach, the thoracic pedicle can be used as a pathway to access anterior spinal column pathology. This approach is an option for excision of noncalcified disc herniations located lateral to the spinal cord. The facet joint at the level and side of the disc herniation is resected. The superior aspect of the pedicle below the herniation is removed with a motorized burr. Sufficient working room is created for the removal of disc material. Limited visualization of the anterior aspect of the spinal cord is provided by this approach. A transpedicular approach is also useful for obtaining a vertebral body biopsy (see Fig. 27.4).

9. **How is the location of the thoracic and lumbar pedicles identified from the posterior midline approach?**
   A rongeur or power burr is used to remove the outer bony cortex and expose the entry site to the pedicle. The entry point for **thoracic pedicle** is located lateral to the midpoint of the superior articular process. The exact location

Laminectomy

Transpedicular

Costotransversectomy

Lateral extracavitary

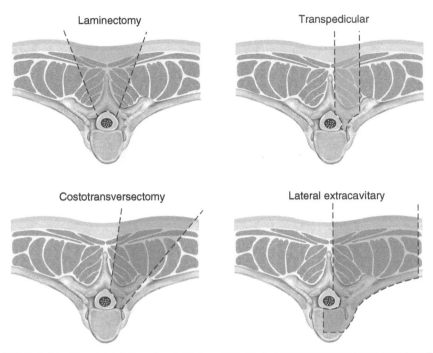

Fig. 27.4 Posterolateral thoracic spinal approaches: laminectomy, transpedicular, costotransversectomy, lateral extracavitary. (From Pacione D, Wilson T, Perin N, et al. Posterolateral approaches to the cervicothoracic junction: Transpedicular, costotransversectomy, lateral extracavitary, and parascapular extrapleural approaches. In: Kim DH, Vaccaro AR, Dickman CA, et al., editors. Surgical Anatomy and Techniques to the Spine. 2nd ed. Philadelphia, PA: Saunders; 2013, pp. 254–266, Fig. 27-10.)

of the pedicle at each thoracic level varies slightly in relation to the transverse process and the lateral border of the pars interarticularis. At the upper and lower extent of the thoracic spine (T1, T2, and T12), the entrance to the pedicle aligns with the midline of the transverse process. In the midthoracic spine (T7, T8, and T9), the entrance to the pedicle overlies the upper margin of the transverse process.

The **lumbar pedicle** is located at the intersection of two lines. The vertical line passes along the lateral aspect of the superior articular process and passes lateral to the pars interarticularis. The horizontal line passes through the middle of the transverse process, where it joins the superior articular process.

10. **What is a thoracic costotransversectomy approach and which procedures are performed using this surgical approach?**
    A costotransversectomy approach is a posterolateral approach to the thoracic spine originally developed for drainage of tuberculous abscesses. It provides unilateral access to the posterior spinal elements, lateral aspect of the vertebral body, and limited access to the anterior aspect of the spinal canal without the need to enter the thoracic cavity (see Fig. 27.4). This surgical approach includes resection of the posteromedial portion of the rib and transverse process. The nerve root may be sacrificed proximal to the dorsal root ganglion to facilitate exposure. When extensive vertebral body resection is required, this approach can be performed bilaterally or combined with a transpedicular approach and posterior spinal instrumentation. The costotransversectomy approach can be used for excision of lateral and paracentral thoracic disc herniations and for placement of an anterior column bone graft or fusion cage. A chest tube may be required with this approach if the pleural cavity is inadvertently entered.

11. **What is a lateral extracavitary approach?**
    A lateral extracavitary approach is a posterolateral extrapleural approach to the thoracic spine and thoracolumbar junction (see Fig. 27.4). It provides greater exposure of the anterior spinal column and anterior aspect of the spinal canal than is achieved with a costotransversectomy. This approach involves removal of portions of the rib, costotransverse joint, facet, and pedicle at the operative level. The exposure achieved is sufficient to permit the excision of central disc herniations, corpectomy, and placement of an anterior strut graft or fusion cage. This approach is generally performed in combination with posterior spinal instrumentation and fusion as it creates significant spinal instability. When this approach is used above T4, mobilization of the scapula improves visualization of the vertebral body.

12. Describe the posterior paraspinal approach to the lumbar spine.

The paraspinal (Wiltse) approach is a posterolateral approach to the lumbar region (Fig. 27.5). This surgical approach utilizes the interval between the multifidus and longissimus muscles. The lumbodorsal fascia is incised two fingerbreadths lateral to the midline. Blunt dissection or tubular dilators are used to expose the facet joint and interlaminar space. This approach provides direct access for the removal of disc herniations and decompression of spinal stenosis located in the extraforaminal zone without the need to resect the pars interarticularis or facet complex. This approach can also be used for placement of pedicle screw instrumentation and for performing lumbar intertransverse fusions. Unilateral resection of the facet complex provides a surgical corridor for direct access to the intervertebral disc for interbody fusion.

13. What is a PLIF approach?

Posterior lumbar interbody fusion (PLIF) refers to a surgical fusion performed by placing structural bone grafts or intervertebral body fusion devices into a lumbar disc space from a midline posterior surgical approach. Retraction of the dural sac and nerve roots are required to prepare the disc space and insert the interbody devices. Procedural steps include laminectomy, bilateral facetectomy, discectomy, restoration of disc space height, and decortication of the vertebral endplates. One interbody device is generally placed on each side of the disc space, and posterior pedicle instrumentation is used to stabilize the spinal segment (Fig. 27.6).

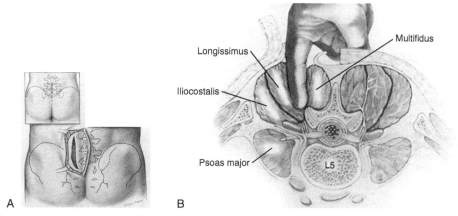

Fig. 27.5 Lumbar paraspinal approach. (From Zindrick MR, Selby D. Lumbar spine fusion: Different types and indications. In: Wiesel SW, Weinstein JN, Herkowitz H, et al., editors. The Lumbar Spine, vol. 2. 2nd ed. Philadelphia, PA: Saunders; 1996, p. 609.)

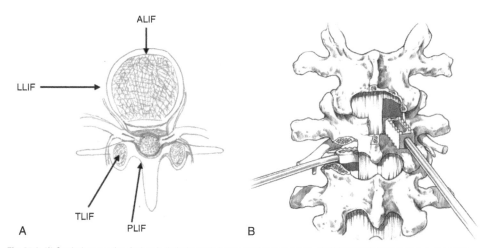

Fig. 27.6 (A) Surgical approaches for interbody fusion: anterior lumbar interbody fusion *(ALIF)*, lateral lumbar interbody fusion *(LLIF)*, transforaminal lumbar interbody fusion *(TLIF)*, and posterior lumbar interbody fusion *(PLIF)*. (B) Placement of an intervertebral body fusion device from a posterior surgical approach with PLIF *(above, right)* versus TLIF *(below, left)*. (From Talia AJ, Wong ML, Lau HC et al. Comparison of different surgical approaches for lumbar interbody fusion. J Clin Neurosci 2015;22:243–251, Fig. 1, p. 244.)

14. What is a TLIF approach?

Transforaminal lumbar interbody fusion (TLIF) refers to placement of structural bone graft(s) or intervertebral body fusion device(s) into a lumbar disc space through a unilateral posterolateral approach (see Fig. 27.6). Unilateral removal of the pars interarticularis and facet complex provides direct posterolateral access to the disc space. This technique does not require significant retraction of the dural sac and preserves the contralateral facet complex. The working space provided by TLIF is sufficient to permit placement of two interbody fusion devices or a single large device through a unilateral approach. Posterior pedicle instrumentation is used to stabilize the operated spine segment. As TLIFs do not require retraction of the thecal sac, TLIFs can be performed safely at the level of the conus medullaris (above L2) and at thoracic spinal cord levels. TLIFs may also be performed bilaterally.

15. What are the various surgical approaches used to provide access to the anterior and lateral aspect of the thoracic spine and thoracolumbar junction?

A. T1–T3 spinal levels
- Low anterior cervical approach
- Median sternotomy
- Transmanubrial approach with or without medial claviculotomy
- Third-rib thoracotomy

B. T4–T12 spinal levels
- Lateral thoracotomy

C. T10–L2 spinal levels
- Transdiaphragmatic thoracolumbar approach

16. What are the indications for the use of an anterior or lateral surgical approach to access the thoracic or lumbar spine?
- Interbody fusion
- Corpectomy for treatment of a tumor, infection, or vertebral body fracture
- Correction of spinal deformity with anterior spinal instrumentation
- Treatment of failed posterior spinal fusions (posterior pseudarthrosis)
- To mobilize a rigid spinal deformity and enhance deformity correction
- To restore anterior column load sharing
- To restore sagittal alignment of the spine
- To eliminate asymmetric spinal growth potential (e.g., in pediatric patients with congenital scoliosis)
- To remove failed or migrated anterior spinal implants

17. List clinical scenarios where an anterior thoracic or lumbar surgical approach may not be advisable.
- Patients who have undergone prior anterior surgery to the same spinal region. Dissection will be difficult because of adhesions and will increase the risk of visceral or vascular injury.
- Patients with compromised pulmonary function who have an unacceptable risk of medical complications associated with an anterior thoracic approach.
- Patients with extensive calcification of the aorta are not ideal candidates for anterior lumbar approaches as extensive mobilization of the great vessels is required and is associated with an increased risk of vascular complications.

18. What anterior surgical approaches may be used to expose the upper thoracic spine (T1–T3)?

Access to the T1 vertebral body is generally possible through a standard anterior cervical approach medial to the sternocleidomastoid muscle. Anterior exposure between T1 and T3 is more challenging. Options for exposure include a transmanubrial approach with or without medial claviculotomy, median sternotomy, or a third-rib thoracotomy. Each approach has advantages and disadvantages, depending on patient anatomy, type of spinal pathology present, number of levels requiring exposure, and type of surgery required.

19. What standard surgical approach is used to expose the anterior and lateral aspect of the thoracic spine between T4 and T12?

The anterior and lateral aspect of the thoracic spine between T4 and T12 is approached by a lateral thoracotomy.

20. What is the preferred method of positioning a patient for a lateral thoracotomy to provide exposure of the thoracic spine?

The lateral decubitus position with an axillary roll under the down-side axilla (Fig. 27.7). Many surgeons prefer approaching the thoracic spine from the left side because it is easier to dissect around the aorta than the vena cava. However, the type of spinal pathology may dictate the side of approach. For example, in the anterior treatment of scoliosis, the surgical approach should be on the convex side of the curve.

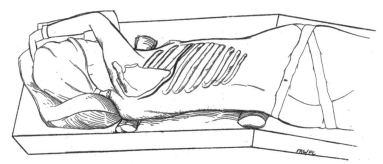

Fig. 27.7 Positioning of the patient for a lateral thoracotomy approach to the thoracic spine. (From Majd ME, Harkess JW, Holt RT et al. Anterior approach to the spine. In: Margulies JY, Aebi M, Farcy JP, editors. Revision Spine Surgery. St. Louis: Mosby; 1999, p. 139.)

21. **What factors determine the level of rib excision when the thoracic spine is exposed through a lateral thoracotomy approach?**

    If the procedure requires exposure of a long segment of the thoracic spine (e.g., for treatment of scoliosis or kyphosis), a rib at the proximal end of the region requiring fusion is removed. For example, removal of the fifth rib allows exposure from T5 to T12.

    If the patient requires treatment of a single vertebral body lesion, the rib two levels proximal to the involved vertebral body is removed. Alternatively, the rib directly horizontal to the target vertebral level at the midaxillary line on the anteroposterior (AP) thoracic spine x-ray is removed.

    If the surgeon requires only a limited exposure (e.g., to excise a thoracic disc herniation), the rib that leads to the disc should be removed (e.g., the eighth rib is removed for a T7–T8 disc herniation).

22. **What are some tips for counting ribs after the chest cavity has been entered during a thoracotomy?**

    The first cephalad palpable rib is the second rib. The first rib is generally located within the space occupied by the second rib and cannot be easily palpated. The distance between the second and third rib is wider than the distance between the other ribs. Application of a marker on a rib with subsequent radiographic verification is one method to identify the level of exposure. It is essential to confirm that the correct spinal level(s) are exposed using fluoroscopy or radiographs prior to initiating discectomy or corpectomy.

23. **During an anterior exposure of the thoracic spine, the parietal pleura is divided longitudinally over the length of the exposed vertebral bodies. What landmarks may be used for identification of critical anatomic structures?**

    The vertebral bodies are located in the depressions, and the discs are located over the prominences (Fig. 27.8). The segmental vessels are identified as they cross the vertebral bodies (depressions). This has been referred to as the *hills-and-valleys concept* (i.e., discs are the hills and vertebral bodies are the valleys).

24. **Are there any risks associated with ligation of the segmental artery and vein as they cross the vertebral bodies?**

    Ligation of the segmental vessels is required to obtain comprehensive exposure of the vertebral body. Unilateral vessel ligation is usually safe. However, ligation too close to the neural foramina risks damage to the segmental feeder vessels to the spinal cord. Temporary and reversible occlusion of segmental vessels may be performed when the risk of paraplegia is high (congenital kyphoscoliosis, severe kyphosis, patients who have undergone prior anterior spinal surgery with vessel ligation). If there is no change in spinal potential monitoring after temporary vessel occlusion, permanent ligation may be carried out safely.

25. **After a standard transpleural thoracotomy for spinal access, placement of a chest tube is necessary. What are the proper placement criteria?**

    The chest tube should be placed at the anterior midaxillary line at least two interspaces from the incision. Placement of the chest tube too posteriorly has the potential for kinking and can cause subsequent blockage of drainage in the supine position. In addition, posterior placement is uncomfortable and painful when the patient lies supine.

26. **What modification of the standard thoracotomy approach allows spinal exposure without the need for use of a chest tube postoperatively?**

    Use of an extrapleural thoracotomy approach can obviate the need to place a chest tube if the pleural cavity is not inadvertently entered during the procedure. After rib excision using this surgical approach, the parietal pleura is

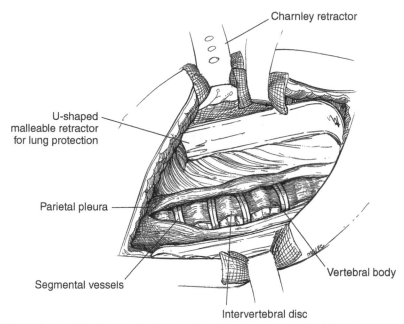

Charnley retractor

U-shaped
malleable retractor
for lung protection

Parietal pleura

Vertebral body

Segmental vessels

Intervertebral disc

Fig. 27.8 Intraoperative view of the anterior and lateral aspect of the vertebral bodies through a lateral thoracotomy approach. (From Majd ME, Harkess JW, Holt RT, et al. Anterior approach to the spine. In: Margulies JY, Aebi M, Farcy JP, editors. Revision Spine Surgery. St. Louis: Mosby; 1999, p.142.)

dissected off the undersurface of the endothoracic fascia and mobilized over the lateral aspect of the vertebral body to the extent required.

27. During a thoracic spinal exposure via thoracotomy, a creamy discharge is noted in the operative field. What anatomic structure has been violated?
The thoracic duct. Thoracic duct injuries are uncommon. Most injuries heal without intervention. Repair or ligation of the area of leakage can be attempted. Leaving a chest tube in place for several additional days can be considered. This strategy may help to avoid a chylothorax by allowing the thoracic duct to heal. If a chylothorax should develop postoperatively, treatment options include chest tube drainage, a low-fat diet, or hyperalimentation.

28. What is the standard surgical approach for exposure of the anterior aspect of the spine between T10 and L2 (thoracolumbar junction)?
Exposure in this region is achieved through a transdiaphragmatic thoracolumbar approach, also termed a *thoraco-phrenolumbotomy* (Fig. 27.9). The patient is positioned as for a thoracotomy. The incision most commonly begins over the tenth rib and extends distally to the costochondral junction, which is transected. The incision extends distally into the abdominal region as required. The layers of the abdominal wall are dissected, and the peritoneum is mobilized from the undersurface of the diaphragm. The diaphragm is then transected from its peripheral insertion. The peritoneal sac and its contents are mobilized off the anterolateral aspect of the lumbar spine. This strategy provides the surgeon with wide continuous exposure of the spine across the two major body cavities (thoracic and abdominal).

29. What are the various surgical approaches used to provide access to the anterior and lateral aspect of the lumbar spine and lumbosacral junction?
A. L2–S1 surgical approaches
   • Paramedian retroperitoneal approach
   • Anterolateral retroperitoneal flank approach
   • Transperitoneal approach
B. Specific surgical approaches for lumbar interbody fusion
   • Lateral lumbar interbody fusion approach
   • Mini-open anterior lumbar interbody fusion approach
   • Oblique lumbar interbody fusion approach

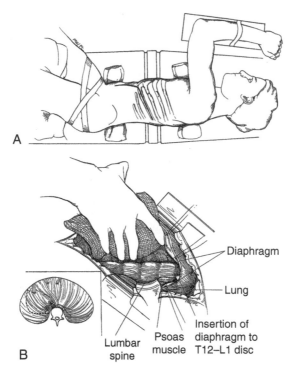

A

B

Diaphragm

Lung

Insertion of
diaphragm to
T12–L1 disc

Lumbar
spine

Psoas
muscle

Fig. 27.9 (A) Positioning of the patient for an anterior surgical approach to the thoracolumbar junction. (B) Intraoperative view of exposure of the thoracolumbar region. Note how the diaphragm requires detachment from its insertion along the lateral chest wall. (From Majd ME, Harkess JW, Holt RT et al. Anterior approach to the spine. In: Margulies JY, Aebi M, Farcy JP, editors. Revision Spine Surgery. St. Louis: Mosby; 1999, pp. 146–147.)

30. Describe the key steps involved in a paramedian retroperitoneal approach to the lumbar spine.

The patient is placed supine and a vertical left paramedian incision is performed. The rectus sheath is incised, and the muscle is retracted to expose the transversalis fascia. The fascia is incised to enter the retroperitoneal space. Alternatively, if exposure of only L5–S1 is required, the retroperitoneal space can be entered below the arcuate line, thus avoiding the need for incising any fascia. The peritoneal sac is swept off the abdominal wall and anterior aspect of the spine to complete initial exposure. Anterior exposure from L2 through S1 can be achieved using this muscle-sparing approach. The direct anterior exposure provided with this approach facilitates placement of an anterior lumbar intervertebral body fusion device. An anterior retroperitoneal approach may also be performed using midline, transverse, or oblique incisions (Fig. 27.10).

31. Describe the key steps involved in the retroperitoneal flank approach to the lower lumbar spine and lumbosacral junction.

In the retroperitoneal flank approach, the patient is most commonly positioned in the lateral decubitus position, with the left side upward. Alternatively, this surgical approach may be performed with the patient in the oblique or supine position. Following incision of the skin and subcutaneous tissues, dissection is carried through the layers of the abdominal wall (external oblique, internal oblique, and transversus abdominis). Next, the transversalis fascia is incised, and the peritoneum is mobilized medially to permit exposure of the psoas muscle, which overlies the anterolateral aspect of the spine. Exposure of the entire lumbar spine and lumbosacral junction can be achieved with this approach after mobilization of vascular structures. Abdominal wall bulging around the surgical incision is commonly reported when this approach is used to expose more than two disc levels and is associated with decreased patient dissatisfaction (Fig. 27.11).

32. What is the most common indication for use of a lumbar transperitoneal approach?

Anterior exposure of the L5–S1 level. The transperitoneal approach is the most direct approach to the anterior L5–S1 disc space. However, this approach requires mobilization of abdominal structures, including the cecum, sigmoid colon, and small bowel to access the anterior spine. It is recommended to open the posterior peritoneum

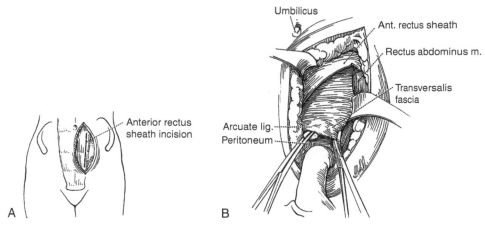

Fig 27.10 Anterior exposure of the lumbar spine through a paramedian retroperitoneal approach. (A) A longitudinal incision is made through the fascia overlying the rectus muscle to expose the muscle belly. (B) The arcuate ligament marks the point of entry into the retroperitoneal space. Using a sponge stick caudad to the ligament in a gentle sweeping motion, the surgeon pushes down and toward the midline to free the peritoneal sac from the fascia and displace it toward the midline, thereby exposing the spine. (From Majd ME, Harkess JW, Holt RT et al. Anterior approach to the spine. In: Margulies JY, Aebi M, Farcy JP, editors. Revision Spine Surgery. St. Louis: Mosby; 1999, p. 151.)

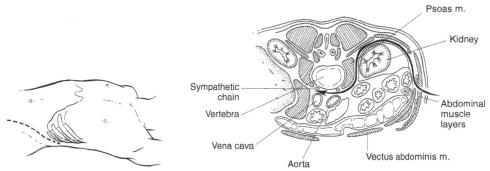

Fig 27.11 The retroperitoneal flank approach to the lumbar spine may be performed with the patient in the lateral or supine position. Dissection passes anterior to the psoas muscle to expose the spine. (From An HS. Surgical exposure and fusion techniques of the spine. In: An HS, editor. Principles and Practice of Spine Surgery. Baltimore: Williams & Wilkins; 1985, p. 56.)

on the right side of the vessel bifurcation, avoid use of electrocautery and perform blunt dissection to gently elevate presacral tissues *en bloc* to minimize the risk of injury to the superior hypogastric plexus which can result in retrograde ejaculation and sterility in males.

33. What is lateral lumbar interbody fusion?

A lateral lumbar interbody fusion (LLIF) is a minimally invasive surgical approach for lumbar interbody graft placement from a lateral approach, which passes through the posterior retroperitoneum and the anterior portion of the psoas muscle. Alternate terms used to describe LLIF include transpsoas interbody fusion, eXtreme Lateral Interbody Fusion (XLIF, NuVasive), and Direct Lateral Interbody Fusion (DLIF, Medtronic). Tubular retractors and electrophysiologic monitoring are integral to these procedures. LLIF is feasible at all lumbar levels except the L5–S1 interspace where the location of the iliac vessels precludes disc space access. LLIF at the L4–L5 disc space may be challenging depending on the height of the iliac crest and is associated with a higher rate of lumbar plexus injury as the nerves of the lumbar plexus are more anteriorly located within the psoas muscle at this level. Advantages of LLIF include the ability to deliver a large interbody device through a minimally invasive approach. Disadvantages associated with LLIF include approach-related neurologic complications including genitofemoral paresthesias, transient or permanent hip flexor and quadriceps weakness, lumbosacral plexus injury, femoral nerve injury, and nerve root injury.

34. What is the mini-open retroperitoneal approach for anterior lumbar interbody fusion?
With the patient in the supine position, a small transverse or oblique incision is performed. Dissection is extended to anterior rectus sheath and the left rectus muscle is mobilized. Retroperitoneal dissection anterior to the psoas muscle is initiated and continued to develop space for insertion of handheld retractors to allow visualization of the anterior aspect of the intervertebral discs and vertebral bodies. Vascular structures including the distal aorta, vena cava, iliac arteries, and iliac veins are identified and protected. Segmental vessels, the middle sacral vessels, and recurrent iliolumbar vessels are identified and ligated depending on the targeted spinal level(s). Radiolucent reverse lip table mounted retractors are used to provide unobstructed exposure of the target intervertebral disc(s) and vertebral bodies (Fig. 27.12).

35. What is an oblique lumbar interbody fusion approach?
An oblique lumbar interbody fusion (OLIF) is a retroperitoneal approach performed through a limited incision with the patient in the right lateral decubitus position. An antepsoas approach is performed with the aid of specialized

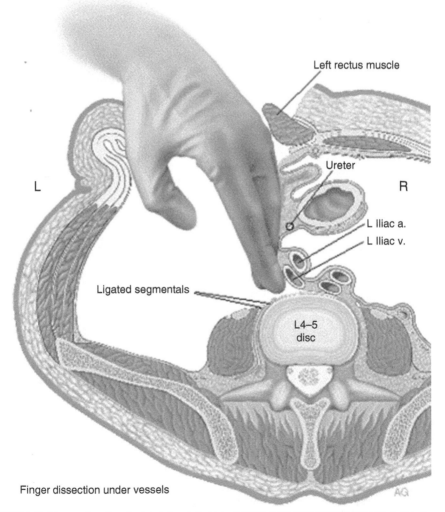

Fig. 27.12 Left mini-open retroperitoneal approach for anterior lumbar interbody fusion. Blunt dissection in the retroperitoneal space anterior to the psoas muscle is performed to expose the anterior aspect of the disc and vertebral body. (From Brau SA. Mini-open approach to the spine for anterior lumbar interbody fusion: Description of the procedure, results and complications. Spine J 2002; 2:216–223, Fig. 5, p. 219.)

lighted retractors and can be used to access spinal levels from L1 to S1. Oblique lateral interbody fusion from L2 to L5 (OLIF25) is performed in the interval between the psoas muscle and the aorta. Oblique lateral interbody fusion at L5–S1 (OLIF51) is performed medial to the left psoas muscle and left common iliac vein at the level of the bifurcation of the great vessels. The OLIF approach is intended to minimize retroperitoneal dissection and the necessity for mobilization of vascular structures.

36. What adverse events have been reported in association with anterior surgical approaches to the lumbar and lumbosacral spine?
    - Direct vascular injury
    - Arterial thrombosis
    - Surgical sympathectomy
    - Retrograde ejaculation
    - Neurologic injury
    - Ureteral injury
    - Bowel injury
    - Deep vein thrombosis
    - Incisional hernia

37. What is the key factor responsible for avoiding vascular injury during anterior and lateral exposures of the lumbosacral spinal region?
    Knowledge of the relationship of vascular structures to the anterior and lateral lumbosacral spine is the key to avoiding vascular complications during anterior and lateral surgical exposures (Figs. 27.13 and 27.14).
    Key factors to consider for open surgical anterior surgical approaches include:
    - The number and location of intervertebral discs requiring exposure. If single-level exposure of the L5–S1 disc is required, the necessary dissection is limited. However, if exposure of the L4–L5 level or multiple disc levels is required, extensive vascular mobilization is necessary and the exposure will be more complex.

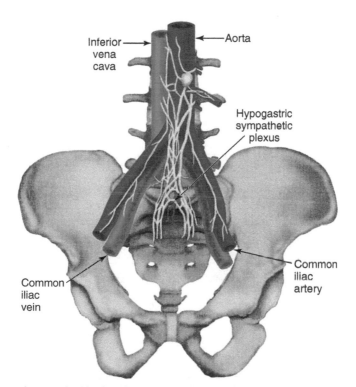

Fig. 27.13 Lumbosacral exposure. Arterial and venous anatomy. Hypogastric sympathetic plexus overlies the L5–S1 disc space. (From Ballard JL, Carlson GD. Spinal operative exposure. In: Sidawy AN, Perler BA, editors. Rutherford's Vascular Surgery and Endovascular Therapy. Philadelphia, PA: Elsevier; 2019, Fig. 58.2, pp. 716–726.)

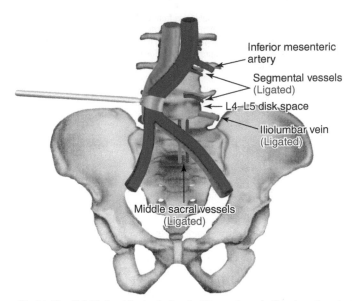

Inferior mesenteric artery

Segmental vessels (Ligated)

L4–L5 disk space

Iliolumbar vein (Ligated)

Middle sacral vessels (Ligated)

Fig. 27.14 Exposure of the L4–L5 and L5–S1 discs following ligation of middle sacral vessels, iliolumbar vein, and segmental vessels. (From Ballard JL, Carlson GD. Spinal operative exposure. In: Sidawy AN, Perler BA, editors. Rutherford's Vascular Surgery and Endovascular Therapy. Philadelphia, PA: Elsevier; 2019, pp. 716–726, Fig. 58.7.)

- The level of the bifurcation of the aorta and vena cava. Although the great vessels most commonly bifurcate at the L4–L5 disc space or at the upper part of the L5 vertebral body, the location of the bifurcation is variable.
- For exposure of the L5–S1 disc, it is necessary to ligate the middle sacral artery and vein, which lie directly over the L5–S1 disc. Exposure of the L5–S1 disc usually involves dissection in the bifurcation between the aorta and vena cava.
- For exposure of the L4–L5 disc it is generally necessary to mobilize vessel branches originating from the distal aorta and vena cava, as well as vessels originating from the external iliac artery and vein. These branches tether the great vessels to the anterior aspect of the spine and limit safe left-to-right retraction of the vascular structures overlying the L4–L5 disc space. It is critical to identify and securely ligate the iliolumbar vein and various ascending lumbar veins. Failure to control the vessels before attempting to retract the great vessels across the L4–L5 disc can result in uncontrolled hemorrhage and even death. The segmental vessels overlying the L4 vertebral body and proximal vertebral levels may also require ligation, depending on how many levels require exposure.

For minimally invasive surgical approaches, key factors to consider include:

- Although vascular structure may not be directly visualized or directly manipulated, vascular structures remain at risk.
- Mortalities following vascular injuries associated with minimally invasive procedures have been reported.
- Surgeons should have a formal preoperative plan and equipment immediately available in the operating room in the event that it becomes necessary to emergently address these extremely rare injuries.

38. A 46-year-old man underwent implantation of an L5–S1 intervertebral body fusion device without the use of supplemental fixation through an anterior retroperitoneal surgical approach. One year later, the surgeon decided to remove the interbody device through a repeat anterior retroperitoneal approach because the fusion did not heal and the interbody device had migrated out of the disc space. During the procedure scar tissue made exposure difficult, and the surgeon was concerned that an injury to the ureter had occurred. What is the best way to evaluate for this problem? What treatment is indicated if a ureteral injury exists?

Urologic consultation for surgical exploration and direct visualization of the ureter is the recommended method for identification of an intraoperative ureteral injury. Repair and/or stenting of the ureter may be performed based on the location and extent of injury. A dye study using intravenous injection of methylene blue or indigo carmine dye may aid identification of the site of ureteral injury. Placement of a ureteral stent prior to surgery can help with identification of the ureter during revision of anterior lumbar surgical procedures.

39. A 40-year-old man underwent a L5–S1 anterior lumbar interbody fusion with implantation of an anterior fusion cage. He complains of erectile dysfunction after the procedure. What should the surgeon advise the patient?

The patient should be advised that prognosis for recovery is good because erection is not controlled by any of the neural structures that course over the anterior aspect of the L5–S1 disc. The patient's difficulty is not related to the anterior approach and other underlying causes should be evaluated.

Erection is predominantly a parasympathetic function through control of the vasculature of the penis. The parasympathetic fibers responsible for erection originate from the L1 to L4 nerve roots and arrive at their target area via the pelvic splanchnic nerves. Somatic function from the S1 to S4 levels is carried through the pudendal nerve.

Anterior spine surgery at the L5–S1 level has the potential to disrupt the superior hypogastric plexus. This sympathetic plexus crosses the anterior aspect of the L5–S1 disc and distal aorta. The superior hypogastric plexus controls bladder neck closure during ejaculation. Failure of closure of the bladder neck during ejaculation causes ejaculate to travel in a retrograde direction into the bladder and can result in sterility.

39. After the left-sided retroperitoneal approach to the lumbar spine, the patient wakes up complaining of coolness in the right lower extremity compared with the left. Palpation of pulses demonstrates strong dorsalis pedis and posterior tibia pulses bilaterally, and the right leg does appear to be cooler than the left leg. How are these clinical findings explained?

The sympathetic chain lies on the lateral border of the vertebral bodies and is often disrupted during an anterior surgical exposure. A sympathectomy effect occurs and allows increased blood flow to the left leg compared with the right. This process explains the temperature increase and occasional swelling noted in the lower extremity on the side of the surgical exposure. Patients should be forewarned of this possible result following an anterior spine procedure and advised that it will not impair the ultimate outcome of surgery.

40. After a left-sided retroperitoneal exposure of the lumbosacral junction, the patient awakens in the recovery room complaining of increased pain in the left lower extremity. The left leg is noted to be cooler than the right leg. What test should be ordered immediately?

An arteriogram should be ordered on an emergent basis. This clinical scenario cannot be explained on the basis of a sympathectomy effect by which the ipsilateral leg on the side of the exposure becomes warmer. When the distal extremity on the side of the exposure becomes cooler, it is usually due to dislodgement of an arteriosclerotic plaque. Thus assessment of the vasculature with an arteriogram is the study of choice to determine whether the plaque has lodged in the trifurcation in the popliteal fossa. Immediate consultation with an experienced vascular surgeon is appropriate.

KEY POINTS

1. Posterior approaches to the thoracic and lumbar spine are extremely versatile and provide surgical access for spinal decompression, fusion, and instrumentation from T1 to the sacrum.
2. The key to avoiding complications during surgical exposures of the anterior spinal column is a detailed knowledge of the relationship of the vascular, visceral, and neurologic structures to the anterior and lateral aspect of the spine.

Websites

1. Complications associated with prone positioning in elective spinal surgery: https://www.wjgnet.com/2218-5836/full/v6/i3/351.htm
2. Anterior exposure of the thoracic and lumbar spine: https://jamanetwork.com/journals/jamasurgery/fullarticle/399156
3. Thoracotomy for exposure of the spine: https://www.ctsnet.org/article/thoracotomy-exposure-spine
4. Methods and complications of anterior exposure of the thoracic and lumbar spine: https://jamanetwork.com/journals/jamasurgery/fullarticle/399156

BIBLIOGRAPHY

1. Ballard, J. L., Carlson, G. D., Chen, J., & White, J. (2014). Anterior thoracolumbar spine exposure: Critical review and analysis. *Annals of Vascular Surgery, 28,* 465–469.
2. Baron, E. M., & Vaccaro, A. R. (2018). *Operative Techniques: Spine Surgery* (3rd ed.). Philadelphia, PA: Elsevier.
3. Brau, S. A. (2002). Mini-open approach to the spine for anterior lumbar interbody fusion: Description of the procedure, results and complications. *Spine Journal, 2,* 216–223.
4. Kim, D. H., Vaccaro, A. R., Dickman, C. A., Cho, D., Lee, S., & Kim, I. (2013). *Surgical Anatomy and Techniques to the Spine* (2nd ed.). Philadelphia, PA: Saunders.
5. Kwon, B., & Kim, D. H. (2016). Lateral lumbar interbody fusion: Indications, outcomes, and complications. *Journal of the American Academy of Orthopaedic Surgeons, 24,* 96–105.
6. Melikian, R., & Rhee, J. M. (2017). The role of anterior interbody fusion (ALIF and XLIF with anterior column release) in the surgical management of adult spinal deformity. *Seminars in Spine Surgery, 29,* 82–90.
7. Miller, M., Chhabra, B. A., Park, J., Shen, F., Weiss, D., & Browne, J. (2015). *Orthopaedic Surgical Exposures* (2nd ed.). Philadelphia, PA: Saunders.
8. Steinmetz, M. P., Benzel, E. C. (2017). *Benzel's Spine Surgery. Techniques, Complication Avoidance, and Management* (4th ed.). Philadelphia, PA: Elsevier.
9. Woods, K. R., Billys, J. B., & Hynes, R. A. (2017). Technical description of oblique lateral interbody fusion at L1–L5 (OLIF25) and at L5–S1 (OLIF51) and evaluation of complications and fusion rates. *Spine Journal, 17,* 545–553.

CHAPTER 28

OCCIPITAL AND CERVICAL SPINE INSTRUMENTATION

Dil B. Patel, BS, Andrew M. Block, BS, Benjamin Khechen, BA, and Kern Singh, BS, MD

1. What are the indications for use of cervical spinal instrumentation?
   - To immobilize an unstable spinal segment
   - To promote bony union
   - To improve soft tissue healing
   - To correct spinal deformity
   - To decrease or eliminate the need for external immobilization

2. How are the various types of cervical spinal implants classified?
   No universal classification exists. Cervical spinal implants may be classified descriptively by:
   - *Location of implant:* anterior spinal column versus posterior spinal column
   - *Spinal region stabilized:* occipitocervical (O–C1); odontoid (C2); atlantoaxial (C1–C2); subaxial (C3–C7); cervicothoracic (C7–T2)
   - *Method of osseous attachment:* screw, hook, wire, cable
   - *Type of longitudinal member:* rod, plate, other (e.g., rib graft)

3. What types of cervical spinal implants are most commonly utilized today?
   Posterior cervical instrumentation most commonly involves use of rod-screw systems. Screws may be placed in the occiput, C1 (lateral mass), and C2 (pedicle vs. pars vs. translaminar screws). In the subaxial cervical region, lateral mass screws are more commonly used compared with pedicle screws at the C3–C6 levels, whereas pedicle screws are typically used at C7 and distally in the thoracic region. Anterior cervical plates are the most commonly used implants in the C3–C7 region. Reconstruction of the anterior spinal column following discectomy or corpectomy may be performed with bone graft or synthetic devices commonly referred to as "fusion cages" (Fig. 28.1A,B).

4. What are the indications for use of spinal instrumentation in the occipitocervical region?
   - Trauma
   - Ligamentous instability
   - Select odontoid fractures
   - Rheumatoid arthritis (basilar invagination)
   - Infection
   - Neoplasm
   - Select skeletal dysplasias
   - Arnold-Chiari malformations
   - Select metabolic bone diseases

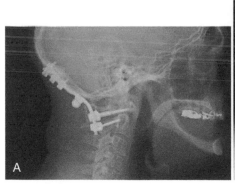
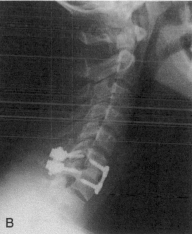

Fig. 28.1 (A) Posterior occiput to C2 spinal instrumentation and fusion. (B) Anterior cervical plate, allograft bone graft, and posterior screw-rod instrumentation.

5. **What implant options are available for use at the occipitocervical junction?**
   - **Anterior options:** Implants are infrequently placed in this region because it is challenging to achieve surgical exposure here. Bone graft or cages are used to reconstruct osseous defects. Occasionally specialized plates (e.g., C2 to clivus plate) or C1-occipital condyle screws are used.
   - **Posterior options:** Rod-screw systems are the most commonly used implant. A hybrid rod-plate combination is an additional option. Contoured rods with wire or cable fixation are an option for special circumstances. Bone grafts and wires may be used in conjunction with other implants but are rarely used in isolation because they are not sufficiently stable to permit patient mobilization without extensive external immobilization, such as a halo device.

6. **Where can a surgeon safely place screws in the occiput when performing posterior occipitocervical instrumentation?**
   Occipital bone is thickest and most dense in the midline below the external occipital protuberance (inion). This region provides an excellent surface for screw purchase. Occipital bone thickness decreases laterally and inferiorly from the inion. Screws should be placed below the superior nuchal line that overlies the transverse sinuses, which can be injured during drilling or screw placement (Fig. 28.2).

7. **How are occipital screws connected to a rod system?**
   The surgeon has several options including:
   - **Modular midline screw plates:** A midline plate permits screw purchase in the thick midline bone and permits minor adjustments to facilitate linkage to an independent dual-rod construct (Fig. 28.3A).
   - **Hybrid rod-plate fixation:** Plates attach laterally to the midline of the occiput and connect with rods for fixation in the cervical spine distally. Specialized implants consisting of a single rod that transitions to a plate are available (see Fig. 28.3B).
   - **Rod with specialized connectors:** Occipital screws are linked to rods via offset screw-rod connectors (see Fig. 28.3C).

8. **How is posterior screw fixation performed at C1?**
   Two basic techniques are utilized:
   - In the first technique, the screw is placed directly in the lateral mass of C1. The entry point is at the junction of the C1 lateral mass with the undersurface of the C1 posterior arch (Fig. 28.4A). The extensive venous plexus in this region makes dissection challenging. In addition, the C2 nerve root is in proximity to the screw entry point

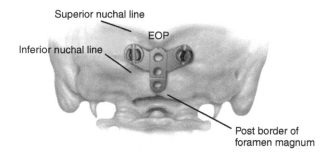

Superior nuchal line
EOP
Inferior nuchal line
Post border of foramen magnum

Fig. 28.2 Safe placement of occipital screws is in the region adjacent to the external occipital protuberance *(EOP)* and below the superior nuchal line. (DePuy Spine, Inc. All rights reserved.)

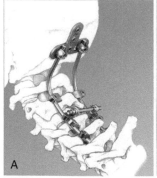
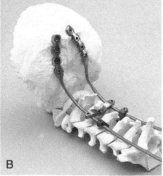
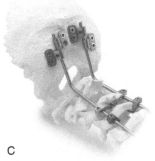

A   B   C

Fig. 28.3 Occipital screw linkage options. (A) Midline screw-plate. (B) Hybrid rod-plate. (C) Rod with specialized connectors. (Synthes Spine. All rights reserved.)

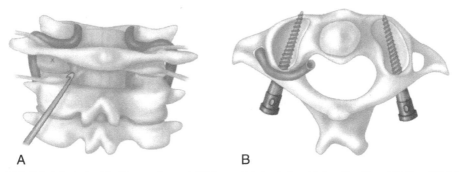

Fig. 28.4 (A) Posterior landmark for C1 screw placement. (B) C1 screw trajectory in the axial plane. (From Vaccaro AR, Baron EM. Spine Surgery: Operative Techniques. Philadelphia, PA: Saunders; 2008, with permission.)

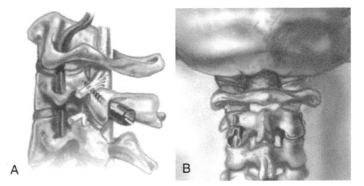

Fig. 28.5 C2 pars screw placement. (A) Lateral view. (B) Anteroposterior view. (From McLaughlin MR, Haid RW, Rodts GE. Atlas of Cervical Spine Surgery. Philadelphia, PA: Saunders; 2005, with permission.)

and must be retracted distally. A modified technique involves creation of a notch on the undersurface of the C1 arch to facilitate drill/screw placement to minimize dissection in the region of this venous plexus. Screws are directed with 5°–10° of convergence and parallel to the C1 arch (see Fig. 28.4B).

• The second technique uses an entry point on the C1 arch and places a screw through the pedicle analog of C1 and into the C1 lateral mass. The vertebral artery is at greater risk with this technique and one must not mistake a common anomaly in which a bony bridge, the arcuate foramen, overlies the vertebral artery or the screw will injure the vertebral artery. This osseous anomaly has been termed the *ponticulus posticus*. With either technique, excessive superior C1 screw angulation will violate the occiput-C1 joint. An excessively long C1 screw may potentially compromise the internal carotid artery or hypoglossal nerve.

9. What are the options for achieving screw fixation in C2?
   Three options exist: C2 pars screws, C2 pedicle screws, and C2 translaminar screws.

10. How is a C2 pars screw placed?
    The *pars interarticularis* is defined as the portion of the C2 vertebra between the superior and inferior articular processes. The screw entry point is 3–4 mm superior and 3–4 mm lateral to the inferior medial aspect of the C2–C3 facet joint. Screw trajectory is parallel to the C2 pars interarticularis with approximately 10° of medial angulation (Fig. 28.5).

11. How is a C2 pedicle screw placed?
    The *C2 pedicle* is defined as the portion of the C2 vertebra connecting the posterior osseous elements with the vertebral body and consists of the narrow area between the pars interarticularis and the vertebral body. The entry point is approximated by the intersection of a vertical line through the center of the C2 pars interarticularis and a horizontal line through the upper edge of the C2 lamina. The screw entry point is 2 mm lateral to the location defined by these landmarks. The screw is placed with 15°–45° of medial angulation and parallel to the superior surface of the C2 pars interarticularis. The medial wall of the C2 pars can be palpated as an additional guide to placement (Fig. 28.6).

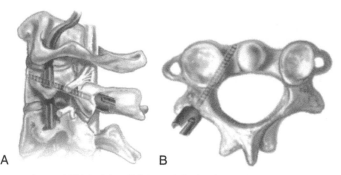

Fig. 28.6 C2 pedicle screw placement. (A) Lateral view. (B) Anteroposterior view. (From McLaughlin MR, Haid RW, Rodts GE. Atlas of Cervical Spine Surgery. Philadelphia, PA: Saunders; 2005, with permission.)

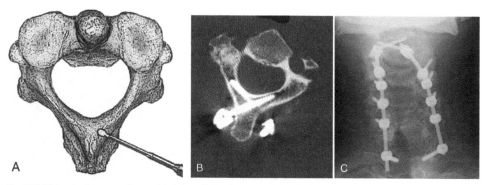

Fig. 28.7 C2 translaminar screw placement technique. (A) Creation of screw tract. (B) Axial computed tomography view after screw placement. (C) Anteroposterior radiograph after screw placement. (A: From Jea A, Sheth RN, Vanni S, et al. Modification of Wright's technique for placement of C2 translaminar screws. Spine J 2008;8:656–660, with permission.)

12. **Compare and contrast a C2 pedicle screw with a C2 pars screw.**
    The C2 pedicle screw trajectory is more superior and medial than the pars screw and has greater risk of injury to a high-riding vertebral artery. A longer screw length may be achieved using a C2 pedicle screw than a C2 pars screw. A C2 pedicle screw can be safely placed with bicortical screw purchase. A C2 pars screw is typically a unicortical screw that stops short of the transverse foramen to prevent potential injury to the vertebral artery.

13. **When might a C2 translaminar screw be preferred over alternative C2 screw fixation methods?**
    A *translaminar screw* is preferred when the trajectory for placement of a C2 pars or pedicle screw is compromised by an aberrantly coursing vertebral artery or aberrant osseous anatomy. The technique is straightforward and consists of creating a small entry window at the junction of the C2 spinous process and lamina. A blunt probe or hand drill is used to create a pathway for screw placement in the cancellous bone of the contralateral lamina. The process is repeated on the opposite side for placement of a second screw that crosses above or below the initial screw. An additional *window* can be created at the facet-laminar junction to visualize *screw-exit* to ensure that the screw has not inadvertently violated the inner cortical surface of the lamina (Fig. 28.7).

14. **What are the indications for spinal implant placement in the atlantoaxial (C1–C2) region?**
    Atlantoaxial instability due to traumatic etiologies (e.g., unstable odontoid fractures), midtransverse ligament disruption, odontoid nonunion, an unstable os odontoideum, or nontraumatic disorders, such as rheumatoid arthritis, congenital malformations, and metabolic disorders.

15. **What are the types of implants most commonly used to stabilize the atlantoaxial joint?**
    C1–C2 stabilization is most commonly performed from a posterior approach using C1–C2 transarticular screws or C1–C2 screw-rod constructs. Posterior wire/cable techniques or rod-clamps are less frequently utilized. Anterior placement of transarticular screws is a specialized technique, which is occasionally used to salvage failed posterior C1–C2 fusions and for unique cases.

16. Describe the technique for posterior C1–C2 transarticular facet screw fixation.

    The starting point for a *transarticular screw* is the same as for a C2 pars screw and is 3–4 mm superior and 3–4 mm lateral to the inferior medial aspect of the C2–C3 facet joint. Screw trajectory should remain as medial as possible without breaking through the medial aspect of the C2 isthmus. Screw insertion can be guided by exposing the posterior C1–C2 facet complex and the isthmus of C2. The transarticular screws traverse the inferior articular process of C2, the isthmus of C2, the superior endplate of C2, the C1–C2 facet joint, and the lateral mass of C1 (Fig. 28.8).

17. What are some complications and challenges associated with transarticular screw placement?

    The technique carries a risk of vertebral artery injury. It cannot be performed in up to 20% of patients due to vertebral artery anomalies. A preoperative computed tomography (CT) scan is required to look for a high-riding vertebral artery whose aberrant path is located along the planned screw trajectory. Proper screw placement requires anatomic reduction of the C1–C2 joints prior to screw placement. Excessively long screws may injure the internal carotid artery or hypoglossal nerve. In addition, screw placement in patients with increased thoracic kyphosis is challenging because it is difficult to achieve the required screw trajectory in this setting.

18. Describe advantages of C1–C2 screw-rod systems versus transarticular screws.

    C1–C2 screw-rod systems have several advantages over transarticular screws for stabilization of the C1–C2 region. C1–C2 screw-rod systems are more versatile. Preoperative reduction of the C1–C2 joints is not required prior to instrumentation. In fact, the independent placement of screws in C1 and C2 can be used as a tool to facilitate reduction, which can be checked with fluoroscopy and modified without the need to replace screws. In addition, C1–C2 screw-rod systems can be used in cases where transarticular screws are contraindicated (e.g., vertebral artery anomalies, severe kyphosis).

19. Why are transarticular screws or screw-rod constructs preferred over posterior wire or cable procedures?

    Transarticular screws and screw-rod techniques provide much greater stability than wire/cable techniques and avoid the need for postoperative external mobilization with a halo vest. In addition, these techniques are associated with higher rates of successful fusion. Screw-based techniques avoid the risk of wire passage adjacent to the spinal cord. Screw-based techniques can be used in the presence of fractured or absent laminae, whereas wire/cable techniques rely on intact posterior elements to provide fixation.

20. Describe two common techniques used to achieve C1–C2 stabilization using wires or cables.

    - The *Gallie technique* begins with sublaminar wire (double-looped) passage from caudal to cranial under the posterior arch of C1. Following wire passage, a structural corticocancellous iliac graft is harvested and shaped to conform to the posterior processes of C1 and C2. The two free ends of the wire are then passed through the leading wire loop, over the graft, and around or through the spinous process of the axis. The free ends of the wire are then twisted in the midline, thereby securing the graft position between C1 and C2 (Fig. 28.9A).

Anteroposterior
landmark

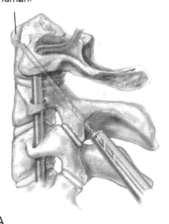
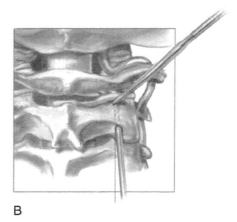

A   B

Fig. 28.8 C1–C2 transarticular screw placement. (A) Lateral view, (B) anteroposterior view. (From McLaughlin MR, Haid RW, Rodts GE. Atlas of Cervical Spine Surgery. Philadelphia, PA: Saunders; 2005, with permission.)

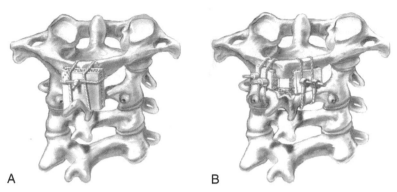

Fig. 28.9 C1–C2 wire techniques. (A) Gallie technique. (B) Brooks technique. (From McLaughlin MR, Haid RW, Rodts GE. Atlas of Cervical Spine Surgery. Philadelphia, PA: Saunders; 2005, with permission.)

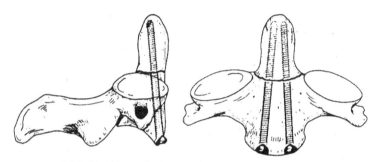

Fig. 28.10 Odontoid screw fixation. *Left,* Lateral view. *Right,* anteroposterior view.

- The *Brooks technique* involves the passage of dual or double sublaminar wires (cables) from caudal to cranial under the arch of C2 and then C1. Following the passage of the wire, two separate triangular or rectangular corticocancellous iliac grafts are harvested and placed over the posterior elements of C1 and C2. The ends of the wires on each side are then tightened together, thereby securing the position of the grafts (see Fig. 28.9B).

21. Describe the fixation of choice for select odontoid fractures treated through an anterior approach.
    One or two screws may be used to stabilize a type 2 odontoid fracture. The critical transverse outer diameter for the placement of two 3.5-mm cortical screws is 9 mm. Cadaveric biomechanical studies have demonstrated that one central screw, which engages the cortical tip of the dens, is just as effective as two screws. Two screws more effectively counter the rotational forces created by the alar ligaments. Single-screw options include the use of a single 4.5-mm cannulated screw or a single 3.5–4.0-mm standard lag screw (Fig. 28.10).

22. What are some contraindications for the use of odontoid screw fixation?
    - Patients who possess anatomic obstructions to appropriate screw placement (e.g., short neck, excessive thoracic kyphosis, barrel chest deformity)
    - Unfavorable fracture patterns (e.g., fracture obliquity in the same direction as screw placement—i.e., a sagittal plane fracture that courses posterosuperiorly to anteroinferiorly, low type 3 odontoid fractures, fractures requiring a flexed neck position to maintain reduction)
    - Poor bone quality (a pathologic fracture with compromised bone quality, significant osteoporosis)

23. What are the indications for posterior subaxial cervical instrumentation?
    Stabilization and fusion of spinal instabilities and deformities (e.g., secondary to trauma, spinal degeneration, tumors, infections), posterior stabilization following an anterior nonunion, adjunctive stabilization following a long segment anterior fusion, or fusion and stabilization following a posterior decompression for cervical myelopathy.

24. Describe three trajectories for placement of lateral mass screws.
    Three commonly employed trajectories for lateral mass screw placement (C3–C6) described by Roy-Camille, Magerl, and An, are summarized in Table 28.1. Laterally directed screws are not utilized at C2 due to concerns regarding vertebral artery proximity.

TECHNIQUE	ROY-CAMILLE	MAGERL	AN
Table 28.1 Recommended Landmarks for Lateral Mass Screw Placement.			
Starting position (lateral mass)	Center	1 mm medial and 1–2 mm cephalad to the center	1 mm medial to the center
Cephalad tilt	0	30	15
Lateral tilt	10	25	30

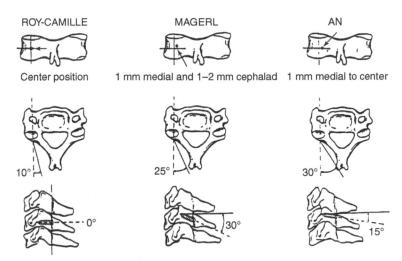

Fig. 28.11 Trajectories for lateral mass screw placement.

At C7, the lateral mass is frequently quite small, and a lateral mass screw risks causing C8 nerve root irritation. For this reason, pedicle screws are more commonly utilized at this level, although C7 lateral mass fixation remains a valid technique depending on individual patient anatomy (Fig. 28.11).

25. What is the role of pedicle screws in the cervical spine?
Pedicle screws are useful and relatively safe at the C2 and C7 levels. In most patients, the vertebral artery enters the foramen transversarium of C6 and is not at risk with C7 pedicle screw placement. Pedicle screws at the C3 through C6 levels are used less frequently than lateral mass screws due to the smaller size of the pedicles at these levels and concern relating to the risk of vertebral artery injury.

26. Describe the placement of C7 pedicle screws.
One technique involves creation of a laminoforaminotomy at C6–C7 to palpate and visualize the medial border of the C7 pedicle. Next, a small drill or pedicle probe can be used to cannulate the C7 pedicle while visualizing a medial pedicle breech. This is followed by screw placement. Alternatively, C7 pedicle screw placement may be guided by fluoroscopy or surgical navigation, or free-hand placement based on anatomic landmarks may be utilized.

27. What are some advantages of lateral mass and pedicle screw fixation versus posterior wire or cable fixation?
Cervical lateral mass and pedicle screw fixation afford significantly increased stability in rotation and extension, compared with posterior wiring or cable fixation. Spinal implant fixation to the lateral masses and pedicles obviates the need for intact laminae or spinous processes, which are necessary for most wire/cable techniques. Rigid postoperative cervical immobilization is not required with screw fixation techniques. Loss of wire fixation, due to wire failure or bony pullout, is the most common complication associated with wire/cable techniques but is rarely seen with screw-based techniques.

28. What techniques have been described for use of wires and cables in the subaxial cervical region?
Wires or cables may be placed beneath the lamina (sublaminar), between adjacent spinous processes (interspinous or *Rogers wiring*), through the facet joints, or between the facet joint and the spinous process. The *Bohlman triple-wire technique* combines midline interspinous wiring with passage of separate wires through adjacent spinous processes, which are used to secure a corticocancellous bone graft to the decorticated posterior elements on each side of the spinous processes.

29. What are the indications for anterior cervical plating?
To decrease the incidence of graft or cage subsidence and dislodgement, minimize kyphotic collapse of the fused interface, improve fusion rates, and minimize the need for postoperative external immobilization.

30. Describe the design features of the first generation anterior cervical plates.
The original Caspar (Aesculap Instrument Company) and Orozco (Synthes Spine) systems were nonconstrained, load-sharing plates that required bicortical screw purchase. Due to the nonconstrained nature of the screw-plate interface, excessive motion at the screw-plate junction occasionally led to screw loosening or pullout. Engagement of the posterior vertebral cortex was required to minimize screw loosening. This is technically challenging and is associated with an increased risk of neurologic injury.

31. What solution was developed to address the difficulties associated with first generation anterior cervical plates requiring bicortical screw purchase?
Because of the technical difficulty associated with bicortical screw purchase, constrained systems that firmly lock the screws to the plate were developed. The first solution was a plate system (cervical spine locking plate [CSLP]) that used a screw with an expandable cross-split head that locks into the plate after insertion of a small central bolt (Synthes Spine). Securing the screws to the plates allows a more direct transfer of the applied forces from the spine to the plate and improved construct stiffness without the need for bicortical screw purchase. Alternative methods were developed to secure the screw to the plate to prevent screw back-out and included a variety of screw head coverage mechanisms (ring locks, blocking heads, screw covers) (Fig. 28.12).

32. How are current anterior cervical plating systems classified?
Anterior cervical plate systems can be broadly classified as either static (constrained) plates or dynamic (semiconstrained) plates.
- **Static plates** rely on screws, which are rigidly locked to the plate. A direct transfer of applied forces from spine to plate is assured, but the theoretical possibility of stress shielding of the anterior spinal column is present.
- **Dynamic plates** utilize screws that are restricted from backing out from the plate but attempt to allow some degree of load sharing between the plate and the anterior spinal column. This load sharing is achieved through various mechanisms that may be used singularly or in combination including: *screw rotation, screw translation,* or *plate shortening. Semiconstrained rotational plates* permit rotation at the plate-screw interface as graft subsidence occurs. *Semiconstrained translational plates* permit screws to slide longitudinally (fixed screws) within slotted holes in the plate. Some designs permit only longitudinal translation (fixed screws), whereas others permit both longitudinal screw translation and screw rotation (variable screws). The last type of plate permits translation by means of plate shortening. The ends of the plate are rigidly fixed to adjacent vertebrae, but the plate itself shortens under physiologic loading (Fig. 28.13).

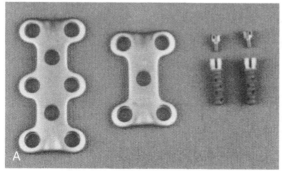
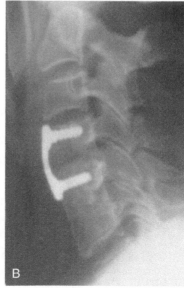

Fig. 28.12 Anterior cervical locking plate (Synthes Spine). (A) The screw head is locked to the plate by insertion of a conical bolt, thereby ensuring angular stability between the plate and the screws. (B) Anterior cervical locking plate application after interbody fusion. Note that penetration of the posterior vertebral body cortex is not required to achieve a stable implant construct.

Rotational vs. Translational

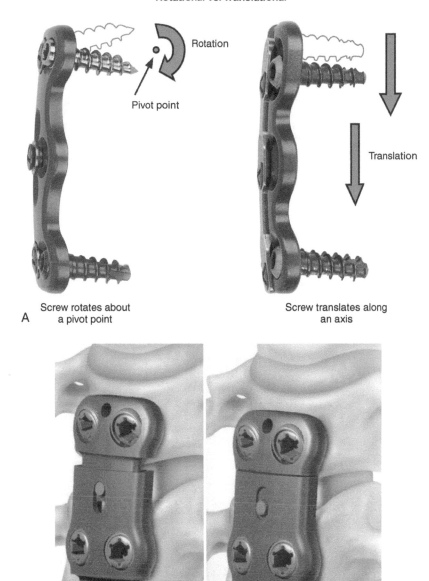

Rotation

Pivot point

Translation

A   Screw rotates about
a pivot point

Screw translates along
an axis

B

C

Fig. 28.13 (A) Rotational versus translational anterior cervical plate. (B) Cervical translation through plate shortening. (C) Note plate length intraoperatively compared with postoperatively. (A: From Medtronic Sofamor Danek, 2005. All rights reserved. B and C: From DePuy Spine, Inc. All rights reserved.)

33. **Which type of anterior cervical plate is superior—a static plate or a dynamic plate?**
This is a controversial area. In the setting of trauma, a *static plate* is preferable because it provides greater immediate stability. In the treatment of degenerative disorders, no studies have established superiority of one particular type of plate. With use of *dynamic plates*, graft settling may lead to segmental kyphosis, foraminal stenosis, and plate impingement on the superior adjacent disc space. However, when multilevel corpectomies are stabilized with anterior plates, graft subsidence may be accommodated by translational plates and potentially decrease the rate of anterior plate fixation failure.

34. **What is a buttress plate?**
A *buttress or junctional plate* is an alternative to a long segment anterior cervical plate, which is subject to large cantilever forces, particularly at the caudal plate-screw-bone junction. A buttress plate spans only the caudal or cephalad graft-host junction, thereby theoretically preventing graft extrusion. The plate is most commonly used at the caudal end of the graft where the cantilever forces are the greatest. A surgeon should use supplemental posterior segmental fixation in the setting of a long anterior strut graft fusion stabilized by a junctional plate stabilization to prevent dislodgement of the plate with potentially catastrophic consequences (Fig. 28.14).

35. **What are cervical intervertebral body fusion devices?**
Cervical intervertebral body fusion devices (i.e., cervical interbody fusion devices, cervical fusion cages) are intended to provide structural support to the anterior spinal column and promote fusion following removal of an intervertebral disc. These devices are made from a variety of materials (e.g., titanium, carbon fiber, polyetheretherketone [PEEK]). These devices possess a hollowed center filled with graft material to promote fusion. Cervical intervertebral body fusion devices are traditionally used in conjunction with supplemental fixation consisting of an anterior cervical plate, which achieves fixation through placement of two screws into the anterior vertebral body surface at each fixated level. An alternative cervical intervertebral body fusion device design incorporates integrated fixation features (e.g., screws, blades) that are deployed through the vertebral endplate and may be used with or without supplemental plate fixation (i.e., "standalone"). Alternative options for reconstruction of the anterior column following cervical discectomy include iliac crest autograft bone graft and structural allograft bone graft (Fig. 28.15A,B).

36. **What are cervical vertebral body replacement devices?**
Cervical vertebral body replacement (VBR) devices are intended to reconstruct the anterior spinal column following corpectomy (i.e., removal of the vertebral body) required for treatment of tumors, fractures, osteomyelitis, or spinal cord compression due to cervical degenerative disorders. These devices may be used with bone graft as an adjunct to spinal fusion, but have the capacity to restore spinal column integrity in the absence of fusion for a limited time period in patients with cervical spine tumors. Cervical VBR designs include static and expandable device types. Static VBRs have fixed dimensions and are placed into a slightly distracted corpectomy defect. Expandable VBRs are inserted at a minimized profile and expanded in situ within the corpectomy defect. Additional options for reconstruction of the anterior spinal column following cervical corpectomy include structural autograft bone graft or allograft bone graft (iliac crest, fibula, and radius) (Fig. 28.16).

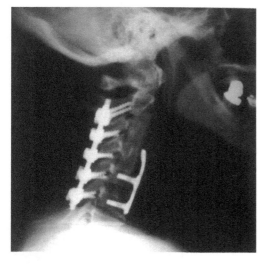

Fig. 28.14 The buttress plate prevents anterior graft dislodgement in combination with posterior cervical instrumentation. (From Vaccaro AR, Baron EM. Spine Surgery: Operative Techniques. Philadelphia, PA: Saunders; 2008, with permission.)

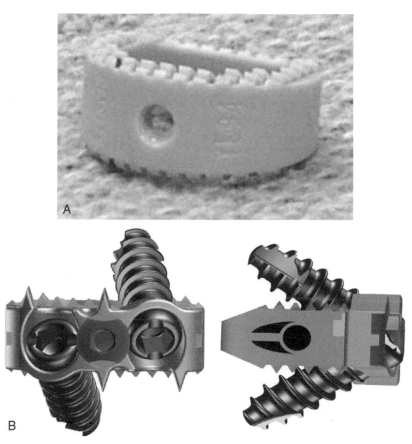

B

Fig. 28.15 (A) Polyetheretherketone interbody spacer for use in conjunction with anterior cervical plate fixation. (B) Interbody device with integrated plate-screw fixation. Frontal view *(left),* lateral view *(right).* (A: From Yson SC, Sembrano JN, Santos ER. Comparison of allograft and polyetheretherketone cage subsidence rates in anterior cervical discectomy and fusion (ACDF). J Clin Neurosci 2017;38: 118–121. B: From Clavenna AL, Beutler WJ, Gudipally M, et al. The biomechanical stability of a novel spacer with integrated plate in contiguous two-level and three-level ACDF models: An in vitro cadaveric study. Spine J 2012;12:157–163.)

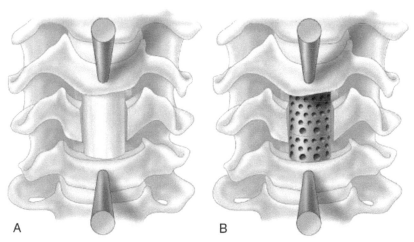

A   B

Fig. 28.16 (A) Fibular graft. (B) Synthetic device. (From Angeles CF, Park J. Procedure 60: Anterior cervical corpectomy and fusion. In: Jandial R, McCormick PC, Black PM, editors. Core Techniques in Operative Neurosurgery. Philadelphia, PA: Saunders; 2011, pp. 422–429.)

KEY POINTS

1. Posterior cervical instrumentation most commonly involves the use of screw-rod systems. Screws may be placed in the occiput, C1 (lateral mass), C2 (pedicle, pars, or translaminar), and from C3–C7 in either the lateral masses or pedicles.
2. Anterior cervical plates are most commonly used in the C3–C7 region and may be classified as static or dynamic plates.
3. The anterior spinal column may be reconstructed with autogenous bone graft (iliac or fibula), allograft bone graft, or synthetic materials (e.g., titanium mesh cages, carbon fiber cages, PEEK cages).

Websites

1. Anterior cervical plate nomenclature of cervical spine study group: http://cme.medscape.com/viewarticle/424941_1
2. Posterior occipital cervical fixation: http://www.spineuniverse.com/displayarticle.php/article288.html
3. The design and evolution of interbody cages in anterior cervical discectomy and fusion: https://www.medscape.com/viewarticle/844633_6

BIBLIOGRAPHY

1. Harms, J., & Melcher, R. P. (2001). Posterior C1–C2 fusion with polyaxial screw and rod fixation. *Spine*, 26:2467–2471.
2. Jea, A., Sheth, R., Vanni, S., Green, B. A., & Levi, A. D. (2008). Modification of Wright's technique for placement of C2 translaminar screws. *Spine Journal, 8*, 656–660.
3. Jeanneret, B., & Magerl, F. (1992). Primary posterior fusion C1–C2 in odontoid fractures: Indications, technique, and results of transarticular screw fixation. *Journal of Spinal Disorders & Techniques, 5*, 464–475.
4. McLaughlin, M. R., Haid, R. W., Rodts, G. E. (2005). *Atlas of Cervical Spine Surgery*. Philadelphia, PA: Saunders.
5. Reilly, T. M., & Sasso, R. C. (2002). Anterior odontoid screw techniques. *Techniques Orthopediques, 17*(3), 306–315.
6. Rhee, J. M., & Riew, K. D. (2007). Dynamic anterior cervical plates. *Journal of the American Academy of Orthopaedic Surgeons, 15*(11), 640–646.
7. Sekhon, L. H. (2005). Posterior cervical lateral mass screw fixation: Analysis of 1026 consecutive screws in 143 patients. *Journal of Spinal Disorders & Techniques, 18*(4), 297–303.
8. Stock, G. H., Vaccaro, A. R., Brown, A. K., & Anderson, P. A. (2006). Contemporary posterior occipital fixation. *Journal of Bone and Joint Surgery American Volume, 88*, 1642–1649.
9. Vaccaro, A. R., & Baron, E. M. (2008). *Spine Surgery: Operative Techniques*. Philadelphia, PA: Saunders.

THORACIC AND LUMBAR SPINE INSTRUMENTATION

Bradley Anderson, D. Greg Anderson, MD, and Vincent J. Devlin, MD

CHAPTER 29

GENERAL CONSIDERATIONS

1. Summarize the functions of spinal instrumentation in thoracic and lumbar fusion procedures.
   - **Enhance fusion**. Spinal implants immobilize spinal segments during the fusion process and thereby increase the rate of successful arthrodesis.
   - **Restore spinal stability**. When pathologic processes (e.g., tumor, infection, fracture) compromise the integrity of the spinal column, spinal implants can restore stability.
   - **Correct spinal deformities**. Spinal instrumentation can provide correction of spinal deformities (e.g., scoliosis, kyphosis, spondylolisthesis).
   - **Permit extensive decompression of the neural elements**. Extensive spinal decompression procedures may create spinal instability. Addition of spinal instrumentation and fusion prevents development of postsurgical spinal deformities and recurrent spinal stenosis.

2. Why is surgical stabilization of the spine considered a two-stage process?
   In the short term, stabilization of the spine is provided by spinal implants. However, in the long term, spinal implants may fail due to repetitive stress unless a spinal fusion is performed to provide long-term stability.

3. What is meant by the terms *tension band principle* and *load-sharing concept*?
   - A tension band is a portion of a construct that is subjected to tensile stresses during loading. In the normal spine, the posterior spinal musculature maintains normal sagittal spinal alignment through application of dorsal tension forces against the intact anterior spinal column. This is termed the **tension band principle**. The posterior spinal musculature can function as a tension band only if the anterior spinal column is structurally intact.
   - Biomechanical studies have shown that in the normal lumbar spine approximately 80% of axial load is carried by the anterior spinal column and the remaining 20% is transmitted through the posterior spinal column. This relationship is termed the **load-sharing concept** (Fig. 29.1).

4. What is the relevance of the load-sharing concept to the selection of appropriate spinal implants?
   Load sharing between an instrumentation construct and the vertebral column is a function of the ratio of the axial stiffness of the spinal instrumentation and the axial stiffness of the vertebral column. If the anterior spinal column is incompetent, the entire axial load must pass through the posterior spinal implant. In the absence of adequate anterior column support, normal physiologic loads exceed the strength of posterior spinal implant systems. In this situation, posterior spinal implants will fail by fatigue, permanent deformation, or implant migration through bone. Thus it is critical to reconstruct an incompetent anterior spinal column when using posterior spinal implant systems.

POSTERIOR SPINAL INSTRUMENTATION

5. Name three posterior spinal instrumentation systems that are considered to be the precursors of contemporary posterior spinal instrumentation systems.
   Harrington instrumentation, Luque instrumentation, and Cotrel-Dubousset instrumentation.

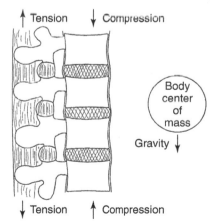

Fig. 29.1 Anterior column load sharing and the posterior tension band principle.

6. **What is Harrington instrumentation?**

The initial instrumentation developed by Dr. Paul Harrington consisted of a single rod with ratchets on one end in combination with a single hook at each end of the rod. Distraction forces were applied to obtain and maintain correction of spinal deformities. This system was introduced in 1960 in Texas for treatment of postpolio scoliosis and was utilized to treat various spinal problems, including idiopathic scoliosis, for more than 25 years. Shortcomings of this system included the need for postoperative immobilization to prevent hook dislodgement and the inability to correct and maintain sagittal plane alignment. Various modifications were introduced to address these problems, including square-ended hooks, use of compression hooks along a convex rod, and use of supplemental wire fixation (Fig. 29.2).

7. **What is Luque instrumentation?**

In the 1980s, Dr. Edwardo Luque from Mexico introduced a system that provided segmental fixation consisting of wires placed beneath the lamina at multiple spinal levels. Wires were tightened around rods placed along both

Fig. 29.2 (A and B) Harrington instrumentation. (A: From Winter RB, Lonstein JE, Denis F, et al. Atlas of Spine Surgery. Philadelphia, PA: Saunders; 1995. B: From Errico TJ, Lonner BS, Moulton AW. Surgical Management of Spinal Deformities. Philadelphia, PA: Saunders; 2009.)

sides of the lamina. Corrective forces were distributed over multiple levels, thereby decreasing the risk of fixation failure. The increased stability provided by this construct eliminated the need for postoperative braces or casts. The ability to translate the spine to a precontoured rod provided improved control of sagittal plane alignment compared with Harrington instrumentation (Fig. 29.3).

8. **What is Cotrel-Dubousset instrumentation?**

In 1984 Drs. Cotrel and Dubousset from France introduced their segmental fixation system, which became known as the CD system. It consisted of multiple hooks and screws placed along a knurled rod. The use of multiple fixation points permitted selective application of compression and distraction forces along the same rod by altering hook direction. A rod rotation maneuver was introduced in an attempt to provide improved three-dimensional correction of scoliosis. Rod contouring permitted improved correction of the sagittal contour of the spine. The stable segmental fixation provided by this system obviated the need for postoperative immobilization (Fig. 29.4).

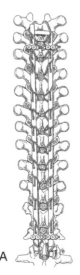
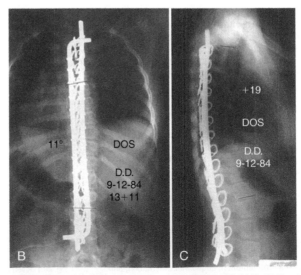

Fig. 29.3 (A–C) Luque instrumentation. (From Winter RB, Lonstein JE, Denis F, et al. Atlas of Spine Surgery. Philadelphia, PA: Saunders; 1995.)

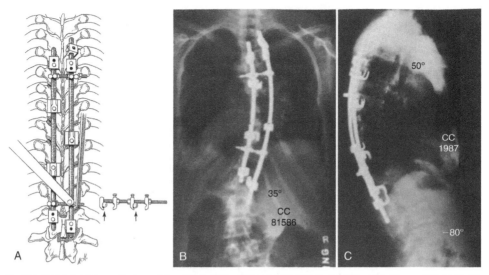

Fig. 29.4 (A–C) Cotrel-Dubousset instrumentation. (A: From Winter RB, Lonstein JE, Denis F, et al. Atlas of Spine Surgery. Philadelphia, PA: Saunders; 1995. B and C: From Lonstein JE, Bradford DS, Winter RB, et al. Moe's Textbook of Scoliosis and Other Spinal Deformities. 3rd ed. Philadelphia, PA: Saunders; 1995.)

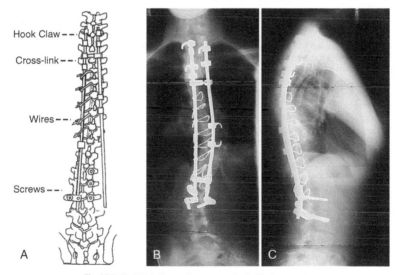

Fig. 29.5 (A–C) Hybrid posterior segmental spinal instrumentation.

9. **What is meant by the term posterior segmental spinal fixation?**

Posterior segmental spinal fixation is a general term used to describe a variety of rod-based posterior spinal instrumentation systems that attach to the spine at multiple anchor points throughout the instrumented spinal segments. Pedicle screws are the most commonly used **anchor type**, but hooks, wires, cables, and bands also play a role in specific clinical scenarios. A complete implant assembly is termed a **spinal construct**. A spinal instrumentation constructs consist of **longitudinal members** (rods, plates, plate/rod combinations) on each side of the spine, which may be connected transversely by cross-linking devices to increase construct stability. Rod-to-rod connectors and offset connectors may be used to longitudinally connect multiple rods within a spinal construct. Various corrective forces can be applied to the spine by means of segmental anchors, including compression, distraction, rotation, cantilever bending, and translation. The Isola system, developed by Dr. Marc Asher and colleagues, popularized the integration of hook, wire, and screw fixation within a single implant construct. Such implant constructs are referred to as **hybrid constructs** (Fig. 29.5).

10. Describe the use of hook anchors in posterior segmental spinal constructs.

Hook anchors may be placed above or below the T1–T10 transverse processes, under the thoracic facet joints, and above or below the thoracic and lumbar laminae. When blades of adjacent hooks face each other, this is termed a **claw configuration**. Compression forces can be applied to adjacent opposing hooks, thereby securing the hooks to the posterior elements. A claw may be composed of hooks at a single spinal level (intrasegmental claw) or adjacent levels (intersegmental claw). Hooks placed in a claw configuration provide more secure fixation than a single hook anchor.

11. Describe the use of flexible anchors such as wires, cables, and bands in posterior segmental spinal constructs.

Wires, cables, and polyethylene bands may be used at any level of the spine. Potential anchorage sites include the base of the spinous process, underneath the lamina (sublaminar position), or underneath the transverse process (subtransverse position). Spinous process and subtransverse anchors remain outside the spinal canal. Sublaminar anchor placement requires careful preparation of the cephalad and caudad interlaminar spaces to minimize the risk of neurologic injury as devices are passed beneath the lamina and dorsal to the neural elements. Specialized clamps may be used to attach polyethylene bands to spinal rods to aid in correction of spinal deformities.

12. Describe the use of pedicle screw anchors in posterior spinal constructs.

Pedicle screw anchors are used throughout the thoracic and lumbar spinal regions and have become the most widely utilized spinal anchor type. Advantages of pedicle screws include secure fixation, the ability to apply forces to both the anterior and posterior columns of the spine from a posterior approach, and the capability to achieve fixation when lamina are deficient. The disadvantages of pedicle screws include technical challenges related to screw placement and the potential for neurologic, vascular, and visceral injury due to misplaced screws. Pedicle screws may be broadly classified as monoaxial (fixed head screws), polyaxial (mobile head screws), uniplanar (screw heads allow cranial-caudal angulation but restrict motion in the medial-lateral direction), or bolts (require a separate connector for attachment to the longitudinal member) (Figs. 29.6 and 29.7).

13. What are the anatomic landmarks for placement of pedicle screws in the thoracic and lumbar spinal regions?

- In the thoracic region, the pedicle entry site is determined by referencing the transverse process, the superior articular process, and the pars interarticularis. The exact position of the entry site is adjusted depending on the specific level of the thoracic spine and whether the screw trajectory is straight-forward (screw trajectory parallels the superior vertebral endplate of the instrumented vertebra) or anatomic (screw trajectory is caudally directed along the sagittal anatomic pedicle axis). Thoracic screws are directed medially, and angulation varies according to spinal level.

- In the lumbar region, the entry site for screw placement is located at the upslope where the transverse process joins the superior articular process just lateral to the pars interarticularis. This site can be approximated by making a line along the midpoint of the transverse process and a second line along the lateral border of the superior articular process. The crossing point of these two lines defines the entry site to the pedicle (Fig. 29.8). Lumbar pedicle screws have a lateral to medial trajectory, with medial angulation increasing from L1 to S1. Recently, a modified trajectory for lumbar screw placement, the cortical bone trajectory, has been introduced. This entry point is more medially located than for a standard pedicle screw and is located at the inferior aspect of the pars interarticularis. The screw trajectory is from medial to lateral in the axial plane and caudal to cranial in the sagittal plane. Those who advocate this approach generally espouse the benefits of reduced lateral dissection to expose the screw entry site.

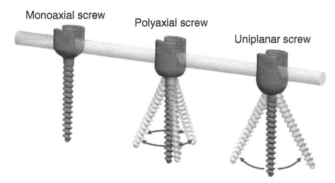

Fig. 29.6 Kinematics of monoaxial, polyaxial, and uniplanar screw constructs. (From Liu PY, Lai PL, Lin CL. A biomechanical investigation of different screw head designs for vertebral derotation in scoliosis surgery. Spine J 2017;17:1171–1179, Fig. 1, p. 1172.)

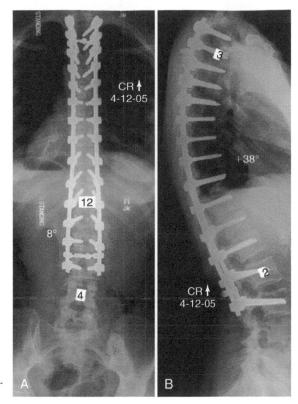

Fig. 29.7 Pedicle screw-based instrumentation construct. (From Buchowksi JM, Kuhns CA, Bridwell KH, et al. Surgical management of posttraumatic thoracolumbar kyphosis. Spine J 2008;8:666–677.)

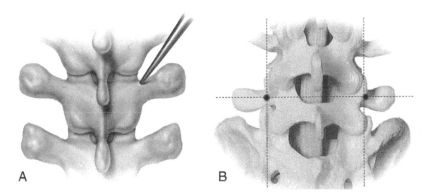

Fig. 29.8 Landmarks for pedicle screw placement. (A) Thoracic spine. (B) Lumbar spine. (Courtesy DePuy Spine, Inc.)

14. **What is dynamic stabilization of the spine?**

    Dynamic stabilization refers to the concept of placing spine anchors (most often pedicle screws) and connecting these anchors with a flexible longitudinal member (e.g., rod, cable, spring, cord, moveable screw head), usually without spinal fusion. The goal of this type of implant is to constrain but not eliminate motion. Proponents of this concept believe this type of implant will produce less stress on the adjacent spinal segments and may prevent some of the complications observed following spinal fusion (e.g., adjacent-level degenerative changes). Opponents worry that, without concurrent spinal arthrodesis, these implants may loosen or fail prematurely and require revision surgery. Currently, there are limited data to prove or disprove the scientific validity of this concept (Fig. 29.9). As spinal nomenclature has evolved, the term dynamic stabilization system has been replaced by **semi-rigid spinal system** to more clearly distinguish these types of implants from traditional rigid pedicle screw systems.

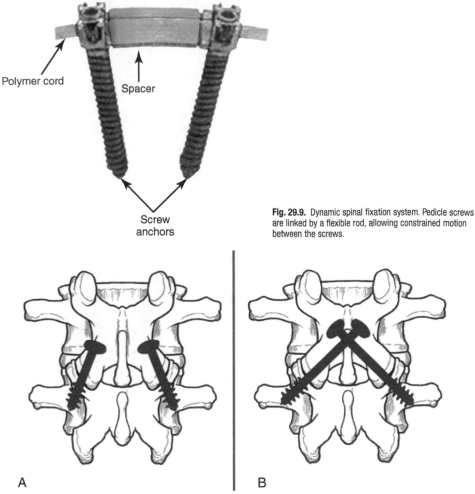

Polymer cord

Spacer

Screw
anchors

Fig. 29.9. Dynamic spinal fixation system. Pedicle screws are linked by a flexible rod, allowing constrained motion between the screws.

A

B

Fig. 29.10 Posterior facet screw fixation. (A) Boucher transfacet technique. (B) Magerl translaminar transfacet technique. (From Bonaldi G, Brembilla C, Cianfoni A. Minimally-invasive posterior lumbar stabilization for degenerative low back pain and sciatica. A review. Eur J Rad 2015;84:789–798, Fig. 5, p. 794.)

15. What is facet-based stabilization?

Facet-based stabilization of lumbar spine motion segments using screws provides an alternative to pedicle screw-rod systems in certain patients. These techniques are most applicable to one- or two-level lumbar fusion procedures in patients with an intact spinous process, lamina, facet joints, and a stable anterior spinal column. For example, facet-based stabilization could provide an option for posterior spinal stabilization following anterior or lateral lumbar interbody fusion in patients who do not require extensive direct posterior spinal decompression. Two common trajectories for lumbar facet screw placement are the Boucher technique and the Magerl technique. In the Boucher technique, one screw is placed on each side entering the lamina to cross the facets in a medial to lateral trajectory and ending in the superior aspect of the inferior pedicle (Fig. 29.10A). In the Magerl technique, screws enter from the side of the spinous process, penetrate the contralateral lamina, cross the facet joint, and end in the base of the transverse process (see Fig. 29.10B). The Magerl technique allows use of a longer length screw and provides increased fixation strength compared to the Boucher technique.

16. What are interspinous implants?

Interspinous implants are used for (1) treatment of symptomatic lumbar spinal stenosis without fusion, and (2) as a method for immobilization and stabilization of spinal segments as an adjunct to fusion. Interspinous implants used for treatment of lumbar spinal stenosis are inserted between adjacent spinous processes to slightly distract

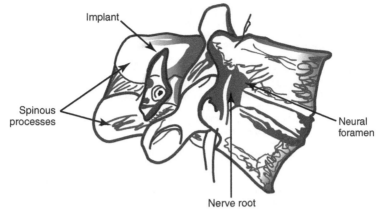

Fig. 29.11 Interspinous implant.

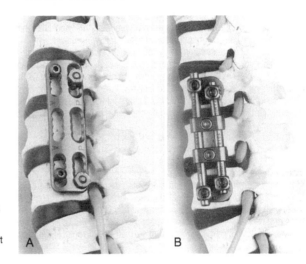

Fig. 29.12 Anterior extracolumnar implants. (A) Plate system and (B) rod system. (From Devlin VJ, Pitt DD. The evolution of surgery of the anterior spinal column. Spine State Art Rev 1998;12:493–528.)

the spinous processes apart and/or limit spinal extension thereby relieving position-dependent spinal stenosis symptoms. Interspinous implants used as an adjunct to fusion attach to the spinous processes by various means and are used at a single spinal level to provide segmental fixation and promote fusion (Fig. 29.11).

ANTERIOR SPINAL INSTRUMENTATION

17. What are the two main categories of anterior spinal instrumentation?
   - Anterior spinal implants may be broadly classified as extracolumnar or intracolumnar implants. **Extracolumnar implants** are located on the external aspect of the vertebral body and span one or more adjacent vertebral motion segments. Extracolumnar implants consist of vertebral body screws connected to a longitudinal member, most commonly consisting of either a plate or a rod. Extracolumnar implants are placed on the lateral aspect of the thoracic and lumbar vertebral bodies with screws directed in a coronal plane trajectory. An exception occurs at the L5–S1 level where extracolumnar implants must be placed in an anterior midline location with screws directed in an anterior to posterior direction due to anatomic constraints created by the vascular structures at this level.
   - **Intracolumnar implants** consist of implants that reside within the contour of the vertebral bodies. Implant options include bone, metal, or other synthetic materials that are capable of bearing loads. Intracolumnar implants may or may not possess potential for biologic incorporation within the anterior spinal column. Two types of intracolumnar implants are intervertebral body fusion devices and vertebral body replacement devices.

18. Contrast the utility of anterior plate systems and anterior rod systems.
   - **Anterior plate systems** (Fig. 29.12A) are useful for short-segment spinal disorders (one or two spinal levels). Tumors, burst fractures, and degenerative spinal disorders requiring anterior fusion over one or two levels are

indications for use of an anterior plate system. The use of a plate system is problematic when significant coronal or sagittal plane deformity exists or when multiple anterior vertebral segments require fixation. Technical difficulties arise because restoration of spinal alignment is required prior to plate application in the presence of significant spinal deformity.

- **Anterior rod systems** (see Fig. 29.12B) offer advantages in comparison to plate systems. In short-segment spinal problems, anterior rod systems permit corrective forces to be applied directly to spinal segments, thereby restoring spinal alignment. For example, in the presence of a kyphotic deformity secondary to a burst fracture, initial distraction provides deformity correction and facilitates placement of an intracolumnar implant. Subsequent compression of the anterior graft or cage restores anterior load sharing and enhances arthrodesis. In long-segment spinal problems (e.g., scoliosis) single or double rod systems can be customized to the specific spinal deformity requiring correction.

19. What are some guidelines for placement of vertebral body screws when using an anterior plate or rod system?
The screws should be parallel to the vertebral endplates. In the axial plane, the screws should be parallel with or angle away from the vertebral canal. The screw tips should purchase the far cortex of the vertebral body but should not protrude more than 5 mm beyond this point (Fig. 29.13).

20. What are some different types of intervertebral body fusion devices and what surgical approaches are used for device insertion?
Intervertebral body fusion devices restore immediate mechanical stability to the anterior spinal column and provide a favorable environment for spinal fusion following discectomy. These devices are filled with a variety of graft materials and are most commonly used in conjunction with some type of supplemental fixation. Intervertebral body fusion devices are available in a range of materials including titanium, carbon fiber, polyetheretherketone (PEEK), and cortical bone. Some cage designs possess integrated fixation or expansion features. Intervertebral body fusion devices are designed to facilitate insertion via specific surgical approaches including posterior lumbar interbody fusion (PLIF), transforaminal lumbar interbody fusion (TLIF), lateral lumbar interbody fusion (LLIF), and anterior lumbar interbody fusion (ALIF) approaches (Figs. 29.14 and 29.15A,B).

21. What are some different types of vertebral body replacement devices and what surgical approaches are used for device insertion?
Vertebral body replacement devices are used to reconstruct the anterior spinal column following corpectomy at one or more spinal levels. Two main design types are available: static and expandable. Vertebral body replacement devices are manufactured from a range of materials including titanium, carbon fiber, and PEEK. Various shapes are available including round, oblong, and rectangular. Vertebral body replacement devices may be inserted through a direct anterior or lateral surgical approach or through a single incision posterolateral approach, which includes resection of the pedicle to provide access to the anterior spinal column. Minimally invasive approaches have been developed for placement of vertebral body replacement devices to limit surgical approach related

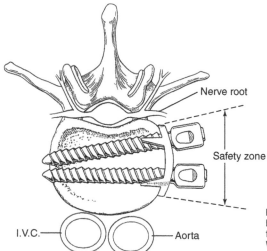

Nerve root

Safety zone

I.V.C.

Aorta

Fig. 29.13 Correct placement of anterior vertebral body screws. (From Zindrick MR, Selby D. Lumbar spine fusion: Different types and indications. In: Wiesel SW, Weinstein JN, Herkowitz H, et al., editors. The Lumbar Spine. 2nd ed. Philadelphia, PA: Saunders; 1996.)

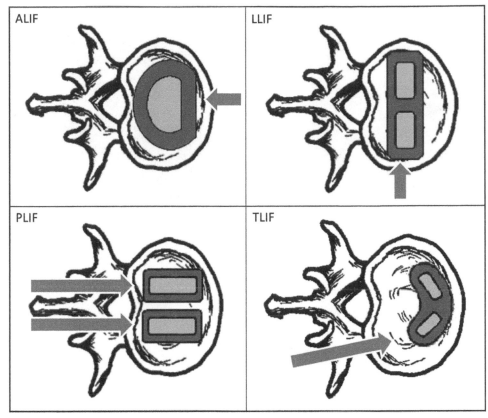

Fig. 29.14 Common surgical approaches for lumbar interbody fusion and typical device designs for each approach. *ALIF,* Anterior lumbar interbody fusion; *PLIF,* posterior lumbar interbody fusion; *LLIF,* lateral lumbar interbody fusion; *TLIF,* transforaminal lumbar interbody fusion. (From Peck JH, Kavlock KD, Showalter BL, et al. Mechanical performance of lumbar intervertebral body fusion devices: An analysis of data submitted to the Food and Drug Administration. J Biomech 2018;78:87–93, Fig. 1, p. 88.)

morbidity. The optimal approach depends on a range of factors including the location and type of spinal pathology requiring treatment and surgeon experience (Fig. 29.16).

22. Describe three potential functions of intracolumnar implants.
    Intracolumnar implants may be differentiated based on their intended function:
    - **Promote fusion**. Intracolumnar implants that have potential for biologic incorporation include autograft bone (e.g., ilium, fibula), structural allograft bone (tibia, femur, humerus), and synthetic cages (titanium mesh, carbon fiber, PEEK) filled with bone graft. Such implants are typically used after discectomy or corpectomy to reconstruct the anterior spinal column and promote spinal fusion.
    - **Function as a spacer**. Certain intracolumnar implants (e.g., polymethylmethacrylate [PMMA]) are intended to function as an anterior column spacer and lack potential for biologic incorporation.
    - **Preserve motion**. Implantation of a total disc arthroplasty device following discectomy is an option for reconstruction of the disc space and can maintain segmental mobility, stability, and disc space height without fusion.

23. When is PMMA used as a spacer to reconstruct an anterior spinal column defect?
    Currently, PMMA is used in two situations:
    - **Anterior spinal reconstruction of metastatic vertebral body lesions in patients with a finite lifespan.** When used for this purpose, PMMA is subject to tensile failure and loosening secondary to development of a fibrous membrane at the cement-bone interface.
    - **Reconstruction of osteoporotic compression fractures.** Vertebroplasty and kyphoplasty procedures involve the injection of PMMA into the vertebral bodies to alleviate pain secondary to acute and subacute fracture.

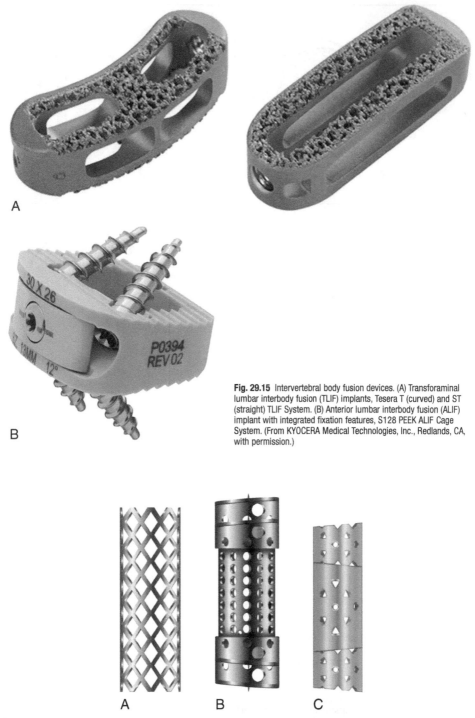

Fig. 29.15 Intervertebral body fusion devices. (A) Transforaminal lumbar interbody fusion (TLIF) implants, Tesera T (curved) and ST (straight) TLIF System. (B) Anterior lumbar interbody fusion (ALIF) implant with integrated fixation features, S128 PEEK ALIF Cage System. (From KYOCERA Medical Technologies, Inc., Redlands, CA, with permission.)

Fig. 29.16 Vertebral body replacement devices. (A) Titanium mesh, (B) expandable titanium cage, and (C) stackable modular polyetheretherketone. (From Kim DH, Henn JS, Vaccaro AR, et al. Surgical Anatomy and Techniques to the Spine. Philadelphia, PA: Saunders; 2006.)

KEY POINTS

1. Spinal implants function to maintain or restore spinal alignment, stabilize spinal segments, and enhance spinal fusion.
2. Short-term stabilization of the spine is provided by spinal implants and long-term stabilization of the spine is traditionally provided by fusion.
3. Components of a contemporary posterior spinal instrumentation construct consist of:
   a. Spinal anchors (screws, hooks, wires, cables, bands)
   b. Longitudinal elements (rods) on each side of the spine
   c. Transverse connectors (cross-linking devices)
   d. Rod-to-rod connectors and offset connectors to longitudinally link multiple rods when necessary
4. Reconstruction of the load-bearing capacity of the anterior spinal column is critical to successful application of spinal instrumentation.

Websites
1. History of surgery for correction of spinal deformity: http://www.medscape.com/viewarticle/448306
2. Thoracic pedicle screw fixation for spinal deformity: http://www.medscape.com/viewarticle/448311

BIBLIOGRAPHY

1. Davis, W., Allouni, A. K., Mankad, K., Prezzi, D., Elias, T., Rankine, J., et al. (2013). Modern spinal instrumentation. Part 1: Normal spinal implants. *Clinical Radiology, 68*, 64–74.
2. Harms, J., Tabasso, G., & Cinanni, R. (1999). *Instrumented Spinal Surgery: Principles and Techniques*. New York, NY: Thieme.
3. Harrington, P. R. (1988). The history and development of Harrington instrumentation. *Clinical Orthopaedics, 227*, 3–5.
4. Vaccaro, D. H., Vaccaro, A. R., Dickman, C. A., Cho, D., Lee, S., & Kim, I. (Eds.). (2013). *Surgical Anatomy and Techniques to the Spine* (2nd ed.). Philadelphia, PA: Saunders.
5. Kim, Y. J., Lenke, L. G., Kim, J., Bridwell, K. H., Cho, S. K., Cheh, G., et al. (2006). Comparative analysis of pedicle screw versus hybrid instrumentation in posterior spinal fusion of adolescent idiopathic scoliosis. *Spine, 31*, 291–298.
6. Steinmetz, M. P., & Benzel, E. C. (Eds.). (2017). *Benzel's Spine Surgery. Techniques, Complication Avoidance, and Management* (4th ed.). Philadelphia, PA: Elsevier.
7. Verma, K., Boniello, A., & Rihn J. (2016). Emerging techniques for posterior fixation of the lumbar spine. *Journal of the American Academy of Orthopaedic Surgeons, 24*, 357–364.

CHAPTER 30

INSTRUMENTATION AND FUSION AT THE LUMBOSACRAL JUNCTION AND PELVIS

Khaled M. Kebaish, MD, FRCSC and Vincent J. Devlin, MD

1. What is the lumbosacral junction?

The lumbosacral junction consists of the L5 vertebra, the sacrum, and the articulations between both segments, consisting of the anteriorly located L5–S1 disc and posteriorly located L5–S1 facet joints. It also includes the ligamentous and muscular structures supporting this important motion segment.

2. Why is the lumbosacral junction important?

- It is the transition between the mobile lumbar spine and the pelvic girdle, which has the main function of transferring the weight from the axial skeleton to the lower appendicular skeleton.
- Substantial biomechanical forces are concentrated at the lumbosacral junction. If fusion is extended to this area, there is a strong lever arm that transmits flexion, extension, and torsional forces from the spine above. These forces cause significant strain that increase the risk of fixation failure and pseudarthrosis.

3. What is the lumbosacral pivot point?

McCord et al (1) introduced the concept of the lumbosacral pivot point, which is defined as the middle of the osteo-oligamentous column at the junction between L5 and S1. The farther that sacropelvic instrumentation progresses anterior to this point, the more stable the construct. Iliac fixation techniques, including traditional iliac screws and S2 alar-iliac (S2AI) screws, provide the most stable method of achieving sacropelvic fixation because they extend fixation for a greater distance anterior to the lumbosacral pivot point than other techniques. S1 screws provide the least resistance to flexion moments compared with other sacropelvic fixation techniques. The addition of a second point of sacral fixation provides improved fixation compared to use of S1 pedicle fixation alone (Fig. 30.1).

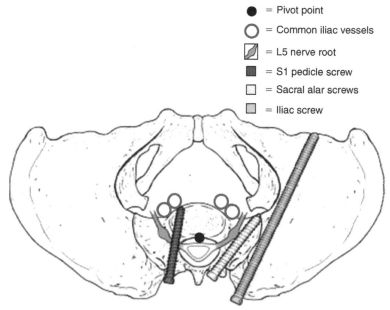

● = Pivot point

○ = Common iliac vessels

▧ = L5 nerve root

■ = S1 pedicle screw

□ = Sacral alar screws

▨ = Iliac screw

Fig. 30.1 Sacropelvic fixation options in relation to the lumbosacral pivot point and adjacent critical structures. (From Polly DW, Latta LL. Spinopelvic fixation biomechanics. Semin Spine Surg 2004;16:101–106.)

4. **What are the most common indications for L5–S1 fusion?**
   - Degenerative disorders involving the L5–S1 level
   - Adult idiopathic or de novo scoliosis
   - Neuromuscular spinal deformities especially when associated with pelvic obliquity
   - L5–S1 spondylolisthesis
   - Infections and tumors requiring lumbosacral spinal reconstruction
   - Fractures involving the lumbosacral junction
   - Revision spinal procedures, especially when significant sagittal and/or coronal correction is required in the lower lumbar or lumbosacral spine

5. **What complications are associated with fusion across the lumbosacral junction?**
   - Pseudarthrosis
   - Loss of lumbar lordosis resulting in sagittal imbalance (flatback syndrome)
   - Recurrent or progressive spinal deformity
   - Instrumentation loosening or failure
   - Sacroiliac joint pain or arthrosis
   - Sacral stress fractures

6. **Why has the L5–S1 fusion traditionally had a higher rate of nonunion and/or instrumentation failure?**
   - An unfavorable biomechanical environment exists here because the lumbosacral junction is a transition zone between the highly mobile L5–S1 disc and the relatively immobile sacropelvis.
   - Tremendous loads are transferred across the lumbosacral junction (up to 11 times body weight) as axial weight-bearing forces are transmitted from the vertebral column to the pelvis.
   - The oblique orientation of the L5–S1 disc results in increased shear forces across this level.
   - The sacrum is mostly cancellous bone, which provides suboptimal fixation.
   - The large diameter and relatively short S1 pedicles provide less secure screw purchase compared with proximal vertebral levels.

7. **What is the 80–20 rule of Professor Harms?**
   Biomechanical studies of the lumbosacral region have demonstrated that approximately 80% of axial load is transmitted through the anterior spinal column and the remaining 20% is transmitted through the posterior column. Spinal fusion and instrumentation procedures that do not restore the anterior column load-sharing property across the lumbosacral junction are destined for failure.

8. **Why is it more difficult to achieve a successful fusion at the L5–S1 level when spinal instrumentation constructs extend from T10 to sacrum compared with L4 to sacrum?**
   Long-segment fusion constructs (i.e., more than four levels) that include the sacrum, especially those that cross the thoracolumbar junction, have a higher rate of failure than short-segment constructs (i.e., L4–S1). Because of the longer lever arm exerted by the proximal spine on the distal sacral instrumentation, the forces placed on the distal sacral fixation are increased. The degree of strain on the S1 screws increases as the number of segments immobilized above the sacrum increases. These biomechanical factors increase the risk of distal fixation failure.

9. **What are the posterior instrumentation options when arthrodesis is performed across the lumbosacral junction?**
   Posterior implant fixation in the sacrum and pelvis can be categorized based on the three anatomic zones (Fig. 30.2) of the sacropelvic unit:
   - **Zone 1:** S1 vertebral body and upper margin of the sacral ala.
   - **Zone 2:** inferior margin of the sacral ala, the middle and lower sacrum, and coccyx.
   - **Zone 3:** composed of the ilium bilaterally.
     Fixation in zone 3 provides the greatest construct stability as it allows placement of instrumentation farthest anterior to the pivot point. Currently, the most common methods used to obtain implant fixation in the sacrum and/or pelvis are sacral pedicle screws and iliac fixation techniques, including iliac screw fixation and S2AI screw fixation. Below is a detailed list of the options for achieving fixation in the sacrum and pelvis, including methods that are of historic value only.

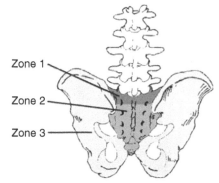

Zone 1

Zone 2

Zone 3

Fig. 30.2 The fixation zones of the sacropelvic unit. (From O'Brien MF, Kuklo TR, Lenke LG. Sacropelvic instrumentation: Anatomic and biomechanical zones of fixation. Semin Spine Surg 2004;16:76–90.)

Zone I options:
- S1 pedicle screws
- S1 tricortical pedicle screws
- L5–S1 transfacet screws
- Dunn-McCarthy S-rod fixation

Zone II options:
- S1 alar screws
- Intrasacral Jackson rod fixation

Zone III options:
- Galveston L-rod fixation
- Iliac screw fixation
- S2AI screw fixation
- Transiliac bar
- Iliosacral screw fixation

10. **Describe the different techniques for S1 pedicle screw placement.**

The dorsal bony cortex at the base of the superior S1 articular process is removed with a rongeur or a burr. A pedicle probe is directed toward the S1 endplate perpendicular to the sacrum and angled medially. Careful penetration of the anterior cortex of the sacrum permits bicortical fixation and increases screw purchase. Screw purchase can be further enhanced by directing the S1 pedicle screw superiorly to engage the anterior margin of the endplate of S1 in the region of the sacral promontory and is termed *tricortical fixation* (posterior sacral cortex, anterior sacral cortex, and superior endplate cortex). Due to the cancellous nature of the S1 pedicle, unicortical screws (short screws that do not engage the anterior sacral cortex) provide less secure fixation and are prone to loosening and failure (Fig. 30.3A).

11. **Describe the technique of laterally directed sacral screw placement.**

Laterally directed sacral screws (alar screws) may be placed at the level of S1 and/or S2. The S1 alar screw entrance point is located just distal to the L5–S1 facet joint in line with the dorsal S1 neural foramen. The S2 alar screw entrance point is located between the dorsal S1 and S2 neural foramina. A starting point is created with a burr or drill in this area. A probe is placed through the sacrum until it contacts the anterior sacral cortex. The ideal trajectory is 35° laterally and parallel with the S1 endplate. Length of this pilot hole is determined with a depth gauge. The anterior sacral cortex is then perforated in a controlled fashion to achieve a bicortical fixation (see Fig. 30.3B).

12. **What structures are at risk when a screw is placed through the anterior cortex of the sacrum?**

S1 pedicle screws that are medially directed and parallel to the upper S1 endplate or directed toward the sacral promontory do not endanger any neurovascular structures with the exception of the middle sacral artery and vein. If an S1 pedicle screw is inserted in a straightforward direction without medial angulation, the L5 nerve root is at risk, where it crosses the anterior sacrum. Screws placed laterally at the S1 level have greater potential to injure critical structures including the lumbosacral trunk, internal iliac vein, and sacroiliac joint. Laterally directed screws at the S2 level have potential to injure the colon, which may be adjacent to the lateral sacrum in this region (see Fig. 30.1).

13. **When is it appropriate to perform a lumbosacral fusion that extends to the sacrum with only bilateral S1 pedicle screw fixation?**

Short-segment instrumented fusion extending from the lower lumbar spine (i.e., L3, L4, or L5) to the sacrum using bilateral S1 pedicle screws as the only distal fixation anchors is likely to be successful in the absence of significant spinal deformity, prior surgery at the L5–S1 level, or osteoporosis. A typical instrumentation construct

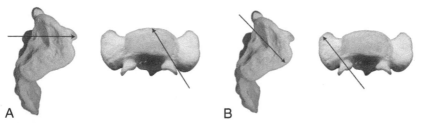

Fig. 30.3 Sacral screw options. (A) S1 pedicle screw and (B) S1 alar screw. (From Kim DH, Henn JS, Vaccaro AR, et al. Surgical Anatomy and Techniques of the Spine. Saunders; 2006, p. 241.)

consists of bilateral lumbar pedicle screws at each proximal level undergoing fusion in addition to bilateral bicortical or tricortical S1 pedicle screws. Intervertebral body fusion using structural allograft or fusion cages is added when restoration of anterior column load sharing is indicated.

14. **What types of spinal implants are used to provide structural support to the anterior spinal column when arthrodesis is performed across the lumbosacral junction?**
Intracolumnar implants are used to reconstruct the anterior spinal column and restore anterior column load sharing when arthrodesis is performed across the lumbosacral junction. Options for interbody support include structural allograft bone (most commonly femoral allograft) or intervertebral body fusion devices (e.g., titanium mesh, carbon fiber, polyetheretherketone [PEEK]) used in combination with bone graft materials, including autograft, allograft, or biologics (e.g., bone morphogenic protein). Intervertebral body fusion devices may be implanted at the lumbosacral junction through a posterior transforaminal approach or an anterior surgical approach. When an anterior surgical approach is performed, supplemental fixation is commonly utilized. Options for supplemental fixation at L5–S1 include large-diameter titanium cancellous retention screws and washers or low-profile anterior plates.

15. **What are the indications for use of S1 pedicle screw fixation in combination with additional iliac fixation?**
Iliac fixation is indicated whenever the biomechanical forces across the lumbosacral junction are expected to exceed the ability of bilateral S1 pedicle screws to provide the stability required to achieve a solid arthrodesis across the lumbosacral junction. Indications for use of iliac fixation in combination with S1 pedicle screw fixation include:
- Long spinal fusions that extend to the sacrum (i.e., four or more fusion levels, any L5–S1 fusion extending to the thoracolumbar junction)
- When correction of pelvic obliquity is required (e.g., neuromuscular scoliosis)
- Stabilization and/or reduction and fusion of high-grade spondylolisthesis (i.e., grade 3 or higher)
- Complex lumbar revision surgery (e.g., osteotomy for sagittal imbalance syndrome; decompression and fusion for distal degeneration and stenosis below a multi-level fusion ending at L5)
- When partial or complete sacrectomy is indicated (e.g., sacral tumors or fractures)
- Sacral fractures with spinopelvic dissociation
- Multilevel fusion procedures in patients with osteopenia/osteoporosis

16. **Describe the technique for placement of the traditional iliac screws.**
In the traditional technique, the posterior superior iliac spine (PSIS) is palpated, and the subcutaneous tissue is dissected off the lumbosacral fascia bilaterally toward the PSIS using Cobb elevators and Bovie electrocautery. A longitudinal or oblique incision is made in the fascia overlying the PSIS. The incision is extended both cephalad and caudad along the ilium with respect to the PSIS. A rongeur or burr is used to breach the cortex overlying the PSIS at the level of S2–S3, approximately 1 cm from the distal ilium. The amount of bone resected depends on the bulkiness of the implant, and the goal should be to minimize implant prominence. A pedicle finder (Fig. 30.4A) is used to develop the path into the ilium, which extends toward the anterior inferior iliac spine (AIIS). This trajectory averages 25° lateral to midsagittal plane and 30°–35° caudal to the transverse plane toward the ASIS. Fluoroscopy can be used to confirm the screw path. Alternatively, placement of a finger into the sciatic notch provides an anatomic landmark to guide placement in the ilium. A blunt probe is used to verify that neither the medial nor lateral iliac crest cortex has been breached. Screw lengths are then measured and screws are inserted. Common screw sizes are 8–10 mm in diameter and 80–100 mm in length. Finally, the iliac screws must then be attached to the longitudinal rods of the main spinal construct, most commonly with the use of a modular connector system (see Fig. 30.4B). The connectors are tunneled anterior to the paraspinal muscles. A modification of the traditional iliac screw placement technique may be used to decrease screw prominence and position the screw head in a more medial position, thereby avoiding the need to use a modular connector to link the iliac screw to the longitudinal rod (see Fig. 30.4C). Minimally invasive iliac screw placement using fluoroscopy to visualize the iliac teardrop as a guide for screw placement has also been described (teardrop technique).

17. **Describe the open S2 alar-iliac (S2AI) technique.**
The placement of the S2AI screw should take place only after all other proximal points of fixation, including the S1 pedicle screws, have been secured. The position of the S1 and S2 dorsal foramina are identified using a Woodson elevator. An awl is used to breach the dorsal cortex over the starting point, located in line with the lateral edge of the S1 foramen and midway between S1 and S2 dorsal foramina (Fig. 30.5A). The most common S2AI trajectory averages 40° of lateral angulation in the transverse plane and 20°–30° of caudal angulation in the sagittal planes directed toward the AIIS. A 2.5-mm pelvic drill bit (extended length) is used to tap drill through the sacral ala, the SI joint, and into the ilium. This distance is roughly 30–45 mm in most patients. At this point, the drill bit is removed and replaced with a 3.2-mm drill bit to reduce the risk of breakage in harder bone and is advanced for a total depth of approximately 90–100 mm. Once the drill has reached the ilium, the drill itself is removed. A depth gauge is then inserted into the hole in order to determine the length of the screw. Next, a 1.45-mm guidewire is placed into the path created. Placement can be confirmed with intraoperative fluoroscopy. The path is then manually tapped over the guidewire using a cannulated tap, and an appropriate length screw size is placed

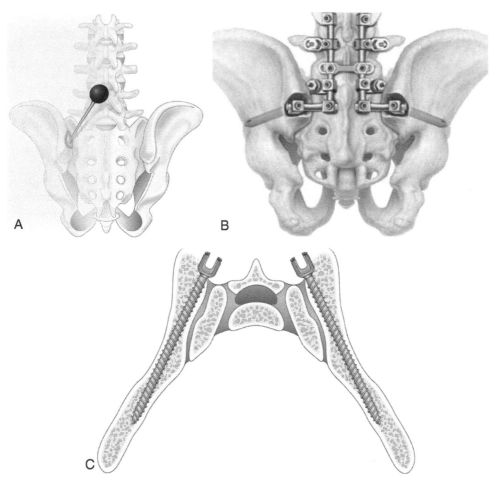

Fig. 30.4 (A) Following removal of bone overlying the posterior superior iliac spine, a blunt probe is introduced to establish the iliac screw pathway. (B) Traditional iliac screws are connected to longitudinal rods using modular connectors. (C) A modified iliac screw insertion technique minimizes screw prominence by medially positioning the screw head to decrease prominence and obviate need for a modular connector. (A and C: From George SG, Lebwohl NH, Pasquotti G, et al. Percutaneous and open iliac screw safety and accuracy using tactile technique with adjunctive anteroposterior fluoroscopy. Spine J 2018;18:1570, Fig. 3, p. 1572; 1577. Fig. 7, p. 1573. B: From Moshirfar A, Kebaish KM, Riley LH. Spinopelvic fixation in spine surgery. Semin Spine Surg 2009;21:55–61, Fig 2, p. 58.)

(see Fig. 30.5B–D). Screw sizes of 8–10 mm in diameter and 80–100 mm in length are most commonly used in adults. Because the screws are in line with the rest of the spinal construct, no additional cross-connectors are required for connection to the main construct (see Fig. 30.5E). Due to the more medial entry point compared to traditional iliac screws, S2AI screws have a lower profile and require less soft tissue dissection. With the S2AI technique, it is possible to place two screws at a single fixation site when necessary to optimize fixation.

18. Describe the percutaneous S2 alar-iliac (S2AI) technique.
   The S2AI technique is amenable to a minimally invasive percutaneous approach, and may be combined with mini-mally invasive percutaneous fixation of the lumbar spine depending on the surgical indication. The approach to the sacrum is a 3-cm midline incision at the level of the S1 and S2 dorsal foramen. The starting point is located in line with the lateral edge of the S1 foramen and midway between the S1 and S2 dorsal foramina. The trajectory is identified using standard anteroposterior (AP) and pelvic inlet fluoroscopic views. A Jamshidi needle is angled toward the AIIS and initially advanced 10–20 mm into the sacral ala. The ideal S2AI trajectory is the same as in the open procedure and averages 40° of lateral angulation in the transverse plane and 20°–30° of caudal angula-tion in the sagittal plane but varies with pelvic obliquity. The C-arm is oriented along the trajectory of the needle to verify its trajectory. Proper needle position is located in the center of the bony teardrop created by the overlap

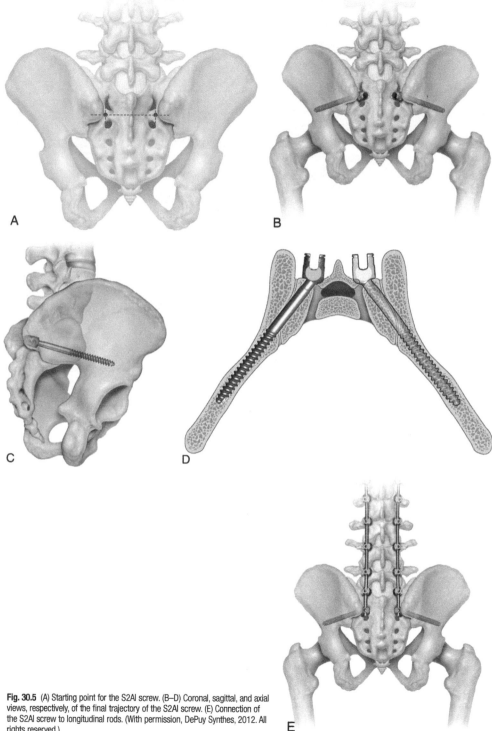

Fig. 30.5 (A) Starting point for the S2AI screw. (B–D) Coronal, sagittal, and axial views, respectively, of the final trajectory of the S2AI screw. (E) Connection of the S2AI screw to longitudinal rods. (With permission, DePuy Synthes, 2012. All rights reserved.)

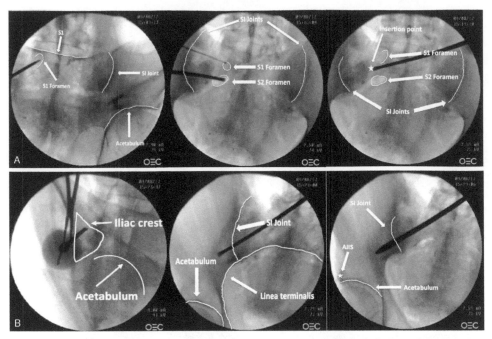

Fig. 30.6 (A) Determination of the insertion site for the S2 alar-iliac screw. *Left:* First, the location of the S1 foramen is identified using a standard probe. *White arrows* identify key anatomic landmarks including the S1 superior endplate, the left sacroiliac joint, and the left acetabulum. *Middle:* A second probe is used to locate the S2 foramen. *Right:* The insertion site *(white star)* is located 10 mm lateral from a midpoint between the previously identified S1 and S2. (B) Fluoroscopic verification of the trajectory and intrailiac screw positioning. *Left:* Once the insertion site has been identified, a probe is advanced so that its tip is centered in the iliac wing (teardrop) identified on the oblique obturator view. *Middle:* The angulation is determined by the anteroposterior view with the probe being directed laterally in the transverse plane and caudally in the sagittal plane. *Right:* The screw is advanced and directed toward the anterior inferior iliac spine *(white star)*. (From Yilmaz E, Abdul-Jabbar A, Tawfik T, et al. S2 alar-iliac screw insertion: Technical note with pictorial guide. World Neurosurg 2018;113:296–301, Fig. 2, p. 297; Fig. 4, p. 298.)

of the AIIS and the PSIS. This teardrop represents the bony channel extending from the PSIS to the ASIS within which the screws are positioned. Subsequent procedural steps are the same as open screw insertion: needle advancement across the sacroiliac joint and into the ilium, guidewire placement, tapping, and screw insertion (Fig. 30.6A,B).

19. **What risks are associated with traditional iliac screw fixation and S2AI screw fixation?**
    - Implant prominence: more common with traditional iliac screws than S2AI screws due to their more superficial location and frequent use of a modular connector
    - Neurovascular injury due to screw misplacement: potential for injury to superior gluteal artery, internal iliac vessels sciatic nerve, obturator nerve, lumbosacral plexus, and cluneal nerves
    - Violation of hip joint by misplaced screw with associated chondral injury
    - Sacroiliac joint pain

20. **What is transsacral fixation?**
    In cases of high-grade isthmic spondylolisthesis (grades 3 and 4), screws and/or bone grafts/cages may be placed obliquely across the L5–S1 disc space and obtain purchase in both the L5 and S1 vertebrae. Traditionally, a fibular graft is placed from either a posterior (from S1 into L5) or anterior approach (from L5 into S1). The addition of screw fixation from the upper sacrum across the L5–S1 disc space and into the L5 vertebral body increases distal screw fixation, increases the fusion rate, and decreases the risk of graft fracture.

21. **What is a transiliac (sacral) bar?**
    This type of fixation uses rod(s) that spans the sacrum passing horizontally from ilium to ilium. Initially, sacral bars were used for fixation of sacral fractures. They have been modified to serve as an anchor within the pelvis to form the basis for complex reconstruction procedures involving fusion across the lumbosacral region. Specialized connectors have been developed to link the transiliac bar with longitudinal rods anchored to proximal spinal levels. This technique is rarely used today.

22. **Describe the technique for placement of an intrasacral rod.**
    This technique is mainly of historic significance as it is rarely used today. A rod is inserted into the lateral sacral mass through the canal of a previously placed S1 pedicle screw. The rod and screw interlock within the sacrum providing secure fixation. The implants are buttressed by the posterior ilium. Fixation provided by this technique is superior to fixation provided by S1 screws alone.

23. **Is an external brace necessary to protect the sacropelvic instrumentation?**
    An external brace is rarely indicated when additional anchors (iliac or S2AI screws) are used in combination with S1 pedicle screws. Sacropelvic instrumentation is sufficiently stable and secure to obviate the need for a cumbersome external brace. However, if the surgeon desires to restrict motion across the lumbosacral junction to protect the S1 pedicle screws fixation, a thoracolumbosacral orthosis (TLSO) with a thigh cuff is required. Lumbar orthoses that do not immobilize the thigh will increase rather than decrease motion across the L5–S1 level.

24. **Summarize the techniques a surgeon can utilize to increase the rate of successful fusion across the L5–S1 segment.**
    - Avoid wide laminectomy at the L5–S1 level whenever possible as it decreases bone surface area available for posterior fusion.
    - Perform meticulous graft site preparation, including thorough decortication of all posterior bony elements, including sacral ala.
    - Use of adequate volumes and types of bone graft materials, including use of autograft and bone graft extenders such as demineralized bone matrices (DBM), as well as select use of bone morphogenic protein in high-risk patients.
    - Perform an L5–S1 interbody fusion with interbody structural support to restore anterior column load sharing and increase fusion surfaces.
    - Use multiple fixation points within the sacropelvic unit (S1 pedicle screws in combination with S2AI or traditional iliac screws).

KEY POINTS

1. S1 pedicle fixation is the most common sacral fixation technique utilized when performing fusion to the sacrum.
2. Some form of iliac fixation should be used to supplement S1 pedicle screws whenever the biomechanical forces across the lumbosacral junction are expected to exceed the ability of the S1 pedicle screws to provide the stable biomechanical environment needed to achieve solid arthrodesis.
3. The S2AI and iliac screws are the most protective and stable forms of sacropelvic fixation.
4. Structural interbody support at the L4–L5 and L5–S1 levels increases fusion rates and decreases the risk of construct failure when performing fusion to the sacrum.

Websites
1. Lumbosacral and sacropelvic fixation strategies: https://thejns.org/focus/view/journals/neurosurg-focus/41/videosuppl1/neurosurg-focus.41.issue-videosuppl1.xml
2. Technique of S2-alar iliac fixation: http://amj.amegroups.com/article/view/4197/4924

REFERENCE

1. McCord, D. H., Cunningham, B. W., Shono, Y., Myers, J. J., McAfee, P. C. (1992). Biomechanical analysis of lumbosacral fixation. *Spine, 17*, 235–243.

BIBLIOGRAPHY

1. Chang, T. L., Sponseller, P. D., Kebaish, K. M., & Fishman, E. K. (2009). Low profile pelvic fixation: Anatomic parameters for sacral alar-iliac fixation versus traditional iliac fixation. *Spine, 34*, 436–440.
2. George, S. G., Lebwohl, N. H., Pasquotti, G., & Williams, S. K. (2018). Percutaneous and open iliac screw safety and accuracy using a tactile technique with adjunctive anteroposterior fluoroscopy. *Spine Journal, 18*, 1570–1577.
3. Kebaish, K. M. (2010). Sacropelvic fixation: Techniques and complications. *Spine, 35*, 2245–2251.
4. Lebwohl, N. H., Cunningham, B. W., Dmitriev, A., Shimamoto, N., Gooch, L., Devlin, V., et al. (2002). Biomechanical comparison of lumbosacral fixation techniques in a calf spine model. *Spine, 27*, 2312–2320.
5. Lehman, R. A., Jr., Kuklo, T. R., Belmont, P. J.. Jr., Andersen, R. C., Polly, D. W., Jr. (2002). Advantage of pedicle screw fixation directed into the apex of the sacral promontory over bicortical fixation: A biomechanical analysis. *Spine, 27*, 806–811.
6. Lombardi, J. M., Shillingford, J. N., Lenke, L. G., & Lehman, R. A. (2018). Sacropelvic fixation: When, why, how? *Neurosurgery Clinics of North America, 29*, 389–397.
7. Martin, C. T., Witham, T. F., & Kebaish, K. M. (2011). Sacropelvic fixation: Two case reports of a new percutaneous technique. *Spine, 36*, 618–621.
8. McCord, D. H., Cunningham, B. W., Shono, Y., Myers, J. J., & McAfee, P. C. (1992). Biomechanical analysis of lumbosacral fixation. *Spine, 17*, 235–243.
9. O'Brien, M. F., Kuklo, T. R., & Lenke, L. G. (2004). Sacropelvic instrumentation: Anatomic and biomechanical zones of fixation. *Seminars in Spine Surgery, 16*, 76–90.
10. Yilmaz, E., Abdul-Jabbar, A., Tawfik, T., Iwanaga, J., Schmidt, C. K., Chapman, J., et al. (2018). S2 alar-iliac screw insertion: Technical note with pictorial guide. *World Neurosurgery, 113*, 296–301.

CHAPTER 31

MINIMALLY INVASIVE SPINE SURGERY

Dil B. Patel, BS, Mundeep S. Bawa, BS, Andrew M. Block, BS, and Kern Singh, BS, MD

1. What is minimally invasive spine surgery?
   Minimally invasive spine (MIS) surgery is a surgical approach or technique intended to provide equivalent or superior outcomes compared with conventional open spine surgery as a result of limiting approach-related surgical morbidity. In spine surgery, as with most other invasive procedures, less is more as long as surgical goals are fully met. Principles shared by MIS procedures include:
   - Small surgical incisions
   - Minimal disruption of musculature compared with standard open approaches
   - Requirement for specialized equipment, retractor systems, and implants
   - Use of intraoperative neurophysiologic monitoring and intraoperative imaging modalities, including fluoroscopy and computerized navigation technologies

2. Have MIS procedures been proven safer or more effective than traditional open spine procedures?
   Despite the fact that MIS procedures are performed through smaller skin incisions, the potential for serious and life-threatening complications is not completely eliminated. All spine procedures are considered *maximally invasive* because neural, visceral, and vascular structures remain at risk for serious injury. Current literature supports that MIS procedures have decreased certain complications such as excessive blood loss and infection compared to traditional open spine procedures. Other complications, such as pseudarthrosis, adjacent level disease, or proximal junctional kyphosis do not seem different between procedure types. However, this may change in the future depending on technological advances, surgeon education, and changes in practice patterns.

3. Are the goals of MIS procedures different from standard open procedures?
   No. The surgeon must be able to achieve the same surgical goals with MIS techniques as with standard open surgical procedures:
   - Adequate neural decompression
   - Stabilization and arthrodesis
   - Balanced correction of spinal deformity
   - Relief of axial and/or radicular pain

4. What are reasonable steps for a surgeon to take in order to overcome the learning curve and maximize patient safety when learning MIS techniques?
   - Attend technique-specific surgical courses
   - Study the anatomy, indications, and potential complications of MIS surgery
   - Rehearse surgical techniques through practice in animal and cadaver laboratory models
   - Visit or train with experienced surgeons currently performing these procedures
   - Perform initial cases in conjunction with an experienced surgeon
   - Develop a game plan for addressing intraoperative problems
   - Maintain competence in MIS techniques through adequate surgical case volume
   - Perform a critical analysis of personal surgical outcomes

MINIMALLY INVASIVE CERVICAL SPINE SURGERY

5. List common applications of MIS techniques for cervical spine pathology.
   Posterior-Based Approaches
   - Tubular laminoforaminotomy
   - Posterior screw-rod fixation and fusion
   Anterior-Based Approaches
   - Endoscopic approaches to the upper cervical spine and craniovertebral junction
   - Anterior cervical foraminotomy

MINIMALLY INVASIVE THORACIC SPINE SURGERY

6. List common applications of MIS techniques for thoracic spine pathology.

Posterior-Based Approaches
- Tubular microdiscectomy
- Percutaneous pedicle screw-rod placement and thoracic posterior fusion via MIS approach

Anterior-Based Approaches
- Thoracoscopic discectomy and corpectomy
- Mini-open thoracoscopic-assisted discectomy and corpectomy
- Anterior instrumentation and fusion for spinal instabilities
- Video-assisted spinal instrumentation and fusion for idiopathic scoliosis

7. What neural structures may be encountered in the thoracoscopic operative field?
- Sympathetic chain
- Greater and lesser splanchnic nerves
- Vagus nerve
- Phrenic nerve
- Intercostal nerves

8. List potential complications of thoracoscopic spinal decompression, fusion, and instrumentation.
- Dural tear
- Direct spinal cord injury
- Pulmonary complications (pneumothorax, hemothorax, mucous plug, pneumonia)
- Intercostal neuralgia
- Vessel injury (segmental artery and vein, azygous vein, aorta, vena cava)
- Pseudarthrosis
- Implant misplacement

9. What are the potential advantages of video-assisted thoracoscopic spinal fusion and instrumentation compared with traditional open thoracotomy approaches for treatment of idiopathic scoliosis?
- Reduced blood loss
- Decreased postoperative pain
- Improved cosmesis due to small incisions
- Diminished length of hospital stay

10. How does video-assisted thoracoscopic spinal instrumentation and fusion compare with standard open posterior spinal instrumentation and fusion using pedicle fixation for treatment of adolescent idiopathic scoliosis?
Similar patient outcomes and complication rates are reported by experienced surgeons for adolescent idiopathic scoliosis patients with single thoracic curves less than 70° treated with either video-assisted thoracoscopic spinal instrumentation and fusion or posterior pedicle instrumentation and fusion. Thoracoscopic surgery is associated with reduced blood loss but has a significant learning curve and requires specialized equipment. In contrast, posterior spinal instrumentation and fusion using pedicle fixation techniques are applicable to all curve types, provide greater curve correction, and require less operative time.

11. Is there a role for posterior MIS techniques in the treatment of pediatric spinal deformities?
Use of posterior MIS techniques has been reported in a range of clinical scenarios including: (1) at the top of long posterior instrumentation constructs as a technique intended to decrease the risk of proximal junctional kyphosis, (2) in the treatment of adolescent idiopathic scoliosis, and (3) for placement of proximal and distal screw anchors in pediatric patients treated with growth-friendly posterior implant systems.

MINIMALLY INVASIVE LUMBAR SPINE SURGERY

12. List common current applications of MIS techniques for lumbar spine pathology.

Posterior-Based Approaches
- Tubular microdiscectomy
- Tubular decompression for spinal stenosis
- Transforaminal lumbar interbody fusion via unilateral or bilateral MIS approach
- Lumbar intertransverse fusion via MIS approach
- Percutaneous pedicle screw-rod placement
- Percutaneous presacral approach

Anterior-Based Approaches
- Mini-open laparotomy retroperitoneal approach

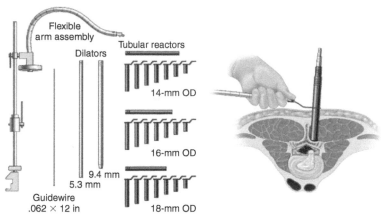

Fig. 31.1 Tubular microdiscectomy. METRx sequential dilator system (Medtronic Sofamor, Danek, Memphis, TN) for minimally invasive lumbar surgery. *OD,* Outer diameter. (From Medtronic Sofamor, Danek, Memphis, TN. From Shen FH, Shaffrey CI:. Arthritis and Arthroplasty: The Spine. Philadelphia, PA: Saunders; 2010.)

Lateral-Based Approaches
- Lateral transpsoas approach

Anterolateral-Based Approaches
- Anterolateral psoas-sparing approach (antepsoas approach)

13. What are the key steps in tubular microdiscectomy?

Using fluoroscopic guidance, a guidewire is inserted through the skin and paraspinous muscles to dock at the spinolaminar junction at the spinal level to be decompressed. A 2.5-cm skin incision is made to permit placement of dilators with sequentially increasing diameter. The tubular retractor is placed over the last dilator. Next, the dilator is removed and the retractor remains in place and is stabilized by attachment to a flexible arm assembly. A laminotomy is created with conventional tools (motorized burr, Kerrison rongeur), and the disc fragment is removed under microscopic or endoscopic visualization. Radiographic confirmation of exposure of the correct surgical level is critical. A tubular microdiscectomy approach is also possible for treatment of disc pathology located lateral to the pedicle. This region is accessed through a more lateral approach to the disc space using the intertransverse window (Fig. 31.1).

14. How is the MIS technique modified for treatment of lumbar spinal stenosis?

The tubular retractor may be angulated (wanded) to provide the enhanced visualization required to perform a bilateral decompression from a unilateral approach. A laminoplasty technique in which contralateral and ipsilateral hemilaminectomies and foraminotomies are performed using a high-speed burr and Kerrison rongeurs has been popularized. Appropriate angulation of the tubular retractor and tilting of the operating room table are used to facilitate contralateral and ipsilateral decompression of the spinal canal.

15. What anatomic principles are used to localize the pedicle during minimally invasive posterior instrumentation procedures?

The percutaneous technique is dependent on the ability to accurately visualize pedicle anatomy with fluoroscopy or surgical navigation technology. When using fluoroscopy, a Jamshidi needle is placed with its tip at the lateral border of the pedicle on a true anteroposterior (AP) view of the vertebra to be instrumented (Fig. 31.2). The needle is advanced from the entry point into bone (position 1) until it reaches the pedicle/vertebral body junction (position 2). The depth from the entry point of the needle into bone to reach the pedicle/vertebral body junction is approximately 20 mm. Therefore, if the tip of the needle remains lateral to the medial border of the pedicle at an insertion depth of 20 mm, the needle is traversing the pedicle and will enter the vertebral body without entering the spinal canal. As the needle is advanced beyond the pedicle/vertebral junction, it will enter into the posterior aspect of the vertebral body (position 3).

16. After localization of the pedicle at each spinal level where screw fixation is indicated, what steps are involved in placement of percutaneous lumbar pedicle screws and rods?

After the correct position of the Jamshidi needle is confirmed (Fig. 31.3A), a guidewire is inserted through the Jamshidi needle into the vertebral body and the Jamshidi needle is removed (Fig. 31.3B). A cannulated tap is placed over the guidewire and used to create a screw channel for placement of a cannulated pedicle screw. Electromyography (EMG) is used to test the tap and/or screw to detect a critical violation of the pedicle wall. After placement of screws, rods are introduced into the screws and secured to complete the construct (Fig. 31.3C). A myriad of innovative techniques have been devised to facilitate percutaneous rod passage and subsequent linkage to pedicle screws.

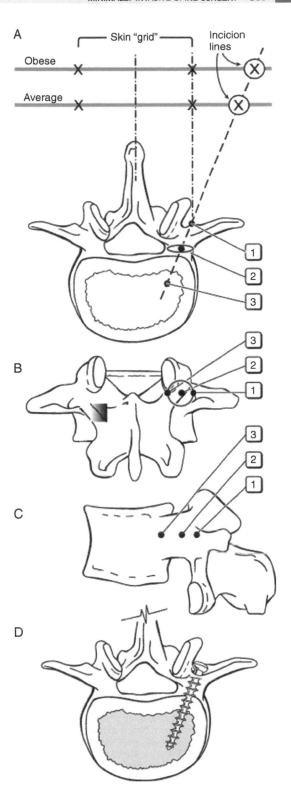

Fig. 31.2. Anatomic principles of percutaneous pedicle localization for screw placement. (A) Axial view. (B) Posteroanterior view. (C) Lateral view. (D) Axial view following pedicle screw placement. The skin entry point is marked and a Jamshidi needle is placed with its tip at the lateral border of the pedicle on a true anteroposterior view of the vertebra to be instrumented. The needle is advanced from the entry point into bone (position 1) until it reaches the pedicle/vertebral body junction (position 2). The depth from the entry point of the needle into bone to reach the pedicle/vertebral body junction is approximately 20 mm. Therefore, if the tip of the needle remains lateral to the medial border of the pedicle at an insertion depth of 20 mm, the needle is traversing the pedicle and will enter the vertebral body without entering the spinal canal. As the needle is advanced beyond the pedicle/vertebral junction, it will enter into the posterior aspect of the vertebral body (position 3). (From Mobbs RJ, Sivabalan P, Li J. Technique, challenges and indications for percutaneous pedicle screw fixation. J Clin Neurosci 2011;18:741–749.)

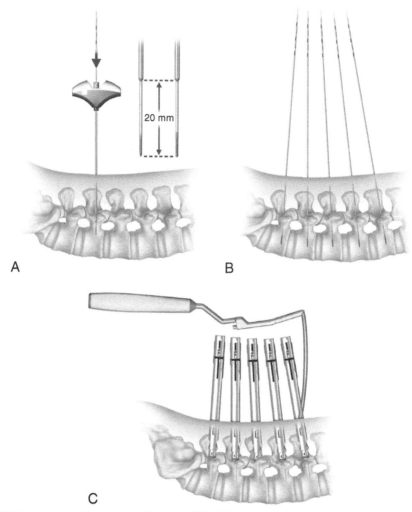

20 mm

A

B

C

Fig. 31.3 Percutaneous pedicle screw and rod placement. (A) Pedicle localization and Jamshidi needle placement. (B) Guidewire placement is followed by use of a cannulated tap and screw placement. (C) Percutaneous rod placement is facilitated by extensions that attach to the top of the pedicle screws. (Courtesy DePuy Spine, Inc. All rights reserved.)

An alternative mini-open technique has evolved aided by development of expandable tubular retractors. The retractor is placed over the pedicle access site, and screws are placed using the identical technique utilized for conventional open pedicle screw placement.

17. What are the key steps involved in minimally invasive interbody fusion from a posterior approach?

The most common technique is to perform a unilateral transforaminal lumbar interbody fusion (TLIF) applying the basic principles of MIS surgery. An expandable tubular retractor is placed over the pedicle region on the side selected for the interbody approach. The facet complex is removed to provide access to the disc space lateral to the traversing nerve root. Disc space preparation is carried out in a similar fashion as for a conventional TLIF. The disc space is packed with bone graft and a structural intervertebral spacer is placed. Pedicle screws are placed on the side of the approach under direct visualization. Pedicle screws on the contralateral side may be placed percutaneously or following placement of a tubular retractor on the opposite side. Finally, rods are placed bilaterally and compression forces are applied across the disc space to interlock the structural spacer between the adjacent vertebral endplates (Fig. 31.4).

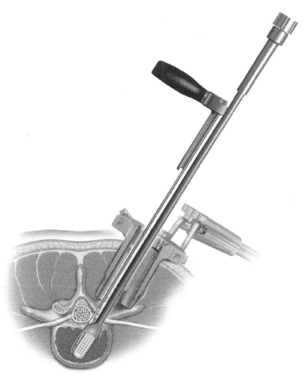

Fig. 31.4 Minimally invasive transforaminal lumbar interbody fusion using an expandable tubular retractor. (Courtesy DePuy Spine, Inc. All rights reserved.)

18. What is the lateral transpsoas approach?

The approach is most commonly performed from the left side with the patient positioned in the right lateral decubitus position. Fluoroscopy is used to mark a small skin incision over the anterior third of the target disc space at the posterior border of the paraspinous muscles. The layers of the lateral abdominal wall are bluntly dissected to enter the retroperitoneal space. The peritoneum is mobilized anteriorly and the psoas muscle is identified. Dissection through the psoas is performed to expose the disc space. Palpation, direct visualization, and neurophysiologic monitoring are used to facilitate safe placement of a specialized expandable tubular retractor. Alternatively, the psoas may be dissected, mobilized, and retracted to expose the disc space (antepsoas approach). While working through the retractor, the disc space is prepared for fusion and a transversely oriented structural interbody spacer containing graft material is inserted.

The lateral transpsoas approach was developed as a less invasive option for achieving anterior fusion from L1 to L5. This approach avoids the need to mobilize the iliac vessels or sympathetic plexus. However, the genitofemoral nerve, lateral femoral cutaneous nerve, and femoral nerve are placed at risk due to their intimate relationship with the psoas muscle. The approach is not feasible at L5–S1 due to the location of the iliac vessels. The approach is challenging at L4–L5 and may not be possible in some patients due to obstruction by the iliac crest or due to the relationship of the lumbosacral plexus to the lateral aspect of the disc space (Fig. 31.5).

19. Explain the presacral surgical approach to the lumbosacral junction and its rationale.

With the patient in the prone position, a small incision is made lateral to the coccyx. A blunt trocar is inserted under biplanar fluoroscopic guidance and advanced into the presacral space while maintaining contact with the anterior surface of the sacrum. A midline position is maintained and a guide pin is inserted into the sacrum at the S1–S2 level and advanced across the L5–S1 disc space into the L5 vertebral body. A series of dilators are used to create an intraosseous working channel. Using specialized instruments, the disc material is removed and the disc prepared for fusion. Finally an axial rod (AxiaLIF+, TranS1; Wilmington, NC) is inserted to stabilize the disc space, and bone graft material is injected.

The presacral approach is intended to provide an option for minimally invasive surgical access to the lumbosacral junction that does not require mobilization of the iliac vessels, limits muscle dissection, and avoids disruption of the autonomic nerves overlying the lumbosacral disc. Potential complications associated with this approach include wound dehiscence, infection, bowel injury, vascular injury, and pseudarthrosis (Fig. 31.6).

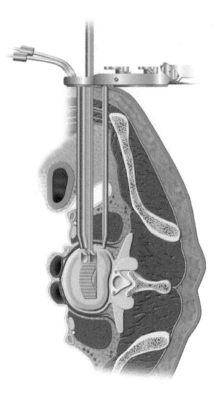

Fig. 31.5 Lateral transpsoas approach. (From Kim DK, Henn JS, Vaccaro AR, et al. Surgical Anatomy and Techniques to the Spine. Philadelphia, PA: Saunders; 2006.)

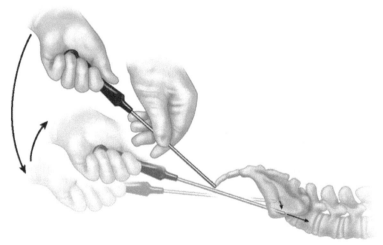

Fig. 31.6. Presacral approach to the lumbosacral spine. A channel is created from inferiorly in the sacrum to allow access to the center of the L5–S1 disc. Discectomy and bone grafting are then performed through this channel. (From Shen FH, Shaffrey CI. Arthritis and Arthroplasty: The Spine. Philadelphia, PA: Saunders; 2010.)

20. Why are mini-open laparotomy approaches preferred by many surgeons for lumbar interbody fusion?

Mini-open laparotomy approaches offer many advantages compared with alternative minimally invasive techniques while avoiding many of their challenges. Mini-open techniques are routinely accomplished through a single small incision and generally require shorter operative times. Extensile exposure of the lumbar spine from L2 to sacrum can be achieved through the surgical plane between the great vessels and the psoas muscle. Complete removal of disc material and meticulous endplate preparation are facilitated by direct visualization of the entire disc space. These approaches are associated with low complication rates and allow relatively rapid patient recovery. Recently described modifications of the traditional mini-open laparotomy approach include the psoas-sparing anterolateral retroperitoneal approach and the oblique lateral interbody fusion (OLIF) procedure.

KEY POINTS

1. Minimally invasive spine procedures intend to limit approach-related surgical morbidity through use of smaller skin incisions and targeted muscle dissection but do not eliminate the potential for serious and life-threatening complications.
2. Use of minimally invasive spine techniques is widespread but claims that MIS procedures are more effective than traditional spine procedures await validation in the current medical literature.

Websites
1. Society for minimally invasive spine surgery: http://www.smiss.org/

BIBLIOGRAPHY

1. Arts, M. P., Brand, R., van den Akker, M. E., Koes, B. W., Bartels, R. H., Tan, W. F., et al. (2011). Tubular diskectomy vs. conventional microdiskectomy for the treatment of lumbar disk herniation: 2-year results of a double-blinded randomized controlled trial. *Neurosurgery, 69*, 135–144.
2. Brau, S. A. (2002). Mini-open approach to the spine for anterior lumbar interbody fusion: Description of the procedure, results, and complications. *Spine Journal, 2*, 216–223.
3. Cragg, A., Carl, A., Casteneda, F., Dickman, C., Guterman, L., & Oliveira, C. (2004). New percutaneous access method for minimally invasive anterior lumbosacral surgery. *Journal of Spinal Disorders & Techniques, 17*, 21–28.
4. Eck, J. C., Hodges, S., & Humphreys, S. C. (2007). Minimally invasive lumbar spinal fusion. *Journal of the American Academy of Orthopaedic Surgeons, 15*, 321–329.
5. Lonner, B. S., Auerbach, J. D., Estreicher, M., Milby, A. H., & Kean, K. E. (2009). Video-assisted thoracoscopic spinal fusion compared with posterior spinal fusion with thoracic pedicle screws for thoracic adolescent idiopathic scoliosis. *Journal of Bone and Joint Surgery, 91*, 398–408.
6. Mobbs, R. J., Sivabalan, P., & Li, J. (2011). Technique, challenges, and indications for percutaneous pedicle screw fixation. *Journal of Clinical Neuroscience, 18*, 741–749.
7. Ozgur, B. M., Aryan, H. E., Pimenta, L., & Taylor, W. R. (2006). Extreme lateral interbody fusion (XLIF): A novel surgical technique for anterior lumbar interbody fusion. *Spine Journal, 6*, 435–443.
8. Samdani, A. F., Asghar, J., Miyanji, F., Haw, J., & Haddix, K. (2011). Minimally invasive treatment of pediatric spinal deformity. *Seminars in Spine Surgery, 23*, 72–75.
9. Woods, K. R., Billys, J. B., & Hynes, R. A. (2017). Technical description of oblique lateral interbody fusion at L1-L5 (OLIF25) and at L5-S1 (OLIF51) and evaluation of complication and fusion rates. *Spine Journal, 17*, 545–553.

CHAPTER 32

ARTIFICIAL DISC REPLACEMENT

Nikhil Jain, MD, Brian W. Su, MD, Adam L. Shimer, MD, and Alexander R. Vaccaro, MD, PhD

1. **Discuss some limitations associated with nonarthroplasty surgical treatment options for degenerative spinal conditions.**

   Neural decompression procedures violate the structural integrity of the spine and may lead to segmental spinal instability unless fusion is performed. Spinal fusion procedures increase stress at adjacent spinal levels and may accelerate the degenerative process leading to adjacent level degeneration, instability, facet joint degeneration, spinal stenosis, and vertebral body fracture. An initial fusion procedure may generate the need for further spinal procedures such as implant removal, pseudarthrosis repair, or debridement of operative site infection. In addition, bone graft harvest for fusion procedures is accompanied by a myriad of problems, including the potential for development of chronic bone graft donor site pain. When the indication for spinal fusion is axial pain without associated neural compression, pain may persist despite achievement of a radiographically healed fusion.

LUMBAR TOTAL DISC ARTHROPLASTY

2. **What is the rationale for development of lumbar total disc arthroplasty?**

   The rationale for development of lumbar total disc replacement (TDR) as an alternative surgical procedure to spinal fusion for treatment of discogenic axial low back pain was based on the following goals:
   - To avoid the negative effects associated with lumbar fusion (e.g., pseudarthrosis, need for additional procedures for implant removal, bone graft donor site problems, adjacent segment pathology)
   - To protect adjacent levels from iatrogenically accelerated degeneration
   - To provide improved treatment outcomes with respect to relief of low back pain
   - To enhance postoperative recovery (earlier return to work and activity)

3. **Discuss the problem of adjacent-level pathology following lumbar fusion.**

   Lumbar fusion results in load transfer to unfused proximal and distal spinal segments resulting in increased intradiscal pressure and increased intersegmental motion at neighboring spinal segments. This may result in the development of radiographic degenerative changes in the adjacent spinal segments (adjacent segment degeneration) and symptoms requiring additional surgical intervention (adjacent segment disease). It has been estimated that the mean annual rate of adjacent segment disease (development of symptoms sufficiently severe to require additional surgery for decompression or arthrodesis) ranges from 0.6% to 4% per year following a lumbar arthrodesis procedure. Estimates of the 5- and 10-year risk of developing adjacent segment disease following lumbar arthrodesis range from 3% to 16.5% and 6% to 26%, respectively. Some factors that increase the risk of development of adjacent segment disease include multilevel fusion, fusions adjacent to but not including L5–S1, and laminectomy adjacent to a fusion. Whether the radiographic and clinical findings are a result of the iatrogenically created rigid spinal segment or progression of the natural history of an underlying degenerative process remains controversial. The term **adjacent segment pathology (ASP)** has been proposed to describe changes that occur adjacent to a previously operated spinal level. Two subtypes are identified: (1) **radiographic ASP (RASP)** is used to describe radiographic changes, including MRI findings which occur at an adjacent motion segment; and (2) **clinical ASP (CASP)** is used to refer to clinical signs and symptoms that occur adjacent to a previously operated spinal motion segment.

4. **What is the current FDA-approved indication for performing lumbar TDR?**

   In the United States, lumbar TDR has received Food and Drug Administration (FDA) approval for treatment of one or two-level degenerative disc disease (DDD) in the lower lumbar spine in skeletally mature patients with no more than grade 1 spondylolisthesis at the involved level. DDD is defined as discogenic back pain due to degeneration of the disc and confirmed by patient history, physical examination, and radiographic studies. Surgery should be reserved for patients who have not responded to at least 6 months of conservative therapy.

5. **What are some of the important contraindications to performing lumbar TDR?**

   Contraindications to lumbar TDR have been divided into four main groups:
   - **Painful lumbar spinal pathology unrelated to the target intervertebral disc or which may respond to less complex treatments.** Pain related to facet joint degeneration, radiculopathy due to disc herniation or spinal

stenosis, multilevel discogenic pain, and poorly defined pain syndromes are unlikely to respond favorably to treatment with single-level lumbar TDR.

- **Conditions that potentially compromise stability of a lumbar disc prosthesis.** Examples include osteoporosis, spinal instability (spondylolysis, lytic spondylolisthesis, degenerative spondylolisthesis > grade 1, prior laminectomy), and spinal deformities.
- **Limited or absent segmental motion at the operative level:** severe spondylosis, disc height <3 mm, prior lumbar fusion, and ankylosing spondylitis or other spinal stiffening diseases.
- **Patient-specific factors:** metal allergy, systemic disease (e.g., diabetes mellitus), malignancy, active infection, morbid obesity, chronic steroid use, abdominal pathology, or prior abdominal surgery that would preclude an anterior retroperitoneal approach, and pregnancy.

Studies investigating the prevalence of contraindications in the population of patients presenting to spine surgeons for surgical treatment of lumbar degenerative pathology have demonstrated that only a small percentage of patients are appropriate candidates for lumbar TDR. One study reported that approximately 14% of lumbar fusion candidates and 5% of all lumbar surgery candidates would meet the criteria for treatment with lumbar TDR.

6. What lumbar TDRs are currently FDA approved for use in the United States?

Two artificial discs are currently approved by the FDA for implantation in the United States: prodisc L (Centinel Spine LLC, West Chester, PA) and activL (Aesculap Implant Systems LLC, Center Valley, PA).

The prodisc L is a semiconstrained articulating metal-on-polyethylene implant composed of two cobalt-chromium-molybdenum alloy endplates and an ultrahigh–molecular-weight polyethylene (UHMWPE) core. The polyethylene core locks into the lower endplate and prevents core extrusion. Small keels and a titanium, plasma-sprayed finish on the device endplates provide for both immediate fixation and long-term fixation by osseous ingrowth (Fig. 32.1).

The activL is a mobile-bearing modular implant consisting of two metal endplates with an UHMWPE core that supports controlled translational and rotational movement. Along with its traditional ball and socket design, it also allows up to 2 mm of anteroposterior (AP) translation. The bone-contacting endplates are coated with Plasmapore μ-CaP, a microporous titanium coating and thin bioactive calcium phosphate surface finish to increase implant stability and bone ingrowth. The activL achieves initial stability through endplate spikes or a keel (Fig. 32.2).

The Charité artificial disc (DePuy Spine, Inc., Raynham, MA), which was the first implant to receive FDA approval for lumbar TDR, was discontinued from the market in 2011. It possessed an unconstrained three-part anatomic design. It is an articulating metal-on-polyethylene implant. It has a mobile core composed of moderately cross-linked UHMWPE. The core is free to move between the two cobalt-chromium-molybdenum alloy endplates. Teeth on the undersurface of the endplates provide anchorage to the vertebrae. A metal wire surrounds the core to aid in imaging. Many alternative lumbar disc replacement designs are currently under study both in the United States and internationally.

7. What particular considerations regarding patient positioning, setup, and surgical technique are important when performing a lumbar TDR compared with an anterior lumbar interbody fusion?

Patient positioning for a lumbar TDR is similar to an anterior lumbar interbody fusion (ALIF). An inflatable bolster may be placed under the sacrum to extend the L5–S1 disc space and to allow adjustment of lumbar lordosis.

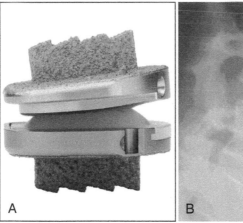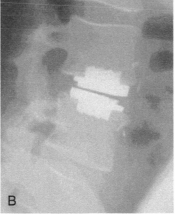

A B

Fig. 32.1 The ProDisc-L artificial disc (Synthes Spine). (A: From Yue JJ, Bertagnoli R, McAfee PC, et al. Motion Preservation of the Spine. Philadelphia, PA: Saunders; 2008. B: From Zigler JE. Lumbar spine arthroplasty using the ProDisc II. Spine J 2004;4:231–238.)

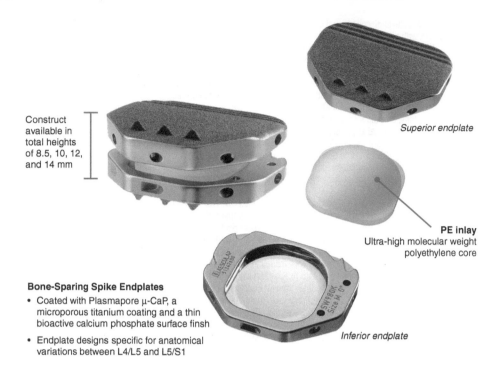

Construct available in total heights of 8.5, 10, 12, and 14 mm

Superior endplate

PE inlay
Ultra-high molecular weight polyethylene core

Bone-Sparing Spike Endplates
- Coated with Plasmapore μ-CaP, a microporous titanium coating and a thin bioactive calcium phosphate surface finsh
- Endplate designs specific for anatomical variations between L4/L5 and L5/S1

Inferior endplate

Fig. 32.2 activL. (activL® Artificial Disc image courtesy of Aesculap Implant Systems, LLC, Center Valley, PA.)

Placement of the bolster directly behind the lumbar spine when performing lumbar TDR should be avoided because it tends to *fish-mouth* the disc space, making critical parallel distraction more difficult. A midline (rectus splitting) surgical approach or paramidline (lateral to rectus) surgical approach may be used to access the lower lumbar disc levels. A retroperitoneal approach is preferred over a transperitoneal approach. As in an ALIF approach, careful identification and retraction of the ureter, peritoneum, sympathetic plexus, and blood vessels are required. Lower extremity pulse oximetry is useful to ensure adequate lower extremity perfusion during and following vessel retraction. Thorough discectomy and accurate midline localization are critical to ensure a technically well-placed lumbar TDR. The anterior, posterior, and lateral margins of the disc space should be clearly delineated. The midline is marked using an intraoperative fluoroscopic AP Ferguson view. A lateral fluoroscopic view is helpful to confirm parallel disc distraction. The lumbar TDR should only recreate the native disc height because *overstuffing* may lead to posterior structure (facet capsule) tension and pain. The bony end plate should be preserved to minimize risk of subsidence or bridging ossification.

8. What complications have been reported in association with lumbar total disc arthroplasty?
   Complications following lumbar TDR may be a result of:
   - **Improper surgical indications:** poor patient selection (e.g., nonorganic pain syndrome, segmental instability, osteoporotic patients, patients with facet arthropathy)
   - **Complications related to the surgical approach:** vascular injury, dural tear, neurologic injury, ureteral injury, retrograde ejaculation, visceral injury, deep vein thrombosis
   - **Complications related to the implant:** migration, dislocation, subsidence, malposition, vertebral body endplate fracture, polyethylene and metal wear, local or systemic adverse reactions to wear debris
   - **Miscellaneous complications:** heterotopic ossification, facet degeneration at the operative or adjacent level, infection

9. How do the results of lumbar total disc arthroplasty compare to other treatments such as lumbar fusion?
   In general, the results of single-level lumbar total disc arthroplasty are at least comparable to outcomes following single-level lumbar fusion. The US FDA Investigational Device Exemption (IDE) study for the Charité

artificial disc supported the conclusion that the Charité disc at one level was not inferior to anterior lumbar interbody fusion with Bagby and Kuslich (BAK) threaded titanium cages augmented with iliac crest autograft. The US IDE study for the ProDisc-L compared total disc arthroplasty with circumferential fusion using anterior femoral ring allograft and instrumented posterolateral fusion with iliac autograft, and showed statistically similar improvement over preoperative status for both study arms at one and two level(s). For the activL device, the control group in the US IDE study that served as the basis for device approval was another lumbar TDR (Charité or ProDisc-L) and comparable results were observed for both study arms for one-level use. The Pro-Disc-L, currently marketed as prodisc L (Centinel Spine) has received marketing approval for use at one or two adjacent vertebral level(s) and the activL (Aesculap Implant Systems) for single-level use.

10. Describe the workup of a patient with persistent or new-onset symptoms following lumbar total disc arthroplasty.

A variety of diagnoses are considered in the patient who presents with continued or new-onset symptoms following lumbar total disc arthroplasty:
- Implant malposition, migration, subsidence, or instability
- Pain due to posterior facet joint arthrosis
- Pain due to neural impingement or excessive elevation of disc space height
- Symptomatic adjacent level pathology
- Infection
- Pain of unknown etiology

After a detailed history and physical examination are completed, imaging is initiated with plain radiography including standing AP and lateral views and flexion-extension views. Fluoroscopy may be helpful to assess the operative level under dynamic loading conditions. CT imaging including axial, sagittal, and coronal views can provide additional information. If neurologic compression is a concern, CT-myelography is indicated because MRI evaluation of currently approved lumbar TDRs is compromised by metal artifact. Injection studies including facet blocks, adjacent level discography, and periprosthetic anesthetic injection may be of value in diagnosis of facet-mediated pain or symptomatic adjacent level disc degeneration, and aid in determining whether the surgical level is the source of pain. Angiography and venography are considered when vessel impingement by displaced prosthetic components is suspected. Periprosthetic infection can be challenging to diagnose, and potentially useful imaging studies include technetium radionuclide scans or positron emission tomography (PET)-CT scans in combination with laboratory studies (complete blood count [CBC], erythrocyte sedimentation rate [ESR], C-reactive protein).

11. What treatment options and challenges are associated with revision surgery following lumbar disc arthroplasty?

Revision surgery options following lumbar total disc arthroplasty include:
- Posterior foraminotomy
- Posterolateral fusion and pedicle screw-rod instrumentation
- Replacement of the prosthesis with a new arthroplasty device
- Device removal, anterior interbody fusion, and posterior instrumentation and fusion

Decision-making regarding revision surgery for a prior lumbar disc arthroplasty depends on various factors including clinical presentation, time from index surgical procedure, failure mode, index surgical approach, operative level, and implant position.

Posterior foraminotomy is considered in the patient with a well-positioned prosthesis who presents with new-onset radiculopathy due to retropulsed disc or endplate material following lumbar TDR.

Posterolateral fusion and pedicle screw-rod fixation is a common revision strategy for patients with persistent pain, subsidence, instability, or facet arthrosis who have failed conservative treatment, and do not require anterior revision surgery. When revision with posterolateral instrumented fusion is performed in a patient with an acceptably placed lumbar artificial disc, prosthesis removal and anterior interbody fusion have not been shown to provide additional clinical benefit.

Anterior surgery for prosthesis revision or conversion to a fusion is indicated for treatment of prosthetic infection, unacceptable implant position, or device migration. Anterior revision surgery is a more complex and challenging procedure compared with posterior revision surgery. Within the first 2 weeks following the index procedure, the difficulty of a revision anterior approach is similar to a primary approach. After this time period, the risk of iatrogenic injury due to scarring around retroperitoneal, vascular, and visceral structures is extremely high and may lead to life-threatening complications during a revision anterior surgical exposure. Suggested measures to minimize complications include placement of ureteral stents to aid in identification and protection of the ureters, placement of balloon catheters in the iliac vessels as an aid to limiting intraoperative blood loss in anticipation of major vessel injury, and use of an alternative approach for surgical exposure. Use of the direct lateral (transpsoas) retroperitoneal approach or use of a contralateral retroperitoneal approach have been suggested.

CERVICAL DISC ARTHROPLASTY

12. What is the rationale for development of cervical total disc arthroplasty?

Anterior cervical discectomy and fusion (ACDF) for treatment of radiculopathy or myelopathy remains one of the most successful procedures in spine surgery. The rationale for development of cervical TDR as an alternative procedure was based on the following goals:

- To avoid the negative effects associated with ACDF (e.g., pseudarthrosis, plate-related complications, bone graft or intervertebral body fusion device-related complications)
- To protect adjacent levels from iatrogenically accelerated degeneration following fusion
- To enhance postoperative recovery (e.g., avoid brace immobilization, permit earlier return to unrestricted activity)

13. Discuss the problem of adjacent-segment pathology in the cervical spine following nonfusion and fusion procedures.

Adjacent segment pathology (ASP) is the current term used to describe changes which occur adjacent to a previously operated spinal level. Current terminology distinguishes between **radiographic ASP (RASP)**, including MRI findings, which are not associated with clinical symptoms, and **clinical ASP (CASP)**, which refers to adjacent level imaging findings associated with clinical signs and symptoms. The risk of developing CASP following an initial ACDF is estimated to range from 1.6% to 4.2% per year. The incidence of CASP after ACDF ranges from 11% to 12% at 5 years, and from 16% to 38% at 10 years. Of patients with CASP, approximately two-thirds will require additional cervical surgery. As the rates of CASP between anterior cervical fusion and nonfusion posterior foraminotomy procedures are similar, it remains uncertain whether the development of CASP reflects a natural progression of cervical spondylosis or results from biomechanical changes following arthrodesis. Risk factors for CASP include age >60 years, fusions adjacent to but not including C5–C6 and/or C6–C7, fusions involving ≤3 levels, preexisting disc herniation or dural compression, and smaller AP spinal canal diameter (≤13 mm).

14. What is the current FDA-approved indication for performing cervical TDR?

The current FDA-approved indication for cervical disc arthroplasty is for reconstruction of the disc space following discectomy for treatment of radiculopathy with or without neck pain or myelopathy due to an abnormality localized to the disc space, with one of the following conditions confirmed by radiographic imaging: herniated nucleus pulposus, spondylosis, and/or visible loss of disc height. Patients are required to be skeletally mature and should have failed to respond 6 weeks of nonoperative treatment or demonstrate progressive signs or symptoms despite nonoperative treatment. Some FDA-approved cervical disc arthroplasty devices are approved for only single-level use, while other devices have received approval for use at both one and two cervical levels.

15. What are some of the major contraindications to performing cervical TDR?

Contraindications to cervical TDR include:

- **Coexistent spinal pathology unrelated to the intervertebral disc:** pain related to facet joint degeneration, cervical or radicular arm pain of unknown etiology
- **Conditions that potentially compromise stability of a cervical disc prosthesis:** spinal instability, osteoporosis, vertebral body deficiency, or deformity (posttrauma, kyphosis)
- **Limited or absent segmental motion at the operative level:** severe spondylosis, severe disc space narrowing, prior anterior cervical fusion
- **Patient-specific factors:** malignancy, active infection, spondyloarthropathy, rheumatoid arthritis, metal allergy, chronic steroid use, systemic diseases (e.g. insulin-dependent diabetes), pregnancy, isolated axial neck pain

Studies investigating the prevalence of contraindications in the population presenting to spine surgeons for surgical treatment of cervical degenerative disorders have documented that the percentage of patients who are appropriate candidates for cervical TDR ranges between 40% and 50%. This is a significantly greater number of patients than the proportion of lumbar surgery candidates who qualify for lumbar TDR.

16. What cervical TDRs are currently FDA approved for use in the United States?

Current FDA-approved cervical TDRs (Table 32.1) include:

- Prestige ST (stainless steel) Cervical Disc (Medtronic Sofamor Danek USA, Inc., Memphis, TN) (Fig. 32.3A)
- Prestige LP (low profile) Cervical Disc (Medtronic Sofamor Danek USA, Inc., Memphis, TN) (see Fig. 32.3B)
- ProDisc-C TDR (Centinel Spine LLC, West Chester, PA) (see Fig. 32.3C)
- Bryan Cervical Disc Prosthesis (Medtronic Sofamor Danek USA, Inc., Memphis, TN) (see Fig. 32.3D)
- Mobi-C Cervical Disc Prosthesis (Zimmer Biomet, Warsaw, IN) (see Fig. 32.3E)
- SECURE-C Artificial Cervical Disc (Globus Medical, Inc., Audubon, PA) (see Fig. 32.3F)
- PCM (porous coated motion) Cervical Disc System (Nuvasive, Inc., San Diego, CA) (see Fig. 32.3G)
- M6-C Artificial Cervical Disc (Spinal Kinetics, LLC, Sunnyvale, CA)

Eight cervical TDRs are currently FDA approved for one-level use. Cervical TDRs approved for use at two levels include the Prestige LP and the Mobi-C Cervical Disc Prosthesis. Many alternative cervical disc replacement designs are currently under study in the United States and internationally.

Table 32.1 Characteristics of FDA-Approved Cervical Arthroplasty Devices.

DEVICE	DESIGN	MOD-ULAR	ARTICULATING METHOD	IMPLANT COMPOSITION	BEARING SURFACE	PRIMARY FIXATION	SECONDARY FIXATION	MANUFAC-TURER
Bryan	Biarticulating contained bearing	No	Biarticulating	Titanium, central polymer	Titanium alloy on polymer	Milled vertebral endplates	Endplate ingrowth	Medtronic
Mobi-C	Superior endplate with ball and socket motion; inferior endplate with sliding constraint	Yes	Biarticulating	Titanium	Titanium on polyethylene modular core	Lateral self-retaining teeth	Endplate ongrowth	Zimmer Biomet
Prestige-LP	Ellipsoid saucer	No	Uniarticulating	Titanium/ceramic composite	Titanium/ceramic composite	Dual rails	Endplate ongrowth	Medtronic
Prestige-ST	Ellipsoid saucer	No	Uniarticulating	316L stainless steel	316L on 316L	Locked vertebral body screws	Locked vertebral body screws	Medtronic
ProDisc-C	Ball and socket	No	Uniarticulating	Cobalt-chromium, UHMWPE	Cobalt-chromium on UHMWPE	Central keel	Endplate ongrowth	Centinel Spine
PCM	Upper endplate translation on fixed UHMWPE	No	Uniarticulating	Cobalt-chromium, UHMWPE	Cobalt-chromium on UHMWPE	Ridged metallic endplates	Endplate ongrowth	NuVasive
SECURE-C	Metal on polyethylene	Yes	Biarticulating	Cobalt-chromium, UHMWPE	Cobalt-chromium on UHMWPE	Ridged central keel	Endplate ongrowth	Globus Medical
M6-C	Titanium endplates, artificial annulus, artificial nucleus	No	Uniarticulating	Titanium, UHMWPE annulus, PCU nucleus	Titanium on PCU and UHMWPE	Serrated fins	Endplate ongrowth	Spinal Kinetics

PCU, Polycarbonate urethane; *UHMWPE*, ultrahigh-molecular-weight polyethylene.

Adapted from Kannan A, Hsu WK, Sasso RC. Cervical disc replacement. In: Garfin SR, Eismont FJ, Bell GR, editors. Rothman-Simeone the Spine. 7th ed. Philadelphia, PA: Elsevier; 2018, pp. 771–783, Table 44.1, p. 776.

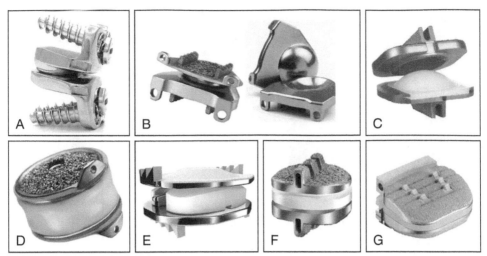

Fig. 32.3 Examples of US Food and Drug Administration approved cervical disc devices. (A) Prestige-ST Cervical Disc (Medtronic Sofamor Danek USA, Inc., Memphis, TN) (B) Prestige LP (Medtronic Sofamor Danek USA, Inc., Memphis, TN) (C) Prodisc-C Total Disc Replacement (Centinel Spine LLC, West Chester, PA) (D) Bryan- Cervical Disc Prosthesis (Medtronic Sofamor Danek USA, Inc., Memphis, TN) (E) Mobi-C Cervical Disc Prosthesis (Zimmer Biomet, Warsaw, IN) (F) SECURE-C Artificial Cervical Disc (Globus Medical, Inc., Audubon, PA) (G) PCM Cervical Disc System (Nuvasive, Inc., San Diego, CA).

17. **What considerations regarding patient positioning, setup, and surgical technique are important when performing a cervical TDR compared with an ACDF?**

    Patient positioning for cervical TDR and ACDF differ. When positioning a patient for a cervical TDR it is important to maintain the neck in a stable and slightly lordotic position by placing a small, rolled towel under the neck. This differs from an ACDF where increased lordosis may be desirable and is achieved by placing a bolster underneath the shoulders. There is routine use of the C-arm for a cervical TDR, and one may consider turning the operating room table 180° to facilitate use of the C-arm and navigation around anesthesia equipment and personnel. Using cloth tape to pull the shoulders inferiorly is particularly important to allow for adequate visualization of the lower cervical levels, particularly at the C6–C7 level. Prior to prepping the operative site for a cervical TDR, it is important to perform a fluoroscopic check to confirm that the operative level is adequately visualized, and that vertebral endplates are parallel on lateral fluoroscopy, and that neutral rotation is present on an AP fluoroscopic view. The position of the neck should be similar to the preoperative neutral lateral radiograph and remain fixed throughout the procedure to avoid improper sagittal alignment of the spine. One should always be prepared to convert the procedure to an ACDF.

    Fluoroscopy may be used to select the appropriate incision location. The surgical approach is similar for both cervical TDR and ACDF and consists of a standard Smith-Robinson anterior approach. However, for cervical TDR, less of each vertebral body needs to be exposed and dissection can be limited to the disc space itself since an anterior plate is not used. Identification of the midline is critical for both procedures and is aided by exposing the longus coli muscles to the lateral aspect of the uncinate joints. A Penfield 4 should be used to verify that the lateral uncinated processes have been adequately exposed. Fluoroscopic guidance is used to ensure midline placement of the distraction pins for cervical TDR. It is critical that the pins are parallel to the disc at the operative level because parallel distraction is important for anatomic placement of the cervical TDR.

    A thorough discectomy, osteophyte removal, and foraminal decompression is especially critical when performing cervical TDR as preservation of motion at the operative level increases the risk of recurrent radiculopathy due to foraminal stenosis compared to ACDF. When performing cervical TDR, minimal bone resection is performed and the endplates are prepared according to the recommended technique for the specific device that is implanted. This differs from an ACDF where a burr is used to create parallel endplates for allograft or cage placement. An appropriately sized cervical TDR should be similar in height to an adjacent normal disc, provide maximal endplate coverage, and be centrally placed in the coronal and sagittal plane. Meticulous hemostasis using bone wax is important in cervical TDR procedures to minimize blood loss and the risk of postoperative heterotopic ossification.

18. **What complications have been reported in association with cervical TDR?**

    Complications following cervical TDR may be a result of:
    - **Improper surgical indications:** poor patient selection (e.g., axial pain syndromes, nonorganic pain syndromes), segmental instability, osteoporotic patients, patients with facet arthropathy
    - **Complications related to the surgical approach:** dysphagia, recurrent laryngeal nerve injury, vertebral artery injury, esophageal injury, hematoma, airway compromise

- **Complications related to the implant:** migration, subsidence, implant loosening, instability, vertebral body endplate fracture, kyphotic deformity, facet-joint overdistraction, polyethylene or metal wear, local or systemic adverse reactions to wear debris
- **Complications related to decompression:** inadequate foraminal decompression leading to radiculopathy, dural tear, neurologic injury
- **Miscellaneous:** heterotopic ossification, facet degeneration at the operative or adjacent level, infection

19. What is the major determinant of MRI clarity of a cervical TDR device following implantation?

The material composition of the device is the most important determinant of its imaging properties. Titanium devices allow satisfactory visualization of neural structures at the index and adjacent levels on postoperative MRI scans. Cobalt-chrome metal alloys and stainless steel cause significant deterioration of MRI quality, and CT-myelography is recommended for evaluation of the neural elements with these devices.

20. What are the outcomes of single-level cervical TDR compared to single-level ACDF?

Longer-term ($\geq$5 years) data from FDA-IDE trials of many approved cervical TDRs and other prospective studies are now available. Systematic reviews and meta-analyses of available data have shown similar to superior patient-reported outcome measures (PROMs), range of motion (ROM), and fewer adverse events and reoperations for one-level cervical TDR as compared with ACDF. Cervical TDR is also associated with a lower rate of adjacent segment degeneration and disease in some systematic reviews and analyses. While TDR and ACDF are both cost-effective, TDR is more cost-effective in the long term (7 years).

21. How do the outcomes of two-level cervical TDR and two-level ACDF compare?

Less data is available for two-level cervical TDR versus one-level cervical TDR, but early data suggest that the advantages of cervical TDR appear to be greater for two-level use as compared with single-level use. Comparison of outcomes for two-level cervical TDR using the Mobi-C (Zimmer Biomet, Warsaw, IN) device versus two-level ACDF performed with allograft and an anterior plate in the FDA-IDE clinical trial showed superiority of cervical TDR at 7 years. Two-level Mobi-C cervical TDR demonstrated a higher overall rate of clinical success as compared with ACDF (60.8% vs. 34.2%), and was mainly attributable to statistically higher improvements in neck disability index (NDI), lower incidence of neurologic failure, and lower risk of subsequent surgery. Two-level Mobi-C cervical TDR showed higher ROM in flexion, extension, and lateral bending at both treated levels as compared with ACDF. Radiographic adjacent segment degeneration was seen at the inferior (Mobi-C 30.3% vs. ACDF 66.7%) and superior (Mobi-C 37.5% vs. ACDF 80.8%) levels. Subsequent surgery for adjacent segment disease occurred in 4.4% of patients after Mobi-C cervical TDR and 11.4% of ACDF patients at 7 years. While PROMs favored two-level cervical TDR, the clinical significance of differences in ROM and adjacent segment disease remains to be seen. The two-level Prestige LP also showed superior results when compared with ACDF with respect to overall success criteria, NDI, and neurologic success.

22. Are there any specific challenges associated with revision of a cervical TDR to ACDF?

The options for revision of a patient with persistent or new-onset symptoms following cervical TDR include:
- Posterior cervical foraminotomy
- Removal of the device in combination with anterior cervical fusion with plate fixation
- Revision with placement of a new cervical TDR

Removal of a cervical disc arthroplasty device requires more extensive exposure compared with primary cervical disc arthroplasty or primary ACDF. It is important to have device-specific instruments to facilitate removal of cervical TDR components. It has been reported that perioperative wound infection, hospital length of stay, and costs are higher for cervical TDR revision compared with revision ACDF.

23. What are the outcomes of cervical TDR when placed adjacent to a prior fusion versus primary cervical TDR or two-level ACDF?

Placement of a cervical TDR adjacent to an ACDF is termed a **hybrid procedure**. The theoretical benefits of such a procedure include the preservation of cervical motion across the operative segments and decrease in the rate of adjacent-level adverse events associated with cervical fusion. While early studies have indicated that a cervical TDR placed adjacent to a fusion leads to similar clinical outcomes compared with a primary cervical TDR or ACDF, data from prospective, randomized controlled trials are necessary to confirm the benefits of this approach.

24. When is cervical TDR an appropriate option for treatment of cervical myelopathy?

Cervical total disc arthroplasty has been shown to be successful for treatment of select patients with cervical myelopathy in whom spinal cord compression is localized to the level of the disc space (retrodiscal). This procedure is not appropriate for patients with severe facet joint degenerative changes at the operative level, severe loss of disc space height, myelopathy due to congenital spinal canal narrowing, and cervical stenosis due to retrovertebral cord compression (e.g., ossification of the posterior longitudinal ligament).

KEY POINTS

1. Cervical total disc arthroplasty is an option for treatment of radiculopathy and/or myelopathy due to neural compression localized to the level of the disc space caused by a disc herniation or spondylotic changes between C3 and C7 that are refractory to nonoperative treatment.
2. Lumbar total disc arthroplasty is an option for treatment of isolated discogenic low back pain caused by degenerative disc disease between L3 and S1 without associated instability that is refractory to nonoperative treatment.
3. Explantation of a failed lumbar total disc arthroplasty is a complex and high-risk procedure compared with revision surgery for a failed cervical total disc arthroplasty.

Websites
1. Cervical total disc arthroplasty: https://www.ncbi.nlm.nih.gov/pmc/articles/PMC6394883/
2. Lumbar total disc arthroplasty: https://www.ncbi.nlm.nih.gov/pmc/articles/PMC5585094/

BIBLIOGRAPHY

1. Abi-Hanna, D., Kerferd, J., Phan, K., Rao, P., & Mobbs, R. (2018). Lumbar disk arthroplasty for degenerative disk disease: Literature review. *World Neurosurgery, 109,* 188–196.
2. Formica, M., Divano, S., Cavagnaro, L., Basso, M., Zanirato, A., Formica, C., et al. (2017). Lumbar total disc arthroplasty: Outdated surgery or here to stay procedure? A systematic review of current literature. *Journal of Orthopaedics and Traumatology, 18*(3), 197–215.
3. Hilibrand, A. S., Carlson, G. D., Palumbo, M. A., Jones, P. K., & Bohlman, H. H. (1999). Radiculopathy and myelopathy at segments adjacent to the site of a previous anterior cervical arthrodesis. *Journal of Bone and Joint Surgery, 81,* 519–528.
4. Laratta, J. L., Shillingford, J. N., Saifi, C., & Riew, K. D. (2018). Cervical disc arthroplasty: A comprehensive review of single-level, multilevel, and hybrid procedures. *Global Spine Journal, 8,* 78–83.
5. Lawrence, B. D., Hilibrand, A. S., Brodt, E. D., Dettori, J. R., & Brodke, D. S. (2012). Predicting the risk of adjacent segment pathology in the cervical spine: A systematic review. *Spine, 37,* 52–64.
6. Lawrence, B. D., Wang, J., Arnold, P., Hermsmeyer, J., Norvell, D. C., & Brodke, D. S. (2012). Predicting the risk of adjacent segment pathology after lumbar fusion: A systematic review. *Spine, 37,* 123–132.
7. Riew, K. D., Buchowski, J. M., Sasso, R., Zdeblick, T., Metcalf, N. H., & Anderson, P. A. (2008). Cervical disc arthroplasty compared with arthrodesis for the treatment of myelopathy. *Journal of Bone and Joint Surgery, 90,* 2354–2364.
8. Zigler, J. E., & Delamarter, R. B. (2012). Five-year results of the prospective, randomized, multicenter, Food and Drug Administration investigational device exemption study of the ProDisc-L total disc replacement versus circumferential arthrodesis for the treatment of single-level degenerative disc disease. *Journal of Neurosurgery Spine, 17,* 493–501.

CHAPTER 33

REVISION SPINE SURGERY

Vincent J. Devlin, MD

GENERAL CONSIDERATIONS

1. Why is the term *failed back surgery syndrome* considered controversial?

   Failed back surgery syndrome is an imprecise term used to refer to patients with unsatisfactory outcomes after spine surgery due to persistent or recurrent pain in the spine and/or extremities. This term does not identify a specific diagnosis responsible for persistent symptoms and implies that additional treatment will not provide benefit. Patients with persistent symptoms following surgical treatment should undergo appropriate assessment to differentiate problems amenable to additional surgical treatment from those problems unlikely to benefit from an operation. Patients unlikely to benefit from additional surgery can then be directed toward appropriate global multidisciplinary nonsurgical management strategies involving specialists with expertise in behavioral health, pain management, rehabilitation medicine, neuromodulation, and other advanced pain therapies.

2. What key elements should be present to support the diagnosis of failed back surgery syndrome?

   An international multidisciplinary panel of experts proposed the following criteria (8):
   - Persistent back and/or leg pain for a minimum duration of 6 months following a recent spine procedure
   - Completion of a thorough clinical and spinal imaging assessment
   - Absence of a clear surgical target based on clinical examination and imaging that is concordant with current symptoms
   - Interdisciplinary agreement that additional surgical intervention for spinal decompression and/or fusion is not appropriate

3. What are some common identifiable causes that may be responsible for poor outcomes following an initial spinal procedure?

   Multiple factors may contribute to a poor outcome following an initial spinal procedure in a specific patient. These causes may occur singularly or in combination. Specific etiologies to consider include:
   - **Negative patient characteristics:** Barriers to successful outcomes may arise as a consequence of medical comorbidities (i.e., diabetes, osteoporosis, smoking), psychosocial factors (litigation, depression, opioid-use disorder, unresolved worker's compensation claims), or a patient's unrealistic expectations and goals regarding surgical treatment.
   - **Inappropriate surgical indications:** An inappropriately indicated procedure will predictably lead to a poor outcome. For example, if a spinal fusion is performed for nonspecific low back pain in the absence of an identified pain generator, improvement in symptoms is unlikely.
   - **Incorrect or incomplete diagnosis:** Surgery is unlikely to benefit a patient when it is based on incomplete preoperative assessment, inadequate imaging studies, or when there is a poor correlation between imaging findings and clinical signs and symptoms.
   - **Inappropriate surgical procedures:** Surgery performed at the incorrect spinal level or surgery that is inadequate to address all aspects of a patient's spinal pathology (i.e., failure to stabilize and fuse when a decompression is performed at an unstable spinal segment) is doomed to failure.
   - **Technical issues related to the index surgical procedure:** An appropriately indicated spine procedure will fail if surgery is not performed with technical expertise. Persistent symptoms may result due to surgical approach-related complications, neural impingement from incorrectly placed spinal implants, incomplete removal of disc fragments, inadequate decompression of spinal stenosis, inadequate instrumentation constructs which dislodge or fail prematurely, or due to failure to maintain or restore lumbar lordosis when multiple lumbar levels undergo spinal instrumentation and fusion.
   - **Persistence or progression of an underlying disease process:** Ongoing spinal degeneration or recurrent tumors may affect the previously operated or adjacent levels and lead to recurrent axial or radicular symptoms.
   - **Epidural, perineural, or intradural fibrosis:** The formation of scar tissue and adhesions following surgery may manifest as chronic neuropathic pain.

- **Postoperative surgical complications:** Prompt recognition and treatment of postoperative complications such as wound infection, epidural hematoma, cerebrospinal fluid (CSF) leakage, implant failure, or pseudarthrosis, are critical to prevent permanent sequalae.
- **Postoperative medical complications:** Major medical complications (i.e., myocardial infarction, pulmonary embolus, stroke, acute kidney injury) are associated with increased patient morbidity and mortality.

4. List some important factors to assess based on the history portion of an initial evaluation of a patient with continuing symptoms after spine surgery.
- What were the indications for the initial or most recent surgery?
- Are the present symptoms predominantly radicular pain, axial pain, or both?
- Are symptoms related to activity and relieved with rest or are symptoms continuous and unrelated to activity?
- Are the present symptoms the same, better, or worse after surgery?
- Was there a period during which the patient had relief of preoperative symptoms (pain-free interval)?
- Are the current symptoms similar to or different from those present before surgery?
- Did intraoperative complications occur? (Review the operative report if possible.)
- Were any complications recognized in the postoperative period?
- Inquire regarding work history, involvement in litigation, substance abuse, tobacco use, and investigate if there are other psychosocial factors that could impact future treatment.
- Is there a history of fever, chills, weight loss, or night sweats?

5. What is the significance of a pain-free interval following spinal surgery? How does the temporal relationship of current symptoms in relation to the index procedure help to inform the differential diagnosis?
The presence or absence of a pain-free interval following surgery and the temporal relationship of symptoms to the index surgical procedure provide a starting point for determining the likely causes of symptoms.
- **When there is no improvement following surgery or recurrent symptoms within 1 month.** Consider wrong level surgery, wrong procedure performed, failure to adequately remove disc fragments or decompress spinal stenosis, iatrogenic nerve root injury, neural impingement by spinal implants, postoperative hematoma or seroma, and surgical site infection.
- **When there is initial symptom relief but pain recurs between 1 and 6 months after surgery.** Consider recurrent disc herniation, implant failure, loosening or migration, iatrogenic spinal instability (i.e., secondary to pars or facet fracture), and surgical site infection.
- **When there is initial symptom relief with pain recurrence after 6 months following surgery.** Consider recurrent pathology at the previously operated segment, new spinal pathology at adjacent segments, epidural, perineural or intradural fibrosis, pseudarthrosis (if spinal fusion was performed), and surgical site infection.

6. What are important points to assess during physical examination of the patient being evaluated for possible revision spine surgery?
A general neurologic assessment and regional spinal assessment are performed. The presence of nonorganic signs (Waddell signs) should be assessed. Global spinal balance in the sagittal and coronal planes is evaluated. The physical examination is tailored to the particular spinal pathology under evaluation. For cervical spine disorders, shoulder pathology, brachial plexus disorders, and conditions involving the peripheral nerves should not be overlooked. For lumbar spine problems, the hip joints, sacroiliac joints, and any prior bone graft sites should be assessed. Examination of peripheral pulses is routinely performed to rule out vascular insufficiency. Depending on clinical symptoms, neurologic disorders such as amyotrophic lateral sclerosis or multiple sclerosis are considered.

7. Are laboratory tests useful in the workup of a patient for possible revision spine surgery?
Yes. Erythrocyte sedimentation rate (ESR) and C-reactive protein (CRP) levels are obtained to rule out an occult infection. Albumin and transferrin levels may be obtained to assess nutritional status.

8. What diagnostic tests are useful in the evaluation of patients following prior spinal surgery?
The sequence of diagnostic studies in the postoperative patient is similar to assessment for primary spine surgery. Imaging studies are indicated to confirm the most likely cause of symptoms based on a comprehensive history and physical examination. Imaging studies performed prior to the most recent surgery should be reviewed if available to better understand details regarding prior surgical treatment. Additional tests that may be considered include diagnostic blocks and electrodiagnostic studies.
- **Radiographs:** Upright posteroanterior (PA) and lateral spine radiographs are the initial imaging study of choice. Lateral flexion-extension radiographs play a role in the diagnosis of postoperative instability and pseudarthrosis. Spinal deformities are assessed using standing PA and lateral radiographs of the entire spine or EOS slot-scanning. An anteroposterior (AP) pelvis radiograph is obtained to assess for hip-joint pathology when indicated. Depending on presenting symptoms, extremity radiographs may be obtained to evaluate for peripheral joint pathologies, which may mimic spine pathology.

- **Magnetic resonance imaging (MRI), computed tomography (CT), and CT-myelography:** The most appropriate study is selected based on the patient's symptoms, the presence or absence of spinal implants, and the specific spinal pathology requiring assessment. MRI with or without gadolinium enhancement is used to visualize the neural elements and associated bony and soft tissue structures. However, MRI is subject to degradation by metal artifact that may arise from microscopic debris remaining at the initial surgical site or from spinal implants (especially nontitanium implants). CT remains the optimal test to assess bone detail and is the most sensitive test for diagnosis of pseudarthrosis. CT-myelography continues to play a role in evaluating the previously operated spine. It provides excellent visualization of the thecal sac and nerve roots in addition to osseous structure, even in the presence of spinal deformity or extensive metallic spinal implants.
- **Nuclear medicine studies:** Technetium bone scans and positron emission tomography (PET) scans are infrequently utilized in planning revision spine procedures, but can provide valuable information to support a diagnosis of infection or metastatic disease.
- **Diagnostic blocks:** Various injection procedures have been described for use in the assessment of anatomic pain generators including discography, medial branch or facet blocks, selective nerve root blocks, and sacroiliac injections.
- **Electrodiagnostic studies:** Electromyograms and nerve conduction velocity studies may be used to assess nerve injury and distinguish between radiculopathy and peripheral neuropathy.

9. What treatment options are available for patients with persistent back or leg symptoms following previous spinal surgery in the absence of a surgically correctable spinal problem?
   - Physical therapy
   - Medication
   - Psychosocial interventions including cognitive behavioral therapy
   - Spinal cord stimulation
   - Intrathecal narcotics (implantable drug pump)
   - Complementary and alternative medicine approaches

10. What surgical options are available for patients who experience persistent symptoms following spine surgery?
    The options for revision surgery may be grouped into the following categories:
    - **Spinal decompression procedures** are performed to relieve encroachment upon the spinal cord and/or nerve roots that has persisted following prior procedures or has developed subsequent to the most recent surgical procedure.
    - **Spinal realignment using spinal instrumentation** with or without adjunctive spinal osteotomies is indicated for treatment of spinal deformities.
    - **Spinal stabilization** is indicated for treatment of spinal instabilities, spinal deformities, and to enhance fusion.
    - **Adjunctive procedures** may be indicated for treatment of related issues including surgery for removal of broken, loose, migrated, or prominent spinal implants, and anterior spinal column reconstruction to restore anterior column load sharing and enhance fusion.

11. What are some basic principles to follow when planning a revision spinal procedure?
    - Perform a comprehensive preoperative patient assessment and risk stratification
    - Optimize the patient prior to revision spine surgery (i.e., smoking cessation, nutritional enhancement, osteoporosis treatment, diabetes management, prehabilitation)
    - Develop a comprehensive preoperative surgical plan which addresses the reason(s) for failure of the previous procedure(s) and provides a definitive surgical solution
    - Ensure adequate neural decompression
    - When fusion is indicated, meticulous preparation of fusion sites and use of an adequate amounts and appropriate types of bone graft materials are critical
    - Maintain or restore sagittal and coronal plane alignment
    - Use biomechanically appropriate spinal implant constructs which achieve fixation using an adequate number of anchor points and reconstruct the anterior spinal column when this is indicated

12. Outline a systematic approach to workup and treatment of a patient who presents with upper or lower extremity radiculopathy following previous spine surgery in terms of an algorithm.
    See Fig. 33.1.

13. Outline a systematic approach to workup and treatment of a patient who presents with axial neck or low back pain following previous spine surgery in terms of an algorithm.
    See Fig. 33.2.

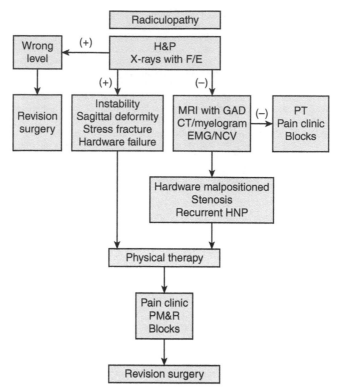

Fig. 33.1 Radiculopathy algorithm. *CT,* Computed tomography; *EMG,* electromyogram; *F/E,* flexion/extension; *GAD,* gadolinium; *H&P,* history and physical examination; *HNP,* herniated nucleus pulposus; *MRI,* magnetic resonance imaging; *NCV,* nerve conduction velocity; *PT,* physical therapy; *PM&R,* physical medicine and rehabilitation. (From Garfin SR, Eismont FJ, Bell GR, editors. Rothman-Simeone The Spine. 7th ed. Philadelphia, PA: Elsevier; 2018, pp. 1851–1863, Fig. 102.14, p. 1860.)

REVISION SURGERY AFTER PRIOR SPINAL DECOMPRESSION PROCEDURES

14. List common causes of failure following spinal decompression procedures according to time of symptom onset in relation to surgery.
    See Table 33.1.

15. What are some factors to consider when treating a recurrent lumbar disc herniation?
    A recurrent lumbar disc herniation is strictly defined as a symptomatic disc herniation occurring at the same spinal level and same side as a previously operated lumbar disc, with a pain-free interval after the primary discectomy that is greater than 3 weeks to 6 months. Alternate definitions include both ipsilateral and contralateral herniations at the previously operated level as recurrent lumbar disc herniations. The absence of a pain-free interval following lumbar discectomy suggests an alternate diagnosis such as wrong-level surgery, persistent symptoms due to incomplete removal of disc material, or unrecognized or residual subarticular or foraminal stenosis. The incidence of recurrent disc herniation following microsurgical lumbar discectomy is estimated to range between 5% and 18%, and is dependent on the criteria used to define recurrence, the extent of operative disc removal, and the size of the posterior annular defect. Higher rates of recurrence (up to 27%) have been reported in patients in whom large annular defects (>6 mm) were present at conclusion of discectomy. It is important to appreciate that although a postoperative MRI may identify the presence of a postoperative disc herniation, the herniation may or may not be associated with symptoms. Surgical treatment for a recurrent lumbar disc herniation is appropriate for patients with correlative symptoms refractory to nonoperative treatment or for patients with neurologic deficits. Revision lumbar microdiscectomy is recommended for patients who present with a first-time symptomatic recurrent disc herniation and radicular pain in the absence of radiographic spinal instability. Patients who present with multiple recurrences, radiographic evidence of spinal instability, or severe chronic low back pain are treated with complete discectomy, interbody fusion, and spinal instrumentation.

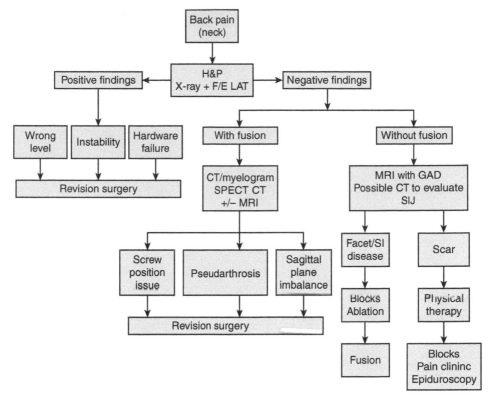

Fig. 33.2 Back pain algorithm. *CT,* Computed tomography; *F/E LAT,* flexion/extension lateral; *GAD,* gadolinium; *H&P,* history and physical examination; *MRI,* magnetic resonance imaging; *SIJ,* sacroiliac joint; *SPECT,* single photon emission computed tomography. (From Easton RW. Failed back surgery syndrome: Historical perspective. In: Garfin SR, Eismont FJ, Bell GR, editors. Rothman-Simeone The Spine. 7th ed. Philadelphia, PA: Elsevier; 2018, pp. 1851–1863, Fig. 102.13, p. 1860.)

16. **What is the most common technique-related factor responsible for persistent radicular pain after lumbar spinal decompression for spinal stenosis?**
    Inadequate neural decompression is the most common technique-related factor responsible for persistent radicular pain following posterior decompression for lumbar spinal stenosis. Surgeons should address all the potential sources of nerve compression including central stenosis, lateral recess stenosis, foraminal stenosis, and extraforaminal compression. When there is a concern about potential instability from excessive bone removal, adequate decompression and concomitant instrumented spinal fusion are indicated.

17. **What preoperative factors increase the risk of developing iatrogenic instability following lumbar decompression for treatment of degenerative lumbar spinal stenosis?**
    Preoperative risk factors that increase the risk of developing iatrogenic instability following lumbar decompression include multilevel decompression, disc height >6 mm, preoperative listhesis, sagittal facet-joint orientation, decreased bone mineral density, and degenerative scoliosis. Surgical techniques that restrict the extent of resection of midline posterior osteoligamentous structures and preserve at least 50% of the facet joint complex and 5 mm of the pars interarticularis bilaterally have been recommended to limit the risk of iatrogenic instability.

18. **Outline the clinical presentation, diagnosis, and treatment of pain attributed to epidural fibrosis and/or arachnoiditis.**
    Scar tissue and adhesions routinely develop after spine surgery, but their relationship to symptoms is inconsistent. In some cases, postoperative inflammation, fibrosis, and adhesions involving the epidural space and intrathecal space (arachnoiditis) are associated with neuropathic pain symptoms involving the spine and extremities. The pain is often described as burning, constant in nature, and worsens with activity. Symptoms may be diffuse or localized to a dermatomal distribution. Radiculopathy and myelopathy may be present. Diagnosis is made with MRI, with and without gadolinium, or with CT-myelography. Imaging findings may include aggregation and clumping of nerve roots or peripheral localization of nerve roots within the thecal sac (empty sac sign). Nonsurgical treatment

Table 33.1 Classification of Failures After Spinal Decompression Procedures.
1. No Improvement in Radicular Symptoms Immediately Following Surgery
A. Wrong Preoperative Diagnosis
1. Tumor
2. Infection
3. Metabolic disease
4. Psychosocial causes
5. Discogenic pain syndrome
6. Decompression performed too late
B. Technical Error
1. Surgery performed at wrong level(s)
2. Inadequate decompression performed
a. Missed disc fragment
b. Failure to treat coexistent spinal stenosis and disc herniation
c. Conjoined nerve root
2. Temporary Relief but Recurrence of Pain
A. Early Recurrence of Symptoms (Within Weeks)
1. Hematoma
2. Infection
3. Meningeal cyst
4. Facet or pars fracture
B. Midterm Failure (Within Weeks to Months)
1. Recurrent disc herniation
2. Stress fracture of pars interarticularis
3. Battered root syndrome
4. Epidural fibrosis or arachnoiditis
5. Unrealistic patient expectations
C. Long-Term Failure (Within Months to Years)
1. Recurrent stenosis
2. Adjacent-level stenosis
3. Segmental spinal instability

Adapted from Kostuik JP. The surgical treatment of failures of laminectomy. Spine State Art Rev 1997;11:509–538.

is recommended and consists of multimodal therapy, which may include anticonvulsants, antidepressants, antiinflammatories, topical medications, oral opioids, spinal cord stimulation, intrathecal morphine pumps, and psychosocial assessment.

REVISION SURGERY AFTER PRIOR SPINAL FUSION

19. List some of the common causes of failure following spinal fusion procedures according to time of symptom onset in relation to surgery and whether the predominant symptoms are axial spine pain or extremity pain.
    See Table 33.2.

20. What is a pseudarthrosis?
    Pseudarthrosis is defined as failure to obtain a solid bony union after an attempted spinal fusion. While this condition may be asymptomatic in some patients, patients with pseudarthrosis often require revision surgery for treatment of related symptoms. The time between initial surgery and the clinical and radiographic presentation of a pseudarthrosis is variable. One year following initial surgery is often cited as an appropriate interval for determining fusion success. However, in some patients pseudarthroses may not present until several years following the index surgery, especially for patients undergoing multilevel spinal instrumentation and fusion procedures. The diagnosis of pseudarthrosis is suggested by the presence of continued or recurrent axial pain and/or neurologic symptoms following surgery and the absence of bridging trabecular bone on plain radiographs or CT scans.

21. What factors influence the rate of pseudarthrosis which is reported following a spinal fusion procedure?
    - The number of levels fused
    - Fusion technique (posterior vs. interbody vs. circumferential techniques)
    - Use and type of spinal instrumentation

Table 33.2 Classification of Failures After Spinal Fusion Procedures.

TIMING	Predominant Symptoms	
	BACK PAIN	LEG SYMPTOMS
Early (weeks)	1. Infection 2. Wrong level fused 3. Insufficient levels fused 4. Psychosocial distress 5. Junctional failure	1. Neural impingement by implants 2. Foraminal stenosis due to change in spinal alignment
Midterm (months)	1. Pseudarthrosis 2. Adjacent-level degeneration 3. Sagittal imbalance 4. Graft donor site pain 5. Inadequate reconditioning 6. Implant failure	1. Neural compression secondary to pseudarthrosis 2. Clinical adjacent segment pathology 3. Graft donor site pain
Long-term (years)	1. Late pseudarthrosis 2. Adjacent-level instability 3. Acquired spondylolysis 4. Compression fracture adjacent to fusion 5. Abutment syndrome	1. Adjacent-level stenosis 2. Adjacent-level disc herniation

Adapted from Kostuik JP. Failures after spinal fusion. Spine State Art Rev 1997;11:589–650.

- Type of bone graft material (autograft, allograft, bone graft substitutes, bone morphogenetic proteins)
- Spinal diagnosis
- Patient-related factors—age, nicotine use, osteoporosis, vitamin D deficiency, medications (e.g., nonsteroidal antiinflammatory drugs)
- Radiographic criteria used to define fusion success

22. **What is the most reliable method for diagnosis of a pseudarthrosis?**
The most reliable method for diagnosis of pseudarthrosis remains surgical exploration of the fusion mass. The most common noninvasive methods used to assess fusion are plain radiography and CT scans. Static radiographs are the most common noninvasive method used to evaluate spinal fusion. Diagnosis of pseudarthrosis is based on the presence of bone bridging, but use of this criteria overestimates the presence of a solid fusion. Flexion-extension radiography may be used to increase diagnostic accuracy, but unfortunately there is a lack of consensus regarding which criteria should be used to define fusion success. In the cervical region, measurement of the interspinous process distance on flexion-extension views is recommended. Interspinous motion ≥1 mm at 150% radiographic magnification with adjacent-level motion of at least 4 mm has been correlated with the diagnosis of pseudarthrosis. In the lumbar region, proposed motion criteria used to define fusion success include <3 mm of translational motion and <5° of angular motion on flexion-extension radiographs. Computerized motion analysis of flexion-extension radiographs may be used to decrease measurement error. Other radiographic observations that suggest the presence of pseudarthrosis include peri-implant radiolucencies, implant failure, and loss of spinal deformity correction. The most accurate imaging method for diagnosis of pseudarthrosis is a thin-section multiplanar CT scan with two-dimensional and three-dimensional reconstructions, but it is associated with significant radiation exposure.

23. **What strategies are recommended for treatment of a pseudarthrosis?**
Asymptomatic patients with pseudarthrosis may be observed for development of symptoms, progressive deformity or implant-related complications. Operative management of a symptomatic pseudarthrosis should only be considered after the patient is optimized for surgery. Revision surgery may require a different surgical approach from that used in the original fusion procedure. Revision surgery often requires the use of additional instrumentation and extension of the fusion to proximal and/or distal spinal levels in combination with use of bone graft materials, including autograft, allograft, bone graft substitutes, and osteoinductive recombinant bone morphogenetic proteins. The overall goals of surgery include achievement of a successful arthrodesis, decompression of concomitant neural compression, and maintenance or restoration of sagittal and coronal plane alignment. Cervical pseudarthroses may be managed through either an anterior or posterior surgical approach, and occasionally circumferential surgery may be necessary. Thoracic pseudarthroses are most often managed through a posterior surgical approach. Circumferential surgery is generally recommended for treatment of lumbar pseudarthroses.

24. Explain what is meant by the term adjacent segment pathology.

The term adjacent segment pathology (ASP) has been proposed as a general term to describe changes that occur adjacent to a previously operated spinal level (5). Radiographic adjacent segment pathology (RASP) refers to asymptomatic radiologic changes that occur at the adjacent segment, and includes findings noted on MRI studies. Clinical adjacent segment pathology (CASP) refers to clinically symptomatic radiologic degenerative changes adjacent to the previously operated motion segment. Whether the radiographic and clinical findings are a result of the iatrogenically created rigid spinal segment or progression of the natural history of an underlying degenerative process remains controversial. Preexisting asymptomatic degenerative changes at spinal levels adjacent to a planned spinal fusion, multilevel fusions, and postoperative sagittal imbalance, are considered among the factors which predispose a patient to CASP.

REVISION SURGERY FOR SPINAL DEFORMITY

25. How common is revision surgery following an initial surgical procedure for adult spinal deformity and what are some common causes for reoperation?

The two-year revision risk following adult spinal deformity is approximately 20% (6). The most common reason for revision surgery is implant failure. Other common reasons for revision include infection, deformity progression, pseudarthrosis, neurologic deficit, miscellaneous implant-related issues, and proximal junctional failure (Box 33.1). Increased age and high comorbidity burden are associated with increased risk of revision.

26. Distinguish between proximal junctional kyphosis and proximal junctional failure.

Increase in the kyphotic angle above the proximal end of a posterior spinal instrumentation construct is a specific form of ASP and occurs along a spectrum ranging from an asymptomatic radiographic observation to a serious complication associated with implant failure, neurologic injury, and revision surgery. The **proximal junctional angle** is most commonly measured as the Cobb angle between the inferior endplate of the upper instrumented vertebra (UIV) and the superior endplate of the second vertebra above the UIV. **Proximal junctional kyphosis** (PJK) is defined as an increase in the proximal junctional angle $\geq 10°$ compared with either the preoperative measurement or by comparing the immediate postoperative and final follow-up radiographs. Postoperative PJK is a common radiographic finding with a rate of occurrence as high as 40%, but is associated with limited clinical impact as most patients do not require revision surgery. **Proximal junctional failure** (PJF) is defined as an increase in the proximal junctional angle due to junctional fracture involving the UIV or the vertebra immediately proximal to the UIV (UIV+1), fixation failure involving the UIV, or posterior osseous or ligamentous disruption requiring proximal extension of the fusion construct. PJF is associated with a major clinical impact as it is often associated with progressive kyphosis, vertebral subluxation, neurologic deficit, implant failure, and the need for unplanned revision surgery. Various strategies have been proposed to prevent PJF including prophylactic vertebroplasty at the UIV and UIV+1 levels, use of hooks rather than pedicle screws at the UIV, tapered transition rods at proximal levels ("soft landing" concept), terminal-rod contouring, percutaneous screw placement at proximal levels, and ligament augmentation.

27. Compare the surgical complication profile, hospital length of stay, and mortality rates for primary and revision surgery procedures for treatment of adult spinal deformity.

Based on US study data from over 10,000 patients undergoing surgery for adult spinal deformity (2), the complication rate in the revision surgery group was higher than in the primary surgery group (66% vs. 52%). Device-related complications were higher in the revision surgery group (44% vs. 6%). Adult spinal deformity patients who underwent revision surgery had an increased risk of nervous system complications, hematoma/seroma, vessel/nerve puncture, postoperative infection, acute respiratory distress syndrome, venous thrombosis events, and wound dehiscence. Revision surgery was associated with increased length of hospital stay compared to primary

---

Box 33.1 Indications for Revision Surgery for Adult Spinal Deformity

1. Implant failure
2. Infection
3. Pseudarthrosis
4. Deformity progression
5. Neurologic deficit
6. Painful or prominent implants
7. Proximal junctional failure
8. Distal junctional failure
9. Sagittal plane imbalance
10. Coronal plane imbalance

surgery. Despite these differences, the mortality rates were similar for primary and revision adult spinal deformity patients.

28. Describe the surgical treatment options for sagittal imbalance following spine surgery.
    Surgery for treatment of sagittal imbalance following prior spine surgery may be accomplished through a variety of surgical strategies, including a single posterior surgical approach or combined anterior and posterior surgical approaches, and often includes use of interbody fusions and spinal osteotomies. Interbody fusions may be performed through a variety of methods including posterior lumbar interbody fusion (PLIF), transforaminal lumbar interbody fusion (TLIF), lateral lumbar interbody fusion (LLIF), and anterior lumbar interbody fusion (ALIF). Nomenclature for the various types of spinal osteotomies has been standardized according to the Schwab anatomical osteotomy classification. Grade 1 osteotomies involve resection of the inferior facet and joint capsule at the osteotomy level, and require mobility of the anterior spinal column. An osteotomy performed through fused articular processes is often referred to as a Smith Peterson osteotomy. Grade 2 osteotomies involve complete facet joint resection and partial resection of the lamina, spinous processes, and ligamentum flavum, and require mobility of the anterior spinal column. A grade 2 osteotomy performed through fused articular processes is often referred to as a Smith Peterson osteotomy. Polysegmental grade 2 osteotomies are referred to as Ponte osteotomies. A grade 3 osteotomy involves resection of the posterior elements in combination with resection of a wedge of bone from the posterior vertebral body and is referred to as a pedicle subtraction osteotomy (PSO). Grade 4 osteotomies are similar to grade 3 osteotomies and also include resection of an adjacent end plate and adjacent intervertebral disc. Grade 5 osteotomies involve resection of one vertebral body and both adjacent discs, while Grade 6 osteotomies involve resection of more than one adjacent vertebral body and discs. Grade 5 and Grade 6 osteotomies are referred to as vertebral column resection procedures (Fig. 33.3).

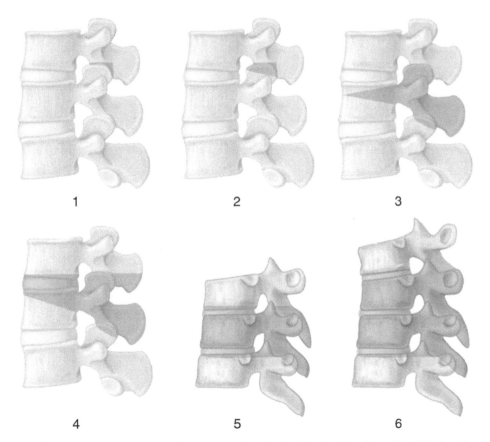

Fig. 33.3 Schwab anatomic classification of spinal osteotomies based on six grades of resection. (From Graham RB, Koski TR. Dorsal thoracic and lumbar combined and complex techniques. In: Steinmetz MP, Benzel EG, editors. Benzel's Spine Surgery. 4th ed. Philadelphia, PA: Elsevier; 2017, pp 742–748, Fig. 86.2.)

KEY POINTS

1. Selection of appropriate candidates for revision spinal surgery depends on comprehensive assessment to determine the factors that led to a less than optimal outcome following initial surgery.
2. For poor surgical outcomes due to errors in surgical strategy or surgical technique associated with the index procedure, appropriate revision surgery may offer a reasonable chance of improved outcome.
3. For surgical failures due to errors in diagnosis or inappropriate patient selection for initial surgery, revision surgery offers little chance for improved outcomes and other treatments are indicated.
4. In the absence of relevant and specific anatomic and pathologic findings, pain itself is not an indication for revision surgery.

Websites
1. Failed back surgery syndrome: https://practicalpainmanagement.com/pain/spine/failed-back-surgery-syndrome2
2. Failed surgery and revision surgery: http://www.wheelessonline.com/ISSLS/content/section-18/
3. The Scoli-RISK-1 Study: https://www.youtube.com/watch?v=B-M1LahuW8o

---

BIBLIOGRAPHY

1. Cerpa, M., Lenke, L. G., Fehlings, M. G., Shaffrey, C. I., Cheung, K. M., & Carreon, L. Y. (2019). Evolution and advancement of adult spinal deformity research and clinical care: An overview of the Scoli-RISK-1 Study. *Global Spine Journal, 9,* 8–14.
2. Diebo, B. G., Passias, P. G., Marascalchi, B. J., Jalai, C. M., Worley, N. J., & Errico, T. J. (2015). Primary versus revision surgery in the setting of adult spinal deformity: A nationwide study on 10,912 patients. *Spine, 40,* 1674–1680.
3. Guyer, R. D., Patterson, M., & Ohnmeiss, D. D. (2006). Failed back surgery syndrome: Diagnostic evaluation. *Journal of the American Academy of Orthopaedic Surgeons, 14,* 534–543.
4. Hill, J. M., Kim, E., Khan, I., & Devin, C. J. (2019). Evaluation and workup in revision spine surgery. *Seminars in Spine Surgery, 31,* 44–52.
5. Norvell, D. C., Dettori, J. R., Skelly, A. C., Riew, K. D., Chapman, J. R., & Anderson, P. A. (2012). Methodology for the systematic reviews on adjacent segment pathology. *Spine, 37,* S10–S17.
6. Pitter, F. T., Lindberg-Larsen, M., Pedersen, A. B., Dahl, B., & Gehrchen, M. (2019). Revision risk after primary adult spinal deformity surgery: A nationwide study with two-year follow-up. *Spine Deformity, 7,* 619–626.
7. Raman, T., Miller, E., Martin, C. T., & Kebaish, K. M. (2017). The effect of prophylactic vertebroplasty on the incidence of proximal junctional kyphosis and proximal junctional failure following posterior spinal fusion in adult spinal deformity: A 5-year follow-up study. *Spine Journal, 17,* 1489–1498.
8. Rigoard, P., Gatzinsky, K., Deneuville, J. P., Duyvendak, W., Naiditch, N., Van Buyten, J. P., et al. (2019). Optimizing the management and outcomes of failed back surgery syndrome: A consensus statement on definition and outlines for patient assessment. *Pain Research and Management, 2019,* 3126464.
9. Schwab, F., Blondel, B., Chay, E., Demakakos, J., Lenke, L., Tropiano, P., et al. (2014). The comprehensive anatomical spinal osteotomy classification. *Neurosurgery, 74,* 112–120.
10. Selby, M. D., Clark, S. R., Hall, D. J., & Freeman, B. J. (2012). Radiologic assessment of spinal fusion. *Journal of the American Academy of Orthopaedic Surgeons, 20,* 694–703.

CHAPTER 34

SPINAL CORD STIMULATION AND IMPLANTABLE DRUG DELIVERY SYSTEMS

Alejandro Carrasquilla, MD, Jonathan J. Rasouli, MD, Fedor E. Panov, MD, and Brian H. Kopell, MD

1. What is neuromodulation?

   Neuromodulation involves the use of both implantable and nonimplantable medical device technologies for treatment of disease through enhancement or suppression of the activity of the nervous system using electrical, pharmacologic, or other agents. Neuromodulation therapies may target the brain, spinal cord, peripheral nerves, and autonomic nervous system. Examples of neuromodulation therapies include spinal cord stimulation, deep brain stimulation, peripheral nerve stimulation, and surgically implanted drug delivery systems.

2. What is the historical basis for the use of electrical impulses for the purpose of neuromodulation?

   Use of electrical impulses for treatment of pain dates back to antiquity when use of torpedo fish to produce numbness was first described. The modern era involving use of electrical impulses for neuromodulation began with deep brain stimulation in the 1960s and was soon followed by application of spinal cord stimulation to the treatment of intractable pain. More recently, electrical stimulation of the central or peripheral nervous system has been applied to the treatment of patients with spinal cord injuries in an attempt to restore various types of functions.

3. What is spinal cord stimulation?

   Modern spinal cord stimulators (SCSs) are neuromodulatory devices that utilize epidural electrodes placed percutaneously, or through a limited open exposure, to deliver electrical impulses to the spinal cord. The epidural electrodes are connected by lead wires to an implanted, programmable pulse generator that can have an internal or external power source. Classically, this stimulation has been used to reduce neuropathic pain, or pain resulting from damage or abnormal activity within the nervous system. By acting on white-matter pathways in the dorsal column of the spinal cord, most modern SCS systems exchange debilitating neuropathic pain with paresthesias, which are considered more tolerable. SCS does not reliably relieve nociceptive pain, or pain from surgery or tissue damage. The location of the stimulation within the vertical axis of the spinal cord targets different areas of the body. Interestingly, SCS have been shown to have angiogenic effects, and have been used to treat diseases such as peripheral artery disease or angina pectoris. Spinal cord stimulation has been further studied for treatment of pain and paralysis resulting from spinal cord injury (SCI).

4. What are the mechanisms by which spinal cord stimulation exerts its effect?

   In the context of treatment of chronic pain, the mechanism of spinal cord stimulation is conceptualized based on the gate control theory of pain. This theory states that peripheral nerve fibers carrying pain to the spinal cord may have their input modified at the spinal cord level prior to transmission to the brain. The synapses in the dorsal horns act as *gates* that can either close to keep impulses from reaching the brain or open to allow impulses to pass. Small-diameter nerve fibers (C-fibers and lightly myelinated A-delta fibers) transmit pain impulses. Excess small fiber activity at the dorsal horn of the spinal cord opens the gate and permits impulse transmission, leading to pain perception. Large nerve fibers (A-beta fibers) carry nonpainful impulses, such as touch and vibratory sensation, and have the capacity to close the gate and inhibit pain transmission. Spinal cord stimulation is thought to preferentially stimulate large nerve fibers because these fibers are myelinated and have a lower depolarization threshold than small-diameter nerve fibers.

   Experimental evidence suggests a mechanism of action for spinal cord stimulation by increasing levels of gamma aminobutyric acid (GABA) within the dorsal horn of the spinal cord. GABA is an inhibitor of neural transmission in the spinal cord and suppresses hyperexcitability of wide-dynamic range interneurons in the dorsal horn. Spinal cord stimulation may also exert a direct effect on brain activity, but this mechanism is not well understood.

5. Describe the two main types of epidural electrodes.
   The two main types of electrodes are catheter-type electrodes and plate-type electrodes.
   - **Catheter-type electrodes** (also known as percutaneous electrodes) are placed via a percutaneous needle approach under fluoroscopic guidance and are ideal for use in trial stimulation to determine whether permanent implantation is appropriate.
   - **Plate-type electrodes** (also known as laminotomy, paddle, or surgical electrodes) require a surgical laminotomy for placement. Advantages of plate-type electrodes include lower risk of migration in the epidural space and increased electrical efficiency. Lead systems have evolved from quadripolar (four electrodes) or octapolar leads (eight electrodes) to current multilead systems (Fig. 34.1).

6. Where are epidural electrodes placed to target pain in the various areas of the body?
   General guidelines regarding initial lead placement are:
   - *Pain involving the posterior occipital region:* place leads near C2
   - *Upper extremity pain not involving the hand:* place leads between C2 and C5
   - *Upper extremity pain involving the hand:* place leads at C5 or C6
   - *Chest wall pain and angina:* place leads between T1 and T4
   - *Pain involving the thigh and knee:* place leads between T9 and T10
   - *Pain involving the lower leg and ankle:* place leads between T10 and T12
   - *Pain involving the foot:* place leads between T11 and L1
     Successful coverage of the soles of the feet is challenging and may require stimulation of the L5 or S1 nerve roots. For axial back pain, one lead is placed at midline and another lead is placed on either side of midline. Final lead position is determined based on patient feedback and lead adjustment following initial lead placement.

7. Describe the two main types of pulse generators.
   The two main types of pulse generator systems are totally implantable pulse generators and radiofrequency-driven pulse generators.
   - **Totally implantable pulse generators** utilize an internal power source (lithium battery). Following activation, these pulse generators are controlled by transcutaneous telemetry and can be switched on-off with a magnet. The battery requires replacement in 2–5 years, while a rechargeable power source may last 10–25 years, or longer. At the end of this life span, the battery must be surgically changed. For this reason, studies have indicated that rechargeable battery systems may offer significant financial savings over long-term use.
   - **Radiofrequency-driven pulse generators** consist of a receiver implanted subcutaneously and a transmitter that is worn outside the body and utilizes an external power source. An antenna is applied to the skin and transmits the stimulation signals to the receiver. The radiofrequency-driven pulse generators have the ability to deliver more power than the totally implantable pulse generators and are appropriate for patients who have greater power requirements.

8. What parameters of neurostimulation are adjusted to optimize pain reduction?
   Four basic parameters of the electrical signal are adjusted to optimize paresthesia and resultant pain reduction:
   - *Amplitude* refers to the strength of the stimulation and is measured in volts.
   - *Pulse width* is the duration of the electric pulse and is measured in microseconds.
   - *Rate* is measured in cycles per second or hertz (Hz).
   - *Electrode selection* is varied by computer-assisted programming with electrons flowing from cathodes (−) to anodes (+).
     Following programming of the device, the patient may adjust intensity and choose between different programs, as well as turn the stimulator on and off. More recently, SCSs that provide higher frequency stimulation than standard SCSs and burst stimulation in conjunction with standard SCS devices provide pain relief with fewer paresthesias.

9. What pain problems are amenable to spinal cord stimulation?
   Spinal cord stimulation has demonstrated effectiveness for many neuropathic pain conditions, including persistent radicular pain following failed spinal surgery, complex regional pain syndrome, chronic inoperable limb ischemia, refractory angina pectoris, and postherpetic neuralgia. Many experts consider the best candidates for spinal cord stimulation following failed spinal surgery are patients with radicular pain greater than axial pain. However, patients with pure neuropathic pain following unsuccessful spine surgery are uncommon. Patients following unsuccessful spine surgery frequently present with mixed nociceptive/neuropathic pain. Advances in programming and electrode technology, including multilead systems, have improved outcomes in this patient population.

10. What are contraindications to spinal cord stimulation?
    Contraindications to spinal cord stimulation include uncontrolled bleeding/anticoagulation, systemic or local infection near the site of implantation, inability to understand or communicate during trial placement, inability to understand and use technology, significant spinal stenosis or myelopathy, implanted cardiac pacemakers or defibrillators, metal allergy, and major psychiatric disease.

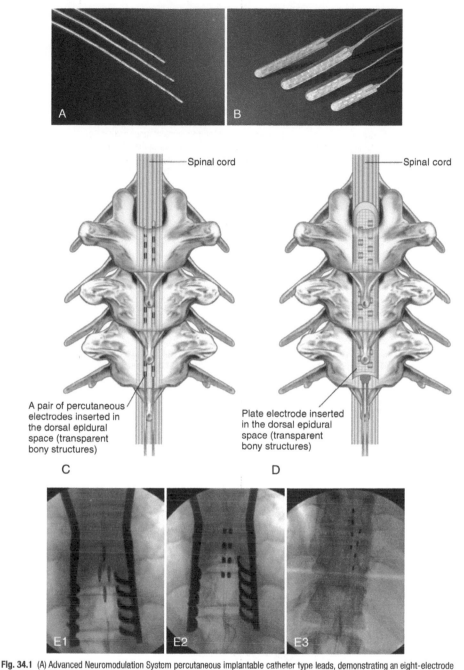

Fig. 34.1 (A) Advanced Neuromodulation System percutaneous implantable catheter type leads, demonstrating an eight-electrode Octrode lead (lower) and two four-electrode leads (upper and middle). The electrodes on all leads are 3 mm long. The eight-electrode lead and one of the four-electrode leads have an interelectrode distance of 4 mm. The other four-electrode lead has an interelectrode distance of 6 mm. (B) Advanced Neuromodulation System plate-type leads which are implanted via laminectomy. There are two wide leads (middle) and two narrow leads (upper and lower). One of the wide leads has 8 electrodes, and the other has 16 electrodes. One of the narrow leads has 8 electrodes, and the other has 16 electrodes. (C) Schematic drawing of two parallel octapolar percutaneous electrodes in the dorsal epidural space. (D) Schematic drawing of a dual-plate electrode in the dorsal epidural space. (E) Radiographs of different types of electrodes. *E1* and *E2*, Electrodes of different configurations which are surgically implanted (Medtronic Inc.); *E3*, percutaneously implanted dual quadripolar electrodes. (A–D: From Slipman CW, Derby R, Simeone FA, et al., editors. Interventional Spine: An Algorithmic Approach. Philadelphia, PA: Saunders; 2007. E1–E3: From McMahon SB. Wall and Melzack's Textbook of Pain. 5th ed. Churchill Livingstone; 2006.)

11. How are trial spinal cord stimulation electrodes placed?

Most trial spinal cord stimulation electrodes are placed into the epidural space through epidural needles utilizing fluoroscopic guidance. The procedure is performed under mild sedation and local anesthetic, as the patient must be awake during electrode placement and testing. The wires from the trial electrode may be left protruding through the skin for direct connection to a trial stimulator. Alternatively, a small incision is made around the epidural needle insertion site and dissection is continued to the level of the thoracolumbar fascia to permit the electrode to be secured to fascia with a silastic anchor. Next, the trial electrode is connected to an extension wire, which is tunneled laterally toward the site where the pulse generator would be implanted if the trial is successful. A small incision is made to permit the extension wire to pass through the skin, allowing the wire to connect to a trial stimulator.

Some physicians prefer placing plate-type electrodes for the trial implant, especially if there is scarring in the epidural space following prior spinal surgery, which can make placement of catheter-type electrodes challenging. Plate-type electrode placement can be performed either under mild sedation in combination with local anesthesia or under general anesthesia with the patient awake during the procedure for testing. The trial period may last days to weeks, but trial periods beyond 3–5 days require that the leads be tunneled under the skin from the insertion site to decrease the risk of infection.

12. How does the patient determine if trial spinal cord stimulation is effective?

The patient's report of subjective pain relief is documented. Spinal cord stimulation is intended to produce a tolerable sensation of tingling, covering the area of pain. To be a candidate for implantation of a permanent stimulator, the patient must experience a minimum of 50% pain relief. Some clinicians prefer a minimum of 60%–70% pain relief, believing such patients experience better long-term outcomes. Other measures of efficacy during a trial period include improved function and decreased medication use.

13. If the spinal cord stimulation trial is successful, how is the implantation of a permanent spinal cord stimulator performed?

The patient undergoes a surgical procedure for placement of a pulse generator, which is most commonly implanted into a *pocket* in the posterior iliac area or lower abdominal region. If a previously placed catheter-type electrode will be used as the *permanent* electrode, the midline incision is reopened and the previously placed extension wire is discarded. The electrode is connected to a new extension wire, which is tunneled and connected to the pulse generator. If a plate-type electrode will be used as the permanent electrode, a midline spinal incision is made and dissection carried onto the lamina at the interspace below the level at which effective trial stimulation was achieved. A laminotomy is created, and the plate-type electrode is inserted over the dura and passed proximally to reach the desired level (usually the lower thoracic cord region for treatment of a lower extremity pain syndrome). The location of the electrode is confirmed with fluoroscopy, and the electrode is secured to the thoracolumbar fascia with a silastic anchor. If the procedure has been performed under general anesthesia, the patient is awakened intraoperatively to confirm electrode position through testing of the pattern of paresthesia generated by stimulation. Finally, extension wires are tunneled for connection to the pulse generator.

14. What complications are associated with spinal cord stimulation?

SCS is a relatively safe procedure and reversible with implant removal. The most common complication of SCS is lead migration. Lead migration is less common with plate-type electrodes. Modern catheter-type electrodes with eight or more electrode contacts per lead are programmable and allow flexibility in programming SCS to maintain effective stimulation should the leads move. Other complications of SCS include spinal cord contusive injury, epidural hematoma, seroma, infection, wound complications, lead breakage, implant malfunction, undesirable pattern/location of stimulation, and cerebrospinal fluid (CSF) leak. Movements may cause the leads to contact the spinal cord, leading to sometimes uncomfortable paresthesias; some patients who experience this turn off their leads at night to prevent being woken up by the sensation while rolling in bed. Paralysis as a result of lead insertion is extremely rare but has been reported.

15. What is the role of SCS in spinal cord injury?

Traumatic SCI can lead to paralysis, paraesthesias, complex pain syndromes, and loss of sphincter control, and can adversely impact on cardiovascular, gastrointestinal, sexual, and psychosocial function. The functions affected by the injury depend on the spinal level and the severity of the injury.

The primary indication for SCS after SCI is to treat complex pain syndromes, which occur frequently in the chronic SCI patient population. Reports on the utility of SCS for SCI-related pain are limited and suggest poorer responses compared with SCS treatment of conditions such as pain due to failed back surgery or peripheral neuropathy.

SCS is also being investigated for the treatment of sensorimotor recovery after SCI. There is preliminary evidence to suggest that epidural SCS may be efficacious in producing electrophysiologic improvements in patients with acute and chronic SCI. Some reports suggest that epidural stimulation (ES) activates both afferent and efferent pathways and helps recruit alpha-motor neurons. In a National Institutes of Health (NIH) sponsored study at the University of Louisville, four patients with paraplegia were able to voluntarily move previously paralyzed muscles after being treated with SCS and physical therapy. Two of these patients had complete motor and sensory loss at the commencement of the study, making the results particularly remarkable. A follow-up study reported that two patients with complete SCI and one with partial SCI regained some voluntary control of previously paralyzed muscles within just a few days. Such results challenge the traditional concept of poor prognosis for patients with complete paralysis. Other technologies under investigation include noninvasive SCS using either electrical or magnetic stimulation.

16. What is the history of implanted spinal catheters and pumps?

The discovery in the 1970s of opioid receptors in the spinal cord and the development of infusion pumps led to injection and infusion of opioids into the epidural and subarachnoid space for acute and chronic pain due to cancer. In 1992 Medicare approved implanted pumps for chronic nonmalignant pain. By infusing opiates directly into the spine, the medication dosages required to treat pain are 30–300 times less than oral dosages.

17. What is an implantable drug delivery system?

An implantable drug delivery system consists of a pump that is surgically inserted into a pocket in the abdomen and delivers medication to the spinal canal through a catheter, which is tunneled under the skin. Pumps have a drug reservoir that can be refilled. Two main types of pumps exist:
- **Constant flow pumps** provide a fixed rate of drug delivery and require changing the drug concentration to adjust the drug dose.
- **Programmable pumps** have the capacity to vary the rate and time of drug delivery to adjust drug dose.

18. Which patients are potential candidates for an implantable drug delivery system?

Potential candidates for an implantable drug delivery system include:
- Patients with spasticity of cerebral or spinal origin
- Patients with nociceptive or neuropathic pain who do not experience relief with medication, SCS, or neuroablative procedures
- Patients who fail SCS trials
- Patients with pain secondary to malignancy, which is not adequately relieved with oral or transdermal analgesics and who have a life expectancy in excess of 3 months

    Potential candidates for an implantable drug delivery system should have failed to respond to treatment with less complex and invasive therapies, including physical and occupational therapy, cognitive and behavioral therapy, and oral/transdermal opioid medications. In addition, documented pathology that correlates with the pain symptoms should exist. Indications for additional surgical intervention should be ruled out. Psychological barriers to successful outcomes should be examined. No absolute contraindications to implantation should be present. Prior to implantation, a trial should be performed to evaluate efficacy and rule out toxicity.

19. What is the role of implantable drug delivery systems in SCI?

Implantable drug delivery systems are used to manage spasticity and neuropathic pain following SCI. Specifically, these systems are employed when patients continue to have severe symptoms despite high doses of medication. Intrathecal baclofen administration is approved for the treatment of medication-resistant spasticity. Similarly, intrathecal opiates or ziconotide may be administered to relieve intractable neuropathic pain following an insult to the nervous system.

20. What are some contraindications for an implantable drug delivery system?

Contraindications to an implantable drug delivery system include:
- Intolerance to the infused medication
- Local or systemic infection
- Bleeding diathesis/anticoagulation
- Titanium allergy
- Pregnancy or desire to become pregnant
- Severe psychopathology

21. What medications are currently approved for infusion via an implantable drug delivery system?

The current Food and Drug Administration (FDA)-approved medications for infusion into the spinal canal are morphine (approved for intrathecal analgesia), ziconotide (Prialt; approved for intrathecal analgesia), and baclofen (approved for spasticity). Other medications have been used off-label, including hydromorphone, fentanyl, sufentanil, bupivacaine, and clonidine. Although opioids are effective for nociceptive pain, they are less effective for neuropathic pain. Pain physicians may combine an opioid with clonidine or bupivacaine to enhance treatment of both nociceptive and neuropathic pain. In addition, combination drug therapy is believed to decrease the development of medication tolerance.

22. What are some risks and complications associated with implantable drug delivery systems?
    - *Device-related complications* may occur and include pump failure, catheter migration or occlusion, catheter dissociation, and catheter breakage. Depending on the type of device failure, reduction in medication dose or overdosage may occur.
    - *Medication-related complications* are related to the specific drug(s) administered intrathecally and may include anaphylaxis, oversedation, or meningitis from use of contaminated solutions. Morphine may cause nausea, pruritus, urinary retention, oversedation, constipation, and confusion. Ziconotide may cause dizziness, nausea, vomiting, urinary retention, and confusion. Baclofen may cause nausea, vomiting, dizziness, urinary retention, paresthesias, and life-threatening withdrawal.
    - *Surgical complications* may occur and include CSF leak, infection, and neurologic injury.
    - *Patient-specific complications* may occur, for example, hormonal changes related to morphine use may lead to fatigue and sexual dysfunction.
    - *Pump refill complications* may occur related to refill with the incorrect medication, incorrect medication concentration, or reprogramming the pump to administer medication at an incorrect rate. Also, the pump can migrate and flip within the surgically created pocket in a manner that prevents convenient access to the reservoir to refill the pump.
    - *A catheter tip granuloma* may develop.

23. What is a catheter tip granuloma? How is this condition diagnosed and treated?
    A catheter tip granuloma is a noninfectious inflammatory mass that can develop on the tip of a catheter following intrathecal drug administration, most commonly following infusion of opioids, especially morphine. The most common symptoms that lead to diagnosis of a catheter tip granuloma are inadequate pain relief or new-onset pain. Granulomas are highly vascular and lead to rapid clearance of administered medications and often present with signs of pump malfunction as the granuloma obstructs the catheter lumen. A catheter tip granuloma may also form space-occupying lesions in the spinal canal and cause a neurologic deficit.

    Diagnosis is by magnetic resonance imaging (MRI) with gadolinium contrast or computed tomography with myelography. Prior to ordering an MRI, it is important to identify the pump model as serious adverse events, including patient injury and death, have been reported in association with the use of implantable infusion pumps in the magnetic resonance (MR) environment. Only patients implanted with MR-conditional pumps can safely undergo MRI examinations, and only under the specified conditions of safe use. Some pump models may automatically stop delivering medication during the MRI examination, and some may need to be reprogrammed before and/or after the examination. Other pump models may need to be completely emptied of drug prior to the MRI examination to prevent unintended over-delivery of medication and drug overdose.

    If imaging confirms the presence of a granuloma and there is no neurologic deficit, treatment options include observation and monitoring for spontaneous resolution of the granuloma, termination of intrathecal drug delivery, or catheter replacement. For patients who present with new-onset neurologic deficits attributed to a catheter-tip granuloma, emergent surgical decompression is indicated.

KEY POINTS

1. Spinal cord stimulation is a minimally invasive treatment in select patients for persistent pain following spinal surgery, chronic regional pain syndrome, and other neuropathic pain syndromes.
2. Implantable drug delivery systems are considered for patients with nociceptive and/or neuropathic pain syndromes who do not experience relief with medication, spinal cord stimulation, or neuroablative procedures.
3. Successful outcomes with spinal cord stimulation or implantable drug delivery systems require careful preoperative evaluation, including a screening trial, to identify patients who are most likely to benefit from the procedure.

Websites
1. International Neuromodulation Society: https://www.neuromodulation.com/about-neuromodulation
2. North American Neuromodulation Society: https://neuromodulation.org/Education/SCSLearningModules.aspx

BIBLIOGRAPHY

1. Angeli, C. A., Boakye, M., Morton, R. A., Vogt, J., Benton, K., Chen, Y., et al. (2018). Recovery of over-ground walking after chronic motor complete spinal cord injury. *New England Journal of Medicine, 379*(13), 1244–1250.
2. Barolat, G. (2007). Spinal cord stimulation for chronic pain management. In C. W. Slipman, R. Derby, F. A. Simeone, (Eds.), *Interventional Spine: An Algorithmic Approach.* Philadelphia, PA: Saunders.
3. Bottros, M. M., & Christo, P. J. (2014). Current perspectives on intrathecal drug delivery. *Journal of Pain Research, 7,* 615–626.
4. Chari, A., Hentall, I. D., Papadopoulos, M. C., & Pereira, E. A. (2017). Surgical neurostimulation for spinal cord injury. *Brain Sciences, 7*(2), 1–18.

5. Harb, M., & Krames, E. S. (2007). Intrathecal therapies and totally implantable drug delivery systems. In C. W. Slipman, R. Derby, & F. A. Simeone (Eds.), *Interventional Spine: An Algorithmic Approach.* Philadelphia, PA: Saunders.
6. North, R. B., Kidd, D. H., Farrokhi, F., & Piantadosi, S. A. (2005). Spinal cord stimulation versus repeated lumbosacral spine surgery for chronic pain: A randomized, controlled trial. *Neurosurgery 56*(1), 98–107.
7. Shamji, M. F., De Vos, C., & Sharan, A. (2017). The advancing role of neuromodulation for the management of chronic treatment refractory pain. *Neurosurgery, 80*(3), 108–113.
8. Song, J. J., Popescu, A., & Bell, R. L. (2014). Present and potential use of spinal cord stimulation to control chronic pain. *Pain Physician, 17*(3), 235–246.

VII

PEDIATRIC SPINAL DEFORMITIES AND SPINAL DISORDERS

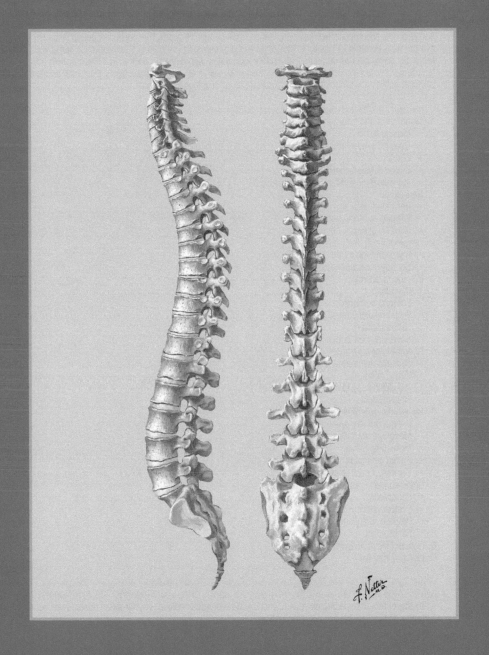

CHAPTER 35

PEDIATRIC BACK PAIN

Vincent J. Devlin, MD

EVALUATION

1. **Discuss the epidemiology of back pain in children compared with adults.**

   Traditionally, back pain in children was considered uncommon, and thought to be associated with a definable cause. Current data show that back pain is a frequent complaint in the pediatric population and that the probability of identifying a specific cause is low. Back pain is much less common before age 10, increases during adolescence, and approaches adult population rates by age 18 years. Diagnosis of a definable cause of back pain symptoms is possible in less than 20% of pediatric patients. Spinal pain in adolescence is considered to be a risk factor for spinal pain as an adult. Risk factors associated with pediatric back pain include growth acceleration, female gender, family history of back pain, backpack use, and previous back injury. Both high and low levels of physical activity are associated with increased risk of developing back pain.

2. **What is the differential diagnosis of back pain in children?**

   1. Mechanical and traumatic disorders
      - Muscle strain
      - Overuse syndrome
      - Fracture
      - Spondylolysis/spondylolisthesis
      - Juvenile degenerative disc disease
   2. Neurologic
      - Herniated disc
      - Slipped vertebral apophysis
      - Congenital spinal stenosis
   3. Developmental disorders
      - Scheuermann kyphosis
      - Spondylolysis/spondylolisthesis
   4. Infectious disorders
      - Discitis
      - Epidural abscess
      - Vertebral osteomyelitis
      - Tuberculosis
      - Sacroiliac joint infection
   5. Rheumatologic disorders
      - Juvenile rheumatoid arthritis
      - Reactive arthritis
      - Ankylosing spondylitis
      - Fibromyalgia
   6. Neoplastic disorders
      - Benign primary spine tumors
      - Malignant primary spine tumors
      - Metastatic tumors
      - Spinal cord/canal tumors
      - Tumors of muscle origin
   7. Referred pain from visceral disorders
      - Pneumonia
      - Pyelonephritis
      - Retrocecal appendicitis
      - Pancreatitis
   8. Nonspecific or idiopathic back pain
   9. Psychogenic pain

3. **What are some of the most common causes of back pain in skeletally immature patients referred to a tertiary pediatric orthopedic clinic or the emergency department?**
   - **In the clinic**: Nonspecific back pain, spondylolysis or spondylolisthesis, herniated nucleus pulposus, Scheuermann disease, spinal tumors, or infection.

- **In the emergency room**: Nonspecific back pain, minor trauma, spine fracture, spine infection, referred pain from visceral disorders, urinary tract infection, sickle cell crises, spondylolysis/spondylolisthesis, rheumatologic disorder, or spine tumors.

4. Why is the child's age often helpful in narrowing the diagnosis of back pain?
No diagnosis is unique to a single age group. However, some generalizations can help in determining the most likely diagnosis:
- **Younger than age 10**: Disc space infection, vertebral osteomyelitis, and tumors (Langerhans cell histiocytosis, leukemia, astrocytoma, neuroblastoma)
- **Older than age 10**: Nonspecific back pain, spondylolysis, spondylolisthesis, Scheuermann kyphosis, fractures, lumbar disc herniation, apophyseal ring injury, osteoid osteoma, tumors, and spinal infections

5. What information should be obtained during a history for evaluation of back pain?
- Duration of pain symptoms (acute, >1 month, chronic)
- Location of pain (cervical vs. thoracic vs. lumbar; axial vs. radicular)
- Frequency of symptoms (intermittent, constant)
- Aggravating and alleviating factors
- Timing
- History of trauma
- Recreational activities, especially sports involving hyperextension
Red flags that should prompt further workup include:
- A history of constitutional symptoms (fever, unintentional weight loss, night sweats, malaise)
- Neurologic symptoms (numbness, weakness, bowel or bladder symptoms, gait difficulty)
- Nonmechanical pain (constant pain, night pain, pain at rest especially if not relieved by nonsteroidal antiinflammatory medications [NSAIDs])
- Pain in a child younger than age 4 years

6. How should the physical examination be performed?
The physical examination must take place with the child undressed and appropriately gowned. All systems should be examined thoroughly. The child should be observed for posture, stance, and gait. The spine should be assessed for tenderness, alignment, and flexibility. A forward bend test should be performed to assess for symmetry and flexibility. Spinal deformity (kyphosis, scoliosis) should prompt further assessment. Suspicion of underlying disease is prompted by spinal tenderness, decreased spinal range of motion, spasticity, hamstring tightness, or skin abnormalities (hemangioma, midline hair patch). The single-leg hyperextension test is a useful provocative test for diagnosis of symptomatic spondylolysis and is performed by instructing the patient to stand on one leg while extending the lumbar spine. The neurologic examination should carefully document motor strength, sensation, deep tendon reflexes, and symmetry of abdominal reflexes. The musculoskeletal examination includes assessment of all muscle groups for tenderness or limited range of joint motion.

7. What laboratory tests are useful during the evaluation of back pain in children?
Useful laboratory tests include a complete blood count (CBC) with differential, erythrocyte sedimentation rate (ESR), and C-reactive protein. These tests are recommended for young children with a history of night pain or constitutional symptoms. A blood smear test may be added to screen for leukemia. Laboratory tests for rheumatologic disorder are not routinely obtained, but when a rheumatologic disorder is considered in the differential diagnosis, additional tests include a rheumatoid factor (RF), anti-cyclic citrullinated peptide (anti-CCP), antinuclear antibody (ANA), and HLA-B27.

8. What imaging studies play a role in evaluation of the child with back pain?
Posteroanterior (PA) and lateral radiographs of the entire spine are the preferred initial imaging study for a child with back pain. If an advanced imaging study is indicated based on clinical assessment and results of initial radiographs, the next study that should be performed is magnetic resonance imaging (MRI). Use of a technetium bone scan and computed tomography (CT) are limited to specific clinical indications due to higher radiation exposure associated with these studies.

9. When are radiographs indicated for evaluation of the child with back pain?
PA and lateral complete spinal radiographs are usually obtained after completion of a detailed history and physical examination. Additional radiographic views such as oblique or flexion-extension views are generally not indicated in the pediatric population as they do not provide additional diagnostic information and result in increased radiation exposure.

10. When is an MRI scan indicated for evaluation of a child with back pain?
MRI is the advanced imaging modality of choice for evaluation of the spinal column and neural axis. Indications for spinal MRI include back pain and an abnormal neurologic examination, radicular pain, constant pain, night

pain, pain lasting >4 weeks, or back pain with constitutional symptoms. MRI is useful for defining spinal patholo-gies such as fracture, tumor, infection, disc herniation, spinal cord abnormalities, spondylolysis, spondylolisthesis, and Scheuermann disease. Use of contrast is indicated when infection, inflammation, or tumors are suspected. As MRI does not deliver ionizing radiation and is noninvasive, it is preferred over CT, CT-myelography, and technetium bone scans whenever possible. Disadvantages associated with MRI include the need for anesthesia when the study is performed in very young children and the danger of attributing symptoms to imaging findings that are clinically irrelevant.

11. When is a CT scan indicated for evaluation of a child with back pain?
Spinal CT provides the clearest three-dimensional depiction of bone detail of any imaging modality. However, CT does not visualize soft tissue as well as MRI, and is associated with significant radiation exposure. As CT is rapidly performed, it is a preferred modality for emergency-room evaluation. It can often be performed in young children without the need for sedation, unlike MRI. CT plays a role in assessment of spinal fractures, spondylolysis, spon-dylolisthesis, and spinal tumors. CT performed in combination with myelography is indicated when visualization of the spinal canal and neural elements are needed and MRI is not feasible.

12. When is a technetium bone scan indicated for evaluation of a child with back pain?
It has been recognized that technetium bone scans expose patients to significantly more ionizing radiation compared to plain radiographs or CT. For this reason, it is recommended that use of technetium bone scans are limited to situations where diagnostic data from plain radiographs, MRI, or CT are inadequate, or when diagnostic data from a bone scan would change clinical management. For example, in a young child with poorly localized pain who requires evaluation of the entire axial skeleton and lower extremities, a technetium bone scan can help to identify the pain source. Single-photon emission computed tomography (SPECT) pro-vides increased sensitivity and specificity compared with a planar bone scan. SPECT is sometimes used in the diagnosis of acute spondylolysis but is less helpful for diagnosis of chronic pars fractures as chronic injuries lack increased bone turnover.

13. Summarize some key recommendations for practitioners regarding how to effectively and systematically evaluate a child with back pain.
Due to the high prevalence of back pain in the pediatric population and the multiple etiologies that may be responsible for clinical symptoms, use of a systematic approach is important. Some general recommendations (1) include:
- All pediatric patients with a history of back pain require evaluation with a detailed history and physical examination.
- Patients with new-onset mechanical or muscular back pain who report activity-related symptoms may be treated with activity restrictions and nonnarcotic medications and return for follow-up in 4–6 weeks. Initial plain radiographs are not always required in this clinical situation, but may be obtained at the discretion of the treating provider.
- PA and lateral radiographs of the entire spine are recommended as the initial imaging study. Positive findings noted on radiographs serve to guide subsequent treatment based on the specific diagnosis.
- Spinal MRI is obtained for pediatric patients with abnormal neurologic findings, constant pain, night pain, or radicular pain. Contrast is added when infection, inflammation, or tumor is suspected.
- Laboratory tests including CBC, ESR, and C-reactive protein are added to the workup to evaluate for a systemic etiology when constitutional symptoms or nonmechanical pain are present and for patients less than age 10 to rule out leukemia.
- A notable percentage of patients (>50%) will not have a specific diagnosis identified as responsible for back pain following appropriate workup and are diagnosed as having nonspecific back pain. Treatment options include NSAIDs, physical therapy with core strengthening and flexibility exercises, hamstring stretching, and interventions directed to specifically address any secondary factors considered to contribute to back pain, including psychosocial issues.

COMMON CONDITIONS ASSOCIATED WITH PEDIATRIC BACK PAIN

14. How is a muscle strain diagnosed in children?
History and physical examination are sufficient to establish the diagnosis of muscle strain. A brief history of localized pain, absence of neurologic findings, and pain onset associated with physical activity are typical. The pain from a muscle strain should resolve within a few weeks. The treatment for muscle strain is activity modification, ice, and NSAIDs. If the pain does not resolve within 1 month, reevaluation and additional workup is needed.

15. Define spondylolysis.
Spondylosis is a defect in the pars interarticularis. The defect is unilateral in 20% and bilateral in 80% of cases.

16. Who is at risk for spondylolysis?

Children engaged in repetitive activities involving hyperextension of the spine are at risk for spondylolysis. Commonly associated sporting activities include gymnastics, diving, dancing, wrestling, and football.

17. How is spondylolysis diagnosed?

History and physical examination are important indicators of spondylolysis. A history of hyperextension activities should alert the clinician to the possibility of the diagnosis. Patients typically present with back pain radiating into the buttocks. Physical examination may reveal tenderness to palpation, hamstring tightness, decreased forward flexion of the lumbar spine, a positive single-leg hyperextension test, or a stiff gait. Lateral radiographs may reveal a pars defect. Oblique views are not indicated as they do not provide additional diagnostic information and result in increased radiation exposure. If a spot lateral L5–S1 radiograph is nondiagnostic, cross-sectional imaging with CT is recommended. MRI is an alternative diagnostic modality and is able to detect inflammation and edema within the pars interarticularis. A technetium bone scan with SPECT imaging is an additional imaging modality but is associated with higher radiation exposure than CT.

18. How is spondylolysis treated?

Activity modification, bracing, physical therapy, and NSAIDs are the basis of nonoperative therapy. Surgical intervention is rarely necessary. Surgical options include repair of the pars defect or a posterolateral fusion.

19. Define spondylolisthesis. How is it diagnosed in children?

Spondylolisthesis is a forward slippage of a vertebra in relation to the adjacent inferior vertebra. The most common type of spondylolisthesis in children is the isthmic type, which occurs when bilateral pars defects allow the upper vertebra to slide forward on the lower vertebra, usually L5 on S1. A standing lateral lumbar radiograph is the preferred test for making this diagnosis. The degree of displacement of the superior vertebra relative to the subjacent vertebra is graded using the Meyerding scale: grade 1 = 1%–24%; grade 2 = 25%–49%; grade 3 = 50%–74%; grade 4 = 75%–100%. MRI is indicated when there is a need to assess the intervertebral disc or if a neurologic deficit is present. CT is indicated when details about formation of the posterior spinal elements (dysplasia) are required for surgical planning.

20. What treatment is recommended for spondylolisthesis?

Low-grade slips (<50%) generally do not require active treatment if the patient is asymptomatic. Such patients should be followed closely for slip progression through skeletal maturity. Symptomatic low-grade slips should undergo initial nonoperative treatment, including activity modification, physical therapy, NSAIDs, and bracing, before considering surgical treatment (spinal fusion). Low-grade slips that are progressive or refractory to nonsurgical treatment and higher-grade slips (>50%) are treated with spinal fusion.

21. How does a lumbar disc herniation present in children?

Lumbar disc herniations are less common in children than adults. In contrast to adults, children commonly report a history of acute injury or chronic repetitive injury, often related to sports activities. Time to diagnosis is often delayed compared to adults as symptoms may be nonspecific and initially attributed to other etiologies. Children present with back pain with or without radicular leg pain. A reactive scoliosis may be present, which develops as the child bends to the side opposite the compressed nerve in an attempt to relieve neural compression. Physical examination commonly shows reduced lumbar range of motion and a positive straight-leg raise test. Neurologic changes and cauda equina symptoms are uncommon in adolescents. Initial treatment options include activity restriction, NSAIDs, ice, physical therapy, and epidural injections. Pediatric patients respond less favorably to nonoperative treatment compared with adults. This is attributed to the increased elasticity and higher water content of the immature disc and the association of disc herniation with an apophyseal ring fracture in up to one-third of cases. Surgery is reserved for prolonged symptoms or neurologic involvement and involves laminotomy and removal of disc and endplate material.

22. What is a slipped vertebral apophysis?

Slipped vertebral apophysis or apophyseal ring fracture is a fracture through the junction of the vertebral body and the cartilaginous ring apophysis. This injury is possible prior to complete fusion of the cartilaginous ring apophysis, which occurs at approximately 18 years of age. Most injuries occur at the L4–L5 or L5–S1 level. This traumatic injury presents most often in males who participate in sports requiring repetitive flexion combined with rotation. Patients present with symptoms similar to a central disc herniation. Surgery is frequently necessary to excise the bone fragment, attached cartilage, and disc material.

23. Should lumbar degenerative disc disease be considered in the differential diagnosis of mechanical back pain in pediatric patients?

Yes; disc degeneration is not unique to the adult population, and has been noted on MRI in pediatric patients, most commonly in adolescents. In many patients, MRI findings are incidental in nature and not related to symptoms. However, in some patients, MRI changes involving the disc, including endplate changes, the loss of disc signal, irregularity of the nucleus, and disc protrusion, are associated with back or lower extremity symptoms. Treatment is generally nonoperative, using NSAIDs, activity modification, and physical therapy with back and abdominal strengthening exercises. Coexistent congenital spinal stenosis has been observed in a subset of adolescent patients with degenerative disc disease and may require surgical decompression. (1) An uncommon condition associated with disc degeneration in pediatric patients is retrograde embolization of nucleus pulposus material into the vessels supplying the spinal cord following minimal stresses to the spine such as bending. This may affect the vascular supply of the spinal cord, resulting in spinal cord infarction and acute myelopathy. (2)

24. **What is Scheuermann disease? How does it present in children?**
Scheuermann disease is a disorder of endochondral ossification that alters the development of the vertebral endplate and ring apophysis. It may lead to intraosseous disc herniations (referred to as a Schmorl's nodes), anterior wedging of the vertebral body, and kyphotic deformity. Scheuermann disease may affect either the thoracic or lumbar region.

In the thoracic region, three consecutive wedged vertebrae ($>5°$), irregular upper and lower vertebral endplates, apparent loss of disc space height, and increased thoracic kyphosis that does not correct when the patient lies supine, are criteria for diagnosis. Patients typically are referred for assessment of the associated kyphotic deformity, which may be associated with pain over the apex of the kyphosis. Scheuermann kyphosis should be differentiated from postural round back, which is a flexible deformity that reduces when the patient lies supine.

Patients with Scheuermann disease in the lumbar region present with back pain. Spinal deformity is generally not a significant problem. Patients generally report a history of previous strenuous physical activity or present with acute injury. Radiographs show vertebral endplate irregularities, intraosseous disc herniation, and disc space narrowing.

25. **What treatment is recommended for Scheuermann disease?**
Most patients with Scheuermann disease involving the thoracic region can be successfully treated with exercise, bracing, and supportive care. Surgical intervention can be considered for persistent pain associated with a kyphotic deformity exceeding 75°. Scheuermann disease involving the lumbar region is generally treated with activity modification and occasionally with an orthosis.

26. **Is adolescent idiopathic scoliosis commonly associated with severe pain?**
No. Idiopathic scoliosis is not typically a cause of severe back pain in adolescents. However, up to one-third of patients with adolescent idiopathic scoliosis report mild, intermittent, and nonspecific back pain. When persistent severe back pain is noted in the presence of a spinal curvature, further workup is indicated to determine the source of pain. Conditions such as infection, tumors, syringomyelia, or disc herniation may cause secondary scoliosis.

27. **What is the difference between discitis and vertebral osteomyelitis?**
In the past, a distinction was made between discitis (infection involving the disc space) and osteomyelitis (infection in the vertebral body). Studies have shown that in children the vascular supply crosses the vertebral endplate from vertebral body to the disc space. As a result, discitis and vertebral osteomyelitis are considered to represent a continuum termed *infectious spondylitis*. Hematogenous seeding of the vertebral endplate leads to direct spread of infection into the disc space. Subsequently, infection involving the disc space and both adjacent vertebral endplates may progress to osteomyelitis. Vertebral fracture and epidural abscess may occur if the infection is permitted to progress without treatment. *Staphylococcus aureus* is the most frequently isolated bacteria. Tuberculosis is prevalent in developing countries and should be considered in children who have migrated or traveled outside of the United States to endemic areas.

28. **Describe the presentation, workup, and initial treatment for spinal infection in a child.**
Children may present with back, abdominal, or leg pain symptoms. The child may limp or refuse to walk. When asked to pick something up from the floor, the child generally avoids bending over and squats in an attempt to keep the spine straight. Some children may appear quite ill with a fever, whereas others are afebrile and report minimal pain.

Radiographs are typically normal during the first month. MRI is the most sensitive and specific imaging test and demonstrates the extent of the lesion, as well as the presence or absence of an epidural abscess. A technetium bone scan may be used to screen the entire skeleton for additional sites of infection. Laboratory studies play a role in diagnosis. The white blood cell count is elevated in less than 50% of cases. The ESR is elevated in more than 90% of patients. C-reactive protein is a more specific indicator of infection and may be useful in diagnosis and evaluation of treatment. Blood cultures should be drawn before starting antibiotics, because 50% will yield an organism. Disc space cultures are not routinely performed as positive results are obtained in only 60% of cases and *S. aureus* is the most commonly isolated organism.

Treatment consists of intravenous antibiotics directed toward *S. aureus.* For early-stage infections with minimal tissue destruction, antibiotic treatment is frequently successful. CT-guided biopsy of the disc space is performed for patients who fail to improve following initial treatment with antibiotics to evaluate for resistant organisms or atypical infections, including tuberculosis and fungal infections. In more advanced cases associated with significant bony destruction, kyphotic deformity, soft tissue abscess, epidural abscess, or neurologic deficit, surgical intervention is indicated.

29. What benign spinal tumors are most commonly found in children?
The most common benign tumors involving the spine in children are osteoid osteoma, osteoblastoma, aneurysmal bone cyst, Langerhans cell histiocytosis, giant cell tumor, hemangioma, and osteochondroma. Aneurysmal bone cyst, osteoid osteoma, osteochondroma, and osteoblastoma typically involve the **posterior spinal column**. Langerhans cell histiocytosis, giant cell tumor, and hemangioma typically involve the **anterior spinal column**. Langerhans cell histiocytosis classically manifests as a vertebra plana.

30. What is the most common malignant condition in the pediatric population?
Acute leukemia is the most common malignancy in children. Back pain may be the presenting symptom. This condition should be suspected in a child younger than age 10 with pain at night. Additional findings include anemia, increased white blood cell count, increased ESR, vertebral compression fractures, diffuse osteopenia, and metaphyseal bands.

31. What primary bone tumors are most likely to involve the spine in the pediatric population?
Osteosarcoma and Ewing sarcoma.

32. What are the most common spinal cord tumors in children?
Astrocytoma and ependymoma.

33. What is the most prevalent malignant condition that produces spinal metastases in children?
Neuroblastoma. Up to 80% of patients develop spinal metastases.

34. What soft tissue sarcoma is most likely to involve the spine in the pediatric population?
Rhabdomyosarcoma.

KEY POINTS

1. The majority of pediatric patients presenting with back pain do not have an identifiable diagnosis.
2. Initial evaluation of the pediatric patient presenting with back pain consists of a detailed history, physical examination, and spinal radiographs.
3. Spinal MRI is obtained for pediatric patients with abnormal neurologic findings, constant pain, night pain, or radicular pain.

Websites
1. Imaging of back pain in children: http://www.ajnr.org/content/ajnr/31/5/787.full.pdf
2. American College of Radiology (ACR) Appropriateness Criteria® Back Pain-Child: https://doi.org/10.1016/j.jacr. 2017.01.039

REFERENCES

1. Dimar, J. R., Glassman, S. D., & Carreon, L. Y. (2007). Juvenile degenerative disc disease: a report of 76 cases identified by magnetic resonance imaging. *The Spine Journal, 7*, 332–337.
2. Quinn, J. N., Breit, H., & Dafer, R. M. (2019). Spinal cord infarction due to fibrocartilaginous embolism: A report of 3 cases. *Journal of Stroke and Cerebrovascular Diseases, 28*, 66–67.

BIBLIOGRAPHY

1. Auerbach, J. D., Ahn, J., Zgonis, M. H., Reddy, S. C., Ecker, M. L., & Flynn, J. M. (2008). Streamlining the evaluation of low back pain in children. *Clinical Orthopaedics and Related Research, 466*, 1971–1977.
2. Biagiarelli, F. S., Piga, S., Reale, A., Parisi, P, Degli Atti, M. L., Aulisa, A. G., et al. (2019). Management of children presenting with low back pain to the emergency department. *American Journal of Emergency Medicine, 37*, 672–679.
3. Dimar, J. R., Glassman, S. D., & Carreon, L. Y. (2007). Juvenile degenerative disc disease: A report of 76 cases identified by magnetic resonance imaging. *The Spine Journal, 7*, 332–337.

4. Feldman, D. S., Straight, J. J., Badra, M. I., Mohaideen, A., & Madan, S. S. (2006). Evaluation of an algorithmic approach to pediatric back pain. *Journal of Pediatric Orthopedics*, *26*, 353–357.

5. Garg, S., & Dormans, J. P. Tumors and tumor-like conditions of the spine in children. *Journal of the American Academy of Orthopedic Surgeons*, *13*, 372–381.

6. Karol, L. A., LaMont, L., & Mignemi, M. (2018). Back pain in children. In S. R. Garfin, F. J. Eismont, G. R. Bell (Eds.), *Rothman-Simeone the Spine* (7th ed., pp. 417–433). Philadelphia, PA: Elsevier.

7. Larson, A. N. (2016). Back pain, disk disease, spondylolysis, and spondylolisthesis. In J. E. Martus (Ed.), *Orthopaedic Knowledge Update: Pediatrics 5* (pp. 415–429). Rosemont: American Academy of Orthopedic Surgeons.

8. MacDonald, J., Stuart, E., & Rodenberg, R. (2017). Musculoskeletal low back pain in school-aged children: A review. *JAMA Pediatrics*, *171*, 280–287.

9. Neuschwander, T. B., Cutrone, J., Macias, B. R., Cutrone, S., Murthy, G., Chambers, H., et al. (2009). The effect of backpacks on the lumbar spine in children: A standing magnetic resonance imaging study. *Spine*, *35*, 83–88.

10. Quinn, J. N., Breit, H., & Dafer, R. M. (2019). Spinal cord infarction due to fibrocartilaginous embolism: A report of 3 cases. *Journal of Stroke and Cerebrovascular Diseases*, *28*, 66–67.

11. Ramirez, N., Flynn, J. M., Hill, B. W., Serrano, J. A., Calvo, C. E., Bredy, R., et al. (2015). Evaluation of a systematic approach to pediatric back pain: The utility of magnetic resonance imaging. *Journal of Pediatric Orthopedics*, *35*, 28–32.

12. Wu, X., Ma, W., Du, H., & Gurung, K. (2013). A review of current treatment of lumbar posterior ring apophyseal fracture with lumbar disc herniation. *European Spine Journal*, *22*, 475–488.

CHAPTER 36

PEDIATRIC CERVICAL DISORDERS

Thomas R. Haher, MD, Margaret McDonnell, and Evan Belanger

DEVELOPMENT OF THE CERVICAL SPINE

1. **What family of genes regulates development of the vertebral column?**
   The *Hox* (homeobox) and *Pax* (paired box) genes regulate embryonic differentiation and segmentation of the developing vertebral column.

2. **Describe the development of the atlas (C1).**
   The atlas is formed from three primary ossification centers: the anterior arch and two neural arches. The anterior arch is not ossified at birth in most patients, which precludes use of the atlantodens interval (ADI) for diagnosis of C1–C2 instability during the first year of life. The neural arches develop into the lateral masses and fuse posteriorly around age 3–5 and fuse to the body anteriorly around age 7–9.

3. **How many primary ossification centers contribute to formation of the axis (C2)?**
   The axis is formed by five primary ossification centers: two neural arches or lateral masses, two halves of the odontoid process, and the body of C2. The body (centrum) is separated from the lateral masses by the neurocentral synchondroses and from the odontoid by the dentocentral synchondrosis. The body and neural arches fuse posteriorly by age 3 and anteriorly by age 6. The body generally fuses to the odontoid by age 6 but can fuse as late as age 11. A secondary ossification center at the tip of the odontoid, the os terminale, appears between ages 3 and 6 and fuses by age 12. Secondary centers of ossification can develop at the tips of the spinous process, transverse processes, and superior and inferior aspects of the vertebral body.

4. **Describe the development of the subaxial cervical vertebrae (C3–C7).**
   The spinal segments from C3 to C7 have a similar pattern of development as the thoracic and lumbar vertebrae and are comprised of a body (centrum) and paired neural arches. The neural arches fuse to the body between ages 2–8 years in the subaxial cervical region, 2–12 years in the lumbar region, and 2.5–18 years in the thoracic region. Secondary centers of ossification develop at the tips of the spinous process, transverse processes, and superior and inferior aspects of the vertebral body. Vertebral bodies grow in height by endochondral ossification, which occurs in a posterior to anterior direction and is responsible for the anterior wedge shape of the vertebra, which persists until approximately age 7 (Fig. 36.1).

5. **When does the immature cervical spine approach adult size and shape?**
   The immature cervical spine approaches adult size and shape around age 8.

6. **What anatomic features differentiate the immature cervical spine from the adult cervical spine?**
   Unique anatomic features of the immature cervical spine include hypermobility, hyperlaxity of ligamentous and capsular structures, presence of epiphyses and synchondroses, incomplete ossification, unique configuration of the vertebral bony elements (e.g., wedge-shaped vertebral bodies, horizontally oriented facet joints), and variable sagittal alignment.

SPECIFIC CONDITIONS AFFECTING THE PEDIATRIC OCCIPITOCERVICAL JUNCTION AND CERVICAL REGION

7. **What are some conditions involving the cervical region in pediatric patients that are important to recognize?**
   Pediatric cervical disorders may be broadly classified by location (occiput-C2, C3–C7), clinical presentation (torticollis, instability, kyphosis, scoliosis), and etiology (e.g., congenital, developmental, acquired). Notable conditions that affect the occipitocervical junction and cervical region in pediatric patients include:
   - Basilar impression (invagination)
   - Arnold-Chiari malformation
   - Occipitocervical anomalies (e.g., occipitalization of C1)
   - Atlas (C1) anomalies (e.g., congenital unilateral absence of C1)
   - Odontoid (C2) anomalies (e.g., aplasia, hypoplasia, os odontoideum)
   - Occiput-C1 and C1–C2 instabilities
   - Atlantoaxial rotatory subluxation

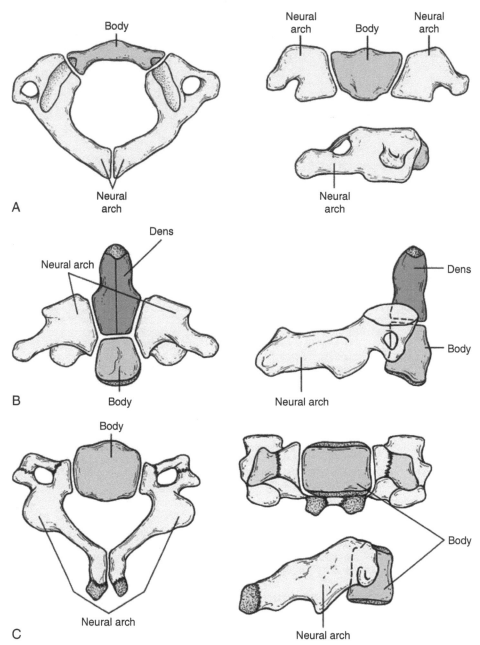

Fig. 36.1 (A) Ossification centers of C1. (B) Ossification centers of C2. (C) Ossification centers of C3–L5 vertebrae. (From Green NE, Swiontkowski M, editors. Skeletal Trauma in Children. 3rd ed. Philadelphia, PA: Saunders; 2003, p. 345, Fig. 11.1.)

- Congenital muscular torticollis
- Syndromic disorders (e.g., Down syndrome, Klippel-Feil syndrome)
- Kyphotic disorders (e.g., iatrogenic, secondary to dysplastic or metabolic disorder)
- Congenital scoliosis (failures of formation and/or segmentation)
- Skeletal dysplasia (e.g., achondroplasia, Larsen syndrome)
- Metabolic disorders (e.g., mucopolysaccharidoses)

- Primary osseous or neural tumors
- Infection
- Inflammatory disorders (e.g., juvenile rheumatoid arthritis)
- Trauma

8. **What is basilar impression?**

Basilar impression (also termed basilar invagination) refers to the prolapse of the vertebral column into the skull base. Upward migration of C2 is associated with narrowing of the foramen magnum. There are two main types of basilar impression: primary and secondary.

Primary basilar impression is the most common type, and is associated with Chiari 1 malformation and syringohydromyelia, as well as vertebral defects including atlanto-occipital fusion, odontoid abnormalities, Klippel-Feil anomaly, hypoplasia of the atlas, and atlantoaxial instability. Vertebral artery abnormalities may also be present. The most significant clinical problems associated with congenital basilar impression are due to compression of the anterior or posterior brainstem. It is the most common congenital anomaly of the upper cervical spine.

Secondary basilar impression arises as the result of softening of osseous structures at the base of the skull. Diseases associated with secondary basilar impression include osteomalacia, rickets, Paget disease, osteogenesis imperfecta, Morquio syndrome, and rheumatoid arthritis.

9. **What clinical findings may be present in patients with basilar impression?**

Clinical manifestations are variable and wide-ranging and result from compression of the brainstem, cervical spinal cord, cranial nerves, cervical nerve roots, and vascular supply. Symptoms may include neck pain, myelopathy, central cord syndrome, and sensory changes. Brainstem compression and vertebrobasilar artery encroachment may manifest as sleep apnea or basilar migraine. Cranial nerve dysfunction may result in problems including hearing loss or dysphagia. Patients with congenital abnormalities may have a visibly shortened neck, painful cervical motion, torticollis, and asymmetry of the skull and face.

10. **How is the diagnosis of basilar impression confirmed with imaging?**

Magnetic resonance imaging (MRI) demonstrates the position of the dens in relation to the foramen magnum with precision and provides the definitive method for diagnosis. A lateral craniocervical radiograph can demonstrate the position of the tip of the dens in relation to the various skull base lines (McGregor, McRae, Chamberlain) but is less precise than MRI or CT. Multiaxial CT is used primarily for presurgical planning.

11. **What treatment is indicated for symptomatic basilar impression?**

Treatment generally involves decompression and stabilization. Options for decompression include anterior transoral odontoid resection or posterior suboccipital craniectomy and C1 laminectomy. Stabilization typically includes posterior occipitocervical fusion with use of rigid internal fixation when anatomically feasible. Associated neurologic conditions, such as hydrocephalus, also require treatment (Fig. 36.2).

12. **What is the Arnold-Chiari malformation?**

The Arnold-Chiari malformation is a developmental anomaly in which the brainstem and cerebellum are displaced caudally into the spinal canal. In Type 1 Arnold-Chiari malformation, the cerebellar tonsils are displaced into the cervical spinal canal. This malformation is associated with other cervical anomalies, including basilar impression

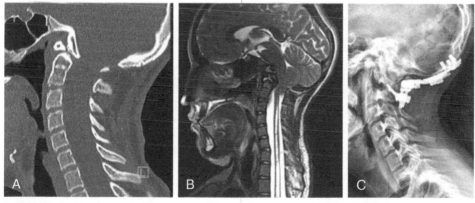

Fig. 36.2 A 14-year-old patient presented with progressive dysphagia and shortness of breath. (A) Sagittal computed tomography and (B) magnetic resonance imaging sequences indicate a pro-atlas segmentation abnormality with a horizontal clivus, atlas assimilation, and a shallow posterior fossa, resulting in ventral medullary compression, tonsillar ectopia, and syringomyelobulbia. (C) The patient experienced neurologic recovery after ventral craniovertebral junction decompression and dorsal occiput–C2 fusion, as shown on postoperative radiograph. (From Winn HR, editor. Youmans & Winn Neurologic Surgery. 7th ed. Philadelphia, PA: Elsevier; 2017, Fig. 233.8.)

and Klippel-Feil syndrome. Dense scarring at the level of the foramen magnum may lead to hydromyelia or syringomyelia. Type 2 Arnold-Chiari malformation is a more complex anomaly and is usually associated with myelomeningocele. Cerebellar displacement is accompanied by elongation of the fourth ventricle, as well as displacement of the fourth ventricle and cervical nerve roots.

13. How is atlanto-occipital instability diagnosed?
Atlanto-occipital instability is defined as greater than 1 mm of translation measured from the basion to the posterior margin of the anterior arch of C1 on lateral flexion-extension radiographs. Atlanto-occipital instability is most commonly due to trauma, but also occurs in association with congenital anomalies and conditions such as Down syndrome or Klippel-Feil syndrome (Fig. 36.3).

14. What is Steel's *rule of thirds*?
Dr. Steel noted that the area of the spinal canal at the C1 level in a normal person could be divided into equal thirds with one-third occupied by the odontoid process, one-third by the spinal cord, and one-third as empty space. The empty space serves as a safe zone into which displacement can occur without neurologic impingement. In the presence of atlantoaxial instability, displacement of the odontoid beyond the safe zone results in spinal cord compression.

15. How is atlantoaxial instability defined based on imaging studies?
Atlantoaxial instability is defined as an increased mobility between C1 and C2. The distance from anterior surface of the odontoid and the posterior aspect of the anterior arch of the atlas is called the atlantodens interval (ADI). The upper limit of normal for the ADI in children is 4 mm (up 5 mm before age 8). The transverse atlantal ligament is the primary ligamentous stabilizer of the atlantoaxial joint. Secondary soft tissue stability is provided by the alar ligaments and joint capsules. An ADI greater than 5 mm is considered pathologic as it represents failure of the transverse ligament. An ADI greater than 10 mm suggests failure of the secondary supporting ligaments, including the alar ligaments, with increased risk of neurologic compromise. In patients with chronic atlantoaxial instability or odontoid anomalies, the odontoid may be hypermobile. In these situations, measurement of the space available for the cord (SAC) is performed to assess for cord compression. The SAC is measured from the posterior margin of the odontoid to the closest posterior structure, either the foramen magnum or the posterior ring of C1. While an SAC of 13 mm or less in adults indicates insufficient space for the spinal cord, measurement in pediatric patients must take into account the age-related diameter of the spinal canal. MRI, although challenging to obtain in young children, is helpful in evaluating complex craniocervical disorders, and may include flexion and extension views to evaluate for dynamic cord compression. If concern remains regarding whether an odontoid anomaly is present, CT is considered (Fig. 36.4).

16. What are some of the major causes of nontraumatic atlantoaxial instability?
The major causes can be categorized as:
1. Anomalies of the odontoid process (e.g., os odontoideum, odontoid hypoplasia)
2. Ligamentous laxity (e.g., Down syndrome, juvenile rheumatoid arthritis, osteochondrodystrophies)

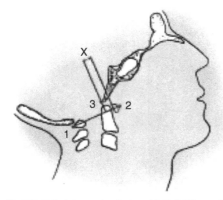

Fig. 36.3 Method of measuring atlanto-occipital instability according to Wiesel and Rothman. These lines are drawn on flexion and extension lateral radiographs, and translation should be no more than 1 mm. Atlantal line joins points 1 and 2. Line drawn perpendicular to atlantal line at posterior margin of anterior arch of atlas. Point 3 is basion. Distance from point 3 to perpendicular line (represented by X) is measured in flexion and extension. Difference represents anteroposterior translation. (From Gabriel KR, Mason DE, Carango P. Occipitoatlantal translation in Down's syndrome. Spine 1990;15:997–1002.)

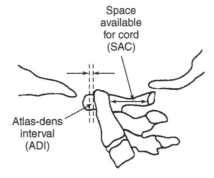

Fig. 36.4 Measurements for atlas-dens interval and the space available for the cord as determined on lateral cervical radiographs. (From Herman MJ, Pizzutillo PD. Cervical spine disorders in children. Orthop Clin North Am 1999;30:457–466, with permission.)

3. Synostosis at adjacent spinal levels (e.g., Klippel-Feil anomaly, occipitalization of the atlas) associated with increased compensatory motion at C1–C2

17. Describe how pediatric patients with atlantoaxial instability may present to clinicians.

Presenting symptoms are variable and may include neck pain, radicular pain, weakness, spasticity, difficulty with ambulation, hyperreflexia, and signs of lower cranial nerve involvement. Some patients present with vague and non-specific symptoms that should not be discounted, such as generalized weakness or lack of physical endurance.

18. Define os odontoideum and explain its etiology.

Os odontoideum is an anomaly of the odontoid process, which appears as an ossicle with smooth cortical margins that is separated from the body of the axis by a radiolucent gap. Recent data support two separate etiologies for os odontoideum: posttraumatic and congenital. Two anatomic types have been described: orthotopic and dystopic. In the orthotopic type, the ossicle is located in the position of the normal dens and moves in conjunction with the C1 arch. In the dystopic type, the ossicle is located adjacent to the clivus and may fuse with the occiput and move in concert with the clivus. The atlantoaxial joint often becomes unstable as the odontoid becomes unable to function as a peg. The direction of instability may be anterior, posterior, or bidirectional. Clinical presentation is variable and ranges from an incidental radiographic finding to mild neck pain with or without myelopathy to sudden death secondary to minor trauma. As the os odontoideum may move in conjunction with the C1 ring, attention should be directed to measurement of both the ADI and SAC when assessing for spinal canal narrowing as the ADI may be unchanged on flexion-extension radiographs.

Surgery is recommended in the presence of neurologic signs or symptoms or C1–C2 instability. Treatment options for asymptomatic patients include clinical and radiographic surveillance versus surgical stabilization. Some experts advise surgical stabilization for all patients with os odontoideum due to the risk of catastrophic spinal cord injury from minor trauma. The most common surgical treatment is posterior C1–C2 fusion with rigid stabilization. Occipitocervical fusion with or without C1 laminectomy is recommended for patients with irreducible posterior cervicomedullary compression or occiput-C1 instability. Anterior decompression is considered for patients with irreducible ventral cervicomedullary compression (Fig. 36.5).

19. What patterns of upper cervical instability are seen in patients with Down syndrome?

Patients with Down syndrome may manifest instability of both the atlanto-occipital and atlantoaxial joints. It is important to rule out atlanto-occipital instability prior to performing fusion of the atlantoaxial joints. In addition, atlanto-occipital instability may develop following a successful atlantoaxial fusion. The underlying problem is generalized ligamentous laxity and congenital abnormalities of the craniocervical junction. Hypoplasia of the posterior arch of C1, occipital condyle hypoplasia, and os odontoideum are prevalent in this population. Caution is advised when surgical treatment is undertaken because of the high risk of surgical complications in this population including nonunion, loss of reduction, neurologic injury, infection, and death.

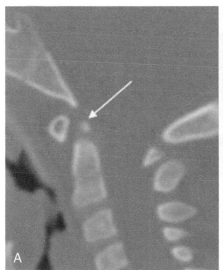
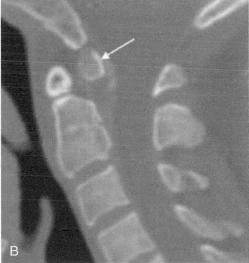

Fig. 36.5 Os odontoideum. Two types: (A) orthotopic and (B) dystopic are shown on the sagittal CT view. The arrow points to the independent ossicle which is separated from the dens by a transverse gap. (From Chong V, editor. Skull Base Imaging. Philadelphia, PA: Elsevier; 2018, Fig. 14.10.)

20. What is the clinical triad described by Klippel-Feil syndrome?

Klippel-Feil syndrome has been classically described as the clinical triad of a short neck, low posterior hairline, and limitation of cervical motion. This classic triad is seen in less than 50% of cases. The spinal anomaly associated with Klippel-Feil syndrome is congenital fusion of the cervical spine. The number of fused segments may vary from two segments to fusion of the entire cervical spine (Fig. 36.6).

21. Why is early recognition of Klippel-Feil syndrome important?

Klippel-Feil anomalies are a marker that should prompt investigation for a wide range of systemic anomalies. Because the embryologic development of cervical spine parallels the development of many other organ systems, a wide range of anomalies may be present, including anomalies involving the genitourinary, cardiovascular, auditory, gastrointestinal, skeletal, and neurologic systems. Associated skeletal system anomalies include scoliosis, Sprengel deformity (failure of descent of the scapula), presence of an omovertebral bone, and cervical ribs. A notable neurologic abnormality present in this population is synkinesis (unconscious mirror movement of one extremity that mimics the opposite extremity). Patients with Klippel-Feil syndrome may develop radiculopathy or myelopathy as the result of spinal cord compression due to a congenitally narrow spinal canal, spinal instability, or basilar invagination.

22. What workup should be performed for a patient diagnosed with Klippel-Feil syndrome?

Diagnosis of a congenital cervical fusion should prompt assessment of the genitourinary system (renal ultrasound), cardiac system (echocardiogram, cardiology referral), and auditory system (hearing test). Neurologic symptoms should be evaluated with an MRI of the brainstem and cervical spine. Cervical instability is evaluated with flexion and extension radiographs.

23. Are any patterns of congenital cervical fusion in Klippel-Feil patients associated with an increased risk of neurologic deficit?

Yes. Specific fusion patterns considered to be associated with an increased risk of neurologic problems are:
1. C2–C3 fusion with occipitalization of the atlas
2. A long cervical fusion in the presence of an abnormal occipitocervical junction
3. A single open interspace between two fused spine segments

24. Define torticollis and outline the differential diagnosis of this condition.

Torticollis is a clinical diagnosis based on head tilt in association with a rotatory deviation of the cranium. Although the differential diagnosis of this condition is wide-ranging, consideration of whether the deformity was present at birth (congenital) versus acquired, and whether this condition is painful versus nonpainful, is suggested to aid in diagnosis. (1)

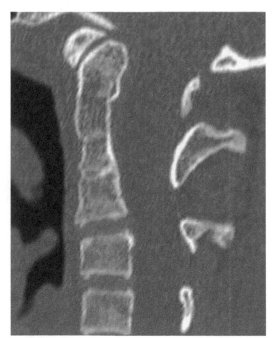

Fig. 36.6 A sagittal reconstruction computed tomography scan shows congenital fusion of C2 and C3 in a young patient with Klippel-Feil syndrome. (From Klimo P, Rao G, Brockmeyer D. Congenital anomalies of the cervical spine. Neurosurg Clin N Am 2007;18:463–478, Fig. 9.)

Congenital Nonpainful Conditions
- Congenital muscular torticollis
- Vertebral anomalies
- Ocular or auditory dysfunction

Acquired Painful Conditions
- Fracture
- Rotatory subluxation of the atlantoaxial joints
- Tumors involving the posterior fossa, brainstem, or spinal cord
- Osseous tumors (osteoid osteoma, aneurysmal bone cyst)
- Infection
- Inflammatory disorders (e.g., juvenile rheumatoid arthritis)
- Sandifer syndrome (gastroesophageal reflux and torticollis)

Acquired Painful or Nonpainful Conditions
- Paroxysmal torticollis of infancy
- Tumors (involving osseous or central nervous systems)
- Syrinx
- Conditions associated with ligamentous laxity
- Dystonic reaction to specific medications (e.g., phenothiazines)

25. What is the most common type of torticollis?

Congenital muscular torticollis is the most common type of torticollis. It presents in the newborn period. Its cause is unknown, but it has been hypothesized to arise from compression of the soft tissues of the neck during delivery, resulting in a compartment syndrome. Clinical examination reveals painless spasm of the sternocleidomastoid muscle on the *same* side ("short side") as the tilt, leading to the typical posture of head tilt toward the tightened muscle and chin rotation to the opposite side. Ultrasound may be used to confirm the diagnosis and shows a homogenous, hyperechoic mass located within the sternocleidomastoid muscle on the affected side. Radiographs of the cervical spine should be obtained to rule out congenital vertebral anomalies. Initial treatment is stretching and is successful in up to 90% of patients during the first year of life. Surgery may be considered for persistent deformity, but is rarely indicated, and may be deferred up to 5 years of age. Common problems noted in patients with congenital muscular torticollis include congenital hip dysplasia and plagiocephaly (facial asymmetry due to flattening of the face on the side of the sternocleidomastoid lesion). Bilateral ultrasound evaluation is recommended to rule out hip dysplasia in this population.

26. What features suggest that torticollis is due to atlantoaxial rotatory subluxation?

Features that suggest that torticollis is due to atlantoaxial rotatory subluxation include prior normal cervical alignment and motion, history of recent upper respiratory infection (Grisel syndrome), normal neurologic examination, and spasm in the sternocleidomastoid muscle on the side *opposite* the head tilt ("long side" of the deformity), and pain with attempted reduction of the deformity. This posture has been termed the "cock robin" deformity. It is distinct from congenital muscular torticollis, in which muscle spasm occurs on the same side as the head tilt. Plain radiographs are frequently difficult to interpret but typically show asymmetry of the C1 lateral masses on the anteroposterior (AP) odontoid view. A cervical MRI or CT scan can be obtained to confirm the diagnosis. Various types of CT studies have been suggested and include a cervical CT scan with standard sagittal and coronal reconstructions, a dynamic rotational CT scan, and a CT scan performed with the patient under general anesthesia.

27. How is atlantoaxial rotatory subluxation classified?

Atlantoaxial rotatory subluxation may be classified according to duration of symptoms as acute (< 1 month), subacute (1–3 months), and chronic (>3 months).

Fielding identified four types of atlantoaxial subluxations based on axial CT scans:

Type 1: Rotatory displacement without anterior shift of C1
Type 2: Rotatory displacement with C1 anterior shift of 5 mm or less
Type 3: Rotatory displacement with C1 anterior shift greater than 5 mm
Type 4: Rotatory displacement with C1 posterior shift

Type 1 is the most common type and represents a unilateral facet subluxation in which the transverse ligament is intact and the dens acts as a pivot. Type 2 is a unilateral facet subluxation with an ADI of 3–5 mm in which the facet joint acts as a pivot and is associated with transverse ligament injury. Types 3 and 4 are rare and represent various degrees of C1–C2 dislocation.

Atlantoaxial rotatory subluxation may also be classified (Ishii classification) based on the presence of facet deformity and lateral angulation of the C1 arch as grade 1 (no facet deformity, no angulation of C1), grade 2 (moderate facet deformity, <20° angulation of C1), and grade 3 (severe facet deformity, >20° angulation of C1).

28. Describe the treatment of atlantoaxial rotatory subluxation.

When the problem is diagnosed early (<1 week), many children respond well to immobilization with a soft cervical collar and stretching exercises. If early follow-up (<1 month) shows persistent subluxation, inpatient treatment with traction via a head halter is indicated. If reduction occurs, immobilization is continued for at least 6 weeks with a cervical collar. For patients presenting with symptoms for over one month or if head halter traction is not tolerated or unsuccessful, halo traction is instituted. If reduction is achieved, immobilization in a halo vest for at least 6 weeks is recommended. Surgery is indicated for failure of reduction following traction treatment, recurrent subluxation, neurologic involvement, and deformities present for more than 3 months. Posterior C1–C2 arthrodesis is the most commonly performed surgical procedure. Various surgical strategies have been described to achieve C1–C2 reduction including skull traction, mobilization of the atlantoaxial joints (from a posterior approach or through a separate transoral or lateral retropharyngeal exposure), C1–C2 intraarticular graft placement, and use of spinal instrumentation. Posterior fusion in conjunction with rigid fixation with C1–C2 screw-rod fixation or transarticular screw fixation is recommended.

29. What etiologies are associated with the development cervical kyphosis in pediatric patients?

Cervical kyphosis is rare in the pediatric population. The most common etiologies include:
- Postlaminectomy kyphosis
- Trauma
- Larsen syndrome (Fig. 36.7)
- Diastrophic dysplasia
- Conradi syndrome (chondrodysplasia punctata)
- Neurofibromatosis

30. What are some examples of skeletal dysplasias associated with specific pediatric cervical spine abnormalities?

Skeletal dysplasias comprise a group of more than 400 genetic disorders associated with abnormal differentiation, development, growth and/or maintenance of bone and cartilage. The impact of these disorders on the function of connective tissue, including bone, cartilage, ligaments, and skin, lead to a diverse range of medical problems. The consequences of skeletal dysplasias include anomalies in the size, shape, and function of the skeleton, as well as adverse impacts on related respiratory, neurologic, craniofacial, and metabolic functions in specific disorders (Table 36.1).

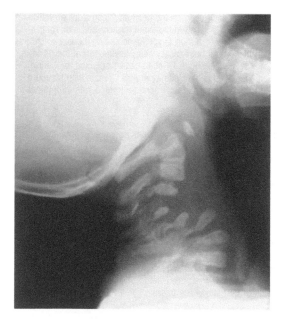

Fig. 36.7 Lateral radiograph of a 10-month-old infant with Larsen syndrome and cervical kyphosis. (From Herring JA, editor. Tachdjian's Pediatric Orthopaedics. 5th ed. Philadelphia, PA: Saunders; 2014, Fig. 11.24.)

Table 36.1 Some Pediatric Cervical Spine Manifestations of Specific Skeletal Dysplasias.	
Achondroplasia	Basilar invagination, subaxial stenosis
Pseudoachondroplasia	Atlantoaxial instability, subaxial stenosis
Spondyloepiphyseal dysplasia	Atlantoaxial instability
Kneist dysplasia	Occipito-atlantal or atlantoaxial instability
Diastrophic dysplasia	Atlantoaxial instability, cervical kyphosis
Hurler syndrome	Atlantoaxial instability, cervical stenosis
Hunter syndrome	Cervical stenosis
Morquio syndrome	Basilar impression, atlantoaxial instability, cervical stenosis
Larsen syndrome	Cervical kyphosis

KEY POINTS

1. A wide range of conditions may cause upper cervical instability.
2. Children younger than age 8 are predisposed to upper cervical injury due to their high head-to-body ratio and horizontal facet orientation.
3. Evaluation of C1–C2 instability should include assessment of both the atlantodens interval (ADI) and the space available for the spinal cord (SAC).
4. The presence of a Klippel-Feil anomaly should prompt investigation for associated organ system anomalies.

Websites
1. Atlantoaxial instability: http://emedicine.medscape.com/article/1265682-overview
2. Klippel-Feil syndrome: http://emedicine.medscape.com/article/1264848-overview
3. International Society for Pediatric Neurosurgery Guide to Pediatric Neurosurgery: https://www.ispn.guide/spinal-diseases-and-anomalies-in-children/cervical-spine-anomalies-in-children/
4. Pediatric Orthopaedic Society of North America, Study Guide, Spine Topics: https://posna.org/Physician-Education/Study-Guide?categoryname=Spine

REFERENCE

1. Copley, L. A. B. (2014). Disorders of the neck. In J. A. Herring (Eds.), *Tachdjian's Pediatric Orthopaedics* (5th ed., pp. 167–205). Philadelphia, PA: Saunders.

BIBLIOGRAPHY

1. Copley, L. A. B. (2014). Disorders of the neck. In J. A. Herring (Eds.), *Tachdjian's Pediatric Orthopaedics* (5th ed., pp. 167–205). Philadelphia, PA: Saunders.
2. Darden, B. V., O'Boynick, C., & Casamitjana, J. M. (2018). Cervical spinal disorders associated with skeletal dysplasias and metabolic bone diseases. In S. R. Garfin, F. J. Eismont, G. R. Bell, et al. (Eds.), *Rothman-Simeone the Spine* (7th ed., pp. 663–675). Philadelphia, PA: Saunders.
3. Menezes, A. H., Ahmed, R., & Dlouhy, B. J. (2017). Developmental anomalies of the craniovertebral junction and surgical management. In H. R. Winn (Ed.), *Youmans & Winn Neurologic Surgery* (7th ed., pp. 1856–1870). Philadelphia, PA: Elsevier.
4. Murphy, R. F., Hedequist, D. J. (2018). Glotzbecker: Congenital anomalies of the cervical spine. In S. R. Garfin, F. J. Eismont, G. R. Bell, et al. (Eds.), *Rothman-Simeone the Spine* (7th ed., pp. 609–640). Philadelphia, PA: Saunders.
5. Neal, K. M., & Mohamed, A. S. (2015). Atlantoaxial rotatory subluxation in children. *Journal of the American Academy of Orthopaedic Surgeons, 23*, 382–392.
6. Rozzelle, C. J., Aarabi, B., Dhall, S. S., Gelb, D. E., Hurlbert, R. J., Ryken, T. C., et al. (2013). Os odontoideum. *Neurosurgery, 72*, 159–169.
7. Samartzis, D. D., Lubicky, J. P., Herman, J., & Shen, F. H. (2006). Classification of congenitally fused cervical patterns in Klippel-Feil patients: Epidemiology and role in the development of cervical spine-related symptoms. *Spine, 31*, E798–E804.
8. Willis, B. P., & Dormans, J. P. (2006). Nontraumatic upper cervical spine instability in children. *Journal of the American Academy of Orthopaedic Surgeons, 14*, 233–246.

CHAPTER 37

EARLY-ONSET SCOLIOSIS

Vincent J. Devlin, MD

BACKGROUND

1. **Why is the age of onset of scoliosis important?**
   Growth and development of the spinal column, thorax, and lungs are interdependent. Deformities affecting the spine and thorax in the first decade of life adversely impact lung development and function. Long-term follow-up of patients with untreated scoliosis (9) has shown increased mortality secondary to respiratory failure and cardiovascular disease in those with infantile scoliosis (birth–3 years) and juvenile scoliosis (4–9 years) but not in patients with adolescent scoliosis (10–16 years).

2. **Briefly outline the different phases of growth of the spine and thorax from birth through adulthood. How is lung development characterized during each growth phase?**
   Lung development and growth of the spine and thorax are interrelated. Rapid growth of the spine and thoracic cage occurs during the first decade of life, a critical period for lung development. During this time, limitation of growth or distortion of the shape of the spine or thorax interferes with lung development and cardiac function. Key aspects regarding the development of the spine, thorax, and lungs have been conceptualized in terms of three phases. (7)
   Early phase (from birth to 5 years)
   - The most rapid period of spinal growth during which length of the T1–S1 segment increases by approximately 10 cm (2 cm/year).
   - The thoracic cage volume increases from approximately 6% of mature size at birth–30% of mature size by age 5.
   - Postnatal lung growth is characterized by rapid alveolar growth during this period, with the greatest increase in alveolar growth between birth and 4 years.
   Middle phase (from 5 to 10 years)
   - Growth of the spine occurs at a slower rate as T1–S1 length increases by approximately 5 cm (1 cm/year).
   - Thoracic cage volume increases from 30% of mature size at age 5 to approximately 50% of mature size by age 10.
   - Lung growth and volume continue at a slower pace with alveolar multiplication markedly slowing after age 8–9.
   Adolescent phase (from age 10 to adulthood)
   - This is a period of increasing spinal growth marked by the adolescent growth spurt but never reaches the rapid velocity of early spine growth. T1–S1 length increases by approximately 10 cm (1.8 cm/year) between age 10 and skeletal maturity.
   - Thoracic volume doubles between age 10 and skeletal maturity.
   - Lung growth and volume increase primarily through increase in alveolar dimensions as few new alveoli form during this phase.

3. **What are some key parameters used to assess spinal growth from birth to maturity?**
   T1–S1 spinal segment length: T1–S1 length is approximately 20 cm at birth and increases to 45 cm at skeletal maturity. T1–S1 length increase is approximately 10 cm from birth to 5 years (2 cm/year), 5 cm between ages 5 and 10 years (1 cm/year), and 10 cm from age 10 to skeletal maturity (1.8 cm/year). The T1–S1 length is a useful measure of overall growth of the spine.

   T1–T12 spinal segment length: T1–T12 length is approximately 12 cm at birth, 18 cm at 5 years, 22 cm at 10 years, and 26.5 cm in adult females and 28 cm in adult males. The T1–T12 growth rate is approximately 1.3 cm/year from birth to 5 years, 0.7 cm/year between ages 5 and 10 years, and 1.1 cm/year during puberty. The T1–T12 segment has been referred to as the "posterior pillar of the thorax" as decreased growth in this region has a definite adverse effect on thoracic growth and lung development. Decreased T1–T12 height following early thoracic spine fusion prior to age 5, especially involving upper thoracic spinal segments, correlates with diminished pulmonary function. A minimum thoracic spine height of 18–22 cm is necessary to avoid respiratory insufficiency. (8)

   L1–L5 spinal segment length: L1–L5 length is approximately 7.5 cm at birth, 10.5 cm at 5 years, 12.5 cm at 10 years, and 15.5 cm in adult females and 16 cm in adult males.

4. **What is thoracic insufficiency syndrome?**
   Thoracic insufficiency syndrome (TIS) is defined as the inability of the thorax to support normal respiration or lung growth. (5) TIS may develop in skeletally immature patients due to a wide range of conditions that restrict lung volume, lung expansion, and postnatal lung growth. Causes of TIS include hypoplastic thorax syndromes such

Jeune syndrome, spinal dysplasias, including spondylocostal and spondylothoracic dysplasia, congenital scoliosis with fused ribs, and early onset spinal deformities associated with distortion of the rib cage.

5. **How is early-onset scoliosis defined?**

Early-onset scoliosis (EOS) is defined as "scoliosis with onset less than the age of 10 years, regardless of etiology." (12) Patients with EOS are at risk for developing progressive deformity involving the spine and thorax, which has the potential to adversely impact normal growth and development of the spinal column, thoracic cavity, and lung parenchyma leading to TIS and early mortality. The four main etiologic categories of EOS are congenital-structural, neuromuscular, syndromic, and idiopathic.

6. **Describe some key features associated with each of the four main etiologic categories of EOS.**

- **Congenital-structural:** These types of early-onset curves arise due to a structural abnormality of the spine or thorax that is present at birth. Congenital spinal anomalies may be classified as failures of vertebral body formation, failures of vertebral body segmentation, and mixed types of anomalies. Structural deformities of the thoracic cage may lead to TIS in patients with conditions such as fused ribs and scoliosis, absence of ribs and scoliosis (i.e., congenital absence of ribs or postsurgical flail chest), hypoplastic thorax (i.e., Jeune asphyxiating thoracic dystrophy), and symmetrically shortened thorax (i.e., spondylothoracic dysplasia). Anomalies associated with these complex conditions include spinal dysraphism, intraspinal anomalies such diastematomyelia and tethered cord, as well as anomalies involving embryologically related organ systems, including **v**ertebral and costal abnormalities, **a**nal atresia, **c**ardiac defects, **t**racheal-**e**sophageal abnormalities, **r**enal and radial anomalies, **l**imb anomalies and **s**ingle umbilical artery, referred to as the "VACTERLS" association.
- **Neuromuscular:** Neuromuscular early-onset curves arise as a consequence of disorders involving the brain, spinal cord, or muscular system, which impair the ability to maintain appropriate spine and trunk alignment, and are often associated with pelvic obliquity and respiratory compromise. A wide range of disorders may cause neuromuscular EOS and are broadly categorized as neuropathic or myopathic. Examples include cerebral palsy, spinal muscular atrophy, Duchenne muscular dystrophy, myelodysplasia, Rett syndrome, Friedreich ataxia, and spinal cord injury.
- **Syndromic:** Syndromic early-onset curves are deformities of the spine or thorax attributed to a systemic disorder or known syndrome in the absence of a congenital-structural or neuromuscular cause. Some examples of conditions considered under the umbrella term "syndromic scoliosis" include neurofibromatosis, Marfan syndrome, Ehlers-Danlos syndrome, Prader-Willi syndrome, and osteogenesis imperfecta. Each syndrome has unique systemic manifestations with the potential to lead to significant morbidity if unrecognized or untreated, and specific knowledge regarding management of these associated conditions is required to optimize treatment outcomes.
- **Idiopathic:** Idiopathic early-onset curves occur in the absence of a known cause. Incompletely identified genetic factors are considered to play an important role. Neural axis abnormalities may be present and are often asymptomatic and detected only with magnetic resonance imaging (MRI). Although infantile idiopathic scoliosis resolves without treatment in the majority of cases, some patients develop progressive curvatures associated with life-threatening deformities.

7. **How is EOS classified?**

EOS is characterized using a consensus-based system (Table 37.1) termed the Classification of Early-Onset Scoliosis (C-EOS) based on the following parameters: age, three core variables (etiology, major curve angle, kyphosis), and an optional modifier to identify annual curve progression. (14)

Age: Patient age at the time of presentation is an important factor in treatment decision-making and is identified by a prefix.

Etiology: Four etiologic subgroups are recognized and designated by a letter. Patients with mixed etiologies are assigned to a single subgroup based on a priority order from high to low: **C**ongenital-structural (C), **N**euromuscular (M), **S**yndromic (S), and **I**diopathic (I).

Table 37.1 Classification of Early-Onset Scoliosis (C-EOS).

ETIOLOGY	SCOLIOSIS (MAJOR CURVE)	KYPHOSIS
C: Congenital or structural	Group 1: <20°	N: Normokyphotic: 20°–50°
M: Neuromuscular	Group 2: 20°–50°	(+) Hyperkyphotic: >50°
S: Syndromic	Group 3: 51°–90°	(−) Hypokyphotic: <20°
I: Idiopathic	Group 4: >90°	

Adapted from Williams BA, Matsumoto H, McCalla DJ, et al. Development and initial validation of the Classification of Early-Onset Scoliosis (C-EOS). J Bone Joint Surg Am 2014;96:1359–1367.

Major curve angle: Four subgroups are identified: group 1: $<20°$, group 2: $20°–50°$, group 3: $51°–90°$, group 4: $>90°$.
Kyphosis: Evaluated as the maximal measurable kyphosis between any two levels and identified as: hypokyphotic: $<20°$ ($-$), normokyphotic: $20°–50°$ (N), or hypokyphotic: $>50°$ ($+$).
Annual progression ratio (APR) modifier: Major curve angle progression is determined based on posteroanterior (PA) spinal radiographs obtained at two distinct time points (t_1, t_2) obtained at a minimum 6-month interval. The APR modifier is calculated from the curve progression measured between t_1 and t_2 multiplied by a time factor (12 months/[$t_2 - t_1$]). The APR modifier subgroups are: P^0: $<10°$/year, P^1: $10°–20°$/year, P^2: $>20°$/year.

8. A 6-year-old nonambulatory child with cerebral palsy presents for follow-up orthopedic evaluation for scoliosis. The most recent prior radiographs obtained 16 months ago showed a 30° major coronal curve and a maximal measurable kyphosis of 35°. Current radiographs show a 46° major coronal curve and a maximal measurable kyphosis of 40°. How would you describe this patient's EOS using the C-EOS classification?
   The **C-EOS classification** for this patient is: **6-year-old M2N** (age=6 years; etiology=M, neuromuscular; major curve angle=2, group 2: $20°–50°$; kyphosis=N, normokyphotic: $20°–50°$).
   This patient's **APR modifier** is **P^1**. To calculate the APR modifier: $(46°–30°) \times$ (12 months/16 months) = $(16° \times 0.75) = 12°$, which denotes an APR modifier P^1 ($10°–20°$/year).

9. What are the goals when treating patients with EOS?
   According to a consensus statement from the Scoliosis Research Society Growing Spine Committee, the treatment goals in EOS are to:
   • Minimize spinal deformity over the life of the patient
   • Maximize thoracic volume and function over the life of the patient
   • Minimize the extent of any final spinal fusion
   • Maximize motion of the chest and spine
   • Minimize complications, procedures, hospitalizations, and burden for the family
   • Consider overall development of the child

NONOPERATIVE TREATMENT

10. What are the nonoperative treatment options for EOS?
    Curves less than 20° are monitored for progression with serial clinical examinations and radiographic follow-up. Nonoperative treatment with serial casting is initiated for EOS curves that progress past 20° or for treatment of patients who initially present with larger curves. Cast treatment can be curative if initiated before 2 years of age in patients with idiopathic EOS $<60°$. Cast treatment is also effective as a delay tactic for nonidiopathic EOS to provide curve control and limit curve progression. This allows time for additional spine and thoracic cage growth and further lung development prior to more definitive treatment with surgery. The role of brace treatment is less known compared with casting and is an area of active investigation. Use of brace treatment is generally limited to older patients with curves that would not be expected to improve with cast treatment, or as an adjunct to cast treatment since bracing has not been proven to result in permanent curve correction in EOS patients. Caution is necessary when treating younger children with bracing due to the risk of iatrogenic chest wall deformity secondary to rib cage compression and sagittal plane spinal deformity. Brace options include use of a Milwaukee brace (cervicothoracolumbosacral orthosis, CTLSO) or an underarm thoracolumbosacral orthosis (TLSO). Halo-gravity traction is an additional nonoperative treatment option and may be used to optimize pulmonary function and improve spinal deformity prior to casting or surgical treatment.

11. What is the significance of the rib-vertebral angle difference and rib phase?
    The rib-vertebral angle difference (**RVAD**) measures the amount of rotation at the apex vertebra and has prognostic value regarding curve progression in patients with idiopathic EOS. This angle is determined by a line perpendicular to the endplate of the apical vertebra and a line drawn through the center of the adjacent rib on both the concave and convex side of the apical vertebra (Fig 37.1). The RVAD equals the difference between the convex and concave angles. If the difference is greater than 20°, curve progression is likely. The **rib phase** is determined by ascertaining whether the head of the convex rib overlaps the apical vertebral body, and is used as an adjunctive measurement. If there is no overlap (phase 1), the RVAD is calculated to determine the likelihood of progression. If there is overlap (phase 2), the risk of progression is high.

12. Describe the modern technique of cast treatment for EOS.
    The elongation, derotation, and flexion (EDF) method of serial casting originally described by Cotrel and Morel and subsequently modified by Mehta is preferred (Fig. 37.2A–C). The cast is most commonly placed with the patient intubated and under general anesthesia. There is also some evidence that casting without anesthesia can be effective, which obviates anesthetic risk in this young EOS population. The patient is positioned on a cast table, which supports the head, arms, and legs and provides circumferential access to the trunk. Tubular stockinette and padding are placed. The feet are placed in a sling and traction is applied to elongate the spine through use of a

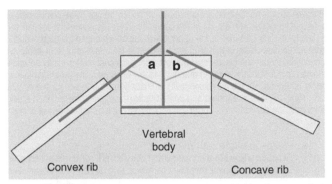

Fig. 37.1 The rib-vertebral angle difference (RVAD). The rib-vertebral angle is determined by a line perpendicular to the endplate of the apical vertebra and a line drawn along the center of the rib. The RVAD is calculated by subtracting the angle of the convex side *(a)* from the concave side *(b)*. (From Choudhury MZB, Tsirikos A, Marks DS. Early-onset scoliosis: Clinical presentation, assessment, and treatment options. Orthop Trauma 2017;31:357–363, Fig. 1, p. 359.)

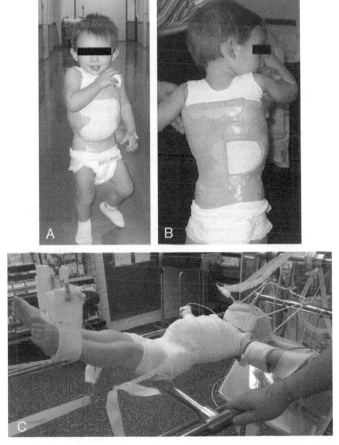

Fig. 37.2 Cast treatment for early-onset scoliosis. (A) The anterior window allows chest and abdominal space while capturing the anterior ribs to prevent their deformity. (B) The posterior window on the concavity allows the curve to settle into the defect and improve the rotation. (C) Cast is applied with traction on specialized table. (A and B: From D'Astous JL, Sanders JO. Casting and traction treatment methods for scoliosis. Orthop Clin N Am 2007;38:477–484, Fig. 4, p. 480. C: From Sanders JO, Johnston CE, D'Astous J. Casting in early-onset scoliosis. Semin Spine Surg 2012;24:144–148, Fig. 1, p. 145.)

head halter and pelvic straps. As the cast is applied, it is important to use three-point molding to apply derotational forces to the posterior ribs at the apex of the curve to correct the posteriorly rotated vertebra. Simultaneously, assistants apply counter pressure to the upper chest and shoulders and simultaneously mold the pelvic portion of the cast at the iliac crests. A mirror at the base of the table is helpful to evaluate and adjust the hand position during derotation. After the plaster cast has set, fiberglass cast material may be applied to strengthen the cast. Next, windows are cut from the cast. An anterior window is cut to allow for abdominal and chest expansion. A posterior window on the side of the curve concavity is created to allow space for the concave ribs and spine to shift posteriorly. Next, the cast is trimmed and upright radiographs are obtained. Cast changes are performed every 8–12 weeks until the desired curve correction is obtained. This treatment phase is typically followed by a period of brace treatment.

13. What is the role of halo-gravity traction in the treatment of EOS?
Halo-gravity traction is a useful adjunct in the treatment of complex EOS deformities and is used to improve respiratory mechanics and provide partial spinal deformity correction prior to operative intervention or cast treatment. A halo ring is applied using a minimum of six to eight pins and traction is initiated with 3–5 pounds and gradually increased by 2–3 pounds per day up to 33%–50% of the patient's bodyweight. During the day, use of an overhead traction unit attached to a wheelchair or standing frame permits patients to mobilize out of bed. At night, traction is reduced but maintained while the patient is sleeping in bed. It is important to monitor upper and lower extremity neurologic and cranial nerve function, as well as perform meticulous pin site cleaning and monitor for pin loosening during treatment. Use of halo-gravity traction has been shown to provide up to 30%–40% nonoperative correction of sagittal and coronal plane deformity and improvement in respiratory function.

SURGICAL TREATMENT

14. What knowledge has led to a paradigm shift in recent years regarding surgical treatment strategies for EOS?
Clinicians recognized that routine treatment of EOS patients with multilevel spinal fusion had an adverse impact on the growth and development of the spine, thoracic cage, and lung function. In addition, early spinal fusion in the growing child was not as effective in controlling spinal deformity as previously thought since recurrent spinal deformity requiring revision surgery was observed. Deformity recurrence was noted following posterior fusion due to continued anterior spine growth, termed the crankshaft phenomenon, as well as following circumferential fusion. These findings have led to a shift toward surgical interventions intended to control spinal deformities and avoid, minimize, or delay the need for spinal fusion. Surgical treatment strategies are directed toward restoration of thoracic volume by thoracic reconstruction and implant stabilization for deformities primarily involving the thorax such as thoracic dysplasias, thoracogenic scoliosis, and multiple fused ribs and congenital scoliosis.

15. What surgical implants currently play a role in the surgical treatment of EOS patients?
Surgical implants used to treat EOS are referred to as "growth-friendly" implants as they are intended to control spine and chest deformities and maximize spinal column growth and thoracic volume and function without spinal fusion. Growth-friendly spinal implants are classified into three main types (11) based on the corrective forces exerted by the implants on the spine and thoracic cage: (1) distraction-based systems, (2) guided growth systems, and (3) compression-based systems. Examples include:
Distraction-based systems
• Vertical Expandable Prosthetic Titanium Rib (VEPTR)
• Traditional growing rods
• Growing rods with proximal rib anchors
• Magnetically controlled growing-rod system
Guided growth systems
• Shilla Growth Guidance System
• Luque trolley and variants
Compression-based systems
• Spinal tethers
• Vertebral body staples

16. What is VEPTR?
The VEPTR is a first-of-a-kind surgically implantable device developed by Robert M. Campbell, Jr., MD, for treatment of skeletally immature patients with severe deformities of the chest, spine, and ribs that prevent normal breathing, lung growth, and development, which he defined as *thoracic insufficiency syndrome* (TIS). The VEPTR device is comprised of curved titanium rods, which attach proximally to ribs and distally to rib, spine, or pelvis anchor sites. Different types of expansion thoracoplasty procedures were developed to allow expansion of a volume-constricted thorax associated with primary rib cage deformity, and stabilization of the thorax through use of VEPTR implants. The VEPTR device also has utility for stabilization of neuromuscular spinal deformities and for use as a

modified growing-rod construct for treatment of complex early-onset spinal deformities. Following the initial VEPTR implantation procedure, the devices are expanded two to three times per year to accommodate growth during a surgical procedure performed with the patient under general anesthesia. Various types of VEPTR constructs (Fig. 37.3A–C) are utilized including rib-to-rib constructs, rib-to-spine constructs, and rib-to-pelvis constructs depending on the specific deformity requiring treatment. (6)

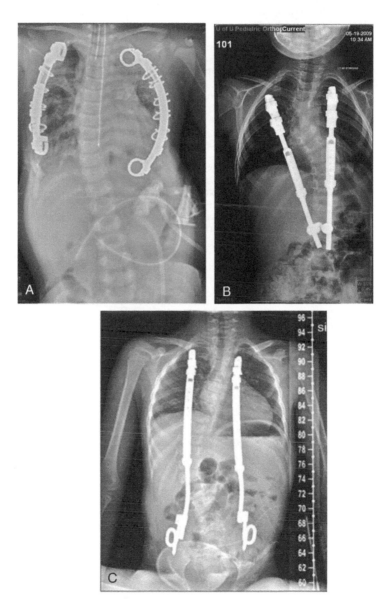

Fig. 37.3 (A) Volume depletion deformity due to global thoracic hypoplasia in a 6-month old patient with Jeune syndrome treated with staged bilateral rib-to-rib vertical expandable prosthetic titanium rib (VEPTR) construct. (B) VEPTR rib-to-spine construct used for treatment of early-onset scoliosis associated with neurofibromatosis type 1. (C) Bilateral VEPTR rib-to-pelvis construct with "S" hook for distal fixation. (A: From Mayer O, Campbell R, Cahill P, et al. Thoracic insufficiency syndrome. Curr Probl Pediatr Adolesc Health Care 2016; 46:72–97, Fig. 8, p. 84. B: From Heflin JA, Cleveland A, Ford SD, et al. Use of rib-based distraction in the treatment of early-onset scoliosis associated with neurofibromatosis Type 1 in the young child. Spine Deform 2015;3:239–245, Fig. 2, p. 241. C: From Campbell RM Jr. Vertical expandable prosthetic titanium rib expansion thoracoplasty. In: Kocher MS, Millis MB, editors. Operative Techniques: Pediatric Orthopaedic Surgery. Philadelphia, PA: Saunders; 2011, pp. 667–698, Fig. 13, p. 685.)

17. What are some advantages and disadvantages of VEPTR constructs?

The major advantage of the VEPTR device is that it provides a treatment for TIS, a life-threatening condition without a method for treatment prior to invention of this device. The VEPTR device provides a technique for surgical correction and stabilization of the deformed thorax and spine that permits adjustment of the device over time to accommodate the growing child. The device is versatile and can be adapted for treatment of both rib-based and spine-based deformities. A disadvantage of the VEPTR device is the need for multiple surgical procedures over time to lengthen the implants by distraction to accommodate growth of the patient. Complications associated with use of VEPTR include wound infection, skin slough, anchor point migration, brachial plexus injury, chest wall scarring, and difficulty controlling the sagittal plane.

18. What is a traditional growing-rod construct?

A traditional growing-rod construct requires exposure of the spine at only the upper and lower ends of the spinal curve requiring treatment. Proximal and distal foundations are created using hook or screw fixation placed over two or three spinal levels. Limited fusions are performed at the proximal and distal foundation sites but spinal growth remains uninterrupted in the region between the foundations as fusion is not performed in this area. Proximal and distal rods are placed extraperiosteally to avoid spontaneous fusion and remain below the fascia (submuscular) to minimize implant prominence. The proximal and distal rods are linked by tandem or side-by-side rod connectors placed in the thoracolumbar region to complete the implant construct (Fig. 37.4A–C). Either unilateral or bilateral rod constructs may be used. Cross-connectors may be added to bilateral rod constructs. Open surgical construct lengthening procedures are performed at the site of the rod connectors at 6-month intervals until adequate spinal growth or thoracic development is achieved at which time the need for definitive spinal instrumentation and fusion is evaluated. Evidence suggests that a final fusion may not be necessary in asymptomatic patients in the absence of curve progression or implant failure following completion of lengthening treatment. Compared with unilateral growing-rod constructs, bilateral growing-rod constructs provide better deformity correction, increased spinal length, lower rates of anchor dislodgement, fewer rod failures, and obviate the need for postoperative bracing, but are more prominent. (1)

19. What are some advantages and disadvantages associated with use of traditional growing-rod constructs?

Single and dual traditional growing rods provide a useful surgical method for controlling progressive thoracic and lumbar spinal deformities without fusion in patients with EOS. However, complications associated with use of this technique remain an unsolved problem. (4) A major disadvantage of this technique is the need for planned multiple staged surgeries for implant lengthening as a 24% increase in complication risk has been reported with each successive procedure. Complications include wound infections, implant prominence, implant dislodgement or

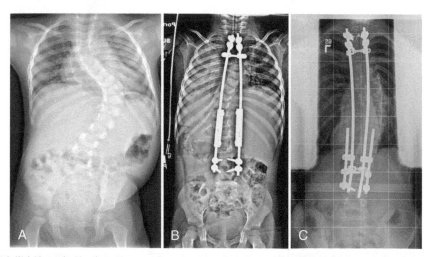

Fig. 37.4 (A) A 29-month-old patient with progressive early-onset scoliosis. Nonoperative treatment failed to control curve progression. (B) Postoperative radiographs following dual growing-rod instrumentation from T2 to L4. Four hooks and a cross connector were used for the upper foundation (T2–T4) and four screws (L3, L4) were used for the lower foundation. A tandem connector was used to connect the proximal and distal rod segments. (C) Example of dual growing-rod construct with overlapping rods and side-to-side connectors in a different patient. A, B: From Mundis GM Jr, Akbarnia BA. Special surgical techniques for the growing spine. In: Devlin VJ, editor. Spine Secrets Plus. 2nd ed. Philadelphia, PA: Mosby; 2012, Fig. 2. pp. 298–303. C: From Oetgen ME, Blakemore LC. Growing rods in early-onset scoliosis. Semin Spine Surg 2012;24:155–163, Fig. 1, p. 157.)

failure, neurologic complications, spinal alignment and balance problems, and spontaneous autofusion. It has been reported that following multiple lengthening procedures, the amount of spinal lengthening achieved per procedure decreases due to increasing spinal stiffness or autofusion and has been termed the "law of diminishing returns." (10) Another issue common to all types of growing-rod techniques is the need for rod exchange to accommodate growth that exceeds the length of the initial implant construct.

20. **What is a hybrid growing-rod construct?**
A hybrid growing-rod construct is a construct with a proximal foundation that achieves fixation through use of rib anchors and a distal foundation that utilizes fixation with screws or hooks. Benefits associated with use of proximal rib anchors include avoidance of exposure of the upper thoracic posterior spinal elements and need for spinal fusion at the proximal foundation site, decreased implant prominence, the opportunity for load-sharing over multiple rib attachment sites, and preservation of the structural integrity of the upper thoracic spine for future surgical instrumentation procedures. Risks associated with upper thoracic rib anchor points include the potential for upper extremity neurologic injury, an increased risk for hook pull out in patients with upper thoracic kyphosis, risk of pleural leak, and intercostal neurovascular injury.

21. **What is a magnetically controlled growing-rod system?**
Magnetically controlled growing-rod constructs are intended to reduce the number of planned open surgical lengthening procedures and thereby reduce associated medical, surgical, anesthetic, and psychologic comorbidities. The magnetically controlled growing rod is a titanium rod with a telescoping, magnetically distractable middle segment. Either a single or dual-rod construct may be used. Implantation is similar to placement of conventional growing-rod constructs (Fig. 37.5). Proximal implant foundation options include rib or spinal anchors and distal implant foundations consist of spinal anchors. Rods are inserted into the proximal and distal implant foundation leaving the spinal segments between the foundations unexposed to allow growth across these intervening spinal segments. The titanium telescoping rods contain a magnetic actuator that is lengthened by coupling with the magnet on an external remote controller to remotely lengthen the rods periodically in the clinic instead of performing an open surgical procedure (Fig. 37.6A,B). The only magnetically controlled rod currently available in the US is the MAGEC System (MAGnetic Expansion Control System, NuVasive, San Diego, CA). By 2016, magnetically controlled growing-rod constructs comprised over 80% of the new growth-friendly implants used in the US.

22. **What are some advantages and disadvantages of magnetically controlled growing-rod constructs?**
In addition to the potential to reduce the number of planned open surgical lengthening procedures and related comorbidities, other advantages of magnetically controlled growing-rod constructs include the ability to directly monitor the patient's neurologic status during outpatient rod distraction procedures. Disadvantages associated with magnetically controlled growing-rod constructs include the need for unplanned reoperations to treat proximal and distal anchor failures, implant prominence, inability to contour the thickened portions of the rod, mechanical failures of the implant, and the need for rod exchange to accommodate growth that exceeds the length of the initial implant construct.

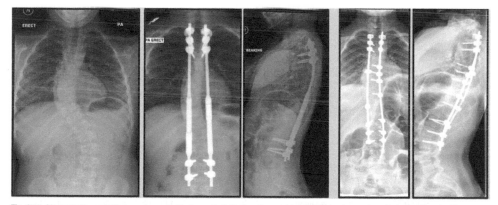

Fig. 37.5 Magnetically controlled growing rods. Radiograph *(left)* of an 8-year-old child with early-onset scoliosis. Treatment with magnetically controlled growing rods *(second and third images)* permitted consecutive lengthenings, which preserved spinal growth and delayed the definitive posterior spinal fusion *(fourth and fifth images)* for 3 years. (From Choudhury MZB, Tsirkos A, Marks DS. Early-onset scoliosis: Clinical presentation, assessment, and treatment options. Orthop Trauma 2017;31:357–363, Fig. 2, p. 362.)

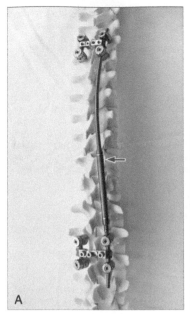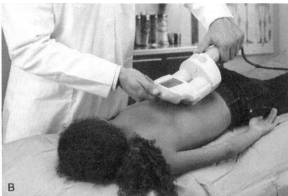

Fig. 37.6 (A) A single magnetically controlled growing rod depicted on a spine model. The enlarged midportion of the rod contains the magnetically controlled distraction mechanism *(red arrow)*. (B) Lengthening of the magnetically controlled growing rod in the office. (A: From Cheung KM, Cheung KP, Samartzis D, et al. Magnetically controlled growing rods for severe spinal curvature in young children: A prospective case series. Lancet 2012;379:1967–1974, Fig. 1, p. 1968. B: Courtesy Behrooz A. Akbarnia, MD, San Diego, CA.)

23. What is the Shilla Growth Guidance System and procedure?

The Shilla procedure is intended to permit curve control and preservation of spinal growth while minimizing the need for subsequent planned rod lengthening procedures. In a Shilla procedure, the apical levels of the deformity are exposed, realigned, and fused, while the proximal and distal spinal levels are left unfused to allow for future spinal growth. The apical levels are instrumented using fixed screws that lock to the rods. The areas above and below the apex are instrumented using specialized pedicle screws, which are placed using a transmuscular extraperiosteal technique and capture the rods without locking to the rods. The specialized screws are able to slide along the two parallel rods that span the spinal curvature and extend at least 2 cm above and below the most proximal and distal screws to accommodate spinal growth (Fig. 37.7A–C). Depending on the magnitude and flexibility of the spinal deformity, correction of the apical region may be performed using a posterior approach with or without osteotomies, or in combination with anterior disc excisions.

24. What are some advantages and disadvantages of a Shilla procedure compared to traditional growing-rod constructs?

An advantage of a Shilla procedure is greater initial correction in Cobb angle compared with traditional growing-rod constructs. However, over the entire course of treatment, patients treated with serial lengthening procedures using traditional growing rods experience greater improvement in Cobb angle and greater increase in T1–S1 length compared with patients treated with a Shilla procedure. Implant complication rates are similar between both procedure types. However, patients treated with Shilla undergo fewer surgical procedures compared with patients treated with traditional growing-rod constructs. (3)

25. What is the role of compression-based correction systems for treatment of EOS?

The role of compression-based implant systems for treatment of EOS has not been clearly defined. Compression-based implants are intended to correct scoliosis by modulating the growth of the vertebral bodies and thereby avoid the need for spinal fusion. This treatment strategy is based on the Heuter-Volkmann principle, which proposes that application of mechanical compression across a growth plate inhibits growth, while reduction of loading accelerates growth. The most commonly utilized technique at present involves placement of vertebral body screws on the convex side of a spinal curve, which are attached to a flexible tether that is tensioned to provide partial curve correction. Additional spontaneous curve correction is observed in patients with remaining growth potential. Compression-based implants have been used primarily in the adolescent idiopathic scoliosis population and limited data regarding use of this technique are currently available for the EOS population.

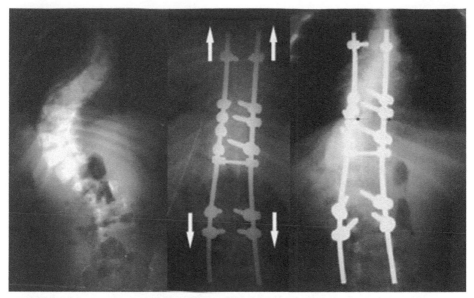

Fig. 37.7 Shilla technique. (A) Preoperative image of a patient with early-onset scoliosis. (B) Rods are secured to the deformity apex, which is fused and instrumented with fixed screws. The vertebrae at the boundaries of the scoliosis remain unfused and special screwheads that are able to slide freely along the rod guide spinal growth *(arrows)*. (C) Note the movement of the proximal and distal sliding screws relative to the rods. (From Cunin V. Early-onset scoliosis: Current treatment. Orthop Traum Sur Res 2015; 101:109–118, Fig. 17, p. 115.)

Table 37.2 Complications Classification System for Growing Spine Surgery.

GRADE	DEVICE-RELATED	DISEASE-RELATED
I	Does not require unplanned surgery	Outpatient medical management only
II		Inpatient medical management
IIA	Requires 1 unplanned surgery	
IIB	Requires multiple unplanned surgeries	
III	Requires abandoning growth-friendly strategy	Requires abandoning growth-friendly strategy
IV	Death	Death

From Smith JT, Johnston C, Skaggs D, et al. A new classification system to report complications in growing spine surgery; A multicenter consensus study. J Pediatr Orthop 2015;35:798–803.

Concerns regarding use of this technique in EOS patients include the potential for overcorrection and morbidity associated with a transthoracic anterior surgical approach.

26. **How are complications associated with growth-friendly spinal implants classified?**
A system for classification of complications related to the treatment of EOS using growth-friendly implants, including traditional growing rods, hybrid growing rods, and VEPTR was developed by Smith and colleagues. (13) A complication is reported as device related or disease related, and graded for severity based on how the complication impacted the overall treatment plan for the patient (Table 37.2). Device-specific complications include those directly related to the device, its anchor sites, or the surgical incisions required for placement of the device. Disease-specific complications include those related to repetitive surgical procedures that are not device related such as pneumonia or sepsis. Reoperations following the index surgical procedure are classified as a planned or unplanned return to the operating room. With introduction of additional instrumentation strategies such as Shilla and magnetically controlled growing-rod constructs directed toward reduction of planned procedures that require return to the operating room, comparison of adverse events across different growth-friendly device types based on **unplanned returns** to the **operating room** (UPROR) has been recommended. (2) Identification of UPROR and related anesthetic exposure is relevant due to concerns regarding the effects of anesthetics on the developing brain.

KEY POINTS

1. Multilevel spinal fusion limits future increase in spinal height and restricts development of the thoracic cage and lung parenchyma in patients with early-onset scoliosis.
2. Thoracic insufficiency syndrome is defined as the inability of the thorax to support normal respiration or lung growth.
3. Growth-friendly surgical treatment options for early-onset scoliosis include the vertical expandable prosthetic titanium rib (VEPTR), traditional and hybrid growing rods, magnetically controlled growing rods, Shilla and other guided-growth implant systems.

Websites
1. Early-Onset Scoliosis Consensus Statement: https://www.srs.org/about-srs/quality-and-safety/position-statements/early-onset-scoliosis-consensus-statement
2. Concerns regarding early childhood exposure to anesthetic agents: https://www.srs.org/about-srs/quality-and-safety/position-statements/response-to-fda-med-watch

---

BIBLIOGRAPHY

1. Akbarnia, B. A., Marks, D. S., Boachie-Adjei, O., Thompson, A. G., & Asher, M. A. (2005). Dual growing rod technique for the treatment of progressive early-onset scoliosis: A multicenter study. *Spine, 30,* 46–57.
2. Anari, J. B., Flynn, J. M., & Cahill, P. J. (2019). Unplanned return to OR (UPROR) for children with early-onset scoliosis (EOS): A comprehensive evaluation of all diagnoses and instrumentation strategies. *Spine Deformity,* 1–7.
3. Andras, L. M., Joiner, E. R., McCarthy, R. E., McCullough, L., Luhmann, S. J., Sponseller, P. D., et al. (2015). Growing rods versus Shilla growth guidance: Better Cobb angle correction and T1-S1 length increase but more surgeries. *Spine Deformity, 3,* 246–252.
4. Bess, S., Akbarnia, B. A., Thompson, G. H., Sponseller, P., Skaggs, D., Shah, S., et al. (2008). Complications in 910 growing rod surgeries: Use of dual rods and submuscular placement of rods decreases complications. *Spine Journal, 8,* 13–14.
5. Campbell, R. M., Jr., Smith, M. D., Mayes, T. C., Mangos, J. A., Willey-Courand, D. B., Kose, N., et al. (2003). The characteristics of thoracic insufficiency syndrome associated with fused ribs and congenital scoliosis. *Journal of Bone and Joint Surgery, 85,* 399–408.
6. Campbell, R. M. Jr., & Smith, M. D. (2007). Thoracic insufficiency syndrome and exotic scoliosis. *Journal of Bone and Joint Surgery, 89,* 108–122.
7. Canavese, F., & Dimeglio, A. (2013). Normal and abnormal spine and thoracic cage development. *World Journal of Orthopedics, 4,* 167–174.
8. Karol, L. A. (2011). Early definitive spinal fusion in young children: What we have learned. *Clinical Orthopaedics and Related Research, 469,* 1323–1329.
9. Pehrsson, K., Larsson, S., Oden, A., & Nachemson, A. (1992). Long-term follow-up of patients with untreated scoliosis. A study of mortality, causes of death, and symptoms. *Spine, 17,* 1091–1096.
10. Sankar, W. N., Skaggs, D. L., Yazici, M., Johnston, C. E., Shah, S. A., Javidan, P., et al. (2011). Lengthening of dual growing rods and the law of diminishing returns. *Spine, 36,* 806–809.
11. Skaggs, D. L., Akbarnia, B. A., Flynn, J. M., Myung, K. S., Sponseller, P. D., Vitale, M. G., et al. (2014). A classification of growth friendly spine implants. *Journal of Pediatric Orthopedics, 34,* 260–274.
12. Skaggs, D. L., Guillaume, T., El-Hawary, R., Emans, J. B., Mendelow, J. M., & Smith, J. W. T. (2015). Early onset scoliosis consensus statement, SRS growing spine committee, 2015. *Spine Deformity, 3,* 107.
13. Smith, J. T., Johnston, C., Skaggs, D., Flynn, J., & Vitale, M. (2015). A new classification system to report complications in growing spine surgery: A multicenter consensus study. *Journal of Pediatric Orthopedics, 35,* 798–803.
14. Williams, B. A., Matsumoto, H., McCalla, D. J., Akbarnia, B. A., Blakemore, L. C., Betz, R. R., et al. (2014). Development and initial validation of the Classification of Early-Onset Scoliosis (C-EOS). *Journal of Bone and Joint Surgery American Volume, 96,* 1359–1367.

IDIOPATHIC SCOLIOSIS

Vincent J. Devlin, MD

CHAPTER 38

1. What is idiopathic scoliosis?
Idiopathic scoliosis is the most common type of scoliosis. At present it is uncertain whether this deformity represents a single disease entity or reflects a similar clinical expression of several different disease states. Idiopathic scoliosis is defined as a spinal deformity characterized by lateral bending and fixed rotation of the spine in the absence of a known cause. The criterion for diagnosis of scoliosis is a coronal plane spinal curvature of 10° or more as measured by the Cobb method. Curves less than 10° are referred to as *spinal asymmetry*. Traditionally, idiopathic scoliosis has been classified according to age at onset as *infantile* (birth–3 years), *juvenile* (4–10 years), and *adolescent* (>10 years) subtypes. Current terminology classifies idiopathic scoliosis that is present before 10 years of age as *early-onset* scoliosis *(EOS)* and idiopathic scoliosis that develops after 10 years of age as *late-onset scoliosis*.

2. What causes idiopathic scoliosis?
The exact cause of idiopathic scoliosis has not been established and remains the focus of ongoing research. A significant challenge associated with this research is distinguishing whether observed changes are secondary to spinal deformity or whether they are the cause of the deformity. Areas under investigation include:
- **Genetic factors:** Genome-wide association studies have identified single-nucleotide polymorphisms, or genetic variations, associated with adolescent idiopathic scoliosis.
- **Neuromuscular factors:** Areas of investigation have included central nervous system asymmetry, vestibular and proprioceptive dysfunction, and impaired paravertebral muscle strength.
- **Hormonal and metabolic influences:** Research has investigated relationships between melatonin, somatomedin, osteopenia, and idiopathic scoliosis.
- **Skeletal growth disturbances:** Anterior spinal column overgrowth and differential growth between the right and left sides of the spinal column have been considered as potential etiologies.
- **Environmental and lifestyle influences:** Diet and calcium and vitamin D intake have been the subject of investigations.

EARLY-ONSET IDIOPATHIC SCOLIOSIS

3. List characteristic features of infantile idiopathic scoliosis.
- More common in Europe than in the United States (<1% of cases in United States)
- Male predominance (vs. adolescent idiopathic scoliosis, which is more common in females)
- Left thoracic curve pattern involving the mid to lower thoracic region is most common (vs. adolescent idiopathic scoliosis, in which right-sided thoracic curves are typical)
- Association with plagiocephaly, developmental delay, congenital heart disease, developmental hip dysplasia, and neural axis abnormalities
- Two types have been identified: a resolving type and a progressive type

4. How are resolving and progressive infantile curve types distinguished?
Resolving and progressive curve types are distinguished by analyzing the relationship between the apical vertebra of the thoracic curve and the adjacent ribs on an anteroposterior (AP) radiograph in order to determine **the rib-vertebral angle difference (RVAD) and rib phase.**
The **RVAD** measures the amount of rotation at the apex vertebra and has prognostic value regarding curve progression in patients with idiopathic EOS. This angle is determined by a line perpendicular to the endplate of the apical vertebra and a line drawn through the center of the adjacent rib on both the concave and convex side of the apical vertebra (Fig. 38.1). The RVAD equals the difference between the convex and concave angles. If the difference is greater than 20°, curve progression is likely.
The **rib phase** is determined by ascertaining whether the head of the convex rib overlaps the apical vertebral body and is used as an adjunctive measurement. If there is no overlap (phase 1), the RVAD is calculated to determine the likelihood of progression. If there is overlap (phase 2), the risk of progression is high.

5. Describe the management of patients with infantile idiopathic scoliosis.
Resolving curves are observed with serial physical examinations and radiographic monitoring. Sleeping in the prone position is recommended because supine positioning has been associated with infantile curves by some investigators. **Progressive curves** are treated with serial casting followed by orthotic treatment. Curves that

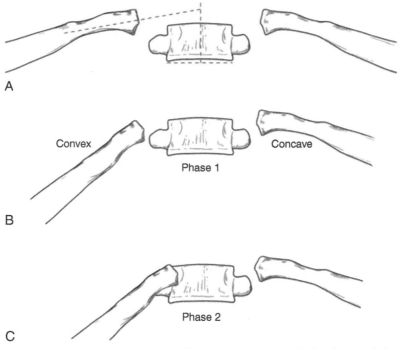

Fig. 38.1 The rib-vertebral angle difference and rib phase. (A) The rib-vertebral angle is determined by a line perpendicular to the endplate of the apical vertebra and a line drawn along the center of the rib. (B) Phase 1, the convex rib does not overlap the vertebral body. (C) Phase 2, the convex rib overlaps the vertebral body. (From Errico TJ, Lonner BS, Moulton AW. Surgical Management of Spinal Deformities. Philadelphia, PA: Saunders; 2009, p. 90.)

continue to progress despite orthotic treatment require surgical treatment with posterior growth-friendly instrumentation techniques such as growing rods, the Shilla technique, or the vertical expandable prosthetic titanium rib (VEPTR). These posterior nonfusion instrumentation strategies attempt to control spinal deformity and delay the need for definitive fusion until the child has achieved additional growth. Posterior spinal fusion is not recommended due to adverse impact on the developing lungs and thoracic cage and lack of effectiveness in controlling spinal deformity in this population.

6. What are the characteristic features of juvenile idiopathic scoliosis?
   Juvenile idiopathic scoliosis represents a gradual transition from the characteristics of infantile idiopathic scoliosis to those of adolescent idiopathic scoliosis. (3) Characteristic features include:
   - Less common than adolescent idiopathic scoliosis (12%–21% of all patients with pediatric idiopathic scoliosis)
   - Increasing female predominance is noted with increasing age (female-to-male ratio is 1:1 from 4 to 6 years and increases to 8–10:1 from 6 to 10 years)
   - Most common curve patterns are right thoracic and double major curve types
   - Approximately 70% of curves progress and require some form of treatment (bracing or surgery)
   - Magnetic resonance imaging (MRI) of the entire spine to visualize from the craniocervical junction to the sacrum is appropriate (also in infantile idiopathic scoliosis) because spinal deformity may be the only clue regarding the presence of a coexistent neural axis abnormality, which may potentially require treatment (e.g., syrinx, Arnold-Chiari malformation, tethered spinal cord)

7. Describe the management of patients with juvenile idiopathic scoliosis.
   Curves less than 20°–25° are observed. Treatment is initiated for curves in the 25°–50° range. Treatment most commonly consists of bracing, although a period of casting may be considered for younger patients or patients with rigid curves. Surgical treatment is considered when curve magnitude exceeds 50°–60°. Surgical decision-making is complex in this heterogeneous population. Growth-friendly treatment strategies such as posterior growing-rod techniques, the Shilla technique, or VEPTR are options that may be used to control deformity and delay spinal fusion to allow for additional growth. While these posterior nonfusion strategies are associated with

advantages compared with early spinal fusion, their disadvantages include the need for multiple operations, device-related complications, wound infections, iatrogenic radiation exposure, and repetitive exposure to anesthesia. Another treatment option for curves less than 65° in older juvenile patients is anterior vertebral body tethering. This involves placement of screws into the vertebral bodies on the convexity of a curve through a thoracoscopic or thoracotomy approach. The screws are connected to a flexible polymer cord, which is tensioned to provide initial curve correction and allows for additional curve correction with continued growth. Patients with severe curves in excess of 80° are considered for treatment with a period of halo-gravity traction ranging from 2 to 6 weeks prior to definitive anterior and/or posterior procedures. Definitive surgical procedures most commonly consist of combined anterior and posterior fusion and attempts are made to defer such procedures until patients approach age 10. Isolated posterior fusions are at risk of the crankshaft phenomenon due to persistent anterior spinal growth in the presence of a posterior fusion, which may lead to recurrence of the spinal deformity.

LATE-ONSET OR ADOLESCENT IDIOPATHIC SCOLIOSIS

8. List characteristic features of adolescent idiopathic scoliosis.
   - Most common type of scoliosis in children and comprises approximately 80% of all pediatric patients with idiopathic scoliosis (prevalence is 3% in the general population)
   - Few adolescent patients (0.3%) develop curves requiring treatment
   - Female predominance, which increases substantially for larger curves requiring treatment
   - Thoracic curve patterns are generally convex to the right (atypical curve patterns are an indication for MRI)
   - Idiopathic scoliosis in adolescence is not typically associated with severe pain

9. Describe the initial evaluation for a patient referred for assessment for adolescent idiopathic scoliosis.
   Patient history
   - Inquire about when and how the deformity was recognized.
   - Inquire regarding history of pain, numbness, weakness, or bowel or bladder symptoms.
   - Discuss with family regarding patient's maturity (include menstrual history in females), growth pattern, birth and developmental history, and family history of scoliosis.
   Physical examination
   - Height and weight assessment.
   - Observation. Assess for shoulder, thorax, or waist asymmetry. Note any cutaneous lesions including café au lait spots, abnormal hair patches, or skin dimpling.
   - Adams forward bend test. The right and left sides of the trunk should be symmetrical. Presence of a thoracic or lumbar prominence suggests scoliosis. Use a scoliometer or digital assessment application on a smartphone to quantitate asymmetry by measuring the apical trunk rotation (ATR). Values ≥7° are considered abnormal.
   - Neurologic evaluation. Assess motor strength, deep tendon reflexes, abdominal reflexes (abnormalities may indicate intraspinal pathology such as syringomyelia), plantar reflexes, clonus testing, cranial nerve function, and balance.
   - Assess ligamentous laxity as a screen for connective tissue disorders.
   - Upper and lower extremity assessment. Evaluate gait and leg lengths.
   Imaging assessment
   - A standing posteroanterior (PA) and lateral full length spinal radiographs or low-dose biplanar slot scan images are obtained.
   - Side-bending radiographs are not required for a routine initial patient evaluation and are reserved for presurgical planning.
   - Standard hand bone age films are obtained to assess skeletal maturity.
   - MRI is not required in the absence of abnormal physical examination findings, atypical radiographic findings, or a history of atypical pain.

10. What radiographic parameters are important to assess when evaluating scoliosis on a full-length PA spinal radiograph?
    Important radiographic parameters to assess in relation to scoliosis (Fig. 38.2A, B) include:
    - **End vertebra:** The upper and lower vertebrae that tilt maximally into the concavity of the curve are termed the end vertebrae. The cephalad end vertebra is the first vertebra in the cephalad direction from the curve apex whose superior endplate is tilted maximally toward the concavity of the curve. The caudad end vertebra is the first vertebra in the caudad direction from the curve apex whose inferior endplate is tilted maximally toward the concavity of the curve.
    - **Apical vertebra:** The apical vertebra is the central vertebra within a curve. It is typically the least tilted, most rotated, and most horizontally displaced vertebra from the central sacral vertical line.

ADOLESCENT IDIOPATHIC SCOLIOSIS

Coronal Cobb measurement technique
Proximal thoracic (PT), main thoracic (MT), and
thoracolumbar/lumbar (TL/L) curves

ADOLESCENT IDIOPATHIC SCOLIOSIS
End, neutral, and stable vertebrae

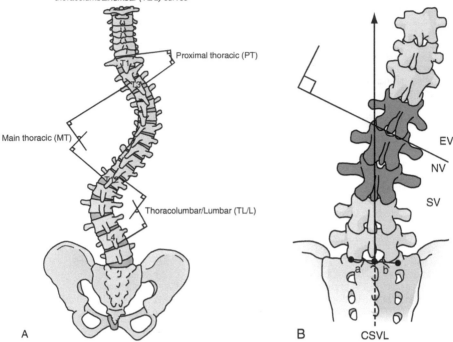

A

B   CSVL

Fig. 38.2 (A) Measurement of the Cobb angle to determine the coronal magnitude of the curve. The two most tilted vertebrae are identified, and a line is drawn marking the angle of the endplate. The angle between the endplates is then measured. To facilitate measurement of the angle, it is also possible to drop a perpendicular line from the endplate and measure the angle subtended by the perpendiculars. (B) End, neutral, and stable vertebrae. The end vertebrae *(EV)* are the most tilted vertebrae, which are selected for measurement of the Cobb angle. The neutral vertebra *(NV)* is the most cephalad vertebral body below the end vertebra with no rotation (pedicles appear symmetrical). The stable vertebra *(SV)* is the most cephalad vertebral body below the end vertebra, which is bisected by the central sacral vertebral line *(CSVL)*. (From Polly DW, Jones KE, Larson AN. Pediatric and adult scoliosis. In: Ellenbogen RG, Sekhar LN, Kitchen ND, et al., editors. Principles of Neurological Surgery. 4th ed. Philadephia, PA: Elsevier; 2018, pp. 561–572, Fig. 37.1, p. 562; Fig. 37.7, p. 567.)

- **Curve location:** The curve location is defined by its apex which may be a vertebral body or an intervertebral disc.

Curve	Apex
Cervicothoracic	C7 or T1
Thoracic	Between T2 and T11–T12 disc
Thoracolumbar	T12 or L1
Lumbar	Between L1–L2 disc and L4
Lumbosacral	L5 or S1

- **Curve direction:** Curve direction is determined by the side of the convexity. Curves convex toward the right are termed right curves, while curves convex to the left are termed left curves.
- **Curve magnitude:** The Cobb technique is used to determine curve magnitude. Perpendicular lines are drawn in relation to reference lines along the superior endplate of the upper end vertebra and along the inferior endplate of the lower end vertebra. The angle created by the intersection of the two perpendicular lines is termed the Cobb angle and defines the magnitude of the curve.
- **Central sacral vertical line (CSVL):** A vertical line on a coronal radiograph that passes through the center of the sacrum.

- **Neutral vertebra:** A vertebra without axial rotation with reference to the most cephalad and caudad vertebra that are not rotated within a curve. Rotation is assessed based on the radiographic appearance of the vertebral pedicle shadow in reference to the lateral margins of the vertebral body (Nash-Moe classification). In a neutrally rotated vertebra the pedicle shadows will be equidistant from the lateral vertebral margins.
- **Stable vertebra:** The vertebra bisected by the CSVL.

11. Define nonstructural curve, structural curve, major curve, minor curve, fractional curve, and full curve.
   Patients typically present with a combination of fixed and flexible spinal deformities. Side-bending radiographs are used to assess the flexibility of curves that comprise a spinal deformity.
   - **Nonstructural curves:** Curves that correct completely when the patient bends toward the convexity of the curve are termed *nonstructural curves*. Nonstructural curves permit the shoulders and pelvis to remain level to the ground and permit the head to remain centered in the midline above the pelvis. For this reason, nonstructural curves are also referred to as compensatory curves. Over time, compensatory curves may develop structural characteristics.
   - **Structural curves:** Curves that do not correct completely on side-bending radiographs are termed *structural curves*.
   - **Major curve:** The *major curve* is the curve with the largest Cobb measurement and is always a structural curve.
   - **Minor curve:** Any curves that do not have the largest Cobb measurement are termed *minor curves* and may be either structural or nonstructural, depending on classification criteria.
   - **Fractional curve:** Curves that have one end vertebra parallel to the ground are termed *fractional curves*. Full curves and fractional curves are distinguished by assessing the angular displacement of the end vertebra of the curve.
   - **Full curves:** Curves in which both end vertebrae are tilted from the horizontal are termed *full curves*.

12. What classification system is most commonly used to describe curves and guide treatment for patients with adolescent idiopathic scoliosis?
   The **Lenke classification** is most commonly used to describe adolescent idiopathic curves and guide treatment. (2, 5) Classification is based on assessment of PA, lateral, and side-bending radiographs. Six curve types and their prevalences are:
   - Main thoracic (51%)
   - Double thoracic (20%)
   - Double major (11%)
   - Triple major (3%)
   - Primary thoracolumbar or lumbar (12%)
   - Primary thoracolumbar or lumbar with a secondary thoracic curve (3%)
        The **basic steps** in curve classification include:
   - **Determine the curve type:** Measure all curves. Identify the major curve. Determine whether the minor curves are structural or nonstructural (Fig. 38.3).
   - **Determine the lumbar spine modifier:** The six main curve types are subclassified as A, B, or C based on relationship of the CSVL to the lumbar spine.
   - **Determine the thoracic sagittal modifier:** "–", "N", or "+" is determined on, the T5–T12 sagittal Cobb angle.
        This **triad** of radiographic information (curve type + lumbar modifier + sagittal modifier) is used to determine the *curve classification* (e.g., 1B+).

13. What are the risk factors for curve progression in skeletally immature patients with adolescent idiopathic scoliosis?
   - Skeletal immaturity and potential for future growth
   - Curve magnitude at the time of diagnosis
   - Curve pattern (double curves progress more frequently than single curves; single thoracic curves progress more frequently than single lumbar curves)
   - Female sex (curves in females are more likely to progress than curves in males)

14. How is skeletal maturity assessed in the adolescent idiopathic scoliosis patient?
   Skeletal maturity status reflects the patient's future growth potential and correlates with the risk of curve progression. Growth during puberty occurs in two stages: an accelerating (ascending) phase followed by peak growth velocity and decelerating (descending) phase (Fig. 38.4). Skeletal maturity is assessed based on a combination of clinical and radiographic parameters. Clinical assessments include age at presentation, Tanner staging, age of menarche, and biometric measurements, including height and weight. Radiographic markers utilized include Risser stage, triradiate physeal closure status, peak height velocity, and the extent of ossification of physes of the bones of the hand, wrist, olecranon, proximal humerus, and calcaneus. (6, 7, 8)

Curve Type				
Type	Proximal Thoracic	Main Thoracic	Thoracolumbar/ Lumbar	Curve Type
1	Non-Structural	Structural (major*)	Non-Structural	Main Thoracic (MT)
2	Structural	Structural (major*)	Non-Structural	Double Thoracic (DT)
3	Non-Structural	Structural (major*)	Structural	Double Major (DM)
4	Structural	Structural (major*)	Structural	Triple Major (TM)
5	Non-Structural	Non-Structural	Structural (major*)	Thoracolumbar/Lumbar (TL/L)
6	Non-Structural	Structural	Structural (major*)	Thoracolumbar/Lumbar-Main Thoracic (TL/L - MT) Lumbar Curve>Thoracic by ≥5°

*Major = Largest Cobb Measurement, always structural
Minor = All other curves with structural criteria applied

STRUCTURAL CRITERIA
(Minor Curves)

Proximal Thoracic: - Side Bending Cobb ≥ 25°
- T2–T5 Kyphosis ≥+20°

Main Thoracic: - Side Bending Cobb ≥ 25°
- T10–L2 Kyphosis ≥20°

Thoracolumbar/Lumbar: - Side Bending Cobb ≥ 25°
- T10–L2 Kyphosis ≥+20°

LOCATION OF APEX
(SRS definition)

CURVE	APEX
THORACIC	T2–T11–12 DISC
THORACOLUMBAR	T12–L1
LUMBAR	L1–L2 DISC–L4

Modifiers				
Lumbar Spine Modifier	CSVL to Lumbar Apex		Thoracic Sagittal Profile T5 - T12	
A	CSVL Between Pedicles		- (Hypo)	< 10°
B	CSVL Touches Apical Body(ies)		N (Normal)	10° - 40°
C	CSVL Completely Medial	A B C	+ (Hyper)	> 40°

Curve Types (1- 6) + Lumbar Spine Modifier (A, B, or C) + Thoracic Sagittal Modifier (-, N, or +)
Classification (e.g. 1B+):_____

Fig. 38.3 Lenke classification system for idiopathic scoliosis. (From Hurley ME, Devlin VJ. Idiopathic scoliosis. In: Fitzgerald RH, Kaufer H, Malkani AL, editors. Orthopaedics. St. Louis: Mosby; 2000, Fig. 8, p. 1347.)

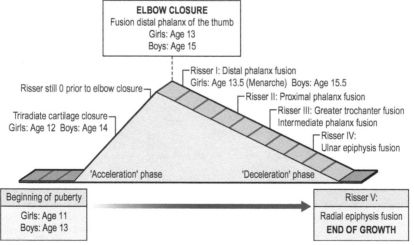

ELBOW CLOSURE
Fusion distal phalanx of the thumb
Girls: Age 13
Boys: Age 15

Risser still 0 prior to elbow closure

Triradiate cartilage closure
Girls: Age 12 Boys: Age 14

Risser I: Distal phalanx fusion
Girls: Age 13.5 (Menarche) Boys: Age 15.5

Risser II: Proximal phalanx fusion

Risser III: Greater trochanter fusion
Intermediate phalanx fusion

Risser IV:
Ulnar epiphysis fusion

'Acceleration' phase   'Deceleration' phase

Beginning of puberty
Girls: Age 11
Boys: Age 13

Risser V:
Radial epiphysis fusion
END OF GROWTH

Fig. 38.4 Pubertal growth diagram. Growth during puberty occurs in two stages: an acceleration phase and a deceleration phase. The triradiate cartilage closes during the midportion of the acceleration phase while the iliac apophysis remains unossified (Risser 0). Peak height velocity occurs after this time during the acceleration phase. The onset of menarche is variable and occurs after closure of the olecranon apophysis, most commonly around the time of Risser stage 1. The deceleration phase continues until skeletal maturity is reached. (From Innocenti M, Baldrighi C. Growth considerations in pediatric upper extremity trauma and reconstruction. In: Chang J, Neligan PC, editors. Plastic Surgery, vol 6. Hand and Upper Extremity. 4th ed. Philadephia, PA: Elsevier; 2018, pp. 670–687, Fig. 30.3, p. 672.)

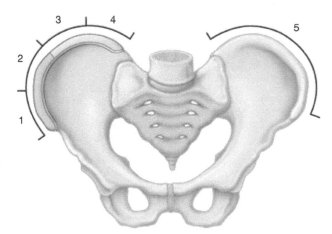

Fig. 38.5 The Risser sign proceeds from grade 0 (no ossification) to grade 4 (all four quadrants show ossification of the iliac apophysis). When the ossified apophysis has fused completely to the ilium (Risser grade 5), the patient is skeletally mature. (From Richards SB, Sucato DJ, Johnston CE. Scoliosis. In: Herring JA, editor. Tachdjian's Pediatric Orthopaedics. 5th ed. Saunders; 2013, Fig. 12.2, p. 208.)

Risser stage: The Risser staging system describes the ossification of the iliac apophysis in terms of six stages (Risser stages 0–5). Ossification begins at the anterior superior iliac spine and progresses posteromedially to the posterior superior iliac spine. In North America, the iliac crest is divided into quarters to serve as a reference, while the European method divides this region into thirds. Risser stage 0 corresponds to the acceleration phase of pubertal growth (Fig. 38.5).

Risser Staging System

Grade 0	Iliac apophysis is not visible due to lack of ossification
Grade 1	1%–25% ossification of the iliac apophysis
Grade 2	26%–50% ossification of the iliac apophysis
Grade 3	51%–75% ossification of the iliac apophysis
Grade 4	76%–100% ossification of the iliac apophysis
Grade 5	Fusion of iliac apophysis to the ilium

Triradiate physeal closure: Closure of the triradiate cartilage of the pelvis occurs at approximately the midpoint of the ascending phase of pubertal growth and provides an additional marker of skeletal maturity.

Peak height velocity: Maximal skeletal growth during the pubertal growth spurt occurs on the ascending phase of pubertal growth and exceeds 8 cm/year. This measurement is determined from serial changes in patient height measurements over time and is not applicable to a patient seen for their initial visit. Risser stage 1 occurs approximately 6 months after peak height velocity.

Sanders Skeletal Maturity Stage (SSMS): Assessment is based on the progressive growth and subsequent fusion of the epiphyses of small long bones of the hand. Parameters evaluated include width, capping, and fusion of the epiphyses. An epiphysis is referred to as "covered" when it is as wide as the metaphysis. An epiphysis is referred to as "capped" when the epiphysis bends or curls over the metaphysis. Epiphyseal fusion is present when a space is absent between the epiphysis and diaphysis, although an epiphyseal scar (transverse line) may be present in a recently fused epiphysis. The Sanders stage is useful for stratification of patients during the ascending phase of pubertal growth as SSMS 1–5 occur during Risser Stage 0. Other notable relationships include: open triradiate cartilages during SSMS 1–4, triradiate cartilage closure during SSMS 5, Risser stage 1 or higher during SSMS 6, Risser stage 4 during SSMS 7, and Risser stage 5 during SSMS 8.

Sanders Skeletal Maturity Stages (SSMS)

1. Juvenile slow	Digital epiphyses are not covered
2. Preadolescent slow	All digital epiphyses are covered
3. Adolescent rapid (early)	Majority of digits are capped and 2nd–5th metacarpal epiphyses are wider than metaphyses
4. Adolescent rapid (late)	Any of the distal phalangeal physes are clearly beginning to close
5. Adolescent steady (early)	All distal phalangeal physes are closed while all remaining physes are open
6. Adolescent steady (late)	Proximal and middle phalangeal physes are closing
7. Early mature	Closure of all phalangeal physes while distal radius physis remains open
8. Mature	Distal radius physis is completely closed

15. **What is the risk of progression of untreated adolescent idiopathic scoliosis in skeletally immature patients?**
Understanding the natural history of untreated scoliosis is important to identify curves that will progress, especially those that are likely to progress into the range where surgery is considered. Early studies analyzed the effect of curve magnitude and Risser grade on curve progression. Lonstein and Carlson (4) noted that for curves <19°, the percentage of curves that progressed ≥10° during Risser stages 0–1 was 22% compared with 1.6% during Risser stages 2–4. For 20°–29° curves, the percentage of curves that progressed ≥5° during Risser stages 0–1 was 68% compared with 23% during Risser stages 2–4. Recent studies have shown that curves ≥30° in patients who are Risser stage 0 with open triradiate cartilages have a high likelihood of progression into the surgical range. Using the SSMS, patients with curves greater than 20°–25° who are SSMS 1–3 have the highest risk of progression into the range where surgery is considered.

16. **Which patients with adolescent idiopathic scoliosis are likely to experience progression of untreated curves in adulthood?**
Approximately two-thirds of adolescent idiopathic curves progress after skeletal maturity. Curves measuring less than 30° at skeletal maturity are unlikely to progress regardless of curve pattern. Curves measuring 30°–50° are likely to progress by an average of 10°–15° over the course of a normal lifetime. Curves measuring 50°–75° at maturity progress steadily, with thoracic curves progressing most rapidly at a rate slightly less than 1° per year. Progression of thoracolumbar and lumbar curves is affected by curve magnitude, apical vertebral rotation, and translatory shifts. For double curves, slightly greater progression is noted in the lumbar curve compared with the thoracic curve. (11)

17. **What are the consequences of untreated adolescent idiopathic scoliosis in adulthood?**
Natural history studies (9) of untreated adolescent idiopathic scoliosis patients provide a benchmark to guide treatment decision-making. Important knowledge gained from these studies includes:
   - **Mortality:** The mortality rate of untreated adult patients with adolescent idiopathic scoliosis is comparable to that of the general population. This contrasts with patients with untreated EOS who may develop severe curves, which can lead to cor pulmonale, right ventricular failure, and premature death.
   - **Impairment of respiratory function:** The risk of respiratory failure is well documented in patients with curves >100°. Patients with curves >80° or curves associated with a large degree of rotation are at risk for shortness of breath. One in five patients with thoracic curves >70° or sagittal plane hypokyphosis (T5–T12 <10°) have respiratory impairment based on pulmonary function tests prior to surgical treatment.
   - **Curve progression:** Curves measuring less than 30° at maturity are unlikely to progress, while curves that measure between 50° and 75° at skeletal maturity, especially thoracic curves, progress most.
   - **Back pain:** The prevalence of back pain in adult idiopathic scoliosis patients is increased compared with the general population but it is not related to curve size or location and is unlikely to interfere with ability to work or perform activities of daily living.
   - **Quality of life and function:** Ability to work and perform daily activities are similar for adult patients with moderate, untreated adolescent idiopathic scoliosis and peers.
   - **Self-image:** Spinal deformity and its negative effect on self-image remain a significant issue for many adult scoliosis patients. These issues are frequently among the reason adult patients seek treatment for idiopathic scoliosis.

18. **Describe the treatment options for patients with adolescent idiopathic scoliosis?**
The traditional treatment options for adolescent idiopathic scoliosis patients include observation, orthoses, and operations *(the three O's)*. Both operative and nonoperative treatments aim to keep curves below the threshold of 50° at skeletal maturity. There is strong interest in alternative treatments for nonsurgical treatments for scoliosis, most notably directed toward physical therapy and scoliosis-specific exercise programs, including the Schroth method from the Barcelona Scoliosis Physical Therapy School and the Scientific Exercise Approach to Scoliosis method from Italy. While such exercise programs have many positive effects for patients, evidence is currently evolving but remains limited regarding their ability to prevent curve progression or correct established curves over the long term.

19. **When is observation indicated for patients with adolescent idiopathic scoliosis?**
Observation is indicated to identify and document curve progression in patients with adolescent idiopathic scoliosis and thereby facilitate timely intervention if this becomes necessary. Patients with idiopathic curves less than 20° are observed. As there is inherent error in the radiographic measurement of spinal curvatures, a criterion for curve progression is most commonly defined as an increased Cobb angle of at least 5°–6°.

20. **What are the indications and contraindications for brace treatment for adolescent idiopathic scoliosis?**
Current indications for brace treatment for adolescent idiopathic scoliosis include curves with a magnitude between 25° and 45°; a Risser stage of 0, 1, or 2; and, for female patients, <1 year postmenarche at the time of

initiation of brace treatment. Contraindications include curves >45°, advanced skeletal maturity, hypokyphosis, and inability to emotionally cope with treatment.

21. **What types of braces are used for treatment of adolescent idiopathic scoliosis?**
    The types of orthoses described for use in adolescent idiopathic scoliosis include:
    - Thoracolumbosacral orthosis (TLSO; e.g., Boston brace, Rigo-Chêneau brace). These low-profile orthoses are the most commonly used types as they are reasonably well accepted by patients and effective for curves with an apex at T7 or below.
    - Bending brace (e.g., Charleston brace). This type of brace holds the patient is an acutely bent position in a direction opposite to the curve apex. It is worn only during sleep. It has been advocated as an alternative to full-time bracing regimens.
    - Dynamic flexible brace (e.g., SpineCor brace). Provides a nonrigid brace option.
    - Cervicothoracolumbosacral orthosis (CTLSO; e.g., Milwaukee brace). Rarely used today due to the cosmetic appearance of its suprastructure. However, for curves with an apex above T7, it remains efficacious.

22. **How effective is brace treatment for preventing progression of high-risk adolescent idiopathic scoliosis into the range where surgery is indicated?**
    A recent prospective trial, the Bracing in Adolescent Idiopathic Scoliosis Trial (BRAIST), evaluated the role of brace treatment versus observation in a population of skeletally immature patients (Risser grade 0, 1, 2) with 20°–40° curves. (10) Brace treatment success, defined as prevention of curve progression beyond the surgical threshold of 50°, was observed in 72% of the brace-treated cohort compared with 48% in the observation cohort. There was a significant association between the average hours of daily brace wear and the likelihood of a successful outcome. The number of patients needed to treat to prevent one operation for scoliosis was three. In a separate study, Karol analyzed the influence of Risser grade on the need for surgery in brace-treated adolescent idiopathic scoliosis patients and noted the highest rate of progression to ≥50° in patients at Risser stage 0 with open triradiate cartilages (Table 38.1).

23. **When is surgery indicated for adolescent idiopathic scoliosis?**
    Factors that enter into decision-making regarding surgery include the coronal Cobb angle, sagittal plane alignment, rotational deformity, natural history of the specific curve, skeletal maturity, and patient and family preferences. In general, for the skeletally immature adolescent patient, surgery is indicated for curves greater than 40°–45° that are progressive despite brace treatment. In the mature adolescent, surgery is considered for curves approaching or greater than 50°.

24. **What surgical treatment options exist when surgery is indicated for adolescent idiopathic scoliosis?**
    - Posterior spinal instrumentation and posterior fusion
    - Anterior spinal instrumentation and anterior fusion
    - Anterior spinal fusion combined with posterior spinal instrumentation and fusion
    - Growth-friendly treatment options such as anterior vertebral body tethering procedures or posterior minimally invasive deformity correction procedures

25. **Describe the key procedural steps involved in a posterior spinal instrumentation and fusion surgery performed for treatment of adolescent idiopathic scoliosis.**
    The posterior surgical approach is applicable to all idiopathic scoliosis curve types. Careful preoperative planning and selection of appropriate vertebral levels for inclusion in the instrumentation and fusion construct are critical for a successful procedural outcome. Patients are positioned prone on a specialized operating table with the

Table 38.1 Progression Rates for Brace Treated Adolescent Idiopathic Scoliosis Patients Based on Initial Curve Magnitude and Risser Sign.

	Curve Magnitude		
RISSER SIGN	25°–29°	30°–39°	40°–45°
Risser 0, Open Triradiate Cartilage	33.3.%	70%	100%
Risser 0, Closed Triradiate Cartilage	4%	42.5%	55.6%
Risser Stage 1	0%	0%	28.6%
Risser Stage 2	0%	0%	0%

Data from Karol LA, Virostek D, Felton K, et al. The effect of Risser stage on bracing outcome in adolescent idiopathic scoliosis. J Bone Joint Surg Am 2016;98:1253–1259.

abdomen hanging free to prevent venous congestion. Tranexamic acid is administered to aid in reduction of intra-operative blood loss. Multimodal intraoperative neurophysiologic monitoring, including transcranial electric motor potentials and somatosensory evoked potentials, is utilized throughout surgery to provide early detection of impending spinal cord injury. During the surgical procedure the posterior spinal structures are exposed, the facet joints are excised, and graft material is packed into the facet joints and over the decorticated posterior spinal elements. Posterior spinal instrumentation is used to realign and stabilize the spinal deformity. The most commonly utilized instrumentation construct consists of two parallel rods attached to multiple pedicle screw anchors. Alternatively, a hybrid instrumentation construct, which achieves fixation to the posterior spinal elements using a combination of hooks, wires or cables, and pedicle screws may be used.

26. **What are some basic principles that guide fusion level selection in patients with adolescent idiopathic scoliosis treated with posterior spinal instrumentation and fusion?**
The Lenke classification is used to guide selection of levels for fusion (Figs. 38.6 and 38.7). Some general principles for fusion-level selection include:
- The major curve and structural minor curves are fused. When T2–T5 or T10–L2 kyphosis is ≥20°, these curves are considered structural and should be included in the fusion.
- Nonstructural minor curves are permitted to correct spontaneously.
- Selection of the appropriate upper instrumented vertebra requires consideration of shoulder balance and flexibility of the upper curve on side-bending radiographs.
- Selection of the appropriate lower end vertebra is based on assessment of curve flexibility, bending radiographs, and the specific lumbar spine modifier defined by the Lenke classification, and is facilitated by accurate identification of the distal end, neutral, and stable vertebra.
- Avoid ending a fusion at the apex of a coronal or sagittal curve.

26. **Describe the key procedural steps involved in an anterior spinal instrumentation and fusion procedure for adolescent idiopathic scoliosis.**
Anterior spinal instrumentation and fusion procedures are most commonly indicated for single thoracic, thoracolumbar, or lumbar curve types. The convex side of the curve is surgically exposed. The thoracic spine is approached via an open thoracotomy or minimally invasive thoracoscopic approach. The thoracolumbar and lumbar spine is approached via an open thoracophrenolumbotomy or a lateral retroperitoneal abdominal approach. The discs, annulus, and cartilaginous vertebral endplates are excised over the levels undergoing instrumentation and

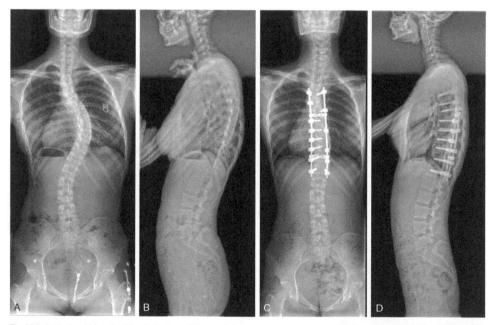

Fig. 38.6 A 15-year old female with a Lenke type 1AN curve that measured 51° preoperatively. (A) Preoperative posteroanterior (PA) radiograph. (B) Preoperative lateral radiograph. The thoracic curve was corrected to 23° with posterior instrumentation and fusion. (C) Postoperative PA radiograph. (D) Postoperative lateral radiograph. (From Yan H, Jiang D, Xu L, et al. Does the full power-assisted technique used in pedical screw placemen affect the safety and efficacy of adolescent idiopathic scoliosis surgery? World Neurosurg 2018;116: 79–85, Fig. 2, p. 81.)

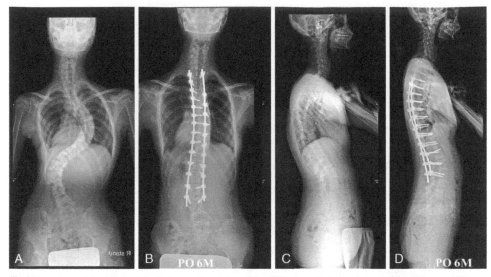

Fig. 38.7 Adolescent idiopathic scoliosis. (A) Preoperative posteroanterior (PA) radiograph shows a 93° Lenke type 4CN curve. (B) PA radiograph 6 months postoperatively. (C) Preoperative lateral radiograph. (D) Postoperative lateral radiograph. (From Hyun SJ, Han S, Kim KJ, et al. Adolescent idiopathic scoliosis surgery by a neurosurgeon: Learning curve for neurosurgeons. World Neurosurg 2018; 110:129–134, Fig. 4, p. 132.)

fusion. The disc spaces are packed with nonstructural bone graft. Structural spacers are often implanted in the disc spaces, especially at the lower end of the construct and in the lumbar region. This structural spacer may be a structural allograft or a synthetic intervertebral body fusion device. Vertebral body screws are placed to engage the opposite vertebral cortex and achieve bicortical fixation. The screws are subsequently linked to rod(s), and corrective forces are applied to the spine. Single- or double-rod systems may be used, depending on a variety of factors, including body habitus and curve location. Minimally invasive approaches utilizing thoracoscopic instrumentation and fusion have been documented to decrease approach-related morbidity in select cases.

27. When are combined anterior and posterior spinal procedures indicated for adolescent idiopathic scoliosis?

Combined anterior and posterior spinal procedures for adolescent idiopathic scoliosis are rarely required for uncomplicated adolescent idiopathic scoliosis. With the use of modern segmental instrumentation, including all pedicle screw constructs and direct vertebral rotation techniques in combination with Smith-Petersen osteotomies, Ponte osteotomies, or a posterior vertebral column resection procedure, most severe curves can be treated with a single-stage posterior approach. Circumstances where combined anterior and posterior procedures are occasionally considered include:
- Extremely large stiff curves (e.g., >100° depending on curve flexibility and location)
- To address coexistent rigid sagittal plane deformities (e.g., excessive thoracic lordosis, hyperkyphosis)
- Revision procedures following unsuccessful prior scoliosis surgery

28. What is the current role of thoracoplasty in the treatment of adolescent idiopathic scoliosis?

Thoracoplasty is a procedure that may be performed in conjunction with a spinal instrumentation and fusion operation for scoliosis to decrease the magnitude of the convex thoracic rib prominence. The medial portions of the convex ribs are excised to restore symmetry to the posterior thoracic cage. The procedure may be performed from either an anterior or posterior surgical approach. The excised rib segments provide an abundant source of bone graft for arthrodesis. Due to the improved correction obtained with pedicle screw instrumentation constructs and the postoperative decline in pulmonary function associated with this procedure, it is much less commonly used in current practice.

29. What potential complications are associated with surgical treatment of adolescent idiopathic scoliosis?

Complications and the need for reoperations are not eliminated despite use of modern techniques of anesthesia, intraoperative neurophysiologic monitoring, improved spinal instrumentation systems, and enhanced postoperative intensive care and pain management. Patients must be informed of the most common complications, including but not exclusively limited to hemorrhage, early and late infection, implant misplacement, construct failure, implant prominence, trunk imbalance, neurologic injury, pseudarthrosis, medical complications, and the possible need for future surgery to treat related problems.

30. **What is the role of vertebral body tethering for treatment of patients with idiopathic scoliosis?**
Vertebral body tethering is a nonfusion growth-modulation technique for surgical treatment of skeletally immature patients with progressive idiopathic scoliosis between 30° and 65°. Vertebral body screws and staples are inserted on the convex side of a curve through a thoracoscopic approach or open lumbar approach and secured to a polyethylene terephthalate cord. Tension is applied to the cord during surgery to partially straighten the curvature. Following surgery, the cord continues to straighten the spine as the patient continues to grow. This technique provides the potential to correct and maintain a spinal curve below the threshold where a spinal fusion is indicated, while preserving spinal motion and potentially avoiding adverse consequences associated with spinal fusion. The degree of correction achieved with this technique is comparable to the correction achieved with posterior spinal instrumentation and fusion (Fig. 38.8). Complications reported following vertebral body tethering include overcorrection of the instrumented curve, tether breakage, bone screw migration, pulmonary complications, and the need for subsequent surgery. In 2019, The Tether-Vertebral Body Tethering System (Zimmer Biomet Spine, Inc.) received FDA approval as a Humanitarian Use Device and is the first device of this type available for use in the United States.

31. **What is the role of a posterior minimally invasive internal brace for treatment of patients with adolescent idiopathic scoliosis?**
A posterior nonfusion minimally invasive instrumentation system has recently been introduced for treatment of adolescent idiopathic scoliosis. The Minimally Invasive Deformity Correction (MID-C) System (ApiFix, Ltd.) received FDA approval as a Humanitarian Use Device and is the first device of this type available for use in the United States. This device consists of a ratchet-based expandable rod attached to pedicle screws placed above and below the curve apex only on the concave side of a curvature. This implant system functions as an internal brace and provides dynamic correction of the curvature over time. (1) Following the initial partial curve correction achieved through intraoperative implant distraction, gradual motion-controlled rod elongation occurs through postoperative spinal exercises, which leads to additional correction of the curvature. This device is indicated for treatment of adolescent idiopathic single curves between 45° and 60° that reduce to ≤30° on side-bending radiographs. Potential advantages of this treatment method include the ability to maintain the curve below the threshold where spinal fusion is indicated. Complications associated with this treatment approach include implant-related problems and the potential need for subsequent surgical procedures.

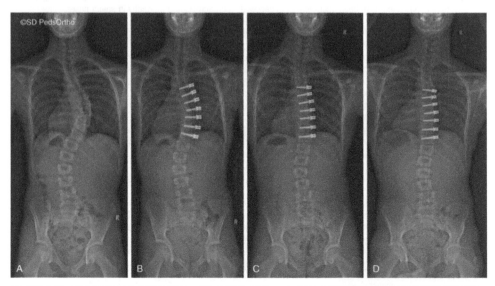

Fig. 38.8 A 13-year-old female with adolescent idiopathic scoliosis. She has a Lenke type 1A curve that measures 53° from T5 to T12 and is Risser stage 0. She underwent spinal growth modulation surgery with vertebral body tethering through an anterior thoracoscopic approach. (A) Preoperative posteroanterior (PA) standing radiograph. (B) PA standing radiograph immediately after surgery. (C) PA standing radiograph 2 years after surgery. (D) PA standing radiograph 3 years after surgery. The scoliotic curve continued to improve over time as the spine grew. (From Newton PO, Wu KW, Yaszay B. Thoracoscopic approach for spinal conditions. In: Garfin SR, Eismont FJ, Bell GR, et al., editors. Rothman-Simeone the Spine. 7th ed. Philadelphia, PA: Saunders; 2018, pp. 509–523, Fig. 29.15, p. 520.)

KEY POINTS

1. Idiopathic scoliosis is a diagnosis of exclusion and requires thorough evaluation to rule out an underlying congenital, neurologic, or syndromic etiology.
2. The management options for patients diagnosed with idiopathic scoliosis include observation, orthoses, exercise, and operative treatment.
3. Patients with idiopathic curves less than 20° are observed.
4. Current indications for brace treatment for adolescent idiopathic scoliosis include curves with a magnitude between 25° and 45°; a Risser stage of 0, 1, or 2; and, for female patients, <1 year postmenarche at the time of initiation of brace treatment.
5. In general, for the immature adolescent patient, surgery is indicated for curves greater than 40°–45° that are progressive despite brace treatment. In the mature adolescent, surgery is considered for curves approaching or greater than 50°.
6. Nonfusion options for surgical treatment of skeletally immature patients with adolescent idiopathic scoliosis include vertebral body tethering and posterior minimally invasive deformity correction.

Websites

1. Adolescent idiopathic scoliosis: https://www.srs.org/professionals/online-education-and-resources/conditions-and-treatments/adolescent-idiopathic-scoliosis
2. Natural history of adolescent idiopathic scoliosis: https://online.boneandjoint.org.uk/doi/epub/10.1007/s11832-012-0462-7
3. Minimally Invasive Deformity Correction (MID-C) System: https://www.fda.gov/medical-devices/recently-approved-devices/minimally-invasive-deformity-correction-mid-c-system-h170001
4. The Tether-Vertebral Body Tethering System: https://www.fda.gov/medical-devices/recently-approved-devices/tethertm-vertebral-body-tethering-system-h190005

BIBLIOGRAPHY

1. Alkhalife, Y. I., Padhye, K. P., & El-Hawary, R. (2019). New technologies in pediatric spine surgery. *Orthopedic Clinics of North America, 50*, 57–67.
2. Lenke, L. G., Betz, R. R., Harms, J., Bridwell, K. H., Clements, D. H., Lowe, T. G., et al. (2001). Adolescent idiopathic scoliosis—a new classification to determine extent of spinal arthrodesis. *Journal of Bone and Joint Surgery, 83*, 1169–1181.
3. Lenke, I. G., & Dobbs, M. B. (2007). Management of juvenile idiopathic scoliosis. *Journal of Bone and Joint Surgery, 89*, 55–63.
4. Lonstein, J. E., & Carlson, J. M. (1984). The prediction of curve progression in untreated idiopathic scoliosis during growth. *Journal of Bone and Joint Surgery, 66*, 1061–1071.
5. Rose, P. S., & Lenke, L. G. (2007). Classification of operative adolescent idiopathic scoliosis: Treatment guidelines. *Orthopedic Clinics of North America, 38*, 521–529.
6. Sanders, J. O. (2007). Maturity indicators in spinal deformity. *Journal of Bone and Joint Surgery, 89*, 14–20.
7. Sitoula, P., Verma, K., Holmes, L., Jr., Gobos, P.G., Sanders, J. O., Yorgova, P., et al. (2015). Prediction of curve progression in idiopathic scoliosis. Validation of the Sanders Skeletal Maturity Staging System. *Spine, 40*, 1006–1013.
8. Sponseller, P. D., Betz, R., Newton, P. O., Lenke, L. G., Lowe, T., Crawford, A., et al. (2009). Differences in curve behavior after fusion in adolescent idiopathic scoliosis patients with open triradiate cartilages. *Spine, 34*, 827–831.
9. Weinstein, S. L., Dolan, L. A., Spratt, K. F., et al. (2003). Health and function of patients with untreated idiopathic scoliosis: A 50-year natural history study. *JAMA, 289*, 559–567.
10. Weinstein, S., Dolan, L. A., Wright, J. G., & Dobbs, M. B. (2013). Effects of bracing in adolescents with idiopathic scoliosis. *New England Journal of Medicine, 369*, 1512–1521.
11. Weinstein, S. L., & Ponseti, I. V. (1983). Curve progression in idiopathic scoliosis. *Journal of Bone and Joint Surgery American, 65*, 447–455.

CHAPTER 39

CONGENITAL SPINAL DEFORMITIES

Lawrence I. Karlin, MD

1. Define congenital scoliosis.
   A lateral curvature of the spine caused by vertebral anomalies that produce a frontal plane growth asymmetry. The anomalies are present at birth, but the curvature may take years to become clinically evident.

2. What genes are thought to be responsible for the congenital spinal malformations?
   Homeobox genes of the Hox class.

3. When do congenital vertebral anomalies form?
   During weeks 4–6 of the embryonic period.

4. What are the two main categories of congenital scoliosis?
   Defects of segmentation and defects of formation. Some congenital abnormalities cannot be placed into this classification scheme.

5. What are the common defects of segmentation?
   Block vertebra, unilateral bar, and unilateral bar and hemivertebra (Fig. 39.1).

6. What are the common defects of formation?
   Hemivertebra and wedge vertebra (Fig. 39.2).

7. What are the types of hemivertebra?
   Fully segmented, semisegmented, nonsegmented, and incarcerated.

8. What is the anatomic cause of progressive spinal deformity?
   Unbalanced growth. The greater the disparity in the number of healthy growth plates between the left and right sides of the spine, the greater the deformity and the more rapidly spinal deformity develops.

9. What factors are used to prognosticate the rate of progression and ultimate deformity due to a congenital spinal anomaly?
   1. The **anatomic type** helps determine the risk and rate of progression.
   2. The **location** of the defect affects spinal balance and difficulty of treatment. A hemivertebra located at the lumbosacral junction causes far more spinal imbalance than one located at the mid-thoracic level. In addition, a hemivertebra at the cervicothoracic junction is more difficult to treat surgically due to limited approach options, and timing of surgical intervention may be altered based on this consideration.

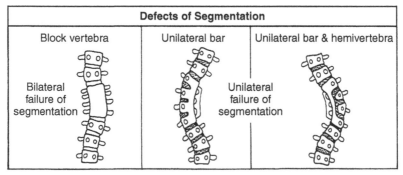

Fig. 39.1 Defects of segmentation. (From McMaster MJ. Congenital scoliosis. In: Weinstein SL, editor. The Pediatric Spine: Principles and Practice. New York: Raven Press; 1994, pp. 227–244.)

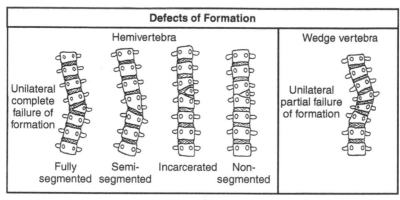

Fig. 39.2 Defects of formation. (From McMaster MJ. Congenital scoliosis. In: Weinstein SL, editor. The Pediatric Spine: Principles and Practice. New York: Raven Press; 1994, pp. 227–244.)

3. The patient **age** determines the risk of progression. Spinal deformities are more likely to progress during times of rapid growth, such as the first 2 years of life and during the adolescent growth spurt.

10. What forms of congenital scoliosis cause the most rapidly progressive deformities?
    • Unilateral unsegmented bar with contralateral hemivertebra (an average of 6° progression per year)
    • Unilateral unsegmented bar (an average of 5° progression per year)

11. What is the accepted initial treatment for a unilateral unsegmented bar?
    Early in-situ fusion, because this deformity can only progress.

12. What is the risk of progression of the various types of hemivertebra?
    • **Fully segmented**. There are two extra growth plates on one side of the spine. Unbalanced growth occurs, producing a scoliosis that worsens at a rate of 1° to 2° per year. Two fully segmented hemivertebrae on the same side of the spine produce a more rapid deterioration (about 3° per year).
    • **Semisegmented**. One border is synostosed to its neighbor, producing a balanced number of growth plates on either side. The hemivertebra produces a tilting of the spine, and a slowly progressive curvature may occur.
    • **Nonsegmented**. No growth plates are associated with this type of hemivertebra, and a progressive deformity does not occur.
    • **Incarcerated**. The vertebral bodies above and below accommodate the hemivertebra, and little or no deformity is produced. The growth plates tend to be narrow with little growth potential. This form of hemivertebra causes little or no deformity.

13. What percentage of people with vertebral malformations have associated anomalies?
    Sixty percent have malformations either within or outside the spine. A relatively benign vertebral abnormality may be associated with a life-threatening (but initially asymptomatic) problem. The importance of a thorough search for associated abnormalities cannot be overemphasized.

14. What common malformations are associated with congenital spinal anomalies?
    • **Vertebral abnormalities at another spinal level**. For example, cervical vertebral anomalies are detected in 25% of people with congenital scoliosis or kyphosis.
    • **Urinary tract structural abnormalities**. Up to 37% of people with congenital vertebral anomalies have urinary tract anomalies, such as renal agenesis, duplication, ectopia, fusion, ureteral anomalies, and reflux.
    • **Intraspinal abnormalities**. Up to 38% of people with congenital vertebral anomalies have intraspinal abnormalities detectable by magnetic resonance imaging (MRI), including tethered cord, diastematomyelia, diplomyelia, and syringomyelia.
    • **Other associated anomalies**. Cranial nerve palsy (11%), upper extremity hypoplasia (10%), clubfoot (9%), dislocated hip (8%), and congenital cardiac disease (7%).

15. Define diastematomyelia.
    A *diastematomyelia* is a congenital bony or fibrocartilaginous septum in the spinal canal that impinges on or splits the neural tissue.

16. What is the incidence of diastematomyelia associated with congenital vertebral abnormalities?
The incidence is 5%–20%.

17. What are the clinical findings in diastematomyelia?
- Cutaneous lesions, such as hair patch, dimple (55%–75%)
- Anisomelia (52%–58%)
- Foot deformities, usually cavus and unilateral (32%–52%)
- Neurologic deficits (58%–88%)
- Scoliosis (60%–100%)

18. What radiographic findings are associated with diastematomyelia?
- Spina bifida occulta (76%–94%)
- Widened interpedicular distance (94%–100%)

19. What is the normal level of the conus in the pediatric population according to age?
The conus medullaris is the distal end of the spinal cord. It is located at the level of the L2–L3 disc in the neonate and the L1–L2 disc or cephalad at 1 year and older.

20. What vertebral malformation is most often associated with an abnormality of the neural axis?
A unilateral unsegmented bar and a same-level contralateral hemivertebra. Approximately 50% of people with this vertebral abnormality have been reported to have an associated neural axis abnormality.

21. What is the VATER association?
VATER is the acronym for the association of the following congenital anomalies: **v**ertebral, **a**norectal, **t**racheo-**e**sophageal fistula, and **r**adial limb dysplasia, and **r**enal anomalies. This acronym has now been expanded to **VAC-TERLS**, adding **c**ardiac and **s**ingle umbilical artery. Trill the *L*, and you will remember lung abnormalities, another associated problem.

22. What tests should be performed to screen a patient with congenital scoliosis for renal abnormalities?
Urinalysis and renal ultrasound are sufficient.

23. When should an MRI be performed to screen for intraspinal abnormalities in a patient presenting with a congenital vertebral anomaly?
Perhaps a controversial answer: A number of studies now place the incidence of associated intraspinal abnormalities in the 30% range. The standard recommendation is to perform an MRI if surgery is planned or when clinical symptoms or physical findings are suggestive of intraspinal pathology. The author believes, as do others, that an MRI should be performed as soon as safety allows. The 30% incidence is too high to ignore when clinical manifestations may be initially absent but not necessarily reversible once they have occurred.

24. What is the accuracy of the Cobb measurement of congenital spinal deformities on plain radiographs?
The abnormally shaped vertebrae make it difficult to be consistent with radiographic measurements. One study revealed an intraobserver variability of ±9.6° and an interobserver variability of ±11.8°. Another study reported an average intraobserver variance of 2.8° and an interobserver variance of 3.4°.

25. What is the role of brace treatment for congenital scoliosis?
The role of brace treatment is limited. Orthoses will not halt the progression of a rigid congenital structural abnormality. A brace may control a compensatory curvature or a long flexible curvature in which the rigid congenital deformity comprises a small section of the entire spinal deformity. Total contact braces may restrict chest wall development and should not be used. A Milwaukee brace (cervicothoracolumbosacral orthosis [CTLSO]) is preferable.

26. What are the goals of surgery for congenital scoliosis?
The goals of surgical treatment for congenital scoliosis include:
1. Achievement of a balanced spine with as much flexibility and length as possible at skeletal maturity
2. Maximization of pulmonary function
3. Minimization of the intrusion of medical care on the lives of the child and family
4. Avoidance of significant major complications
The key to success is to consider the full armamentarium of treatment techniques and to customize the most expeditious treatment program for the highly variable clinical presentation of each patient.

27. Surgical treatment options for congenital scoliosis include various types of spinal fusion procedures and growth-sparing surgical techniques. What are the indications for each type of treatment? What surgical options are available for spinal fusion and growth-sparing treatment?
Spinal fusion surgery is indicated to prevent predicted or documented progression of spinal deformity, or to correct problematic established deformity. Spinal fusion should be designed and/or timed to avoid stunting spinal growth to the extent that pulmonary function is adversely affected. *Growth-sparing surgical techniques* are best reserved for young children with significant remaining growth and spinal deformities such as multiple hemivertebrae that involve a large segment of spine. Fusion of the entire deformity in these cases would adversely affect pulmonary function and should be avoided.
    The various fusion and growth-sparing surgical options include:
Spinal fusion techniques: (a) posterior in-situ fusion, (b) combined anterior and posterior fusion, (c) convex growth arrest, (d) hemivertebra excision, (e) posterior fusion with instrumentation and correction
Growth-sparing techniques: (a) growing spinal instrumentation, (b) vertical expandable prosthetic titanium rib (VEPTR)

28. What is the indication for in-situ posterior spinal arthrodesis without spinal instrumentation for treatment of congenital scoliosis?
This procedure is indicated for a small curvature ($<25°$, limited to $\leqslant5$ vertebrae) that is anticipated to worsen (e.g., scoliosis due to a unilateral unsegmented bar). In-situ posterior fusion should be avoided across lordotic spinal segments as continued anterior spinal growth will lead to worsening of lordosis over time. It should be recognized that bending of the fusion (crankshaft) can occur with significant anterior growth and may require treatment with anterior fusion.

29. What is the crankshaft deformity and why does it occur after the surgical treatment of congenital scoliosis?
The crankshaft deformity results when anterior growth occurs following a successful posterior arthrodesis performed for scoliosis and manifests as a worsened rotational deformity. This phenomenon has been documented in children with idiopathic scoliosis and congenital scoliosis who are treated before age 10 years by posterior fusion alone. It has not been reported when combined anterior and posterior arthrodesis is performed.

30. What is the indication for combined anterior and posterior fusion for treatment of congenital scoliosis?
Anterior and posterior arthrodesis is indicated in the very young patient or when significant anterior growth (i.e., presence of healthy anterior growth plates) is anticipated. An example where a combined anterior and posterior fusion is an option is a young patient with mild curvature secondary to a unilateral bar with a contralateral hemivertebra. The addition of instrumentation may limit the need for postoperative immobilization.

31. What is the indication for convex hemiepiphysiodesis and hemiarthrodesis for treatment of congenital scoliosis? What levels should be fused?
This procedure is designed to produce a gradual correction of curvatures due to hemivertebra. The prerequisites for success include a curvature with concave growth potential, limited length of involvement (five or fewer vertebral bodies), limited curve magnitude ($<70°$), no kyphosis, and young age (<5 years). The entire curvature should be fused anteriorly and posteriorly, only on the convex side. Fusion is performed at the level of the hemivertebra and also at one intervertebral level above and below. The benefit of the procedure is safety; the disadvantage is the unpredictability of final curve correction that is achieved. The procedure can be performed via (1) an open or thoracoscopic anterior approach and open posterior approach, or (2) through an entirely posterior approach with a transpedicular access to the anterior spinal column. The transpedicular approach is especially helpful for regions of the spine that are difficult to access through an anterior surgical approach, such as the upper thoracic spine.

32. What is the indication for hemivertebra excision for treatment of congenital scoliosis?
Hemivertebra excision is indicated for treatment of a fully segmented hemivertebra which causes significant trunk imbalance (Fig. 39.3). This is theoretically a more dangerous procedure than in-situ fusion or hemiepiphysiodesis. However, it produces dramatic curve correction while maintaining maximal spinal flexibility. It is the treatment of choice for a lumbosacral hemivertebra that causes significant oblique take-off of the lumbar spine above the sacrum. The safety and efficacy of sequential and simultaneous anterior and posterior approaches for hemivertebra excision are well documented. More recently, posterior-only techniques have been developed as an alternative to combined approaches and have documented favorable outcomes.

33. What is the indication for posterior fusion with instrumentation and deformity correction for treatment of congenital scoliosis?
This procedure is indicated in the older child as a definitive procedure to stop the growth of the spine and thereby achieve permanent correction of the spinal deformity. Prior to planning fusion of multiple spinal segments, the patient should be assessed to ensure that an adequate thoracic volume has been attained and their spine has reached an

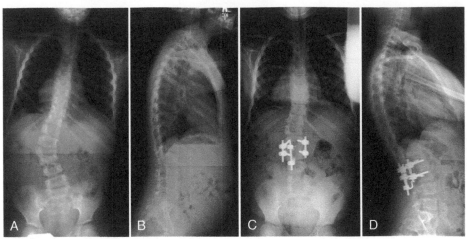

Fig. 39.3 (A and B) This 2-year-old boy with scoliosis, secondary to a fully segmented hemivertebra, progressed 12° in 1 year. (C and D) A hemivertebra resection performed through a single-stage posterior approach produced a significant improvement in both the curvature and coronal balance without an appreciable loss of flexibility or growth. In a small child, the bones may not tolerate the stresses produced by instrumented manipulation, and fixation to maintain the correction may be lost. Here the correction was obtained by manual pressure over the ribs and flank and compression of the laminar hooks. The correction was then fine-tuned and maintained by the pedicle screw-rod construct.

acceptable length so as not to adversely affect pulmonary function. In general, deformity correction will not occur through the rigid congenital deformity but rather through adjacent flexible spine segments. For complex congenital deformities with significant trunk imbalance or prior surgery, adjunctive procedures, including anterior and posterior spinal osteotomies or vertebral column resection, may be considered.

34. **What is the role of growth-friendly spinal instrumentation for treatment of congenital scoliosis?**
   For children with select congenital spinal deformities without chest wall abnormalities, spinal-based extensible rods (i.e., growing rods) have been shown to effectively correct and control deformity, allow for continued spinal growth and improve the space available for the lungs. Nonfusion growth-enabling spinal implant constructs require lengthening on a periodic basis as the child grows. Traditional growing rods require an open surgical procedure to adjust the implant construct. Magnetic-controlled growing rods have been developed that allow noninvasive rod lengthening, reducing the number of surgeries required in the course of treatment.

35. **What is the role of the VEPTR procedure in congenital spinal deformity?**
   The vertical expandable prosthetic titanium rib (VEPTR) was developed to treat thoracic insufficiency syndrome (defined as the inability of the thorax to support normal respiration and lung growth) associated with fused ribs. Following thoracoplasty of the fused ribs, the device lengthens and expands the hypoplastic hemithorax. When used in congenital scoliosis associated with fused ribs, growth of the concave and convex sides of the spine, including growth through unilateral unsegmented bars, may occur in addition to hemithorax enlargement (Fig. 39.4).

36. **How is congenital kyphosis classified (Fig. 39.5)?**
   Type I: Failure of formation
   Type II: Failure of segmentation
   Type III: Mixed anomalies

37. **What forms of congenital kyphosis are associated with spontaneous neurologic deterioration?**
   Type I (failure of formation) and type III (mixed anomalies).

38. **In congenital kyphosis, when is posterior surgery alone sufficient?**
   Posterior fusion surgery is reasonable in the absence of anterior neural compression, kyphosis correcting to 50° or less on supine radiographs, and age younger than 5 years.

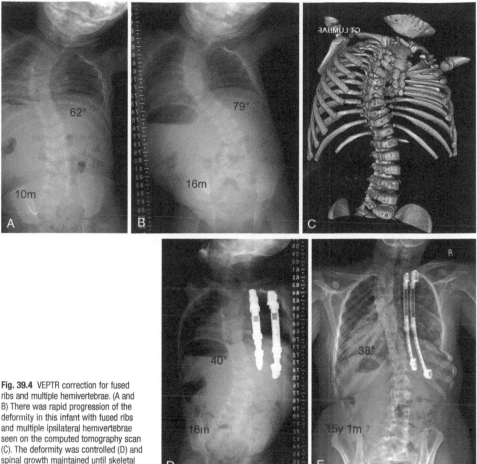

Fig. 39.4 VEPTR correction for fused ribs and multiple hemivertebrae. (A and B) There was rapid progression of the deformity in this infant with fused ribs and multiple ipsilateral hemivertebrae seen on the computed tomography scan (C). The deformity was controlled (D) and spinal growth maintained until skeletal maturity (E). (Courtesy John Emans, MD.)

39. What is the treatment of type I congenital kyphosis?

Arthrodesis by age 5 years. An aggressive surgical approach is indicated due to the substantial risk of neurologic deficit without treatment.

40. What is the treatment for type II congenital kyphosis?

Observation. Fusion should be performed if deformity progression is noted. The prognosis for deformity progression is greater when there is an anterolateral bar producing kyphoscoliosis than when a midline bar produces a pure kyphotic deformity.

41. What is the treatment for type III congenital kyphosis?

Arthrodesis by age 5 years.

42. Lumbar hypoplasia is an unusual cause of congenital thoracolumbar kyphosis. Define this entity and describe the clinical significance of this deformity.

Lumbar hypoplasia is a kyphotic deformity of the upper lumbar spine in which the anatomic defect is limited to the superior aspect of the anterior half of a single affected vertebral body. Unlike congenital kyphosis due to anterior failure of formation, the natural history of lumbar hypoplasia is spontaneous resolution (Fig. 39.6).

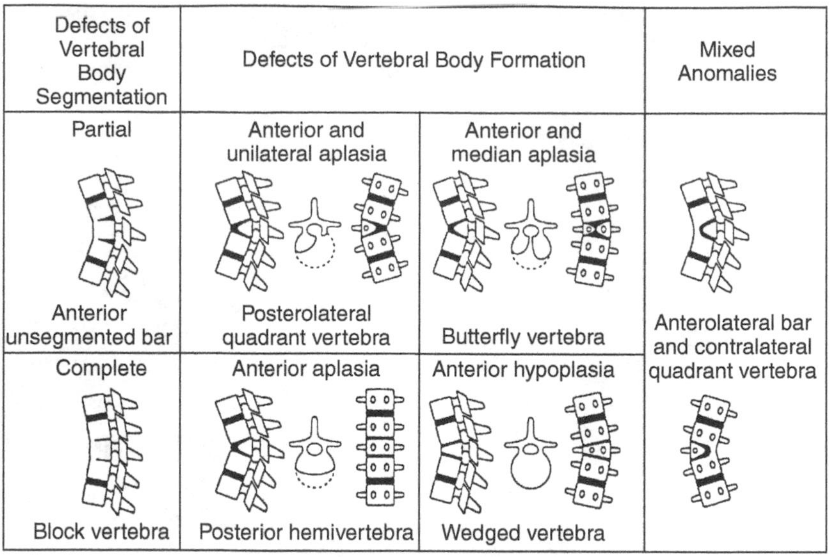

Defects of Vertebral Body Segmentation	Defects of Vertebral Body Formation		Mixed Anomalies
Partial	Anterior and unilateral aplasia	Anterior and median aplasia	
Anterior unsegmented bar	Posterolateral quadrant vertebra	Butterfly vertebra	Anterolateral bar and contralateral quadrant vertebra
Complete	Anterior aplasia	Anterior hypoplasia	
Block vertebra	Posterior hemivertebra	Wedged vertebra	

Fig. 39.5 Classification of congenital kyphosis. (From McMaster MJ, Singh H. Natural history of kyphosis and kyphoscoliosis. A study of one hundred and twelve patients. J Bone Joint Surg 1999;81[10]:1367–1383.)

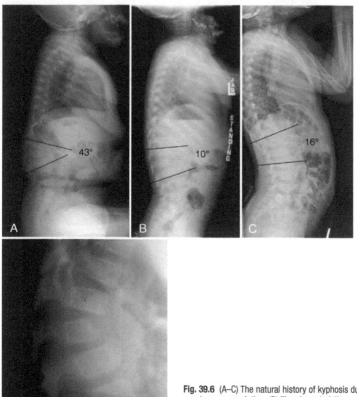

43°

10°

16°

Fig. 39.6 (A–C) The natural history of kyphosis due to lumbar hypoplasia is spontaneous resolution. (D) The characteristic anatomic finding is a defect limited to the anterior half of the superior portion of the single affected vertebral body. (From Campos MD, Fernandes P, Dolan LA, et al. Infantile thoracolumbar kyphosis secondary to lumbar hypoplasia. J Bone Joint Surgery 2008;90[8]:1726–1729.)

43. **What characteristics distinguish congenital spinal dislocation from congenital kyphosis?**
The *congenitally dislocated spine* is the most severe form of congenital kyphosis and is distinguished by a sudden sagittal vertebral displacement designated as the *step-off* sign. Multiplanar displacements have been reported. The deformity is frequently associated with instability and neurologic compromise. Stabilization by circumferential fusion at the time of diagnosis is recommended.

44. **Define segmental spinal dysgenesis and describe treatment of this deformity.**
Segmental spinal dysgenesis is a congenital spinal deformity characterized by focal dysgenesis or agenesis of the lumbar or thoracolumbar spine, and a focal abnormality of the underlying spinal cord and nerve roots. The bony defects include canal stenosis, hypoplastic vertebrae, spinal column subluxation, and instability. Neural pathology includes narrowing of the thecal sac and absent nerve roots. Early spinal stabilization, usually by anterior and posterior arthrodesis, is required to prevent progressive deformity and neurologic deterioration.

KEY POINTS

1. The prognosis for a congenital spinal deformity depends on three factors: type of anomaly, patient age, and location of the defect.
2. A wide range of intraspinal and extraspinal anomalies are associated with congenital spinal deformities, and a thorough evaluation for associated abnormalities is critical.
3. MRI of the spine is an integral part of the evaluation of a patient with congenital spinal deformity.
4. Orthoses have little effect on progression of congenital spinal deformities.
5. Early surgical intervention is advised for progressive congenital spinal deformities to balance spinal growth and avoid development of rigid deformities and secondary structural curvatures.
6. Treatment timing and technique should be selected to minimize deformity and maximize spinal growth and pulmonary function.

Websites
1. Classification of congenital scoliosis and kyphosis: http://www.medscape.com/viewarticle/707687
2. Congenital scoliosis: https://www.srs.org/professionals/online-education-and-resources/conditions-and-treatments/congenital-scoliosis
3. Congenital spinal deformity: http://members.medscape.com/article/1260442-overview

---

BIBLIOGRAPHY

1. Andrew, T. E., & Piggott, H. A. (1985). Growth arrest for progressive scoliosis. Combined anterior and posterior fusion of the convexity. *Journal of Bone and Joint Surgery, 67*(2), 193–197.
2. Campbell, R. M., Jr., Smith, M. D., Mayes, T. C., Mangos, J. A., Willey-Courand, D. B., Kose, N., et al. (2004). The effect of opening wedge thoracostomy on thoracic insufficiency syndrome associated with fused ribs and congenital scoliosis. *Journal of Bone and Joint Surgery, 86*(8), 1659–1674.
3. Campos, M. A., Fernandes, P., Dolan, L. A., & Weinstein, S. L. (2008). Infantile thoracolumbar kyphosis secondary to lumbar hypoplasia. *Journal of Bone and Joint Surgery, 90*(8), 1726–1729.
4. Elsebai, H. B., Yazici, M., Thompson, G. H., Emans, J. B., Skaggs, D. L., Crawford, A. H., et al. (2011). Safety and efficacy of growing rod technique for pediatric congenital spinal deformities. *Journal of Pediatric Orthopaedics, 31*(1), 1–5.
5. Flynn, J. M., Emans, J. B., Smith, J. T., Betz, R. R., Deeney, V. F., Patel, N. M., et al. (2013). VEPTR to treat nonsyndromic congenital scoliosis: A multicenter, mid-term follow-up study. *Journal of Pediatric Orthopedics, 33*(7), 679–684.
6. Hedequist, D. J. (2009). Instrumentation and fusion for congenital spine deformities. *Spine, 34*(17), 1783–1790.
7. Hughes, L. O., McCarthy, R. E., & Glasier, C. M. (1998). Segmental spinal dysgenesis: A report of three cases. *Journal of Pediatric Orthopedics, 18*(2), 227–232.
8. Keller, P. M., Lindseth, R. E., & DeRosa, G. P. (1994). Progressive congenital scoliosis treatment using a transpedicular anterior and posterior convex hemiepiphyseodesis and hemiarthrodesis. A preliminary report. *Spine, 19*(17), 1933–1939.
9. Lazar, R. D., & Hall, J. E. (1999). Simultaneous anterior and posterior hemivertebra excision. *Clinical Orthopaedics and Related Research*, (364), 76–84.
10. McMaster, M. J., & Singh, H. (2001). The surgical management of congenital kyphosis and kyphoscoliosis. *Spine, 26*(19), 2146–2154.
11. Ruf M, Jensen R, Letko L, & Harms J. (2009). Hemivertebra resection and osteotomies in congenital spine deformity. *Spine, 34*(17), 1791–1799.
12. Terek, R. M., Wehner, J., & Lubicky, J. P. (1991). Crankshaft phenomenon in congenital scoliosis: A preliminary report. *Journal of Pediatric Orthopedics, 11*(4), 527–532.
13. Yazici, M., & Emans, J. (2009). Fusionless instrumentation systems for congenital scoliosis: Expandable spinal rods and vertical expandable prosthetic titanium rib in the management of congenital spine deformities in the growing child. *Spine, 34*, 1800–1807.
14. Zeller, R. D., Ghanem, I., & Dubousset, J. (1996). The congenital dislocated spine. *Spine, 21*(10), 1235–1240.

CHAPTER 40

NEUROMUSCULAR SPINAL DEFORMITIES

Vincent J. Devlin, MD

GENERAL CONCEPTS

1. **Why do patients with neuromuscular disorders develop spinal deformities?**

   Neuromuscular spinal deformities develop in patients with underlying neuropathic or myopathic disorders due to trunk muscle weakness, spasticity, or spinal imbalance, which compromise the ability to maintain normal alignment of the spine and pelvis. Asymmetric spinal column loading of the immature spine leads to asymmetric vertebral body growth due to the Hueter-Volkmann principle, which states that increased loading across an epiphyseal growth plate inhibits growth while decreased loading accelerates growth. The severity of a deformity is influenced by a range of patient-specific factors, including the underlying diagnosis, the type and extent of neuromuscular involvement, ambulatory status, and skeletal maturity. A broad spectrum of spinal deformities may develop, including scoliosis, hyperkyphosis, hyperlordosis, and complex multiplanar deformities.

2. **How are neuromuscular spinal deformities classified?**

   Neuromuscular spinal deformities referred for evaluation and treatment include cerebral palsy, Duchenne muscular dystrophy, spinal muscular atrophy, myelodysplasia, posttraumatic deformities, and Rett syndrome. Neuromuscular disorders may be classified as **neuropathic** (affecting either the upper or lower motor neurons) or **myopathic**. Certain conditions such as myelodysplasia and posttraumatic deformities may present with both upper and lower motor neuron involvement.

   MYOPATHIC DISORDERS
   1. Muscular dystrophy
      - Duchenne type
      - Limb-girdle
      - Facioscapulohumeral
   2. Arthrogryposis multiplex congenita
   3. Congenital hypotonia
   4. Myotonia dystrophica

   NEUROPATHIC DISORDERS
   A. Upper motor neuron lesions
      1. Cerebral palsy
      2. Spinocerebellar degeneration
         - Friedreich ataxia
         - Charcot-Marie-Tooth disease
         - Roussy-Lévy disease
      3. Syringomyelia
      4. Quadriplegia secondary to spinal cord trauma or tumor
      5. Rett syndrome
   B. Lower motor neuron lesions
      1. Spinal muscular atrophy
      2. Poliomyelitis
      3. Dysautonomia (Riley-Day syndrome)
      4. Traumatic

3. **How common are neuromuscular spinal deformities?**

   The incidence of spinal deformities varies across different neuromuscular disorders and is dependent on patient-specific factors such as the extent neuromuscular involvement and the criteria used to define a spinal deformity. Some general incidence ranges for neuromuscular scoliosis include: cerebral palsy (25%–100%), myelodysplasia (60%–100%), spinal muscular atrophy (67%), Friedreich ataxia (80%), Duchenne muscular dystrophy (90%), and spinal cord injury before 10 years of age (100%).

4. **List important differences between neuromuscular scoliosis and idiopathic scoliosis.**

   - Evaluation of neuromuscular scoliosis requires assessment of the underlying neuromuscular disease in combination with the spinal deformity. In contrast, idiopathic scoliosis is a spinal deformity occurring in an otherwise normal patient.
   - Multidisciplinary evaluation is required for problems associated with the underlying neuromuscular disease in patients with neuromuscular scoliosis (e.g., contractures, hip dislocations, seizures, malnutrition, cardiac and pulmonary disease, urinary tract dysfunction, developmental delay, pressure sores, insensate skin).
   - Neuromuscular scoliosis usually develops at an earlier age than most cases of idiopathic scoliosis, often before age 10, and is more likely to progress.
   - Neuromuscular curves tend to be longer, more rigid, and involve more vertebrae than idiopathic curves.
   - Neuromuscular scoliosis often presents in combination with sagittal plane deformities.
   - Neuromuscular curves are frequently accompanied by pelvic obliquity, which may compromise sitting ability and upper extremity function.

- Brace or cast treatment does not provide a long-term solution for most neuromuscular curves, although such treatments are helpful to improve sitting posture and provide temporary curve control in specific circumstances.

5. **What are some key steps in the initial evaluation of neuromuscular spinal deformities?**
   A general clinical examination is the first step in evaluation and includes a detailed birth, developmental, and family history. Physical examination includes detailed assessment of the spine, extremities, and thorax, including neurologic function, pelvic obliquity, trunk balance, chest wall excursion, and inspection for cutaneous markers of systemic disorders. Initial imaging evaluation consists of biplanar radiographs or slot-scanning radiography, which includes the entire spine and pelvis. Upright radiographs are obtained in patients who are able to stand. Patients who are able to sit without hand support are assessed in the sitting position. Patients who are unable to sit are evaluated with recumbent anteroposterior and lateral radiographs. The examiner should assess curve magnitude, curve progression, spinal balance, pelvic obliquity (if present), and curve flexibility. Spinal magnetic resonance imaging (MRI) is required if intraspinal problems (e.g., syrinx, tethered cord) are suspected. Additional testing may include blood tests, computed tomography, ultrasound, bone density scans, muscle biopsy, pulmonary function tests, and electromyogram. Patients and families diagnosed with neuromuscular spinal deformities benefit from coordination of care by a multidisciplinary team and in some cases referral for genetic and family counseling.

6. **What radiographic features are characteristic of typical neuromuscular curves?**
   Neuromuscular curves are often S-shaped curves or long, sweeping C-shaped curves with a curve apex in the thoracolumbar or lumbar region that extends to the pelvic region. Significant sagittal plane deformity often accompanies coronal plane deformity. Pelvic obliquity is common and poses a major problem because it creates an uneven sitting base.

7. **What are options for nonoperative treatment of neuromuscular spinal deformities?**
   Nonoperative treatment options include observation, serial casts, orthoses, wheelchair and seating modifications, and specific medical treatments directed toward the underlying neuromuscular disorder. Observation is considered for patients with small nonprogressive curves, patients with severe developmental disability and large curves without associated functional loss, and patients with contraindications for major spinal reconstructive surgery. Although brace treatment does not positively affect the natural history of neuromuscular curves, in select patients it is used to improve sitting posture and control spinal curves temporarily to allow additional spinal growth prior to definitive surgery. Wheelchair and seating modifications can also be used to improve seating for patients with severe deformities. Orthotic management is challenging due to poor muscle control, impaired sensation, pulmonary compromise, impaired gastrointestinal function, obesity, and cognitive impairment.

8. **What are the indications and treatment options for neuromuscular spinal deformities?**
   The decision to intervene surgically for treatment of a neuromuscular spinal deformity depends on a range of factors, including etiology of the underlying neuromuscular disorder, deformity magnitude, skeletal maturity, and associated medical comorbidities. The operative treatment options for neuromuscular spinal deformities include both nonfusion and fusion surgical techniques.
   Nonfusion or "growth-friendly" surgical techniques are considered for patients with early-onset neuromuscular scoliosis (<10 years of age) to treat curves that are not adequately controlled with bracing. Various strategies are used to control such curves and can prevent or limit progression without adversely affecting future lung growth and function. These include use of various devices implanted through a posterior surgical approach such as expandable rod systems, which require periodic open surgical lengthening; magnetically controlled expandable rod systems, which allow for noninvasive lengthening; growth-guidance systems; and the vertical expandable prosthetic titanium rib (VEPTR).
   Surgical techniques intended to achieve fusion are considered for patients who are not candidates for growth-friendly surgery to treat progressive deformity, unacceptable trunk shift, or pelvic obliquity that affects standing or sitting balance or positioning. Operative treatment has been suggested when progressive curves exceed 50° or when patients develop trunk decompensation. Earlier surgical treatment is advised for patients with Duchenne muscular dystrophy (when curves reach 20°) due to predictable pulmonary deterioration associated with further curve progression. Neuromuscular curves up to approximately 90° are most commonly treated with posterior spinal instrumentation and fusion, while larger or rigid curves require more complex anterior and posterior procedures that are associated with higher morbidity. The most common procedure for neuromuscular scoliosis is a long posterior fusion with posterior instrumentation extending from T2 to the pelvis, although fixation ending at L5 distally is considered in ambulatory patients with a level pelvis whose deformity ends proximal to L5.

9. **List some important preoperative considerations in evaluation of patients with neuromuscular spinal deformity.**
   Assessment by a multidisciplinary team is critical and includes assessment of:
   - **Functional status:** Assess ambulatory ability, sitting ability, hand function, cognitive ability.
   - **Pulmonary function:** Inquire regarding a history of upper respiratory infection or pneumonia; assess for chronic aspiration; perform pulmonary function testing if possible.

- **Gastrointestinal function:** Assess for gastroesophageal reflux and intraabdominal volume compromise.
- **Cardiac assessment:** Evaluation is critical in disorders such as Duchenne muscular dystrophy or Friedreich ataxia due to associated cardiac anomalies.
- **Nutritional status:** Address deficits to help prevent impaired wound healing and decrease infection risk.
- **Hematologic assessment:** Evaluation and correction for preoperative coagulopathies and planning to optimize anticipated blood loss is an important part of preoperative assessment.
- **Seizure disorders:** Require assessment by a neurologist and includes confirmation of appropriate levels of antiseizure medications.
- **Metabolic bone disease:** Osteopenia is common secondary to disuse, poor nutrition, and anticonvulsants, and benefits from preoperative optimization.

10. What are some important technologic innovations that have advanced the surgical treatment of neuromuscular spinal deformities?
    - **Pedicle screw and hybrid posterior implant constructs:** Pedicle screws provide fixation across all three spinal columns and are biomechanically advantageous compared with hook or sublaminar wire fixation, and provide a means for achieving secure fixation in patients with congenital or acquired laminectomy defects. Hybrid posterior instrumentation constructs, which combine hooks, wires, and screws, permit customization to optimize spinal fixation and maximize deformity correction.
    - **Sacropelvic fixation with S2 alar-iliac or iliac screws:** Improved techniques for attaining secure sacropelvic fixation eliminates the need for complex rod bends and provides a secure foundation for correction of severe neuromuscular deformities associated with pelvic obliquity.
    - **Osteotomies and vertebral column resection procedures for rigid deformities:** Various types of posterior osteotomies and excision of vertebrae in the apical region of a severe rigid curve can enhance multiplanar correction of severe spinal deformities.
    - **Preoperative halo-gravity traction, intraoperative halo-femoral traction, and temporary intraoperative internal distraction techniques:** Use of these adjunctive techniques have been shown to optimize and facilitate posterior surgical approaches for treatment of severe neuromuscular spinal deformities.
    - **Intraoperative use of antifibrinolytic agents:** Use of antifibrinolytics such as tranexamic acid (TXA) have been shown to reduce intraoperative blood loss in patients undergoing surgery for neuromuscular spinal deformities.
    - **Intraoperative neurophysiologic spinal monitoring:** Evidence supports use of multimodality intraoperative spinal monitoring to protect existing neurologic function during surgical treatment of neuromuscular spinal deformities.

11. What intraoperative problems should be anticipated during spinal procedures for neuromuscular spinal deformity?
    Problems encountered during operative procedures for children with neuromuscular spinal deformities include excessive blood loss, malignant hyperthermia, cardiac dysfunction, hypotension, coagulopathy, latex allergy, and difficulty with monitoring neurologic function.

12. What postoperative problems should be anticipated after spinal procedures for neuromuscular spinal deformities?
    Pulmonary dysfunction (atelectasis, pneumonia, aspiration, and the need for postoperative ventilator support), intravascular fluid shifts, gastrointestinal dysfunction, poor wound healing, and postoperative wound infection.

SPECIFIC NEUROMUSCULAR DISORDERS

CEREBRAL PALSY

13. Explain how cerebral palsy is defined and outline some important factors associated with the development of scoliosis in this disorder.
    Cerebral palsy is the most common neuromuscular disorder in children and the most common cause of neuromuscular scoliosis. Cerebral palsy is defined as a group of permanent disorders that affect the development of movement and posture, causing activity limitation, which are attributed to nonprogressive disturbances that occurred in the developing fetal or infant brain. The motor disorders of cerebral palsy are often accompanied by disturbances of sensation, perception, cognition, communication, and behavior, epilepsy, and secondary musculoskeletal problems, which manifest throughout life. (1) Various criteria are used for classification of cerebral palsy, including the pattern of limb involvement (monoplegia, hemiplegia, quadriplegia, diplegia, triplegia, double hemiplegia), muscle tone and movement pattern (spastic, athetoid, ataxic, mixed types), and motor impairment based on assessment of self-initiated movement according to the five-level Gross Motor Function Classification System (GMFCS):
    GMFCS I: Walk without limitations
    GMFCS II: Walk with limitations

GMFCS III: Walk using a handheld mobility device
GMFCS IV: Self-mobility with limitations; may use powered mobility
GMFCS V: Transported in a manual wheelchair

The incidence and degree of scoliosis correlates with patient age and GMFCS. At age 10, the incidence of moderate or severe scoliosis has been reported as: GMFCS I or II, 1%; GMFCS III, 5%; GMFCS IV, 10%; and GMFCS V, 30%. At age 20, the incidence of moderate or severe scoliosis has been reported as: GMFCS I or II, 5%; GMFCS III, 30%; GMFCS IV, 45%; and GMFCS V, 80%. (2)

14. **Discuss some important considerations regarding surgical treatment of scoliosis secondary to cerebral palsy.**
Surgical intervention is generally considered for patients with scoliosis secondary to cerebral palsy with curves between 50° and 70°. Recent data for patients with cerebral palsy scoliosis showed no clear benefits to operating on curves less than 70° compared with 70°–90°, although delaying surgery beyond 90° is associated with increased risks. (3) Curves are classified based on curve pattern (single vs. double curve) and the presence or absence of pelvic obliquity. The most commonly performed surgical procedure is a long posterior fusion with segmental fixation from T2 to the pelvis. Instrumentation options include pedicle screw-based constructs or posterior hybrid constructs comprised of a combination of hooks, sublaminar wires or bands, and pedicle screws. Distal pelvic fixation options include iliac bolts or S2 alar-iliac screws. If the deformity fails to correct on side-bending or traction radiograph to less than 70°, an anterior release is considered. Curves that remain rigid following anterior release are candidates for an apical vertebral resection. Curves greater than 90° often require complex surgery, including combined anterior and posterior approaches, Ponte osteotomies, and vertebral column resections (Fig. 40.1).

DUCHENNE MUSCULAR DYSTROPHY

15. **What is Duchenne muscular dystrophy?**
Duchenne muscular dystrophy is the most common form of muscular dystrophy and is the most common hereditary neuromuscular disorder. It is an X-linked recessive disorder resulting from mutation in the dystrophin gene. Progressive muscle weakness develops in affected males between 3 and 5 years of age leading to inability to ambulate. Patients typically become wheelchair bound between 10 and 12 years of age and develop scoliosis due to muscle weakness during this time.

16. **What is the role of surgery for scoliosis associated with Duchenne muscular dystrophy?**
Because scoliosis is rapidly progressive and is associated with loss of vital capacity in patients with Duchenne muscular dystrophy, surgical correction and stabilization is advised to prevent pulmonary impairment once the curve is greater than 20°. Treatment consists of posterior spinal instrumentation and fusion from T2 to L5 or the

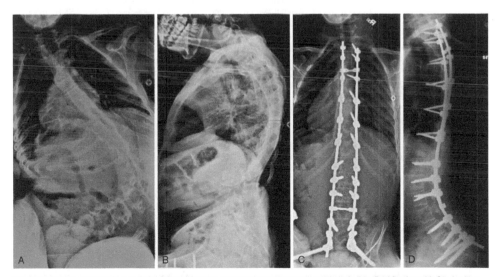

Fig. 40.1 This 13-year-old with cerebral palsy underwent posterior fusion and instrumentation, including distal fixation with S2 alar-iliac screws. (A) Preoperative posteroanterior (PA) and (B) lateral radiographs. (C) Postoperative PA and (D) lateral radiographs. Pelvic obliquity was corrected from 27° to 3° and the coronal curve was corrected from 100° to 8°. (From Jain A, Kebaish KM, Sponseller PD. Sacral-alar-iliac fixation in pediatric deformity: Radiographic outcomes and complications. Spine Deform 2016;4:224–229, Fig. 1, p. 226.)

pelvis with segmental fixation. The distal extent of instrumentation and fusion is limited to L5 in patients with mild curves without significant pelvic obliquity (<10°–15°). Patients with larger curves (>40°) or significant pelvic obliquity are instrumented and fused to the pelvis. Recent studies support the administration of glucocorticoids to prolong ambulatory ability and decrease the need for surgery for treatment of scoliosis. Comorbidities associated with Duchenne muscular dystrophy include cardiomyopathy, cardiac arrhythmias, nutritional compromise, risk of malignant hyperthermia, and preoperative respiratory compromise.

SPINAL MUSCULAR ATROPHY

17. What is spinal muscular atrophy?

Spinal muscular atrophy (SMA) is an autosomal recessive disorder associated with loss of anterior horn cells in the spinal cord and brain stem. It is the most common genetic cause of mortality during childhood with an incidence of 1:10,000 births. SMA is caused by a deletion or mutation of the survival motor neuron (SMN) 1 gene located on chromosome 5q, which leads to inadequate levels of SMN protein, which is critical to the maintenance and survival of motor neurons. Characteristic clinical features of SMA include proximal muscle weakness, progressive muscle atrophy, respiratory and swallowing difficulty, scoliosis, joint contractures, and difficulty with activities, including sitting, standing, and walking. Patients generally have normal intelligence and preservation of sensory function.

SMA is classified into various subtypes based on age at symptom onset and disease severity:

- **SMA type I** (Werdnig Hoffmann disease, acute infantile form): This is the most common (60%) and most severe form. Disease onset occurs by 6 months of age. Symptoms include muscle weakness, lack of development of head control, and inability to sit unassisted. Death usually occurs within the second year of life due to respiratory problems.
- **SMA type II** (Dubowitz intermediate or chronic infantile form): Responsible for approximately 30% of cases. Disease onset occurs between 6 and 18 months of age. Symptoms are less severe compared with SMA type 1. Patients develop the ability to sit without support but do not ambulate. Hip dislocations, scoliosis, and respiratory complications are common, but life expectancy can extend to the fifth decade depending on the degree of respiratory compromise.
- **SMA type III** (Kugelberg-Welander disease, chronic juvenile form): Less common (<15%) with disease onset after 18 months but before 3 years of age. Initial symptoms include proximal muscle weakness. Patients are initially able to stand and walk during childhood but progress to use of a wheelchair during adolescence. Complications include joint contractures, scoliosis, and respiratory issues. Life expectancy is normal.
- **SMA type IV** (adult form): Rare condition with onset in second or third decade of life. Presents with mild to moderate proximal leg muscle weakness. Life expectancy is usually not affected.

18. What medical treatments are available for treatment of spinal muscular atrophy?

Identification of the SMN protein has led to the development of new medical treatments. Two SMN genes code for SMN protein and are identified as SMN1 and SMN2. The SMN1 gene codes for a full-length version of SMN protein, which is integral to maintenance of motor neurons. Although the SMN2 gene also codes for SMN protein, the majority of the SMN2 pre-mRNA lacks exon 7, which leads to production of an unstable, nonfunctional, truncated variant of the SMN protein. However, a small amount of functional SMN protein is still produced by SMN2. The amount of functional SMN protein that is produced is not adequate to avoid SMA but is sufficient to affect the type and severity of SMA. In the absence of SMN1, the number of SMN2 gene copies influences the presentation of SMA by acting as a phenotypic modifier. The more copies of SMN2, the less severe the phenotype. Approximately 90% of SMA type I patients have two copies of SMN2, 85% of SMA type II patients have three SMN2 copies, while SMA type III patients present with three or four SMN2 copies, and SMA type IV patients present with four SMN2 copies. Two new medical therapies have been introduced for SMA: SPINRAZA (nusinersen) and ZOLGENSMA (onasemnogene abeparvovec-xioi).

SPINRAZA is a SMN2-directed antisense oligonucleotide (ASO) administered by intrathecal injection (four initial doses administered over 2 months followed by maintenance doses every 4 months) and indicated for the treatment of pediatric and adult patients with SMA. SPINRAZA binds to the SMN2 pre-mRNA and promotes the inclusion of exon 7 in the mRNA transcript, with the goal of increasing the production of functional SMN protein.

ZOLGENSMA is an adeno-associated virus vector-based gene therapy designed to deliver a functional copy of the SMN1 gene, which encodes SMN protein. A single dose is administered intravenously as a one-time treatment for pediatric SMA patients less than 2 years of age. Presently, this gene therapy treatment is considered the most expensive drug therapy in the world.

19. Discuss important aspects regarding management of scoliosis associated with spinal muscular atrophy.

Development of scoliosis is common in patients with SMA and linked to the severity and type of SMA. All patients with type I or type II SMA and 50% of patients with type III SMA develop scoliosis. Scoliosis in type II SMA patients generally develops between 2 and 4 years of age, while type III SMA patients who become nonambulators develop scoliosis during adolescence. The most common curve type is a single C-shaped thoracolumbar curve. Brace treatment and wheelchair supports are prescribed for progressive curves to provide trunk support and improve sitting. Brace treatment is also used to delay progression of scoliosis and allow for additional trunk and lung growth prior to spinal fusion surgery, especially in type II patients who develop scoliosis at a very young age. However, brace treatment may not be well tolerated because of underlying respiratory dysfunction due to intercostal muscle and diaphragm weakness and the restrictive effect of bracing on respiratory function. Surgical treatment is indicated for patients with progressive curves greater than 50° despite brace treatment. If possible, surgery is delayed until the patient reaches 10–12 years of age and consists of a long posterior spinal instrumentation and fusion from T2 to the pelvis. For younger patients with spinal deformities that are not adequately controlled with brace treatment or wheelchair modifications, growth-friendly spinal instrumentation techniques may be used to control spinal curvatures and pelvic obliquity while allowing for additional thoracic growth, but are unable to improve the associated collapsing rib cage deformity, termed "parasol rib" deformity because of its similarity to the closing of an umbrella.

MYELODYSPLASIA

20. What is myelomeningocele?
    Myelomeningocele, the most common form of neural tube defect, occurs in approximately one in 3000 live births in the US. Failure of posterior closure of the embryonic neural tube (primary neurulation) results in a persistent neural plate, referred to as the *neural placode*, with protrusion of neural tissue through a defect in the posterior spinal elements with associated cerebrospinal fluid leakage. Etiology is multifactorial, with both genetic and environmental factors associated with this condition. Some identified risk factors include folic acid deficiency, diabetes, obesity, and antiseizure medications. Screening is performed with an ultrasound evaluation. The two treatment options are fetal surgery during pregnancy or postnatal spinal bifida repair, which should be performed within 72 hours following birth. Myelomeningocele is a multisystem problem that is associated with specific central nervous system abnormalities, including hydrocephalus, requiring placement of a ventriculoperitoneal shunt, Arnold-Chiari malformation, syringomyelia, and spinal cord tethering. Neurologic assessment demonstrates sensory and motor deficits related to the location of the lesion, and neurologic status may change over time due to problems such as hydrocephalus resulting from shunt malfunction or the development of spinal cord tethering. Ambulatory potential is related to the neurologic level of involvement. Neurogenic bladder and bowel dysfunction are common. Associated orthopedic problems involving the spine and extremities are ubiquitous. Additional problems in this population include latex allergy, endocrine disorders, osteoporosis, and cognitive deficits.

21. What types of spinal deformities may develop in patients with myelomeningocele?
    Spinal deformities are common in myelomeningocele patients and include scoliosis and kyphotic deformities. Spinal deformities may be developmental (paralytic, occurrence due to the underlying neuromuscular disorder) or congenital (due to anomalous vertebral segmentation or formation).

22. Describe the options for surgical treatment of scoliosis in patients with myelomeningocele.
    Scoliosis occurs in 50%–80% of patients with myelomeningocele, with congenital anomalies responsible for approximately one-third of curves. Bracing is challenging in this population due to multiple factors, including obesity and insensate skin. Bracing does not provide definitive treatment but may be used as a temporizing measure to delay surgery and improve sitting posture. Surgery is often suggested for curve magnitudes greater than 50°. Progressive scoliosis in a child with myelomeningocele warrants further workup, including spinal and brain MRI to rule out problems such as a tethered cord, syringomyelia, or decompensated hydrocephalus. The lack of normal posterior vertebral elements makes achievement of a solid spinal fusion difficult. As a general principle, both anterior and posterior fusion are recommended in regions of the spine where the posterior elements are deficient to maximize fusion success when a definitive fusion is performed. In specific circumstances, successful outcomes are reported with single-stage anterior instrumentation and anterior fusion for treatment of thoracolumbar curves less than 75° in the absence of significant kyphosis or pelvic obliquity. Success with single-stage posterior instrumentation and fusion is challenging due to deficient posterior spinal elements and compromised skin quality. Growth-preserving posterior instrumentation is an option for myelodysplasia patients with early onset spinal deformities.

23. Describe the options for surgical treatment of a rigid thoracolumbar or lumbar kyphotic deformity in a patient with myelomeningocele.
    A rigid kyphotic deformity or gibbus deformity develops in the thoracolumbar or upper lumbar region in approximately 10%–20% of patients with myelomeningocele. Skin breakdown over the apex of the kyphotic deformity, sitting difficulty, and respiratory impairment are indications for treatment with kyphectomy. The procedure involves resection of vertebrae in the region of the apex of the deformity, segmental fixation to any remaining posterior bony structures, and insertion of rods through the S1 foramina on each side, which are contoured with two distal 90° bends to rest on the anterior aspect of the sacrum (Warner-Fackler technique). As the rods are levered downward and secured to the posterior spinal elements with sublaminar wires or screws, the kyphotic deformity is corrected and the pelvis is rotated posteriorly into a more anatomic position. In patients whose spines are still growing, a limited fusion is performed at the apex of the kyphosis and the adjacent spinal regions may be left unfused to allow growth to continue cranially and caudally (modified Fackler or sagittal Shilla technique). Growth-friendly management of gibbus deformity in myelodysplasia has also been described using rib-based distraction to the pelvis without kyphectomy (Figs. 40.2 and 40.3).

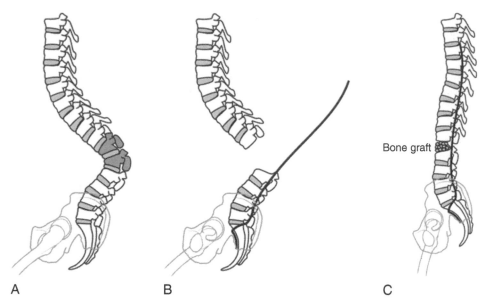

Fig. 40.2 Sagittal diagram describing the sequence for performing kyphectomy. (A) The spine is exposed, the dural sac is mobilized or tied off, and the kyphotic segment of the spine is excised. (B) To improve mobility of the remaining segments, the discs can be excised and the lower two or three pairs of ribs sectioned from their origins. (C) The two segments of the spine are then "folded inward," bone grafted (from the excised segments), and wired to previously contoured rods. (From Newton PO, Faro F, Wenger D, et al. Neuromuscular scoliosis. In: Herkowitz HN, Garfin SR, Eismont FJ, et al., editors. Rothman and Simeone the Spine. 5th ed. Philadelphia, PA: Saunders; 2009, p. 557.)

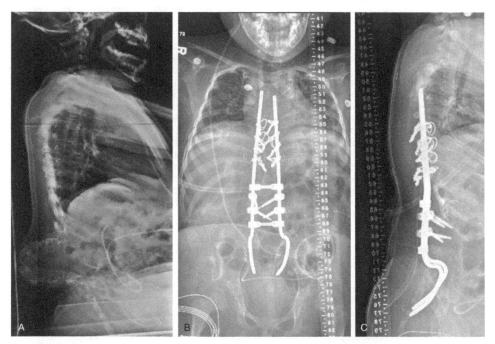

Fig. 40.3 A 6-year-old female patient with myelomeningocele. (A) Preoperative lateral radiograph shows a 135° myelokyphotic curve. (B) Postoperative anteroposterior and (C) lateral radiographs following resection of the L1 and L2 vertebrae and instrumentation using the Fackler or sagittal Shilla technique. (From Margalit A, Sponseller PD. Myelokyphectomy in spina bifida: The modified Fackler or sagittal Shilla technique. Oper Tech Orthop 2016;26:222–228, Fig. 6, p. 226.)

MISCELLANEOUS NEUROMUSCULAR DISORDERS

24. A 6-year-old female patient presents for evaluation to the spine deformity clinic for scoliosis assessment. Her parents describe a history of normal early development over the first year of life but she failed to progress with respect to speech, cognitive development, and ambulation. What genetic disorder should be considered in the differential diagnosis?

Rett syndrome. Rett syndrome is a neurodevelopmental X-linked dominant genetic syndrome affecting females and attributed to a mutation in the methylcytosine-binding protein 2 (MECP2) gene, which is required for normal brain development. Patients appear to initially grow and develop normally until approximately 6–18 months followed by the development of problems related to language, learning, coordination, and movement. Scoliosis is the most common orthopedic condition in Rett syndrome and develops in 75% of patients by age 15 years. Brace treatment is often used initially but does not positively affect the long-term history of scoliosis. A long posterior spinal instrumentation and fusion from the upper thoracic spine to the pelvis is commonly performed for curves that progress to 40°–50°.

25. What curve patterns are most commonly noted in patients with Friedreich ataxia who develop scoliosis?

Friedreich ataxia is a spinal cerebellar degenerative disorder resulting from a mutation in the gene on chromosome 9, which encodes for the protein *frataxin* and is responsible for normal mitochondrial function. Disease transmission occurs in an autosomal recessive pattern. Preoperative assessment of cardiac and respiratory function is important due to an association with cardiomyopathy and restrictive lung disease. Scoliosis develops in a large percentage of patients (63%–100%) and appears similar to idiopathic scoliosis in many patients. Posterior spinal instrumentation and fusion are performed for curves that progress to 40°–50°.

26. A teenager presents with a painful 45° left thoracic curve pattern associated with thoracic kyphosis of 50°. Neurologic examination reveals asymmetric abdominal reflexes and dissociated pain and temperature loss in the extremities. What is the most likely diagnosis?

The radiographic and clinical findings are typical for syringomyelia. Syringomyelia, a fluid-filled cavity within the spinal cord, may lead to a spinal curvature that can be mistakenly attributed to idiopathic scoliosis. Idiopathic thoracic curves are not typically associated with severe pain in adolescence, are convex to the right, and are associated with normal or decreased thoracic kyphosis. MRI is indicated to confirm this diagnosis. A symptomatic syrinx requires surgical treatment, which may improve neurologic deficits and prevent curve progression. Severe curves require surgical correction and fusion.

27. What is the most significant risk factor for the development of spinal deformity in a patient who sustains a traumatic complete spinal cord injury?

The *age at injury* is the most significant risk factor for development of spinal deformity. The incidence of spinal deformity after spinal cord injury has been reported as 100% in patients injured before 10 years of age. Various studies have reported that scoliosis developed in 97% of patients injured before the adolescent growth spurt and in 50% of those injured after their growth spurt. Prophylactic bracing should be used to attempt to slow deformity progression in young patients. Surgical treatment utilizing the surgical principles for treatment of neuromuscular spinal deformities is indicated for large or progressive deformities.

KEY POINTS

1. Neuromuscular disorders frequently result in severe spinal deformities that are challenging to treat and associated with high complication rates following surgical treatment.
2. Evaluation of the patient with a neuromuscular spinal deformity requires assessment of the underlying disease process in combination with the spinal deformity.
3. Surgical treatment of neuromuscular spinal deformities has the potential to improve the patient's functional ability and quality of life, as well as provide improved caregiver satisfaction.

Websites
1. Neuromuscular scoliosis: https://emedicine.medscape.com/article/1266097-overview
2. Neuromuscular scoliosis: https://www.srs.org/patients-and-families/conditions-and-treatments/parents/scoliosis/neuromuscular-scoliosis

REFERENCES

1. Rosenbaum, P., Paneth, N., Leviton, A., Goldstein, M., Bax, M., Damiano, D., et al. A report: The definition and classification of cerebral palsy April 2006. (2007). *Developmental medicine and child neurology Supplement, 109*, 8–14.
2. Hägglund, G., Pettersson, K., Czuba, T., Persson-Bunke, M., & Rodby-Bousquet, E. (2018). Incidence of scoliosis in cerebral palsy: A population-based study of 962 young individuals. *Acta Orthopaedica, 89*, 443–447.
3. Hollenbeck, S. M., Yaszay, B., Sponseller, P. D., et al. (2019). The pros and cons of operating early versus late in the progression of cerebral palsy scoliosis. *Spine Deformity, 7*, 489–493.

BIBLIOGRAPHY

1. Buchowski, J. M., Bhatnagar, R., Skaggs, D. L., & Sponseller, P. D. (2006). Temporary internal distraction as an aid to correction of severe scoliosis. *Journal of Bone and Joint Surgery American, 88*, 2035–2041.
2. Hägglund, G., Pettersson, K., Czuba, T., Persson-Bunke, M., Rodby-Bousquet, E. (2018). Incidence of scoliosis in cerebral palsy: A population-based study of 962 young individuals. *Acta Orthopaedica, 89*, 443–447.
3. Hollenbeck, S. M., Yaszay, B., Sponseller, P. D., Bartley, C. E., Shah, S. A., Asghar, J., et al. (2019). The pros and cons of operating early versus late in the progression of cerebral palsy scoliosis. *Spine Deformity, 7*, 489–493.
4. Keeler, K. A., Lenke, L. G., Good, C. R., Bridwell, K. H., Sides, B., Luhmann, S. J. (2010). Spinal fusion for spastic neuromuscular scoliosis—is anterior releasing necessary when intraoperative halo-femoral traction is used? *Spine, 35*, 427–433.
5. Lebel, D. E., Corston, J. A., McAdam, L. C., Bigger, W. D., & Alman, B. A. (2013). Glucocorticoid treatment for the prevention of scoliosis in children with Duchenne muscular dystrophy. *Journal of Bone and Joint Surg American, 95*, 1057–1061.
6. McElroy, M. J., Sponseller, P. D., Dattilo, J. R., Thompson, G. H., Akbarnia, B. A., Shah, S. A., et al. (2012). Growing rods for the treatment of scoliosis in children with cerebral palsy. *Spine, 37*, 1504–1510.
7. Newton, P. O., Jankowski, P. P., & Yaszay, B. Neuromuscular scoliosis. In S. R. Garfin, F. J. Eismont, G. R. Bell, et al. (Eds.), *Rothman-Simeone The Spine* (pp. 469–507). 7th ed. Philadelphia, PA: Saunders; 2018.
8. Rosenbaum, P., Paneth, N., Leviton, A., Goldstein, M., Bax, M., Damiano, D., et al. (2007). A report: The definition and classification of cerebral palsy April 2006. *Developmental Medicine and Child Neurology Supplement, 109*, 8–14.

CHAPTER 41

SAGITTAL PLANE DEFORMITIES IN PEDIATRIC PATIENTS

Owoicho Adogwa, MD, MPH, Munish C. Gupta, MD, and Vincent J. Devlin, MD

BACKGROUND

1. **Describe how sagittal plane alignment of the cervical, thoracic, and lumbar spine changes from birth to adulthood.**

   The sagittal alignment of the spine is dynamic and changes with age. In newborns the spinal column possesses a single C-shaped sagittal curve. Cervical lordosis develops as an infant gains independent head control and lumbar lordosis develops with progression to standing and walking. Young children have positive sagittal balance as noted by the forward displacement of the C7 plumb line relative to the anterior-superior corner of the S1 vertebral body. As lumbar lordosis increases during growth, progressive posterior displacement of the C7 plumb line occurs. Additional interactions between spinal and sacropelvic sagittal parameters occur as the child matures toward an adult sagittal alignment profile. In the adult, cervical lordosis measured from the inferior endplate of C2 to inferior endplate of C7 ranges from 30° to 45° and adjusts to maintain the head over the sacrum in the sagittal plane. Thoracic kyphosis measured from T2 to T12 ranges from 20° to 45°. The thoracolumbar junction (T10–L2) is neutrally aligned in the sagittal plane in adults as compared with children who have a slightly kyphotic alignment in this region. Lumbar lordosis measured from the superior endplate of L1 to superior endplate of S1 ranges between 30° and 60°, with most of the curvature occurring between L4 vertebra and the sacrum. In a balanced spine, a line from the center of the C7 vertebral body passes anterior to the thoracic spine, through the center of the L1 vertebral body, posterior to the lumbar spine, through the lumbosacral disc, and between S2 and the femoral heads.

2. **What are the causes of pediatric sagittal plane deformities?**

   A wide range of conditions are responsible for pediatric sagittal plane deformities (Table 41.1).

3. **What factors are used to classify the various types of thoracolumbar kyphotic deformities and guide surgical treatment?**

   Thoracolumbar kyphotic deformities have been classified by Rajasekaran et al. (1) based on the structural integrity of the anterior and posterior spinal columns.

Table 41.1 Causes of Pediatric Sagittal Plane Deformities.

1. Postural	10. Skeletal dysplasias
2. Scheuermann disease	a. Achondroplasia
3. Congenital	b. Neurofibromatosis
a. Failure of formation	c. Mucopolysaccharidosis
b. Failure of segmentation	11. Collagen diseases
c. Mixed failure	a. Marfan syndrome
4. Posttraumatic	12. Rheumatologic
5. Postsurgical	a. Ankylosing spondylitis
a. Postlaminectomy	13. Postinfectious
b. Junctional kyphosis	a. Bacterial
6. Neuromuscular	b. Fungal
7. Myelomeningocele	c. Tuberculosis
a. Congenital (present at birth)	14. Tumor
b. Developmental (secondary to paralysis)	a. Benign
8. Postirradiation	b. Malignant
9. Metabolic	i. Primary
a. Osteoporosis	ii. Metastatic
b. Osteogenesis imperfecta	

Type I kyphosis is present when both the anterior and posterior spinal columns are intact. Type I kyphosis may present with mobile disc spaces (type IA) as seen in Scheuermann kyphosis or with fused disc spaces (type IB) as seen in ankylosing spondylitis.

Type II kyphosis arises due to deficiency of either the anterior (type IIA) or posterior (type IIB) columns. Type IIA kyphosis develops secondary to spinal pathologies such as tumors, infections, and traumatic fractures. Type IIB kyphosis develops due to spinal pathologies such as surgical laminectomy or congenital deformities such as myelomeningocele.

Type III kyphosis is associated with deficiency of both columns and is stratified according to severity as ≤60° (type IIIA), >60° (type IIIB), or severe kyphosis associated with buckling collapse of the spinal column (type IIIC). Etiologies associated with type III kyphosis include congenital anomalies, trauma, neurofibromatosis, and prior spine surgery.

The kyphosis type may be used to guide selection among various surgical osteotomies for treatment of kyphotic deformities, including Ponte osteotomy, pedicle subtraction osteotomy, disc bone osteotomy, single-level vertebrectomy, and multiple-level vertebrectomy.

4. What is the deformity angular ratio?
The **deformity angular ratio (DAR)** is defined as the curve magnitude divided by the number of involved vertebral segments. (2) Patients with a longer, more gradual curve have a lower DAR. Sharp angular deformities, either in the coronal or sagittal plane, are associated with a higher DAR, and are generally more rigid deformities and are often accompanied by neural compression.

POSTURAL KYPHOSIS

5. What is postural kyphosis?
Postural kyphosis is common in adolescence and arises due to slouching or poor posture. The deformity may be corrected by voluntary contraction of back musculature or by lying supine. Patients often report mild backache. Lateral radiographs often show a mildly increased thoracic kyphosis (<60°) without any pathologic vertebral changes such as focal wedging or endplate changes as seen in Scheuermann disease. Treatment consists of reassurance and education of the patient and family as the condition is a cosmetic concern and does not result in long-term problems. Physical therapy for postural and core-strengthening exercises is a treatment option.

SCHEUERMANN KYPHOSIS

6. What is Scheuermann kyphosis and how is this condition diagnosed?
Scheuermann disease is the most common cause of structural thoracic or thoracolumbar hyperkyphosis in adolescents. Onset occurs during the prepubertal growth spurt in 0.4%–10% of adolescents, with males and females affected at similar rates. Although Scheuermann disease was originally attributed to abnormal development of the vertebral ring apophysis, true etiology remains unknown and proposed causes include disordered vertebral endplate endochondral ossification, endocrine abnormalities, genetic factors, and juvenile osteoporosis.

Patients present with thoracic or thoracolumbar deformity and/or back pain. Forward bending will increase kyphotic deformity and patients will be unable to correct the deformity with active trunk extension. A compensatory increase in cervical and lumbar lordosis is common. Patients often have tight hamstrings. Approximately one-third of patients have mild scoliosis in addition to increased kyphosis. The incidence of spondylolysis is also increased in this population.

Radiographic evaluation includes full-length standing posteroanterior (PA) and lateral images and a lateral hyperextension radiograph performed over a radiolucent bolster to assess kyphosis flexibility. On lateral radiographs, characteristic imaging features of Scheuermann disease include: thoracic kyphosis >45°, thoracolumbar kyphosis >30°, anterior wedging of three or more adjacent thoracic vertebrae >5°, vertebral endplate irregularities, Schmorl nodes, and disc space narrowing. The most common deformity pattern (type 1, typical pattern) involves the mid-thoracic region (T7–T9 apex) and is associated with multilevel vertebral wedging. Less commonly, the apex of the kyphotic deformity is located at the thoracolumbar junction (type 2, atypical pattern) and may involve the lumbar spinal region. The term lumbar Scheuermann disease is used to refer to a pattern of involvement limited to the lumbar spine and associated with endplate irregularities, Schmorl nodes, disc space narrowing, and wedging limited to one or two vertebrae. Magnetic resonance imaging (MRI) is not routinely obtained in the absence of neurologic symptoms, or rapidly progressive kyphosis, unless surgical correction of kyphosis is planned (Fig. 41.1).

7. What are the nonsurgical treatment options for Scheuermann kyphosis?
Nonsurgical treatment options include observation, physical therapy, and orthotic treatment. Physical therapy consists of postural, core-strengthening, and hamstring stretching exercises directed toward improving posture and flexibility, and decreasing pain. Brace treatment is considered for patients who are skeletally immature with at least 1 year of growth remaining and a kyphotic deformity <70°, but is poorly tolerated by patients. A deformity

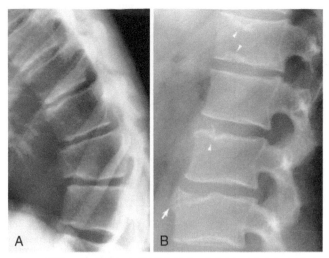

Fig. 41.1 Scheuermann disease. (A) Thoracic spine lateral radiograph. Findings include irregularity in vertebral contour, reactive sclerosis, intervertebral disc space narrowing, anterior vertebral wedging, and kyphosis. (B) Lumbar spine lateral radiograph. Observe the cartilaginous nodes *(arrowheads)* creating surface irregularity, lucent areas, and reactive sclerosis. Anterior disc displacement *(arrow)* has produced an irregular anterosuperior corner of a vertebral body, which is termed a *limbus vertebra.* (From Resnick D, Kransdorf MJ. Bone and Joint Imaging. 3rd ed. Philadelphia, PA: Saunders; 2005.)

with an apex at T9 or above is traditionally treated with a Milwaukee type brace (cervicothoracolumbosacral orthosis [CTLSO]). A thoracolumbar orthosis (TLSO) is considered if the apex is below T9. A period of cast treatment prior to brace treatment may be considered for patients with rigid deformities that show limited passive correction on hyperextension lateral radiographs performed over a bolster.

8. When is surgical treatment indicated for treatment of Scheuermann kyphosis?
   Surgical treatment is considered for thoracic kyphotic deformities >70°–75°, thoracolumbar kyphotic deformities >55°, and for treatment of neurologic deficits due to disc herniation or cord compression. Additional indications for surgery include kyphosis progression despite brace treatment, painful deformities, and deformities associated with an unacceptable cosmetic appearance.

9. What are the surgical options for treatment of Scheuermann kyphosis?
   Current surgical treatment options include single-stage posterior spinal instrumentation and fusion or combined anterior and posterior fusion. A single-stage posterior surgical procedure with multilevel posterior column shortening osteotomies, termed Ponte osteotomies (Fig. 41.2), in combination with pedicle screw-based instrumentation (Fig. 41.3) is commonly performed as this approach avoids the morbidity associated with combined anterior and posterior surgical procedures. In rigid kyphotic deformities, more advanced osteotomy techniques including pedicle subtraction osteotomy or posterior vertebral column resection may be needed if single-stage posterior procedure is performed. Alternatively, for very large or rigid kyphotic deformities, a combined anterior and posterior approach may be utilized and consists of a first-stage anterior release and fusion performed by a transthoracic or thoracoscopic approach prior to posterior fusion and instrumentation.

10. Describe some of the important principles to consider when performing posterior instrumentation and fusion for treatment of Scheuermann kyphosis. What levels should be treated? How much deformity correction should be obtained?
    The instrumentation and fusion should include the entire measured kyphotic deformity. The proximal instrumented vertebra is the proximal vertebra that is most tilted into the kyphosis. The lower instrumented vertebra incorporates the first lordotic disc below the end vertebra of the measured kyphotic deformity and also includes the vertebra touched by a vertical line drawn from the posterior sacrum, termed the *sagittal stable vertebra*. The goal for kyphosis correction is to reduce kyphosis to the upper end of the normal range (45°) and avoid greater than 50% correction of the baseline kyphotic deformity. Following spinal exposure and completion of multilevel Ponte osteotomies around the apex of the kyphotic deformity, correction is performed by applying sequential compression to close the osteotomies and by cantilevering proximally anchored rods into the screws below the apex of the deformity. Avoidance of overcorrection and disruption of soft tissue, ligaments, and facet joints at the

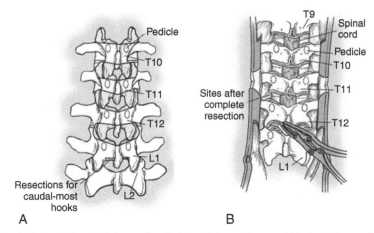

Fig. 41.2 Ponte osteotomies. (A) Broad posterior resection *(shaded parts)* at every intersegmental level extending over the entire area of fusion and instrumentation. (B) Posterior view showing levels of completed resections. Correction is achieved by closing gaps. (From Canale ST, Beaty JH. Campbell's Operative Orthopaedics. 11th ed. Philadelphia, PA: Mosby; 2008. [Redrawn from Ponte A. Posterior column shortening for scheuermann kyphosis. An innovative one-stage technique. In: Haher TR, Merola AA, editors. Surgical Techniques for the Spine. New York: Thieme; 2003.])

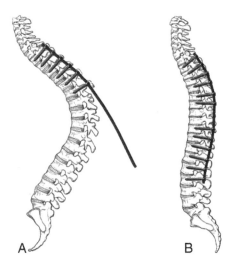

Fig. 41.3 Correction of Scheuermann kyphosis. (A) Rods are contoured to reflect the degree of kyphosis correction desired and connected to screws in the vertebra above the apex of the deformity. (B) Rods are cantilevered into screws in the vertebra distal to the deformity apex to achieve correction. (From Errico TJ, Lonner BS, Moulton AW. Surgical Management of Spinal Deformities. Philadelphia, PA: Saunders; 2009.)

transition between instrumented and noninstrumented spinal levels are important technique-related factors that decrease the risk of junctional deformities (Fig. 41.4).

11. What complications are associated with surgical treatment of Scheuermann kyphosis?
Surgical treatment of Scheuermann kyphosis is associated with major complications. Studies have reported a complication rate of 14% in conjunction with the operative treatment of Scheuermann kyphosis. Complications include:
- Surgical site infection
- Instrumentation-related complications
- Neurologic complications
- Reoperations
- Proximal junctional kyphosis
- Distal junctional kyphosis
- Pseudarthrosis

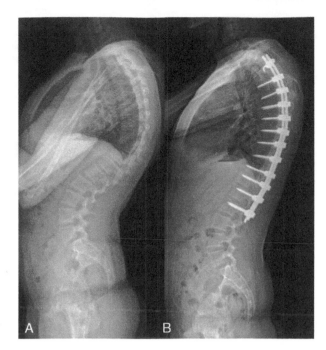

Fig. 41.4 (A) Preoperative standing lateral radiograph of a 17-year-old boy with a painful thoracic kyphosis due to Scheuermann disease (B) Postoperative standing lateral radiograph following treatment with multiple Ponte osteotomies and posterior spinal instrumentation.

CONGENITAL KYPHOSIS

12. Describe the different types of congenital kyphosis.

Congenital kyphosis is due to abnormal embryologic development of the spine leading to vertebral anomalies, which, although present at birth, may not be clinically evident. Three types of deformities are identified. **Type I** is a failure of formation of part or all of the vertebral body. Types of vertebral malformations include posterolateral quadrant vertebrae, posterior hemivertebrae, butterfly vertebrae, and anterior or anterolateral wedged vertebrae. Type I deformities are most common, and occur most frequently in the upper thoracic and thoracolumbar region. **Type II** is a failure of vertebral body segmentation resulting in an anterior unsegmented bar or block vertebra, and occur most commonly in the lower thoracic or thoracolumbar region. **Type III** is a mixed failure of formation and segmentation. Depending on the pattern of vertebral involvement, kyphosis or a combination of kyphosis and scoliosis may develop. Type I deformities are attributed to incomplete vascularization of the cartilaginous centrum of the vertebral body during its development. Type II deformities are attributed to anomalous ossification involving the anterior portion of the annulus fibrosus (see Chapter 39).

13. What is the natural history of congenital kyphosis?

The natural history of congenital kyphosis depends on several factors, including the type of deformity, number of vertebral levels involved, location of deformity, patient age, and amount of growth remaining. Type I deformities progress rapidly (6°–7° per year) and have a higher risk of neurologic deterioration and worse prognosis than type II deformities. If left untreated, type I deformities may result in paraplegia as they lead to an acute angular deformity and spinal cord compression. Neurologic deficits develop most commonly during the adolescent growth spurt, although paraplegia may occur earlier. Type II deformities progress more slowly (4°–5° per year) and rarely cause neurologic compromise as the deformity is less acutely angulated. Type III deformities may also progress rapidly and lead to neurologic compromise.

14. Why is it important to perform a systematic and comprehensive evaluation and follow-up of a patient with congenital kyphosis?

As with other types of congenital spinal deformities, patients often have other associated anomalies within or outside the spinal column. These include cardiac, chest, and renal anomalies, Klippel-Feil syndrome, and intraspinal anomalies, including diastematomyelia, tethered cord, and syringomyelia. In addition to a thorough neurologic examination, MRI of the entire neural axis, cardiac echocardiogram, and renal ultrasound are indicated. Patients require serial radiographic monitoring as deformity progression is insidious, and detection requires comparison of current radiographs with previous and initial radiographs. During periods of rapid spinal growth, more frequent evaluations are prudent as deformity progression is more likely.

15. **What is the role of nonoperative treatment in management of congenital kyphosis?**
    Nonoperative treatment plays a limited role in management of congenital kyphosis and consists of serial observation to monitor for deformity progression and development of neurologic symptoms. Brace or cast treatment are ineffective as these treatments do not prevent deformity progression or provide long-term correction. Surgery is the primary treatment for congenital kyphosis.

16. **What surgical procedures are indicated for treatment of congenital kyphosis?**
    Decisions regarding surgery depend on multiple factors, including the type of malformation, patient age, deformity magnitude, and whether spinal cord compression or neurologic symptoms are present.
    For type I deformities, early surgery is indicated. Posterior in-situ fusion is an option for children under 5 years of age with a kyphosis measuring less than 50°. Postoperatively, patients may be immobilized in a hyperextension cast for several months followed by a period of brace immobilization. For more severe deformities, anterior and posterior fusion is performed with or without resection of the vertebral malformation, and may include use of spinal instrumentation. For older children and adults, anterior and posterior fusion is performed. Symptomatic neural decompression at the apex of the kyphosis requires decompression. One option is to perform separate anterior and posterior procedures. The anterior surgery involves anterior resection and strut grafting, and is followed by posterior surgery with posterior fusion and spinal instrumentation. Alternatively, a circumferential decompression and fusion, resection of the anomalous vertebra, and posterior instrumentation may be performed through a single-stage posterior surgical approach (Fig. 41.5). This technique is referred to as a vertebral column resection (VCR).
    Type II deformities progress at a slower rate and are associated with a lower risk of neurologic injury compared with type I deformities. Young patients with mild deformities are treated with posterior fusion while older children with larger deformities may be treated with anterior osteotomy and fusion in combination with posterior instrumentation and fusion, or by a single-stage posterior resection and fusion procedure.

MISCELLANEOUS PEDIATRIC SAGITTAL PLANE DEFORMITIES

17. **What is the cause of congenital lordosis?**
    Congenital lordosis is a rare disorder caused by failure of posterior segmentation, typically spanning multiple segments, which develops in an immature patient due to continued anterior spinal growth. When this anomaly occurs

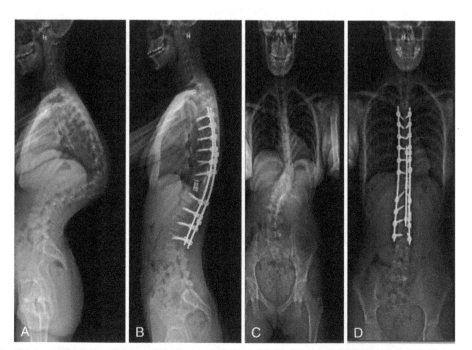

Fig. 41.5 Preoperative and postoperative radiographs of a 14-year-old female with severe congenital kyphoscoliosis of the thoracolumbar spine with an apex at T9. Treatment consisted of posterior vertebral column resection and posterior spinal instrumentation and fusion. (A) Preoperative lateral radiograph. (B) Postoperative lateral radiograph. (C) Preoperative PA radiograph. (D) Postoperative PA radiograph.

in the thoracic region, it may lead to a deformity that causes decrease of the spine-sternal distance and restriction of pulmonary function. Depending on the location of the posterior segmentation anomaly, lordosis, or lordoscoliosis may develop. Congenital lordosis is less common than congenital scoliosis or congenital kyphosis and less frequently associated with neurologic deficits.

18. Describe treatment options for congenital lordosis.

When congenital lordosis is diagnosed early in life, surgical treatment consists of anterior spinal fusion to eliminate anterior growth potential. Patients presenting later in life require more complex surgery. Moderate deformities may be treated with wide posterior release followed by segmental instrumentation and fusion. Severe deformities require circumferential surgery. One option is to perform separate anterior and posterior procedures. This option includes anterior closing-wedge osteotomies and posterior segmental spinal instrumentation and fusion with or without rib resections to enhance correction. Alternatively, a single-stage posterior VCR is an option for select deformities. Preoperative assessment of pulmonary function is important as associated pulmonary hypertension increases mortality and may be a contraindication to surgery.

19. Is thoracic hypokyphosis commonly present in adolescent idiopathic scoliosis?

Yes. Loss of thoracic kyphosis has been identified as an early finding in patients with adolescent idiopathic scoliosis. However, sagittal plane analysis using PA and lateral spine radiographs is limited by distortion caused by malrotation of vertebrae out of the imaging plane. With the introduction of three-dimensional (3D) upright imaging using biplanar slot scanning (EOS imaging), it is possible to adequately evaluate the spine in 3D. Sullivan and colleagues (3) reported that increasing curvature in the coronal plane is correlated with progressive loss of thoracic kyphosis in patients with idiopathic scoliosis. There is a subgroup of patients with severe hypokyphosis or actual lordosis of the thoracic spine. Thoracic lordosis is a contraindication to brace treatment of idiopathic scoliosis. In patients with progressive thoracic lordosis or lordosis in excess of −10°, with or without scoliosis, surgical treatment is considered, even if the coronal plane Cobb measurement is less than 40°.

20. What are the indications for surgical correction of a gibbus associated with myelomeningocele?

A sharply angulated short-segment kyphotic deformity involving the thoracolumbar or lumbar region, referred to as a gibbus deformity, develops in approximately 15% of pediatric patients with myelomeningocele. Surgical treatment is indicated for skin breakdown over the apex of the gibbus, difficulty maintaining an upright sitting posture, respiratory compromise due to abdominal cavity compression and/or impaired diaphragm function, pain attributed to rib impingement on the iliac crests, and progressive kyphotic deformity. Surgical treatment options include kyphectomy or vertebral decancellation in combination with posterior spinal instrumentation with or without fusion. In young children, minimally invasive surgery using the vertical expandable prosthetic titanium rib (VEPTR) device as a rib-to-pelvis construct is an option for treatment of the growing child with flexible deformities.

21. What is the most common sagittal plane deformity associated with achondroplasia?

Thoracolumbar kyphosis is the most common sagittal plane deformity in patients with achondroplasia. Achondroplasia is the most common skeletal dysplasia and the most common form of dwarfism. Its cause is a mutation in the fibroblast growth factor receptor (FGFR) gene on chromosome 4p and leads to impairment of endochondral ossification. Achondroplasia manifests as a rhizomelic pattern of limb shortening associated with lower extremity angular deformities, elbow deformities, thoracolumbar kyphosis, foramen magnum stenosis, lumbar spinal stenosis, and hyperlordosis. Increased kyphosis is often evident at birth, progresses as the child begins to sit, and resolves in approximately 70% of cases with ambulation. Radiographs show anterior wedging at the apex of the deformity. Progression can lead to a focal kyphosis and neural compression, which may be masked by associated lumbar spinal stenosis.

22. What are the nonoperative and surgical options for management of achondroplastic thoracolumbar kyphosis?

Newborn infants with achondroplasia commonly demonstrate a thoracolumbar kyphosis in the range of 20° that resolves in many patients by age 12–18 months. Parents are advised to avoid unsupported sitting as this is associated with progressive kyphosis. A thoracolumbar orthosis is considered for children aged 3 years and older in whom the kyphosis does not resolve with ambulation. Surgical treatment is reserved for children with progressive deformity, thoracolumbar kyphosis greater than 50° at age 5 years and older, or neural compromise attributed to compression in the kyphotic region. Surgical treatment options include posterior spinal instrumentation and fusion using pedicle fixation with or without anterior fusion and decompression of symptomatic neural compression. Spinal implants that enter the spinal canal (hooks, wires) are contraindicated due to associated spinal stenosis and lack of space within the spinal canal.

23. What factors contribute to the development of postlaminectomy kyphosis?

In the pediatric population, laminectomies are performed most commonly for treatment of children with tumors and dysraphism. Instability after facetectomy, hypermobility associated with removal of the posterior osteoligamentous structures, and growth disturbance contribute to the development of postlaminectomy kyphosis.

Postlaminectomy kyphosis is associated with younger age, multilevel laminectomies, and surgery in the upper thoracic and cervical spine.

24. **How can postlaminectomy deformity be avoided or treated?**
Maintenance of the facet joints, laminoplasty in lieu of laminectomy, and postoperative bracing may help stabilize the spine following posterior surgery. If wide decompression is required or if progressive spinal deformity develops, posterior fusion and stabilization are required.

25. **How is tuberculosis of the spine uniquely associated with thoracolumbar kyphosis in children?**
The three patterns of spinal involvement by tuberculosis are central, peridiscal, and anterior. Among those, central lesions are most common in children while peridiscal involvement is most common among adults. Central lesions generally involve the whole vertebral body and lead to bony collapse and kyphotic deformity. The thoracolumbar junction is the most common location affected by spinal tuberculosis. When multiple levels are involved, healing can lead to anterior bony bridging and worsening of the kyphotic deformity with growth.

26. **What types of fractures may lead to posttraumatic kyphosis in children?**
Flexion-compression, burst, and flexion-distraction (seat-belt) type injuries can cause acute kyphosis in the pediatric spine patient. Growth disturbances may lead to late deformity. The risk of disrupting growth potential must be considered in planning operative versus nonsurgical treatment. Traumatic paralysis often results in neuromuscular kyphosis that does not respond to brace treatment and requires spinal instrumentation and fusion.

KEY POINTS

1. The sagittal alignment of the spine is dynamic and changes from birth to maturity.
2. The causes of pediatric kyphotic deformities are wide-ranging and include poor posture, Scheuermann disease, congenital anomalies, skeletal dysplasias, neuromuscular disorders, trauma, infections, and tumors.

Websites
1. Pediatric Orthopaedic Society of North America, Study Guide, Spine Topics: https://posna.org/Physician-Education/Study-Guide?categoryname=Spine
2. Lenke LG, Makhni MC: Lumbar Spine Online Textbook. Osteotomies for rigid spinal deformity: evaluation, indications and technique: http://www.wheelessonline.com/ISSLS/section-9-chapter-8-osteotomies-for-rigid-spinal-deformity-evaluation-indications-and-techniques/

REFERENCES
1. Rajasekaran, S., Rajoli, S. R., Aiyer, S. N., Kanna, R., & Shetty, A. P. (2018). A classification for kyphosis based on column deficiency, curve magnitude, and osteotomy requirement. *Journal of Bone and Joint Surgery American, 100*(13), 1147–1156.
2. Lewis, N. D., Keshen, S. G., Lenke, L. G., Zywiel, M. G., Skaggs, D. L., Dear, T. E., et al. (2015). The deformity angular ratio: Does it correlate with high-risk cases for potential spinal cord monitoring alerts in pediatric 3-column thoracic spinal deformity corrective surgery? *Spine, 40*(15), E879–E885.
3. Sullivan, T. B., Reighard, F. G., Osborn, E. J., Parvaresh, K. C., & Newton, P. O. (2017). Thoracic idiopathic scoliosis severity is highly correlated with 3D measures of thoracic kyphosis. *Journal of Bone and Joint Surgery American, 99*(11), e54.

BIBLIOGRAPHY
1. Agabegi, S. S., Thawrani, D. P., & Crawford, A. H. (2018). Pediatric Kyphosis: Scheuermann Disease and Congenital Deformity. In S. R. Garfin, F. J. Eismont, G. R. Bell, et al, (Eds.), *Rothman-Simeone the Spine* (7th ed., pp. 525–547). Philadelphia, PA: Saunders.
2. Johnston, C. E. (2014). Kyphosis. In J. A. Herring (Ed.), *Tachdjian's Pediatric Orthopaedics* (5th ed., pp. 308–327). Philadelphia, PA: Saunders.
3. Lonner, B. S., Toombs, C. S., Guss, M., Braaksma, B., Shah, S. A., Samdani, A., et al. (2015). Complications in operative Scheuermann kyphosis: Do the pitfalls differ from operative adolescent idiopathic scoliosis? *Spine, 40*(5), 305–311.
4. Lewis, N. D., Keshen, S. G., Lenke, L. G., Zywiel, M. G., Skaggs, D. L., Dear, T. E., et al. (2015). The deformity angular ratio: Does it correlate with high-risk cases for potential spinal cord monitoring alerts in pediatric 3-column thoracic spinal deformity corrective surgery? *Spine, 40*(15), E879–E885.
5. McMaster, M. J., & Singh, H. (2001). The surgical management of congenital kyphosis and kyphoscoliosis. *Spine, 26*(19), 2146–2154.
6. Murray, P. M., Weinstein, S. L., & Spratt, K. F. (1993). The natural history and long-term follow-up of Scheuermann kyphosis. *Journal of Bone and Joint Surgery, 75*(2), 236–248.

7. Sardar, Z. M., Ames, R. J., & Lenke, L. (2019). Scheuermann kyphosis: diagnosis, management, and selecting fusion levels. *Journal of the American Academy of Orthopaedic Surgeons, 27*(10), e462–e472.
8. Rajasekaran, S., Rajoli, S. R., Aiyer, S. N., Kanna, R., & Shetty, A. P. (2018). A classification for kyphosis based on column deficiency, curve magnitude, and osteotomy requirement. *Journal of Bone and Joint Surgery American, 100*(13), 1147–1156.
9. Shirley, E. D., & Ain, M. C. (2009). Achondroplasia: manifestations and treatment. *Journal of the American Academy of Orthopaedic Surgeons, 17*(4), 231–241.
10. Sullivan, T. B., Reighard, F. G., Osborn, E. J., Parvaresh, K. C., & Newton, P. O. (2017). Thoracic idiopathic scoliosis severity is highly correlated with 3D measures of thoracic kyphosis. *Journal of Bone and Joint Surgery American, 99*(11), E54.

CHAPTER 42

SPONDYLOLYSIS AND SPONDYLOLISTHESIS IN PEDIATRIC PATIENTS

Vincent J. Devlin, MD

DEFINITIONS

1. Define spondylolysis.
   Spondylolysis is a unilateral or bilateral defect in the region of the pars interarticularis that may or may not be accompanied by vertebral displacement. The origin of the term *spondylolysis* is from the Greek words *spondylo* (vertebra) and *lysis* (break or defect).

2. Define spondylolisthesis.
   Spondylolisthesis refers to anterior displacement of the cranial vertebral body in relation to the subjacent vertebral body. The origin of the term is from the Greek words *spondylo* (vertebra) and *olisthesis* (movement or slippage). The deformity not only involves the olisthetic vertebra but affects the entire spinal column above the level of slippage as the entire trunk moves forward with the displaced vertebra. Slippages <50% are referred to as low-grade spondylolisthesis while slippages ≥50% are referred to as high-grade spondylolisthesis.

3. Define spondyloptosis.
   Spondyloptosis refers to a slippage of the L5 vertebra in which the entire vertebral body of L5 is located below the top of S1. It is the most severe degree of slippage possible. Fortunately, this condition is quite rare. The origin of the term is from the Greek words *spondylo* (vertebra) and *ptosis* (to fall).

SPONDYLOLYSIS

4. What is the current state of evidence regarding the etiology and prevalence of pediatric lumbar spondylolysis?
   Evidence supports that pediatric spondylolysis is an acquired fracture of the pars interarticularis, which may occur unilaterally or bilaterally. The prevalence of spondylolysis in the general pediatric population is between 3% and 7%. Variability exists in the prevalence of spondylolysis. Spondylolysis does not occur in a uniform distribution across populations and is more common in males than females, in the offspring of first-degree relatives with the condition, and in certain ethnic groups, with the highest prevalence in the Eskimo population (28%). Spondylolysis is the most common diagnosis in pediatric athletes presenting with low back pain, especially those who participate in sports requiring repetitive hyperextension.

5. Describe common symptoms and physical examination findings in a pediatric patient who presents with symptomatic spondylolysis.
   Patients may present with localized acute or chronic low back pain. Pain is usually exacerbated with activity and hyperextension. Pain may radiate to the buttocks or posterior thighs. Radicular symptoms are uncommon, but may occur. Findings that may be present on physical examination include localized tenderness to palpation, back pain exacerbated by hyperextension and rotation, and a positive single-leg hyperextension test.

6. What imaging studies are indicated for evaluation of a patient with suspected spondylolysis?
   Initial radiographic assessment should consist of standing posteroanterior (PA) and lateral lumbosacral radiographs or low-dose slot scanner images. Oblique views of the lumbosacral region are not indicated as they do not improve diagnostic sensitivity or specificity and increase radiation exposure. For patients who require additional imaging studies, magnetic resonance imaging (MRI) or computed tomography (CT) are preferred as the next imaging test after radiographs rather than a bone scan with single-photon emission CT (SPECT), which is associated with substantial radiation exposure. Literature recommends choosing the subsequent imaging modality based on the time course of symptoms, and supports use of MRI in patients with early symptoms, and CT in patients with persistent symptoms.

7. **What are the advantages and disadvantages of CT for the assessment of spondylolysis?**
CT plays a role when a pars defect is suspected on a clinical basis but is not evident on plain radiographs or MRI. CT remains the optimal test for assessment of osseous anatomy. However, CT is unable to identify early-stage acute stress reactions involving the pars interarticularis associated with marrow edema or microtrabecular fracture. A limited-window CT scan provides a lower radiation dose than a bone scan and similar radiation dose to oblique lumbar radiographs. However, to minimize radiation exposure from CT for the pediatric patient it is necessary to utilize a low-dose protocol and restrict the scan to the anatomic region of interest.

8. **What are the advantages and disadvantages of MRI in the assessment of spondylolysis?**
Advantages of MRI compared with plain radiography include increased sensitivity, ability to visualize soft tissue and neural structures in multiple planes, and lack of exposure to ionizing radiation. MRI is able to identify early stress reactions involving the pars region, as well as chronic pars defects, evaluate associated lumbar disc pathology, and can rule out other serious causes of back pain, such as tumors or infection. However, the sensitivity of MRI is highly dependent on the specific imaging protocol utilized and may fail to detect spondylolysis unless sagittal thin section T1- and T2-weighted sequences, as well as T1 and T2 fat-suppression sequences, are obtained.

9. **What are the advantages and disadvantages of nuclear imaging studies for the assessment of spondylolysis?**
Technetium bone scan, SPECT, or SPECT-CT are imaging options when clinical findings suggest a pars defect but radiographs are negative. Nuclear imaging studies are helpful for diagnosis of stress reactions in the pars region and acute fractures, but less helpful for chronic lesions. As bone scans deliver seven to nine times the effective radiation dose compared to AP and lateral lumbar radiographs, these modalities are utilized less frequently today than MRI or CT.

10. **What are the nonsurgical treatment options for an adolescent with spondylolysis?**
Asymptomatic spondylolysis discovered as an incidental radiographic finding requires no specific treatment. Treatment of symptomatic patients begins with rest, physical therapy, including core strengthening and lumbar flexion-based exercises and hamstring stretching, and activity restriction from sports for 2–6 months. Use of a rigid antilordotic orthosis is an option, especially for patients with a pars stress reaction or acute pars fracture.

11. **What is the natural history of pediatric spondylolysis?**
Current evidence suggests that early-stage unilateral or incomplete pars lesions achieve bone union in 80% of patients. However, chronic unilateral pars defects and bilateral pars defects do not achieve bone union in the majority of patients. In addition, 43%–74% of patients with chronic bilateral pars defects will progress to grade 1 or 2 spondylolisthesis. In the short term, resolution of pain and return to activity occurs in 80% of patients following nonsurgical treatment. In the long term, some patients develop pain and activity restriction in adulthood, which requires surgical treatment.

12. **When is surgery considered for spondylolysis?**
Indications to consider surgical treatment include persistent or increasing pain lasting more than 6–12 months despite nonsurgical treatment.

13. **What are the surgical treatment options for treatment of spondylolysis?**
The surgical treatment options for spondylolysis are (1) a direct repair of the pars interarticularis, or (2) a single-level intertransverse fusion. In general, a **pars repair** is considered for defects between L1 and L4. An **intertransverse fusion** is most often considered for L5 pars defects, although pars repair remains an option at the L5 level.

14. **What are the prerequisites for successful outcome with a pars repair? How is this procedure performed?**
Patients who are best suited for pars repair are younger than age 25, have no evidence of disc or facet pathology at the level of spondylolysis, and have a slippage less than 2 mm. The procedure requires careful debridement of the pars pseudarthrosis and application of autogenous bone graft to this region. Internal fixation across the pars defect is required (Fig. 42.1). Fixation options include:
- Direct screw fixation across the pars defect (Buck technique)
- Wire fixation between the transverse process and spinous process (Scott technique)
- Wire-screw or cable-screw construct (connects a pedicle screw via a wire or cable passing under the lamina and tightened around the spinous process)
- Screw-hook-rod fixation (ipsilateral pedicle screw and infralaminar hook are connected by a rod)
- An intralaminar link construct (U-shaped rod passes over the posterior aspect of the right and left lamina and underneath the spinous process to connect screws in the right and left pedicles)
- Pedicle screw-intralaminar screw-rod construct

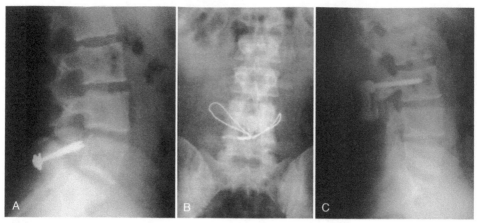

Fig. 42.1 Techniques for repair of the pars interarticularis. (A) Direct screw fixation. (B) Scott wire technique. (C) Screw-hook-rod fixation. (A: From Reitman CA, Esses SI. Direct repair of spondylolytic defects in young competitive athletes. Spine J 2002;2:142–144. B: From Ginsburg GM. Spondylolysis and spondylolisthesis. In: Brown DE, Neumann RD, editors. Orthopedic Secrets. 2nd ed. Philadelphia, PA: Hanley & Belfus; 1999, pp. 200–204, with permission. C: From Benzon HT, Rathmell JP, Wu CL, et al. Raj's Practical Management of Pain. 4th ed. St. Louis: Mosby; 2008.)

SPONDYLOLISTHESIS

15. Discuss the current state of evidence regarding the etiology and prevalence of pediatric lumbar spondylolisthesis?

Spondylolisthesis refers to anterior displacement of the cranial vertebral body in relation to the subjacent vertebral body. Displacement <50% is referred to as low-grade spondylolisthesis while displacement ≥50% is referred to as high-grade spondylolisthesis. The prevalence of spondylolisthesis in the general pediatric population is not clearly defined and is estimated as 6%. In pediatric patients, isthmic and dysplastic spondylolisthesis are the most common subtypes of spondylolisthesis, accounting for 85% and 15% of cases respectively. Both types occur most commonly at the L5–S1 level. Isthmic spondylolisthesis is due to an acquired defect in the region of the pars interarticularis and is more common in males. Over half of patients with persistent bilateral spondylolysis develop grade 1 or 2 spondylolisthesis. Dysplastic spondylolisthesis is a developmental disorder that results from deficiencies in the formation of the posterior osseous structures (L5 laminae, pars interarticularis, lumbosacral facet joints, transverse processes) in combination with sacral growth plate abnormalities, which render the lumbosacral junction unable to resist loads associated with upright posture. Dysplastic spondylolisthesis is more common in females, more likely to progress to high-grade spondylolisthesis, and more likely to require surgical treatment. Slip progression most commonly occurs during adolescence and less commonly in the adult population.

16. Describe the range of symptoms and physical examination findings that may be present in a pediatric patient who presents for evaluation and is diagnosed with spondylolisthesis.

The presentation of patients with spondylolysis and spondylolisthesis is variable. Symptomatic patients most commonly present with low back pain, which may radiate into the buttocks and thighs. Hamstring tightness or spasm is common. Occasionally a patient will report radicular symptoms due to nerve compression at the level of the slippage. Patients with high-grade spondylolisthesis may present with additional symptoms, including postural deformity, scoliosis, gait abnormality, or cauda equina symptoms. In some cases, spondylolisthesis is diagnosed as incidental findings on lumbar or pelvic radiographs obtained for unrelated reasons or during lumbar MRI in asymptomatic patients.

17. What imaging studies are indicated for evaluation of a pediatric patient with spondylolisthesis?

The initial radiographic assessment should consist of AP and lateral lumbosacral radiographs obtained in the standing position to assess spinal alignment under physiologic loading. The lateral image is assessed for the presence of a pars defect. Patients being considered for surgical treatment undergo additional imaging studies. A lateral full-length radiograph or slot scanner image is used to assess the sagittal vertical axis (SVA) and pelvic parameters. A Ferguson view (supine AP view with the x-ray beam angled 30°–35° cephalad) is obtained to provide a true AP view of the L5–S1 segment and to assess transverse process size. Flexion-extension radiographs may be obtained to assess for translational instability. Patients with neurologic symptoms are evaluated with MRI. A CT scan is obtained when detailed evaluation of osseous anatomy is indicated.

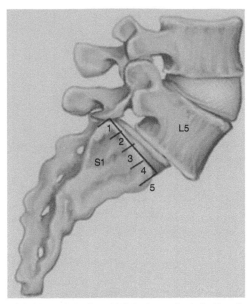

Fig. 42.2 Measurement of the translational component of spondylolisthesis according to the Meyerding grade. (From Kasliwal MK, Smith JS, Kanter A, et al. Management of high-grade spondylolisthesis. Neurosurg Clin 2013;24:275–291, Fig. 1, p. 276.)

18. **What radiographic parameters are important to assess in a patient with spondylolisthesis?**
    The most useful radiographic measurements for describing spondylolisthesis are the *degree of slip* and the *slip angle*. Additional important radiographic parameters to assess include spinopelvic parameters (pelvic incidence, pelvic tilt, and sacral slope) and global sagittal spinal alignment (C7 plumb line).
    The **degree of slip** refers to the amount of translation of the superior vertebra relative to the inferior vertebra (Fig. 42.2). Translation is quantified into five grades (Meyerding system): grade 1, 1%–25%; grade 2, 26%–50%; grade 3, 51%–75%; grade 4, 76%–100%; and grade 5, slippage of the L5 vertebra anterior and distal to the superior S1 endplate (spondyloptosis)
    The **slip angle** measures the degree of lumbosacral kyphosis or angular deformity. It is calculated by measuring the angle between a line perpendicular with the posterior aspect of S1 and a line parallel to either the superior or inferior endplate of L5 (Fig. 42.3). Increased lumbosacral kyphosis is a risk factor for deformity progression prior to or following fusion.
    The **sacropelvic parameters** measured are pelvic incidence (PI), sacral slope (SS), and pelvic tilt (PT). PI is a fixed anatomic parameter unique to the individual. SS and PT are variable parameters. The relationship among the parameters determines the overall alignment of the sacropelvic unit according to the formula PI = PT + SS. PI is the angle defined by a line perpendicular to the sacral endplate line at its midpoint and a line connecting this point to the femoral rotational axis (line connecting the centers of the femoral heads). PT is defined by a vertical reference line and a line from the midpoint of the sacral endplate to the femoral rotational axis. SS is the angle defined by a line along the sacral end plate line and a horizontal reference line (Fig. 42.4).
    Global sagittal alignment is assessed by measuring the SVA by constructing a plumb line dropped from the center of C7. SVA is considered negative when the C7 plumb line falls behind the posterosuperior margin of the sacrum, and positive when the C7 plumb line falls anterior to the posterosuperior margin of the sacrum.

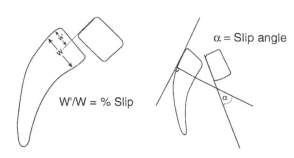

Fig. 42.3 Radiographic measurements of spondylolisthesis. (From Ginsburg GM. Spondylolysis and spondylolisthesis. In: Brown DE, Neumann RD, editors. Orthopedic Secrets. 2nd ed. Philadelphia, PA: Hanley & Belfus; 1999, pp. 200–204, with permission.)

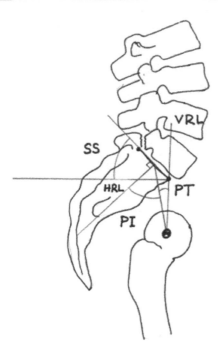

Fig. 42.4 Sacropelvic radiographic parameters. Pelvic incidence *(PI)*, sacral slope *(SS)*, pelvic tilt *(PT)*, horizontal reference line *(HRL)*, vertical reference line *(VRL)*. (From Marawar SV. The radiographic parameters for prediction of spondylolysis and spondylolisthesis. Semin Spine Surg 2014 26:219–224, Fig. 2, p. 221.)

19. Describe the Wiltse classification of spondylolisthesis.

The Wiltse classification (Fig. 42.5) identifies type of spondylolisthesis based on a combination of etiologic and anatomic features:

- **Type I:** *Dysplastic:* Associated with a congenital deficiency of the L5–S1 articulation
- **Type II:** *Isthmic:* Associated with a lesion in the pars interarticularis
  - Subtype IIA: Lytic defect (stress fracture) of the pars
  - Subtype IIB: An elongated or attenuated pars
  - Subtype IIC: An acute pars fracture
- **Type III:** *Degenerative:* Disc degeneration and facet arthrosis lead to spondylolisthesis and associated spinal stenosis and occurs in adults.
- **Type IV:** *Traumatic:* An acute fracture in a region of the posterior elements other than the pars interarticularis (e.g., facets, pedicle, lamina) leads to spondylolisthesis.
- **Type V:** *Pathologic:* Generalized bone disease (e.g., metabolic, neoplastic) results in attenuation of the pars and/or pedicle region leading to spondylolisthesis.
- **Type VI:** *Postsurgical:* Spondylolisthesis that develops following lumbar laminotomy or laminectomy.

20. What is the Marchetti and Bartolozzi classification of spondylolisthesis?

Marchetti and Bartolozzi classified spondylolisthesis into two major subgroups, developmental and acquired. **Developmental spondylolisthesis** is associated with dysplasia at the level of the spondylolisthesis and is subdivided into high- and low-dysplastic types. Dysplastic changes may include lumbosacral facet anomalies, deficient L5 and S1 laminae, elongation of the pars interarticularis, rounding of the dome of the sacrum, sacral endplate abnormalities, a trapezoidal-shaped L5 vertebra, and hypoplastic L5 transverse processes. **Acquired** types of spondylolisthesis include traumatic, degenerative, postsurgical and pathologic etiologies. The traumatic type may be secondary to an acute fracture or result from chronic repetitive stress through a normally developed pars interarticularis. Marchetti and Bartolozzi recognized that the presence or absence of a pars defect could not be used to reliably define the spondylolisthesis type, as slip progression in a dysplastic spondylolisthesis with an initially intact pars interarticularis may lead to subsequent development of a pars defect. The categories of spondylolisthesis identified by Marchetti and Bartolozzi include:

Developmental
  - High dysplasia
  - Low dysplasia

Acquired
  - Traumatic
  - Degenerative
  - Postsurgical
  - Pathologic

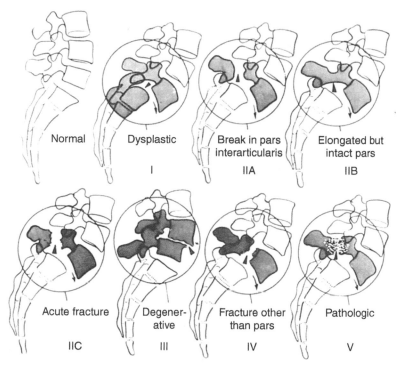

Fig. 42.5 Wiltse classification of spondylolisthesis. (From Neuwirth MG. Spondylolysis and spondylolisthesis in children and adults. In: Comins M, O'Leary P, editors. The Lumbar Spine. New York: Raven Press; 1987, pp. 258, with permission.)

21. **What is the Spinal Deformity Study Group classification of spondylolisthesis?**
    The Spinal Deformity Study Group classification (Fig. 42.6) was developed to incorporate current understanding of sacropelvic and global spinal balance as a guide for treatment decision-making. Classification is based on three factors: (1) degree of slip (low grade, <50%; high grade, ≥50%), (2) sacropelvic balance, and (3) global spinal balance. In a balanced pelvis, sacral slope exceeds pelvic tilt (high SS/low PT). In contrast, in an unbalanced pelvis, there is a low sacral slope and a high pelvic tilt (low SS/high PT) and the pelvis becomes retroverted and the sacrum becomes vertically oriented. Global spinal balance is assessed by the position of the C7 plumb line. The spine is considered balanced when the C7 plumb line is located through or behind the femoral heads, and unbalanced when the C7 plumb line is located anterior to the femoral heads.

    Low-grade spondylolisthesis is stratified into three types based on pelvic incidence: type 1 (low PI, <45°), type 2 (normal PI, 45°–60°), and type 3 (high PI, >60°). Type 3 patients with high PI have increased shear stress across the lumbosacral junction and are at increased risk of spondylolisthesis progression compared with type 1 or type 2 patients.

    High-grade spondylolisthesis is divided into three types based on sacropelvic balance and global spinal balance. If the patient is able to increase lumbar lordosis adequately to compensate for high sacral slope and the patient's PI, sacropelvic balance is maintained and the spondylolisthesis is classified as type 4. In type 5 patients, the compensation provided by increasing lordosis is inadequate, and sacropelvic imbalance (low SS/high PT) develops due to pelvic retroversion and verticalization of the sacrum, although global spinal balance is still maintained as the C7 plumb line remains located behind the femoral heads. In type 6, patients present with combined sacropelvic imbalance and global spinal imbalance as the C7 plumb line falls in front of the femoral heads.

22. **What clinical and radiographic factors suggest that a child with spondylolisthesis is likely to have persistent symptoms, slip progression, and spinal deformity?**
    Clinical risk factors for symptomatic or progressive spondylolisthesis include:
    - Young age at presentation
    - Female sex
    - Presence of back pain symptoms

    Radiographic risk factors for symptomatic or progressive spondylolisthesis include:
    - Dysplastic type of spondylolisthesis
    - Unstable radiographic contour (dome-shaped sacrum, trapezoidal-shaped L5 vertebra)

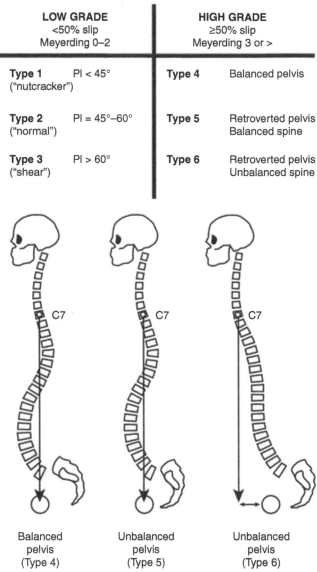

LOW GRADE <50% slip Meyerding 0–2		HIGH GRADE ≥50% slip Meyerding 3 or >	
Type 1 ("nutcracker")	PI < 45°	**Type 4**	Balanced pelvis
Type 2 ("normal")	PI = 45°–60°	**Type 5**	Retroverted pelvis Balanced spine
Type 3 ("shear")	PI > 60°	**Type 6**	Retroverted pelvis Unbalanced spine

Balanced pelvis (Type 4) — C7

Unbalanced pelvis (Type 5) — C7

Unbalanced pelvis (Type 6) — C7

Fig. 42.6 Classification of spondylolisthesis according to the Spinal Deformity Study Group. (From Johnston CE, Ramo BA. Other anatomic disorders of the spine. In: Herring JA, editor. Tachdjian's Pediatric Orthopaedics. 5th ed. Philadelphia, PA: Saunders; 2014, Fig. 14.1, p. 329.

- High PI (>60°)
- Instability on dynamic radiographs
- Degree of slip >50%
- Slip angle >40°

23. **What is the role of nonsurgical treatment for pediatric spondylolisthesis?**
Pediatric patients with asymptomatic low-grade slips are observed. Symptomatic patients with low-grade slips are initially treated nonoperatively with physical therapy, activity modification, and a spinal orthosis. Patients with low-grade slips with dysplastic features without spondylolysis are more likely to fail to respond nonoperative treatment compared with isthmic spondylolisthesis patients due to back pain, leg pain, or neurologic deficit related to cauda equina compression by the intact neural arch. Patients with high-grade slips are generally symptomatic and usually considered for surgical treatment.

24. What are the indications to consider surgical treatment for pediatric patients with spondylolisthesis?

Surgical indications include progressive slippage, intractable low back or radicular pain, neurologic deficits, including cauda equina symptoms, gait abnormality, and severe sagittal plane spinal deformity.

25. What surgical treatment is recommended for pediatric patients with symptomatic low-grade spondylolisthesis?

Surgical treatment for grade 1 and grade 2 spondylolisthesis is an in situ posterolateral L5–S1 spinal fusion. Posterior spinal instrumentation consisting of pedicle screws and rods are commonly utilized as an adjunct to fusion to increase union rates. The procedure can be performed through either a midline approach or a paraspinal approach. Spinal decompression is performed for symptomatic neural compression, which occurs most commonly in patients with dysplastic spondylolisthesis.

26. What are the surgical options for treatment of pediatric patients with high-grade spondylolisthesis?

Options for treatment of pediatric patients with high-grade spondylolisthesis include:
- In situ posterolateral L4–S1 spinal fusion and posterior spinal instrumentation
- Circumferential fusion consisting of posterolateral L4–S1 fusion and posterior spinal instrumentation, spinal decompression, L5–S1 interbody fusion, and partial or complete reduction of spondylolisthesis.
- Circumferential fusion consisting of posterolateral L4–S1 spinal fusion and instrumentation, spinal decompression, and transsacral interbody fusion and fixation ± partial reduction of spondylolisthesis.

27. What are some important considerations regarding surgical treatment of high-grade spondylolisthesis with in situ posterolateral spinal fusion?

When in situ posterolateral spinal fusion is performed for high-grade spondylolisthesis, proximal extension of the posterior fusion to L4 is recommended by many surgeons. Use of spinal instrumentation and addition of interbody fusion are recommended to increase fusion rates. Complications associated with in situ fusion for patients with high-grade spondylolisthesis include pseudarthrosis, progressive slippage, persistent lumbosacral deformity, and cauda equina syndrome.

28. What are some important considerations regarding surgical treatment of high-grade spondylolisthesis with a circumferential fusion, spinal decompression, and partial or complete reduction?

Treatment with reduction, posterior spinal instrumentation, and circumferential fusion of high-grade spondylolisthesis is associated with a lower rate of pseudarthrosis compared with in situ posterior fusion and allows for correction of sacropelvic and global spinopelvic sagittal deformity. Spondylolisthesis reduction and realignment are recommended for type 5 and type 6 deformities. Important considerations (Fig. 42.7) include:
- Posterior instrumentation typically includes bilateral L4, L5, and S1 pedicle screws supplemented by sacropelvic fixation with iliac screws or S2 alar-iliac screws.
- Early identification, decompression, and protection of the L5 nerve roots in combination with wide surgical decompression are critical procedural steps.
- A posterior approach for L5–S1 interbody fusion is often preferred due to challenges associated with access to the L5–S1 disc space in the presence of severe L5–S1 spondylolisthesis.
- Temporary intraoperative distraction is used to facilitate L5–S1 disc space access and preparation, sacral dome osteotomy, intervertebral grafting, placement of intervertebral body fusion devices or structural bone grafts, and gradual intraoperative reduction of the translational deformity.
- Reduction of spondylolisthesis provides correction of sacropelvic imbalance and global spinopelvic imbalance.
- Partial rather than complete reduction of the amount of slippage is often desirable and is safer as the majority of strain on the L5 nerve root occurs with reduction of the last 25% of slippage.
- Correction of the slip angle is important as this leads to improvement in global sagittal alignment.
- Intraoperative neurophysiologic monitoring, including somatosensory evoked potential monitoring, motor evoked potential monitoring, and electromyographic monitoring techniques are used throughout the procedure to reduce the risk of neurologic injury.

29. What is the role of transsacral interbody fusion and L5–S1 transfixation in combination with posterior decompression in the treatment of high-grade spondylolisthesis?

When reduction of a high-grade spondylolisthesis is not performed or when placement of an interbody device is challenging, a procedure consisting of posterior decompression, partial reduction, transvertebral screw fixation, and placement of a transsacral fibula graft or fusion cage provides an alternative method to achieve circumferential fusion. This technique permits reduction of the slip angle, which is the major component of the deformity. It minimizes the risks associated with attempting major correction of vertebral translation (spondylolisthesis reduction) and provides a circumferential fusion through a single-stage posterior approach (Fig. 42.8A, B).

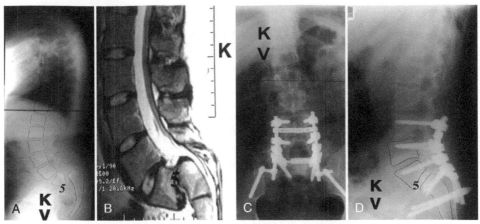

Fig. 42.7 Treatment of high-grade isthmic spondylolisthesis with reduction and circumferential fusion from a posterior approach. (A) Lateral radiograph. (B) Magnetic resonance imaging shows grade 4 developmental spondylolisthesis. Treatment included reduction of the spondylolisthesis utilizing bilateral S1 and iliac screws; reduction screws in L3, L4, and L5; sacral dome osteotomy; and posterior lumbar interbody fusion with cortical bone interbody spacers and iliac crest autograft. (C) Postoperative anteroposterior radiograph. (D) Lateral radiograph (postoperative). (From O'Brien MF, Kuklo TR, Mardjetko SJ, et al. The sacropelvic unit: Creative solutions to complex fixation and reconstruction problems. Semin Spine Surg 2004;16:134–149.)

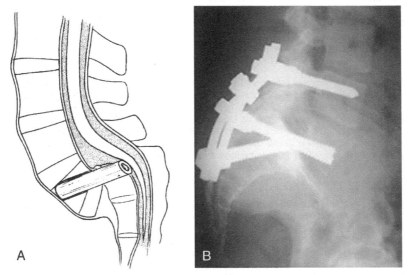

Fig. 42.8 Decompression, transfixation, and transsacral interbody fusion. (A) A fibula graft is placed across the sacrum, L5–S1 disc, and into the L5 vertebral body. (B) Pedicle screws are subsequently placed via the S1 pedicle from S1 into L5. (A: From Winter RB, Lonstein JW, Denis F, et al., editors. Atlas of Spine Surgery. Philadelphia, PA: Saunders; 1995, p. 461, with permission B: From Devlin VJ, with permission.)

30. **What are the surgical treatment options for spondyloptosis?**
    Fortunately, spondyloptosis is a rare condition. Treatment options include a reduction procedure or L5 vertebrectomy. A combined anterior and posterior approach, often performed in two stages, is referred to as a Gaines procedure. In the first stage, an anterior approach to the spine is performed and the L4–L5 disc, L5–S1 disc, and L5 vertebra are removed. In the second stage, the lamina and pedicles of L5 are removed to complete the L5 resection and the L4 vertebra is realigned with the sacrum and stabilized with pedicle fixation (Fig. 42.9). A single stage posterior-only vertebral column resection has been recently reported and provides an alternative technique for treatment of this complex deformity.

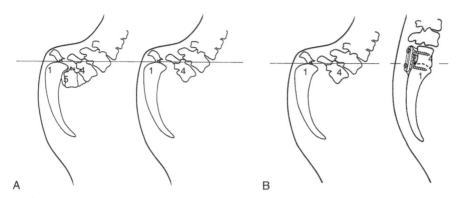

Fig. 42.9 Gaines procedure. (A) First stage. (B) Second stage. (From Grobler LJ, Wiltse LL. Classification and nonoperative treatment of spondylolisthesis. In: Fryomer JW, editor. The Adult Spine: Principles and Practice. 2nd ed. Philadelphia, PA: Lippincott-Raven; 1997, pp. 1889, with permission.)

KEY POINTS

1. Spondylolysis is a unilateral or bilateral defect in the region of the pars interarticularis and is a common cause of low back pain in pediatric patients.
2. Surgical treatment for low grade pediatric spondylolisthesis is an in situ posterolateral L5–S1 spinal fusion and is usually performed in conjunction with posterior spinal instrumentation.
3. Circumferential fusion provides the highest likelihood of successful arthrodesis in patients with high-grade spondylolisthesis.

Websites
1. Spondylolysis and spondylolisthesis: http://orthokids.org/Condition/Spondylolysis-Spondylolisthesis

BIBLIOGRPAHY

1. Abdu, W. A., Wilber, R. G., & Emery, S. E. (1994). Pedicular transvertebral screw fixation of the lumbosacral spine in spondylolisthesis. *Spine, 19,* 710–715.
2. Crawford, C. H., Ledonio, C. G. T., Bess, R. S., Buchowski, J. M., Burton, D. C., Hu, S. S., et al. (2015). Current evidence regarding the etiology, prevalence, natural history and prognosis of pediatric lumbar spondylolysis: A report from the Scoliosis Research Society Evidence-Based Medicine Committee. *Spine Deformity, 3,* 12–29.
3. Crawford, C. H., Ledonio, C. G. T., Bess, R. S., Buchowski, J. M., Burton, D. C., Hu, S. S., et al. (2015). Current evidence regarding the surgical and nonsurgical treatment of pediatric lumbar spondylolysis: A report from the Scoliosis Research Society Evidence-Based Medicine Committee. *Spine Deformity, 3,* 30–44.
4. Crawford, C. H., Larson, A. N., Gates, M. G., Bess, R. S., Guillaume, T. J., Kim, H. J., et al. (2017). Current evidence regarding the treatment of pediatric lumbar spondylolisthesis: A report from the Scoliosis Research Society Evidence Based Medicine Committee. *Spine Deformity, 5,* 284–302.
5. Gaines, R. W. (2005). L5 vertebrectomy for the surgical treatment of spondyloptosis: Thirty cases in 25 years. *Spine, 30,* S66–S70.
6. Johnston, C. E., & Ramo, B. A. (2014). Chapter 14: Other anatomic disorders of the spine. In J. A. Herring (Ed.), *Tachdjian's Pediatric Orthopaedics* (5th ed., pp. 328–355). Philadelphia, PA: Saunders.
7. Kasliwal, M. K., Smith, J. S., Kanter, A., Chen, C. J., Mummaneni, P. V., Hart, R. A., et al. (2013). Management of high grade spondylolisthesis. *Neurosurgery Clinics of North America, 24,* 275–291.
8. Kim, H. J., Crawford, C. H., Ledonio, C. G. T., Bess, S., Larson, A. N., Gates, M., et al. (2018). Current evidence regarding the diagnostic methods for pediatric lumbar spondylolisthesis: A report from the Scoliosis Research Society Evidence-Based Medicine Committee. *Spine Deformity, 6,* 185–188.
9. Larson, A. N., Schueler, B. A., & Dubousset, J. (2019). Radiation in spine deformity: State-of-the-art reviews. *Spine Deformity, 7,* 386–394.
10. Ruf, M., Koch, H., Melcher, R. P., & Harms, J. (2006). Anatomic reduction and monosegmental fusion in high-grade developmental spondylolisthesis. *Spine, 31,* 269–274.
11. Schoenleber, S. J., Shufflebarger, H. L., & Shah, S. A. (2015). The assessment and treatment of high-grade lumbosacral spondyloptosis in children and young adults. *JBJS Reviews, 3*(12), e3.

CHAPTER 43

PEDIATRIC SPINAL TRAUMA

Eric S. Varley, DO

GENERAL CONSIDERATIONS

1. **Why is it important to consider the normal growth and development of the spine when evaluating a child with a suspected spinal injury?**
   Knowledge of the developmental anatomy of the spine is important to avoid misdiagnosis of anatomic differences such as normal physes, synchondroses, and secondary ossification centers as acute fractures.
   - The **atlas (C1)** is formed from three ossification centers: the anterior arch and two posterior neural arches. The anterior arch is ossified in only 20% of newborns.
   - The **axis (C2)** is formed from five primary ossification centers. The area between the odontoid process and C2 body (dentocentral synchondrosis) commonly fuses by 6 years of age and may be confused with a fracture before this age. The secondary ossification center at the tip of the odontoid, the ossiculum terminale, typically fuses by age 12.
   - The **subaxial cervical spine (C3–C7)** and the **thoracic** and **lumbar spine** develop in a similar pattern from three primary ossification centers. Secondary ossification centers can form at the tips of the spinous processes, transverse processes, and superior and inferior vertebral margins and may be misdiagnosed as fractures.

2. **What are some anatomic differences between the immature and the adult spine that influence patterns of spinal injury that occur in the pediatric population?**
   The capacity for growth and the potential for injury to the growth plate differentiate pediatric and adult spine trauma patients and contribute to the complexity of evaluation of the pediatric spine trauma patient. Unique anatomic features of the immature spine include:
   - Hypermobility
   - Hyperlaxity of ligamentous and capsular structures
   - Presence of epiphyses and synchondroses
   - Incomplete ossification
   - Unique configuration of the vertebral bony elements (e.g., wedge-shaped vertebral bodies, horizontal cervical facet joints)

3. **What are the most common injury mechanisms in children who sustain significant spine trauma?**
   Motor vehicle accidents, falls, and sports-associated injuries. Birth injuries and nonaccidental injury (child abuse) are less common but important injury mechanisms to consider.

4. **What are the relative strengths and weaknesses of plain radiographs, computed tomography (CT) scan, and magnetic resonance imaging (MRI) in the detection of spine injuries in pediatric patients?**
   Radiographs: Plain radiographs play a role in the initial imaging evaluation of the spine-injured pediatric patient. A cervical spine series consists of anteroposterior (AP) and lateral views. The lateral radiograph must clearly visualize the C7–T1 level. The open-mouth AP odontoid view is difficult to obtain in an uncooperative child and has not been shown to provide important additional information in children less than age 9. AP and lateral radiographs of the thoracic and lumbar spine are obtained if there is concern regarding injury to these spinal regions. If faced with equivocal findings or an uncooperative child with a mechanism of injury or physical examination that is suspicious for spinal injury, more advanced imaging is indicated as studies have documented that plain radiographs fail to diagnose 25%–75% of pediatric spinal injuries, especially injuries involving unossified tissues and soft tissues such as ligaments, joint capsules, intervertebral discs, and cartilaginous endplates.
   CT scans: The use of helical CT scanning for screening for spinal injury in the pediatric polytrauma patient has increased due to the high sensitivity of CT compared to plain radiography for detection of osseous injury. However, radiation exposure and future cancer risk due to organ sensitivity and longer life expectancy of pediatric patients are important concerns that limit widespread use of CT in the pediatric population.
   MRI: Advantages of MRI include lack of exposure to ionizing radiation and the ability to assess neurologic structures and detect injuries to soft tissue and unossified structures that are not detected with plain radiographs or CT scan. However, it may be challenging to obtain an expeditious MRI for evaluation of the pediatric polytrauma patient due to logistical considerations, including the frequent need for sedation during image acquisition.

5. **How does a child's age affect the pattern of traumatic spine injury?**

In neonates, birth trauma is the most common cause of spinal injury. In infants and young children (<3 years), nonaccidental (child abuse) and accidental trauma are common causes of injury. Prior to 8 years of age, pediatric patients have a high head-to-body ratio that predisposes children to upper cervical injury (C3 or above). These injuries are associated with a notable rate of neurologic injury and fatality. After age 8 years, injury patterns most commonly involve the subaxial cervical region and the thoracic and lumbar regions, with the most commonly injured region of the vertebral column located between L2 and the sacrum.

6. **What characteristic findings are noted in a child who has sustained a spine injury as a result of child abuse?**

Spine fractures due to nonaccidental trauma are most commonly reported in patients less than 2 years of age. These injuries may involve all regions of the spine, but are more common in the upper cervical region. Multilevel spinal injuries and neurologic injury are present in over half of these patients. Spinal injuries most often involve the vertebral bodies, with varying degrees of anterior compression, frequently involving multiple spinal levels. Avulsion fractures of the spinous processes, pars fractures, pedicle fractures, ligament injuries, anterior notching of the vertebral body near the superior endplate, decreased disc height caused by disc herniation and fracture-dislocation may be present (Fig. 43.1). Other stigmata that suggest child abuse include fractures involving the skull, ribs, and long bones, as well as soft tissue injuries.

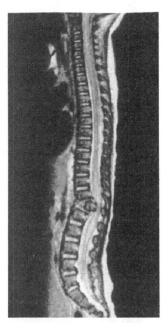

Fig. 43.1 Magnetic resonance image of a fracture-dislocation of the spine occurring in a 10-month-old infant who was the victim of child abuse. The image reveals cord compression in this patient with incomplete paraplegia. (From Akbarnia BA. Pediatric spine fractures. Orthop Clin North Am 1999; 30:531, with permission.)

7. **What maternal risk factors are related to neonatal spinal cord injury?**

The risk factors include small pelvic dimensions, obesity, prolonged delivery, forceps use, and shoulder dystocia. Early clinical findings that suggest a spinal cord injury include severe respiratory compromise and profound hypotonia. It should be noted that brachial plexus injury is far more common than spinal cord injury (i.e., Erb [C5/C6] or Klumpke [C7/T1] palsy). Detailed physical examination and MRI are critical in making this distinction.

8. **What is SCIWORA?**

SCIWORA is an acronym for spinal cord injury without radiographic abnormality, and is defined as an injury to the spinal cord without visible changes on plain radiographs or CT. Due to the variable elasticity of the spinal column in children, forces applied to the spine may be accommodated by the spinal column but exceed the elastic limit of the spinal cord and manifest as a stretch injury to the spinal cord. It has been demonstrated that the spinal column of an infant can be stretched up to 2 inches, whereas the spinal cord can be stretched only 0.25 inches before rupturing. MRI is the imaging study of choice to diagnose patients with suspected SCIWORA as this imaging modality can demonstrate injury to the spinal cord and unossified tissues. Characteristic MRI findings include acute hemorrhage and edema of the spinal cord, ligamentous injury, disc herniation, and physeal injuries. SCIWORA most commonly involves the cervical region and cervicothoracic junction. Thoracolumbar involvement is less common but may occur in association with high-energy trauma, and typically involves the watershed region of the cord. SCIWORA injuries are treated as potentially unstable injuries as initial spinal column displacement may spontaneously reduce. Delayed-onset SCIWORA may be seen up to 4 days after injury in the setting of ligamentous instability. Brace immobilization up to 12 weeks is recommended for patients with SCIWORA. Although uncommon, recurrent SCIWORA after an initial period of neurologic stabilization may occur days to weeks after injury and may be prevented with immobilization.

9. **How does the addition of a shoulder harness to a lap belt influence the type of spinal injury sustained by a pediatric motor vehicle passenger?**

Use of a lap belt in isolation permits the belt to act as an anterior fulcrum leading to a flexion-distraction injury mechanism in the thoracolumbar spine. The addition of a shoulder harness to a lap belt reduces this injury pattern by limiting forward flexion of the thorax during impact and reducing flexion-distraction forces on the lumbar spine. However, by restraining the thorax, a shoulder harness can increase the risk of cervical spine injuries in severe accidents. Less commonly, the shoulder harness of seat belts may be associated with injuries to the supraaortic vessels (carotid and subclavian) in association with first and second rib fractures.

CERVICAL SPINE

10. What is the correct way to immobilize a child during initial evaluation of a suspected traumatic cervical spine injury?

Because children have a large cranium in relation to their thorax, immobilization on a standard spine board will place the cervical spine in a flexed position. Use of a double mattress to elevate the thorax or use of a pediatric spine board with a recess for the occiput is recommended to avoid undesirable displacement of cervical injuries.

11. What unique anatomic features of the immature cervical spine can lead to confusion during the evaluation of cervical radiographs following spine trauma?

Ten anatomic features of the pediatric cervical spine commonly cause confusion during spine trauma evaluation (Fig. 43.2).

12. How does a child's age affect the pattern of traumatic cervical spine injury?

Before age 8 years, most cervical injuries occur at *C3 or above* and are associated with a high risk of fatality. After age 8, cervical injury patterns are similar to adults, occur *below C3*, and are less likely to be fatal.

13. How are pediatric cervical spine injuries classified according to anatomic location?

Occiput-C2 Region
- Occipital condyle fracture
- Atlanto-occipital dissociation
- Atlas (C1) fractures
- Axis (C2) fractures
  - Odontoid fractures
  - Traumatic spondylolisthesis (Hangman's fracture)
- Atlantoaxial instability
  - Secondary to ligament injury
  - Secondary to C1 ring fracture
  - Atlantoaxial rotatory subluxation

Subaxial Cervical Region
- Compression fracture
- Facet injuries (unilateral or bilateral fracture, subluxation, dislocation)
- Burst fracture
- Flexion teardrop fracture
- Vertebral apophyseal fracture
- Ligament injury

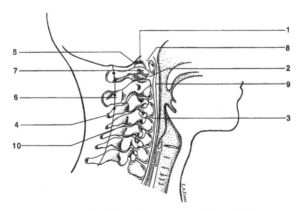

Fig. 43.2 Ten unique features of the pediatric cervical spine that can cause confusion during the trauma evaluation: *(1)* the apical ossification center can be mistaken for a fracture; *(2)* the synchondrosis at the base of the odontoid can be mistaken for a fracture; *(3)* vertebral bodies appear rounded off or wedged, simulating a fracture; *(4)* secondary centers of ossification at the tips of the spinous processes can be mistaken for a fracture; *(5)* the odontoid may angulate posteriorly in 4% of children; *(6)* C2–C3 pseudosubluxation (can be assessed with Swischuk's line); *(7)* the ossification center of the anterior arch of C1 may be absent in the first year of life; *(8)* the atlantodens interval may be as wide as 4.5 mm and still be normal; *(9)* the width of the prevertebral soft tissues varies widely, especially with crying, and may be mistaken for swelling; and *(10)* horizontal facets in young children can be mistake for a fracture. (From Flynn JM. Spine trauma in the pediatric population. Spine State Art Rev 2000;14:249–262, with permission.)

14. **How is an occipitoatlantal dissociation diagnosed and treated?**
     This is often a catastrophic and fatal injury, although survival is possible with early diagnosis and treatment. The dislocation may spontaneously reduce and remain unrecognized until traction is applied to the skull. Neurologic deficits are present in up to 80% of patients. Halo immobilization is recommended as soon as this injury is recognized. Definitive treatment consists of a posterior occipitocervical fusion (Fig. 43.3).

     Diagnosis is not always straightforward. Positive MRI findings include occiput-C1 (O-C1) subluxation, distraction between O-C1 or C1-C2, and soft tissue swelling or abnormal signal involving O-C1-C2 ligamentous structures. Various radiographic measurements have been described for identification of occipitoatlantal dislocation including **Powers ratio**, **X-lines**, **Harris lines**, and the **occipital condyle-C1 interval** (Fig. 43.4). Although Powers ratio is useful for diagnosis of an anterior occipitoatlantal dislocation, it is insensitive to posterior dislocation. It should be noted that measurement of the distance between the basion and the dens (basion-dens interval, BDI) is unreliable in children <13 years due to incomplete ossification of the odontoid.

15. **Are fractures of C1 common in pediatric patients?**
     Fractures of the atlas are less common than other types of cervical fractures in children. Various fracture types have been described including posterior arch fractures, lateral mass fractures, isolated anterior ring fractures, and burst fractures (Jefferson fractures). Instability is identified by the presence of an avulsion of the transverse atlantal ligament or wide displacement (>7 mm) of the lateral masses of C1 beyond the lateral border of the lateral masses of C2. Most C1 fractures are treated nonoperatively in the absence of major instability.

16. **What is the most common cervical spine injury in children?**
     Odontoid fractures are the most common cervical spine injuries in children, with 4 years being the mean age of injury. The injury usually occurs as an epiphyseal separation of the growth plate at the base of the odontoid. Minimally displaced fractures are difficult to diagnose on plain film, making MRI and CT scan with reconstructions important diagnostic studies (Fig. 43.5).

17. **What is an os odontoideum?**
     An *os odontoideum* appears as a rounded piece of bone at the apex of the odontoid with a radiolucent gap separating it from the remainder of the axis and body of C2. Many consider os odontoideum to arise from a previously unrecognized injury. Unrestricted motion following this initial fracture leads to the development of a pseudarthrosis. Clinical presentation may mimic an acute fracture.

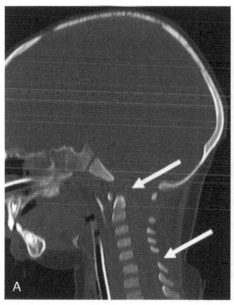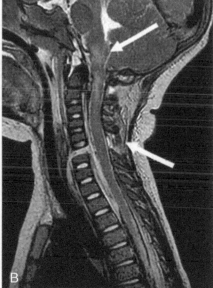

Fig. 43.3 (A) Sagittal CT and (B) MRI scans in a 5-year-old patient show atlanto-occipital (*upper arrows*) and C5–C6 (*lower arrows*) injuries following a motor vehicle accident. (From Fournier J, Tsirkos Al. Paediatric spinal trauma: Patterns of injury, clinical assessment, and principles of treatment. Orthop Trauma 2016;30:421–429, Fig. 1.)

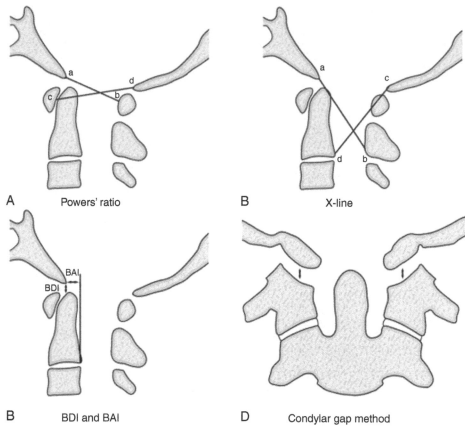

A   Powers' ratio   **B**   X-line

B   BDI and BAI   **D**   Condylar gap method

Fig. 43.4 Occipitocervical injuries. (A) Powers ratio is the ratio of the distance from the basion *(a)* to the posterior cortex of the atlas *(b)*, and the distance from the opisthion *(d)* to the anterior arch of the atlas *(c)*. Powers ratio is considered abnormal if the ratio of AB/CD is >1. (B) In the X-line method, two lines are drawn. The first line is drawn from the basion to the axis spinolaminar junction *(ab)*. The second line is drawn from the opisthion to the posteroinferior corner of the axis body. The examination is considered abnormal if the first line *(ab)* does not intersect with the C2 vertebra, or the second line *(cd)* does not intersect with the C1 vertebra. (C) The basion-dens interval *(BDI)* is considered abnormal when the distance from the basion to the upper tip of the odontoid is >12 mm in adults. The basion-axis interval *(BAI)* is considered abnormal when the basion lies >4 mm anterior or 12 mm posterior to a line projecting cranially from the posterior cortex of the C2 vertebral body (when the BDI and BAI are used together they are known as Harris lines). (D) Occipital condyle–C1 interval or the condylar gap method is considered abnormal if the distance between the occipital condyle and the superior articular facet of the atlas *(arrows)* is >2 mm in adults or 5 mm in children. (From Smorgick Y, Fischgrund JS. Occipitocervical injuries. Semin Spine Surg 2013; 25:14–22, Fig. 2.)

18. **Injury to what spinal ligament will result in atlantoaxial instability?**

    Injury to the transverse atlantal ligament will result in atlantoaxial (C1–C2) instability. This injury is suspected if the **atlanto-dens interval** is greater than 5 mm on a lateral cervical radiograph. There are two types: ligamentous tear (type I) and bony avulsion injury (type II).

    A trial of nonoperative treatment for 10–12 weeks consisting of immobilization in a Minerva brace or halo may be considered for type II injuries. Some experts advocate immediate C1–C2 fusion for both injury types. Fusion is required for patients with persistent instability despite orthotic treatment.

19. **What is a Hangman's fracture?**

    A Hangman's fracture, also referred to as traumatic spondylolisthesis, is a bilateral fracture involving the pars interarticularis region of C2. A modification of the Effendi classification is used to guide treatment of Hangman's fractures:

    - Type I injuries consist of a fracture through the neural arch with no angulation and up to 3 mm of displacement. Treatment involves use of a rigid cervical orthosis.
    - Type II fractures have both significant angulation and fracture displacement (>3 mm). Initial treatment involves traction realignment followed by immobilization in a halo vest or rigid cervical orthosis.

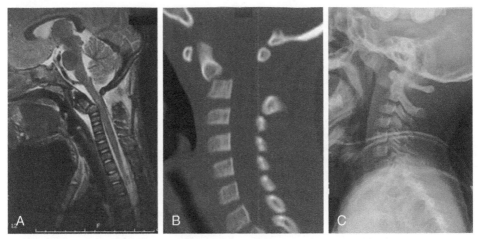

Fig. 43.5 Odontoid fracture in a 3-year-old child involved in a motor vehicle accident. (A) Sagittal magnetic resonance image and (B) computed tomography scans show the fracture through the dentocentral synchondrosis with the characteristic forward angulation and subluxation of the dens. There is subtle cord signal change at the C2 level. (C) The fracture was reduced and successfully treated with a halo for 8 weeks. (From Klimo P Jr, Ware ML, Gupta N, et al. Cervical spine trauma in the pediatric patient. Neursurg Clin N Am 2007;18:599–620, Fig. 6.)

- Type IIA injuries show minimal displacement but are associated with severe angulation as a result of a flexion-distraction injury mechanism. Treatment involves closed reduction by positioning in extension followed by treatment with a halo vest.
- Type III injuries combine severe angulation and displacement with a unilateral or bilateral facet dislocation between C2 and C3. Surgical treatment is required for reduction of the facet dislocation followed by surgical stabilization.

    Images should be carefully scrutinized to avoid misinterpretation of a persistent synchondrosis of C2 or pseudosubluxation of C2–C3 as a Hangman's fracture.

20. **What is pseudosubluxation?**
    This refers to normal anterior translation that can occur between C2 and C3, and less frequently between C3 and C4, in patients younger than 8 years. This displacement is secondary to the increased ligamentous laxity and transverse facet orientation seen in young children. The *posterior cervical line (spinolaminar line of Swischuk)* is used to distinguish pathologic displacement from normal anterior displacement. A line is constructed connecting the anterior aspect of the spinous processes of C1–C3. If the anterior aspect of the spinous process of C2 is more than 1.5 mm from this line, an injury should be suspected (Fig. 43.6).

21. **What factors guide treatment decision making regarding pediatric subaxial spine injuries?**
    Treatment decision making regarding pediatric subaxial spine injuries takes into account the injury pattern, fracture stability, presence or absence of a neurologic deficit, and whether spinal cord compression is present on imaging studies. Stable injuries are treated with a rigid cervical collar. Unstable injuries are stabilized and fused using rigid segmental instrumentation. Spinal decompression is performed as needed based on clinical findings and the results of imaging studies.

22. **What special measures should be taken when considering halo placement in a pediatric patient?**
    Special considerations are necessary, especially in very young patients, and include:
    - **Appropriate size halo ring:** a custom ring is often required and should be 2 cm larger than skull diameter
    - **Appropriate size halo vest or halo cast:** custom fabrication is often necessary
    - **Preapplication skull CT scan:** to assess skull thickness and location of cranial suture lines
    - **General anesthesia:** frequently required in the very young patient
    - **Appropriate number of pins:** less than 2 years, use 10–12 pins; 2–7 years, use 6–8 pins; 8 years and older, use 4 pins
    - **Appropriate pin torque:** less than 2 years, use 2 in-lbs; 2–7 years, use 4–5 in-lbs; 8 years and older, use 8 in-lbs.

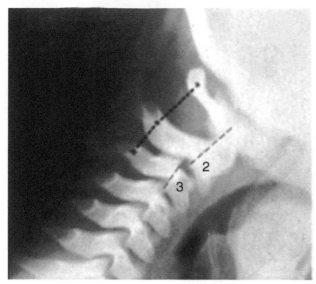

Fig. 43.6 Pseudosubluxation. Swischuk described the posterior cervical line (spinolaminar line), which is drawn from the anterior aspect of the spinous process of C1 to the anterior aspect of the spinous process of C3. If the line does not pass within 1.5 mm of the anterior aspect of the spinous process of C2 on flexion–extension radiographs, a true injury should be suspected. (Martus JE, Mencio GA. Fractures of the spine. In: Mencio GA, Swiontkowski MF, editors. Green's Skeletal Trauma in Children. 5th ed. Philadelphia, PA: Saunders; 2015, pp. 270–310, Fig. 12.10.)

THORACIC AND LUMBAR SPINE

23. **What are the common injury mechanisms and types of thoracic and lumbar fractures seen in the pediatric population?**

    Thoracic and lumbar fractures are uncommon in the pediatric population. Motor vehicle accidents, pedestrian-vehicle accidents, falls, and sports-associated injuries are the most common injury mechanisms. The common fracture types are described as:

    - **Compression fractures:** comprise the largest subgroup of pediatric thoracolumbar fractures. Present with isolated loss of anterior vertebral body height due to an injury mechanism associated with flexion and axial loading. Majority of fractures present with less than 20% height loss. Injuries with greater than 50% height loss are suspicious for posterior column involvement and instability and warrant MRI.
    - **Burst fractures:** present with loss of anterior and posterior vertebral body height due to an injury mechanism associated with axial loading. Retropulsion of bone into the spinal canal, posterior element fractures, posterior ligamentous injuries, and neurologic deficits may occur depending on the severity of injury.
    - **Flexion-distraction injuries:** present as a three-column spinal injury due to application of flexion-distraction forces relative to a fixed axis (e.g., seat-belt). Neurologic injury (40% of patients overall, 15% present with paraplegia) and intraabdominal injury (up to two-thirds of patients) are frequently associated with this injury pattern. Associated injuries may involve the small bowel, colon, stomach and duodenum, pancreas, kidney, diaphragm, and aorta.
    - **Fracture-dislocations:** present as the result of high-energy injury that completely disrupts the integrity of all three spinal columns and results in displacement of the spine in one or more planes. Severe neurologic injuries are associated with this fracture pattern.

24. **What is the appropriate treatment for a child with a Risser sign of 0 or 1 who sustains multiple compression fractures with less than 10° of deformity in each vertebra and no neurologic compromise?**

    Studies following these patients to skeletal maturity have shown that no treatment is necessary in such patients. Children, especially those younger than 10 years of age, have excellent healing potential and usually reconstitute lost vertebral height in the sagittal plane in mild compression fractures. Patients who are older, have more than 10° of deformity per vertebra, or have deformity in the coronal plane usually require treatment.

25. How are flexion-distraction injuries treated in children?

Injuries confined to bone both anteriorly and posteriorly generally heal without instability if treated nonoperatively in a thoracolumbosacral orthosis (TLSO) for 2–3 months. Bracing is usually successful if the initial kyphosis is less than 20°. Surgical treatment is indicated for:
- Unstable, purely ligamentous injuries
- Very unstable fractures that cannot be managed in a brace
- Fractures with significant kyphosis that cannot be reduced or maintained in a brace
- Fractures associated with neurologic injury or abdominal injury

The guiding surgical principle is to reconstitute a sufficient posterior tension band either with posterior wiring in small children or posterior compression constructs using rigid segmental instrumentation in older or larger children.

26. What are the two primary surgical indications for the treatment of pediatric burst fractures?

The first indication is partial or progressive neurologic deficit caused by spinal canal compromise. The mere presence of bone in the canal is not a sufficient indication for surgery because bone remodeling and reabsorption occur over time. The second indication is the prevention of late kyphotic deformity. More than 25° of localized kyphosis is generally accepted as an indication for surgery.

27. How does the treatment of burst fractures differ in children and adults?

Children and adolescents have strong bones with excellent healing potential. Late kyphotic deformity is less likely in children. Combined anterior and posterior fusions, which are commonly used for highly comminuted adult burst fractures, are rarely necessary in children. Children also have greater potential to remodel bone within the spinal canal than adults. In addition, children are less likely to suffer the detrimental effects of immobilization compared with adults. Otherwise, the basic principles of adult burst fracture treatment can be applied to children and adolescents.

28. What is the treatment for a fracture-dislocation of the thoracic or lumbar spine?

Posterior spinal instrumentation and fusion is the treatment of choice for all fracture-dislocations with or without neurologic deficit.

29. What is the risk of scoliosis following pediatric spinal cord injury?

The risk of scoliosis is dependent on the patient's age at the time of spinal cord injury and the timing of the injury in relation to the adolescent growth spurt. The prevalence of spinal deformity approaches 100% in patients who sustain a spinal cord injury prior to age 10. Surgical treatment typically involves a long spinopelvic fusion.

30. What is a limbus fracture? Where does it occur?

Fractures crossing the vertebral endplate in the immature spine are called **limbus fractures**. These fractures often traverse through the growth plate (hypertrophic zone) of the physis, in the same pattern seen in immature long bone injuries. This region is biomechanically weak and thus susceptible to injury. A limbus fracture should not be confused with a limbus vertebra, which represents herniation of nucleus pulposus through the vertebral endplate and beneath the ring apophysis.

31. What are the most common clinical and imaging findings in children with limbus fractures?

Most limbus (vertebral end plate) fractures occur in the lumbar spine at the L4–L5 and L5–S1 levels. Clinical presentation is similar to that of a herniated nucleus pulposus. Most patients have symptoms of stiffness and spasm, numbness, weakness, and occasionally neurogenic claudication. Infrequently, limbus fractures present with a cauda equina syndrome. Many patients have a positive Lasègue sign. Limbus fractures are difficult to visualize on plain radiographs. MRI, CT, or CT-myelography can be used to confirm the diagnosis.

32. What are the four types of vertebral end plate fractures? (Fig. 43.7)
- **Type I:** Pure cartilage avulsion of the entire posterior cortical vertebral margin without attendant osseous defect
- **Type II:** Large central fracture of portions of the posterior cortical margin and cancellous bony rim
- **Type III:** More localized, lateral fracture of the posterior cortical margin of the vertebral body
- **Type IV:** Fracture that involves the entire length and breadth of the posterior vertebral body

33. What treatment is advised for acute traumatic spondylolysis?

Treatment of traumatic spondylolysis is usually nonoperative. Nonoperative treatment consists of immobilization with a corset or TLSO, restriction from vigorous activity, and physical therapy for stretching of the hamstring muscles and strengthening of the abdominal musculature. If nonoperative treatment fails, various surgical options exist, including posterolateral fusion or direct bony repair of the pars defect supplemented with screw, wire, or screw-rod fixation.

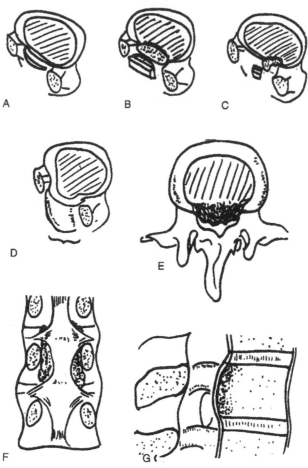

Fig. 43.7 Fractures of the vertebral limbus. (A) Type I—pure cartilage avulsion of the entire posterior cortical vertebral margin without attendant osseous defect. (B) Type II—large central fracture of portions of the posterior cortical margin and cancellous bony rim. (C) Type III—more localized, lateral fracture of the posterior cortical margin of the posterior vertebral body. (D–G) Type IV—fracture that involves the entire length and breadth of the posterior vertebral body. The type IV fracture effectively displaces bone in the posterior direction, filling the floor of the spinal canal with a combination of reconstituted cortical bone and cancellous bone accompanied in part by scar formation. (From Akbarnia BA. Pediatric spine fractures. Orthop Clin North Am 1999;30:525, with permission.)

KEY POINTS

1. Up to the age of 8 years, children have a large cranium in relation to their thorax. The size of the cranium must be accommodated when pediatric patients are immobilized on a spine board to prevent excessive cervical flexion.
2. Normal variation and development must be considered when evaluating pediatric spine radiographs to avoid interpreting these findings as spinal injuries.
3. The elasticity of the immature spinal column exceeds the elasticity of the spinal cord. Pediatric spinal trauma may lead to tension-distraction injury with associated neurologic deficit.
4. Odontoid fractures are the most common pediatric cervical spine fracture.
5. In pediatric patients with symptoms suggestive of a disc herniation, the diagnosis of an apophyseal ring fracture should be considered.
6. Skeletally immature patients who sustain a spinal cord injury require surveillance for the development of spinal deformities.

Websites
1. Lumbar fractures: http://www.posna.org/education/StudyGuide/lumbarFractures.asp
2. Pediatric cervical spine: http://radiographics.rsnajnls.org/cgi/content/full/23/3/539?maxtoshow=&HITS=10&hits=10&RESULTFORMAT=&fulltext=spine&andorexactfulltext=and&searchid=1&FIRSTINDEX=0&sortspec=relevance&resourcetype=HWCIT
3. Pediatric spinal cord and spinal column trauma: http://www.neurosurgery.org/sections/section.aspx?Section=PD&Page=ped_spine.asp
4. Pediatric spine trauma: http://www.orthonurse.org/portals/0/spinal%20cord%20injury%208.pdf
5. Thoracolumbar spine fractures: http://www.posna.org/education/StudyGuide/thoracicFractures.asp

BIBLIOGRAPHY

1. Akbarnia, B. A. (1999). Pediatric spine fractures. *Orthopedic Clinics of North America, 30*, 521–536.
2. Arlet, V., & Fassier, F. (2001). Herniated nucleus pulposus and slipped vertebral apophysis. In S. L. Weinstein (Ed.), *The Pediatric Spine: Principles and Practice* (2nd ed., pp. 576–583). Philadelphia, PA: Lippincott Williams & Wilkins.
3. Bible, J. E., Sielatycki, J. A., & Lee, J. Y. (2018). Cervical, thoracic, and lumbar trauma of the immature spine. In S. R. Garfin, F. J. Eismont, G. R. Bell, et al., (Eds.), *Rothman-Simeone the Spine* (7th ed., pp. 565–588). Philadelphia, PA: Saunders.
4. Daniels, A. H., Sobel, A. D., Eberson, & C. P. (2013). Pediatric thoracolumbar spine trauma. Journal of the American Academy of Orthopaedic Surgeons, 21, 707–716.
5. Flynn, J. M. (2000). *Spine Trauma in the Pediatric Population. Spine State Art Reviews, 14*(1), 249–262.
6. Fournier, J., & Tsirkos, A. I. (2016). Paediatric spinal trauma: Patterns of injury, clinical assessment, and principles of treatment. *Orthopaedics and Trauma, 30*, 421–429.
7. Klimo P., Jr., Ware, M. L., Gupta, N., & Brockmeyer. D. (2007). Cervical spine trauma in the pediatric patient. *Neurosurgery Clinics of North America, 18*, 599–620.
8. Limbrick, D. D., Leonard, J. C., & Wright, N. M. Cervical spine trauma in children including spinal cord injury without radiographic abnormality. In D. H. Kim, R. R. Betz, S. L. Huhn, et al., (Eds.), *Surgery of the Pediatric Spine* (pp. 489–500). New York, NY: Thieme Medical Publishers; 2008.
9. Martus, J. E., & Mencio, G. A. (2015). Fractures of the spine. In G. A. & Mencio, M. F. Swiontkowski (Eds.), *Green's Skeletal Trauma in Children* (5th ed., pp. 270–310). Philadelphia, PA: Saunders.
10. Pouliquen, J. C., Kassis, B., Glorion, C., & Langlais, J. (1997). Vertebral growth after thoracic or lumbar fracture of the spine in children. *Journal of Pediatric Orthopedics, 17*(1), 115–120.

DEGENERATIVE DISORDERS OF THE ADULT SPINE

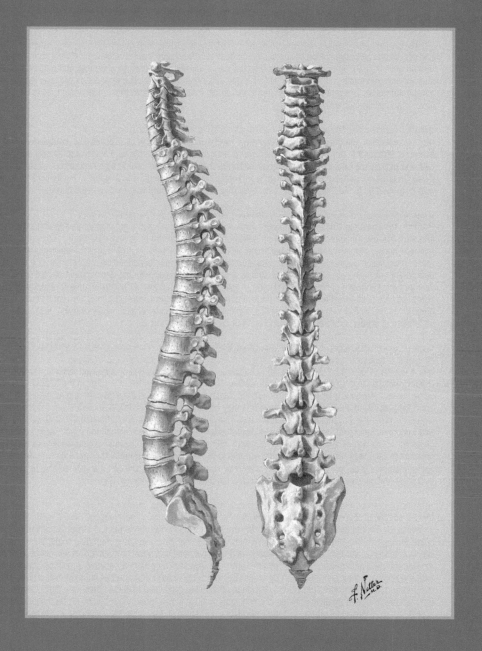

CHAPTER 44

PATHOPHYSIOLOGY AND PATHOANATOMY OF DEGENERATIVE DISORDERS OF THE ADULT SPINE

Vincent J. Devlin, MD

1. What factors play a role in the development of degenerative disorders of the spine?

The prevalence and progression of spinal column degenerative changes are associated with increasing age, but remain asymptomatic in many individuals. Mechanical, traumatic, nutritional, biochemical, and genetic factors interact and contribute to the development of spinal degeneration. The relative importance of these factors varies among individuals and remains incompletely understood. Evidence suggests that spinal degenerative conditions have important genetic influences.

2. What mechanical factors have been associated with disc degeneration?

Disc degeneration has traditionally been linked to mechanical factors such as excessive or repetitive loading resulting in structural injury and subsequent development of axial pain symptoms. Factors traditionally associated with the occurrence of disc degeneration according to this *injury model* include age, occupation, male gender, cigarette smoking, and exposure to vehicular vibration. An observation cited to support a mechanical basis for disc degeneration is the development of degenerative changes adjacent to previous spinal fusions.

3. How does genetics influence the development of disc degeneration?

Findings from multiple studies including the *Twin Spine Study* have shown a substantial genetic influence on intervertebral disc degeneration and the presence of pathoanatomic findings including Modic endplate changes, Schmorl nodes, endplate defects, lumbar spinal stenosis, and back pain. (1) The traditional environmental and mechanical factors associated with disc degeneration in an injury model had only a modest influence on disc degeneration and back pain in more recent studies. Gene loci associated with the development of disc degeneration include type 1 collagen genes *(COL1A1)*, type IX collagen genes *(COL9A1, COL9A2)*, vitamin D receptor genes *(Taq1 and Fok1)*, interleukin-1 and interleukin-6 genes, and metalloproteinase-3 genes. Current thinking is that genetic factors, with or without the presence of other risk factors such as spine injury or aging, lead to the development of intervertebral disc degeneration in specific populations. (5)

4. Can psychosocial factors influence a patient's perception of axial pain associated with degenerative spinal disorders?

Yes. A variety of factors have been shown to influence a patient's perception of axial pain associated with degenerative spinal disorders. When pathologic processes stimulate pain-sensitive structures in the lumbar spine and pelvis, neural signals are transmitted through the dorsal root ganglion to the spinal cord and ultimately to the brain for processing. Perception of these stimuli may be modulated by a variety of factors along the pathway of signal transmission. Psychologic and social factors have been demonstrated to influence this process. Such factors include chronic pain illness, depression, somatization (expression of emotional and psychologic symptoms in physical terms), and secondary gain (e.g., worker's compensation claims, litigation claims following motor vehicle accidents). (3) One of the most challenging aspects in the evaluation and treatment of patients with degenerative spinal disorders is our poor understanding of why similar appearing degenerative changes may be asymptomatic in one patient but cause severe pain and impaired function in other individuals. (7)

5. Is it accurate to classify degenerative spinal disorders as diseases?

Strictly speaking, degenerative changes involving the intervertebral discs and zygapophyseal (facet) joints are not a disease in the traditional sense, but rather the natural consequences of mechanical stresses applied to the spine throughout life. Although disc and facet joint degeneration are universal in the aging spine, these changes are inconsistently and only occasionally associated with pain and functional limitation. There is concern that labeling patients with a diagnosis such as "degenerative disc disease" may have a negative impact on certain patients who may perceive their diagnosis as a progressive, irreversible disease that may not improve over time. Caution is recommended in interpreting the clinical relevance of spinal degeneration features noted on imaging studies due to the high prevalence of imaging findings of spinal degeneration in asymptomatic subjects. (2) Data show that the prevalence of degenerative findings observed on spinal imaging studies increases with age and exceeds 90% in

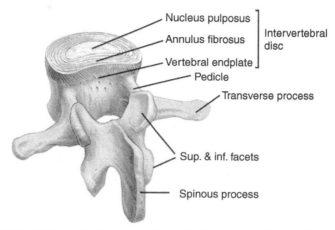

Fig. 44.1 Lumbar vertebrae. The intervertebral disc comprises the annulus fibrosus, nucleus pulposus, and superior (Sup.) and inferior (Inf.) facet joints. Only the superior vertebral endplate is shown. (From Wills BPD, Mohr A, Zdeblick TA. Current status of imaging of the intervertebral disc. Semin Spine Surg 2007; 19:58–64, Fig. 1, p. 59.)

individuals >50 years of age who are evaluated with magnetic resonance imaging (MRI). It is critical that imaging findings of spinal degeneration are interpreted in the context of the individual patient's clinical condition.

6. Describe the morphology of the normal intervertebral disc.
   The intervertebral disc consists of **three distinct regions**:
   - The **annulus fibrosus** comprises the outer aspect of the disc and is composed of concentric rings (lamellae) of predominantly type 1 collagen. Fibroblast-like cells and elastin fibers are located between adjacent lamellae. Collagen fibers penetrate the endplate and attach the disc to the vertebral body.
   - The **nucleus pulposus** comprises the central disc region and consists of type 2 collagen and elastin embedded in a hydrated proteoglycan matrix that contains chondrocytes.
   - The **vertebral endplate** is the interface between the disc and the adjacent vertebral body and consists of a layer of condensed cancellous bone and an adjacent thin layer of hyaline cartilage. Disc metabolism and nutrition is dependent on diffusion of nutrients across the vertebral endplate (Fig. 44.1).

7. What pathoanatomic changes occur within the intervertebral disc in association with the degenerative process?
   There is loss of distinctness between the nuclear and annular regions in the disc. Loss of hydration of the nucleus pulposus occurs. Fissures develop in the annulus fibrosus. Thinning of the vertebral endplate occurs. Disc resorption and loss of disc space height develop. Disc function is compromised as the disc is no longer able to function hydrostatically under load resulting in abnormal force distribution across the spinal segment. This may lead to an increase in loading of the facet joints and may ultimately result in facet arthrosis. (10)

8. What biochemical changes occur within the disc in association with the degenerative process?
   - **Annulus:** The ratio and relative distribution of type 1 to type 2 collagen changes in the outer annulus. A decrease in collagen cross-links occurs, making the annulus more susceptible to mechanical failure.
   - **Nucleus:** Matrix changes occur, including fragmentation of proteoglycans (mainly aggrecan), increase in the ratio of keratin sulfate to chondroitin sulfate, decreases in proteoglycan and water concentrations, and decrease in number of viable cells.
   - **Endplate:** Decrease in proteoglycan, type 1 collagen and water content occur and lead to decreased blood supply, impaired disc nutrition, and communication between the disc nucleus and vertebral bone marrow. These changes contribute to tissue breakdown in the endplate region and nucleus and development of bone marrow lesions detectable on MRI termed Modic changes (Fig. 44.2).

9. How is the severity of lumbar disc degeneration described on MRI?
   The **Pfirrmann classification** is commonly used to describe the severity of lumbar disc degeneration on MRI (see Chapter 48). This five-grade system considers disc structure, the distinction between the nucleus pulposus and annulus fibrosus, signal intensity of the disc nucleus, and intervertebral disc height. (6)
   - **Grade 1:** Defined as a homogenous nucleus pulposus, high T2 signal intensity, clear distinction of the nucleus and annulus and normal disc height.

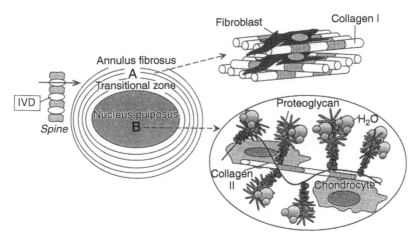

Fig. 44.2 Microstructure of the intervertebral disc (IVD). The annulus fibrosus (A) consists of densely packed layers of collagen type 1 fibers maintained by fibroblast cells. The fiber direction of each layer is perpendicular to the adjacent layer. The nucleus pulposus (B) contains collagen type 2 fibers providing support, proteoglycan aggregates that attach water molecules, and chondrocytes that maintain the type 2 collagen and the proteoglycan matrix in which it is embedded. (From Chung SA, Khan SN, Diwan AD. The molecular basis of disc degeneration. Orthop Clin North Am 2003;34:209–219, Fig. 1, p. 210.)

- **Grade 2:** Defined as an inhomogenous nucleus pulposus with or without horizontal bands, high T2 signal intensity, and clear distinction of the nucleus and annulus, and normal disc height.
- **Grade 3:** Defined as an inhomogenous, gray nucleus pulposus, intermediate T2 signal intensity, unclear distinction of the nucleus and annulus, and normal to slightly decreased disc height.
- **Grade 4:** Defined as an inhomogenous, gray to black nucleus pulposus, intermediate to low T2 signal intensity, loss of distinction of the nucleus and annulus, and normal to moderately decreased disc height.
- **Grade 5:** Defined as an inhomogenous, black nucleus pulposus, low T2 signal intensity, loss of distinction of the nucleus and annulus, and a severe loss of disc height.

10. Describe the morphology of the zygapophyseal joints.
    At each spinal level, bilateral zygapophyseal joints, also referred to as facet joints or z-joints, connect adjacent vertebral arches and function to transfer load and guide spinal motion. The orientation and configuration of the facet joints varies across different spinal regions. The facet joints are synovial (diarthrodial) joints and are surrounded by a multilayered joint capsule: outer layer (dense fibroelastic tissue), middle layer (areolar and loose connective tissue), and inner layer (synovial membrane). Hyaline cartilage covers the joint surfaces, which are nourished and lubricated by synovial fluid produced by the synovial membrane. Synovial folds comprised of synovial-lined extensions of the capsule protrude into the joint space and partially cover the hyaline cartilage articular surfaces and protect the articular cartilage during joint motion. The capsule, subchondral bone, synovium, and synovial folds are innervated with mechanoreceptors, proprioceptors, and nociceptors (Fig. 44.3).

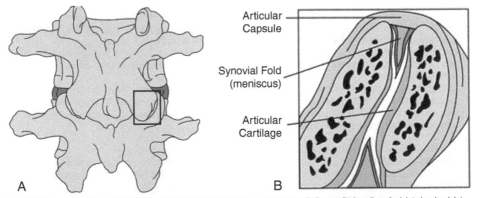

Fig. 44.3 Zygapophyseal (facet) joint. (A) Posterior view of z-joints *(right z-joint in box)*. (B) Parasagittal section of z-joint showing joint capsule, articular fold, and articular cartilage. (From Cramer GD, Ross K, Pocius J, et al. Evaluating the relationship among cavitation, zygapophyseal joint gapping, and spinal manipulation: An exploratory case series. J Manipulative Physiol Ther 2011;34:2–14, Fig. 2, p. 4.)

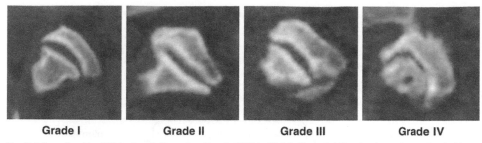

| Grade I | Grade II | Grade III | Grade IV |

Fig. 44.4 Examples of facet joint osteoarthritis grading. (From Suri P, Katz JN, Rainville J, et al. Vascular disease is associated with facet joint osteoarthritis. Osteoarthritis Cartilage 2010;18:1127–1132, Fig. 1, p. 1129.)

11. What pathoanatomic changes occur within the zygapophyseal joints in association with the degenerative process?

Facet joint cartilage thinning, facet capsule laxity, hypermobility, facet subluxation, and facet joint hypertrophy may develop. Altered loading of the facet joints occurs and may ultimately lead to facet arthrosis. For many years, it was assumed that spinal motion segment degeneration began in the intervertebral disc and led to subsequent facet joint degeneration due to altered patterns of vertebral loading. However, more recent evidence has challenged this assumption and suggests that facet and disc degeneration may proceed simultaneously, or in some cases, facet degeneration may precede development of degenerative changes in the disc. (4)

12. How is the severity of facet joint degeneration described on computed tomography (CT) and MRI studies?

A four-grade system (normal, mild, moderate, severe) (Fig. 44.4) is most commonly used to grade the severity of facet joint degeneration due to osteoarthritis, as described by Suri et al (9):

Grade I (normal): No joint space narrowing (joint space >2 mm); no osteophytes or possible small osteophytes; no articular process hypertrophy; no sclerosis or doubtful sclerosis; no subchondral erosions; no subchondral cysts; no joint space vacuum phenomenon.

Grade II (mild): Joint space 1–2 mm; and/or definite small osteophytes; and/or mild articular process hypertrophy; and/or definite sclerosis; no subchondral erosions; no subchondral cysts; no joint space vacuum phenomenon.

Grade III (moderate): Joint space <1 mm; and/or moderate osteophytes; and/or moderate articular process hypertrophy; and/or mild subchondral erosions; and/or mild subchondral cysts; and/or joint space vacuum phenomenon.

Grade IV (severe): Severe joint space narrowing (bone to bone); and/or large osteophytes; and/or severe articular process hypertrophy; and/or severe articular erosions; and/or severe subchondral cysts.

13. What are some of the important clinical manifestations of degenerative spinal disorders?

The clinical manifestations of degenerative spinal disorders include axial pain syndromes, radiculopathy, myelopathy, symptomatic spinal instabilities including degenerative spondylolisthesis, as well as spinal deformities such as adult-onset degenerative scoliosis and kyphotic deformities.

14. What is the degenerative cascade?

The term **degenerative cascade** was introduced by Dr. Kirkaldy-Willis to explain the development and progression of lumbar spine degeneration and serves as a useful framework for understanding the evolution and consequences of spinal degeneration across all spinal regions. (8) Spinal degeneration is conceptualized in terms of a **three-joint complex** composed of the intervertebral disc and two zygapophyseal joints that comprise a **functional spinal unit**, the smallest anatomic unit of the spinal column that demonstrates its basic functional characteristics. The progression of degenerative changes involving the three-joint complex is conceptualized in terms of **three phases**: dysfunction, instability, and stabilization.

In the **first phase, dysfunction**, minor trauma or unusual activity leads to back pain. Segmental spinal muscles become tender and spastic. Circumferential tears in the annulus and degeneration of the nucleus occur. Synovitis and cartilage degeneration in the facet joints develop. Disc material may herniate into the spinal canal through an annular tear.

In the **second phase, instability**, progressive facet capsule laxity and internal disc disruption lead to segmental instability. Degenerative spondylolisthesis and dynamic lateral nerve root entrapment may develop during this phase.

In the **third phase, stabilization**, osteophytes develop around and within the facet joints and intervertebral disc. The ligamentum flavum may thicken and cause narrowing of the spinal canal. Central spinal stenosis and fixed lateral nerve root entrapment may occur (Fig. 44.5).

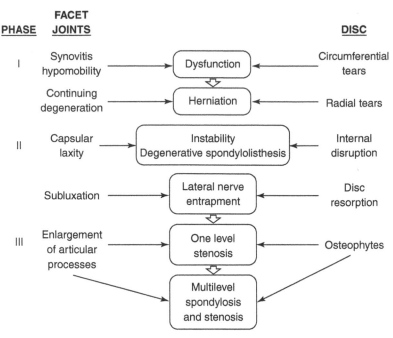

Fig. 44.5 The degenerative cascade. Interactions between the facet joints and intervertebral disc during the three phases of degenerative spondylosis. (Adapted from Kirkaldy-Willis WH, Bernard TH. Managing Low Back Pain. 4th ed. Philadelphia, PA: Churchill Livingstone; 1999, Fig. 13.2, p. 250.)

15. **What important anatomic structures are affected by spinal degeneration involving the cervical region and what clinical syndromes result?**
    The important anatomic structures in the cervical spine affected by the degenerative process include the intervertebral disc, facet joints, neurocentral joints of Luschka, and ligamentum flavum. The adverse effects of the degenerative process may be exacerbated by abnormal motion segment mobility, congenital narrowing of the cervical spinal canal, ossification of the posterior longitudinal ligament, and kyphotic deformity. The degree and extent of neurologic compression requires detailed evaluation with high-quality neurodiagnostic imaging studies. The common clinical syndromes associated with cervical degenerative disease include neck pain, radiculopathy, and myelopathy.

16. **Why are symptomatic thoracic disc herniations less common compared with cervical or lumbar disc herniations?**
    Symptomatic thoracic disc herniations represent less than 1% of all symptomatic disc herniations. Less than 2% of operations performed for disc herniation involve the thoracic spine. The low rate of symptomatic disc herniation is attributed to the limited mobility of the thoracic spine. Stability provided by the rib cage, costovertebral joints, and vertical orientation of the thoracic facet joints limits force application to the thoracic region and decreases the risk of disc degeneration. Thoracic disc herniations most commonly occur at the thoracolumbar junction, where the transition from a stiffer thoracic spine to a more mobile lumbar spine occurs.

17. **Explain why spinal deformities develop in the aging thoracic and lumbar spine?**
    As an individual patient's spine passes through the degenerative cascade, the rate of degeneration may exceed the patient's ability to autostabilize the spinal column by formation of osteophytes around the facet joints and intervertebral discs. Risk factors remain incompletely understood but include osteoporosis, female sex, poor connective tissue quality, diabetes, and obesity. Disc height loss, facet subluxation, asymmetric disc space collapse, anterolisthesis, lateral listhesis, and rotatory subluxations may develop. Spinal deformities develop as the structural integrity of the motion segment is compromised by the degenerative process and include unisegmental spinal deformities (e.g., degenerative spondylolisthesis) or multisegmental spinal deformities (e.g., degenerative scoliosis or kyphosis). Narrowing of the central and lateral spinal canal may lead to lower extremity symptoms due to spinal stenosis. Deformity magnitude ranges from mild curvatures causing minimal symptoms to major deformities presenting with severe coronal and sagittal imbalance with symptomatic spinal stenosis.

KEY POINTS

1. Mechanical, traumatic, nutritional, biochemical, and genetic factors interact and contribute to development of spinal degeneration.
2. Spinal degeneration occurs in all individuals and remains asymptomatic in many patients.
3. There is a poor correlation between the severity of degenerative changes on spinal imaging studies and the severity of spine-related symptoms.
4. The clinical manifestations of degenerative spinal disorders may include axial pain syndromes, radiculopathy, myelopathy, spinal instabilities, and spinal deformities.

Websites
1. Lumbar facet arthropathy: http://emedicine.medscape.com/article/310069-overview
2. Intervertebral disc degeneration: http://www.biomedcentral.com/content/pdf/ar629.pdf

---

BIBLIOGRAPHY

1. Battié, M. C., Videman, T., Kaprio, J., Gibbons, L. E., Gill, K., Manninen, H., et al. (2009). The twin spine study: Contributions to a changing view of disc degeneration. *Spine Journal, 9*, 47–59.
2. Brinjikji, W., Luetmer, P. H., Comstock, B., Bresnahan, B. W., Chen, L. E., Deyo, R. A., et al. (2015). Systematic literature review of imaging features of spinal degeneration in asymptomatic populations. *American Journal of Neuroradiology, 36*, 811–816.
3. Carragee, E. J., Alamin, T. F., Miller, J. L., & Caragee, J. M. (2005). Discographic, MRI and psychosocial determinant of low back pain disability and remission: A prospective study in subjects with benign persistent back pain. *Spine Journal, 5*, 24–35.
4. Eubanks, J. D., Lee, M. J., Cassinelli, E., & Ahn, N. U. (2007). Does lumbar facet arthrosis precede disc degeneration? A postmortem study. *Clinical Orthopaedics and Related Research, 464*, 184–189.
5. Feng, Y., Egan, B., & Wang, J. (2016). Genetic factors in intervertebral disc degeneration. *Genes & Diseases, 3*, 178–185.
6. Kettler, A., & Wilke, H. J. (2006). Review of existing grading systems for cervical or lumbar disc and facet joint degeneration. *European Spine Journal, 15*, 705–718.
7. Polatin, P. B., Kinney, R. K., Gatchel, R. J., Lillo, E., & Mayer, T. G. (1993). Psychiatric illness and chronic low back pain: The mind and the spine—which goes first? *Spine, 18*, 66–71.
8. Singh, K., & Phillips, F. M. (2005). The biomechanics and biology of the spinal degenerative cascade. *Seminars in Spine Surgery, 17*, 128–136.
9. Suri, P., Katz, J. N., Rainville, J., Kalichman, L., Guermazi, A., & Hunter, D. J. (2010). Vascular disease is associated with facet joint osteoarthritis. *Osteoarthritis and Cartilage, 18*, 1127–1132.
10. Urban, J. P. G., & Roberts, S. (2003). Degeneration of the intervertebral disc. *Arthritis Research and Therapy, 5*, 120–130.

CHAPTER 45

CERVICAL DEGENERATIVE DISORDERS

Vincent J. Devlin, MD

1. **Define cervical spondylosis. How does this condition present in clinical practice?**
   Cervical spondylosis is a nonspecific term that refers to age-related degenerative changes within the cervical spinal column. The degenerative process can affect the intervertebral discs, facet joints, uncovertebral joints, and associated soft tissue supporting structures. Often patients with cervical spondylosis have little or no pain. Positive radiographic findings in asymptomatic patients have been reported in approximately 25% of adults under age 40, 50% of adults over age 40, and 85% of adults over age 60. Similarly, abnormal magnetic resonance imaging (MRI) findings in asymptomatic individuals are quite common with disc degeneration reported in more than 25% of adults less than age 40 and 60% of adults older than age 40. Symptomatic patients with cervical spondylosis are often categorized into three clinical syndromes: axial neck pain, cervical radiculopathy, or degenerative cervical myelopathy (see Chapter 13 for details regarding initial evaluation and nonoperative treatment).

AXIAL NECK PAIN

2. **What is known about the epidemiology, risk factors, and natural history of axial neck pain in adults?**
   Self-reported neck pain is very common and is experienced by 30%–50% of the adult population annually. The precise location and source of neck pain is often unidentified. Half to three-quarters of patients with neck pain continue to report neck pain 1–5 years later. The prevalence of neck pain peaks during middle age and is higher among women, who are more likely to experience persistent neck pain and less likely to experience pain resolution compared with men. Risk factors for neck pain are multifactorial in nature and include genetic factors, advanced age, female gender, physical activity participation, poor psychological health, tobacco use, history of neck or low back pain, and rear-end automobile accidents. The presence of cervical spinal degeneration on imaging studies is not considered a risk factor for neck pain. The natural history of neck pain in adults is favorable overall, but pain recurrence and chronicity are reported in a substantial number of patients. For patients with acute neck pain, recovery is most rapid in the first 6–12 weeks and gradually slows with little recovery noted after 1 year. Up to 30% of patients with acute neck pain will develop chronic symptoms. Patients with chronic neck pain may experience a stable or fluctuating course with episodes of remission and exacerbation over time.

3. **What nonoperative treatments are recommended for chronic axial neck pain?**
   Patients should be reassessed for red flags (serious underlying conditions) and yellow flags (barriers to recovery) at the time of initial evaluation. Treatment of chronic neck pain is directed toward specific cervical structural pathology, as well as any psychosocial factors that contribute to pain and disability. Evidence-based treatments for chronic neck pain includes active rehabilitation therapy with supervised exercise. Components of an active treatment program include stretching, strengthening with isometric and/or dynamic exercises, cervicothoracic stabilization, and aerobic conditioning. Pharmacologic treatment options include nonsteroidal anti-inflammatory drugs (NSAIDs) or serotonin-norepinephrine reuptake inhibitors (SNRIs) such as duloxetine. Alternatively, a short course (few weeks) of a nonbenzodiazepine muscle relaxant may be considered. Opioid medications are not recommended for treatment of chronic musculoskeletal cervical pain. Alternative therapies supported by randomized controlled evidence include qigong (a holistic system of coordinated body posture and movement) and Iyengar yoga (emphasizes precision and alignment in all postures). Select patients may benefit from cognitive behavioral therapy or a functional restoration program. For patients with presumed zygapophyseal joint pain, diagnosis may be confirmed with nerve blocks performed by anesthetizing the medial branch nerves innervating the target facet joint(s). Anesthetic agents of varying duration of effect are utilized during two separate injection sessions. If the diagnosis is confirmed, percutaneous radiofrequency neurotomy to ablate the medial branch nerves innervating the target facet joint(s) is a treatment option. Although cervical disc degeneration is a cause of neck pain in some patients, distinguishing painful from nonpainful cervical discs remains challenging.

4. **How does cervical spondylosis lead to degenerative cervical spinal instability?**
   Instability is present when the spine is unable to withstand physiologic loads, resulting in significant risk for neurologic injury, progressive deformity, and long-term pain and disability. Cervical degenerative instability presents most commonly as spondylolisthesis. Cervical degenerative instability is less common compared to lumbar instability. Cervical degenerative instability may occur at the C1–C2 level or in the subaxial cervical region.
   C1–C2 instability occasionally develops secondary to chronic degeneration involving the atlantodental joint and atlantoaxial joints in association with incompetence of the transverse ligament. Symptoms may include

chronic unilateral or bilateral neck pain or pain radiating toward the skull. Retroodontoid ligamentous hypertrophy and pannus formation can lead to symptomatic neural compression. Surgical treatment is instrumented C1–C2 posterior fusion and decompression.

Subaxial cervical instability may develop at a mobile cervical level adjacent to stiff spondylotic segments or between spondylotic segments. Subaxial cervical instability develops most commonly in patients with spondylotic stiffening of middle and lower cervical regions due to compensatory hypermobility at an adjacent mobile segment, most commonly C3–C4 or C4–C5. Cervical degenerative spondylolisthesis presents as neck pain with or without cervical radiculopathy and/or myelopathy. Treatment options include spinal decompression and instrumented fusion through posterior, anterior, or combined approaches. Cervical spinal instability may be diagnosed according to the radiographic criteria of White (>11° angulation, >3.5 mm translation of adjacent subaxial cervical spine segments).

5. **When is surgery indicated for chronic neck pain in the absence of radiculopathy or myelopathy?**
   Indications for surgical treatment of patients with axial neck pain without radicular or myelopathic symptoms are not clearly defined. There is limited evidence in the literature to support anterior cervical discectomy and fusion or cervical disc arthroplasty for this indication. It has been suggested that surgical treatment with single-level anterior cervical fusion be considered after a minimum 1-year course of appropriate nonoperative treatment, in the absence of secondary gain or other factors that could adversely affect outcomes for patients with advanced degenerative changes at one level and relatively normal adjacent levels. The role of cervical discography in this setting remains controversial.

CERVICAL RADICULOPATHY

6. **What signs and symptoms may be present in a patient with cervical radiculopathy due to a cervical disc herniation?**
   Cervical radiculopathy most commonly presents with unilateral pain that is most intense in the upper arm below the deltoid insertion and extends below the elbow to involve the thumbs or fingers of the hand according to the specific pattern of dorsal root ganglion or cervical nerve root involvement. Arm pain may be constant and aggravated by neck movement, coughing, or sneezing. Scapular pain is often present. Symptoms are generally worsened by extension of the head or lateral rotation of the head towards the side of the arm pain. Some combination of sensory loss, motor weakness, or impaired reflexes occurs in a dermatomal distribution. Upper cervical radiculopathy may present with occipital pain with radiation. Other symptoms that may occasionally occur include anterior chest pain and headaches.

7. **Which nonoperative treatment options are effective for cervical disc herniations?**
   The majority of patients with cervical radiculopathy improve with nonoperative treatment. Supervised active physical therapy is recommended. Medication options include NSAIDs, SNRIs such as duloxetine, or a short course of oral corticosteroids. Epidural and selective nerve root steroid injections may be considered. Intermittent cervical traction or resting the neck by use of an orthosis, such as a soft collar and reduction of activities, may provide benefit.

8. **When is surgery indicated for treatment of a symptomatic cervical disc herniation?**
   Indications for surgical treatment for a symptomatic cervical disc herniation include intractable radicular symptoms that have not improved with at least 6 weeks of nonoperative treatment, a progressive neurologic deficit, or a neurologic deficit that is associated with significant radicular pain. Neuroimaging studies should correlate with clinical symptoms.

9. **What are the options for surgical treatment of a patient with a single-level cervical disc herniation who presents with radiculopathy refractory to nonsurgical treatment?**
   Surgical treatment options for single-level disc pathology include:
   - Posterior foraminotomy with discectomy
   - Anterior discectomy and fusion
   - Cervical disc arthroplasty

10. **Discuss the indications and results of posterior foraminotomy and discectomy for a herniated cervical disc.**
    Patients who have acute radiculopathy without long-standing chronic neck pain and posterolateral or intraforaminal soft tissue disc herniation are appropriate candidates for posterior cervical foraminotomy. The disc space height should be well preserved, and there should be no associated spinal instability. The advantages of this technique are avoidance of fusion and early return to function. The disadvantages are difficulty in removing pathology ventral to the nerve root, especially an osteophyte, and the potential for instability if more than 50% of the facet is removed. Satisfactory outcomes are seen in 85%–90% of properly selected cases (Fig. 45.1).

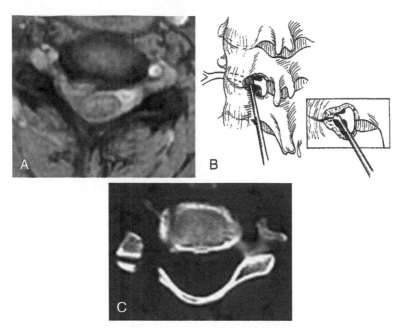

Fig. 45.1 (A) Magnetic resonance imaging shows a lateral C5–C6 disc herniation. (B) Posterior foraminotomy and discectomy were performed. (C) Postoperative computed tomography scan shows extent of foraminotomy. (B and C: From Herkowitz HN, Garfin SR, Eismont FJ, et al. The Spine. 5th ed. Philadelphia, PA: Saunders; 2006, pp. 843–844).

11. **How does anterior cervical discectomy, fusion, and plate fixation compare with cervical disc arthroplasty for treatment of single-level cervical disc pathology?**
    Anterior cervical discectomy and fusion (ACDF) in combination with plate fixation for treatment of radiculopathy secondary to cervical disc herniation is an effective option for treatment of single-level cervical disc pathology. It provides predictable relief of arm pain, neck pain, and neurologic deficits. Placement of an interbody graft or spacer provides indirect decompression of foraminal stenosis and restores cervical lordosis. Plate fixation is used to maintain alignment, decrease risk of graft collapse or subsidence, and minimize or eliminate postoperative brace use. Complications associated with ACDF include pseudarthrosis, implant or graft-related complications, and adjacent-level degeneration. Cervical disc arthroplasty provides comparable clinical outcomes to ACDF but is contraindicated in patients with poor bone quality, kyphotic alignment, narrowed disc spaces, segmental instability, facet joint degeneration, or infection. Complications associated with cervical disc arthroplasty include heterotopic ossification and potential for occurrence of same segment pathology as the motion segment is not fused. Cervical disc arthroplasty is associated with a lower rate of secondary revision surgery compared to ACDF (Fig. 45.2).

12. **What are the options for surgical treatment for a patient with cervical disc pathology involving two adjacent levels that is refractory to nonsurgical treatment?**
    Surgical options for treatment of adjacent two-level cervical disc pathology (Fig. 45.3) include:
    - Two-level posterior foraminotomies ± discectomy
    - Two-level anterior discectomy, fusion, and plate fixation
    - Two-level cervical disc arthroplasty
    - Anterior corpectomy, fusion, and plate fixation
    - Hybrid anterior cervical fusion-cervical disc arthroplasty

13. **Compare various surgical options for treatment of cervical disc pathology involving two adjacent cervical disc levels.**
    Two-level posterior cervical foraminotomy is an option for patients with posterolateral or foraminal pathology involving two adjacent levels but is not indicated for treatment of a centrally located disc herniation. Two-level ACDF and plating is an effective option for treatment of all types of cervical disc pathology and provides predictable relief of arm pain, neck pain, and neurologic deficits. Drawbacks of ACDF include pseudarthrosis, motion restriction, and adjacent-level degeneration. Two-level cervical disc arthroplasty has shown comparable or even better

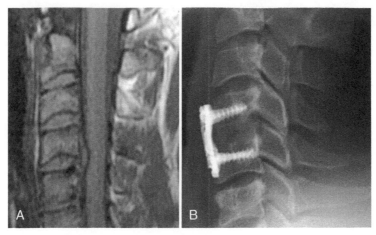

Fig. 45.2 (A) Sagittal magnetic resonance imaging shows a C4–C5 disc herniation. (B) Surgical treatment with C4–C5 anterior cervical discectomy and fusion with allograft bone graft and anterior cervical plate.

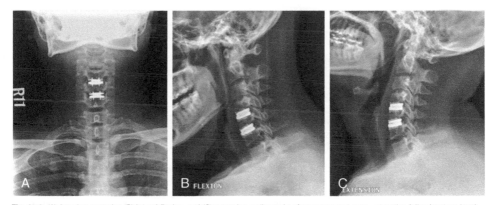

Fig. 45.3 (A) Anterior–posterior, (B) lateral flexion, and (C) extension radiographs show preserved range of motion following two-level PRESTIGE LP arthroplasty. (From Wu JC, Meyer SA, Gandhoke G, et al. PRESTIGE cervical arthroplasty: Past, present, and future. Semin Spine Surg 2012;24:14 19, Fig. 2, p 16.)

clinical success when compared with ACDF, and has a lower rate of subsequent surgery compared with ACDF. Anterior cervical corpectomy and fusion is necessary when retrovertebral decompression is required and is recommended to enhance safety during removal of disc and osseous pathology from a narrow spinal canal. An advantage of corpectomy is the decreased number of bone interfaces that require union, which decreases pseudarthrosis risk. However, biomechanical studies strongly favor two-level discectomy over corpectomy. Clinical advantages of multilevel interbody fusion compared with corpectomy include improved ability to restore sagittal alignment and improved fixation due to the ability to achieve screw fixation in the intervening vertebral body. Use of hybrid ACDF-cervical disc arthroplasty has been reported, but limited data exist to assess the role of this option for treatment of two-level cervical disc pathology.

14. **What is the rate of pseudarthrosis after an anterior cervical discectomy and fusion procedure?**
    Pseudarthrosis rates correlate to number of levels arthrodesed and whether anterior cervical fusion is performed with or without anterior plate fixation. No consistently reported differences in fusion rates have been identified for use of allograft versus iliac crest bone graft. Pseudarthrosis rates are significantly higher in patients treated without plate fixation. The rates of pseudarthrosis reported in the literature for ACDF performed with plating range widely for one-level (0%–10%), two-level (0%–28%), three-level (7%–37%), and four-level (6%–53%) fusions.

However, the pseudarthrosis rates for two-level fusions are consistently higher than for one-level fusions, and pseudarthrosis rates for three- and four-level fusions are consistently higher than for either one- or two-level fusions across studies.

15. List some of the complications reported in association with anterior cervical procedures.
Some complications associated with anterior cervical procedures include:
- Dysphagia (acute, chronic)
- Graft or interbody device-related complications
  - Collapse
  - Migration
  - Dislodgement
  - Nonunion
- Other implant-related complications
- Neurologic complications
  - Spinal cord or nerve root injury
  - Recurrent laryngeal nerve injury
  - Superior laryngeal nerve injury
  - C5 palsy
  - Hypoglossal nerve injury
  - Horner syndrome
- Vertebral artery injury
- Airway obstruction
- Esophageal injury
- Thoracic duct injury
- Adjacent segment degeneration or disease

16. Why does motion segment degeneration occur at spinal segments adjacent to a prior cervical fusion?
The causes of adjacent segment degeneration are:
1. Progression of the underlying degenerative disease process, which would occur regardless of whether spinal surgery was performed.
2. Increased load and stress transfer, resulting in accelerated degeneration of the motion segment adjacent to a cervical fusion.
No clear evidence determines which process is the more important one.

17. What is the potential for development of degenerative changes adjacent to fused cervical spine segments?
Long-term studies after anterior cervical discectomy and fusion indicate that progressive radiographic degenerative changes occur in up to 50% of cases. The incidence of degenerative changes after anterior cervical fusion has been reported to exceed the rate predicted if fusion was not performed. Hilibrand and Morrissey (1) documented development of new symptomatic radiculopathy or myelopathy in adjacent segments at a rate of approximately 3% per year. Within 10 years after anterior cervical decompression and fusion, 26% of patients developed symptomatic radiculopathy or myelopathy.

DEGENERATIVE CERVICAL MYELOPATHY

18. What is degenerative cervical myelopathy?
Degenerative cervical myelopathy (DCM) is an umbrella term (2) that has recently been defined to encompass the various types of degenerative cervical spine pathologies that lead to myelopathy due to compression of the spinal cord including:
- Cervical spondylotic myelopathy
- Ossification of the posterior longitudinal ligament (OPLL) and ligamentum flavum
- Congenital conditions (i.e., congenital stenosis, Klippel-Feil anomaly, Down syndrome, skeletal dysplasias)
- Occupational factors (i.e., professional athletes in collision sports, military pilots)

19. How common is DCM and how does it develop?
DCM is the most common cause of spinal cord dysfunction in patients older than age 55. In North America the estimated annual incidence is 41 million cases per year and the estimated prevalence is 605 cases per million inhabitants. Age-related spinal column tissue degeneration leads to spinal cord compression and foraminal narrowing due to disc narrowing and protrusion, osteophyte formation, facet degeneration, and uncinate and ligamentous hypertrophy. Static neural compression is exacerbated by dynamic factors that may lead to segmental instability (e.g., spondylolisthesis, especially at C3–C4 or C4–C5) and kyphotic deformities. In some patients, the effects of

spinal cord compression are exacerbated due to the presence of a congenitally narrowed spinal canal, OPLL, or other cervical anomalies. The end result is spinal cord dysfunction secondary to spinal cord compression, a diminished vascular supply, or both.

20. What are the clinical findings in patients with DCM?
DCM typically has an insidious onset and is slowly progressive. The diagnosis of DCM is often delayed as it is associated with nonspecific symptoms such as neck pain and stiffness, generalized fatigue, weakness, clumsiness of hands, arm or hand pain or numbness, loss of balance, gait disturbance, and bladder or bowel impairment. Pain may be lacking or minimal. Physical findings include reduced neck motion, especially in extension; atrophy and weakness of muscles; muscle fasciculation; poor hand coordination; upper extremity numbness; increased muscle tone; ataxia of gait; and the Romberg sign. Reflexes in the upper extremity are variable but are usually increased in the legs. Pathologic reflexes (e.g., Hoffman sign, Babinski sign) and clonus may be present. Lhermitte sign may be present (shock-like paresthesias with neck flexion).

21. Discuss the natural history of DCM.
The natural history of patients with established cervical myelopathy is poor. Often there is a slow, stepwise worsening with periods of neurologic plateau preceding another episode of deterioration. Rarely, patients present with acute deterioration or even quadriplegia. Current literature shows that 20%–62% of patients with DCM will deteriorate over a follow-up period of 3–6 years based on assessment of modified Japanese Orthopedic Association (mJOA) scores. The severity of DCM is graded objectively using the mJOA assessment scale, an investigator-administered tool that provides scores for upper extremity motor function (0–5), lower extremity motor function (0–7), sensation (0–3), and bladder function (0–3), which are combined in a composite score. Severity of myelopathy is graded as mild ($\geq$15 points), moderate (12–14 points), or severe ($<$12 points).

22. Describe the typical radiographic and imaging findings associated with DCM.
MRI is the preferred imaging modality for diagnosis of DCM. A variety of spinal pathologies may result in cord compression and lead to subsequent development of myelopathy. Spinal pathology may occur at a single level or, more commonly, involve multiple spinal levels. Patterns of cord encroachment vary and include anterior-based compression, posterior-based compression, or circumferential compression. Many patients with myelopathy have a congenitally small spinal canal with a midsagittal diameter measuring less than 10 mm. Associated imaging findings may include anterior and posterior osteophytes, retrolisthesis (especially at C5–C6 and C6–C7), anterolisthesis (most common at C3–C4 and C4–C5), and acute soft tissue disc herniation. MRI may demonstrate focal or diffuse cord compression. Deformation of the cord with decreased anteroposterior diameter and increased medial-lateral diameter may be noted. In 20%–40% of cases, signal changes in the cord are present on MRI. If focal high signal is present only on T2-weighted images, this represents a broad range of pathologies and may be reversible (e.g., edema). It does not necessarily indicate a poor potential for recovery following surgery. If high signal is present on T2-weighted images and low signal is present on T1-weighted images, this represents a severe gray matter lesion with a poor prognosis. Also, patients with multiple levels of high signal involvement on T2-weighted images are associated with a worse prognosis compared with patients with focal involvement on T2-weighted images.

23. What are the indications for surgical treatment for patients with DCM?
Most patients with cervical myelopathy should be treated surgically, unless intervention is contraindicated by age or medical conditions. Increasing numbers of patients with cord compression on MRI, but without neurologic symptoms or evidence of myelopathy, are being evaluated. In the absence of objective findings or symptoms of myelopathy, such patients are best treated nonoperatively. However, these patients should be educated about cervical myelopathy and monitored with periodic examinations for the future development of cervical myelopathy.

24. List the surgical treatment options for patients with DCM.
Posterior Procedures
• Laminectomy
• Laminectomy and instrumented posterior fusion
• Laminoplasty
Anterior Procedures
• Anterior cervical discectomy and fusion
• Anterior cervical corpectomy and fusion
• Hybrid anterior cervical discectomy and corpectomy procedures
• Cervical disc arthroplasty
Combined Anterior and Posterior Procedures
• Anterior cervical discectomies and/or corpectomies and fusion $\pm$ plate fixation in combination with posterior instrumented fusion $\pm$ posterior decompression

25. What are some of the factors that enter into surgical decision-making for DCM? What are the indications for anterior versus posterior versus circumferential surgical procedures?

Both anterior and posterior surgical approaches are safe and effective for treatment of cervical myelopathy. Sagittal alignment, anatomic location of compressive pathology, number of levels of compression, type of compressive pathology (spondylosis, OPLL), presence of spinal instability or deformity, and bone quality are among the factors that enter into decision making. An **anterior approach** is optimal for treatment of anterior-based compressive pathology involving three or fewer intervertebral segments, especially in the presence of kyphotic deformity. A **posterior approach** is optimal for treatment of multilevel compression involving more than three intervertebral segments in patients with neutral or lordotic cervical alignment. A posterior approach is also preferable for treatment of posterior-based compressive pathology and for treatment of OPLL. **Circumferential approaches** are less commonly utilized but play an important role in treatment of patients with complex conditions such as rigid kyphotic deformities treated with three-level corpectomies, as well as revision surgery for treatment of conditions such as postlaminectomy deformities or in treatment of severely osteoporotic patients.

26. Compare the various posterior surgical options for treatment of DCM.

The two primary posterior surgical options for treatment of DCM are laminoplasty and laminectomy in combination with instrumented posterior fusion. Both are safe and effective treatments for DCM in patients with neutral or lordotic cervical alignment. Multilevel laminectomy is no longer recommended due to high rates of postlaminectomy kyphotic deformity and the availability of better treatment options. Laminoplasty procedures preserve the posterior osseous structures and decompress the spinal cord by elevating the lamina *en bloc* using a variety of techniques. Preservation of the posterior spinal elements decreases the likelihood of postoperative spinal instability and extensive postoperative epidural scar formation, and preserves cervical motion. Laminoplasty should be avoided in patients with severe neck pain, spinal instability, and kyphotic cervical alignment. Laminectomy performed in conjunction with instrumented posterior fusion is recommended for treatment of patients with severe neck pain, spinal instability, or flexible kyphotic deformities that are correctable with intraoperative repositioning. Disadvantages of laminectomy and fusion include loss of cervical motion and the complexity of the procedure (see Chapter 24 for additional information about spinal decompression procedures) (Figs. 45.4 and 45.5).

27. What is the role of different anterior surgical decompression techniques in the treatment of DCM? Multilevel anterior cervical discectomies? Hybrid discectomy-corpectomy? Corpectomy?

Advantages of multilevel discectomy approaches compared with corpectomy approaches include decreased intraoperative blood loss, greater ability to correct sagittal alignment, and enhanced construct stability due to the ability to achieve segmental fixation. Advantages of corpectomy approaches include the ability to decompress retrovertebral stenosis, a lesser number of bone graft interfaces requiring union, and the possibility for side-to-side bone healing within the corpectomy trough. Based on existing literature, when there is minimal retrovertebral stenosis, a multilevel discectomy approach is recommended over a hybrid discectomy-corpectomy or corpectomy approach due to more favorable clinical outcomes, improved sagittal correction, and lower rates of C5 palsy. When decompression of retrovertebral stenosis is required, discectomy–corpectomy approaches are recommended over multiple corpectomy approaches (Fig. 45.6).

28. What is the role of cervical disc arthroplasty for treatment of patients with DCM?

Cervical disc arthroplasty is indicated for a specific subset of patients with cervical degenerative myelopathy involving one or two spinal levels in whom stenosis is limited to the level of the disc space in the absence of congenital stenosis, instability, facet arthropathy, posterior-based neural compression, or osteoporosis.

29. When are combined anterior and posterior procedures indicated for the treatment of DCM?

Indications for combined anterior and posterior procedures include:
1. Postlaminectomy kyphotic deformities
2. Complex spinal deformities and instabilities
3. All three-level corpectomies and some two-level corpectomies (e.g., corpectomies ending at C7, patients with osteopenia)
4. Treatment of complex pseudarthroses

(Fig. 45.7)

30. What are the most common intraoperative and postoperative adverse events associated with patients undergoing surgical treatment for DCM using anterior, posterior, or circumferential surgical approaches?

Based on a recent large prospective case series (3), the most common intraoperative adverse events were instrumentation malposition requiring revision, instrumentation malposition not requiring revision, and dural tear. Additional intraoperative adverse events included spinal cord injury, surgical approach-related adverse events,

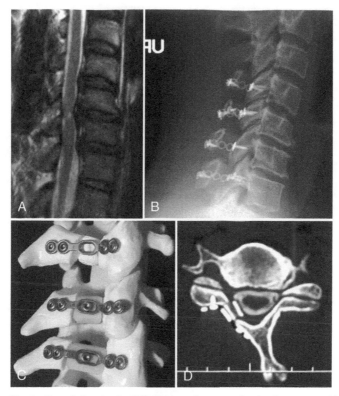

Fig. 45.4 A 55-year-old male with cervical myelopathy. (A) Sagittal magnetic resonance imaging shows severe multilevel stenosis due to congenital spinal canal narrowing and superimposed multilevel disc herniations. (B) Lateral radiograph following C4–C7 laminoplasty. (C) Model demonstrates use of laminoplasty miniplates and allograft spacers that are used to hold open the hinge and maintain expansion of the spinal canal. (D) Postoperative computed tomography myelogram demonstrates expansion of the spinal canal via allograft bone spacers and miniplate fixation. (C and D: From Feigenbaum F, Henderson FC. A decade of experience with expansile laminoplasty: Lessons learned. Semin Spine Surg 2006;18[4]:207–210.)

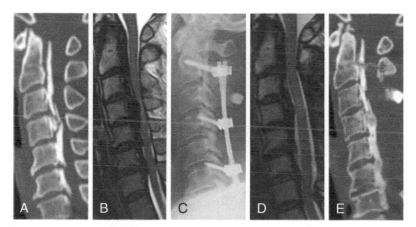

Fig. 45.5 (A) Preoperative midsagittal computed tomography (CT) image of a 49-year-old man with mixed type ossification of the posterior longitudinal ligament (OPLL). (B) A preoperative T2-weighted magnetic resonance image (MRI) shows multilevel spinal cord compression and a high-intensity area at C4–C5 and C5–C6. (C) Postoperative radiographs show posterior decompression and instrumented fusion from C2 to C7. (D) MRI at 1 year postoperatively shows posterior shift of the spinal cord at C4–C5 and C5–C6. (E) CT at 6 years postoperatively shows that the mixed-type OPLL had changed to the continuous type. (From Katsumi K, Hirano T, Watanabe K, et al. Perioperative factors associated with favorable outcomes of posterior decompression and instrumented fusion for cervical ossification of the posterior longitudinal ligament: A retrospective multicenter study. J Clin Neurosci 2018;57:74–78, Fig. 3, p. 78.)

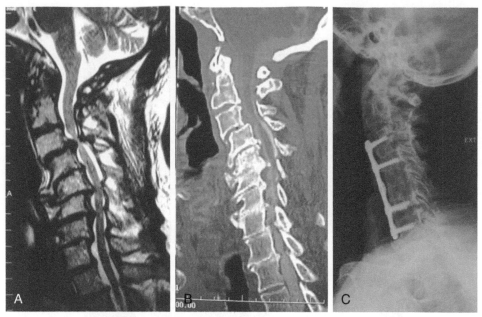

Fig. 45.6 (A) Severe multilevel cervical spondylotic myelopathy. Note the classic imaging findings consistent with degenerative cervical stenosis on T2-weighted sagittal magnetic resonance imaging. (B) Sagittal reconstruction of computed tomography myelogram. (C) This complex compressive pathology was treated with a hybrid anterior technique consisting of C3–C4 and C6–C7 anterior cervical discectomy and fusion, and C5 corpectomy with strut allograft. (From Yoon TS, Freedman BA. Cervical spinal stenosis. In: Miller MD, Hart JA, MacKnight JM, editors. Essential Orthopaedics. Philadelphia, PA: Saunders; 2010, pp. 479–483, Fig. 114.4, p. 482.)

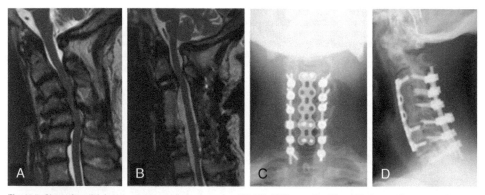

Fig. 45.7 Circumferential decompression and fusion procedure (C3–T1). (A) Preoperative T2-weighted magnetic resonance imaging (MRI) sagittal image. (B) Postoperative T2-weighted MRI sagittal image. (C) Postoperative anteroposterior radiograph. (D) Postoperative lateral radiograph. (From Kato S, Ganau M, Fehlings MG. Surgical decision-making in degenerative cervical myelopathy–anterior versus posterior approach. J Clin Neurosci 2018;58:7–12, Fig. 3, p. 9.)

airway/ventilation issues, and iatrogenic dental injury. The most common postoperative adverse events were dysphagia, urinary tract infection, delirium, postoperative neuropathic pain, and cardiac adverse events. Additional postoperative adverse events included wound infection, wound hematoma, wound dehiscence, dysphonia, neurologic deterioration, pneumonia, renal failure, and electrolyte imbalance. Other adverse events reported in association with surgical procedures for treatment of DCM include C5 nerve root palsy, pseudarthrosis, adjacent level degeneration, and adjacent segment disease.

KEY POINTS

1. Cervical spondylotic changes are common with increasing age and may or may not be responsible for clinical symptoms.
2. To ensure optimal results for the surgical treatment of radiculopathy, it is important that the patient's history, physical findings, and imaging studies correlate.
3. Surgical treatment is indicated for moderate or severe degenerative cervical myelopathy unless medically contraindicated because there is no good nonsurgical treatment.

Websites

1. Cervical stenosis, myelopathy and radiculopathy: https://www.spine.org/KnowYourBack/Conditions/Degenerative-Conditions/Cervical-Stenosis-Myelopathy-and-Radiculopathy
2. Herniated cervical disc: https://www.spine.org/KnowYourBack/Conditions/Degenerative-Conditions/Herniated-Cervical-Disc
3. Degenerative cervical myelopathy: https://www.bmj.com/content/360/bmj.k186

REFERENCES

1. Hilibrand, A. S., Morrissey, P. B. (2017). Chapter 15: Cervical degenerative disease. In E. Truumees & H. Prather (Eds.), *Orthopaedic Knowledge Update 5—Spine* (pp. 211–227). Rosemont, IL: American Academy of Orthopaedic Surgeons.
2. Yamaguchi, S., Mitsuhara, T., Abiko, M., Takeda, M., & Kurisu, S. (2018). Epidemiology and overview of the clinical spectrum of degenerative cervical myelopathy. *Neurosurgery Clinics of North America, 29,* 1–12.
3. Hartig, D., Batke, J., Dea, N., Kelly, A., Fisher, C., & Street, J. (2015). Adverse events in surgically treated cervical spondylopathic myelopathy: A prospective validated observational study. *Spine, 40,* 292–298.

BIBLIOGRAPHY

1. Badhiwala, J. H., & Wilson, J. R. (2018). The natural history of degenerative cervical myelopathy. *Neurosurgery Clinics of North America, 29,* 21–32.
2. Boselie, T. F., Willems, P. C., van Mameren, H., de Bie, R. A., Benzel, E. C., & van Santbrink, H. (2013). Arthroplasty versus fusion in single-level cervical degenerative disc disease: A Cochrane review. *Spine (Phila Pa 1976), 38,* E1096–E1107.
3. Davis, R. J., Nunley, P. D., Kim, K. D., Hisey, M. S., Jackson, R. J., Bae, H. W., et al. (2015). Two-level total disc replacement with Mobi-C cervical artificial disc versus anterior cervical discectomy and fusion: A prospective, randomized, controlled multicenter clinical trial with 4-year follow-up results. *Journal of Neurosurgery Spine, 22,* 15–25.
4. Fehlings, M. G., Santaguida, C., Tetreault, L., Arnold, P., Barbagallo, G., Defino, H., et al. (2017). Laminectomy and fusion versus laminoplasty for the treatment of degenerative cervical myelopathy: Results from the AOSpine North America and International prospective multicenter studies. *The Spine Journal, 17,* 102–108.
5. Hartig, D., Batke, J., Dea, N., Kelly, A., Fisher, C., & Street, J. (2015). Adverse events in surgically treated cervical spondylopathic myelopathy: A prospective validated observational study. *Spine (Phila Pa 1976), 40,* 292–298.
6. Hilibrand, A. S., & Morrissey, P. B. (2017). Chapter 15: Cervical degenerative disease. In E. Truumees & H. Prather (Eds.), *Orthopaedic Knowledge Update 5—Spine* (pp. 211–227). Rosemont, IL: American Academy of Orthopaedic Surgeons.
7. Shamji, M. F., Massicotte, E. M., Traynelis, V. C., Norvell, D. C., Hermsmoyer, J. T., & Fehlings, M. G. (2013). Comparison of anterior surgical options for the treatment of multilevel cervical spondylotic myelopathy—A systematic review. *Spine (Phila Pa 1976), 38* (22 Suppl. 1), S195–S209.
8. Wilson, J. R., Tetreault, L. A., Kim, J., Shamji, M. F., Harrop, J. S., Mroz, T., et al. (2017). State of the art in degenerative cervical myelopathy: An update on current clinical evidence. *Neurosurgery, 80*(3S), S33–S45.
9. Yamaguchi, S., Mitsuhara, T., Abiko, M., Takeda, M., & Kurisu, K. (2018). Epidemiology and overview of the clinical spectrum of degenerative cervical myelopathy. *Neurosurgery Clinics of North America, 29,* 1–12.
10. Zahrai, A., & Rhee, J. M. (2013). Cervical and thoracic degenerative spinal instability. *Seminars in Spine Surgery, 25,* 83–91.

CHAPTER 46

THORACIC DISC HERNIATION AND STENOSIS

Vincent J. Devlin, MD

1. **Is thoracic disc herniation a common clinical problem?**

   No. The incidence of symptomatic thoracic disc herniation has been reported as 1 per million patients. It is estimated that 0.15%–4% of all symptomatic disc protrusions occur in the thoracic spine. The lower rate of symptomatic disc herniation in the thoracic region compared with the cervical and lumbar regions is attributed to the stability provided by the rib cage. However, magnetic resonance imaging (MRI) and computed tomography (CT) myelogram studies have shown a prevalence of thoracic disc herniation ranging between 11% and 37% based on imaging studies performed in asymptomatic patients. Imaging studies alone cannot be used to select patients for operative treatment because more than 70% of asymptomatic adults will have abnormal anatomic findings on thoracic spine MRI studies (disc herniation, disc bulging, annular tear, spinal cord deformation, or end-plate irregularities).

2. **Describe the clinical presentation of a symptomatic thoracic disc herniation.**

   Peak incidence occurs in the fifth decade. Males and females are equally affected. Degenerative changes are considered to be the major factor responsible for thoracic disc herniation. An association between Scheuermann disease and thoracic disc herniation has been reported. Trauma plays a role as a precipitating or aggravating factor in a small percentage of cases. The clinical presentation is variable and can include axial pain, radicular pain, and/or myelopathy. Axial thoracic pain is typically mechanical in nature but is sometimes confused with cardiac, pulmonary, or abdominal pathology, or referred pain from the cervical spine. Radicular complaints most commonly consist of pain radiating around the chest wall along the path of an intercostal nerve but occasionally may include groin pain or lower extremity pain. Myelopathy may develop as a result of spinal cord compression. Careful examination for upper motor neuron signs can lead to the diagnosis of myelopathy. Findings may include a Romberg sign, Babinski reflex, clonus, ataxic gait, lower extremity motor weakness, loss of rectal tone, or decreased perianal sensation. T1–T2 disc herniations may mimic a cervical disc herniation and lead to intrinsic hand weakness and Horner syndrome. Tandem stenosis with involvement of both the thoracic and lumbar region should be suspected in patients with lumbar stenosis who present with neurogenic claudication and subtle signs or symptoms that suggest myelopathy.

3. **At what spinal level do thoracic disc herniations most commonly occur?**

   Thoracic disc herniation can occur at any level in the thoracic spine. Disc herniation is most common in the lower third of the thoracic spine (T9–10 through T12–L1), less common in the middle third (between T5–T6 and T8–T9), and least common in the upper thoracic region (T1–T2 through T4–T5). The level with the highest percentage of reported thoracic disc herniations is the T11–T12 level. The increased occurrence of thoracic disc herniation below T8 is attributed to the decreased stability provided to the spinal column by the rib cage in this area. Ribs 8–10 do not directly attach to the sternum but instead attach to proximal ribs by a fibrocartilaginous connection, and ribs 11 and 12 lack an anterior attachment to the sternum and are termed "free-floating" ribs.

4. **Which imaging modalities are useful in the diagnosis of a thoracic disc herniation?**

   Standard plain radiographs should be performed to rule out osseous abnormalities such as spinal tumors, deformities, or fractures. In addition, plain radiographs are essential as an intraoperative reference to help determine if the surgeon is operating at the correct level. MRI is the best imaging modality for assessment of the thoracic vertebra, intervertebral discs, and neural elements. CT can complement MRI as it has utility for determining whether calcification of the disc or posterior longitudinal ligament is present. CT-myelography is useful for assessment of patients who are unable to undergo MRI, and provides accurate assessment of the degree of spinal cord compression, disc calcification, and identification of intradural disc herniation in patients who require surgical intervention.

5. **What are some important features of thoracic disc herniations to describe when reviewing a thoracic MRI?**

   A thoracic disc herniation is present when disc material extends beyond the posterior margin of the vertebral endplate and encroaches on the space available for the spinal cord and/or nerve roots. Important features to describe include level of herniation, disc location with respect to the spinal canal (central, paracentral, lateral), presence/absence and degree of spinal cord compression, and the presence/absence of calcification within the disc herniation. See Fig. 46.1.

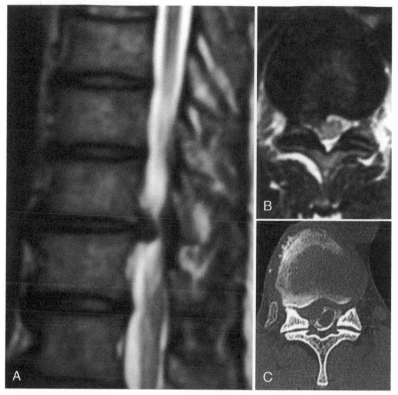

Fig. 46.1 Preoperative imaging demonstrating a right paracentral disc herniation at the T11–T12 level. (A) T2-weighted sagittal view of magnetic resonance imaging (MRI). (B) T2-weighted axial view of MRI. (C) Computed tomography myelogram. (From Sasai K, Adachi T, Togano K, et al. Two-level disc herniation in the cervical and thoracic spine presenting with spastic paresis in the lower extremities without clinical symptoms or signs in the upper extremities. Spine J 2006;6[4]:464–467.)

6. How is treatment for a thoracic disc herniation determined?
   Treatment of a thoracic disc herniation is individualized based on the patient's symptoms, physical examination, imaging findings, and patient preference.

7. What treatment is recommended for an asymptomatic thoracic disc herniation noted on thoracic MRI?
   Asymptomatic disc herniations require no treatment. It is important to realize that thoracic disc herniations are common findings on MRI studies in asymptomatic adults, and imaging findings require correlation with the patient's medical history and physical examination to guide treatment. The natural history of asymptomatic disc herniations is not fully defined.

8. What treatment is recommended for a symptomatic thoracic disc herniation without myelopathy?
   Symptomatic disc herniations without myelopathy are initially treated nonoperatively. Clinical presentations vary, and symptoms are often vague. Acute disc herniations resulting in axial pain may be treated with activity modification and medication such as nonsteroidal antiinflammatory medication, a short-term course of muscle relaxants, or other analgesics. As acute symptoms subside, patients may be transitioned to active physical therapy approaches, including low-impact aerobics and strengthening exercises with emphasis on extension exercises. In patients with radicular complaints, gabapentinoids, nerve blocks, and/or epidural steroid injections may be considered. This approach often provides sufficient pain relief to permit initiation of physical therapy.

9. When is surgical treatment considered for thoracic disc herniation?
   Surgery is indicated for thoracic disc herniations associated with myelopathy, lower extremity weakness, or bowel/bladder dysfunction, and for thoracic disc herniations associated with radiculopathy in patients who fail

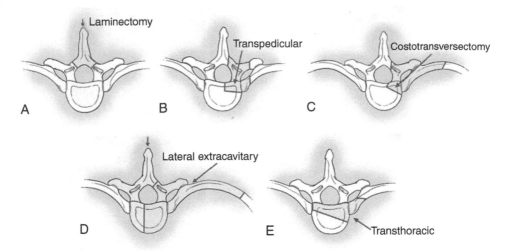

Fig. 46.2 (A) Exposure of thoracic disc provided by standard laminectomy. (B) Transpedicular approach. (C) Costotransversectomy approach. (D) Lateral extracavitary approach. (E) Transthoracic approach. (Redrawn from Fessler RG, Sturgill M. Complications of surgery for thoracic disc disease. Surg Neurol 1998;49[6]:609–618. From Canale ST, Beaty JH, editors. Campbell's Operative Orthopaedics. 11th ed. St. Louis: Mosby; 2007, Fig. 39.90.)

to improve with nonoperative treatment. Surgery for axial back pain associated with thoracic disc disease is controversial.

10. **What are the surgical approach options for treatment of a symptomatic thoracic disc herniation?**
   Surgical approach options include:
   - **Anterior transthoracic surgical approaches,** including transpleural thoracotomy, retropleural mini-open thoracotomy and video-assisted thoracoscopic approaches.
   - **Posterolateral surgical approaches,** including transfacet, transpedicular, transforaminal, and costotransversectomy approaches.
   - **Lateral surgical approaches,** including the lateral extracavitary approach and laterally based minimally invasive approaches using tubular or dual-blade retractors.
   The extent of exposure of the thoracic disc provided by each approach is shown in Fig. 46.2. The posterior laminectomy approach has been abandoned due to poor outcomes and associated high rate of neurologic injury.

11. **What factors are considered when selecting the most appropriate approach for treatment of a thoracic disc herniation?**
   Various factors are considered when selecting the most appropriate surgical approach for a thoracic disc herniation including:
   1. Location of the herniation in relation to the spinal cord (central, paracentral, lateral)
   2. Level of the herniation (the upper and lower ends of the thoracic region are more challenging to approach via thoracotomy)
   3. Size of the disc herniation and extent of neural compression
   4. Calcification of the disc herniation
   5. Patient's underlying medical condition
   6. Number of disc levels requiring treatment
   7. Surgeon's familiarity with various spinal approaches
   An anterior approach is preferred for a central disc herniation, especially if the herniation is calcified. This approach allows the creation of a working corridor by removing a portion of the posterior vertebral bodies adjacent to the target disc space. This permits disc excision to be performed by working in a direction away from the spinal cord, which decreases the risk of neurologic injury. Anterior approaches can be used for any type of thoracic disc herniation as direct access to the entire disc space is possible. In the midthoracic and lower thoracic regions, a standard or mini-open thoracotomy approaches or video-assisted thoracoscopic surgery (VATS) are options. Exposure of the upper thoracic spine is more challenging through an anterior transthoracic exposure. The T1–T2 and T2–T3 discs are typically exposed via a low anterior cervical approach, but modifications such as resection of the medial clavicle or manubrium may be necessary depending on body habitus. Other anterior approach

options in the upper thoracic region include a third rib thoracotomy or a transsternal approach. Video-assisted thoracoscopic surgery (VATS) is an additional approach option for appropriately trained and experienced surgeons. For discectomies involving spinal levels at the thoracolumbar junction, incision of the ipsilateral hemidiaphragm is required.

Posterolateral and lateral approaches are an option for lateral or paracentral disc herniations but are not optimal for central disc herniations because the spinal cord cannot be retracted or mobilized without risk of injury. Surgical approach options include transfacet, transpedicular, transforaminal, costotransversectomy, and lateral extracavitary approaches. Minimally invasive techniques which utilize tubular or dual blade retractors are additional options.

12. How does the surgeon determine the correct thoracic surgical level intraoperatively?

Intraoperative determination of the correct thoracic surgical level is crucial. Spinal MRI scout films are often numbered from C1 downward. However, intraoperatively it is often easier to count vertebrae upward from the sacrum or to use the ribs as a reference. Preoperatively, an MRI scout film of the entire spine should be performed and counting from the lumbar spine upward should be utilized to identify the level of interest. In addition, anteroposterior and lateral radiographs of the thoracic and lumbar spine should be obtained to determine the number of thoracic and lumbar vertebrae present. The ribs should be numbered to correspond with appropriate thoracic levels and the number of non–rib-bearing vertebrae should be documented. In the thoracic spine, the first, eleventh, and twelfth ribs usually only articulate with their corresponding vertebral bodies. Between T2 and T10, the rib heads articulate with the corresponding vertebral body, as well as the proximal vertebral body, and overlie the intervening disc space. Localization of the correct surgical level during thoracic discectomy may be challenging. Innovative methods to assist intraoperative localization using fluoroscopy include preoperative percutaneous placement of intravertebral polymethylmethacrylate or metal coils, or percutaneous temporary placement of a K-wire or Jamshidi needle into a pedicle at the desired surgical level or into the most cranial lumbar vertebra that can be visualized on the same fluoroscopic image as the sacrum immediately prior to positioning for thoracic discectomy procedure.

13. At which level should a thoracotomy be performed for a transthoracic disc resection?

A chest radiograph can be used to determine the slope of the ribs in the thoracic spine. Usually, a standard thoracotomy is performed one or two levels above the target disc space. This strategy allows a parallel approach to the disc space, thus permitting the use of a microscope if desired. Alternatively, a minithoracotomy can be performed to minimize approach-related morbidity. The posterior portion of the rib leading to the target disc space is removed (e.g., remove the posterior portion of the ninth rib to access a T8–T9 disc herniation).

14. When is spinal fusion or spinal instrumentation indicated following thoracic discectomy?

Addition of a fusion should be considered in cases of multilevel discectomy, underlying Scheuermann disease with kyphosis, when a significant amount of the vertebral body is resected to facilitate decompression of the spinal cord, or when extensive facet joint resection is performed to access the anterior aspect of the spinal canal from a posterior surgical approach.

Use of spinal instrumentation provides immediate spinal stability and enhances fusion. For anterior-based surgical approaches, fusion may be performed with a section of rib without use of supplemental instrumentation. Alternatively, a structural interbody bone graft or intervertebral body fusion device in combination with an anterior rod-screw or plate system can be used. When a posterior-based surgical approaches are utilized, posterior unilateral or bilateral transfacet pedicle-sparing decompression in combination with segmental pedicle screw-rod fixation and interbody fusion can provide circumferential decompression, segmental stabilization, and fusion while avoiding the approach-related complications associated with transthoracic surgical approaches.

15. What complications can occur after surgery for thoracic disc herniation?

Complications can include death, deterioration of neurologic function (including complete paralysis), dural tear, cerebrospinal fluid leak, infection, kyphotic deformity, pseudarthrosis, and instrumentation failure, as well as medical-, anesthetic-, and surgical approach-related complications. Concerns regarding complications specific to anterior transthoracic approaches, including atelectasis, lung contusion, intercostal neuralgia, pneumothorax, hemothorax, and the potential need for a chest tube, have led to a shift toward posterior-based surgical approaches for treatment of thoracic disc herniations.

16. Does spinal stenosis occur in the thoracic region?

Yes. Spinal stenosis can occur in the thoracic region although it is less common than cervical or lumbar spinal stenosis. Thoracic spinal stenosis occurs most commonly in the T10–T12 region due to acquired degenerative changes superimposed on preexisting developmental canal narrowing. Hypertrophic spondylosis and ossification of the posterior longitudinal ligament and ligamentum flavum may lead to circumferential narrowing of the lower thoracic spinal canal. A wide range of neurologic dysfunction, may occur as the lower thoracic spinal canal contents include the lumbosacral spinal cord segments, conus medullaris, as well as the lower thoracic and lumbosacral nerve roots. Symptoms may include both upper and lower motor neuron lesions, claudication, lower extremity pain, back pain, and cauda equina symptoms. Tandem stenosis involving both the thoracic and lumbar spine, although rare, may occur and is a cause of neurologic deterioration following decompression surgery for lumbar spinal stenosis.

17. What are the surgical treatment options for thoracic spinal stenosis?

Surgical treatment requires decompression of all stenotic levels diagnosed on preoperative imaging studies. If stenosis is the result of predominantly anterior pathology (e.g., disc-based osteophytes) and limited to one or two spinal segments, anterior decompression and fusion is an option. If stenosis is predominantly due to facet and/or ligamentum hypertrophy or extends over multiple levels, a posterior approach with laminectomy is reasonable. Posterior fusion and instrumentation, with or without interbody fusion, are added when posterior decompression involves multiple levels, especially when decompression crosses the thoracolumbar junction, and for patients who require circumferential decompression.

KEY POINTS

1. Thoracic disc herniations associated with neurologic deficit are rare lesions with an estimated incidence of 1 per million population.
2. A high prevalence of anatomic abnormalities is noted on thoracic spine MRI studies in asymptomatic patients.
3. An anterior transthoracic surgical approach is preferred for central thoracic disc herniations, especially if the herniation is large and calcified.
4. Posterolateral and lateral surgical approaches are an option for paracentral and lateral thoracic disc herniations.
5. Posterior thoracic transfacet pedicle-sparing decompression in combination with segmental pedicle screw-rod fixation and interbody fusion provides an efficient approach for achievement of circumferential decompression, segmental stabilization, and fusion for patients with thoracic disc herniation or stenosis.
6. Spinal stenosis can present in the thoracic region and most commonly occurs at the thoracolumbar junction.

Websites

1. Diagnosis and treatment of thoracic disc herniation: https://www.bcmj.org/worksafebc/diagnosis-and-treatment-thoracic-disc-herniation
2. Thoracic discogenic pain: https://emedicine.medscape.com/article/96284-overview

BIBLIOGRAPHY

1. Anand, N., & Regan, J. J. (2002). Video-assisted thoracoscopic surgery for thoracic disc disease: Classification and outcome study of 100 consecutive cases with a 2-year minimum follow-up period. *Spine, 27*(8), 871–879.
2. Angevin, P. D., & McCormick, P. C. (2001). Retropleural thoracotomy. *Neurosurgical Focus, 10*(1), 1–5.
3. Arts, M. P., & Bartels, R. H. (2014). Anterior or posterior approach of thoracic disc herniation? A comparative cohort of mini-trans-thoracic versus transpedicular discectomies. *The Spine Journal, 14*(8), 1654–1662.
4. Carr, D. A., Volkov, A. A., Rhoiney, D. L., Setty, P., Barrett, R. J., Claybrooks, R., et al. (2017). Management of thoracic disc herniations via posterior unilateral modified transfacet pedicle-sparing decompression with segmental instrumentation and interbody fusion. *Global Spine Journal, 7*(6), 506–513.
5. Fushimi, K., Miyamoto, K., Hioki, A., Hosoe, H., Takeuchi, A., & Shimizu, K. (2013). Neurological deterioration due to missed thoracic spinal stenosis after decompressive lumbar surgery: A report of six cases of tandem thoracic and lumbar stenosis. *Bone and Joint Journal, 95*(10), 1388–1391.
6. Jain, A., Menga, E. N., Hassanzadeh, H., Jain, P., Lemma, M. A., & Mesfin, A. (2014). Thoracic disc disorders with myelopathy: Treatment trends, patient characteristics, and complications. *Spine, 39*(20), E1233–E1238.
7. Palumbo, M. A., Hilibrand, A. S., Hart, R. A., & Bohlman, H. H. (2001). Surgical treatment of thoracic spinal stenosis: A 2- to 9-year follow-up. *Spine, 26*(5), 558–566.
8. Simpson, J. M., Silveri, C. P., Simeone, F. A., Balderston, R. A., & An, H. S. (1993). Thoracic disc herniation: Re-evaluation of the posterior approach using a modified costotransversectomy. *Spine, 18*(13), 1872–1877.
9. Wood, K. B., Blair, J. M., Aepple, D., Schendel, M. J., Garvey, T. A., Gundry, C. R., et al. (1997). The natural history of asymptomatic thoracic disc herniations. *Spine, 22*(5), 525–529.

CHAPTER 47

LUMBAR DISC HERNIATION

Vincent J. Devlin, MD

1. **Describe the prevalence and natural history of lumbar disc herniation. Contrast the prevalence and natural history of lumbar disc herniation and low back pain.**
   The lifetime prevalence of a *symptomatic lumbar disc herniation* in the adult population is approximately 2%. The natural history of sciatica secondary to lumbar disc herniation is spontaneous improvement in the majority of cases. Among patients with radiculopathy secondary to lumbar disc herniation, approximately 10%–25% (0.5% of the population) experience persistent symptoms. These statistics are in sharp contrast to *low back pain*, which has a lifetime prevalence of 60%–80% in the adult population. Although the natural history of acute low back pain is favorable in many patients, recurrent pain is common, and successful management of patients with chronic symptoms remains an enigma.

2. **What is the typical history of a patient with a lumbar disc herniation?**
   Often there is an attempt to link the onset of back and leg pain with a traumatic event, but many patients will report experiencing intermittent episodes of back and leg pain for months or years. Factors that tend to exacerbate symptoms include physical exertion, repetitive bending, torsion, and heavy lifting. Pain most commonly originates in the lumbar area and radiates to the sacroiliac and buttock regions. Radicular pain typically becomes dominant and extends below the knee in the distribution of the involved nerve root. Radicular pain may be accompanied by paresthesia, weakness, and/or reflex changes in the distribution of the involved nerve root. Patients with a disc herniation commonly report that pain in the leg is worse than low back pain, although patients may occasionally present with substantial low back pain. Pain tends to be exacerbated by sitting, straining, sneezing, and coughing, and relieved with standing or bed rest.

3. **Define cauda equina syndrome.**
   Cauda equina syndrome is defined as a complex of low back pain, sciatica, saddle hypoesthesia, and lower extremity motor weakness in association with bowel or bladder dysfunction. The mode of onset may be slow or rapidly progressive. The most common cause of cauda equina syndrome is a central lumbar disc herniation at the L4–L5 level. Prompt surgical treatment is advised.

4. **Outline key points in the physical examination of a patient with a suspected lumbar disc herniation.**
   The patient should be undressed. Observation may reveal the presence of a limp or a list (sciatic scoliosis). Spinal range of motion is assessed. A complete neurologic examination (sensory, motor, reflex testing) is performed to identify the involved nerve root. Nerve root tension signs are evaluated. Hip and knee range of motion are assessed to rule out pathology involving these joints. Peripheral pulses (dorsalis pedis and posterior tibial) are assessed to rule out peripheral vascular problems. A rectal examination is performed in patients suspected of having cauda equina syndrome.

5. **What are nerve root tension signs?**
   Tension signs are maneuvers that stretch the sciatic or femoral nerve and in doing so further compress an inflamed nerve root against a lumbar disc herniation. Both the symptomatic and contralateral lower extremities should be examined. The supine straight leg raise test (Lasègue test) and its variants (sitting straight leg raise test, bowstring test) increase tension along the *sciatic nerve* in the symptomatic lower extremity and are used to assess the L5 and S1 nerve roots. A positive supine straight leg test reproduces symptoms between 30° and 70° of hip flexion. Tests involving the symptomatic lower extremity are sensitive but not specific for diagnosis of sciatica. The contralateral straight leg raise test (crossed straight leg test) reproduces pain in the symptomatic leg by raising the unaffected leg, and is a highly specific test for diagnosis of lumbar disc herniation. The femoral nerve stretch test (reverse straight leg raise test) increases tension along the *femoral nerve* and is used to assess the L2, L3, and L4 nerve roots.

6. **Compare and contrast sciatica with other common clinical syndromes presenting with low back and/or lower extremity pain symptoms.**
   - **Sciatica:** Leg pain rather than low back pain is typically the predominant symptom, although some patients may also present with substantial low back pain. Neurologic symptoms and signs are found in a specific nerve root distribution. Nerve root tension signs are present.

- **Nonmechanical back and/or leg pain:** Pain is constant and minimally affected by activity and unrelieved with rest. Pain is usually worse at night or early morning (e.g., spinal tumor, infection).
- **Mechanical back and/or leg pain:** Pain is exacerbated by activity, changes in position, or prolonged sitting. Pain is relieved with rest, especially in the supine position (e.g., degenerative disc pathology, spondylolisthesis).
- **Neurogenic claudication:** Low back and buttock pain, radiating leg or calf pain, worse with ambulation, worse with spinal extension, and relieved with flexion maneuvers, with absent nerve root tension signs (e.g., spinal stenosis).

7. When clinical examination suggests the presence of an acute lumbar disc herniation, what is the preferred imaging test to confirm the diagnosis?

Magnetic resonance imaging (MRI) is the preferred imaging test because it provides the greatest amount of information about the lumbar region. It is unparalleled in its ability to visualize pathologic processes involving the disc, thecal sac, epidural space, neural elements, paraspinal soft tissue, and bone marrow. However, caution is indicated when interpreting results of MRI scans due to the high frequency of disc abnormalities in asymptomatic patients. It is critical to correlate imaging findings with clinical examination. Although lumbar radiographs cannot show a lumbar disc herniation, standing radiographs are advised prior to referral for MRI in order to define regional lumbar anatomy and diagnose other potential pathologies such as spondylolisthesis.

8. At what spinal level are symptomatic lumbar disc herniations most commonly diagnosed?

Most lumbar disc herniations occur at the L4–L5 and L5–S1 levels (90%). The L3–L4 level is the next most common level for a symptomatic lumbar disc herniation.

9. What terms are used to describe lumbar disc pathology noted on MRI?

Terms used to describe lumbar disc pathology noted on MRI include degeneration, bulge, protrusion, extrusion, and sequestration (Fig. 47.1).

- **Degeneration:** Decreased or absent T2-weighted signal is noted from the intervertebral disc. It is not possible to distinguish symptomatic from asymptomatic degeneration based on MRI.
- **Disc bulge:** Disc material is noted to extend beyond the disc space with a diffuse, circumferential, nonfocal contour. Disc bulges are caused by early disc degeneration and infrequently cause symptoms in the absence of spinal stenosis.

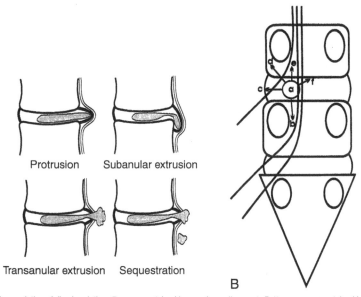

Protrusion   Subanular extrusion

Transanular extrusion   Sequestration

A   **B**

Fig. 47.1 (A) The four varieties of disc herniation. *Top row,* contained by annulus or ligament. *Bottom row,* noncontained by annulus or ligament. (B) Potential patterns of migration of disc material away from typical posterior/lateral position *(a).* Migratory positions include: *(b)* distal beside the pedicle of the level below; *(c)* lateral; *(d)* upward into neural foramen; *(e)* upward into axilla of exiting nerve root; and *(f)* medial. (From McCulloch JA. Least invasive spine surgery at the L5–S1 level in adults. Spine State Art Rev 1997;11:215–238, with permission.)

- **Protrusion:** Displaced disc material extends focally and asymmetrically beyond the disc space. The displaced disc material is in continuity with the disc of origin. The diameter of the base of the displaced portion, where it is continuous with the disc material within the disc space of origin, has a greater diameter than the largest diameter of the disc tissue extending beyond the disc space.
- **Extrusion:** Displaced disc material extends focally and asymmetrically beyond the disc space. The displaced disc material has a greater diameter than the disc material maintaining continuity (if any) with the disc of origin.
- **Sequestration:** Refers to a disc fragment that has no continuity with the disc of origin. By definition all sequestered discs are extruded. However, not all extruded discs are sequestered.

10. How is the location of a disc herniation within the spinal canal described?
    The location of a disc herniation within the spinal canal is described in terms of a *three-floor anatomic house* (story 1 = disc space level, story 2 = foraminal level, story 3 = pedicle level) (Fig. 47.2). The spinal canal is also divided in terms of *zones*—central, foraminal, and extraforaminal. The *central zone* is located between the pedicles. The *foraminal zone* is located between the medial and lateral pedicle borders. The *extraforaminal zone* is located beyond the lateral pedicle border. This anatomic scheme is applicable to lumbar disc herniations, as well as lumbar spinal stenosis syndromes.

11. How does the location of a disc herniation along the circumference of the annulus of the disc determine the pattern of nerve root compression?
    Discs herniations are described by their relationship along the circumference of the annulus fibrosus as *central* (midline), *posterolateral* (most common), *foraminal*, or *extraforaminal*. The location of the disc herniation

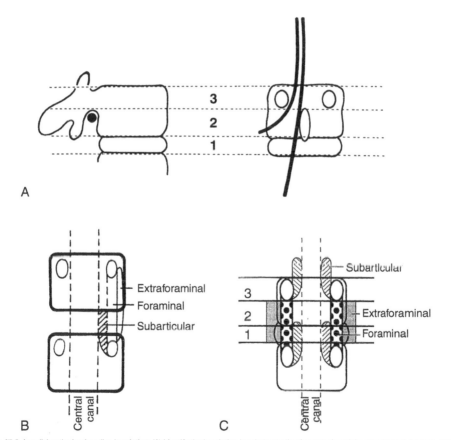

Fig. 47.2 Localizing the lumbar disc herniation. (A) Identify the herniation in relation to the three stories of the spinal canal (story 1, disc space level; story 2, foraminal level; story 3, pedicle level). (B) Determine if the pathology lies within the central spinal canal or the lateral zone. (C) Identify the pathology on the anatomic grid for the involved spinal segment and determine the surgical plan. (From McCulloch JA. Microdiscectomy: The gold standard for minimally invasive disc surgery. Spine State Art Rev 1997;11:373–396, with permission.)

determines the pattern of nerve root compression. The nerve roots of the lumbar spine exit the spinal canal beneath the pedicle of the corresponding numbered vertebra and above the caudad intervertebral disc. A posterolateral L4–L5 disc herniation compresses the L5 nerve root (the traversing nerve root of the L4–L5 motion segment). An L4–L5 foraminal or extraforaminal disc herniation compresses the L4 nerve root (the exiting nerve root of the L4–L5 motion segment). A central disc herniation compresses one or more of the caudal nerve roots.

12. **What initial treatment is advised for patients with a suspected acute lumbar disc herniation?**
Initial treatment options include a short period of bedrest (not to exceed 3 days), oral medications (nonsteroidal antiinflammatory drugs), progressive ambulation, return to activity, and patient reassurance. Epidural injections can be considered if pain is severe or refractory to other treatments. As acute pain subsides, physical therapy and aerobic conditioning are advised. If a patient fails to improve with 4–6 weeks of nonsurgical care, further evaluation including MRI is indicated. The optimal time for nonsurgical treatment ranges from a minimum of 4 weeks to a maximum of 6 months.

13. **What are the indications for surgical treatment for a lumbar disc herniation?**
Occasionally an acute massive central disc herniation can result in cauda equina syndrome, which is appropriately managed by emergent surgical treatment. However, most patients with lumbar disc herniations do not develop a cauda equina syndrome and instead undergo elective surgical treatment due to failure of radicular pain to improve with nonsurgical treatment. Lumbar discectomy is directed at improving the patient's leg pain. However, some patients with lumbar radicular pain due to lumbar disc herniation also present with substantial preoperative low back pain and are likely to experience significant improvement in low back pain symptoms following lumbar disc excision without the need for lumbar fusion. Appropriate criteria for surgical intervention include:
- Functionally incapacitating leg pain extending below the knee within a nerve root distribution
- Nerve root tension signs with or without neurologic deficit
- Failure to improve with 4–8 weeks of nonsurgical treatment
- Confirmatory imaging study (preferably MRI), which correlates with the patient's physical findings and pain distribution

14. **How does surgery compare with nonoperative treatment for a symptomatic lumbar disc herniation?**
Surgery has been shown to lead to a more rapid and greater degree of improvement compared with nonoperative treatment. Operative treatment is associated with a low rate of complications. However, patients who prefer nonoperative treatment and are able to tolerate their symptoms often improve and achieve an acceptable level of pain and function.

15. **What surgical procedure is recommended for treatment of a symptomatic lumbar disc herniation?**
Open lumbar discectomy using microsurgical technique remains the gold standard for the treatment of a symptomatic lumbar disc herniation (Fig. 47.3). Important technical points include use of a small incision, limited muscle and bone dissection, and limited removal of displaced or loose disc material. A surgical microscope or headlight and loupe magnification is used to enhance intraoperative visualization. Uncomplicated patients typically go home within 24 hours of surgery and are able to return to work in 1 month. The success rate for relief of leg pain exceeds 90% in appropriately selected patients. Transmuscular tubular microdiscectomy has been popularized as an alternative surgical technique, but superior long-term functional and clinical outcomes have not been substantiated.

16. **How much disc material should be removed during a lumbar discectomy procedure?**
The optimal amount of intraoperative disc removal is controversial. **Sequestrectomy** restricts disc removal to free disc fragments located posterior to the vertebral body that are compressing the neural elements and avoids probing of the annulus or removal of nucleus pulposus material. **Limited discectomy** removes any herniated fragments in addition to the removal of any loose fragments located inside the disc space. **Subtotal discectomy** includes a formal annulotomy, end plate curettage, and removal of all accessible disc fragments in the disc space. Studies suggest that sequestrectomy and limited discectomy may be associated with a decreased incidence of long-term recurrent low back pain but result in a higher incidence of recurrent disc herniation compared with subtotal discectomy.

17. **How does the location of a disc herniation influence selection of the appropriate surgical approach?**
Disc herniations in a central or subarticular location are treated through an **interlaminar** surgical approach. Disc herniations located in the extraforaminal zone are treated through an **intertransverse** surgical approach. The surgical approach for disc herniations located in the foraminal zone is determined based on a combination of factors,

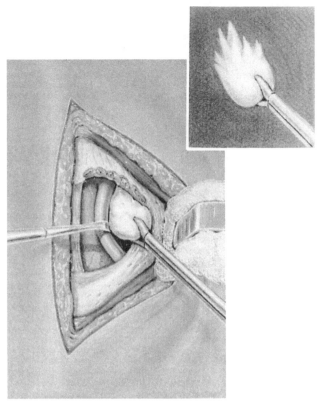

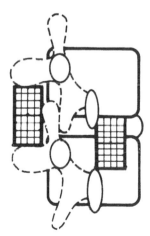

Fig. 47.3 Lumbar disc fragment excision. (From McCulloch JA. The lateral approach to the lumbar spine. Oper Tech Orthop 1991;1:27, 55, with permission.)

including whether or not a portion of the disc herniation extends into the subarticular zone (Fig. 47.4). At the L5–S1 level, an interlaminar approach to foraminal herniations is facilitated by its unique anatomic features including the large size and more oblique orientation of the pedicles and the location of the lateral border of the pars interarticularis at the midpedicle sagittal plane.

18. **What are the surgical alternatives to microsurgical lumbar discectomy?**
A variety of alternative procedures have been proposed. However, no procedure has demonstrated superior surgical outcomes compared with microsurgical lumbar discectomy. Alternative procedures include chymopapain injection, percutaneous automated discectomy, laser discectomy, and a variety of endoscopic surgical techniques.

19. **What are some complications reported in association with microsurgical lumbar discectomy?**
Surgical complications are rare but may include:
- Vascular injury
- Nerve root injury
- Dural tear
- Infection
- Increased back pain
- Recurrent disc herniation
- Cauda equina syndrome

Fig. 47.4 The two windows of opportunity into the spinal canal: interlaminar *(right)* and intertransverse *(left)*. (From McCulloch JA. The lateral approach to the lumbar spine. Oper Tech Orthop 1991;1:27, 55, with permission.)

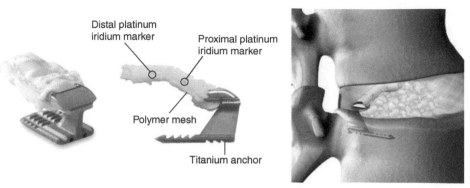

Fig. 47.5 Barricaid annular closure device. (From Trummer M, Eustacchio S, Barth M, et al. Protecting facet joints post-lumbar discectomy: Barricaid annular closure device reduces risk of facet degeneration. Clin Neurol Neurosurg 2013;115:1440–1445, Fig. 1.)

- Spinal instability
- Medical complications (e.g., thrombophlebitis, urinary tract infection)

20. **What is the most common cause of surgical failure after lumbar disc excision?**
Poor patient selection is the most common cause of treatment failure following lumbar discectomy. Other factors that may contribute to a poor surgical outcome include prolonged symptoms (>6–12 months), abnormal pain behavior, workers' compensation situation, litigation, and tobacco use.

21. **What is the incidence of recurrent disc herniation after microsurgical lumbar discectomy?**
The incidence of recurrent disc herniation following microsurgical lumbar discectomy is estimated to range between 5% and 18%, and is dependent on the criteria used to define recurrence, the extent of operative disc removal, and the size of the posterior annular defect. Higher rates of recurrence (up to 27%) have been reported in patients in whom large annular defects (>6 mm) were present at the conclusion of a discectomy. An annular closure device, Barricaid (Intrinsic Therapeutics Inc., Woburn, MA), which anchors into the vertebral body adjacent to the annular defect, has been shown to decrease the rate of recurrent disc herniations in patients with large annular defects (Fig. 47.5).

22. **What surgical treatment is recommended for patients with symptomatic recurrent disc herniations who do not improve with nonoperative treatment?**
For patients who present with a first-time symptomatic recurrent disc herniation, if symptoms are predominantly radicular in nature and radiographic spinal instability is not present, revision lumbar microdiscectomy is recommended. For patients who present with second-time recurrences, radiographic evidence of spinal instability, or severe chronic low back pain, spinal fusion and instrumentation are considered.

KEY POINTS

1. The majority of patients with a lumbar disc herniation improve with nonoperative treatment.
2. Relief of leg pain is the primary goal of lumbar discectomy.

Websites
1. Lumbar disc nomenclature: version 2.0: https://www.ncbi.nlm.nih.gov/pubmed/24768732
2. Herniated disc in the lower back: https://orthoinfo.aaos.org/en/diseases-conditions/herniated-disk-in-the-lower-back/
3. Disc pathology: http://www.nlm.nih.gov/medlineplus/herniateddisk.html#cat3

BIBLIOGRAPHY

1. Atlas, S. J., Keller, R. B., Wu, Y. A., Deyo, R. A., & Singer, D. E. (2005). Long-term outcomes of surgical and nonsurgical management of sciatica secondary to a lumbar disc herniation: 10 year results from the Maine Lumbar Spine Study. *Spine, 30*, 927–935.
2. Carragee, E. J., Han, M. Y., Suen, P. W., & Kim, D. (2003). Clinical outcomes after lumbar discectomy for sciatica: The effects of fragment type and anular competence. *Journal of Bone and Joint Surgery, 85*, 102–108.
3. Kreiner, D. S., Hwang, S. W., Easa, J. E., Resnick, D. K., Baisden, J. L., & Bess, S. (2014). North American Spine Society: An evidence-based clinical guideline for the diagnosis and treatment of lumbar disc herniation with radiculopathy. *Spine Journal, 14*, 180–191.
4. Lurie, J. D., Tosteson, T. D., Tosteson, A. N., Zhao, W., Morgan, T. S., & Abdu, W. A. (2014). Surgical versus nonoperative treatment for lumbar disc herniation: Eight-year results for the Spine Patient Outcomes Research Trial. *Spine, 39*, 3–16.
5. McCulloch, J. A., & Young, P. A. (1998). *Essentials of spinal microsurgery.* Philadelphia, PA: Lippincott-Raven.
6. McGirt, M. J., Eustacchio, S., Varga, P., Vilendecic, M., Trummer, M., & Gorensek, M. A. (2009). Prospective cohort study of close in-terval computed tomography and magnetic resonance imaging after primary lumbar discectomy: Factors associated with recurrent disc herniation and disc height loss. *Spine, 34*, 2044–2051.
7. Mroz, T. E., Lubelski, D., Williams, S. K., O'Rourke, C., Obuchowski, N. A., Wang, J. C., et al. (2014). Differences in the surgical treat-ment of recurrent lumbar disc herniation among spine surgeons in the United States. *Spine Journal, 14*, 2334–2343.
8. Owens, R. K., Carreon, L. Y., Bisson, E. F., Bydon, M., Potts, E. A., & Glassman, S. D. (2018). Back pain improves significantly following discectomy for lumbar disc herniation. *Spine Journal, 18*, 1632–1636.

CHAPTER 48

DISCOGENIC LOW BACK PAIN

Eeric Truumees, MD

1. **Define lumbar disc degeneration.**
   Lumbar disc degeneration has been defined by the North American Spine Society Consensus Committee on Nomenclature in terms of morphologic changes involving the anatomic components of the lumbar disc. These changes may include:
   - Desiccation, fibrosis, vacuum changes, or cleft formation in the *nucleus*
   - Fissuring, mucinous degeneration, or calcification in the *annulus*
   - Defects and sclerosis of the *vertebral endplates*
   - Osteophytes at the *vertebral apophysis*

2. **What is lumbar degenerative disc disease?**
   Although disc degeneration is virtually universal in the aging spine, disc degeneration is inconsistently and only occasionally associated with pain and functional limitation. *Degenerative disc disease (DDD)* is broadly defined as a clinical syndrome characterized by manifestations of disc degeneration and symptoms attributed to these changes. Causal connections between degenerative changes and symptoms are often difficult clinical distinctions. No evidence-based consensus exists for differentiating pathologic degenerative disc changes from disc changes associated with normal aging.

3. **How is the clinical syndrome of lumbar DDD characterized?**
   Lumbar DDD refers to a continuum of nonradicular pain disorders of degenerative origin. Specifically excluded are symptoms related to disc impingement on neural elements, facet-mediated back pain, and spinal deformities secondary to lumbar DDD (e.g., spondylolisthesis, degenerative scoliosis).
   Clinical presentation is characterized by low back pain, which may radiate to the sacroiliac and/or buttock region. Common physical examination findings include tenderness with palpation over the lumbar region and limited lumbar range of motion. In the absence of concomitant facet joint degeneration, discogenic back pain is often more severe with flexion and less severe with extension.
   Radiographic findings include disc height loss, decreased lumbar lordosis, vacuum phenomena, osteophytes, and endplate sclerosis. Similar degenerative changes are frequently noted in asymptomatic patients. A change in radiographic alignment, such as retrolisthesis, from supine to standing or from flexion to extension may occur.
   Magnetic resonance imaging (MRI) findings include disc desiccation, annular fissures, high-intensity zones (HIZ), loss of disc space height, and changes in vertebral endplate morphology. No pathognomonic findings have been identified that permit distinction of asymptomatic age-related changes from symptomatic lumbar DDD, though the Pfirrmann classification system is often used to describe the severity of these changes.
   Lumbar discography has been utilized as a provocative test to assess patients with DDD. Although controversial, this test attempts to directly identify a cause and effect relationship between MRI findings of DDD and clinical symptoms. Findings that support a diagnosis of discogenic pain include concordant pain on injection of a specific disc level with absent or minimal pain on injection of adjacent control levels. Additional criteria for diagnosis include pain reproduction with a low pressure/low volume injection and presence of abnormal disc morphology. Discography can accelerate degeneration, especially at otherwise normal "control" levels and should not be obtained in patients with abnormal psychometric profiles, chronic pain illness, worker's compensation claims, and secondary gain issues.

4. **What is a high-intensity zone?**
   Annular fissures commonly occur as the structural integrity of the annulus of the intervertebral disc is compromised by the degenerative process, but may not always be detected with MRI or discography. Annular fissures are classified as concentric, transverse, or radial types. When fluid or granulation tissue infiltrates an annular fissure, this region may be visualized as an area of increased signal intensity in the posterior annular region on T2-weighted MRI and is termed a high-intensity zone (HIZ). Initial reports suggested that a HIZ was a marker for symptomatic internal disc disruption and concordant pain reproduction with discography. However, additional studies have demonstrated that a HIZ is not a specific marker for symptomatic disc disruption as this finding may be present in many asymptomatic individuals (Fig. 48.1).

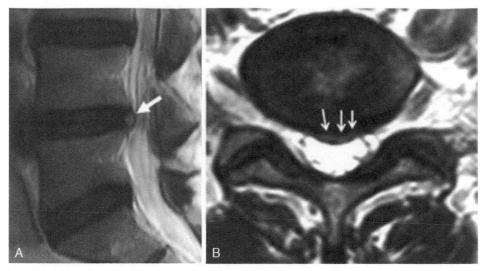

Fig. 48.1 High-intensity zone (HIZ). (A) Sagittal and (B) axial views of a HIZ in the posterior aspect of a lumbar disc representing fissures and granulation tissue (note *arrows* in A. and B.). (From Bonaldi G, Brembilla C, Cianfoni A. Minimally-invasive posterior lumbar stabilization for degenerative low back pain and sciatica. A review. Eur J Radiol 2015;84:789–798, Fig. 9.)

5. Explain how to use the Pfirrmann classification to describe the severity of lumbar disc degeneration noted on MRI.

The **Pfirrmann classification** is a five-grade system, which considers disc structure, the distinction between the nucleus pulposus and annulus fibrosus, signal intensity of the disc nucleus, and intervertebral disc height.
- **Grade 1:** Defined as a homogenous nucleus pulposus, high T2 signal intensity, clear distinction of the nucleus and annulus, and normal disc height.
- **Grade 2:** Defined as an inhomogenous nucleus pulposus with or without horizontal bands, high T2 signal intensity, clear distinction of the nucleus and annulus, and normal disc height.
- **Grade 3:** Defined as an inhomogenous, gray nucleus pulposus, intermediate T2 signal intensity, unclear distinction of the nucleus and annulus, and normal to slightly decreased disc height.
- **Grade 4:** Defined as an inhomogenous, gray to black nucleus pulposus, intermediate to low T2 signal intensity, loss of distinction of the nucleus and annulus, and normal to moderately decreased disc height.
- **Grade 5:** Defined as an inhomogenous, black nucleus pulposus, low T2 signal intensity, loss of distinction of the nucleus and annulus, and severe loss of disc height (Fig. 48.2).

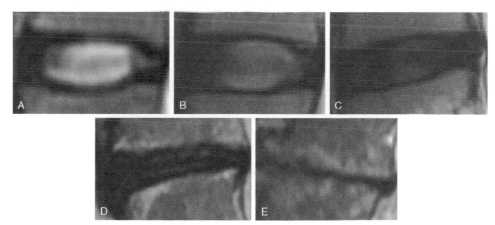

Fig. 48.2 The five Pfirrmann magnetic resonance classification grades of lumbar intervertebral disc degeneration. (From Kim JY, Ryu DS, Paik HK, et al. Paraspinal muscle, facet joint and disc problems: Risk factors for adjacent segment degeneration after lumbar fusion. Spine J 2016;16:867–875, Fig. 4.)

6. What is the significance of endplate changes on lumbar MRI?

Changes in vertebral endplate morphology adjacent to degenerating discs are frequently observed on MRI. These changes have been classified by Modic into three types based on T1- and T2-weighted MRI:

- **Type I** changes reflect acute disruption and fissuring of vertebral endplates, which leads to growth of vascularized fibrous tissue into the adjacent vertebral body marrow. This tissue exhibits a diminished T1 and increased T2 signal pattern and represents bone marrow edema and inflammation.
- **Type II** changes develop in the context of chronic degeneration as the normal red hematopoietic peridiscal marrow undergoes fatty degeneration. A type II pattern exhibits increased T1 signal and an isointense or slightly hyperintense T2 signal.
- **Type III** changes reflect extrinsic bone sclerosis as seen on plain radiographs. Dense bone in the vertebral endplates yields a hypointense signal on both T1 and T2 images.

Modic changes have been conceptualized as dynamic markers of the degenerative process. Modic changes are more prevalent in patients with low back pain compared to the general population (46% vs. 6%). Type I changes have been most strongly correlated with low back pain symptoms and segmental hypermobility. Type II changes are less strongly correlated with low back pain and considered to represent a more stable state. The significance of type III changes is unclear. Modic changes may convert from one type to another, and type I changes may sometimes resolve.

Recent clinical research has identified a potential correlation between Modic type I changes and infection with low-virulence anaerobic organisms *(Propionibacterium acnes)* in some patients, and identified a potential new treatment method for this specific patient subgroup. Antibiotic treatment (amoxicillin-clavulanate, 500 mg/125 mg) in patients with Modic type I changes, which developed in the adjacent vertebra following a previous disc herniation, was shown to provide statistically significant improvement compared to placebo in a double-blinded randomized controlled trial. (1) Additional confirmatory studies are necessary to define the role of Modic antibiotic spine therapy (MAST) (Fig. 48.3).

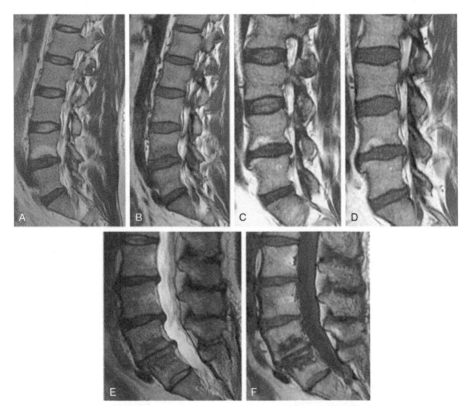

Fig. 48.3 Endplate (Modic) changes. Type I: (A) Sagittal T2-weighted magnetic resonance imaging (MRI) shows hyperintense signal in marrow adjacent to L4 inferior endplate. Note loss of T2 signal in L4–L5 and L5–S1 discs. (B) Matched sagittal T1-weighted MRI in same patient shows hypointense T1 signal adjacent to L4 inferior endplate consistent with type I endplate changes. Type II: (C) Sagittal T2-weighted MRI shows increased T2 signal in the anterior aspect of L4. (D) Matched sagittal T1-weighted MRI in same patient shows increased T1 signal adjacent to the L4 inferior endplate consistent with type II endplate changes. Type III: (E) Sagittal T2-weighted MRI shows low T2 signal adjacent to the L4–L5 disc. (F) Matched sagittal T1-weighted MRI in same patient shows low T1 signal adjacent to the L4–L5 disc consistent with type III endplate change. (From Maus T. Imaging the back pain patient. Phys Med Rehab Clin N Am 2010;21:725–766, Fig. 2.)

7. **What is the cause of the pain associated with lumbar DDD?**

The answer to this question remains elusive. The outer layers of the annulus fibrosis are innervated by sympathetic pain fibers via the sinuvertebral nerve. Theories that have evolved to explain the painful symptoms associated with disc degeneration include:

- **Chemical:** The disc releases inflammatory mediators, which irritate the annular nerve fibers.
- **Disc nociception:** Motion and loading of a degenerated disc becomes painful following nerve fiber ingrowth into the outer annular region.
- **Instability:** The degenerative process leads to excessive and abnormal painful motion of the degenerative lumbar segment.
- **Neutral zone:** The *neutral zone* is conceptualized as a region of intervertebral motion around the neutral posture where little or no resistance to motion exists due to the passive structures of the spinal motion segment. Although the overall flexion-extension arc of motion may decrease with DDD, the types of motion and force required to produce motion may change. In early DDD, disc dehydration and nuclear resorption cause the peripheral annulus to become lax. This laxity increases translatory motion in the motion segment's *neutral zone*. Abnormal motion or laxity may cause pain by abnormally loading the annulus or by inducing lumbar extensor muscle spasticity to control abnormal motion.
- ***Stone in the shoe* hypothesis:** Focal abnormal loads (the *stone in the shoe*) cause areas of focal endplate overloading resulting in pain.

8. **Are there easily defined subtypes of DDD?**

A variety of terms have been applied to patients with nonradicular lumbar pain disorders of a degenerative origin including discogenic pain syndrome, annular tear syndrome, *dark disc disease*, internal disc disruption (IDD), isolated disc resorption, and lumbar spondylosis (LS). Currently, no level I evidence supports subsegregation of DDD, and no universally accepted classification exists. Patients with chronic low back pain of discogenic origin with decreased signal within the disc on T2-weighted MR images and relative preservation of disc height (IDD) are often contrasted with patients with marked disc space collapse, osteophyte formation, and vacuum disc changes (LS). These disease subgroups may be associated with varied responses to operative and nonoperative interventions. For example, stand-alone anterior fusion procedures may fail at a higher rate in IDD. LS patients may not respond as well to lumbar disc replacement.

9. **How much is known about the natural history of DDD?**

Understanding of the natural history of DDD is limited. The available natural history data yield the following conclusions:

- The natural history of lumbar DDD is, for the most part, benign.
- There are more elements at work than mechanical factors alone.
- Patients with fewer radiographic abnormalities may have more pain and functional limitation than ones with much "worse" radiographic change.
- Similarly, a patient's pain may worsen without concomitant change on imaging or may improve despite radiographic progression.
- The subjective nature of these pain complaints makes objective grading of disease state severity impossible.

10. **Discuss common nonsurgical treatment options for chronic low back pain due to lumbar DDD.**

Nonsurgical treatment options for chronic low back pain due to lumbar DDD include:

- **Observation:** For patients with limited symptoms, reasonable function, and good core strength, observation is an appropriate treatment.
- **Medication:** Nonsteroidal antiinflammatory medications are effective for short-term relief of symptoms. Muscle relaxants (benzodiazepine and nonbenzodiazepine) and anticonvulsant medications are considered second-line medication options. Tricyclic antidepressants are a useful adjunct. Tramadol, a synthetic analgesic, has been shown to significantly reduce pain and improve physical function in chronic low back pain patients, but has significant abuse potential. Long-term use of opioids is discouraged due to decreasing efficacy over time and high rates of substance abuse. Corticosteroids are not recommended in treatment of lumbar DDD.
- **Physical therapy:** Exercise therapy with emphasis on core muscle strengthening (abdominal wall muscles, lumbar muscles), stretching, and endurance training have shown benefit.
- **Injections:** Facet and epidural injections may provide short-term relief of symptoms, but are not typically recommended for axial pain due to DDD. More recently, a variety of stem cell and other injections have been offered based on minimal evidence of safety or efficacy.
- **Miscellaneous:** A myriad of traditional (e.g., chiropractic, orthoses, traction, laser, transcutaneous electrical nerve stimulation), as well as complementary and alternative medicine treatments (e.g., acupuncture, massage, herbs, meditation), have been advocated based on varying levels of supportive medical evidence.

11. **What is the most important component of an exercise program for the treatment of low back pain due to lumbar DDD?**

The most important component of a low back exercise program is to address fear-avoidance behavior of the patient by reassuring the patient that it is safe to exercise despite the chronic pain he or she may experience. The appropriate exercise program is a supervised active physical therapy program that uses progressive, non–pain-contingent exercise (i.e., the patient is encouraged to exercise despite their pain) to increase strength and endurance. Successful outcomes may be achieved with a variety of exercise programs, including core strengthening, McKenzie therapy, Pilates, and aerobic conditioning. It is counterproductive to tell patients, "Let pain be your guide." Patients with lumbar DDD must be reassured that they will not do any damage to their spine, even if exercise is painful.

12. **What surgical options are available for treatment of lumbar DDD?**
    A wide range of surgical procedures have been advocated (Table 48.1). Surgical procedures which directly address the pain generator in the intervertebral disc such as lumbar interbody fusion or artificial disc replacement are preferred by many surgeons compared to posterior fusion procedures.
    - **Interbody fusion procedures** are favored by many surgeons as they directly address the pain generator (lumbar disc). Interbody fusion can be performed through various approaches:
      Anterior approach (trans- or retroperitoneal anterior lumbar interbody fusion [ALIF])
      Posterior approach (posterior lumbar interbody fusion [PLIF], transforaminal lumbar interbody fusion [TLIF])

Table 48.1 Common Treatment Options for Lumbar Degenerative Disc Disease.

TYPE OF MANAGEMENT	ADVANTAGES	DISADVANTAGES	COMMENTS
Nonoperative management	• Least costly • Least morbid	• Some patients will not respond	• Trial of nonoperative treatment for all patients
Disc decompression procedures (e.g. laser, nucleoplasty)	• Low initial morbidity • Motion preserving	• High rates of failure in patients with mechanical back pain	• Lack of evidence to support efficacy
Posterior motion preserving implants	• Less invasive • May be revised to fusion	• Success rates unknown	• Theoretical advantages remain unproven
Posterolateral fusion (PLF)	• Decreases axial pain • Breakdown unlikely after successful healing	• Increased surgical morbidity • Adjacent segment degeneration (ASD) • Painful micromotion may persist due to unfused anterior column	• Appropriate for some patients
Noninstrumented PLF	• Less morbidity and cost than instrumented fusion	• High pseudarthrosis risk	• Appropriate in select cases
Instrumented PLF	• Higher fusion rates • No brace required • Sagittal alignment may be improved	• Increased morbidity and costs • Increased ASD risk, especially if cranial screws violate facets • Screw misplacement may injure nerves • Fixation failures in osteoporotic bone	• Used in most cases • Increased fusion rates may not be associated with improved outcomes
Anterior lumbar interbody fusion (ALIF)	• Direct removal of pain generator • Avoids disruption of posterior extensor muscles • Avoids manipulation of neural structures	• Access surgeon available • Difficult if prior abdominal surgery • More difficult at L4-L5 • Exposure-related complications	• Stand-alone ALIF controversial due to complications especially in multilevel cases
Circumferential fusion, separate anterior + posterior surgical approaches	• Higher fusion rate and superior functional outcomes compared to posterior fusion	• Exposure-related complications due to anterior approach • ASD risk	• Recent studies show better outcomes and less cost to society compared with posterior fusion

Table 48.1 Common Treatment Options for Lumbar Degenerative Disc Disease. *(Continued)*

TYPE OF MANAGEMENT	ADVANTAGES	DISADVANTAGES	COMMENTS
Posterior lumbar inter-body fusion (PLIF); transforaminal lumbar interbody fusion (TLIF) techniques	• Allows circumferen-tial fusion via single incision • Provides advantages of ALIF and PLF	• ASD risk • Autologous bone graft frequently utilized	• Many different techniques • Outcome is more technique dependent compared with circum-ferential fusion
Artificial disc replacement	• Motion preservation • Removal of pain generator	• Difficult to revise • Long-term stability unknown • Strict indications	• Potentially useful for select patients in absence of facet joint arthropathy

Lateral and/or oblique approaches (direct lateral interbody fusion [DLIF], extreme lateral interbody fusion [XLIF]—not indicated at the L5–S1 level, oblique lateral interbody fusion [OLIF]—may be utilized at L5–S1; note: some are medical device manufacturer-specific surgical approaches)

Combined circumferential approaches

A variety of implants can be used to promote interbody fusion including autograft, allograft, or fusion cages used in combination with autograft, allograft, synthetic graft material, or bone morphogenetic protein. Posterior spinal instrumentation with or without posterolateral fusion are commonly performed in conjunction with interbody fusion. Minimally invasive and percutaneous approaches have been popularized to decrease exposure-related surgical morbidity.

- **Artificial disc replacement** is an alternative to fusion. However, candidates for artificial disc replacement represent a much narrower group of patients than those considered for fusion. For example, patients with facet joint arthrosis or severe disc space narrowing (<4 mm) are not candidates for artificial disc replacement (Fig. 48.4).

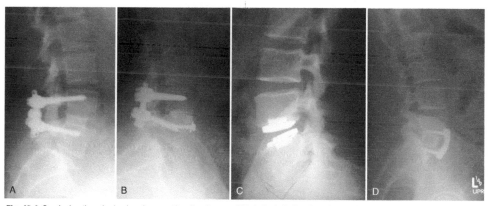

Fig. 48.4 Surgical options for lumbar degenerative disc disease. (A) Interbody fusion through a posterior approach using cortical allograft combined with posterior spinal instrumentation and fusion. (B) Interbody fusion through an anterior approach using femoral allograft combined with posterior spinal instrumentation and fusion. (C) Artificial disc replacement with the ProDisc-L implant. (D) Anterior lumbar interbody fusion with plate fixation. (A: From Herkowitz HN, Garfin SR, Eismont FJ, et al., editors. Rothman Simeone The Spine. 5th ed. Philadelphia, PA: Saunders; 2006, Fig. 91.10, p. 1531. B: From Devlin VJ. C: From Yue JJ, Bertagnoli R, McAfee PC, et al., editors. Motion Preservation Surgery of the Spine. Philadelphia, PA: Saunders; 2008, Fig. 39.2A, p. 321. D: From Daubs, MD. Chapter 39. Anterior lumbar interbody fusion. In: Baron EM, Vaccaro AR, editors. Operative Techniques: Spine Surgery. Philadelphia, PA: Elsevier; 2018, Fig. 39.13, pp. 340–346.)

13. **How does surgical treatment compare with nonoperative treatment for patients with discogenic low back pain?**

Data from randomized controlled trials permit comparison of nonoperative and operative treatment for patients with discogenic low back pain. Conclusions drawn include:

- Spinal fusion is superior to nonstructured nonoperative treatment.
- Spinal fusion outcomes are similar to outcomes obtained with a structured nonoperative treatment program consisting of intensive outpatient physical rehabilitation.

- Outcomes of artificial disc replacement are similar or slightly better than outcomes of spinal fusion, but arthroplasty is indicated for a more highly selected population compared with fusion.

14. **Which patients are the most appropriate candidates for surgical treatment for lumbar DDD?**
It is challenging to successfully identify candidates for surgical procedures for discogenic back pain. Surgery may be considered for treatment of low back pain of discogenic origin in patients who fail to improve after a minimum of 6–12 months of appropriate nonsurgical care. Appropriate surgical criteria include:
- Patients with pain and disability for more than 1 year
- Failure of aggressive physical conditioning and conservative treatment for more than 6 months
- Marked, single-level degeneration on MRI
- Absence of psychiatric or secondary gain issues
  Patients with multilevel disc degeneration (greater than two levels) are poor candidates for surgery because outcome studies fail to document reliable benefit. Use of discography to identify surgical candidates is controversial.

15. **Which patients are less than ideal candidates for surgical treatment for lumbar DDD?**
Surgical treatment is associated with poor outcomes in patients with unresolved secondary gain issues, worker's compensation claims, litigation, multiple emergency department visits, high levels of opioid usage, abnormal psychometrics, chronic pain illness, and exaggerated pain behaviors. Patients off work for greater than 3 months tend to have worse results. To have any sense that surgery might benefit the patient, the surgeon must get to know the patient. Overreliance on MRI or discography data will lead to a high rate of clinical failures. Motivated patients with clear, provocative, and palliating factors, and without psychosocial overlay are likely to do well. Deviation from these strict criteria exposes the patient to significant operative risks with much less potential benefit.

16. **Are there any new or emerging treatments for lumbar DDD?**
Given the frustration many patients and clinicians feel regarding our poor understanding and limited treatment options for DDD, there have always been a wide array of complementary and alternative therapies. These range from chiropractic treatment to acupuncture and all have a limited evidence base. More recently, some physicians have begun to offer stem cell and other injections into the lumbar discs in hopes of "regenerating" these tissues. Unfortunately, there is a lack of high-level clinical evidence to support the use of stem cell therapies in humans, except for indications such as hematopoietic reconstitution for treatment of certain disorders of the blood and immune system and acquired loss of bone marrow function.
  One notable development is the use of radiofrequency (RF) energy to ablate the basivertebral nerve as a treatment for chronic lumbar pain (Intracept Procedure, Relievant Medsystems, Minneapolis, MN). The basivertebral nerve originates from the sinuvertebral nerve and follows the course of the basivertebral artery and vein to enter the posterior cortex of the vertebral body through the paired basivertebral foramen. The basivertebral nerve branches repeatedly and spreads throughout the vertebral body, to include the regions near the superior and inferior vertebral endplates. Early data regarding this treatment includes a 3-month report of a significantly greater decrease in Oswestry Disability Index scores (decrease in patient functional limitations due to back pain) when compared with a sham procedure.

KEY POINTS

1. The pathophysiology of lumbar degenerative disc disease and its relation to low back pain symptoms is poorly understood.
2. Mechanical, traumatic, chemical, psychosocial, and genetic factors may interact and play a role in the development of symptomatic disc degeneration.
3. Evidence-based treatment options for symptomatic lumbar degenerative disc disease include a structured outpatient physical rehabilitation program, spinal fusion, and artificial disc replacement.

Websites
1. North American Spine Society Consensus Committee on Nomenclature: https://www.thespinejournalonline.com/article/S1529-9430(14)00409-4/fulltext#sec3.3
2. Lumbar degenerative disc disease: http://emedicine.medscape.com/article/309767-overview
3. Degenerative disc disease condition center: http://www.spineuniverse.com/conditions/degenerative-disc/degenerative-disc-disease-condition-center
4. FDA warns about stem cell therapies: https://www.fda.gov/ForConsumers/ConsumerUpdates/ucm286155.htm

REFERENCE

1. Albert HB, Sorenson JS, Christensen BS, et al. Antibiotic treatment in patients with chronic low back pain and vertebral bone edema (Modic Type I changes): A double-blind randomized clinical controlled trial of efficacy. *Eur Spine J* 2013;22:697–707.

BIBLIOGRAPHY

1. Albert HB, Sorenson JS, Christensen BS, et al. Antibiotic treatment in patients with chronic low back pain and vertebral bone edema (Modic Type I changes): A double-blind randomized clinical controlled trial of efficacy. *Eur Spine J* 2013;22:697–707.
2. Coe M, Mirza S, Sengupta D. The role of fusion for discogenic axial back pain without associated leg pain, spondylolisthesis or stenosis: An evidence-based review. *Semin Spine Surg* 2009;21:246–256.
3. Fardon DF, Williams AL, Dohring EJ, et al. Lumbar disc nomenclature: Version 2.0: Recommendations of the combined task forces of the North American Spine Society, the American Society of Spine Radiology and the American Society of Neuroradiology. *Spine J* 2014;14:2525–2545.
4. Fischgrund JS, Rhyne A, Franke J, et al. Intraosseous basivertebral nerve ablation for the treatment of chronic low back pain: A prospective randomized double-blind sham-controlled multi-center study. *Eur Spine J* 2018;27:1146–1156.
5. Marks PW, Witten CM, Califf RM. Clarifying stem-cell therapy's benefits and risks. *N Engl J Med* 2017;376:1007–1009.
6. Rainville J, Nguyen R, Suri, P. Effective conservative treatment for chronic low back pain. *Semin Spine Surg* 2009;21:257–263.
7. Risbud MV, Andersson GB. Lumbar disc disease. In: Garfin SR, Eismont FJ, Bell GR, et al., editors. Rothman-Simeone and Herkowitz's The Spine. 7th ed. Philadelphia, PA: Saunders, pp. 807–838.
8. Truumees E, Fischgrund J. Axial low back pain. *Semin Spine Surg* 2008;20:73–160.
9. Yavin D, Casha S, Wiebe S, et al. Lumbar fusion for degenerative disease: A systematic review and meta-analysis. *Neurosurgery* 2017;80:701–715.

CHAPTER 49

LUMBAR SPINAL STENOSIS

Vincent J. Devlin, MD

1. **What is lumbar spinal stenosis?**

   Lumbar spinal stenosis is defined as any type of narrowing of the spinal canal, nerve root canals, or intervertebral foramen. This narrowing can be caused by soft tissue, bone, or a combination of both. The resultant nerve root compression leads to nerve root ischemia and a clinical syndrome associated with variable degrees of low back, buttock, and leg pain.

2. **What are the two main types of lumbar spinal stenosis?**

   The two main types of spinal stenosis are (1) congenital-developmental and (2) acquired spinal stenosis. In the most widely accepted classification, spinal stenosis is subdivided into two congenital-developmental subtypes and six acquired subtypes.

   CONGENITAL-DEVELOPMENTAL STENOSIS
   - Idiopathic
   - Achondroplastic

   ACQUIRED STENOSIS
   - Degenerative
   - Combined congenital and degenerative stenosis
   - Spondylolytic or spondylolisthetic
   - Iatrogenic (e.g., following laminectomy or spinal fusion)
   - Posttraumatic
   - Metabolic (e.g., Paget disease, fluorosis)

3. **What is the most common type of lumbar spinal stenosis?**

   Acquired degenerative spinal stenosis is the most common type.

4. **How does degenerative lumbar spinal stenosis develop?**

   Pathologic changes in the lumbar disc and facet joints are responsible for the development of spinal stenosis. With the passage of time, biochemical and mechanical changes in the intervertebral disc decrease its ability to withstand cyclic loading. These changes predispose the disc to annular tears, loss of disc height, annular bulging, and osteophyte formation. A degenerative sequence also occurs posteriorly in the facet joint complex. Disc space narrowing increases loading on posterior facet and capsular structures leading to joint erosion, loss of cartilage, and capsular laxity. Ultimately, facet hypertrophy and osteophyte formation occur.

   Osteophytes on the inferior articular process encroach medially resulting in **central spinal canal stenosis**. Ligamentum flavum hypertrophy and annular bulging further contribute to stenosis involving the central spinal canal.

   Osteophytes on the superior articular process enlarge, resulting in **lateral zone stenosis**. Osteophytes may also form circumferentially at the vertebral margins at the attachment of the anulus in an attempt to autostabilize the motion segment. Portions of these osteophytes, termed uncinate spurs, may protrude from the subjacent vertebral endplate or disc margin into the lateral nerve root canal above and provide an additional source of lateral nerve root entrapment. Loss of disc space height can also decrease the cross-sectional area of the neural foramen and lead to symptomatic lateral zone stenosis.

   Spinal instability may develop as a result of the degenerative process and lead to the development of degenerative spondylolisthesis, lateral listhesis, scoliosis, and complex spinal deformities.

5. **What is the epidemiology of lumbar spinal stenosis?**

   Spinal stenosis may present at any age (e.g., congenital type). However, the acquired degenerative type of spinal stenosis typically becomes symptomatic in the sixth and seventh decades of life. The most common levels of involvement in the lumbar region are L3–L4 and L4–L5. Up to 15% of patients with degenerative lumbar spinal stenosis have coexistent cervical spinal stenosis (tandem stenosis).

6. **Describe the typical history reported by a patient with acquired lumbar degenerative spinal stenosis.**

   The typical patient reports the gradual onset of low back, buttock, thigh, and calf pain. Patients may report numbness, burning, heaviness, or weakness in the lower extremities. The lower extremity symptoms may be unilateral or bilateral. Symptoms are exacerbated by activities that promote spinal extension such as prolonged standing or walking (neurogenic claudication). Maneuvers that permit spinal flexion such as sitting, lying down, or leaning forward on a shopping cart tend to relieve symptoms as these positions increase spinal canal diameter. Changes in bowel or bladder function due to lumbar spinal stenosis are uncommon but occasionally noted.

7. **What common conditions should be considered in the differential diagnosis of lumbar spinal stenosis?**
   Common conditions that should be ruled out during assessment include:
   - Degenerative arthritis involving the hip joints
   - Peripheral neuropathy
   - Vascular insufficiency
   - Metastatic tumor

8. **Compare and contrast the presentation of neurogenic claudication and vascular claudication.**
   Patients with **neurogenic claudication** report tiredness, heaviness, and discomfort in the lower extremities with ambulation. The distance walked until symptoms begin and the maximum distance that the patient can walk without stopping varies from day to day, and even during the same walk. Patients report that leaning forward relieves symptoms. These patients may not experience symptoms during activities performed in a flexed posture such as riding a bicycle or walking uphill. In contrast, activities performed in extension such as walking downhill tend to worsen symptoms. Patients with **vascular claudication** describe cramping or tightness in the calf associated with ambulation. The distance they are able to walk before symptoms occur is constant. Their symptoms are not affected by posture. They are unable to tolerate walking uphill or downhill, or cycling.

9. **What findings are typically noted on physical examination of the patient with lumbar spinal stenosis?**
   Although most patients with lumbar spinal stenosis have significant subjective complaints, physical examination generally reveals few objective findings. The most frequent physical examination findings include reproduction of pain with lumbar extension, weakness of the extensor hallucis longus muscle, and sensory deficits over the lower extremities. Neurologic findings not otherwise detectable are sometimes demonstrated by performing a stress test (walking until symptoms occur and repeating the neurologic examination).

10. **Contrast the role of radiographs, magnetic resonance imaging, computed tomography, and CT-myelography in the assessment of lumbar spinal stenosis.**
    - **Radiographs:** Useful to diagnose spinal deformities (scoliosis, spondylolisthesis, lateral listhesis). Flexion-extension radiographs are useful to diagnose spinal instabilities. Radiographs can also exclude pathologic processes such as neoplasm, infection, or hip osteoarthritis.
    - **Magnetic resonance imaging (MRI):** The best initial study for the diagnosis of spinal stenosis. In many cases it provides sufficient diagnostic information to eliminate the need for further advanced diagnostic studies when interpreted in conjunction with upright lumbar spine radiographs. However, imaging findings must be correlated with clinical signs and symptoms as more than 20% of asymptomatic patients over age 60 have spinal stenosis on lumbar MRI studies.
    - **Computed tomography (CT):** Its strength is assessment of osseous anatomy in relation to spinal stenosis syndromes. CT does not provide optimal soft tissue detail or visualization of neural structures.
    - **CT-myelography:** This is generally limited to the presurgical patient whose spinal canal is not adequately visualized with MRI due to its invasive nature. It may be used to visualize postural-dependent stenosis of the lumbar spinal canal.

11. **What are the options for nonsurgical management of lumbar spinal stenosis?**
    The majority of patients with lumbar spinal stenosis do well with nonsurgical management. The nonsurgical treatment options for lumbar spinal stenosis include:
    - Medication (nonsteroidal antiinflammatory drugs, anticonvulsants)
    - Physical therapy (flexion exercises, functional stabilization exercises)
    - General fitness and conditioning (cycling, pool exercise)
    - Injections (epidural corticosteroid injections)
    - Manual therapy

12. **What are the indications for surgical treatment for patients with lumbar spinal stenosis?**
    Surgical treatment is indicated for patients with moderate or severe spinal stenosis accompanied by intractable pain or significant neurogenic claudication, or patients who fail to improve with appropriate nonsurgical treatment. Surgical treatment for spinal stenosis is elective in nature except in the presence of bowel or bladder dysfunction (cauda equina syndrome). It is recommended that the decision whether to pursue surgical treatment is based on shared decision making and considers individual patient factors, including symptom severity, degree of activity limitation, activity goals, age, medical comorbidities, and patient preference.

13. **What are the surgical treatment options for lumbar spinal stenosis?**
    The basic surgical treatment for spinal stenosis is spinal **decompression**, which involves removal of portions of those structures (lamina, ligamentum flavum, hypertrophied facet joints, uncinate spurs) responsible for compression of the dural sac and/or nerve roots. Decompression of the neural elements may be achieved by **laminectomy** (removal of the midline osseous and ligamentous structures, including the lamina, spinous processes, interspinous ligaments, ligamentum flavum, and portions of the facet joints) or **laminotomy** (partial removal of the lamina, facet complex, and ligamentum flavum with preservation of midline structures including

the spinous processes and interspinous ligaments). A variety of minimally invasive decompression techniques have been popularized as alternatives to standard laminectomy and laminotomy. In certain situations (e.g., spondylolisthesis), a spinal fusion should be considered in conjunction with spinal decompression. Other proposed treatment alternatives include insertion of an **interspinous process spacer** to provide indirect decompression of the spinal canal as an alternative to direct surgical decompression and insertion of an interspinous or interlaminar device as a nonfusion adjunct to surgical decompression.

14. Explain the basic steps involved in a laminectomy procedure to treat central spinal stenosis between L4 and S1.
A skin incision is made between L3 and S1. The paraspinal muscles are elevated from the lamina between L3 and S1. The L4 and L5 spinous processes are resected. The pars interarticularis is identified at each level to ensure that bone removal does not compromise its integrity. The hypertrophic laminae of L4 and L5 are thinned with a motorized burr or osteotome to facilitate removal with angled Kerrison rongeurs. Adhesions between the dural sac and surrounding tissue are released with a Penfield elevator. Starting to the L5–S1 interspace, lamina and hypertrophic ligamentum flavum are resected between L4 and S1. The midline decompression is widened to permit visualization of the lateral border of the dural sac, as well as the medial border of the pedicle at each level to ensure adequate decompression (Fig. 49.1).

15. Explain the basic steps involved in decompression of lumbar lateral zone stenosis.
Clinical evaluation and preoperative imaging studies are reviewed to determine the extent of lateral zone stenosis. Potential sources of neural compression include:
- **Zone 1** (also called the subarticular zone, entrance zone, or lateral recess). Osteophytes from the superior articular process may compress the exiting nerve root in this zone.
- **Zone 2** (also called the foraminal zone, midzone, pedicle zone, or hidden zone). A variety of pathologies may cause nerve root impingement including facet and ligamentum flavum hypertrophy, disc bulges, and uncinate spurs.
- **Zone 3** (also called the extraforaminal zone, exit zone, or far-lateral zone). Nerve root compression may result from disc protrusion, uncinate spurs, facet subluxation, and ligamentous structures.

After the midline decompression is completed, each nerve root in the surgical field must be inspected and decompressed. Each nerve root is identified along the medial border of its respective pedicle. Medial facet overgrowth and ligamentum flavum hypertrophy are resected with a Kerrison rongeur. The goal is to undercut the facet joint without sacrificing its integrity. The intervertebral disc is palpated or visualized to ensure the disc is not causing significant nerve root compression. Resection of disc and/or uncinate spurs is performed as needed to enlarge the foramen. Adequacy of decompression is checked by assessing the ability to retract the nerve root 1 cm medially and laterally without tension at the entrance zone. In addition, it should be possible to pass a blunt probe dorsal and volar to the nerve root through the neural foramen (zone 3) without resistance (Fig. 49.2).

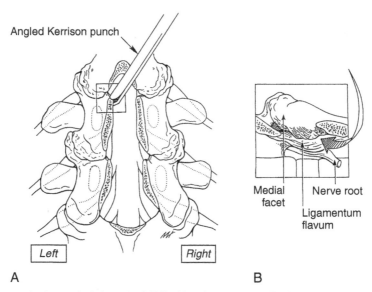

Angled Kerrison punch

Left | Right

A | B

Medial facet | **Nerve root** | **Ligamentum flavum**

Fig. 49.1 Decompression for central spinal stenosis. (A) Midline bilateral laminectomy provides decompression of the cauda equina. (B) Removal of the medial aspect of hypertrophic facet joints and infolded ligamentum flavum. (From Stambough JL. Technique for lumbar decompression of spinal stenosis. Oper Tech Orthop 1997;7(1):36–43.)

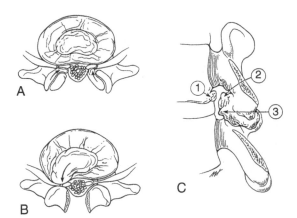

Fig. 49.2 Decompression for lateral zone stenosis. (A) Zone 1—stenosis due to hypertrophy of the superior articular process. (B) Zone 2—stenosis due to lateral disc bulging and uncinate spurs. (C) Zone 3—stenosis due to uncinate spur *(1)* and superior articular process hypertrophy *(2, 3)*. (From Stambough JL. Technique for lumbar decompression of spinal stenosis. Oper Tech Orthop 1997;7(1):36–43.)

16. What complications may occur with lumbar decompression procedures for spinal stenosis?
Some commonly encountered complications include:
- Dural tear
- Arachnoiditis
- Infection
- Nerve root injury
- Spinal instability
- Inadequate decompression
- Persistent symptoms
- Recurrent stenosis

17. Compare and contrast laminectomy and laminotomy for treatment of lumbar spinal stenosis.
Laminectomy is the traditional procedure for surgical decompression for lumbar stenosis. It involves removal of the midline osseous and ligamentous structures, including the lamina, spinous processes, interspinous ligaments, and portions of the facet joints. It provides excellent visualization of neural structures and facilitates complete decompression of involved neural structures. However, spinal instability may develop following laminectomy and require treatment with spinal instrumentation and fusion. **Laminotomy** involves partial removal of the lamina and facet complex but preserves the midline structures, including the spinous processes and interspinous ligaments. Preservation of the midline structures decreases the risk of developing spinal instability. When bilateral decompression is indicated, procedure options include a bilateral laminotomy technique or bilateral decompression through a unilateral laminotomy approach. Disadvantages of laminotomy include technical difficulty of the procedure and risk of inadequate decompression due to limited exposure. An intermediate approach between laminotomy and laminectomy is an **interlaminar decompression**, which enhances visualization of the neural elements for decompression but minimizes bone resection and is potentially less destabilizing than laminectomy. Laminotomies are most appropriate for treatment of patients with spinal stenosis limited to the level of the facet joints and disc space involving one or two spinal levels. Laminectomies are most appropriate for patients with congenital stenosis or multi-level severe spinal stenosis. Regardless of which procedure is utilized, preservation of pars interarticularis and at least 50% of the facet joints bilaterally is recommended to prevent iatrogenic spinal instability.

18. What are the indications for fusion in lumbar spinal stenosis procedures?
The indications for fusion in patients with lumbar spinal stenosis fall into two broad categories:
PREOPERATIVE STRUCTURAL CONDITIONS ASSOCIATED WITH SPINAL INSTABILITY
- Degenerative spondylolisthesis or lateral listhesis
- Progressive scoliosis or kyphosis
- Recurrent spinal stenosis requiring repeat decompression at the same level
INTRAOPERATIVE STRUCTURAL ALTERATIONS THAT PREDISPOSE TO POSTOPERATIVE INSTABILITY
- Excess facet joint removal (>50%)
- Pars interarticularis fracture or removal
- Radical disc excision with resultant destabilization of the anterior spinal column

19. **What types of fusion procedures are performed for unstable lumbar spinal stenosis syndromes?**
The most common type of fusion procedure is a posterior fusion combined with posterior pedicle screw fixation. Interbody fusion may be added for patients with severe coronal and/or sagittal imbalance, rotatory subluxations, severe foraminal stenosis (to provide indirect decompression through restoration of foraminal height), deficient posterior facet joints, or biologic factors that negatively affect fusion success.

20. **How does an interspinous process device improve lumbar spinal stenosis symptoms if direct neural decompression is not performed?**
Insertion of a rigid device between adjacent spinous processes creates segmental distraction at the operative level. This indirectly increases the cross-sectional area of the stenotic spinal canal and neural foramina and may potentially provide relief of neurogenic claudication due to lumbar spinal stenosis without the need for concomitant direct spinal decompression or spinal fusion. An example of a contemporary interspinous process device is the Superion Indirect Decompression System (Vertiflex, Inc., Carlsbad, CA), which is indicated for implantation at one or two adjacent lumbar levels in patients with moderate spinal stenosis and no greater than grade 1 degenerative spondylolisthesis whose symptoms are relieved with sitting and flexion maneuvers. Superion consists of a titanium alloy implant with deployable superior and inferior projections that engage the spinous processes to prevent dislodgement. This device is implanted via a cannula and deployed under fluoroscopy to provide distraction at the target spinal level while preserving motion. The rigid implant maintains interspinous distraction and limits spinal extension thereby preventing repetitive compression of neural elements responsible for symptoms of intermittent neurogenic claudication in patients with lumbar spinal stenosis.

21. **What is the role of a posterior spacer in patients who undergo posterior spinal decompression for treatment of neurogenic claudication?**
Posterior spinal column spacer devices have been advocated as an adjunct to lumbar decompression surgery to provide stability to the operated spinal segment, while avoiding the rigidity and loss of motion associated with an instrumented spinal fusion. An example of this device type is Coflex (Paradigm Spine, New York, NY), an interlaminar stabilization device, which is inserted in the midline between adjacent laminae following decompression of 1- or 2-level lumbar spinal stenosis. This device is indicated for use in patients with at least moderate impairment in function, who experience relief in flexion from symptoms of buttock, leg, or groin pain and no greater than grade 1 degenerative spondylolisthesis. This U-shaped titanium alloy device has vertical wing extensions on the superior and inferior ends of the "U" that anchor on the superior and inferior spinous processes. It is a functionally dynamic implant as it is not only compressible with lumbar extension but also allows lumbar flexion, while providing distraction of the posterior elements throughout the range of motion.

KEY POINTS

1. Lumbar spinal stenosis is defined as any type of narrowing of the spinal canal, nerve root canals, or intervertebral foramen.
2. Lumbar spinal stenosis symptoms are typically position dependent and exacerbated by activities that promote spinal, extension such as prolonged standing, or walking and relieved with spinal flexion maneuvers.
3. The majority of patients with lumbar spinal stenosis improve with nonsurgical management.
4. In the absence of spinal instability, lumbar decompression (laminotomy or laminectomy) without arthrodesis is the recommended surgical treatment for symptomatic lumbar spinal stenosis.

Websites
1. Lumbar spinal stenosis: http://www.aafp.org/afp/980415ap/alvarez.html
2. Lumbar spinal stenosis:http://orthoinfo.aaos.org/topic.cfm?topic=A00329
3. Spinal stenosis: http://www.nlm.nih.gov/medlineplus/spinalstenosis.html

BIBLIOGRAPHY

1. Arnoldi CC, Brodsky AE, Cauchoix J, Crock HV, Dommisse GF, Edgar MA, et al. Lumbar spinal stenosis and nerve root entrapment syndromes: Definition and classification. *Clin Orthop Relat Res* 1976;(115):4–5.
2. Atlas SJ, Keller RB, Wu YA, Deyo RA, Singer DE. Long-term outcomes of surgical and nonsurgical management of lumbar spinal stenosis: 8–10 year results from the Maine Lumbar Spine Study. *Spine* 2005;30(8):936–943.
3. Derman PB, Rihm J, Albert TJ. Surgical management of lumbar spinal stenosis. In: Garfin SR, Eismont FJ, Bell GR, et al, editors. Rothman-Simeone the Spine. 7th ed. Philadelphia, PA: Saunders; 2018, pp. 1039–1057.
4. Herkowitz HN, Sidhu KS. Lumbar spine fusion in the treatment of degenerative conditions: current indications and recommendations. *J Am Acad Orthop Surg* 1995;3(3):123–135.
5. Kebaish KM, Elder BD, Lo SL, Witham TF. Sublaminar decompression: a new technique for spinal canal decompression in the treatment of stenosis in degenerative conditions. *Clin Spine Surg* 2017;30(1):14–19.
6. Gala RJ, Russo GS, Whang PG. Interspinous implants to treat spinal stenosis. *Curr Rev Musculoskel Med* 2017;10(2):182–188.

7. Lurie JD, Tosteson TD, Tosteson A, Abdu WA, Zhao W, Morgan TS, et al. Long-term outcomes of lumbar spinal stenosis: Eight-year results of the Spine Patient Outcomes Research Trial. *Spine* 2015;40(2):63–76.
8. O'Leary PF, McCance SE. Distraction laminoplasty for decompression of lumbar spinal stenosis. *Clin Orthop Relat Res* 2001;(384):26–34.
9. Overdevest GM, Jacobs W, Vleggeert-Lankamp C, Thomé C, Gunzburg R, Peul W. Effectiveness of posterior decompression techniques compared with conventional laminectomy for lumbar stenosis. *Cochrane Database Syst Rev* 2015;(3):CD010036.

CHAPTER 50

DISORDERS OF THE SACROILIAC JOINT

Philip J. York, MD, David C. Ou-Yang, MD, and Vikas V. Patel, MD

BACKGROUND

1. Why has the sacroiliac joint historically been neglected as part of the history, physical examination, and diagnostic workup of low back pain?
   - As sacroiliac joint (SIJ) pain presents with symptoms similar to hip and lumbar spine pathology, the SIJ is often overlooked as a pain generator.
   - Historically, poor outcomes have been reported with surgical intervention for SIJ pain due to high complication rates and inadequate pain relief.
   - Imaging studies that assess the SIJ are difficult to interpret and have low sensitivity and specificity for identifying symptomatic pathology.

2. What percentage of patients who present to a spine clinic for evaluation of low back pain have SIJ pain?
   Up to 15% of patients presenting to a spine clinic for evaluation for low back pain will have SIJ pain. (1) Pain originating from the lumbar spine, hip joints, and SIJ may be difficult to distinguish and more than one pain generator may be present in the same patient. In a study of patients evaluated in a spine surgery clinic, 82% had spine pathology but only 65% of patients had pathology limited to the lumbar spine—17.5% had a combination of spine and hip and/or SIJ pathology, 18% had hip and/or SIJ pathology without spine pathology, and 10% had pain from an unidentified source.

3. What is the disease burden of SIJ dysfunction?
   SIJ dysfunction is associated with a high burden of disease quantified at 0.5 quality-adjusted life years (QALYs). This burden is lower than chronic obstructive pulmonary disorder, coronary artery disease, angina, asthma, and mild heart failure, but comparable with other orthopedic conditions such as hip or knee osteoarthritis, degenerative spondylolisthesis, and spinal stenosis. Those with SIJ dysfunction report lower functional and utility scores and health-related quality of life (HRQoL) scores, compared to controls. (2)

ANATOMY

4. What are the functions of the SIJ?
   - The SIJ connects the sacrum to the ilium.
   - It is an integral part of the pelvic ring.
   - It transmits the body weight of the torso from the spine to the pelvis and subsequently the legs.

5. How is the SIJ morphology different from other synovial joints?
   - It is an amphiarthrosis (75% synovial, 25% fibrocartilaginous) and permits only minimal motion. The anterior or intracapsular portion of the joint contains articular cartilage, while the posterior or extracapsular portion is mainly ligamentous.
   - Structural changes occur from childhood to adulthood. The SIJ is flat through adolescence with changes in topography after puberty.
   - The sacral portion of the joint includes the fused portions of S1, S2, and variably S3.
   - The adult SIJ has variable morphology but is generally auricular shaped with the apex of the joint pointed anteriorly at approximately S2 (Fig. 50.1).

6. Describe the motions of the SIJ and explain how it is stabilized.
   - SIJ motion is limited and is reported as less than 4° of rotation and less than 1.6 mm of translation. The primary motion of the SIJ is rotation of the sacrum around its transverse axis at S2 and is described as nutation (anterior rotation of the sacrum in relation to the ilium) and counternutation (posterior rotation of the sacrum in relation to the ilium).
   - Normal aging is considered to have a deleterious effect on SIJ mobility due to increasing fibrous connections and decreasing proportion of synovial joint surface to syndesmosis.
   - In pregnancy, the SIJ stabilizing ligaments become more flexible and allow for opening of the pelvis for delivery. Asymmetric laxity of the SIJ has been linked to pregnancy-related pelvic pain.

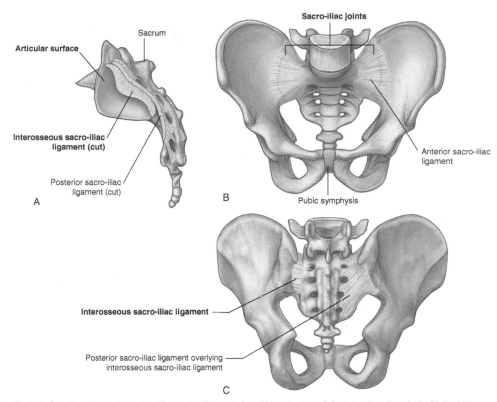

Fig. 50.1 Sacroiliac joints and associated ligaments. (A) Lateral view. (B) Anterior view. (C) Posterior view. (From Drake RL, Vogl AW, Mitchell AWM. Pelvis and perineum. In: Drake RL, Vogl AW, Mitchell AWM, editors. Gray's Anatomy for Students. 3rd ed. Philadelphia, PA: Churchill Livingstone; 2015, pp. 413–524, Fig. 5.24.)

- Ligaments (passive stabilizers)—the primary stabilizers of the SIJ include the sacroiliac, sacrotuberous, and sacrospinous ligaments. Joint load is resisted by deep anterior, posterior, and interosseous ligaments.
- Muscles (active/dynamic stabilizers) include the gluteus maximus and gluteus medius, erector spinae, latissimus dorsi, biceps femoris, iliacus, psoas, piriformis, and oblique and transversus abdominus muscles (Fig. 50.2).

7. **Which nerves provide innervation to the SIJ?**
Nociceptors have been identified within the SIJ capsule, ligaments, and subchondral bone. Innervation of the anterior intracapsular portion of the SIJ derives from multiple sources, including anterior contributions from the L2–S1 ventral rami, lumbosacral plexus, and superior gluteal nerve. The posterior aspect of the joint and surrounding ligaments are innervated by lateral branches of the dorsal rami of S1–S3, with additional innervation from L5 and S4 dorsal rami in some individuals.

DIAGNOSIS

8. **Describe the typical pain pattern for SIJ dysfunction.**
SIJ dysfunction is a term commonly used to describe pain related to poor functioning of the SIJ. Symptoms that suggest SIJ-related pain include:
- Pain with positional changes (sitting to standing, turning in bed), which often improves when lying down
- Pain when sitting on hard surfaces
- Pain localized to the region between the posterior superior iliac spine (PSIS) and the sacral sulcus, known as Fortin's area
- Pain with radiation to the groin, buttock, and posterior thigh
- Pain above L5 suggests another pain source
- Approximately 20% of patients with SIJ pain report radiation of pain distal to the knee

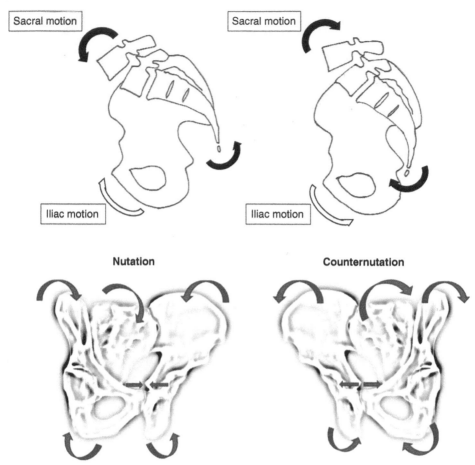

Fig. 50.2 Motion of the sacroiliac has been termed nutation and counternutation. Simplified depiction of relative motion of the sacrum to the ilium in the sagittal plane *(top)*. Depiction of the complex three-dimensional relative motions of the sacrum to the ilium *(bottom)*.

9. **What are potential etiologies of SIJ pain?**
   A wide range of etiologies may be responsible for SIJ pain and may involve the intraarticular or extraarticular portions of the joint or both. Etiologies include:
   • Direct trauma such as a fall on the buttocks or a motor vehicle accident
   • Repetitive microtrauma
   • Disorders of joint hyperlaxity such as Ehlers-Danlos syndrome
   • Pregnancy-related laxity of the pelvic ligaments
   • Inflammatory arthropathies such as ankylosing spondylitis
   • Major trauma
   • Degenerative arthritis
   • Infection
   • Tumors
   • Idiopathic
   • Iatrogenic (secondary to iliac bone graft harvest, after lumbar or lumbosacral fusion)

10. **What effect does lumbar fusion have on the development of SIJ dysfunction?**
    Rates of radiographically appreciable SIJ degeneration following lumbar fusion have been reported as high as 75%. Fusion to the sacrum, as opposed to stopping at L5, has been linked to increased rates of radiographic degeneration. However, the clinical impact of this radiographic degeneration is unclear. In terms of symptomatic SIJ dysfunction, 10.7% of patients who underwent lumbar or lumbosacral fusion in a retrospective study developed SIJ pain diagnosed via examination followed by intraarticular injection. The incidence of SIJ pain increased with increasing numbers of fused segments and was significantly more common in patients with at least three fused segments.

11. Is there a correlation between lumbosacral transitional vertebrae and SIJ dysfunction?
    Yes. The prevalence of SIJ dysfunction has been reported as significantly higher in patients who present with low back pain and a transitional vertebra compared with those with low back pain without the transitional vertebra (28.5% vs. 10.8%).

12. How is SIJ dysfunction evaluated by physical examination?
    The presumptive diagnosis of SIJ dysfunction on physical examination is based on localizing and provocative maneuvers (Table 50.1). A positive provocation test requires reproduction of SIJ pain. Three or more positive tests in a patient whose symptoms cannot be made to centralize on physical examination support a diagnosis of SIJ pain.
    - **Fortin finger test:** A positive test requires that the patient localize pain with one finger immediately inferomedial to the PSIS within 1 cm (Fig. 50.3).
    - **Provocative tests:** Gaenslen, distraction, compression, sacral thrust, thigh thrust, and Patrick or FABER (flexion-abduction-external rotation) tests (Fig. 50.4).

Table 50.1 Clinical Tests for Sacroiliac Joint Pain.

CLINICAL TEST	DESCRIPTION
Gaenslen	Torsional force is applied with the patient supine or side lying as the hip and knee joints of the unaffected leg are flexed toward the chest, and the leg on the affected side is extended.
Distraction	With the patient supine, a vertically oriented pressure is applied bilaterally to the anterior superior iliac spinous processes to distract the sacroiliac joints.
Compression	With the patient either supine or in the lateral position, the iliac crests are pushed toward the midline in an attempt to elicit pain in the sacroiliac joint.
Sacral Thrust	With the patient prone, the examiner applies anteriorly directed pressure over the sacrum.
Thigh Thrust	With the patient supine, the hip flexed to 90°, and the knee bent, the examiner applies a posteriorly directed force through the femur at varying angles of abduction/adduction.
Patrick (FABER)	With the patient supine, the knee on the affected side is flexed and the foot placed on the opposite patella. The flexed knee is then pushed laterally to stress the sacroiliac joint. Also called the FABER test (flexion-abduction-external rotation).

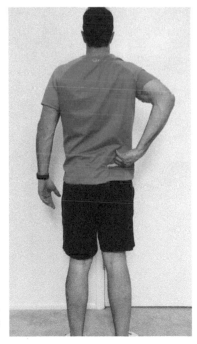

Fig. 50.3 Fortin finger test. Have the patient point with one finger to the point of maximal pain. Patients with sacroiliac pain will often localize the pain to the area of the sacroiliac joint.

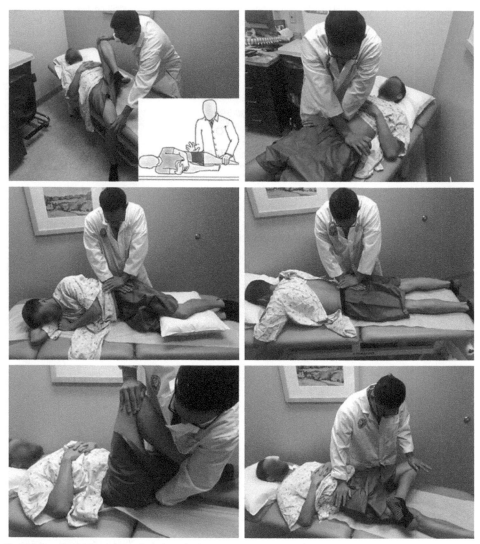

Fig. 50.4 Sacroiliac joint provocative physical examination maneuvers. Top row: The Gaenslen maneuver, which applies torsional stress and can be performed with the patient in the supine or lateral position *(left)*, the distraction test *(middle)*, and the compression test *(right)*. Bottom row: The sacral thrust test *(left)*, the thigh thrust or femoral shear test *(middle)*, and the Patrick or FABER (flexion, abduction, and external rotation) test *(right)*. (Reprinted with permission from Ou-Yang D, York PJ, Kleck CJ, Patel VV. Diagnosis and management of sacroiliac joint dysfunction. J Bone Joint Surg 2017;99:2027–2036.)

13. **What radiographic techniques are useful for diagnosis of SIJ dysfunction?**
Imaging is rarely diagnostic of SIJ dysfunction but is often used to rule out other pathology that may be responsible for SIJ pain such as infection, inflammatory arthropathy, fracture, or neoplasm. Instead, history, physical examination, and diagnostic injections are the basis for diagnosis of SIJ dysfunction. Degenerative change can be seen on radiographs in up to 65% of asymptomatic individuals. Computed tomography (CT), magnetic resonance imaging, single-photon emission CT, and bone scintigraphy can be used to further evaluate anomalies if identified, but are not routinely used to evaluate SIJ dysfunction.

14. **When is a diagnostic intraarticular SIJ injection indicated?**
A diagnostic intraarticular SIJ injection is indicated in a patient with a history consistent with SIJ pathology, in the presence of three or more positive findings on SIJ provocative testing, and after initial conservative treatments have failed.

15. **How is an intraarticular SIJ injection performed?**
An intraarticular injection of 1–2 mL of a contrast agent and local anesthetic is most commonly performed with imaging using either fluoroscopic (Fig. 50.5) or CT (Fig. 50.6) guidance. A false-positive rate of up to 20% has been reported with uncontrolled SIJ blocks. It is suggested that at least one CT-guided injection be considered to ensure intraarticular delivery and diagnostic validity.

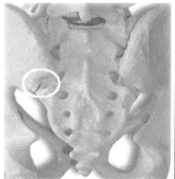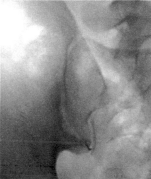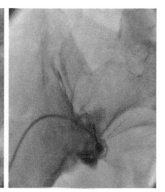

Fig. 50.5 Procedural images from a fluoroscopic-guided sacroiliac joint injection. Posterior location for needle insertion *(left)*. Needle placement in the inferior aspect of the sacroiliac joint *(middle)*. Injection of contrast medium to confirm intraarticular placement *(right)*. (From Le Heuc JC, Tsoupras A, Leglise A et al. The sacro-iliac joint: A potentially painful enigma. Update on the diagnosis and treatment of pain from micro-trauma. Ortho trauma: Surg and research. 2019;105:S31-S42, Fig. 11, p. S38.)

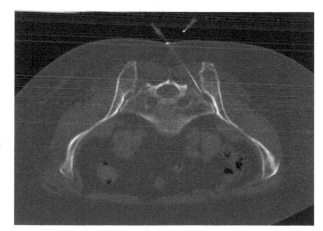

Fig. 50.6 Procedural images from a computed tomography–guided sacroiliac joint injection. Shown is the path of two spinal needles placed at different levels toward the right and left sacroiliac joints. (From D'Orazio F, Gregori LM, Gallucci M. Spinal epidural and sacroiliac joints injections—when and how to perform. Eur J Rad 2015;84:777–782, Fig. 6, p. 781.)

16. What is considered a positive response (in terms of percent-reported pain improvement) following a diagnostic intraarticular injection in the SIJ?

There is controversy regarding what threshold for improvement following an injection should be considered a positive response. Many practitioners suggest that >75% improvement should be used as a cutoff. Others report that the degree of improvement following an SIJ injection does not correlate with the degree of improvement following fusion, and a cutoff of >75% would exclude some patients that would benefit from fusion and therefore suggest using a cutoff of >50%.

NONSURGICAL TREATMENTS

17. What are some commonly utilized noninvasive treatments of the SIJ?
- Physical therapy for strengthening of SIJ muscle stabilizers
- Ultrasound, iontophoresis treatment, and stretching
- Manual manipulation performed by physical therapists and/or chiropractors
- Antiinflammatory medication as SIJ pain may have a significant inflammatory component
- Pelvic belts or supports

18. Describe the role of manual manipulation for sacroiliac dysfunction.

Manual manipulation provides a low-risk option for nonsurgical treatment of SIJ pain. However, literature provides only limited guidance regarding this treatment due to variable diagnostic criteria for SIJ dysfunction in published studies, unclear indications for intervention, and limited follow-up duration. A recent systematic review reported positive outcomes regarding decreased pain scores with the following physiotherapy modalities: manipulation along with guided isotonic exercises directed toward increasing pelvic stability, manipulation alone, and kinesiotaping (KT).

19. What interventional pain management techniques are utilized for treatment of SIJ pain?
- Intraarticular injections
- Extraarticular injections
- Prolotherapy
- Radiofrequency ablation (RFA)

20. In addition to the use of intraarticular injections for diagnostic purposes, can intraarticular injections of corticosteroid be used to provide a therapeutic effect in SIJ dysfunction?

Evidence supporting intraarticular SIJ injections for definitive treatment is limited. Patients with three out of five positive provocative maneuvers will likely have some benefit following intraarticular SIJ injections. Approximately 43%–67% of patients can expect 50% pain improvement that lasts between 4 and 6 weeks.

21. Describe prolotherapy and explain the theory behind its use for treatment of sacroiliac dysfunction.

Prolotherapy is a procedural intervention that involves injection of irritant solution into soft tissue structures to stimulate inflammation and subsequent scarring. Patients with presumed instability based on physical examination (i.e., glide test, posterior pelvic pain provocation test, active straight leg test, external manual compression test, Gillet test) would be expected to benefit. When compared with intraarticular injections, prolotherapy has been reported to provide more sustained relief, but requires significantly more injections than with corticosteroids. (3)

22. What is radiofrequency ablation and what is its role for treatment of SIJ dysfunction?

Radiofrequency ablation (RFA) is a percutaneous procedural intervention for treatment of SIJ dysfunction that is performed under fluoroscopic-guidance and places radiofrequency probes adjacent to the dorsal rami of L4–S4 to denervate the sensory nerve branches (Fig. 50.7). As RFA is directed toward the posterior nerve supply, it does not directly treat pain that originates from the ventral aspect of the SIJ. Conventional RFA utilizes a single probe and provides a circumferential treatment effect. Bipolar RFA allows for more focal tissue ablation in which only the tissue between the two probes is affected. Cooled RFA probes allow for water cooling of the probe to decrease the temperature of the probe during the procedure (60 degrees Celsius compared to 90 degrees with conventional probes) resulting in a larger lesion diameter, which could potentially increase success rates. As RFA affects the dorsal sensory branches to the SIJ, it has been suggested that RFA is more likely to provide benefit in patients with a positive response to dorsal, extraarticular injections targeting the L4–S1 rami in contrast to patients with pain identified with an intraarticular block.

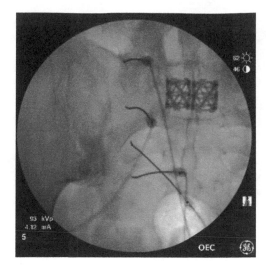

Fig. 50.7 Procedural images from a radiofrequency ablation of the sacral dorsal rami. The L5–S3 dorsal rami were targeted using fluoroscopy after which sensory and motor testing was performed prior to heating the probes to 80 degrees Celsius for 95 seconds.

23. What is the effectiveness of RFA for treatment of SIJ pain?

Based on a multicenter study, 52% of patients continued to experience 50% or greater pain relief for 6 months following RFA. Patient characteristics found to negatively affect RFA outcomes included a long duration of pain, higher preprocedure pain scores, regular opioid use, age >65 years, and pain radiating below the knee. (4) Data is not available reporting RFA outcomes for periods longer than 1 year.

SURGICAL TREATMENT

24. What open surgical approaches to the SIJ have been utilized for SIJ fusion?

Posterolateral approach: Placement of bone graft into the SIJ through a surgical window in the ilium was initially described in 1921 by Smith-Petersen. Subsequent procedural modifications included the addition of screws with or without plate fixation.

Posterior approach: Various types of posterior surgical approaches to the SIJ were described early in the 20th century. Some utilized a direct midline incision with elevation of the paraspinal musculature, others utilized dual incisions directly over the SIJs to denude cartilage. Stabilization techniques included spanning one or both SIJs with dorsal plates, other types of sacral-spanning implants or allografts, as well as the use of screws or screw-rod systems.

Open anterior approach: This approach was used to provide surgical access for bone graft harvest from the ilium and anterior access to the SIJ for denudation of the cartilage, bone grafting, and plate fixation.

Open transiliac approach: This approach utilizes a midline posterior approach with paraspinal elevation followed by osteotomy of the posterior ilium to access the SIJ for fusion and has been described in combination with the use of pedicle screws and a rod for stabilization.

25. What are some complications reported in association with open SIJ fusion?

The most common complications reported include implant-related pain, implant revisions and removals, deep wound infections, pseudarthrosis, and nerve root injury or nerve irritation. Other complications include graft site issues, intraoperative iliac crest fracture, and approach-related complications.

26. What minimally invasive surgical techniques are available for SIJ fusion?

The development of minimally invasive surgical (MIS) SIJ fusion began initially in 1998 with the first endoscopically-assisted anterior SIJ fusion. (5) In 2004 Giannakis et al. (6) described the next advancement in which autologous iliac bone plugs were impacted across drill holes from lateral to medial across the SIJ via small lateral incisions.

Current MIS SIJ fusion techniques typically use biplanar fluoroscopy or three-dimensional image-guided navigation to place two to three implants into or across the SIJ. Some implants aim to promote fusion around the implant itself, while others aim to provide adequate stability combined with some form of joint decortication to promote fusion across the joint. Current MIS SIJ fusion techniques include:

A. Placement of implants from lateral to medial across SIJ via small lateral incisions (Fig. 50.8). Examples include:
  - Triangular porous-coated implants (e.g., iFuse Implant System; SI-BONE, Inc., Santa Clara, CA, USA)
  - Standard, partially-threaded screws (e.g., SImmetry; RTI Surgical Holdings, Inc., Alachua, FL, USA)

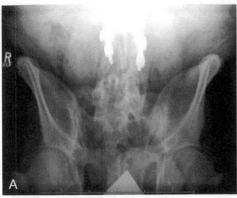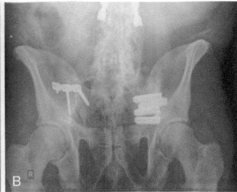

Fig. 50.8 Open and minimally invasive sacroiliac joint fusion. (A) Preoperative radiograph of a patient with bilateral sacroiliac pain following spinal fusion. Note the transitional lumbosacral vertebra. (B) Patient underwent a right-sided open anterior ilioinguinal approach fusion and plating. During a different operative session the patient underwent a minimally invasive left-sided sacroiliac fusion with triangular titanium implants. (From Polly DW. The sacroiliac joint. Neurosurg Clin N Am 2017;28:301–312, Fig. 9, p. 305.)

- Hollow cages or fenestrated screws (e.g., TriCor; Zimmer Biomet Spine, Warsaw, IN, USA) packed with bone graft and/or biologics
- Machined allograft implants (e.g., SIFlx; NuTech Spine, Inc., Birmingham, AL, USA)
- Hydroxyapatite-coated compression screws (e.g., SI-LOK; Globus Medical) Audubon, PA, USA
B. Placement of implants directly into the SIJ or using an oblique approach from posterior to anterior across the SIJ. Examples include:
  - Cylindrical threaded fusion devices (e.g., Rialto SI Fusion System; Medtronic) Sofamor Danek, Memphis, TN, USA

27. List some of the benefits of MIS SIJ fusion compared with open SIJ fusion techniques.
- Higher proportion of patients reaching a minimal clinically important difference (MCID) in functional scales
- Decreased surgical time
- Decreased blood loss
- Decreased hospitalization time
- Enhanced recovery
- Greater decrease in pain

28. What are some of the complications reported in association with MIS SIJ fusion?
Reported complications include trochanteric bursitis, hematoma, deep infection, implant malposition requiring revision, neural or vascular injury, and pseudarthrosis.

29. How do the results of MIS SIJ fusion compare to nonsurgical treatment outcomes?
Most data exists for triangular porous-coated implants (iFuse Implant System; SI-BONE) inserted from a lateral transarticular approach. Results show superior pain, disability, and quality of life improvement after surgery compared with nonsurgical treatment based on two prospective randomized controlled trials, large prospective multicenter studies, long-term comparative cohorts, case series, prospective and retrospective single-center case series, and systematic reviews.

KEY POINTS

1. The sacroiliac joint is a common cause of chronic axial low back pain.
2. Diagnosis of sacroiliac joint pain relies on patient history, specific physical examination findings, and diagnostic injections, as imaging tests are unreliable for identification of a symptomatic sacroiliac joint.
3. Various nonsurgical treatments may be beneficial for treatment of sacroiliac joint pain including physical therapy, manual manipulation, periarticular and intraarticular injections, and radiofrequency denervation.
4. Minimally invasive sacroiliac joint arthrodesis has been shown to improve pain and function in patients with sacroiliac pain confirmed by physical examination and image-guided diagnostic intraarticular sacroiliac joint blocks.

Websites
1. Sacroiliac joint anatomy: https://www.ncbi.nlm.nih.gov/pmc/articles/PMC3512279/
2. Sacroiliac joint pain: https://www.spine.org/KnowYourBack/Conditions/Low-Back-Pain/SI-Joint-Pain

REFERENCES

1. Sembrano JN, Polly DW. How often is low back pain not coming from the back? *Spine* 2009;34:27–32.
2. Cher D, Polly D, Berven S. Sacroiliac joint pain: Burden of disease. *Med Devices (Auckl)* 2014;7:73–81.
3. Kim WM, Lee HG, Jeong CW, et al. A randomized controlled trial of intra-articular prolotherapy versus steroid injection for sacroiliac joint pain. *J Altern Complement Med* 2010;16:1285–1290.
4. Cohen SP, Strassels SA, Kurihara C, et al. Outcome predictors for sacroiliac joint (lateral branch) radiofrequency denervation. *Reg Anesth Pain Med* 2009;34:206–214.
5. Güner G, Gürer S, Elmali N, et al. Anterior sacroiliac fusion: A new video-assisted endoscopic technique. *Surg Laparosc Endosc* 1998;8:233–236.
6. Giannikas KA, Khan AM, Karski MT, et al. Sacroiliac joint fusion for chronic pain: A simple technique avoiding the use of metalwork. *Eur Spine J* 2004;13:253–256.

BIBLIOGRAPHY

1. Al-Subahi M, Alayat M, Alshehri MA, et al. The effectiveness of physiotherapy interventions for sacroiliac joint dysfunction: A systematic review. *J Phys Ther Sci* 2017;29:1689–1694.
2. Buchowski JM, Kebaish KM, Sinkov V, et al. Functional and radiographic outcome of sacroiliac arthrodesis for the disorders of the sacroiliac joint. *Spine J* 2005;5:520–528.
3. Cher D, Polly D, Berven S. Sacroiliac joint pain: Burden of disease. *Med Devices (Auckl)* 2014;7:73–81.
4. Cohen SP, Strassels SA, Kurihara C, et al. Outcome predictors for sacroiliac joint (lateral branch) radiofrequency denervation. *Reg Anesth Pain Med* 2009;34:206–214.
5. Dengler J, Duhon B, Whang P, et al. Predictors of outcome in conservative and minimally invasive surgical management of pain originating from the sacroiliac joint: A pooled analysis. *Spine* 2017;42:1664–1673.
6. Giannikas KA, Khan AM, Karski MT, et al. Sacroiliac joint fusion for chronic pain: A simple technique avoiding the use of metalwork. *Eur Spine J* 2004;13:253–256.
7. Güner G, Gürer S, Elmali N, et al. Anterior sacroiliac fusion: A new video-assisted endoscopic technique. *Surg Laparosc Endosc* 1998;8:233–236.
8. Kim WM, Lee HG, Jeong CW, et al. A randomized controlled trial of intra-articular prolotherapy versus steroid injection for sacroiliac joint pain. *J Altern Complement Med* 2010;16:1285–1290.
9. Ou-Yang D, York PJ, Kleck CJ, et al. Current concepts review: Diagnosis and management of sacroiliac joint disease. *J Bone Joint Surg Am* 2017;99:2027–2036.
10. Sembrano JN, Polly DW. How often is low back pain not coming from the back? *Spine* 2009;34:27–32.
11. Zaidi HA, Montoure AJ, Dickman CA. Surgical and clinical efficacy of sacroiliac joint fusion: A systematic review of the literature. *J Neurosurg Spine* 2015;23:59–66.

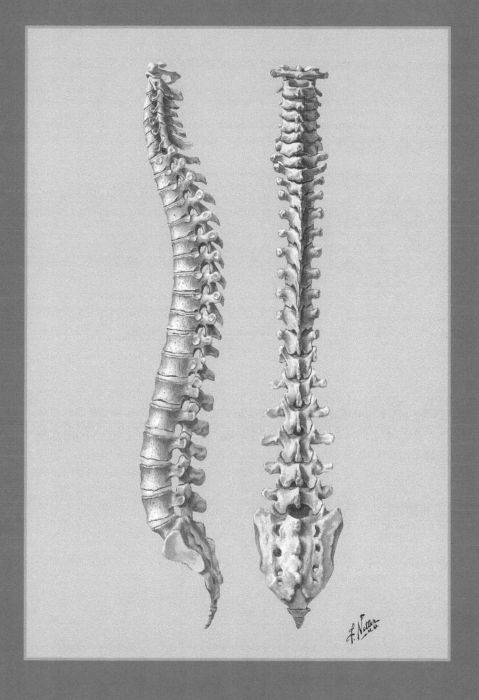

CHAPTER 51

ADULT IDIOPATHIC AND DEGENERATIVE SCOLIOSIS

Floreana N. Kebaish, MD and Khaled M. Kebaish, MD, FRCSC

1. Define adult scoliosis and describe the prevalence and incidence of this condition.

Adult scoliosis is a spinal deformity characterized by a Cobb angle in excess of 10° in the coronal plane that is present in a skeletally mature patient. Recent estimates regarding the prevalence of scoliosis in adults range from 2.5% to 25% of the population, and increasing age is associated with higher prevalence rates. Kebaish et al (1) reported a prevalence of 9% in adults aged 40 years and older, and a prevalence as high as 68% in a population of adults aged 60 years and older. According to 2010 US Census data, the incidence of adult scoliosis is 5.9 million adults, based on a conservative prevalence rate of 2.5%, with 1.6 million adults receiving treatment either on an inpatient or outpatient basis.

2. What are the major types of scoliosis identified in adults?

Three types of scoliosis in adults are identified according to the Aebi classification system:

- **Type 1: Primary degenerative or de novo scoliosis** develops after age 40 in patients with a previously straight spine, as the result of multilevel asymmetric disc and facet joint degeneration. It is the most common type of adult scoliosis and involves the thoracolumbar and lumbar spinal regions.
- **Type 2: Progressive idiopathic scoliosis** consists mainly of adult patients who developed idiopathic scoliosis during adolescence, which was unrecognized or left untreated. Coronal plane curvatures may involve the thoracic, thoracolumbar, or lumbar spinal regions, and may be associated with spinal degenerative changes.
- **Type 3: Secondary adult scoliosis** consists of two subtypes:
  - **Type 3A** deformities result from conditions within the spine such as an adjacent idiopathic, neuromuscular, or congenital curve; a lumbosacral anomaly; or from conditions outside the spine such as pelvic obliquity, leg length inequality, or hip pathology.
  - **Type 3B** deformities develop as a consequence of metabolic bone disease or osteoporotic fractures.

3. Compare and contrast de novo adult scoliosis and idiopathic scoliosis in adulthood.

See Table 51.1.

Table 51.1 Factors Used to Distinguish De novo Scoliosis from Adult Idiopathic Scoliosis.

FACTOR	DE NOVO SCOLIOSIS	ADULT IDIOPATHIC SCOLIOSIS
History of prior curve	No	Yes
Age	Older (6th decade)	Younger (3rd–4th decade)
Sex	Male > Female	Female > Male
Curve magnitude	Smaller (15°–50°)	Larger (35°–80°)
Curve location	L	T, TL, L
Curve length	<5 spinal levels	>5 spinal levels
Rotatory deformity	Limited to curve apex	Throughout entire curve
Neurologic dysfunction	50%–90%	7%–30%
Coronal imbalance	Less common	More common
Sagittal imbalance	More common	Less common

L, Lumbar; *T*, thoracic; *TL*, thoracolumbar.

Data from Sciubba DM. Management of degenerative scoliosis. In: Quiones-Hinojosa A, editor. Schmidek and Sweet: Operative Neurosurgical Techniques. 6th ed. Philadelphia, PA: Saunders; 2012, Table 185.1, p. 2102.)

4. **What are some factors associated with curve progression in patients with adult scoliosis?**
Patients with adult scoliosis may experience curve progression. Curve progression occurs in a high percentage of adult patients with degenerative scoliosis. Reported curve progression rates in degenerative scoliosis patients vary from 1° to 6° per year and average 3° per year. Multiple rotatory subluxations, curve magnitude >30°, and a relative lack of osteophyte formation are factors associated with curve progression. In adult idiopathic scoliosis patients, curves in excess of 50° are estimated to progress at a mean rate of slightly less than 1° per year. A relatively small percentage of curves between 30° and 50° progress, and progression of thoracic curves less than 30° is unlikely. Each patient, however, is unique, and one cannot always predict whether lumbar or thoracic curves will progress in adulthood.

5. **Outline some key components involved in the evaluation of an adult patient with scoliosis.**
   - **Detailed patient history:** Inquire when spinal deformity was first observed. Identify the main reason for seeking medical treatment (pain? neurologic symptoms? impaired function in activities of daily living? increasing deformity? cardiorespiratory symptoms?). If pain is present, describe its location, severity, duration, frequency, exacerbating and relieving factors, and whether pain is related to activity or present at rest.
   - **Medical history:** Have prior diagnostic studies or spine treatments been performed? Are there any associated or general medical problems? Are risk factors for osteoporosis present?
   - **Medications:** Record dose, route, and frequency for each medication
   - **Allergies**
   - **Review of major organ systems**
   - **Family history:** Is there a family history of spinal deformity?
   - **Social history:** Record occupation, history of use of tobacco, alcohol, or narcotics
   - **Comprehensive physical examination:**
     - *Inspection.* Assess for asymmetry of the neckline, shoulder height, rib cage, waistline, flank, pelvis, and lower extremities. Observe the patient's gait.
     - *Palpation.* Palpate the spinous processes and paraspinous region for tenderness, deviation in spinous process alignment, or a palpable step-off.
     - *Spinal range of motion.* Test spinal flexion-extension, side-bending, and rotation.
     - *Neurologic examination.* Assess sensory, motor, and reflex function of the upper and lower extremities.
     - *Spinal alignment and balance assessment in the coronal plane.* Normally the head should be centered over the sacrum and pelvis. A plumb line dropped from C7 should fall through the gluteal crease.
     - *Spinal alignment and balance assessment in the sagittal plane.* When the patient is observed from the side, assess the four physiologic sagittal curves (cervical and lumbar lordosis, thoracic and sacral kyphosis). When the patient is standing with the hips and knees fully extended, the head should be aligned over the sacrum.
     - *Extremity assessment.* Assess leg lengths. Assess joint range of motion in the upper and lower extremities.

6. **What imaging studies are necessary to comprehensively assess a patient with adult scoliosis?**
Standing full-length posteroanterior (PA) and lateral radiographs are required and should permit visualization from the occiput proximally to atleast the level of the femoral heads distally. If neurologic symptoms are present or if surgery is considered, spinal magnetic resonance imaging is obtained. Computed tomography is obtained to assist with surgical planning on a case-by-case basis. Assessment of bone mineral density (BMD) with dual-energy x-ray absorptiometry (DFXA) is performed for patients with risk factors for osteoporosis.

7. **Why is it important to visualize the femoral heads on the lateral standing spine radiograph?**
There is an interrelationship between the orientation of the distal lumbar spine, sacrum, and the pelvic unit, which influences sagittal alignment of the spine. Three pelvic parameters are measured: pelvic incidence (PI), sacral slope (SS), and pelvic tilt (PT). Pelvic incidence (PI) is a fixed anatomic parameter unique to the individual. Sacral slope (SS) and pelvic tilt (PT) are variable parameters. The relationship among the parameters determines the overall alignment of the sacropelvic unit according to the formula $PI = PT + SS$. Increased pelvic tilt is a compensatory mechanism for a positive shift in sagittal vertical axis (SVA) and should be considered when planning reconstructive spinal surgery for sagittal imbalance.

8. **Summarize the basic radiographic parameters that should be assessed in patients with adult scoliosis.**
   - Coronal plane
     - Magnitude of each curve (Cobb angle)
     - Central Sacral Line
     - C7 plumb line
     - Fractional lumbar curve (if present)
   - Sagittal plane
     - Thoracic kyphosis (TK)
     - Thoracolumbar kyphosis (TLK)

- Lumbar lordosis (LL)
- Sagittal vertical axis (SVA)
- Pelvic parameters
  - Pelvic incidence (PI)
  - Pelvic tilt (PT)
  - Sacral slope (SS)
- Curve flexibility in the coronal and sagittal planes
  - Comparison of standing and supine radiographs
  - Side-bending radiographs

(Fig. 51.1A, B)

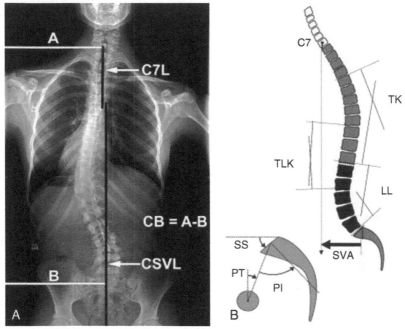

Fig. 51.1 (A) Coronal balance. A line, perpendicular to the floor, is drawn through the middle of the C7 vertebral body *(C7L)*. The central sacral vertical line *(CSVL)* is obtained by drawing a line, perpendicular to the floor, through the midline of the sacrum. Distance from the left edge of the radiograph to the C7L *(A)* is measured, as well as from the left edge of the radiograph to the CSVL *(B)*. Coronal balance *(CB)* = A − B. (B) Sagittal plane radiographic parameters: C7 sagittal vertical axis *(SVA)*; thoracic kyphosis *(TK)*, T5–T12; thoracolumbar kyphosis *(TLK)*, T10–L2; lumbar lordosis *(LL)*, T12–S1. Pelvic incidence *(PI)*, pelvic tilt *(PT)*, and sacral slope *(SS)*. (A: From Fenton DS. Lumbar scoliosis. In: Czervionke LF, Fenton DS, editors. Imaging Painful Spinal Disorders. Philadelphia, PA: Saunders; 2011, p. 505, Fig. 66.5. From Wantanabe K, Hirano T, Katsumi K, et al. Characteristics of spinopelvic alignment in Parkinson's disease: Comparison with adult spinal deformity. J Ortho Sci 2017;22:16–21, Fig. 1B, p. 18.)

9. **Is coronal or sagittal plane spinal alignment most closely correlated with functional status in patients with adult scoliosis?**
Spinal deformity in the coronal plane has not been strongly correlated with patient-reported pain or disability. In contrast, sagittal plane parameters have been highly correlated with adverse health status outcomes. Patients with adult scoliosis involving the lumbar spine generally have coexistent disc degeneration over multiple levels. This results in loss of anterior disc space height, segmental kyphosis, and positive sagittal malalignment. To maximize health-related quality of life following reconstructive surgery for adult scoliosis, ideal sagittal alignment goals have been identified as: sagittal vertical axis (SVA) <50 mm, pelvic tilt (PT) <20°, and pelvic incidence (PI) minus lumbar lordosis (LL) <10°.

10. **Explain the Scoliosis Research Society-Schwab Adult Spinal Deformity Classification.**
The Scoliosis Research Society-Schwab Adult Spinal Deformity Classification separates coronal curves into **four types** and assigns **three sagittal plane modifiers** that have been highly correlated with pain and disability. The **curve types** are classified based on the location of the major coronal curve (>30°): **thoracic** (curve apex at T9 or above), **thoraco-lumbar or lumbar** (curve apex at T10 or below), **double curves**, or **type N** (no curve >30°) (Table 51.2).

Table 51.2 Scoliosis Research Society-Schwab Adult Spinal Deformity Classification.

Curve Type	
T	Thoracic major curve >30°, lumbar curve <30°
TL/L	Thoracolumbar or lumbar major curve >30°, thoracic curve <30°
D	Double major curves each >30°
N	No coronal curve >30°
Sagittal Modifiers	
1. Pelvic Incidence − Lumbar Lordosis	
Grade 0	Within 10°
Grade +	Moderate 10°–20°
Grade ++	Marked >20°
2. Global Alignment	
Grade 0	SVA <4 cm
Grade +	SVA 4–9.5 cm
Grade ++	SVA >9.5 cm
3. Pelvic Tilt	
Grade 0	PT <20°
Grade +	PT 20°–30°
Grade ++	PT >30°

D, Double; *L*, lumbar; *N*, no curve; *PT*, pelvic tilt; *SVA*, sagittal vertical axis; *T*, thoracic; *TL*, thoracolumbar.
Data from Schwab F, Ungar B, Blondel B, et al. Scoliosis Research Society—Schwab Adult Spinal Deformity Classification: A validation study. Spine 2012;37:1077–1082.

11. **What is a fractional lumbar curve and why is it an important consideration when planning surgical treatment of adult scoliosis?**
    A compensatory curve at the level of the lumbosacral junction below a major lumbar curve is called a fractional lumbar curve. It is characteristically located between L4 and S1. Important points to consider regarding surgical treatment of adult scoliosis patients with a fractional curve include:
    • The concave side of a fractional curve is the most common site of foraminal stenosis and is the most common cause of radicular pain in this population.
    • Ending a spinal instrumentation construct in a patient with adult scoliosis above a fractional curve is associated with a high likelihood of development of adjacent segment breakdown requiring extension of the instrumentation and fusion to the sacropelvis.
    • Inadequate correction of a rigid fractional curve at the time of surgery will lead to iatrogenic coronal malalignment.

12. **What is the role of nonoperative treatment for patients with adult scoliosis?**
    Nonoperative treatment is appropriate for patients without disabling spine-related symptoms. Physical therapy, activity modification, traction, aquatic therapy, and oral medications (e.g., antiinflammatory medication, muscle relaxants, pregabalin, or gabapentin) may be considered. Epidural injections are occasionally considered for treatment of patients with radiculopathy. Spinal orthoses may provide temporary relief of back pain, but long-term use has been associated with spinal deconditioning. However, nonoperative treatment is unlikely to provide significant long-term improvement in pain and function. Patients who are dissatisfied with their current spine condition should be counseled regarding surgical options.

13. **What are the indications for surgical treatment in patients with adult scoliosis?**
    When the benefits are expected to outweigh the risks in an individual patient with adult scoliosis, given his/her age, function, and health status, surgery is indicated for treatment of:
    • Axial or radicular pain unresponsive to nonsurgical treatment
    • Progressive deformity that is unacceptable to the patient
    • Major coronal and/or sagittal malalignment
    • Neurologic deficit
    • Neurogenic claudication

14. What are the surgical treatment options for patients with degenerative scoliosis?

A range of surgical options exist for treatment of patients with adult scoliosis and have been grouped into six levels by Silva and Lenke (2):

I. Decompression

II. Decompression and limited posterior instrumented fusion of only the decompressed levels

III. Decompression and instrumented posterior fusion of the entire lumbar curve

IV. Decompression with instrumented anterior and posterior lumber fusion

V. Decompression, anterior/posterior instrumented fusion which includes thoracic and lumbar levels

VI. Inclusion of osteotomies

15. When is a decompression without fusion an option for treatment of adult degenerative scoliosis?

A single-level decompression procedure without fusion (level I) is appropriate for patients with radicular pain or neurogenic claudication and small curves (<30°) with stabilizing osteophytes. Patients treated with decompression alone should not have major back pain, spinal instability, lateral subluxation (<2 mm), progressive deformity, or major coronal or sagittal malalignment. It is critical to preserve stability following decompression by limiting facet joint resection to less than 50% at the operative level and avoid excessive resection of the pars interarticularis. Failure of this approach may occur due to deformity progression or postsurgical instability leading to recurrent neural compression and the need for posterior spinal fusion and instrumentation.

16. When is a decompression and instrumented spinal fusion limited to the decompressed spinal levels an option for treatment of adult degenerative scoliosis?

Spinal decompression and instrumented spinal fusion limited to the decompressed spinal level(s) (level II) is a treatment option for patients with mild degenerative curves (<30°) and radicular pain or neurogenic claudication in the absence of severe back pain. Patients who require extensive decompression, lack stabilizing osteophytes, or have subluxations >2 mm are candidates for this procedure. Patients treated with this approach should have well-preserved regional and global spinal alignment.

17. When is decompression and posterior instrumented fusion of the entire lumbar curve indicated for treatment of patients with degenerative scoliosis? When is the addition of an anterior column fusion considered?

Decompression and posterior instrumented fusion of the entire lumbar curve (level III) is indicated for treatment of degenerative scoliosis patients with acceptable coronal and sagittal balance who present with back pain and spinal stenosis. Such patients generally present with curves >30°, subluxations >2 mm, and often lack stabilizing osteophytes. Addition of an anterior fusion (level IV) is considered for patients with mild sagittal imbalance, risk factors for pseudarthrosis, or severe foraminal stenosis. Anterior column fusion may be performed through an anterior or lateral interbody approach, or more commonly through a posterior transforaminal approach.

18. When should lumbar instrumentation and fusion be extended into the thoracic spine in patients with degenerative scoliosis? When are osteotomies necessary?

In patients with degenerative scoliosis, lumbar spinal instrumentation and fusion should be extended into the thoracic spine (level V) in patients with thoracic hyperkyphosis, sagittal imbalance, or coronal imbalance. Osteotomies (level VI) are indicated for treatment of patients with rigid spinal deformities and marked global spinal imbalance.

19. What is the most common curve pattern in patients with lumbar degenerative scoliosis? What nerve root is most commonly affected when spinal stenosis is present?

A double lumbar curve is the most common pattern in which one curve, usually left-sided, is from T12 to L3, and the second curve is right-sided, from L3 to the sacrum. At L3–L4, there is usually a rotatory subluxation with lateral listhesis, which forms the transitional segment between the two curves. The distal curve from L3 to S1 is referred to as the fractional curve. When foraminal stenosis develops in the lower lumbar spine, the L5 nerve root, which exits between the L5 and S1 pedicles, is most commonly involved. The most common location for nerve root compression is in the concavity of the fractional curve. As the fractional curve is usually convex to the right and the concavity of the fractional curve is on the left, the left L5 nerve root is most commonly affected (Fig. 51.2A–D).

20. What are the surgical treatment options for patients with idiopathic scoliosis in adulthood?

Adult idiopathic scoliosis patients who have not undergone prior surgical treatment present differently based on age. Young adults (age 30–40 years) present due to trunk asymmetry, mild mechanical back pain, or progressive deformity. Severe back or radicular pain in the absence of advanced lumbar degenerative changes should prompt a workup to rule out unsuspected pathology. When spinal instrumentation and fusion are performed in these younger patients, level selection is similar to surgical treatment of adolescent idiopathic patients. In older adults (age 50–70), superimposed lumbar degenerative changes and a rigid fractional curve are often present and are accompanied by low back and radicular pain symptoms, and surgical treatment requires instrumentation and fusion of these additional spinal levels.

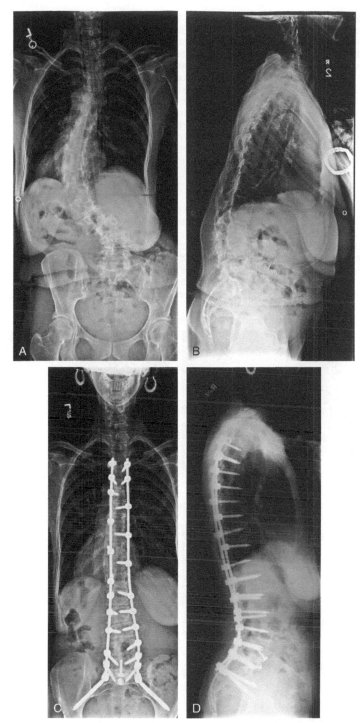

Fig. 51.2 73-year-old female with degenerative (de novo) scoliosis with significant coronal (A) and sagittal (B) malalignment. Treatment consisted of posterior segmental instrumentation and fusion and use of multiple Ponte osteotomies to achieve coronal correction. Postoperative radiographs show coronal (C) and sagittal (D) deformity correction with restoration of physiologic sagittal and coronal alignment. Anterior fusion at L5–S1 was also performed to provide anterior structural support and enhance fusion.

In general, patients with flexible idiopathic curves of less than 70° without significant kyphosis or decompensation are treated with posterior instrumentation and fusion alone. Spinal osteotomies are added for curves >70°, rigid curves, and curves associated with sagittal and/or coronal imbalance. The goal of surgery is a balanced spine with the head centered over the pelvis in the sagittal and coronal planes rather than maximal correction of spinal deformity. Structural curves are instrumented and fused, usually from the cephalad stable and neutral vertebra to the distal stable and neutral vertebra. In the presence of superimposed degenerative changes in the lower lumbar spine or the presence of a rigid fractional curve, fusion should not end at L4, and extension of the fusion to L5, or more commonly S1 is necessary. Although it is uncommon to see a substantial amount of central spinal stenosis in patients who have preexisting idiopathic scoliosis with superimposed degenerative changes, it is common to see either lateral recess stenosis or foraminal stenosis on the concavity of the fractional curve. At L3–L4, stenosis often accompanies a rotatory subluxation. At L4–L5, lateral recess stenosis is most common, and at L5–S1, foraminal stenosis is most common. The stenosis at L4–L5 and L5–S1 is usually on the concavity of the fractional curve (Fig. 51.3A–D).

21. **What are some general principles used to guide selection of proximal and distal fusion levels in patients with adult scoliosis?**
  - Avoid ending a fusion at the apex of a sagittal or coronal curve.
  - Avoid ending a fusion adjacent to a severely degenerated or unstable motion segment.
  - Avoid ending a fusion at a spinal level with rotatory subluxation, lateral listhesis, retrolisthesis, or anterolisthesis.
  - Avoid ending a fusion at a kyphotic spinal segment.
  - The upper and lower instrumented vertebra should be stable (bisected by a vertically directed central sacral line), neutral (without axial rotation), and horizontal.
  - When an instrumented fusion extends from the lower thoracic region to the lumbosacral junction, T10 is considered a more stable proximal end vertebra compared with T11 or T12 as the T10 segment is

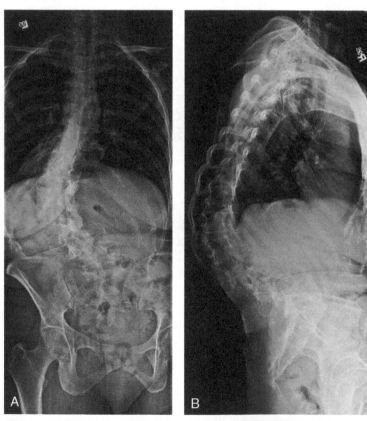

Fig. 51.3 Posteroanterior (A) and lateral (B) radiographs of a 68-year-old female with adult idiopathic scoliosis, severe spinal canal stenosis related to her deformity, and superimposed degenerative changes. Note the rigid deformity due to bony ankylosis and a fractional lumbosacral curve causing coronal malalignment. Patient underwent posterior instrumentation and fusion from T3 to pelvis.

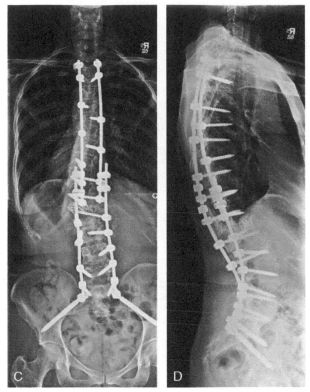

Fig. 51.3, cont'd Posteroanterior (C) and lateral (D) radiographs show the operative correction that was achieved through a combination of multiple Ponte osteotomies in lumbar spine and a three-column osteotomy at L1.

supported by true ribs, while T11 and T12 are associated with floating ribs which lack costosternal attachment.
- Long posterior instrumented fusions performed to correct sagittal imbalance that extends distally from the thoracic region should extend to the sacrum rather than stopping at L5 due to the high risk of failure associated with constructs that end at L5 because of subsequent L5–S1 degeneration.
- When selecting the upper instrumented vertebra in a long posterior fusion from the thoracic spine to the sacrum, extending fixation to the upper thoracic region reduces the incidence of revision surgery related to proximal junctional kyphosis but increases operative time and blood loss.

22. What are the most important surgical principles that should be followed to achieve fusion success when performing a long instrumented spinal fusion that extends from the thoracic region to the sacrum?

Principles to optimize success when performing long instrumented posterior spinal fusions extending from the thoracic region to the sacrum include:
- Use segmental pedicle fixation at all levels of the lumbar spine
- Use four-point fixation of the sacrum and pelvis
- Use structural interbody support at L5–S1 (also L4–L5 if a wide laminectomy is performed)
- Preserve the posterior osseous elements by avoiding wide laminectomies whenever feasible to provide additional surface area for posterior fusion
- Achieve neutral or slightly negative sagittal balance
- Identify and treat patients with osteoporosis whenever possible prior to surgery

23. What are some options used to provide structural support to the interbody space at the lower end of a long instrumented spinal fusion extending from the thoracic region to the sacrum?
1. Fresh frozen femoral rings packed with nonstructural autogenous bone or allograft
2. Titanium mesh or three-dimensional–printed titanium cages packed with graft material
3. Polyetheretherketone (PEEK) or carbon fiber cages packed with bone graft material

Autogenous tricortical iliac bone graft is rarely used to provide lumbar structural support due its suboptimal mechanical properties, donor site morbidity, and limited quantity. Alternative graft materials are used in combination with interbody structural allografts or cages and include recombinant human bone morphogenetic protein-2 (rhBMP-2), nonstructural allograft, nonstructural autogenous iliac crest bone graft, or local autogenous bone graft.

24. **What is the current role of extensile anterior surgical approaches in the treatment of adult scoliosis?**
Extensile anterior surgical approaches are less commonly performed today for treatment of adult scoliosis due to recognition of the morbidity associated with anterior surgical approaches and recent data which suggests that similar correction and fusion rates are achievable with interbody fusions performed through a posterior-only approach. A *mini-open* anterior retroperitoneal approach is, however, still commonly performed to achieve anterior column structural interbody grafting at the caudal segments of a long fusion extending to the sacrum. Minimally invasive surgical approaches have been introduced and provide an alternative approach for anterior release and interbody structural support. Options include minimally invasive lateral interbody fusion, oblique lumbar interbody fusion (OLIF), as well as anterior column realignment (ACR) procedures. However, controversy exists as to whether these minimally invasive procedures improve fusion rates or patient outcomes.

25. **What types of spinal osteotomies play a role in treatment of adult scoliosis?**
1. Ponte osteotomy
2. Pedicle subtraction osteotomy
3. Vertebral column resection

26. **What is a Ponte osteotomy?**
The **Ponte osteotomy**, originally described for treatment of Scheuermann kyphosis, involves removal of the inferior part of the spinous process, lamina, facet joints, and ligamentum flavum. The superior and inferior facets are resected in their entirety. Correction is achieved by compression of the posterior elements and pivots around the center of the disc space without disruption of the anterior longitudinal ligament. Between 4° and 8° of correction is achieved per level of osteotomy. Ponte osteotomies are frequently performed over multiple levels. In contrast, the **Smith-Petersen osteotomy** was originally described for use in ankylosing spondylitis and involved a narrow resection of facet joints without laminar resection and obtained correction by wide opening of the anterior disc space. Despite the differences between the Ponte osteotomies and Smith-Petersen osteotomies, these terms are sometimes used interchangeably (Fig. 51.4A,B).

27. **What is a pedicle subtraction osteotomy?**
A pedicle subtraction osteotomy (PSO) includes surgical resection of the posterior elements, pedicles, and a portion of the vertebral body. Deformity correction is achieved by closure of the osteotomy by posterior compression. A PSO hinges on the anterior column and closes the middle and posterior columns and provides 25°–35° of correction at the osteotomy level (Fig. 51.5).

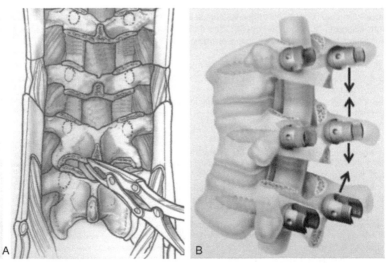

Fig. 51.4 (A) Ponte osteotomy. (B) Ponte osteotomy from pedicle to pedicle. (From Ponte A, Orlando G, Siccardi GL. The true Ponte osteotomy: By the one who developed it. Spine Deform 2018;6:2–11, Fig. 4, p. 5.)

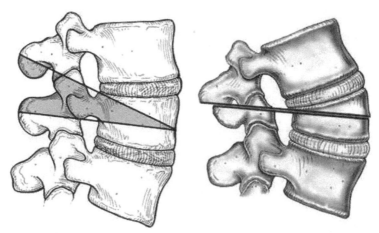

Fig. 51.5 Three-column pedicle subtraction osteotomy. (From Kebaish KM. Spinal sagittal plane deformities: Etiology, Evaluation, and management. Semin Spine Surg 2009;21:41–48, Fig. 6, p. 44.)

28. What is a vertebral column resection and how does this procedure differ from a pedicle subtraction osteotomy?

A vertebral column resection (VCR) is an osteotomy that involves removal of the entire vertebral body and adjacent intervertebral discs. It is most commonly performed through a single posterior approach, but may be performed through separate anterior and posterior surgical approaches. Both PSO and VCR can be performed in the thoracic and lumbar spine; however, most commonly for fixed deformity, a PSO is performed in the lumbar spine and a VCR is carried out in the thoracic spine. The most distinguishing feature that differentiates a PSO from VCR is correction mechanics. In a PSO, a fixed angle of closure is determined by the size of the wedge resection. In a VCR, the spine is dissociated in two separate segments and the arc of correction falls anterior to the spinal column with no fixed closure angle. For this reason, VCR is often best suited for sharp, angular deformities that can be significantly corrected, provided that the spinal cord can tolerate the configurational change the osteotomy affords (Fig. 51.6). A VCR is able to provide a greater degree of correction than either multiple Ponte osteotomies or a PSO, and enables treatment of severe scoliosis and multiplanar rigid spinal deformities through an all-posterior surgical approach.

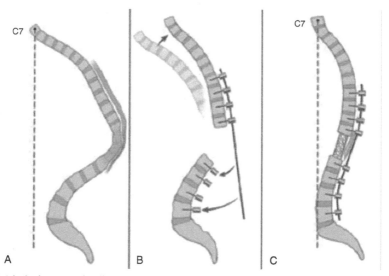

Fig. 51.6 Vertebral column resection. (A) Thoracolumbar kyphotic deformity with sagittal imbalance as identified by the location of the C7 plumb line. (B) Vertebral column resection is performed and correction of the kyphotic deformity is initiated. (C) A cage is placed in the anterior column defect and correction of the kyphotic deformity is completed as depicted by the location of the C7 plumb line. (From Daubs MD. Osteotomies for adult deformity: Surgical techniques. Oper Tech Orthop 2011;21:213–224, Fig. 14, p. 223.)

29. What are some common complications encountered in relation to surgical treatment of adult scoliosis patients?
    1. Medical complications
    2. Pseudarthrosis and instrumentation failure
    3. Surgical site infection (deep and superficial)
    4. Neurologic deficit
    5. Iatrogenic sagittal and/or coronal malalignment
    6. Adjacent level degeneration, proximal junctional kyphosis, and proximal junction failure

KEY POINTS

1. The two most common types of scoliosis in adults are degenerative scoliosis and idiopathic scoliosis.
2. Degenerative scoliosis, also called de novo scoliosis, develops after age 40 in patients with previously straight spines as a result of multilevel asymmetric disc and facet joint degeneration.
3. Scoliosis presenting in adulthood may represent *idiopathic scoliosis*, which initially developed in adolescence and was unrecognized or left untreated.
4. Nonoperative treatment is appropriate for patients without disabling spine-related symptoms but is unlikely to provide significant long-term improvement in pain and function.
5. Surgical indications for adult scoliosis include progressive deformity, pain, and symptomatic neural compression.
6. The goals of surgical treatment in adult scoliosis patients include achievement of optimal sagittal and coronal plane balance, solid and durable arthrodesis, decompression of symptomatic neural compression, and improvement in pain and function.
7. Successful surgical treatment of adult scoliosis involves appropriate patient selection, sound preoperative surgical planning, and use of a range of techniques including segmental pedicular fixation, pelvic fixation, osteotomies, and anterior column structural support.

Websites
1. Scoliosis Research Society: https://www.srs.org/patients-and-families/conditions-and-treatments/adults
2. United States Bone and Joint Initiative: The Burden of Musculoskeletal Diseases in the United States (BMUS), Fourth Edition, forthcoming. Rosemont, IL: https://www.boneandjointburden.org/2014-report/iiid21/prevalence-adult-scoliosis

---

REFERENCES

1. Kebaish KM, Neubauer PR, Voros GD, et al. Scoliosis in adults aged forty years and older: Prevalence and relationship to age, race, and gender. *Spine* 2011;36:731–736.
2. Silva FE, Lenke LG. Adult degenerative scoliosis: Evaluation and management. *Neurosurg Focus* 2010;28:E1–E10.

BIBLIOGRAPHY

1. Aebi M. The adult scoliosis. *Eur Spine J* 2005;14:925–948.
2. Bridwell KH, DeWald RL, editors. The Textbook of Spinal Surgery. 3rd ed. Philadelphia, PA: Lippincott-Raven; 2011.
3. Campbell PG, Nunley PD. The challenge of the lumbosacral fractional curve in the setting of adult degenerative scoliosis. *Neurosurg Clin N Am* 2018;29:467–474.
4. Cho KJ, Kim YT, Shin SH, et al. Surgical treatment of adult degenerative scoliosis. *Asian Spine J* 2014;8:371–381.
5. Fu X, Sun XL, Harris JA, et al. Long fusion correction of degenerative adult spinal deformity and the selection of the upper or lower thoracic region as the site of proximal instrumentation: A systematic review and meta-analysis. *BMJ Open* 2016;6:e012103.
6. Glassman SD, Bridwell K, Dimar JR, et al. The impact of positive sagittal balance in adult spinal deformity. *Spine* 2005;30:2024–2029.
7. Kebaish KM, Neubauer PR, Voros GD, et al. Scoliosis in adults aged forty years and older: Prevalence and relationship to age, race, and gender. *Spine* 2011;36:731–736.
8. Kelly MP, Lurie JD, Yanik EL, et al. Operative versus nonoperative treatment for adult symptomatic lumbar scoliosis. *J Bone Joint Surg* 2019;101:338–352.
9. Silva FE, Lenke LG. Adult degenerative scoliosis: Evaluation and management. *Neurosurg Focus* 2010;28:E1–E10.
10. Weinstein SL, Ponseti IV. Curve progression in idiopathic scoliosis. *J Bone Joint Surg* 1983;65:447–455.
11. York PJ, Kim HJ. Degenerative scoliosis. *Curr Rev Musculoskelet Med* 2017;10:547–558.

CHAPTER 52

SAGITTAL PLANE DEFORMITIES IN ADULTS

Mostafa H. El Dafrawy, MD, Munish C. Gupta, MD, and Vincent J. Devlin, MD

GENERAL PRINCIPLES

1. What is the "cone of economy" concept?

   The concept of the **"cone of economy"** was introduced by Dr. Jean Dubousset and describes a cone-shaped region extending from the feet upward around the trunk. When the body's center of gravity is maintained within this region, energy expenditure is minimized. Deviation outside this cone increases the energy expenditure required to maintain an erect posture. Sagittal balance of the spine is dependent on the relationship of the four curves of the spine, as well as the position of the sacrum and pelvis, which serve as an intercalary "pelvic vertebra" between the trunk and lower extremities. A balanced spine is able to maintain the standing position and horizontal gaze with minimal muscular effort. Spinal balance is an active process that reflects the harmony between posture and motion and is imperfectly represented by static radiographs alone. In contrast, spinal alignment is a radiographic concept, evaluated on static standing radiographs, and serves as the basis for the preoperative and postoperative assessment of posture in patients with spinal deformity (Fig. 52.1).

2. Describe the normal sagittal alignment of the adult spine.

   The **sagittal alignment** of the spine may be described on a **segmental** level (i.e., alignment between adjacent vertebrae), **regional** level (i.e., cervical, thoracic, lumbar, sacral alignment), and **global** level (i.e., alignment of C7 relative to the sacrum). In the sagittal plane, the normal spine possesses four curves, which interact to balance

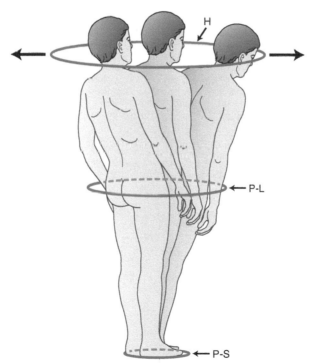

Fig. 52.1 Cone of economy. H, head; P-L, pelvic level; P-S, polygon of sustentation. (From Nelles D, Majid K. Adult scoliosis. In: Garfin SR, Eismont FJ, Bell GR, et al., editors. Rothman-Simeone The Spine. 7th ed. Philadelphia, PA: Saunders; 2018, pp. 1239–1259, Fig. 72.1, p. 1240.)

the occiput above the sacrum (Fig. 52.2). The kyphotic thoracic and sacral regions are balanced by the lordotic cervical and lumbar regions. The thoracolumbar junction is the transitional region between thoracic kyphosis and lumbar lordosis and is neutrally aligned in the sagittal plane. The **sagittal vertical axis (SVA)** is determined by dropping a plumb line from the center of the C7 vertebral body and normally passes anterior to the thoracic spine, through the center of the L1 vertebral body, posterior to the lumbar spine, and through the lumbosacral disc. A positive SVA is present when this line passes in front of the posterior superior corner of S1. A negative SVA is present when this line passes behind the posterior superior corner of S1.

3. **What are normal values for thoracic kyphosis, lumbar lordosis, and SVA in adults?**
   There is a wide range of normal values in adults. Thoracic kyphosis (T2–T12) varies between 30° and 50°. Lumbar lordosis varies between 45° and 70°. Normally, two-thirds of lumbar lordosis is located between L4 and S1 and one-third between L1 and L3. The SVA normally passes within 2–5 cm of the posterior superior corner of S1. In general, lumbar lordosis must exceed thoracic kyphosis by 20°–30° to maintain spinal balance and normal position of the sagittal vertical axis.

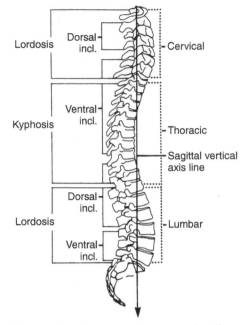

Fig. 52.2 Normal sagittal alignment of the spinal column. Note the sagittal vertical axis line and the orientation of each individual vertebrae. (From DeWald RL. Revision surgery for spinal deformity. In: Instructional Course Lectures, Vol. 41. Park Ride, IL: American Academy of Orthopaedic Surgeons; 1992.)

4. **How does sagittal alignment change with age?**
   Aging is associated with loss of anterior spinal column height secondary to degenerative disc changes, vertebral body compression, and decreased posterior muscular and ligamentous tone. These changes result in increased thoracic kyphosis and decreased lumbar lordosis. The SVA moves anterior relative to the sacrum as thoracic kyphosis increases and lumbar lordosis decreases. SVA in asymptomatic normal adolescents and young adults is negative. SVA becomes progressively positive with normal aging but this change is not always associated with symptoms. Although a general target for correction of SVA within 50 mm of the posterior superior sacrum is useful for initial surgical planning, treatment of an individual patient requires consideration of the patient's age in addition to other radiographic and clinical parameters.

5. **What are some of the causes of sagittal plane spinal deformity that require surgical treatment in the adult population?**
   Any adult spinal deformity of sufficient severity to warrant surgical intervention requires analysis of preoperative sagittal plane alignment. Spinal pathologies associated with sagittal spinal deformities in adult patients include:
   - Degenerative spinal disorders
   - Posttraumatic kyphotic deformities
   - Ankylosing spondylitis
   - Scheuermann kyphosis
   - Adult scoliosis
   - Congenital vertebral anomalies
   - Spinal column infections
   - Primary and metastatic spinal tumors
   - Osteoporotic compression fractures
   - Iatrogenic spinal disorders
     - Postlaminectomy deformity
     - Flatback syndrome
     - Sagittal malalignment following lumbar spinal fusions performed to treat degenerative spinal conditions
     - Kyphotic decompensation syndrome
     - Adjacent segment spinal pathology

6. **Why is sagittal alignment an important consideration in treatment of coronal plane spinal deformities such as adult scoliosis?**
Although the coronal plane deformity is often the most obvious radiographic finding on initial assessment of a patient with adult scoliosis, studies have not shown a correlation between the magnitude of coronal plane deformity and health-related quality of life. Disability in adults with adult scoliosis has been identified primarily as a problem involving the sagittal plane, and restoration of sagittal alignment is crucial in achieving treatment success.

7. **What are the initial steps in evaluation of an adult patient who presents with a sagittal plane spinal deformity?**
   - **Perform a detailed patient history.** Identify the main reason for seeking medical treatment. Inquire about back pain, leg pain, lower extremity weakness or numbness, symptoms suggestive of neurogenic claudication, bowel or bladder dysfunction, postural abnormalities, and limitations of activities of daily living. Review prior treatment and relevant medical and surgical history.
   - **Perform a comprehensive physical examination.** Evaluate range of motion in the cervical, thoracic, and lumbar regions. Check range of motion in the major joints of both upper and lower extremities. Assess for hip flexion contractures and pelvic obliquity. Perform a detailed neurologic examination. Assess balance in the coronal and sagittal planes with the hips and knees extended. Perform an assessment of sagittal alignment with the patient standing, sitting, and supine.
   - **Obtain and review adequate quality spinal deformity radiographs.** A systematic analysis of radiographs is required and should include quantification of the spinal deformity in the sagittal and coronal planes.

8. **What initial radiographs are required for evaluation of an adult patient who presents with sagittal plane spinal deformity?**
Posteroanterior (PA) and lateral full-length standing spine radiographs are required. Images should provide visualization from the occiput to the level of the proximal femurs and clearly visualize the femoral heads. Patients should stand with the hips and knees fully extended if possible. The elbows should be flexed and the patient's hands should rest in the supraclavicular fossa. Lateral flexion-extension radiographs, comparison of upright and supine imaging studies, as well as supine cross-table lateral hyperextension radiographs performed over a radiolucent bolster, are methods that may be used to assess whether a sagittal deformity is flexible or rigid. If coronal plane curvatures are present, supine AP radiographs and side-bending films are useful to determine curve flexibility. Although not available in all spinal centers, EOS imaging (EOS Imaging, Inc., Cambridge, MA) offers advantages compared with conventional radiography. EOS imaging provides full-body biplanar imaging from the head to the feet in the weight-bearing position with a reduced radiation dose, and allows the creation of three-dimensional images of the spine and lower extremities. Analysis of a spinal deformity should include assessment of the following parameters:
   - **Segmental alignment:** identify segmental abnormalities involving adjacent vertebrae, including spondylolisthesis, lateral listhesis, retrolisthesis, and rotatory subluxation.
   - **Regional alignment parameters:** thoracic kyphosis, thoracolumbar junction alignment, and lumbar lordosis
   - **Pelvic alignment parameters:** pelvic incidence, pelvic tilt, and sacral slope
   - **Global alignment parameters:** sagittal vertical axis (SVA), coronal plane vertical axis, spinopelvic inclination (T1 and T9 sagittal tilt), T1 pelvic angle (TPA), and global tilt angle.
   - **Curve flexibility in the sagittal and coronal planes:** comparison of standing radiographs with supine imaging studies (radiographs, computed tomography, magnetic resonance imaging), side-bending radiographs, flexion-extension or hyperextension radiographs.

9. **What are some terms used to describe kyphotic deformities observed on imaging studies?**
   - **Segmental or local kyphosis:** kyphosis that involves one or two spinal motion segments (i.e., lumbar spondylolisthesis, thoracolumbar burst fracture with kyphotic deformity)
   - **Regional kyphosis:** kyphosis that involves multiple spinal motion segments within a spinal region but overall balance of C7 with respect to the sacropelvis is maintained in the sagittal and coronal planes (i.e., Scheuermann kyphosis)
   - **Kyphosis with global sagittal plane malalignment:** a kyphotic deformity that is accompanied by an inability to balance the head and C7 over the sacropelvis and inability to maintain the body's center of gravity within the cone of economy despite use of compensatory mechanisms (i.e., flatback syndrome)
   - **Kyphosis with combined global sagittal and coronal plane malalignment:** less commonly, a kyphotic deformity may be associated with global imbalance in both the sagittal and coronal planes
   - **Flexible kyphosis:** kyphosis that corrects within the normal range with hyperextension or prone positioning
   - **Rigid kyphosis:** kyphotic deformity that resists correction with hyperextension or prone positioning
   - **Rotational kyphosis:** the vertebral bodies rotate out of the sagittal plane and a complex spinal deformity develops simultaneously affecting the sagittal, axial, and coronal planes.

10. **What is meant by spinopelvic alignment?**

An interrelationship between the orientation of the distal lumbar spine, sacrum, and the pelvic unit influences sagittal alignment of the spine (Fig. 52.3). Three pelvic parameters are measured: pelvic incidence (PI), sacral slope (SS), and pelvic tilt (PT). PI is a fixed anatomic parameter unique to the individual. SS and PT are variable parameters. The relationship among the parameters determines the overall alignment of the sacropelvic unit according to the formula **PI = PT + SS**.

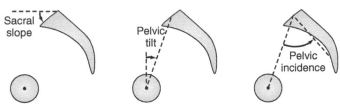

Fig. 52.3 Pelvic parameters: sacral slope (SS), pelvic tilt (PT), and pelvic incidence (PI). PI = PT + SS. (From Polly DW, Jones KE, Larson AN. Pediatric and adult scoliosis. In: Ellenbogen RG, Sekhar LN, Kitchen ND, editors. Principles of Neurological Surgery. 4th ed. Philadelphia, PA: Elsevier; 2018, Fig. 37.8, pp. 561–572.)

11. **How is PI measured and why is it important?**

PI is measured by the angle between a line drawn perpendicular to the midpoint of the sacral endplate and a line from the femoral head axis to this point. PI is a morphological parameter that is fixed and independent of position. A high PI is associated with increased sacral slope and increased lumbar lordosis. A low PI is associated with decreased sacral slope and decreased lordosis. In other words, a patient with high PI has a more vertically oriented superior sacral endplate and requires more lumbar lordosis to maintain sagittal balance compared with a patient with a low PI. Average PI in asymptomatic individuals is approximately 50°–55° but may range between 30° and 80° across individuals. Normal PI is within 10° of lumbar lordosis. Mismatch of PI and lumbar lordosis >10° has been correlated with disability.

12. **How is PT measured and why is it important?**

PT is measured by the angle between a vertical line drawn upwards from the center of the femoral head axis and a line drawn from the center of the femoral heads to the midpoint of the sacral endplate. PT is a variable parameter and is altered by pelvic retroversion. As sagittal balance increases, patients attempt to maintain sagittal alignment by rotating the pelvis posteriorly, which extends the hip joints leading to an increase in PT and a corresponding decrease in SS. Additional compensation for sagittal malalignment may be provided by flexion of the knee joints. As hip extension and knee flexion are not energy efficient compensatory mechanisms, muscular fatigue and disability result from this posture. A normal value for PT is approximately 12°, and PT beyond 20° is associated with severe disability.

13. **How is SS measured and why is it important?**

SS is measured by the angle between a line drawn along the sacral endplate and a horizontal reference line. SS is a variable parameter that determines the position of the lumbar spine. Sacral slope decreases and the sacral endplate becomes more horizontal as pelvic tilt increases according to the formula PI = PT + SS.

14. **What are the major mechanisms used by the body to compensate for sagittal plane malalignment?**

The body has its own compensatory mechanisms to adjust posture and optimize energy expenditure to maintain balance as the SVA increases. These compensatory mechanisms involve the spine, pelvis, and lower extremities.

- **Spine:** An early compensation mechanism involves hyperextension of mobile spinal segments adjacent to the spinal deformity and commonly manifest as increased cervical lordosis and decreased thoracic kyphosis.
- **Pelvis:** Compensation at the level of the pelvis may occur by pelvic retroversion, which increases pelvic tilt leading to hip hyperextension, and by posterior shift of the sacrum in the sagittal plane.
- **Lower extremities:** Compensation occurs through knee flexion and ankle dorsiflexion. Patients adopt a flexed-knee–flexed-hip posture.

15. **What are some limitations associated with the use of SVA to assess global sagittal plane alignment?**

Some limitations regarding the use of SVA to measure global sagittal plane alignment are listed here:

- The use of SVA in isolation may underestimate the true extent of sagittal plane malalignment as it does not take into account the effect of pelvic parameters and lower-extremity compensatory mechanisms on sagittal alignment.

- SVA is a linear measurement and is dependent on radiographic calibration.
- As SVA is measured in the standing position, it is not useful for the assessment of global sagittal alignment intraoperatively.

Alternative parameters for use in measurement of sagittal spinal alignment developed to address the limitations associated with use of SVA include: spinopelvic inclination (SPI), T1 pelvic angle (TPA), and global tilt.

16. What is SPI?

SPI is measured as the angle between a vertical plumb line and a second line drawn from the center of the femoral head axis to the center of either the T1 vertebral body (T1–SPI) or T9 vertebral body (T9–SPI). The T1–SPI quantifies T1 offset relative to the femoral head axis, unlike SVA, which is measured relative to the posterior sacrum. As T1–SPI is an angular measurement, it is not necessary to adjust for radiographic magnification when recording this measurement (Fig. 52.4).

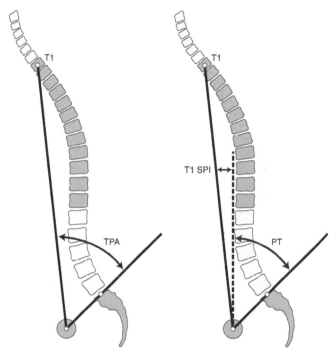

Fig. 52.4 T1 and T9 spinopelvic inclination *(SPI)*. Pelvic tilt *(PT)*. T2 pelvic angle *(TPA)*. (From Nelles D, Majid K. Adult scoliosis. In: Garfin SR, Eismont FJ, Bell GR, et al., editors. Rothman-Simeone the Spine. 7th ed. Philadelphia, PA: Saunders; 2018, pp. 1239–1259, Fig. 72.4, p. 1244.)

17. What is the T1 pelvic angle?

The **T1 pelvic angle (TPA)** is measured as the angle between a line from the femoral head axis to the center of T1 and a line from the center of the femoral head axis to the center of the superior endplate of S1 (Fig. 52.4). The TPA reflects the sum of the T1–SPI and PT. Advantages of this measurement include (1) TPA is an angular measure and does not require adjustment for radiographic magnification, (2) TPA can be measured intraoperatively with the patient in the prone position, and (3) TPA values correlate with health outcomes. A surgical target of 10° has been recommended and TPA of 20° has been identified as the threshold for severe deformity and related disability.

18. What is global tilt angle and how is it measured?

Global tilt (GT) is another recently described parameter that combines spinal alignment and pelvic compensation into a single measurement. GT is the angle formed by the intersection of a line drawn from the center of C7 to the center of the sacral endplate and a second line drawn from the center of the femoral heads to the center of the sacral endplate. GT is the sum of PT and C7 vertical tilt (angular value of SVA).

19. What is the Global Alignment and Proportion Score?

The Global Alignment and Proportion (GAP) Score is a newly validated score derived from pelvic incidence-based proportional parameters and can be used to predict mechanical complications following surgery for adult spinal deformity. Using the GAP score, optimal sagittal alignment is calculated based on four factors as they deviate from their ideal values, and these factors are related proportionally to the PI measure. The four parameters are: relative pelvic version (the measured minus the ideal sacral slope), relative lumbar lordosis (the measured minus the ideal lumbar lordosis), lordosis distribution index (the L4–S1 lordosis divided by the L1–S1 lordosis multiplied by 100), relative spinopelvic alignment (the measured minus the ideal GT), and an age factor (<60 or >60 years).

SURGICAL TREATMENT

20. Describe the principles of surgical treatment for posttraumatic kyphosis.
   Posttraumatic kyphosis most commonly arises due to injury involving one or two adjacent spinal motion segments. Posttraumatic kyphosis typically presents as a short-radius kyphotic deformity that may be either flexible or rigid. Surgical treatment of posttraumatic kyphosis is individualized based on a variety of factors, including neurologic status, deformity magnitude, whether the deformity is flexible or rigid, and the extent of injury to the anterior and posterior spinal columns. Treatment options include: (1) surgery through an entirely posterior approach consisting of posterior release with or without osteotomies and posterior instrumentation and fusion, (2) anterior reconstruction with corpectomy, anterior fusion, and anterior spinal instrumentation, or (3) combined anterior and posterior instrumentation and fusion (Fig. 52.5).

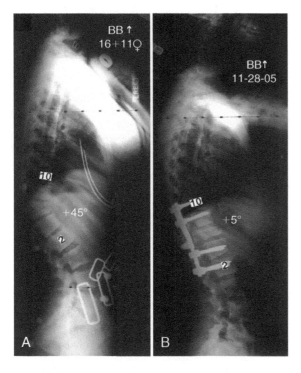

Fig. 52.5 (A) Lateral x-ray films of a 16-year-old female who sustained a three-column–flexion-distraction injury during a motor vehicle accident. She was treated with a posterior spinal fusion from T10 to L2 with a T12 pedicle subtraction osteotomy with correction of her deformity and restoration of normal sagittal balance as seen in (B) the postoperative lateral x-ray. (From Buchowski JM, Kuhns CA, Bridwell KH, et al. Surgical management of posttraumatic thoracolumbar kyphosis. Spine J 2008;8: 666–677.)

21. Describe the principles of surgical treatment for Scheuermann kyphosis.
   Scheuermann kyphosis is a regional kyphotic deformity that presents as a long-radius kyphotic deformity, which may be flexible or rigid. Adult deformities of sufficient severity to require surgical treatment tend to be rigid. Surgery is considered for treatment of pain refractory to nonsurgical treatment, severe deformity, and cosmesis. Surgical correction is most commonly performed through a single-stage posterior surgical approach, which includes multilevel interlaminar closing-wedge resections (Ponte osteotomies) and posterior spinal column shortening by application of compression forces using posterior spinal instrumentation. In severe rigid deformities, a pedicle subtraction osteotomy may be added to obtain additional sagittal plane correction. Alternatively, a first-stage anterior approach to release contracted anterior spinal column structures, including the anterior longitudinal ligament, annulus, and intervertebral disc, followed by a second-stage procedure for correction of the deformity with posterior segmental spinal instrumentation with or without posterior osteotomies, may be performed.

22. **What principles guide surgical treatment of spinal deformities associated with global sagittal malalignment?**

General principles used to guide surgical treatment of spinal deformities associated with global sagittal malalignment include:

- Intervertebral body fusion devices, vertebral body replacement devices, and structural allografts restore sagittal alignment by lengthening the anterior spinal column.
- Posterior spinal implants achieve correction of sagittal plane deformities by shortening the posterior spinal column.
- Flexible spinal deformities are treated using posterior spinal instrumentation and wide posterior releases. Transforaminal lumbar interbody fusions or anterior interbody fusions are added to restore the intervertebral disc height and segmental lordosis, especially at the lower end of an implant construct that extends to the sacrum.
- In rigid spinal deformities or previously fused spines, osteotomies are performed to achieve spinal realignment. Various types of osteotomies are used and include Ponte osteotomies, pedicle subtraction osteotomies, and vertebral column resections.
- Experienced spinal deformity surgeons use a structured framework to plan their approach to surgery for treatment of complex sagittal and multiplanar spinal deformities, which includes the following steps:
  1. Determine the driver of the spinal deformity and quantify the deformity.
  2. Evaluate the impact of the spinal deformity on global spinal alignment.
  3. Set alignment targets.
  4. Determine spinal flexibility.
  5. Decide on a surgical strategy.
  6. Execute the intraoperative surgical strategy in a controlled fashion and use intraoperative imaging to confirm achievement of the planned deformity correction. If initial spinal alignment is inadequate, obtain the necessary correction prior to leaving the operating room.

23. **What general alignment targets are recommended when planning correction of sagittal spinal deformity?**

General alignment targets (Fig. 52.6) recommended when planning correction of sagittal spinal deformity include:

- Match lumbar lordosis to within 11° of PI
- Decrease PT to less than 25°, and
- Decrease SVA to less than 5 cm

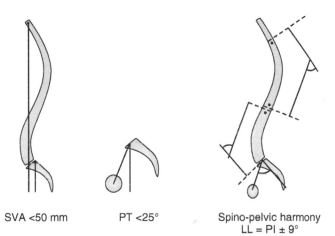

SVA <50 mm   PT <25°   Spino-pelvic harmony
                                          LL = PI ± 9°

Fig. 52.6 Sagittal realignment surgical goals. *LL,* lumbar lordosis; *PI,* pelvic incidence; *PT,* pelvic tilt; *SVA,* Sagittal vertical axis. (From Polly DW, Jones KE, Larson AN. Pediatric and adult scoliosis. In: Ellenbogen RG, Sekhar LN, Kitchen ND, editors. Principles of Neurological Surgery. 4th ed. Philadelphia, PA: Elsevier; 2018, Fig. 37.9, pp. 561–572.)

24. **What is a flatback deformity?**

Flatback deformity describes the symptomatic loss of normal sagittal plane alignment due to decreased lumbar lordosis. This results in a posture in which the head and trunk shift to an anterior position relative to the sacrum and is associated with low back pain and difficulty maintaining an erect posture. This deformity was initially reported in association with the use of Harrington instrumentation to correct scoliosis by application of posterior distraction forces. Harrington instrumentation had the unintended consequence of decreasing the normal lordotic alignment of the lumbar region and created an iatrogenic spinal deformity, which is also referred to as fixed sagittal imbalance or sagittal plane malalignment (Fig. 52.7). Other causes of sagittal plane malalignment include lumbar fusions performed for degenerative spinal disorders when adequate lumbar lordosis is not restored during the initial surgery. Transition syndrome (breakdown of spinal segments above or below a solid spinal fusion) is another frequent cause of sagittal malalignment. Autofusion of the spine as a result of conditions such as Forestier disease (diffuse idiopathic skeletal hyperostosis [DISH]) or ankylosing spondylitis may also lead to sagittal malalignment. Osteoporotic compression fractures are an additional cause of sagittal imbalance. Other etiologies that may lead to fixed sagittal malalignment include spinal tumors, spinal trauma, spinal infections, and iatrogenic deformities following instrumented spinal fusion surgery.

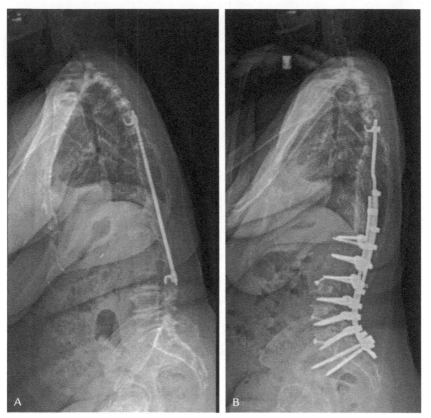

Fig. 52.7 (A) Preoperative lateral 36-inch radiograph demonstrating flatblack syndrome with loss of lumbar lordosis and sagittal plane malalignment caused by Harrington rod instrumentation. (B) The patient underwent staged anterior interbody fusions (L3–S1) and posterior instrumentation and fusion to restore lumbar lordosis and correct the sagittal plane malalignment.

25. How is sagittal plane alignment altered in ankylosing spondylitis?

Patients with ankylosing spondylitis may develop fixed flexion deformities of the hips and spine. Over time, these patients may develop cervical and thoracic hyperkyphosis, as well as the flattening of lumbar lordosis (Fig. 52.8). Cervicothoracic hyperkyphosis may progress to a rigid chin-on-chest deformity. Patients with severe deformities due to ankylosing spondylitis are unable to look straight ahead and experience extreme difficulties carrying out activities of daily living. Surgical treatment for hip involvement consists of total hip arthroplasty. Severe spinal deformities require spinal osteotomies to restore sagittal alignment.

26. What types of osteotomies are used to correct sagittal plane deformities?

The major types of spinal osteotomies that are used to correct sagittal plane spinal deformities are Ponte osteotomies, pedicle subtraction osteotomies, and vertebral column resection procedures.

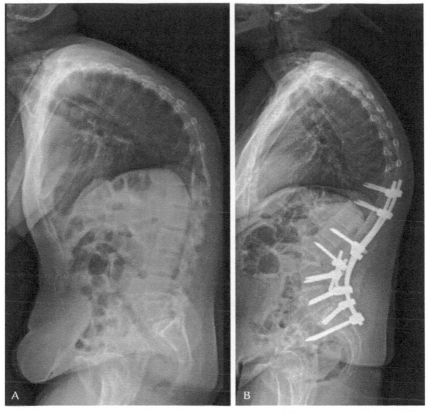

Fig. 52.8 (A) Preoperative lateral radiograph of 39-year-old male with ankylosing spondylitis and severe sagittal plane malalignment, loss of lumbar lordosis, and increased thoracic kyphosis. (B) Lateral 36-inch standing radiograph showing improved sagittal alignment after posterior instrumented fusion from T10 to pelvis with a pedicle subtraction osteotomy at L3 to restore lumbar lordosis.

The **Ponte osteotomy**, originally described for treatment of Scheuermann kyphosis, involves removal of the inferior part of the spinous process, lamina, facet joints, and ligamentum flavum. The superior and inferior facets are resected in their entirety. Correction is achieved by compression of the posterior elements and pivots around the center of the disc space without disruption of the anterior longitudinal ligament. Between 4° and 8° of correction is achieved per level of osteotomy Ponte osteotomies are frequently performed over multiple levels.

A **pedicle subtraction osteotomy (PSO)** includes surgical resection of the posterior elements, pedicles, and a portion of the vertebral body. Deformity correction is achieved by closure of the osteotomy by posterior compression. A PSO hinges on the anterior column and closes the middle and posterior columns and provides 25°–35° of correction at the osteotomy level.

A **vertebral column resection (VCR)** is an osteotomy that involves removal of the entire vertebral body and adjacent intervertebral discs. It is most commonly performed through a single posterior approach, but may be performed through separate anterior and posterior surgical approaches. A VCR can correct both sagittal and coronal plane deformities while simultaneously decompressing the neural elements.

KEY POINTS

1. Any adult spinal deformity patient considered for surgical treatment involving multilevel spinal instrumentation and fusion requires a detailed preoperative analysis of sagittal plane alignment.
2. Surgical techniques that play a role in restoration of sagittal alignment include sagittal rod contouring, restoration of segmental sagittal alignment by use of wide posterior releases or interbody fusions, and spinal osteotomies.
3. Surgical options for treatment of sagittal plane malalignment in the previously fused spine include Smith-Petersen osteotomies, Ponte osteotomies, pedicle subtraction osteotomy, combined anterior and posterior osteotomies, and vertebral column resection.

Websites
1. Kyphosis: https://www.srs.org/patients-and-families/conditions-and-treatments/adults/kyphosis
2. Spinal osteotomies: https://online.boneandjoint.org.uk/doi/full/10.1302/2058-5241.2.160069

BIBLIOGRAPHY

1. Bernhardt M, Bridwell KH. Segmental analysis of the sagittal plane alignment of the normal thoracic and lumbar spines and thoracolumbar junction. *Spine* 1989;14:717–721.
2. Buchowski JM, Kuhns CA, Bridwell KH, et al. Surgical management of posttraumatic thoracolumbar kyphosis. *Spine J* 2008;8:666–677.
3. Dubousset J. Three-dimensional analysis of the scoliotic deformity. In: Weinstein SL, editors. The Pediatric Spine: Principles and Practice. New York: Raven Press Ltd.; 1994, pp. 479–496.
4. Glassman SD, Bridwell K, Dimar JR, et al. The impact of positive sagittal balance in adult spinal deformity. *Spine* 2005;30:2024–2029.
5. Iyer S, Sheha E, Fu MC, et al. Sagittal spinal alignment in adult spinal deformity: An overview of current concepts and a critical analysis review. *JBJS Rev* 2018;6:e2.
6. Lafage V, Schwab F, Patel A, et al. Pelvic tilt and truncal inclination: Two key radiographic parameters in the setting of adults with spinal deformity. *Spine* 2009;34:599–606.
7. Legaye J, Duval-Beaupère G, Hecquet J, et al. Pelvic incidence: A fundamental pelvic parameter for three-dimensional regulation of spinal sagittal curves. *Eur Spine J* 1998;7:99–103.
8. Nelles D, Majid K. Adult scoliosis. In: Garfin SR, Eismont FJ, Bell GR, editors. Rothman-Simeone The Spine. 7th ed. Philadelphia, PA: Saunders; 2018, pp. 1239–1259.
9. Obeid I, Boissière L, Yilgor C, et al. Global tilt: A single parameter incorporating spinal and pelvic sagittal parameters and least affected by patient positioning. *Eur Spine J* 2016;25:3644–3649.
10. Protopsaltis T, Schwab F, Bronsard N, et al. The T1 pelvic angle, a novel radiographic measure of global sagittal deformity, accounts for both spinal inclination and pelvic tilt and correlates with health-related quality of life. *J Bone Joint Surg* 2014;96:1631–1640.
11. Yilgor C, Sogunmez N, Boissiere L, et al. Global Alignment and Proportion Score: Development and validation of a new method of analyzing spinopelvic alignment to predict mechanical complications after adult spinal deformity surgery. *J Bone Joint Surg* 2017;99:1661–1672.

CHAPTER 53

SPONDYLOLYSIS AND SPONDYLOLISTHESIS IN ADULTS

Vincent J. Devlin, MD

1. **What are the different types of spondylolisthesis and how are they classified?**

Spondylolisthesis refers to ventral displacement of the proximal spinal column in relation to the distal spinal column. The degree of slip is determined by measuring the amount of anterior translation of the displaced vertebra relative to the superior aspect of the inferior vertebra and is expressed as a percentage. The **Meyerding Classification** grades translational displacement as:

- Grade 1: 1%–25%
- Grade 2: 26%–50%
- Grade 3: 51%–75%
- Grade 4: 76%–100%
- Grade 5: slippage of the L5 vertebra anterior and distal to the superior S1 endplate (spondyloptosis)

   Slippages <50% are referred to as low-grade spondylolisthesis, while slippages >50% are referred to as high-grade spondylolisthesis.

   The **Wiltse Classification** identifies type of spondylolisthesis based on a combination of etiologic and anatomic features:

- Type 1: *Dysplastic.* Associated with a congenital deficiency of the L5–S1 articulation
- Type 2: *Isthmic.* Associated with a lesion in the pars interarticularis (type 2A: stress fracture; type 2B: elongated but intact pars interarticularis; type 2C: acute pars fracture)
- Type 3: *Degenerative.* Disc degeneration and facet arthrosis lead to spondylolisthesis and associated spinal stenosis in adults
- Type 4: *Traumatic.* An acute fracture in a region of the posterior elements other than the pars interarticularis (e.g., facets, pedicle, lamina)
- Type 5: *Pathologic.* Generalized bone disease (e.g., metabolic, neoplastic) results in attenuation of the pars and/or pedicle region leading to spondylolisthesis
- Type 6: *Postsurgical.* Spondylolisthesis that develops following lumbar laminotomy or laminectomy

   The **Marchetti and Bartolozzi Classification** identifies two major types of spondylolisthesis: developmental and acquired. **Developmental** spondylolisthesis is associated with dysplasia at the level of the spondylolisthesis and is subdivided into high- and low-dysplastic types. **Acquired** types of spondylolisthesis include traumatic, degenerative, pathologic, and postsurgical etiologies.

   The **Spinal Deformity Study Group Classification of Spondylolisthesis** was developed to incorporate the current understanding of sacropelvic and global spinopelvic balance as a guide to treatment decision making. Classification of L5–S1 spondylolisthesis is based on three factors:

- Degree of slip (low grade or high grade),
- Sacropelvic alignment and balance, and,
- Global spinopelvic balance.

   Low-grade spondylolisthesis is stratified into three types based on pelvic incidence (PI):

- Type 1 (low PI, <45°),
- Type 2 (normal PI, 45°–60°) and
- Type 3 (high PI, >60°).

   Type 1 patients have low PI, which results in low shear stress across the lumbosacral junction and low risk of slip progression. In contrast, type 3 patients have high PI, which increases shear stress across the lumbosacral junction and increases the risk of spondylolisthesis progression.

   High-grade spondylolisthesis is subdivided into three types:

- Type 4 (balanced pelvis)
- Type 5 (retroverted pelvis with a balanced spine)
- Type 6 (retroverted pelvis with an unbalanced spine)

   In a balanced pelvis, sacral slope (SS) exceeds pelvic tilt (PT) (i.e., high SS/low PT). In contrast, in an unbalanced pelvis, there is a low sacral slope and a high pelvic tilt (i.e., low SS/high PT) and the pelvis becomes retroverted and the sacrum becomes vertically oriented. Global spinopelvic balance is assessed by the position of the C7 plumb line. The spine is considered balanced when the C7 plumb line is located through or behind the femoral heads and unbalanced when the C7 plumb line is located anterior to the femoral heads. Surgery to restore sagittal alignment through reduction and realignment procedures is recommended for type 5 and type 6 deformities (Table 53-1; Fig. 42.6).

Table 53.1 Spinal Deformity Study Group Classification of Lumbosacral Spondylolisthesis.

SLIP GRADE	SACROPELVIC ALIGNMENT/BALANCE	SPINOPELVIC BALANCE	SPONDYLOLISTHESIS TYPE
Low grade	Low pelvic incidence (<45°)	-	Type 1
	Normal pelvic incidence (45°-60°)	-	Type 2
	High pelvic incidence (>60°)	-	Type 3
High grade	Balanced sacropelvis	-	Type 4
	Unbalanced (retroverted) sacropelvis	Balanced	Type 5
	Unbalanced (retroverted) sacropelvis	Unbalanced	Type 6

Note: A balanced sacropelvis has high sacral slope/low pelvic tilt. An unbalanced sacropelvis has low sacral slope/high pelvic tilt. Spinopelvic balance is usually relevant only in high grade slips with an unbalanced sacropelvis as the spine remains balanced in low grade slips and high grade slips with a balanced sacropelvis.

From Kasliwal MK, Smith JS, Kanter A, et al. Management of high-grade spondylolisthesis. Neurosurg Clin N Am 2013;24:275–291; Labelle H, Mac-Thiong JM, Roussouly. Spino-pelvic sagittal balance of spondylolisthesis: A review and classification. Eur Spine J 2011;20:641–646.

ISTHMIC SPONDYLOLISTHESIS

2. What level of the spine is most commonly involved in isthmic spondylolisthesis?
   Ninety percent of cases of isthmic spondylolisthesis occur at the L5–S1 level. The next most commonly affected level is L4–L5.

3. What is the most common clinical presentation of adult isthmic spondylolisthesis?
   The clinical presentation of adults with isthmic spondylolisthesis is quite variable. Adult isthmic spondylolisthesis occurs more commonly in males than females. The prevalence of isthmic spondylolisthesis in adults with and without low back pain has been reported as 10.8% and 7.3%, respectively. Symptomatic adult patients with isthmic spondylolisthesis most commonly present with low back pain and over half of patients present with lower extremity radicular pain. Symptomatic adults present most commonly with low-grade slips. Patients with high-grade slips are more commonly encountered during adolescence, but occasionally present in adulthood due to new-onset or worsening symptoms or for evaluation following prior surgical treatment. Spondylolysis and low-grade isthmic spondylolisthesis that have been asymptomatic since childhood may become symptomatic in later life in the absence of precipitating trauma. As the ability of the intervertebral disc to resist shear forces at the level of the pars defect is compromised, spondylolisthesis progression may occur as degenerative disc changes develop, most often during the fourth and fifth decades of life.
   It is critical to precisely localize the pain generator in adult patients with spondylolisthesis because pain may not be related to the level of the spondylolisthesis, but rather due to degenerative spinal pathology at adjacent spinal levels, or extraspinal causes such as hip or knee arthritis.

4. What are the most appropriate imaging studies for diagnosis and evaluation of adult lumbar isthmic spondylolisthesis?
   A standing lateral spinal radiograph is the initial imaging study required for diagnosis of spondylolisthesis in adult patients. Magnetic resonance imaging (MRI) is used to evaluate neural compression and assess the status of the lumbar discs. Computed tomography (CT) is the method of choice for assessing osseous anatomy. Patients who are surgical candidates require a standing lateral full-length spinal radiograph to assess sagittal alignment and global balance.

5. What nonoperative treatment options are considered for adults with spondylolysis or isthmic spondylolisthesis?
   Nonsurgical treatment options include active physical therapy, education, and instruction in a home exercise program, nonsteroidal antiinflammatory medication, and bracing. Epidural injections are a treatment option for patients with isthmic spondylolisthesis and clinically significant lower extremity radicular symptoms.

6. When is surgery considered for an adult patient with spondylolysis or isthmic spondylolisthesis?
   Surgery is infrequently required for adult patients with spondylolysis or isthmic spondylolisthesis. General indications to consider surgical intervention include:
   - Failure of nonsurgical treatment for disabling back and/or leg pain
   - Patients with symptomatic and radiographically unstable isthmic spondylolisthesis
   - Documented slip progression (> grade 2 slip)
   - Symptomatic grade 3 or 4 spondylolisthesis or spondyloptosis

- Associated symptomatic spinal stenosis or progressive neurologic deficit
- Cauda equina syndrome related to spondylolisthesis

7. **What patterns of neural compression are associated with L5–S1 isthmic spondylolisthesis?**
L5 nerve root compression (exiting nerve root of the L5–S1 motion segment) is the type of neural compression most commonly associated with L5–S1 isthmic spondylolisthesis. L5 nerve root compression may occur secondary to:
- Hypertrophy of fibrocartilage at the site of the pars defect
- Compression in the foraminal zone as the L5 nerve root is compressed between a disc protrusion or osteophyte and the inferior aspect of the L5 pedicle
- Compression between the inferior aspect of the L5 transverse process and the superior aspect of the sacral ala
- Increased tension within the L5 nerve root may occcur due to forward displacement of the L5 vertebra when the L5 nerve root is tethered by a hook-like projection from the lamina at the inlet to the intervertebral foramen.
     The sacral nerve roots can become involved in high-grade isthmic spondylolisthesis as these nerves become stretched over the L5–S1 disc and posterior aspect of the sacrum.

8. **Is repair of the pars interarticularis recommended for treatment of adult patients with spondylolysis?**
No. Adult patients with symptomatic spondylolysis have poorer healing potential compared with pediatric patients, and additional pain generators within the spinal motion segment other than the pars interarticularis are often responsible for back and/or leg pain symptoms. Spinal fusion is recommended for treatment of symptomatic spondylolysis that does not respond to nonoperative treatment.

9. **What are the options for surgical treatment of low-grade L5–S1 isthmic spondylolisthesis in adult patients?**
Potential surgical treatment options for low-grade isthmic spondylolisthesis include:
- L5–S1 decompression
- Decompression and in situ posterolateral fusion with or without posterior pedicle fixation
- Decompression, posterolateral fusion, and posterior pedicle fixation combined with interbody fusion
     Lack of consensus exists regarding the optimal procedure for treatment of low-grade L5–S1 isthmic spondylolisthesis. Posterior decompression without fusion is rarely performed due to the high risk of postoperative slip progression. Adult patients are frequently treated with posterior spinal fusion in combination with pedicle fixation and direct neural decompression. The rationale for use of posterior spinal instrumentation is to decrease the risk of postoperative slip progression and increase fusion rates. Some surgeons prefer to perform posterior fusion without direct neural decompression in the absence of severe neurologic deficits to preserve greater osseous surface area for posterior fusion. Other surgeons advocate posterior fusion without use of instrumentation for low-grade slips. The addition of an L5–S1 interbody fusion is advocated by many surgeons and may be performed through a variety of approaches including transforaminal lumbar interbody fusion (TLIF), posterior lumbar inter-body fusion (PLIF), and anterior lumbar interbody fusion (ALIF). Rationale for use of interbody fusion includes in-creased fusion surface area, which is expected to increase fusion rates; restoration of disc space height, which increases neuroforaminal height and provides indirect neural decompression; and increased segmental stability provided by anterior column support, which reduces stress on posterior spinal implants and promotes early patient mobilization (Fig. 53.1). Use of stand-alone anterior lumbar interbody fusion and supplemental anterior fix-ation is reported for treatment of adult low grade isthmic spondylolisthesis. However, notable complications have been described with this strategy including pseudarthrosis, instrumentation failure and sacral fracture due to the coexistence of high anterior column shear forces in the presence of a posterior tension band defect.

10. **What are the options for surgical treatment of high-grade L5–S1 isthmic spondylolisthesis in adult patients?**
Surgical treatment options for high-grade isthmic spondylolisthesis include:
- In situ posterolateral L4–S1 spinal fusion in combination with posterior spinal instrumentation and spinal decompression.
- Circumferential fusion consisting of posterolateral L4–S1 fusion and posterior spinal instrumentation, spinal decompression, L5–S1 interbody fusion, and partial or complete reduction of spondylolisthesis.
- Circumferential fusion consisting of posterolateral L4–S1 spinal fusion and instrumentation, spinal decompression and transsacral interbody fusion and fixation ± partial reduction of spondylolisthesis.
- L5 vertebrectomy (Gaines procedure) for spondyloptosis
     Surgery that restores sagittal alignment through reduction and realignment procedures is recommended for type 5 and type 6 deformities based on the Spinal Deformity Study Group Classification of Spondylolisthesis. Inter-body fusion through either an anterior or posterior approach and use of distal fixation consisting of either S2 alar-iliac screw fixation or iliac screw fixation are integral to the success of reduction procedures.

11. **Is it necessary to achieve a complete reduction of a high-grade spondylolisthesis to obtain a successful clinical outcome following surgical treatment?**
No. The factors associated with a successful outcome in high-grade spondylolisthesis surgery are maintenance or restoration of sagittal balance and achievement of a solid fusion. It has been demonstrated that reduction of the

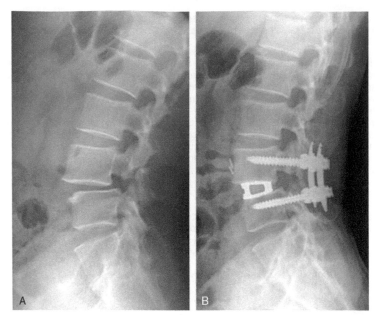

Fig. 53.1 Low-grade adult isthmic spondylolisthesis. (A) Standing lateral radiograph. (B) Postoperative lateral radiograph following treatment with anterior lumbar interbody fusion and posterior percutaneous pedicle screw-rod instrumentation. (From Kim JS, Kim DH, Lee SH, et al. Comparison study of the instrumented circumferential fusion with instrumented anterior lumbar interbody fusion as a surgical procedure for adult low-grade isthmic spondylolisthesis. World Neursurg 2010;73:565–571, Fig. 2, p. 568.)

slip angle (lumbosacral kyphosis) is more important than complete reduction of the degree of slip for restoration of sagittal alignment. Complete reduction of a high-grade spondylolisthesis is associated with a high rate of L5 nerve root injury. Circumferential fusion is associated with the highest rate of successful arthrodesis, and surgical techniques have evolved to permit a circumferential fusion construct without the need to achieve complete reduction of spondylolisthesis. However, in extreme cases with severe deformity, complex procedures including complete reduction, sacral osteotomy, or L5 vertebrectomy remain valid treatment options.

12. What is the rationale for transsacral interbody fusion and transvertebral screw fixation?
    - **Secure implant fixation:** It is challenging to place L5 pedicle screws in a high-grade L5–S1 spondylolisthesis without reduction of listhesis. Secure fixation of L5 can be achieved by placing medially directed S1 screws across the anterior sacral cortex and across the L5–S1 disc and into the adjacent L5 vertebra.
    - **Simplified technique for anterior column fusion:** Placement of a fibular graft or axial fusion cage can be achieved from either a posterior or anterior approach without the need for anatomic reduction of spondylolisthesis.
    - **Potential for deformity correction:** Partial correction of the slip angle is feasible using this technique when indicated (see Fig. 42.8).

DEGENERATIVE SPONDYLOLISTHESIS

13. Define degenerative spondylolisthesis.
    Degenerative spondylolisthesis is an acquired anterior subluxation of the proximal vertebra and spinal column relative to the adjacent distal vertebra and spinal column in the presence of an intact posterior neural arch as a consequence of degenerative changes. It is the most common type of spondylolisthesis in adults.

14. Who is most likely to develop degenerative spondylolisthesis?
    Degenerative spondylolisthesis generally occurs in patients over 40 years of age. It is most common in the sixth decade. Risk factors include female sex (female-to-male ratio: 4:1), diabetes, osteoporosis, and sacralization of the L5 vertebra.

15. What level of the spine is most commonly involved in degenerative spondylolisthesis?
    Ninety percent of cases of degenerative spondylolisthesis occur at L4–L5, and 10% of cases occur at L3–L4 or L5–S1.

16. **What are the common presenting symptoms of degenerative spondylolisthesis?**

Degenerative spondylolisthesis may be diagnosed as an incidental radiographic finding in an asymptomatic patient or may present due to clinical symptoms. Symptoms may include low back pain, intermittent neurogenic claudication, and/or radicular pain. Low back pain is mechanical in nature. Neurogenic claudication most commonly presents as bilateral buttock and thigh pain with cramping associated with prolonged standing or walking. Patients may report numbness, heaviness, or weakness in the lower extremities. Symptoms are exacerbated by spinal extension and relieved by sitting or leaning forward to position the lumbar spine in a flexed posture, such as leaning on a shopping cart. Radicular symptoms occur most commonly in an L5 nerve root pattern due to lateral recess stenosis and may also involve the L4 nerve root when foraminal stenosis is present. Occasionally, bowel or bladder dysfunction is reported due to cauda equina compression.

17. **What are some common nonspinal conditions that can mimic the clinical presentation of degenerative spondylolisthesis with spinal stenosis?**

Degenerative arthritis involving the hip joints and lower extremity peripheral vascular disease are two common conditions that may present with restricted walking ability and lower extremity pain. Hip joint arthrosis often causes buttock and thigh pain that mimics symptoms of spinal stenosis. Assessment of hip joint range of motion can determine whether radiographs are necessary to evaluate the hip joints for arthritis. If both hip arthritis and degenerative spondylolisthesis are present, injection of the hip joint under fluoroscopic or ultrasound guidance can aid in identifying which problem is more symptomatic. Peripheral vascular disease can also cause lower extremity claudication. Assessment of lower extremity peripheral pulses should be routinely documented during the assessment of patients with adult spinal disorders. Vascular claudication is associated with increased muscular exertion independent of trunk position. Symptoms due to vascular claudication typically occur in the distal calf and foot and are not associated with back pain. In contrast, symptoms of neurogenic claudication are exacerbated by standing, relieved with sitting, typically occur above the level of the knees, and are associated with a positive "shopping cart sign." Other conditions to consider in the differential diagnosis include greater trochanteric bursitis, piriformis syndrome, diabetic peripheral neuropathy, and sacroiliac joint degeneration.

18. **What are the most appropriate imaging studies for diagnosis and evaluation of lumbar degenerative spondylolisthesis?**

The most important imaging test for diagnosis of lumbar degenerative spondylolisthesis is a lateral lumbar radiograph obtained with the patient in the standing position. Lateral flexion–extension radiographs are an option for diagnosis of translational instability. Similar information may be provided by comparing spinal alignment on a standing lateral lumbar radiograph with the alignment on a supine sagittal MRI image, thereby avoiding the necessity of flexion–extension radiographs and additional radiation exposure. A lumbar MRI is most commonly used to evaluate the spinal canal for neural compression in patients with degenerative spondylolisthesis. In patients with a contraindication to MRI or patients with associated severe scoliosis and spondylolisthesis, a CT or CT-myelogram is the next most appropriate study. Patients who are surgical candidates require a standing lateral full-length spinal radiograph to assess sagittal alignment and global balance (Fig. 53.2).

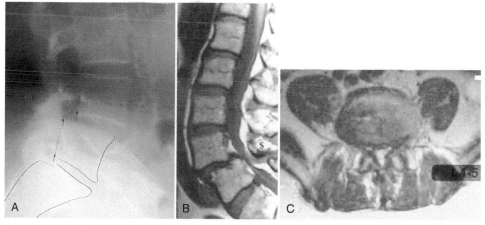

Fig. 53.2 Imaging studies for degenerative spondylolisthesis. (A) Standing lateral radiograph. (B) Magnetic resonance imaging (MRI), sagittal view. (C) MRI, axial view. (B: From Barckhausen RR, Math KR. Lumbar spine disease. In: Katz DS, Math KR, Groskin SA, editors. Radiology Secrets. Philadelphia, PA: Hanley & Belfus; 1998.)

19. **What clinical and radiographic criteria are used to diagnose spinal instability in patients with degenerative spondylolisthesis?"**

    Lack of consensus exists regarding a universally accepted reference standard for the diagnosis of spinal instability in patients with degenerative spondylolisthesis. Recently, a classification for identification of spinal stability in patients with degenerative spondylolisthesis has been proposed. (1) Preoperative parameters considered predictive of stability included absence of low back pain, restabilization signs (disc height loss, osteophyte formation, vertebral endplate sclerosis, ligament ossification), no disc angle change or less than 3 mm of translation on dynamic radiographs, and absence of facet joint effusions on MRI (Table 53.2).

Table 53.2 Degenerative Spondylolisthesis Instability Classification.			
PARAMETER	**TYPE I, STABLE**	**TYPE II, POTENTIALLY UNSTABLE**	**TYPE III, UNSTABLE**
LBP	None or very mild	Primary or secondary symptom	Primary or secondary symptom
Restablization	Restabilization signs, grossly narrowed disc height	Some restabilization signs, reduced disc height	No restabilization signs, normal to slightly reduced disc height
Disc angle	Lordotic disc angle on flexion radiographs or <3 mm translation on dynamic films[a]	Neutral disc angle on flexion radiographs or 3–5 mm of translation on dynamic films[a]	Kyphotic disc angle on flexion radiographs or >5 mm translation on dynamic films[a]
Joint effusion	No facet joint effusion on MRI	Facet joint effusion on MRI without joint distraction	Large facet joint effusion on MRI

[a]Dynamic films include flexion and extension radiographs or supine to standing radiographs.

MRI, magnetic resonance imaging.

From Simmonds AM, Rampersaud YR, Dvorak MF, et al. Defining the inherent stability of degenerative spondylolisthesis: A systematic review. J Neurosurg Spine 2015;23:178–189.

20. **What MRI finding suggests the presence of lumbar degenerative spondylolisthesis despite normal spinal alignment on MRI?**

    Facet joint effusion. As degenerative spondylolisthesis may be position dependent and evident only under physiologic loading, MRI performed in the supine position may fail to detect this condition. Fluid in the facet joints is a helpful diagnostic marker of a degenerative spondylolisthesis that is not evident on an imaging study performed in the supine position (Fig. 53.3).

21. **What pattern of neural compression is most commonly associated with L4–L5 degenerative spondylolisthesis?**

    Degenerative spondylolisthesis at the L4–L5 level leads to central spinal stenosis and associated compression of the cauda equina, as well as subarticular stenosis, which causes compression of the L5 nerve roots (traversing

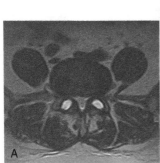
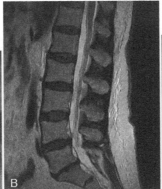
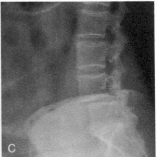

Fig. 53.3 Dynamic degenerative spondylolisthesis. (A) Axial magnetic resonance imaging (MRI) shows facet joint effusions, which suggest segmental instability. (B) MRI sagittal view shows normal alignment at L4–L5 in the supine position. (C) Standing lateral radiograph documents spinal instability with L4–L5 degenerative spondylolisthesis.

nerve roots of the L4–L5 motion segment). The L4 nerve roots (exiting nerve roots of the L4–L5 motion segment) may be compressed when there is loss of disc space height, which results in narrowing of the neural foramen.

22. **What degree of subluxation is associated with degenerative spondylolisthesis?**
In a patient who has not undergone prior spine surgery, degenerative spondylolisthesis presents with a subluxation less than 50% (grade 1 or grade 2 slips). Further slippage is limited by the intact neural arch.

23. **What are the nonsurgical treatment options for degenerative spondylolisthesis?**
Nonsurgical treatment options include active physical therapy, education and instruction in a home exercise program, nonsteroidal antiinflammatory medication, and bracing. Epidural injections are an option for the treatment of patients with degenerative spondylolisthesis and clinically significant lower extremity symptoms secondary to spinal stenosis.

24. **When is surgery considered for degenerative spondylolisthesis?**
Surgery is recommended for treatment of patients with persistent or recurrent symptoms despite adequate nonsurgical management. Surgical candidates should have confirmatory imaging studies that are consistent with their symptoms and diagnosis.

25. **What are the surgical treatment options for degenerative spondylolisthesis and spinal stenosis?**
Surgical treatment options for patients with degenerative spondylolisthesis and spinal stenosis include:
- Decompression (laminotomies, interlaminar decompression, laminectomy)
- Decompression and posterolateral fusion without spinal instrumentation
- Decompression, posterolateral fusion, and posterior spinal instrumentation
- Decompression, posterolateral fusion, posterior spinal instrumentation, and interbody fusion
- Minimally invasive approaches for decompression with or without fusion
- Innovative device technologies such as interspinous and interlaminar devices

26. **Describe some recent classifications that have been proposed for stratification of patients with degenerative spondylolisthesis.**
The **Clinical and Radiographic Degenerative Spondylolisthesis (CARDS) classification** (2) was developed to identify subgroups of degenerative spondylolisthesis based on radiographic morphology (types A, B, C, D) and leg pain symptoms (modifiers 0, 1, 2), and results in 12 subgroups. This classification was developed for communication and research but was not intended to guide treatment. Radiographic morphologies include:
Type A: advanced disc space collapse without kyphosis
Type B: disc partially preserved with translation of 5 mm or less
Type C: disc partially preserved with translation of more than 5 mm
Type D: kyphotic alignment
Leg pain modifiers include: 0, without leg pain; 1, unilateral leg pain; 2, bilateral leg pain
    The **Degenerative Lumbar Spinal Instability Classification** defined grades of stability and proposed a surgical treatment algorithm. (1) Preoperative parameters considered predictive of stability (Table 53.2, above) included absence of low back pain, restabilization signs (disc height loss, osteophyte formation, vertebral endplate sclerosis, ligament ossification), no disc angle change or less than 3 mm of translation on dynamic radiographs, and absence facet joint effusions on MRI. Selection of surgical treatment is stratified according to three stability grades:
Grade 1, stable: treatment with decompression alone
Grade 2, potentially unstable: treatment with decompression and posterior fusion
Grade 3, unstable: treatment with decompression and posterior fusion and interbody fusion
    The **French Society for Spine Surgery** proposed a classification for treatment of degenerative spondylolisthesis and identified five subtypes based on segmental lordosis, lumbar lordosis, PI, PT, and sagittal vertical axis. These factors were used to select among various surgical options, including posterior instrumentation and fusion, posterior instrumentation and fusion in combination with interbody fusion, use of an extended instrumentation construct from L3 to S1, and sagittal spinal deformity correction in combination with surgery for degenerative spondylolisthesis.

27. **Describe some of the challenges and factors that influence selection of an optimal surgical procedure for treatment of patients with degenerative spondylolisthesis with spinal stenosis?**
Patients with degenerative spondylolisthesis are a heterogeneous population comprised of poorly defined subgroups with variable clinical presentations, radiographic features, and medical comorbidities. Selection of an appropriate surgical procedure for a specific patient is challenging due to the absence of consensus regarding a treatment-based classification to guide surgical decision making and lack of consensus regarding the diagnosis and definition of spinal instability. In general, outcome studies support posterior decompression and fusion compared with decompression alone for treatment of patients with degenerative spondylolisthesis and

spinal stenosis. The addition of posterior spinal instrumentation is recommended to improve fusion rates, although the addition of instrumentation may not improve outcomes based on the literature. Interbody fusion is considered in addition to posterior instrumentation and fusion in patients with instability. Surgical decompression alone with preservation of midline structures is reported to provide equivalent outcomes compared to decompression with fusion for treatment of symptomatic single-level stable low-grade (<20%) degenerative spondylolisthesis with central stenosis, especially in the absence of lateral foraminal stenosis, and has become more widely utilized.

28. What are the advantages and disadvantages of laminectomy versus laminotomy for decompression of L4–L5 spinal stenosis in patients with degenerative spondylolisthesis? What are the key steps in each procedure?
Options for direct decompression of spinal stenosis associated with L4–L5 spondylolisthesis include midline laminectomy and laminotomy approaches. A **midline laminectomy** involves removal of the midline osseous and ligamentous structures including the lamina, spinous processes, interspinous ligaments, and portions of the facet joints. This approach provides excellent visualization of neural structures and facilitates complete decompression of involved neural structures. However, as a laminectomy further destabilized the spine in a patient with degenerative spondylolisthesis, it is most commonly performed in conjunction with posterior spinal instrumentation and fusion. **Laminotomy** involves partial removal of the lamina and facet complex but preserves the midline structures, including the spinous processes and the supraspinous and interspinous ligaments. Preservation of the midline structures decreases the risk of worsening of preexistent spinal instability. Bilateral L4–L5 decompression of central and lateral recess stenosis may be performed through bilateral laminotomies or an extended unilateral laminotomy approach.

The key procedural steps involved in lumbar decompression for L4–L5 spinal stenosis include either complete removal of the laminae of L4 and L5 (laminectomy), or partial removal of the inferior portion of the L4 lamina, superior portion of the L5 lamina, and intervening ligamentum flavum (laminotomy) to decompress the central spinal canal. Midline structures including the spinous processes, interspinous ligaments, and supraspinous ligaments are either removed or preserved depending on whether laminectomy or laminotomy are performed. Next, the L5 nerve roots are decompressed by removing the medial one-half of the L4–L5 facet joints and accompanying ligamentum flavum. The decompression of the L5 nerve root is continued until the L5 nerve root is mobile and a probe passes without restriction through the neural foramen. The L4 nerve root and foramen is also checked for potential compression. In many cases, it is feasible to perform a bilateral decompression through a unilateral laminotomy approach if desired.

29. What are the key steps involved in an intertransverse fusion procedure for treatment of L4–L5 degenerative spondylolisthesis. What is the role of posterior spinal instrumentation?
After completion of the decompression, the transverse processes of L4 and L5 are carefully exposed and soft tissue is removed from the intertransverse membrane extending between the transverse processes. The transverse processes are decorticated with a curette or burr to expose their cancellous surface. Next, bone graft material is applied to the intertransverse region to complete the fusion procedure. If posterior pedicle screws and rods are utilized, a facet fusion is also performed. However, if no instrumentation is used, facet disruption may increase the risk of postoperative instability and is not routinely performed.

The addition of posterior instrumentation at the level of listhesis has several advantages. Pedicle fixation has been shown to increase the rate of successful fusion, decrease the risk of progressive postoperative slippage and recurrent stenosis, and facilitates early patient mobilization following surgery. However, noninstrumented single-level posterolateral fusion is an option in the elderly patient with a narrow L4–L5 disc space, with little or no motion on flexion–extension radiographs, and mild degenerative spondylolisthesis (Fig. 53.4).

30. What are some indications for performing an interbody fusion as part of the surgical procedure for treatment of L4–L5 degenerative spondylolisthesis?
Various surgical techniques may be used to perform an interbody fusion as part of a surgical procedure for treatment of degenerative spondylolisthesis, including lateral lumbar interbody fusion (LLIF), TLIF, PLIF, and ALIF. Indication for interbody fusion in the treatment of degenerative spondylolisthesis include:
• Degenerative spondylolisthesis with segmental L4–L5 kyphotic alignment
• Mobile L4–L5 degenerative spondylolisthesis with marked translational instability
• Degenerative spondylolisthesis with severe disc space narrowing and L4 foraminal stenosis. In this situation, addition of an interbody fusion will increase the dimensions of the neural foramen between L4 and L5 resulting in indirect decompression of the L4 nerve roots.
• Degenerative spondylolisthesis in which the required decompression has compromised the amount of remaining posterior bone surface available for posterior fusion. For example, if one or both facet joints are completely resected and/or the pars interarticularis is violated, an isolated posterior fusion is less likely to heal.
• Degenerative spondylolisthesis associated with degenerative scoliosis and sagittal imbalance.

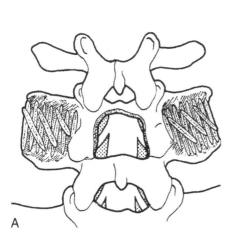
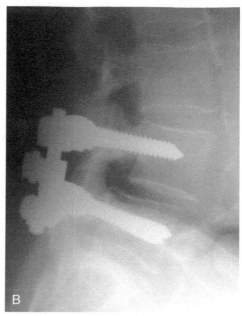

A   B

Fig. 53.4 Posterolateral L4–L5 decompression and fusion. (A) Without spinal instrumentation. (B) With pedicle screw fixation. (A: From Grobbler LJ, Wiltse LL. Classification, non-operative, and operative treatment of spondylolisthesis. In: Frymoyer JW, editor. The Adult Spine: Principles and Practice. New York: Raven Press; 1991, p. 1696, with permission.)

KEY POINTS

1. Radiculopathy most commonly involves the exiting nerve root in isthmic spondylolisthesis, while the traversing nerve root is most commonly involved in degenerative spondylolisthesis.
2. Treatment options for degenerative spondylolisthesis include decompression, decompression and posterior fusion with or without instrumentation, and decompression and posterior instrumented fusion in combination with interbody fusion.
3. Circumferential fusion performed in conjunction with posterior spinal instrumentation provides the highest fusion rate in adult patients with isthmic spondylolisthesis.

Websites
1. Spinal Deformity Study Group Radiographic Measurement Manual: https://www.oref.org/docs/default-source/default-document-library/sdsg-radiographic-measuremnt-manual.pdf?sfvrsn=2&sfvrsn=2
2. Diagnosis and treatment of adult isthmic spondylolisthesis: https://www.spine.org/Portals/0/assets/downloads/ResearchClinicalCare/Guidelines/AdultIsthmicSpondylolisthesis.pdf
3. Diagnosis and treatment of degenerative spondylolisthesis: https://www.spine.org/Portals/0/assets/downloads/ResearchClinicalCare/Guidelines/Spondylolisthesis.pdf

REFERENCES

1. Simmonds AM, Rampersaud YR, Dvorak MF, et al. Defining the inherent stability of degenerative spondylolisthesis: A systematic review. *J Neurosurg Spine* 2015;23:178–189.
2. Kepler CK, Hilibrand AS, Sayadipour A, et al. Clinical and radiographic degenerative spondylolisthesis classification. *Spine J* 2015;15:1804–1811.

BIBLIOGRAPHY

1. Floman Y. Progression of lumbosacral isthmic spondylolisthesis in adults. *Spine* 2000;25:342–347.
2. Gille O, Challier V, Parent H, et al. Degenerative spondylolisthesis: Cohort of 670 patients, and proposal of a new classification. *Orthop Traumatol Surg Res* 2014;100:311–315.
3. Kasliwal MK, Smith JS, Kanter A, et al. Management of high-grade spondylolisthesis. *Neurosurg Clin N Am* 2013;24:275–291.
4. Kepler CK, Hilibrand AS, Sayadipour A, et al. Clinical and radiographic degenerative spondylolisthesis classification. *Spine J* 2015;15:1804–1811.

5. Kwon BK, Albert TJ. Adult low-grade acquired spondylolytic spondylolisthesis: Evaluation and management. Spine 2005;30, 35–41.
6. Labelle H, Mac-Thiong JM, Roussouly P. Spinopelvic sagittal balance of spondylolisthesis: A review and classification. *Eur Spine J* 2011;20:641–646.
7. Matz PG, Meagher RJ, Lamer T, et al. Guideline summary review: An evidence-based clinical guideline for the diagnosis and treatment of degenerative lumbar spondylolisthesis. *Spine J* 2016;16:439–448.
8. Noorian S, Sorensen K, Cho W. A systematic review of clinical outcomes in surgical treatment of adult isthmic spondylolisthesis. *Spine J* 2018;18:1441–1454.
9. Simmonds AM, Rampersaud YR, Dvorak MF, et al. Defining the inherent stability of degenerative spondylolisthesis: A systematic review. *J Neurosurg Spine* 2015;23:178–189.
10. Smith JA, Deviren V, Berven S, et al. Clinical outcome of trans-sacral interbody fusion after partial reduction for high-grade L5–S1 spondylolisthesis. *Spine* 2001;26:2227–2234.
11. Swan J, Hurwitz E, Malek F, et al. Surgical treatment for unstable low-grade isthmic spondylolisthesis in adults: A prospective controlled study of posterior instrumented fusion compared with anterior-posterior fusion. *Spine J* 2006;6:606–614.

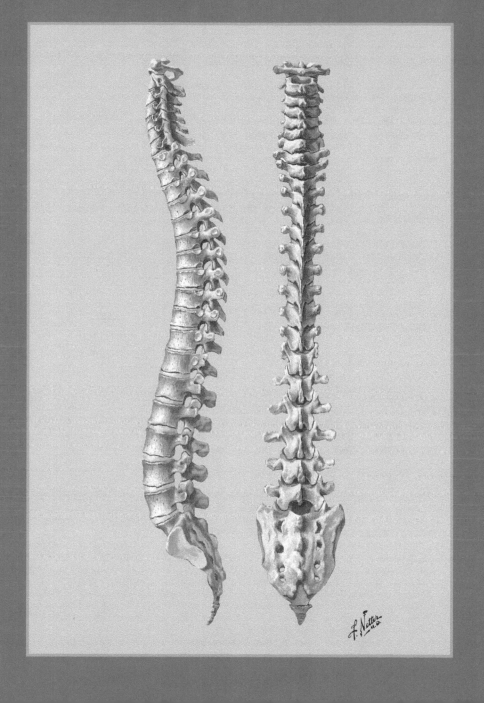

CHAPTER 54

EVALUATION OF THE SPINE TRAUMA PATIENT

Vincent J. Devlin, MD

1. **How many traumatic spinal column and spinal cord injuries occur in the United States each year?**
   It is estimated that over 50,000 traumatic spinal column fractures occur per year in the United States. (1) According to the National Spinal Cord Injury Statistical Center, 17,730 new cases of spinal cord injury occur each year in the United States. This equates to approximately 54 cases per million population annually. Neurologic injury occurs in approximately 25% of all spine fractures but in up to 40% of cervical fractures. There are two peaks of injury with a first peak occurring in young men aged between 15 and 29, and a second peak occurring in adults over age 65 years. The average age of spinal cord injury in the United States during 2015–2018 was 42.9 years, which is consistent with a slow steady increase in the average age of patients sustaining spinal cord injuries.

2. **What is the distribution of spinal injuries according to spinal region?**
   It is estimated that 20% of spinal injuries occur in the cervical region, 30% in the thoracic region, and 50% in the lumbar and sacral region. More than 15% of patients with traumatic spines fracture have a second, noncontiguous vertebral column fracture. (2, 3)

3. **What are the most common causes of spinal cord injury?**
   The leading causes of spinal cord injury are:
   - Vehicular accidents (39.3%)
   - Falls (31.8%)
   - Acts of violence, including gunshot wounds and stabbings (13.5%)
   - Sport-related injuries (8%)
   - Medical/surgical causes (4.3%)
   - Miscellaneous causes (3.1%)

4. **What is the distribution of spinal cord injuries according to neurologic level and extent of neurologic involvement?**
   The distribution of spinal cord injuries by neurologic level and extent of involvement is:
   - Incomplete tetraplegia: 47.2%
   - Incomplete paraplegia: 20.4%
   - Complete paraplegic: 20.2%
   - Complete tetraplegic: 11.5%
     Less than 1% of persons with an initial spinal cord injury experience complete neurologic recovery by the time of hospital discharge.

5. **Summarize the key principles that guide the initial evaluation and management of a trauma patient with a potential spine injury.**
   - Patients are triaged according to treatment needs and available resources. Initial assessment includes a rapid primary survey, resuscitation, detailed secondary survey, and initiation of definitive care in accordance with Advanced Trauma Life Support (ATLS) principles (American College of Surgeons, The Committee on Trauma).
   - All trauma patients are assumed to have a spine injury until proven otherwise
   - The injured patient should be immobilized at the accident scene with a rigid cervical collar supplemented with lateral bolsters and straps secured to a long spine board to immobilize the entire spine. Pediatric patients less than 8 years of age require immobilization on a backboard with an occipital recess or placement of a pad underneath the torso to maintain neutral neck position and avoid neck flexion due to their larger head to body ratio. Special precautions are necessary in patients with ankylosed spines such as those with ankylosing spondylitis or diffuse idiopathic skeletal hyperostosis (DISH) as they are at risk of neurologic deterioration with supine positioning on a rigid spine board or placement of a cervical collar and should be splinted in the position of injury with pillows.
   - The cervical spine should remain immobilized and the spine protected by maintaining strict log-roll precautions until spinal injury is ruled out.

- Long backboards should be used only during patient transportation, and should be removed promptly following arrival at the hospital.

6. **What are the components of the primary survey?**
The primary survey is performed simultaneously with resuscitation and includes the "A, B, C, D, Es" of trauma care:
A: Airway maintenance while taking care to protect the cervical spine
B: Breathing and ventilation
C: Circulation and control of hemorrhage
D: Disability assessment including a brief evaluation of neurologic status and Glasgow Coma Scale (GCS)
E: Exposure and environmental control, which includes fully exposing the patient and measures to prevent hypothermia.

7. **What are the components of the Glasgow Coma Scale?**
The GCS is a 15-point scale to assess traumatic brain injury and impaired consciousness. It is comprised of three components that rate the stimulus intensity required for an eye-opening response (E), verbal response (V), and motor response (M). A final score results from the sum of each of the three components and the injury is categorized based on this score as mild (13–15), moderate (9–12), or severe (3–8) (Table 54.1).

Table 54.1 Glasgow Coma Scale.

Eye Opening Response		Verbal Response		Motor Response	
SCORE	RESPONSE	SCORE	RESPONSE	SCORE	RESPONSE
4	Spontaneous	5	Oriented	6	Obeys commands
3	To voice	4	Confused	5	Localizes
2	To pain	3	Inappropriate	4	Normal flexion withdrawal
1	None	2	Incomprehensible	3	Abnormal flexion
		1	None	2	Extension
				1	None

8. **Distinguish between hemorrhagic shock, neurogenic shock, and spinal shock.**
Hemorrhagic shock is the most common cause of posttraumatic shock. Early recognition and treatment of intravascular volume loss is critical. An injured patient with tachycardia who is cool to touch is presumed in shock. As compensatory mechanisms maintain blood pressure until blood loss exceeds 30% of circulating blood volume, hypotension is an insensitive indicator of shock. Additional early clinical manifestations of hemorrhagic shock include tachypnea, weak peripheral pulses, pale or mottled skin, narrow pulse pressure, anxiety, and decreased urine output.
Neurogenic shock results from disruption of the descending sympathetic tracts after spinal cord injuries above the T6. Loss of sympathetic tone causes vasodilation and blood pooling leading to hypotension, bradycardia, preserved urine output, and warm extremities. Neurogenic shock should be considered only after hemorrhagic shock has been ruled out. Fluid resuscitation should be utilized judiciously, and vasopressors should be used to maintain mean arterial pressure >85 mm Hg to optimize spinal cord perfusion.
Spinal shock is a temporary depolarization of the spinal cord below the level of an injury. Spinal shock is characterized by the loss of reflexes, bladder function, and flaccid paralysis below the level of a spinal cord injury. Loss of sympathetic outflow results in hypotension and bradycardia. Although spinal shock may last for days or weeks, duration is often less than 72 hours depending on the criteria used to define resolution of spinal shock. Recovery from spinal shock occurs in four phases: areflexia or hyporeflexia, initial reflex return, early hyperreflexia, and spasticity. The end of spinal shock is commonly defined as the return of the bulbocavernosus reflex, which is mediated by the S1–S3 nerve roots and elicited by gently pulling on a Foley catheter or squeezing the glans penis or clitoris and assessing for contraction of the external anal sphincter.

9. **What are some of the key elements assessed in a patient with a suspected spinal injury during the secondary trauma survey?**
History: Information regarding allergies, current medications, past illnesses/pregnancy, last meal, and events/environment related to the injury (mnemonic is "AMPLE") is recorded. Specific questions are directed toward the mechanism of injury, location and time of injury, presence and location of pain, whether loss of consciousness occurred, and any occurrences of transient or persistent neurologic symptoms and previously known spinal conditions such as ankylosing spondylitis, prior spine surgery, or congenital anomalies.
Physical examination: The patient is log-rolled with assistance to inspect and palpate the posterior spine from skull to coccyx looking for tenderness, spinous process step-off, bruising, fluid collections, or abrasions. Suspicion of a

spinal injury is increased in the presence of concomitant head, neck, or facial injuries (cervical injury), lap or seat belt injuries (thoracolumbar flexion-distraction injury), or pelvic fractures (lumbosacral injury). The back portion of the cervical collar is temporarily removed, while the neck is stabilized by an assistant to allow assessment of the posterior cervical spine. A detailed **neurologic assessment** is performed and includes the following elements:

- Motor evaluation (grade as 0–5 in key upper and lower extremity muscle groups)
- Sensory assessment (pinprick, light touch)
- Reflex assessment (deep tendon reflexes, bulbocavernosus reflex, clonus, Babinski)
- Rectal examination (perianal sensation for pinprick and light touch, deep anal pressure, maximal voluntary anal sphincter contractility, perianal wink reflex)

10. Distinguish between skeletal and neurologic level of injury in the assessment of a person with a traumatic spinal cord injury?

The **skeletal level of injury** is defined as the level in the spine where the greatest vertebral damage is found on radiographic examination. The **neurologic level of injury** is defined as the most caudal segment of the spinal cord with normal sensory function and antigravity (grade 3 or more) motor function bilaterally, provided that sensory and motor function proximal to this segment is intact.

11. How is the neurologic status of a patient described following a spinal column injury? Patients are stratified into the following categories:

Complete spinal cord injury. Defined as the total absence of sensory and motor function below the anatomic level of injury in the absence of spinal shock. In a complete spinal injury there is no sensory or motor function present in the lowest sacral segment, S4–S5 (i.e., no light touch or pinprick sensation near the anal mucocutaneous junction, no deep anal pressure sensation during digital rectal examination, and no voluntary contraction of the external anal sphincter during digital rectal exam).

Incomplete spinal cord injury. Present when residual spinal cord and/or nerve root function exists below the anatomic level of injury, including partial preservation of sensory and/or motor function at S4–S5 (termed "sacral sparing"). Incomplete neurologic injuries are broadly classified by pattern of neurologic deficit into one of several syndromes: (A) cruciate paralysis, (B) central cord syndrome, (C) anterior cord syndrome, (D) Brown-Séquard syndrome, (E) posterior cord syndrome, and (F) conus medullaris syndrome.

Injuries involving one or more lumbar nerve roots. These injuries include: (A) cauda equina syndrome and (B) isolated lumbar nerve root injuries.

Neurologically intact. Patient is awake, alert, and demonstrates normal motor, sensory, reflex, bowel, and bladder function.

12. What is the ASIA Impairment Scale for assessment of the spinal cord-injured patient?

The American Spinal Injury Association (ASIA) Impairment Scale (AIS) is a five-grade scale used to identify the severity of a spinal cord injury:

A = **Complete:** No sensory or motor function is preserved in the sacral segments S4–S5

B = **Sensory Incomplete:** Sensory but not motor function is preserved below the neurologic level and includes the sacral segments S4–S5 (light touch or pinprick at S4–S5 or deep anal pressure sensation) AND no motor function is preserved more than three levels below the motor level on either side of the body and no voluntary anal sphincter contraction is present.

C = **Motor Incomplete:** Motor function is preserved at the most caudal sacral segments for voluntary anal contraction OR the patient meets the criteria for sensory incomplete status (i.e., light touch or pinprick at S4–S5 or deep anal pressure sensation is present) and has some sparing of motor function more than three levels below the ipsilateral motor level on either side of the body and more than half of key muscles below the neurologic level have a muscle grade less than 3. This includes key or non-key muscle functions to determine motor incomplete status.

D = **Motor Incomplete:** Motor incomplete status as defined above and at least half of key muscles below the single neurologic level of injury have a muscle grade 3 or greater.

E = **Normal:** Sensory and motor function are normal in a patient with prior deficit. Someone without an initial spinal cord injury does not receive an AIS grade.

13. Outline the steps involved in determining the classification of a patient with a spinal cord injury according to the International Standards for Neurological Classification of Spinal Cord Injury.

See Fig. 54.1A,B.

14. Briefly explain the common injury mechanisms and clinical presentations of the various types of incomplete spinal cord and nerve root injury syndromes.

Central cord syndrome is the most common incomplete spinal cord injury syndrome. It is often seen in elderly patients with preexisting cervical stenosis who sustain a hyperextension injury. Patients present with tetraparesis with bilateral sensory and motor deficits more severe in the upper extremities than the lower extremities, and greater dysfunction in the distal extremities compared with proximally. Lower extremity hyperreflexia, sacral

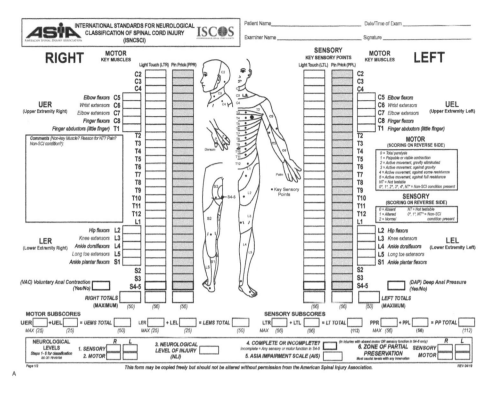

A

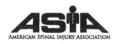

Fig. 54.1 (A and B): International Standards for Neurological Classification of Spinal Cord Injury (ISNCSCI)—American Spinal Injury Association (ASIA) Worksheet 2019. (© 2019 American Spinal Injury Association. Reprinted with permission.)

sparing, and variable bowel and bladder involvement are noted. The prognosis is variable, with return of bowel and bladder function, ambulation, and improvement in hand function, in approximately 50% of patients.

Brown-Séquard syndrome is caused by a hemisection of the spinal cord. The clinical presentation includes ipsilateral motor and proprioception loss with contralateral pain and temperature sensation loss distal to the level of injury. The prognosis for recovery is good, with most patients recovering some degree of ambulatory capacity and bowel and bladder function. Injury mechanisms include penetrating injuries, missile wounds, unilateral laminar or pedicle fractures, and rotational injuries with subluxations.

Anterior cord syndrome results from compression of the anterior cord and/or anterior spinal artery by bone or disc or as the result of vascular ischemia. Typically, neural function is absent in the anterior two-thirds of the spinal cord. Findings include complete loss of motor function and pain and temperature sensation distal to the site of injury and sparing of dorsal column function with preservation of vibration and proprioception. Common etiologies include vertebral body fractures associated with retropulsed bone or disc or intraoperative hypotension during procedures in patients with cervical myelopathy. The prognosis for recovery is poor.

Posterior cord syndrome presents with loss of discriminative touch, as well as position and vibratory sense, but preservation of motor function and other sensory functions. This syndrome is uncommon but may occur in association with an extension injury mechanism. Other potential causes include vitamin B12 deficiency and syphilis.

Conus medullaris syndrome may result due to injury of the T12–L2 vertebrae associated with damage to the sacral segments of the spinal cord located in the conus medullaris, which typically results in an areflexic bowel and bladder, saddle anesthesia, lower extremity sensory loss, and incomplete paraplegia. It has been noted that lower extremity muscle weakness and sensory loss is symmetrical in most cases.

Cauda equina syndrome may result due to injury of the L3–L5 vertebrae associated with damage to lumbosacral nerve roots within the neural canal, which results in variable lower extremity motor and sensory function, bowel and bladder dysfunction, and saddle anesthesia. It has been noted that lower extremity muscle weakness and sensory loss is often asymmetrical.

15. What is spine clearance?

Spine clearance is the process of accurately confirming the absence of a spine injury. Following blunt trauma, patients are assumed to have a spine injury and are immobilized until clearance is performed.

16. What are the NEXUS Criteria and Canadian C-Spine Rule?

The National Emergency X-Radiography Utilization Study (NEXUS) Low-Risk Criteria and The Canadian C-Spine Rule (CCR) are decision rules used to guide clinical clearance and the need for cervical spine radiography in low-risk, awake, alert, symptomatic patients following a blunt traumatic injury.

According to the **NEXUS Criteria**, patients with a suspected cervical spine injury can be clinically cleared and do not require radiographs if they exhibit all of the following criteria:
1. No posterior midline cervical spine tenderness
2. No evidence of intoxication
3. Normal level of alertness
4. No focal neurologic deficit
5. No painful distracting injuries

Addition of a functional evaluation of cervical range of motion to the NEXUS criteria has been recommended to further improve its accuracy.

According to the **CCR,** a patient with a suspected cervical spine injury can be clinically cleared if they are alert (GCS 15), not intoxicated, and do not have a distracting injury, and meet the following criteria:
1. The patient does not have high-risk factors that mandate radiography (age >65 years or dangerous injury mechanism or paresthesias in extremities).
2. A low-risk factor that allows safe assessment of range of motion exists (simple rear-end motor vehicle collision, seated position in the emergency department, ambulation at any time posttrauma, delayed onset of neck pain, and the absence of midline cervical spine tenderness).
3. The patient is able to actively rotate their neck 45° left and right.

Cervical spine clearance in pediatric patients following blunt trauma is especially challenging due to a variety of factors, including the unique injury patterns in the immature spine and the increased lifetime risks for cancer related to radiation exposure, and has recently been addressed through a consensus statement and algorithm published by the Pediatric Cervical Spine Clearance Working Group. (4)

17. Describe the current recommended approach to clearance of the cervical spine following blunt trauma in an adult patient.

Following initial clinical examination, the cervical clearance process is initiated by assigning the patient to one of four groups:
1. **Asymptomatic** (i.e., alert, oriented, absent cervical pain/midline tenderness, normal neurologic examination, no intoxication, no distracting injuries). These patients may be cleared based on clinical assessment without obtaining imaging studies based on NEXUS criteria or the CCR.

2. **Temporarily unable to assess** (i.e., presence of intoxication or distracting injuries that impair clinical examination and that are expected to improve over 24–48 hours). These patients are initially immobilized in a cervical collar. Reevaluation at 24–48 hours may permit patient clearance based on clinical criteria if the patient is assessable and asymptomatic. Alternatively, if the patient is assessable and symptomatic, the protocol for symptomatic patients is followed. If the patient cannot be assessed clinically, the patient should remain immobilized in a collar and is evaluated according to the protocol for an obtunded patient.

3. **Symptomatic** (i.e., presence of pain, tenderness, neurologic symptoms). Such patients are maintained in a cervical collar until spinal imaging studies are obtained. Multidetector computed tomography (CT) has replaced plain radiography in the initial evaluation of the adult trauma patient. Magnetic resonance imaging (MRI) is performed as an adjunctive study in patients with neurologic injury, suspected ligamentous injury, potential disc herniations associated with facet injuries, and for assessment prior to surgery, but not as a primary modality for clearance due to its high false-positive rate.

4. **Obtunded**. No consensus exists regarding an optimal clearance protocol. At a minimum, an obtunded trauma patient requires a cervical CT scan. Evidence supports cervical clearance based on a negative CT alone. Others recommend a combination of CT and MRI for clearance as MRI has been shown to identify clinically important injuries in patients following a negative CT finding.

18. Describe the recommended approach to clearance of the thoracic and lumbar spine in an adult patient following blunt trauma.
Following blunt trauma, an awake, alert patient without back pain or tenderness may be excluded from thoracolumbar injury based on clinical assessment without radiographic evaluation in the absence of a high-energy injury mechanism, a distracting injury, or another spine fracture. CT is the first choice imaging modality for evaluation of traumatic spinal injuries and should include review of sagittal and coronal reformatted images. If a spine injury is identified, the entire spine requires radiographic imaging. Standard chest, abdomen, and pelvic CT scans obtained during the initial trauma workup provide adequate visualization of the spine and obviate the need for a dedicated CT to specifically evaluate the spinal column. Patients with back pain or tenderness, neurologic deficit, altered mental status, distracting injuries, or high-energy injury mechanisms require imaging of the spine with CT. Plain radiography is not sufficiently sensitive for use in screening the thoracic and lumbar spine. MRI is not indicated for use in screening but plays an important role in the subsequent evaluation of patients, including those with abnormalities identified on CT, patients with neurologic symptoms, and for evaluation of ligamentous disruption.

19. What is the role of cervical traction in the acute management of patients with cervical spine injuries?
Skeletal traction with either tongs or a halo ring is commonly used to provide initial temporary stabilization of the spine as a bridging measure until definitive care is performed. Cervical traction also plays a role in the initial treatment of patients with a wide range of cervical injuries, including displaced odontoid fractures, select C2 hangman's fractures, facet dislocations, and cervical fractures with displacement.
Emergent closed reduction is considered in patients with cervical canal compromise and a neurologic deficit, especially spinal cord injuries. Common fractures requiring immediate reduction include burst fractures and facet dislocations. If the patient is alert and neurologic status can be assessed clinically, traction reduction can commence without MRI. If the patient is obtunded or uncooperative, MRI is obtained prior to proceeding with closed reduction. Contraindications to closed reduction using skull traction include patients with skull fractures, distraction injuries (e.g., atlantoaxial dislocations), and concomitant subaxial and upper cervical injuries (e.g., odontoid fracture).

20. In a patient with a traumatic spinal cord injury, what medical treatments have proven beneficial?
Initial resuscitation to raise and maintain blood pressure to a mean arterial blood pressure of 85 mm Hg is beneficial to the injured spinal cord. In an acute spinal cord injured-patient, this usually requires the addition of pressor agents. Hypoxemia must be avoided. Supplemental oxygen is routinely administered, and ventilatory support is utilized as indicated. The use of neuroprotective agents such as methylprednisolone has been controversial. Current guidelines suggest offering a 24-hour infusion of high-dose methylprednisolone sodium succinate (MPSS) to adult patients within 8 hours of an acute spinal cord injury, but not to those patients who present after 8 hours. In addition, it is suggested not offering a 48-hour infusion of high-dose MPSS to adult patients with acute spinal cord injury. (5)

21. What factors are considered when selecting the best treatment approach for a specific spine injury?
Factors considered in treatment decision making regarding nonoperative versus operative treatment for spine injuries include injury location, spinal stability, the necessity for surgical decompression of the neural elements, and specific patient characteristics and comorbidities.

KEY POINTS

1. Patients with high-energy injury mechanisms or altered mental status should be assumed to have sustained a significant spinal injury and undergo immediate spinal immobilization during extrication, transport, and initial evaluation.
2. The potentially spinal-injured patient is assessed according to Advanced Trauma Life Support (ATLS) protocols.
3. Patients with neurologic injury are assessed according to the Standards for Neurologic Classification established by the American Spinal Injury Association (ASIA).
4. Hypotension and hypoxemia require aggressive treatment in the spinal cord-injured patient.
5. The clinical syndromes resulting from spinal cord injury depend on the level of injury and the anatomic tracts involved by the injury.

Websites
1. ASIA e-Learning Center: https://asia-spinalinjury.org/learning/
2. Landmark papers in trauma and acute care surgery. Eastern Association for the Surgery of Trauma: https://www.east.org/education/publications/landmark-papers-in-trauma-and-acute-care-surgery
3. The International Standards for Neurological Classification of Spinal Cord Injury (ISNCSCI)—American Spinal Injury Association (ASIA) Worksheet: https://asia-spinalinjury.org/wp-content/uploads/2019/04/ASIA-ISCOS-IntlWorksheet_2019.pdf
4. National Spinal Cord Injury Statistical Center: https://www.nscisc.uab.edu/
5. The Burden of Musculoskeletal Diseases in the United States: Traumatic Spine Fractures: https://www.boneandjointburden.org/2014-report/iiia12/traumatic-spine-fractures

---

REFERENCES

1. Ju KL, Harris MB. Chapter 10: Initial evaluation of the spine in trauma patients. In: Browner BD, Jupiter JB, Krettek C, editors. Skeletal Trauma: Basic Science, Management, and Reconstruction. 5th ed. Philadelphia, PA: Saunders; 2015, pp. 303–314.
2. Henderson RL, Reid DC, Saboe LA. Multiple noncontiguous spine fractures. *Spine* 1991;16:128–131.
3. Hu R, Mustard CA, Burns C. Epidemiology of incident spinal fracture in a complete population. *Spine* 1996;21:492–499.
4. Herman MJ, Brown KO, Sponseller PD, et al. Pediatric cervical spine clearance: A consensus statement and algorithm from the Pediatric Cervical Spine Clearance Working Group. *J Bone Joint Surg* 2019;101:e1.
5. Fehlings MG, Wilson JR, Tetreault LA, et al. A clinical practice guideline for the management of patients with acute spinal cord in-jury: Recommendations on the use of methylprednisolone sodium succinate. *Global Spine J* 2017;7:203–211.

BIBLIOGRAPHY

1. Henry S. Advanced Trauma Life Support Student Course Manual. 10th ed. Chicago: American College of Surgeons.
2. Ditunno JF, Little JW, Tessler A, et al. Spinal shock revisited: A four-phase model. *Spinal Cord* 2004;42:383–395.
3. Dvorak MF, Noonan VK, Fallah N, et al. The influence of time from injury to surgery on motor recovery and length of hospital stay in acute traumatic spinal cord injury: An observational Canadian cohort study. *J Neurotr* 2015;32:645–654.
4. Fehlings MG, Wilson JR, Tetreault LA, et al. A clinical practice guideline for the management of patients with acute spinal cord in-jury: Recommendations on the use of methylprednisolone sodium succinate. *Global Spine J* 2017;7:203–211.
5. Henderson RL, Reid DC, Saboe LA. Multiple noncontiguous spine fractures. *Spine* 1991;16:128–131.
6. Herman MJ, Brown KO, Sponseller PD, et al. Pediatric cervical spine clearance: A consensus statement and algorithm from the Pediatric Cervical Spine Clearance Working Group. *J Bone Joint Surg* 2019;101:e1.
7. Hu R, Mustard CA, Burns C. Epidemiology of incident spinal fracture in a complete population. *Spine* 1996;21:492–499.
8. Ju KL, Harris MB. Chapter 10: Initial evaluation of the spine in trauma patients. In: Browner BD, Jupiter JB, Krettek C, editors. Skeletal Trauma: Basic Science, Management, and Reconstruction. 5th ed. Philadelphia, PA: Saunders; 2015, pp. 303–314.
9. Peetz AB, Salim A. Clearance of the spine. *Curr Trauma Rep* 2015;1:160–168.
10. Schoenfeld AJ, Beck AW, Harris MB, et al. Evaluating the cervical spine in the blunt trauma patient. *J Am Acad Orthop Surg* 2019;27:633–641.

CHAPTER 55

SPINAL CORD INJURY

Vincent Huang, MD and Thomas N. Bryce, MD

1. **Which of the following terms are currently favored to describe impairment or loss of motor and/or sensory function due to damage of neural elements within the spinal canal: (1) tetra-plegia, (2) paraplegia, (3) quadriplegia, (4) quadriparesis, and/or (5) paraparesis?**
   Tetraplegia refers to the impairments resulting from damage to neural elements within the cervical spinal canal, whereas **paraplegia** refers to the impairments resulting from damage to neural elements within the thoracic, lumbar, or sacral spinal canal. As *tetra*, *para*, and *plegia* are of Greek origin and *quadri* is of Latin origin, to maintain uniformity in word root origins, tetraplegia is preferred over quadriplegia. Because the American Spinal Injury Association (ASIA) Impairment Scale (or AIS) more precisely defines incomplete tetraplegia and paraplegia (see Question 7) than the terms quadriparesis and paraparesis; the use of the latter terms is discouraged.

2. **What is the difference between a skeletal level and a neurologic level of injury in assessing a person with a traumatic spinal cord injury?**
   - The **skeletal level of injury** is defined as the level in the spine where the greatest vertebral damage is found on radiographic examination.
   - The **neurologic level of injury** (NLI) is defined as the most caudal segment of the spinal cord with normal sensory function and antigravity (grade 3 or more) motor function bilaterally, provided there is intact sensory and motor function proximal to this segment.

3. **How are the sensory and motor components assessed in the determination of a neurologic level of spinal cord injury?**
   Sensory and motor functions are assessed according to the *International Standards for Neurological Classification of Spinal Cord Injury (ISNCSCI)*:
   - **Sensory component**: Light touch and pinprick sensation are tested for each dermatome and graded on a three-point scale:
   Light touch:
   - 0 = Absent
   - 1 = Impaired (partial or altered appreciation, including hyperesthesia)
   - 2 = Normal
   Pinprick:
   - 0 = Absent or inability to distinguish sharp/dull
   - 1 = Impaired (partial or altered appreciation, including hyperesthesia) and can reliably distinguish sharp/dull 80% of the time
   - 2 = Normal
   The **sensory level** is the most caudal dermatome where both light touch and pinprick are normal and where all rostral dermatomes are also normal
   - **Motor component**: A key muscle is tested from each myotome in a rostral-caudal sequence by manual muscle test and graded on a six-point scale:
   - 0 = Total paralysis, no palpable or visible contraction
   - 1 = Palpable or visible contraction
   - 2 = Active movement, full range of motion (ROM) with gravity eliminated
   - 3 = Active movement, full ROM against gravity only
   - 4 = Active movement, full ROM against resistance
   - 5 = Normal
   The **motor level** is the most caudal muscle having grade 3 or better strength where all muscles above are grade 5. If the level of injury is at a site where there is no key muscle (e.g., C2–C4, T2–L1, S2–S4/5), the motor level is defined by the sensory level.

4. **Identify the key muscles that are tested in determining the motor level.**
   Upper extremities:
   - C5 = Elbow flexors (biceps, brachialis)
   - C6 = Wrist extensors (extensor carpi radialis longus and brevis)
   - C7 = Elbow extensors (triceps)
   - C8 = Finger flexors (flexor digitorum profundus) to the middle finger
   - T1 = Small finger abductors (abductor digiti minimi)

Lower extremities:
  L2 = Hip flexors (iliopsoas)
  L3 = Knee extensors (quadriceps)
  L4 = Ankle dorsiflexors (tibialis anterior)
  L5 = Long toe extensors (extensor hallucis longus)
  S1 = Ankle plantar flexors (gastrocnemius, soleus)

5. Identify the key point for each sensory dermatome that is tested in determining the sensory level.
  C2 = Occipital protuberance
  C3 = Supraclavicular fossa
  C4 = Top of acromioclavicular joint
  C5 = Lateral side of antecubital fossa
  C6 = Thumb
  C7 = Middle finger
  C8 = Little finger
  T1 = Medial (ulnar) side of antecubital fossa
  T2 = Apex of the axilla
  T3 = Third intercostal space (IS)
  T4 = Fourth IS (nipple line)
  T5 = Fifth IS (midway between T4 and T6)
  T6 = Sixth IS (level of xiphisternum)
  T7 = Seventh IS (midway between T6 and T8)
  T8 = Eighth IS (midway between T6 and T10)
  T9 = Ninth IS (midway between T8 and T10)
  T10 = Tenth IS (umbilicus)
  T11 = Eleventh IS (midway between T10 and T12)
  T12 = Inguinal ligament at mid-point
  L1 = Half the distance between T12 and L2
  L2 = Mid-anterior thigh
  L3 = Medial femoral condyle
  L4 = Medial malleolus
  L5 = Dorsum of the foot at the third metatarsal phalangeal joint
  S1 = Lateral heel
  S2 = Popliteal fossa in the midline
  S3 = Ischial tuberosity
  S4–S5 = Perianal area (taken as one level)

6. What is the difference between a complete and an incomplete spinal cord injury?
   - **Complete spinal cord injury** is defined by the total absence of sensory and motor function below the anatomic level of injury in the absence of spinal shock. Recovery from spinal shock typically occurs within 48 hours following an acute spine injury. In a complete spinal injury there is no sensory or motor function present in the lowest sacral segment, S4–S5 (i.e., no light touch or pin prick sensation near the anal mucocutaneous junction, no deep anal pressure sensation during digital rectal examination, and no voluntary contraction of the external anal sphincter during digital rectal examination).
   - **Incomplete spinal cord injury** is present when residual spinal cord and/or nerve root function exists below the anatomic level of injury, including partial preservation of sensory and/or motor function at S4–S5 (termed "sacral sparing"). Incomplete neurologic injuries are broadly classified by pattern of neurologic deficit into one of several syndromes, which is helpful in determining prognosis.

7. How is the severity of a spinal cord injury classified?
   The AIS, a component of the ISNCSCI, is a five-point scale (A, B, C, D, E) used to specify the severity of injury. It includes definitions of complete and incomplete injuries.
   - A = Complete: No sensory or motor function is preserved in the sacral segments S4–S5.
   - B = Sensory Incomplete: Sensory but not motor function is preserved below the neurologic level and includes the sacral segments S4–S5 (light touch or pin prick at S4–S5 or deep anal pressure sensation) AND no motor function is preserved more than three levels below the motor level on either side of the body, and no voluntary anal sphincter contraction is present.
   - C = Motor Incomplete: Motor function is preserved at the most caudal sacral segments for voluntary anal contraction OR the patient meets the criteria for sensory incomplete status (i.e., light touch or pin prick at S4–S5 or deep anal pressure sensation is present) and has some sparing of motor function more than three levels below the ipsilateral motor level on either side of the body and more than half of key muscles below the neurologic level have a muscle grade less than 3. This includes key or non-key muscle functions to determine motor incomplete status.

- D = Motor Incomplete: Motor incomplete status as defined above and at least half of key muscles below the neurologic level have a muscle grade 3 or greater.
- E = Normal: Sensory and motor function are normal in a patient with prior deficit. Someone without an initial spinal cord injury does not receive an AIS grade.

8. Identify and describe six different patterns of incomplete neurologic injury that may be present following a traumatic spinal injury.
   - **Cruciate paralysis**: damage to the anterior spinal cord at the C2 level (level of corticospinal tract decussation) with greater loss of motor function in upper compared with lower extremities, variable sensory loss, and variable cranial nerve deficits.
   - **Central cord syndrome**: damage to the central spinal cord below the C2 level with greater loss of motor function in upper extremities (especially in the hands) compared with lower extremities with variable sensory loss, at least partial sacral sparing, and variable bowel and bladder involvement.
   - **Anterior cord syndrome**: damage to the anterior spinal cord with relative preservation of proprioception and variable loss of pain sensation, temperature sensation, and motor function.
   - **Brown-Séquard syndrome**: damage to the lateral half of the spinal cord with relative ipsilateral proprioception and motor function loss and contralateral pain and temperature sensation loss.
   - **Conus medullaris syndrome**: damage to the sacral segments of the spinal cord located in the conus medullaris, which typically results in an areflexic bowel and bladder, lower extremity sensory loss, and incomplete paraplegia.
   - **Cauda equina syndrome**: damage to lumbosacral nerve roots within the neural canal results in variable lower extremity motor and sensory function, bowel and bladder dysfunction, and saddle anesthesia.

9. What is the current guideline for managing mean arterial pressure (MAP) following an acute spinal cord injury?
   The pathophysiology of acute spinal cord injury involves both primary and secondary injury mechanisms.
   - **Primary injury** to the spinal cord results from mechanical forces applied to the spinal column at the time of injury and is not correctable.
   - **Secondary injury** to uninvolved neurologic tissue in the vicinity of the primary injury may occur due to a variety of mechanisms and can potentially be modified via blood pressure augmentation with volume support and vasopressors. Hypotension and diminished spinal cord perfusion may contribute to secondary injury and exacerbate central nervous system injury.

   Current recommendations, according to the guidelines of the American Association of Neurological Surgeons/Congress of Neurological Surgeons Joint Section of Spine and Peripheral Nerves, advise correcting hypotension and maintaining a MAP goal of 85–90 mmHg for the first 7 days after spinal cord injury.

10. What is the difference between neurogenic shock and spinal shock?
    See Table 55.1.

11. Identify six complications of spinal cord injury that may manifest within the first 2 days after injury.
    Hypotension, bradycardia, hypothermia, hypoventilation, gastrointestinal bleeding, and ileus.

12. What causes hypotension, bradycardia, and hypothermia?
    Acute cervical or upper thoracic spinal cord injuries are associated with a functional total sympathectomy with resultant loss of vasoconstrictor tone in the trunk and extremities and loss of beta-adrenergic cardiostimulation, leading to a clinical picture of hypotension with paradoxical bradycardia. The loss of sympathetic tone also leads to an inability to regulate body temperature. After it is clearly established that no visceral or extremity injury is causing occult hemorrhage and blood loss, hypotension is best treated with sympathomimetic agents (e.g., dopamine).

Table 55.1 Neurogenic and Spinal Shock.

NEUROGENIC SHOCK	SPINAL SHOCK
• Severe hypotension and bradycardia following spinal cord injury • Due to disruption of the supraspinal control immediately following injury and loss of sympathetic tone to the smooth muscle of the blood vessels and imbalance in autonomic control • Requires vasopressive therapy, is associated with the severity of the spinal cord injury, and can last up to 5 weeks postinjury	• Temporary loss of motor and sensory reflexes following spinal cord injury • Reflexes in spinal cord caudal to the spinal cord injury are depressed (hyporeflexia) or absent (areflexia) • Reflexes rostral to the spinal cord injury remain unaffected • Lasts days to months

13. **What causes hypoventilation?**

The innervation to the diaphragm, the major muscle responsible for inspiration, is C3–C5 ("3, 4, 5 keeps you alive"). The innervation to the internal intercostals and the abdominal muscles, the major muscles responsible for forced expiration (e.g., cough) are local thoracic and abdominal segmental nerves. Thus a cervical or thoracic spinal cord injury can affect inspiration, cough, or both, depending on the level of injury. Patients with a C1–C2 complete SCI have no volitional diaphragmatic function and require mechanical ventilation or placement of a diaphragm/phrenic pacer. Patients with a C3–C4 complete spinal cord injury have severe diaphragmatic weakness and commonly require mechanical ventilation, at least temporarily. Patients with C5–T1 complete spinal cord injury are usually able to maintain independent breathing but remain at high risk for pulmonary complications due to loss of innervation to the intercostal and abdominal muscles.

Pneumonia is the most common cause of early death in persons with tetraplegia and is often related to aspiration of stomach or oropharyngeal contents, commonly occurring at or shortly after the initial injury. Atelectasis may result from hypoexpansion of the chest due to either pain or muscle weakness or to inadequate cough predisposing to inadequate clearing of secretions. Respiratory failure may develop immediately after spinal cord injury or over several days. Close monitoring of respiratory function is warranted in persons with cervical spinal cord injury during the first week after injury. See Table 55.2.

14. **What causes gastrointestinal bleeding/ulcer?**

Risk is increased with any physical or psychologic trauma. It is recommended to initiate peptic ulcer prophylaxis after traumatic SCI. Most peptic ulcers happen within the first 4 weeks, and prolonged use of proton pump inhibitors has been associated with increased rate of *Clostridium difficile* infections. Therefore, 4 weeks of peptic ulcer prophylaxis is indicated in most uncomplicated situations.

15. **What causes ileus?**

Adynamic (paralytic) ileus occurs after acute spinal cord injury in 8% of cases. Place a nasogastric tube for abdominal decompression if needed. After its resolution, usually within 2–3 days, a bowel routine of stool softeners, stimulant laxatives, and bowel evacuants is initiated to facilitate regularly timed evacuations of the bowel. Bowel distention and inadequate evacuation can lead to nausea and vomiting, high gastric residuals, anorexia, poor lung expansion, and inadequate venous return. Therefore, attention to bowel evacuation early after injury can prevent these complications.

16. **When should anticoagulant prophylaxis against venous thromboembolism (VTE) be started after spinal cord injury?**

Venous thromboembolism (VTE) is found in one-half to three-quarters of persons with traumatic spinal cord injury who are not receiving anticoagulant prophylaxis. The highest risk is within the first 2 weeks after spinal cord injury. Therefore, anticoagulant prophylaxis should be started as soon as hemostasis has been achieved, unless there is a contraindication. Low-molecular-weight heparin (LMWH) is the recommended anticoagulant for use after spinal cord injury. Use of subcutaneously administered unfractionated heparin has been shown to be inferior to LMWH for the prevention of VTE and should only be used if LMWH is unavailable or contraindicated. Direct oral anticoagulants (DOACs) may be considered for postacute thromboprophylaxis in patients with spinal cord injury. Mechanical compression devices have been shown to decrease the risk of VTE when used in conjunction with anticoagulant prophylaxis.

17. **When should anticoagulant VTE prophylaxis to prevent VTE in individuals with spinal cord injury be discontinued?**

The majority of VTE events occur during the first 2 weeks after spinal cord injury with a substantial decrease after 8 weeks after injury. Therefore, thromboprophylaxis is recommended for a minimum of 8 weeks after spinal cord injury. Factors to consider for initiating longer duration prophylaxis include motor complete spinal cord injury, lower extremity fractures, older age, previous VTE, cancer, and obesity.

Table 55.2 Respiratory Function and Spinal Injury.

INJURY LEVEL	RESPIRATORY SYSTEM CHANGES	MECHANICAL VENTILATION
Occiput–C2	(–) Diaphragm, (–) intercostals	Always needed
C3–C4	(+/–) Diaphragm, (–) intercostals	Often needed acutely
C5–T1	(+) Diaphragm, (–) intercostals	Only needed if there are associated pulmonary complications
T2–T12	(+) Diaphragm, (+/–) intercostals	Usually not needed

–, Loss of function; +, normal function.

18. When should a filter be placed?

A retrievable IVC filter should only be placed in spinal cord injured patients with an acute proximal deep vein thrombosis (DVT) and an absolute contraindication to therapeutic anticoagulation. In this circumstance, placement of a temporary inferior vena cava (IVC) filter is appropriate until the contraindication resolves.

19. What is orthostatic hypotension and what are potential physical and pharmacologic treatments?

Orthostatic hypotension (OH) is a decrease in systolic blood pressure of >20 mmHg and/or a decrease in diastolic pressure of >10 mmHg, when changing from the supine to an upright position. OH occurs due to a disruption of efferent sympathetic activity resulting in loss of vascular resistance with resultant accumulation of blood within the venous system and reduced return to the heart. Symptoms include light headedness, feeling faint, syncope, nausea, fatigue, pallor, perioral, and facial numbness and poor tolerance of an upright position. OH tends to improve gradually over time in the early rehabilitation period due to restoration of fluid balance, improved auto-regulation of cerebral circulation, improved sensitivity of baroreceptor walls, adaptation of the plasma renin-angiotensin system, and development of spasticity, which improves venous return. Initial physical treatment of OH includes: use of an elastic abdominal binder; use of lower limb compression stockings; changing the degree of upright positioning in a recliner or tilt-in-space wheelchair from near supine to fully upright as tolerated; and raising the head of the bed gradually before getting the patient out of bed. Pharmacologic treatments of OH include: salt tablets (1–2 grams two to three times daily before meals); fludrocortisone (synthetic corticosteroid with much greater mineralocorticoid than glucocorticoid potency; 0.1–0.2 mg once or twice per day); midodrine (alpha-1 receptor agonist; 5–20 mg one to three times per day); and droxidopa (synthetic amino acid analog that is directly metabolized to norepinephrine by dopa decarboxylase; 100–600 mg one to three times per day).

20. What are the signs and symptoms of autonomic dysreflexia?

Autonomic dysreflexia (AD) is a potentially dangerous clinical syndrome that develops in individuals with spinal cord injury at thoracic level T6 or above, resulting in acute uncontrolled hypertension. Common causes include bladder distension (e.g., due to a kinked or blocked catheter) or bowel distension (e.g., due to fecal impaction). Signs and symptoms of AD are:

- A sudden, significant increase in blood pressure, above the normal levels, frequently associated with bradycardia, although tachycardia may also occur. Systolic blood pressure elevations more than 15–20 mmHg above baseline may occur, and may reach over 200 mmHg.
- Pounding headache
- Profuse sweating above the level of the lesion
- Piloerection or goose bumps above the level of lesion
- Cardiac arrhythmias, atrial fibrillation, premature ventricular contractions, and atrioventricular conduction abnormalities
- Flushing of the skin above the level of lesion
- Blurred vision
- Appearance of spots in the visual fields
- Nasal congestion
- Feelings of apprehension or anxiety over an impending physical problem
- Minimal or no symptoms, despite a significantly elevated blood pressure (silent AD)

AD is due to an imbalance between the sympathetic and parasympathetic nervous systems in an individual with spinal cord injury at thoracic level T6 or above. In response to noxious stimuli, uninhibited sympathetic tone constricts the splanchnic vascular bed and results in elevated blood pressure. Descending inhibitory parasympathetic-mediated signals are unable to travel past the level of neurologic injury and mitigate the rise in blood pressure. Unopposed parasympathetic activity above the level of spinal cord injury is responsible for the occurrence of bradycardia, facial flushing, pupillary constriction, nasal congestion, and other related symptoms.

21. What is the management of autonomic dysreflexia?

Once diagnosed, the first step in the management of AD is to sit the patient up, if supine, and loosen any restrictive clothing. If the blood pressure remains elevated, the urinary system should be evaluated. If the blood pressure continues to be elevated after bladder distention has been ruled out, the lower bowels should be evaluated for fecal impaction, but only after systolic blood pressure is reduced to less than 150 mmHg, using antihypertensive medication if necessary. Medications, such as nitroglycerin paste (nitropaste), should be used only after the first three steps are taken. If the precipitating cause of AD has not yet been determined, check for less frequent causes. The patient may require admission to the hospital for monitoring in order to maintain pharmacologic control of the blood pressure and to investigate the cause.

22. How can incontinence of stool be prevented after spinal cord injury?

A neurogenic bowel after spinal cord injury affects mainly the colon and rectum distal to the splenic flexure and can be classified as an upper motor neuron (UMN) type if sacral reflexes are present (e.g., bulbocavernosus or anocutaneous) or lower motor neuron (LMN) type if these reflexes are absent. Institution of a bowel routine or daily timed evacuation of the colon can prevent incontinence by allowing predictable evacuations in nearly everyone with SCI.

During a UMN-type bowel routine, digital stimulation of the rectum triggers reflex evacuation of stool. This can be further facilitated by inserting an irritant suppository or mini-enema into the rectum and performing this routinely after a meal to take advantage of the gastrocolic reflex.

During a LMN-type bowel routine, digital evacuation of the rectum empties the rectum of stool. Stool-bulking agents or fiber are useful in maintaining an optimal consistency of stool, because water absorption is usually impaired within an areflexic colon. Oral irritant or osmotic laxatives given 8–12 hours before the routine may be necessary to help propel the stool through the colon to the distal portion where it can be evacuated.

23. **How should a neurogenic lower urinary tract dysfunction be initially managed after a spinal cord injury?**
An indwelling transurethral catheter (or suprapubic tube if indicated) should be placed as soon as feasible and should remain in place until the patient's fluid status has stabilized. Once stabilized and when medically appropriate, intermittent catheterization should be initiated for patients who have the potential to catheterize themselves to minimize the risk of catheter-associated urinary tract infection.

24. **Identify six interventions that can help prevent the development of pressure ulcers after acute spinal cord injury.**
    1. The length of time spent on a spine board should be minimized, and pressure relief should be provided every 30 minutes for patients maintained on the board.
    2. Patients in spinal traction should be immobilized on rotating kinetic beds.
    3. Patients must be turned from side to side (30°–45° from supine) every 2 hours around-the-clock while in bed to prevent prolonged pressure over bony prominences.
    4. All patients with sensory and motor impairments should be placed on pressure-reducing mattresses in the acute setting.
    5. Bowel and bladder incontinence should be managed with timed bowel evacuations and catheter drainage of the bladder.
    6. Shear pressure on the skin should be avoided by lifting rather than dragging immobile patients.

25. **Identify six reasons for transferring a patient with tetraplegia to a specialized spinal cord injury center.**
    • Overall survival rates increase
    • Complication rates (e.g., incidence of new pressure ulcers) decrease
    • Length of hospital stay decreases
    • Functional gains during rehabilitation are greater
    • Home discharge is more likely
    • Rehospitalization rates are lower

26. **What is the prognosis for neurologic recovery of a patient with a complete tetraplegia?**
Only **22%–30%** of patients who have an initial **AIS grade A convert to AIS B or better** by 1 year, with 8% converting to AIS grade C and 7% converting to grade D. However, 30%–80% of patients with motor complete tetraplegia recover a single motor level (gaining functional motor strength at that level) within 1 year of injury. The average spontaneous improvement in bilateral upper extremity motor score is 10 motor points. Regardless of initial cervical motor level, most individuals recover a similar number of motor points and levels.

A muscle with grade 1 or 2 strength at 1 month has a 90% chance of reaching grade 3 by 1 year, whereas a muscle with grade 0 strength has only a 25% chance to reach grade 3 or better by 1 year. The chance of functional recovery of a muscle two levels below the motor level of injury, when the first muscle below the motor level is grade 0, is exceedingly rare.

27. **What is the prognosis for neurologic recovery for patients with incomplete tetraplegia?**
Among patients who are initially **sensory incomplete** (AIS grade B), 34% remain unchanged with respect to AIS grade, 30% become AIS grade C, and 37% become AIS grade D by 1 year. Among sensory incomplete patients, the type of sensation preserved below the level of injury is prognostically important. Patients with preservation of perianal pinprick sensation have a greater than 70% chance of regaining ambulatory ability, whereas those who have spared light touch sensation only in the same region are unlikely to regain ambulatory ability.

Among patients with **motor incomplete** spinal cord injury, over 80% of those who are initially AIS grade C convert to AIS grade D or E by 1 year. Among those who are initially AIS grade D, 14% become AIS grade E by 1 year.

28. **What are the prognostic clinical predictors of ambulation for patients with traumatic spinal cord injury?**
Early prognostication of a patient's ability to walk at 1 year postinjury is possible using a simple clinical prediction rule based on age and four neurologic tests. This clinical model considers age ($<$ 65 vs. $\geq$ 65 years), motor scores of the quadriceps femoris (L3) and gastrocsoleus (S1) muscles, and light touch sensation of dermatomes L3 and S1 to accurately predict ambulation outcomes following traumatic spinal cord injury.
   Among patients with **motor incomplete spinal cord injury,** age and initial motor strength seem to be major determinants of ambulation. In one study of 105 patients with incomplete motor tetraplegia, in which age 50 was arbitrarily chosen as a cutoff, 91% of all patients younger than age 50 years, either AIS C or D, ambulated at 1 year; all persons older than 50 years and AIS D ambulated; while only 40% of patients older than 50 years and AIS C ambulated.

29. **What is the prognosis for neurologic recovery for patients with paraplegia?**
Among patients with **complete paraplegia,** 75% retain the same NLI at 1 year that they had at 1 month postinjury, 20% gain a single level, and 5% gain two neurologic levels. Patients with T1–T8 complete paraplegia do not recover lower limb voluntary movement. Fifteen percent of those with T9–T11 complete paraplegia recover some lower limb function, while 55% of patients with T12 or below complete paraplegia recover some lower limb function.
   Patients with **incomplete paraplegia** have the best prognosis for ambulation among all groups with traumatic spinal cord injury. Eighty percent of individuals with incomplete paraplegia regain functional hip flexion and knee extension within 1 year of injury, making both indoor and community-based ambulation possible.

30. **What typical lower extremity motor function is required for community ambulation?**
Typically, community ambulation requires bilateral grade 3 hip flexor strength and at least one knee with grade 3 knee extensor strength.

31. **Compare the expected patterns of muscular weakness for patients with C1–C3, C4, C5, C6, C7–C8, T1–T9, and T10–L1 neurologic levels.**
See Table 55.3.

32. **What is the expected functional outcome for eating, dressing, transfers, wheelchair propulsion, and ambulation for patients with C1–C3, C4, C5, C6, C7–C8, T1–T9, and T10–L1 neurologic levels?**
See Table 55.4.

33. **What is spasticity and what peripheral factors can cause an exacerbation of spasticity?**
Spasticity is a motor disorder characterized by a velocity-dependent increase in tonic stretch reflexes (muscle tone) with exaggerated tendon jerks, resulting from hyperexcitability of the stretch reflex as one component of the UMN syndrome. Peripheral factors that may exacerbate spasticity include heterotopic ossification, urolithiasis, urinary tract infections, stool impaction, pressure ulcers, fracture/dislocations, and ingrown toenails.

34. **Name six pathologic changes associated with late neurologic deterioration after spinal cord injury.**
   1. Posttraumatic cysts
   2. Delayed spinal deformity

Table 55.3 Patterns of Muscular Weakness Associated With Spinal Cord Injury.

INJURY LEVEL	PATTERN OF MUSCULAR WEAKNESS
C1–C3	Total paralysis of trunk, upper extremities, lower extremities; dependent on ventilator
C4	Paralysis of trunk, upper extremities, lower extremities; inability to cough, endurance and respiratory reserve low secondary to paralysis of intercostals
C5	Absence of elbow extension, pronation, all wrist and hand movement; total paralysis of trunk and lower extremities
C6	Absence of wrist flexion, elbow extension, hand movement; total paralysis of trunk and lower extremities
C7–C8	Paralysis of trunk and lower extremities; limited grasp release and dexterity secondary to partial intrinsic muscles of hand
T1–T9	Lower trunk paralysis; total paralysis of lower extremities
T10–L1	Paralysis of lower extremities

Table 55.4 Functional Outcomes for C1–L1 Spinal Cord Injuries.

	C1–3	C4	C5	C6	C7–C8	T1–T9	T10–L1
Eating	D	D	IA	IA	I	I	I
Upper body/lower body dressing	D/D	D/D	A/D	I/A	I/I or A	I	I
Level/uneven transfers	D	D	D	A or I/ A or D	I/I or A	I	I
Wheelchair propulsion	IP	IP	IP	IP/IM indoors	IM	IM	IM
Standing/ambulation	D/NI	D/NI	D/NI	D/NI	I or A/NI	I/NF	I/A to I

A, Assistance needed; *D,* dependent; *I,* independent; *IA,* independent with adaptive equipment; *IM,* independent manual wheelchair; *IP,* independent power wheelchair; *NF,* not functional; *NI,* not indicated.

3. Residual cord compression
4. Tethering
5. Fibrosis
6. Subarachnoid cysts

35. List some common musculoskeletal conditions that affect persons with spinal cord injury.
    1. Spasticity and contractures
    2. Extremity fractures
    3. Heterotopic ossification
    4. Musculoskeletal pain
    5. Imbalance between bone formation and bone resorption, which may lead to adverse clinical effects including osteoporosis, hypercalcemia, and renal calculi
    6. Hip and spinal deformities in growing children with SCI

36. A tetraplegic patient develops an L2–L3 destructive spinal lesion 10 years after a C5–C6 fracture-dislocation. Workup reveals no evidence of a spinal tumor or infection. What is the most likely cause of this lesion?
    Neuropathic spinal arthropathy (Charcot spine). Destructive spinal lesions can develop in spinal cord–injured patients due to repetitive loads placed on the denervated spine during daily activities. The most common clinical presentation is a spinal deformity. Patients may present with audible clicking or crepitus due to spinal instability, loss of sitting balance, cauda equina syndrome, nerve root compression, or obstructive uropathy.

37. What are the three most common causes of death after spinal cord injury?
    1. Diseases of the respiratory system
    2. Infective and parasitic diseases
    3. Neoplasms

KEY POINTS

1. Perform baseline and serial neurologic assessments using the International Standards for Neurological Classification of Spinal Cord Injury to detect neurologic changes, as well as to define the severity of injury.
2. Patients with spinal cord injury should be initially managed in an intensive care unit due to the high risk of respiratory complications and hypotension.
3. Early surgical stabilization allows earlier mobilization, enables more intensive rehabilitation, and results in a shorter hospital stay.
4. Correcting hypotension and maintaining mean arterial pressure goal of 85–90 mmHg for the first 7 days after spinal cord injury may modify secondary spinal cord injury.
5. A simple clinical prediction rule based on age (<65 vs. ≥65 years) and four neurologic tests (motor scores of the quadriceps femoris [L3] and gastrocsoleus [S1] muscles, light touch sensation of dermatomes L3 and S1) can be used to prognosticate a patient's ability to walk independently at 1 year following traumatic spinal cord injury.

Websites
1. International Standards and Spinal Cord Independence Measure are available at http://www.iscos.org.uk/resources/international-standards-and-spinal-cord-independence-measure-scim
2. International Spinal Cord Society developed a web-based teaching and educational resource for comprehensive management of SCI, available at www.elearnSCI.org
3. Clinical practice guidelines, developed by the Consortium for Spinal Cord Medicine, are available for download at www.pva.org
4. Bladder Management for Adults with Spinal Cord Injury
5. Preservation of Upper Limb Function Following Spinal Cord Injury
6. Respiratory Management Following Spinal Cord Injury
7. Early Acute Management in Adults with Spinal Cord Injury
8. Depression Following Spinal Cord Injury
9. Neurogenic Bowel Management in Adults with Spinal Cord Injury
10. Outcomes Following Traumatic Spinal Cord Injury
11. Acute Management of Autonomic Dysreflexia
12. Pressure Ulcer Prevention and Treatment Following Spinal Cord Injury
13. Prevention of Thromboembolism in Spinal Cord Injury

BIBLIOGRAPHY

1. Bryce, T. N. (2016). Spinal cord injury. In D. X. Cifu (Ed.), *Braddom's Physical Medicine and Rehabilitation* (5th ed., pp. 1095–1136). Philadelphia, PA: Elsevior.
2. Consortium for Spinal Cord Medicine. (2008). Early acute management in adults with spinal cord injury: A clinical practice guideline for health-care professionals. *Journal of Spinal Cord Medicine, 31*(4), 403–479.
3. Consortium for Spinal Cord Medicine. (1998). Neurogenic bowel management in adults with spinal cord injury. *Journal of Spinal Cord Medicine, 21*(3), 248–293.
4. Consortium for Spinal Cord Medicine. (2000). Outcomes following traumatic spinal cord injury: Clinical practice guidelines for health-care professionals. *Journal of Spinal Cord Medicine, 23*(4), 289–316.
5. Consortium of Spinal Cord Medicine. (2016). Prevention of venous thromboembolism in individuals with spinal cord injury: Clinical practice guidelines for health care providers, 3rd ed. *Topics in Spinal Cord Injury Rehabilitation, 22*(3), 209–240.
6. Consortium of Spinal Cord Medicine. (2002). Acute management of autonomic dysreflexia: Individuals with spinal cord injury presenting to health-care facilities. 2nd ed. *Journal of Spinal Cord Medicine, 25*(1), S67–S88.
7. Heary, R. F., Zouzias, A. D., & Campagnolo, D. I. (2011). Acute medical and surgical management of spinal cord injury. In S. Kirshblum & D. I. Campagnolo (Eds.), *Spinal cord medicine* (2nd ed., pp. 106–118). Philadelphia, PA: Lippincott Williams & Wilkins.
8. Kirshblum, S. C., Burns, S. P., Biering-Sorensen, F., Donovan, W., Graves, D. E., Jha, A., et al. (2011). International standards for neurological classification of spinal cord injury (revised 2011). *Journal of Spinal Cord Medicine, 34*(6), 535–546.
9. National Spinal Cord Injury Statistical Center. *Annual statistical report*. University of Alabama: Birmingham; 2017. Retrieved from https://www.nscisc.uab.edu/public/2017%20Annual%20Report%20-%20Complete%20Public%20Version.pdf.
10. Steeves, J. D., Kramer, J. K., Fawcet, J. W., Cragg, J., Lammertse, D. P., & Blight, A. R., et al. (2011). Extent of spontaneous motor recovery after traumatic cervical sensorimotor complete spinal cord injury. *Spinal Cord, 49*(2), 257–265.
11. van Middendorp, J. J., Hosman, A. J., Donders, A. R., Pouw, M. H., Ditunno, Jr., J. F., Curt, A., et al. (2011). A clinical prediction rule for ambulation outcomes after traumatic spinal cord injury: A longitudinal cohort study. *Lancet, 377*(9770), 1004–1010.
12. Waters, B. C., Hadley, M. N., Hurlbert, R. J., Aarabi, B., Dhall, S. S., Gelb, D. E., et al. (2013). Guidelines for the management of acute cervical spine and spinal cord injuries: 2013 update. *Neurosurgery, 60*(1), 82–91.

CHAPTER 56

UPPER CERVICAL SPINE TRAUMA

Jens R. Chapman, MD and Rod J. Oskouian, MD

1. **What are the major types of injuries involving the upper cervical (occiput–C2) region?**
   The major types of injuries can be classified based on anatomic location as:
   1. Occipitocervical articulation
      - Occipital condyle fractures
      - Craniocervical dissociation
   2. Atlas (C1) and atlantoaxial joints
      - Atlas fractures
      - Transverse atlantal ligament (TAL) injuries
      - Atlantoaxial instabilities
   3. Axis (C2) and C2–C3 joints
      - Odontoid fractures
      - Traumatic spondylolisthesis of the axis
      - Axis body fractures
      - C2 body fractures and C2–C3 dislocations

2. **How common are upper cervical spine injuries and who is most affected?**
   It is estimated that one-third of cervical spine trauma involves the upper cervical region (occiput-C2) and two-thirds involves the subaxial cervical region (C3–T1). There is a clear bimodal distribution of upper cervical injuries in adults with younger, mainly male, patients aged 25–40 years affected by road traffic accidents and falls from a height, while the second spike affects patients 65 years and older and mainly results from ground-level falls. In patients over 65 years of age, odontoid fractures are the most common isolated spine fracture and have the highest morbidity and mortality of any spine fracture—up to 50% depending upon age and comorbidities. In the pediatric population, upper cervical injuries are more common in patients less than 8 years of age due to their high head-to-body ratio while subaxial injuries are more common in older patients. Of special importance is the association between head injuries and upper cervical spine injuries. Approximately 5% of patients with moderate or severe head injuries can be expected to have an upper cervical spine injury, while 20% of patients with an established cervical spine fracture-dislocation may also have a concomitant head injury. Up to one-third of upper cervical spine injuries are associated with spinal cord, cranial nerve or cervical nerve root injuries.

3. **How are upper cervical spine injuries diagnosed?**
   It can be relatively easy to miss upper cervical spine injuries due to initial clinical focus on head injury or other trauma, as well as the relative subtlety of these injuries. Frequently, no specific symptoms or findings on physical examination strongly point to the presence of a significant osseous or ligamentous injury involving the upper cervical region. Symptoms are notoriously vague and may include headaches, suboccipital pain, greater occipital neuralgia, neck pain, local tenderness and swelling, or neurologic deficits, including cranial nerve deficits, myelopathy or spinal cord injury. Not infrequently, the patient may be unconscious or intubated following trauma. A neurologic evaluation following the American Spinal Injury Association (ASIA) guidelines is recommended, and should include assessment and documentation of bilateral lower cranial nerve function. Use of clinical risk profiling based on injury mechanism (i.e., fall from 10 feet or higher, motor vehicle crash at 35 mph or higher, presence of head injury, facial trauma, pelvis fracture, multiple rib fractures, or focal neurologic deficits) can increase injury awareness and highlight the necessity for obtaining neuroimaging studies. Pediatric patients less than 8 years of age present as a particularly concerning subgroup due to their relatively large head size relative to their torso, relatively lax ligaments, and poorly matured cervical joint contours. Victims of child abuse and pediatric patients who were struck by a vehicle or were involved in car crashes while being restrained in a modern car seat with a four-point torso restraint system should raise high suspicions for such possible injuries.

   Computed tomography (CT) with sagittal and coronal plane reformatted views is required to assess the full magnitude of injury, and is the imaging modality of choice for initial evaluation of cervical trauma in severely injured patients. Plain radiographs remain important as they can show over 90% of upper cervical spine injuries and can assess craniocervical alignment and instability. Magnetic resonance imaging (MRI) is indicated for patients with cervical spinal cord injury, suspected ligament injuries that are not evident with other imaging modalities, and to assess related pathologies such as vertebral artery injuries. T2 fat-suppressed images are especially useful to assess ligamentous injuries, hemorrhage, as well as cord signal changes. If CT documents a cervical spine fracture with displacement of transverse foramina, an additional study to confirm vertebral artery integrity is indicated, such as a CT-angiogram or MR angiography. During the acute injury evaluation phase, the patient should remain immobilized with a rigid cervical collar.

4. **What are some special considerations related to injuries involving the upper cervical (occiput–C2) region that are a consequence of the unique anatomic features of this spinal region?**

A wide range of injury mechanisms exist: Because of the fragile nature of the bony and ligamentous components of the upper cervical spine, injuries are relatively common, especially in the setting of closed head trauma. Typical injury mechanisms include flexion, extension, or compressive forces applied to the head during motor vehicle accidents, falls from a height, or sporting injuries, but also include injuries due to low-energy injury mechanisms in the aging population.

Upper cervical spine stability and mobility are dependent upon the integrity of both osseous and ligamentous structures: Suspicion regarding the presence of occult upper cervical ligament injuries is vital as missed injuries may lead to serious complications, including secondary dislocations. As in other regions of the spine, capsuloligamentous injuries have a much poorer chance for stable healing with nonsurgical means compared with osseous fractures. Small bone fragments at joint edges provide an important tip-off regarding the presence of an underlying more profound ligamentous disruption ("tip of the iceberg fragment"). It is important to recognize that certain injuries such as craniocervical dislocations may spontaneously reduce, leaving deficient structural stability, which is not apparent on imaging.

Concomitant and noncontiguous spinal injuries often occur: The upper cervical spine is unique in that it functions as an "integrated motion unit" and an injury in one area may adversely affect another spinal segment or region. Combination injuries involving the upper cervical spine are common. For instance, more than 50% of C1 posterior arch fractures are associated with a second injury in the cervical region ("indicator fracture"), which may include odontoid fractures, traumatic spondylolisthesis of the axis, occipital condyle fractures, C2 teardrop fractures, cervical burst fractures, and lateral mass fractures. Close scrutiny for noncontiguous injuries or related pathology is therefore important in patients with upper cervical spine injuries.

Atypical neurologic injury patterns may be encountered: From a neurologic injury perspective, the relatively large size of the spinal canal provides some protection from spinal cord injury as the majority of upper cervical injuries are not associated with neurologic deficit. However, major dislocations of the upper cervical spine are usually not survivable injuries due to compromise of the respiratory and cardiac centers in the medulla and upper cervical cord. Disruption of the craniocervical ligaments is reported as the leading cause of fatal motor vehicle occupant trauma. In survivors, high-energy incomplete upper cervical spinal cord injuries may present as cervicomedullary syndromes or cranial nerve injuries. Part of routine neurologic assessment for patients with upper cervical spine injuries includes cranial nerve evaluation with documentation of any abnormal findings. In addition, traumatic brain injury is noted more commonly following upper cervical spine injuries compared with injuries in other spinal regions.

Upper cervical spine injuries may be associated with vascular injuries: Vertebral artery injuries, as well as carotid injuries, are increasingly diagnosed through use of imaging protocols that are routinely activated in the presence of fractures involving the transverse processes or distractive spine injuries. The vertebral artery regions that are susceptible to injury include the V3 and V4 sections of the artery where it is positioned laterally in relation to the atlantoaxial joints (V3) and on the superior aspect of the atlas arch (V4). Vertebral artery injuries in these regions can be diagnosed with CT-angiography or MRI.

5. **How is upper cervical spine stability determined in an acute injury setting?**
Certain injuries are clearly recognized by their appearance as "unstable" based on clinical and/or imaging criteria. For instance, any patient with a neurologic and/or vascular injury in combination with an upper cervical spine fracture-dislocation has an unstable injury. Most craniocervical ligamentous disruptions are unstable. Upper cervical spine fractures with more than 3 mm displacement or 5° of angulation are likely unstable. Note that a determination of instability does not necessarily equate to a need for surgical intervention, but recognition of instability does necessitate that extra precautions are taken when choosing potential nonsurgical treatment options. In some patients it may be challenging to determine whether the spine is stable even after conclusion of comprehensive neuroimaging studies. For patients who remain neurologically intact and show minimal or no upper cervical bony displacement but are considered at risk of harm due to potential osteoligamentous instability, some additional studies that may potentially inform treatment decision making include:

Two-step lateral radiographs: For a patient who is a reasonable candidate for potential treatment with a rigid collar, the first step is to obtain a lateral radiograph centered on the upper cervical spine with the patient in the recumbent lateral position. If there is no concerning displacement noted, the patient is assisted to the upright position and clinically reassessed. If the patient's clinical status is unchanged, the second step is to repeat the lateral radiograph with the patient upright in the collar and compare this radiograph to the supine imaging study. If the patient remains comfortable and reports no new neurologic symptoms, and radiographic alignment and injury displacement are unchanged, it is reasonable to conclude that the injury is relatively stable and can undergo a trial of physician-supervised brace treatment.

Traction test: In the uncommon clinical scenario where CT and MRI are nondiagnostic and there is ongoing concern regarding the presence of a possible craniocervical dislocation that has spontaneously reduced, a traction test can be performed. This test is only indicated if all conventional imaging studies do not allow for a conclusive determination of stability. With the patient in the supine position, an image intensifier is used to obtain a baseline lateral radiographic image of the cervical spine. Traction weights are added in 5-lb increments (20-lb limit) using a head halter or Gardner-Wells tongs as the cervical region is monitored radiographically. If distraction of more than 2 mm between the occipital condyles and atlas or between the atlas and axis occurs, the test is considered positive for a spontaneously reduced craniocervical dislocation.

Flexion–extension radiographs: Although flexion–extension radiographs can effectively document cervical instability, these studies are of limited value and even potentially dangerous in the acute trauma setting. It is usually unadvisable to perform flexion–extension radiographs in the presence of known fractures and/or ligament injuries. Pain and muscle spasms may limit the actual motion excursion and convey a false sense of reassurance. In a subacute setting however, roughly definable as 2–3 weeks after an injury, or for the assessment of final healing of an injury 2–3 months following initiation of nonoperative treatment or following surgical reconstruction, flexion–extension radiographs remain a mainstay for determination of cervical spine stability. As in any diagnostic spine study, the patient should be instructed to stop any movement if they notice the onset of neurologic symptoms or undue pain.

6. What systems exist for classification of upper cervical spine injuries?
Historically there have been a large number of empirically based and eponymous classifications and subclassifications for injuries involving each segment of the upper cervical spine. These classifications are notoriously difficult to remember and some are of dubious clinical merit. However, as related terminology persists in current literature, familiarity with these classifications is needed until a comprehensive spine injury classification is widely adopted. Based on a series of international studies, AOSpine proposed a validated classification (Fig. 56.1) that provides a more systematic description and stability assessment for all spine injuries, including the upper cervical spine using an A, B, C system. The AOSpine classification subdivides the upper cervical spine into three general regions. Each region is defined by an osseous element and the articulation below:

Upper cervical spine regions
- Region 1: Occipital condyle and craniocervical junction (Occ, 0–C1)
- Region 2: Atlas and atlantoaxial joints (C1, C1–C2)
- Region 3: Axis and C2–C3 joints (C2 and C2–C3)

The AOSpine classification applies the A, B, C system to injuries in each region. This classification is hierarchical, progressing from least to most unstable, and is based on injury morphology. Two sets of modifiers are applied to each injury. One modifier classifies neurologic injury and the other identifies specific factors that may affect treatment, prognosis or adversely affect healing.

A. **Injury types**
- Type A injuries: Bone injuries without significant ligamentous, tension band, or discal injuries. These are stable injuries.
- Type B injuries: Tension band/ligamentous injuries without complete separation of anatomic integrity. These may be either stable or unstable injuries.
- Type C injuries: These are injuries with significant translation in any directional plane and separation of anatomic integrity. These are unstable injuries.

B. **Neurologic status modifiers**
- N0: neurologically normal
- N1: Transient neurologic deficit
- N2: Radiculopathy or cranial nerve injury
- N3: Incomplete spinal cord injury
- N4: Complete spinal cord injury
- N5: Unexaminable patient
- N+: Ongoing spinal cord compression

C. **Case-specific modifiers**
- M1: Injuries at high risk of nonunion with nonoperative treatment
- M2: Injury with significant potential for instability
- M3: Patient-specific factors adversely affecting healing potential
- M4: Vascular injury or abnormality affecting treatment

OCCIPITAL CONDYLE AND CRANIOCERVICAL JUNCTION

7. What is the mechanism for occipital condyle fractures and how are these injuries classified?
Occipital condyle fractures typically result from a direct blow to the head or from a rapid deceleration injury. These injuries are frequently associated with C1 fractures and cranial nerve injuries. CT is used to classify these injuries according to the AOSpine classification or the Anderson and Montesano classification (below):
- Type 1: A stable comminuted fracture resulting from an axial loading injury.
- Type 2: A stable skull base fracture that extends into the occipital condyle.
- Type 3: An avulsion fracture of the condyle at the attachment of the alar ligament, either unilateral or bilateral. This fracture type may be stable or unstable and may be associated with craniocervical dissociation.

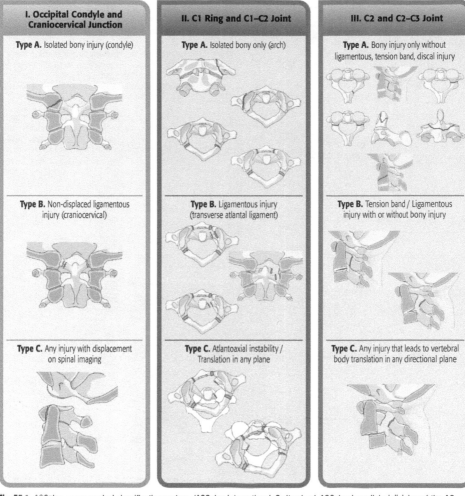

I. Occipital Condyle and Craniocervical Junction	II. C1 Ring and C1–C2 Joint	III. C2 and C2–C3 Joint
Type A. Isolated bony injury (condyle)	**Type A.** Isolated bony only (arch)	**Type A.** Bony injury only without ligamentous, tension band, discal injury
Type B. Non-displaced ligamentous injury (craniocervical)	**Type B.** Ligamentous injury (transverse atlantal ligament)	**Type B.** Tension band / Ligamentous injury with or without bony injury
Type C. Any injury with displacement on spinal imaging	**Type C.** Atlantoaxial instability / Translation in any plane	**Type C.** Any injury that leads to vertebral body translation in any directional plane

Fig. 56.1 AOSpine upper cervical classification system. (AOSpine International, Switzerland. AOSpine is a clinical division of the AO Foundation—an independent medically guided nonprofit organization.)

8. **How are occipital condyle fractures treated?**
   Stable injuries are treated with a rigid cervical orthosis, or less commonly with a halo orthosis. Unstable injuries include those associated with displacement or craniocervical dissociation and require treatment with posterior occipitocervical fusion.

9. **What is a craniocervical dissociation?**
   A craniocervical dissociation is an injury which involves the complex articulation between the occiput and C2 comprised by the occiput, atlas, axis and ligaments that span from C2 to the occiput. A range of injury patterns with various degrees of stability may occur and include isolated bony injuries, non-displaced incomplete or complete ligamentous injuries, atlanto-occipital dislocations and C1–C2 vertical distraction injuries. (Fig. 56.2).

10. **How is the craniocervical junction evaluated on imaging studies?**
    The craniocervical junction may be evaluated with plain radiography, CT or MRI. Important imaging parameters to evaluate include:
    - **Soft tissue swelling** adjacent to the upper cervical vertebral bodies (>6 mm)
    - **Diastasis or subluxation** of atlanto-occipital articulation (Fig. 56.3A)

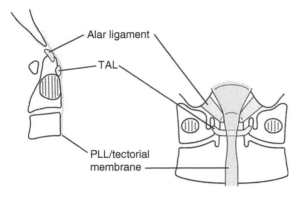

Fig. 56.2 Craniocervical ligaments. The tectorial membrane is the uppermost extension of the posterior longitudinal ligament *(PLL)* and attaches to the occipital condyles providing for stability against cranial traction and flexion forces. The alar ligaments extend from the tip of the odontoid process and attach to the anterior aspect of the foramen magnum serving as checkreins against rotation and distraction. These ligaments run from the occiput to C2 without attaching directly to C1, which serves as a bushing. The transverse atlantal ligament *(TAL)* restricts translation of C1 on C2. (Jens R. Chapman.)

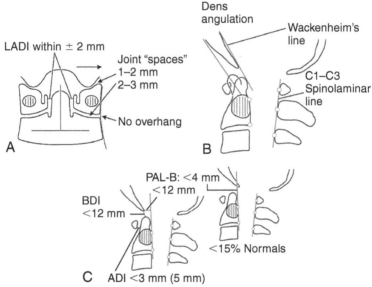

Fig. 56.3 (A) The lateral masses of the atlas should closely articulate with the superior articular processes of the atlas. The odontoid should be centered symmetrically between the lateral masses of the atlas (lateral atlantodens interval *[LADI]*). (B) Additional screening lines include Wackenheim's line and the C1–C3 spinolaminar line. (C) The tip of the odontoid should remain in close proximity to the basion, as shown with the reference lines described by Harris. *ADI,* Atlantodens interval; *BDI,* basion-dens interval; *PAL-B,* posterior axis line. (Jens R. Chapman.)

- Disruption of **Harris lines**—this is a combination of two measurements that have been termed the *rule of twelve* (Fig. 56.3C):
  - **Basion-dens interval (BDI):** The distance from the dens to the basion should be less than 12 mm.
  - **Basion-atlantal interval (BAI):** A measurement from a perpendicular line extending along the posterior margin of the C2 vertebral body (posterior axis line [PAL-B]) should not be more than 4 mm anterior and less than 12 mm posterior to the basion.
  Additional measurements have been described but are less reliable than Harris lines. These include **Wackenheim's line** (Fig. 56.3B) and **Powers ratio**, which is defined as the ratio between the distance from the basion to the posterior arch of C1 divided by the distance from the opisthion to the anterior arch of C1 and is usually less than 1. A Powers ratio greater than 1 suggests an anterior dislocation of the atlanto-occipital joint. Note that use of the Powers ratio is limited to anterior dislocations of the occiput and is not applicable for other displacements.
  The diagnosis of suspected craniocervical injury based on radiographs may be confirmed with a CT scan with sagittal and coronal reformatted images and/or MRI. Occasionally, a cervical traction test is necessary to confirm the presence of an occult craniocervical instability.

11. **How are craniocervical dissociations classified?**
    The Traynelis classification assessed unstable injuries according to the direction of displacement of the head rela-
    tive to the cervical spine and described anterior, vertical, posterior, and oblique dislocations. However, classifica-
    tion according to displacement in the presence of global ligamentous failure is somewhat arbitrary as displace-
    ment can be altered by patient positioning. In addition, such a classification does not grade injury severity or the
    potential for spontaneously reduced dislocations, which would be overlooked if the sole criterion for injury is dis-
    placement. It is important to distinguish incomplete injuries that retain partial meaningful craniocervical ligamen-
    tous integrity from occult injuries in which a rebound phenomenon led to partial or complete deformity reduction.
    Spontaneously reduced injuries are easily overlooked yet may have catastrophic consequences if left untreated.
        The **Harborview classification** stratifies injuries according to severity:
    - **Type I:** MRI shows edema or hemorrhage at the craniocervical junction, but normal cervical alignment is pre-
      sent on CT. A traction test performed to rule out a spontaneously reduced injury is normal (≤2 mm distraction).
    - **Type II:** MRI shows edema or hemorrhage at the craniocervical junction, but borderline normal screening mea-
      surement values are noted on CT. A traction test shows sufficient distraction or displacement to meet cranio-
      cervical instability criteria. A spontaneous partial reduction of the cranium to its cervical location, through re-
      maining residual ligamentous attachments, has occurred and is potentially misleading without this test.
    - **Type III:** These injuries demonstrate obvious major craniocervical displacement >2 mm on static plain radio-
      graphs.
    The AOSpine classification identifies occipital condyle and craniocervical junction injury types as A (isolated bony
    injury, stable), B (ligamentous injury, stable or unstable) or C (displaced injury, unstable).

12. **What is the treatment for craniocervical dissociation?**
    Stable injuries are treated in a rigid collar or halo vest for 8–12 weeks. Unstable injuries are temporarily immobi-
    lized using a neck collar and sandbags or a halo vest while awaiting surgical treatment. Definitive treatment of
    unstable craniocervical injuries consists of posterior occipitocervical arthrodesis with rigid segmental spinal
    instrumentation with screw-rod systems (Fig. 56.8A). Attempts at occiput to C1 fusion are unwarranted because
    this treatment does not address the disrupted alar ligaments and tectorial membrane, which extend between C2
    and the occiput. Significant ethical challenges, in terms of sustaining life-preserving support measures, may arise
    in cases of patients with associated anoxic or traumatic brain injury.

ATLAS FRACTURES AND C1–C2 JOINT INJURIES

13. **How are atlas fractures classified?**
    Several classifications stratify atlas fractures based on fracture location and pattern. (Fig. 56.4) Landells described
    three main fracture types:
    - **Type 1:** Fractures involve either the posterior arch or anterior arch but not both.
    - **Type 2:** Fractures involve both the anterior and posterior arch, and include burst fractures (Jefferson
      fracture), which may consist of three or four parts. These injuries may occur with or without an associated
      TAL disruption.
    - **Type 3:** Fractures primarily involve the lateral mass. These injuries may occur with or without an associated
      TAL disruption.
        Type 1 fractures are considered stable. Type 2 and 3 fractures may be stable or unstable. For type 2 and
    3 fractures, one of the most important determinants of stability is the integrity of the TAL. Other criteria that factor
    into decision making include fracture comminution, fracture line orientation, and fracture displacement. Fractures
    that involve the transverse process are not included in the Landells classification but are considered stable inju-
    ries that require evaluation to rule out a vertebral artery injury.
        Atlas fractures also may be classified according to the AOSpine classification for atlas and atlantoaxial joint
    injuries which defines the following injury types: A (isolated bony injury, stable), B (ligamentous injury, stable or
    unstable) or C (displaced injury, unstable).

14. **How are atlas fractures treated?**
    - Type 1 injuries that occur as an isolated injury are considered stable injuries and are treated with a collar.
      Transverse process fractures are treated similarly.
    - Type 2 injuries are treated with a cervical collar if they are stable (intact TAL) and minimally displaced. For
      unstable fractures with TAL disruption as evident by lateral mass displacement or an increased atlantodens
      interval (ADI), surgery is generally considered and may consist of either C1 osteosynthesis or arthrodesis
      (C1–C2 or occiput–C2).
    - Type 3 injuries that are minimally displaced (intact TAL) are treated with a collar, while fractures with dis-
      placement are generally considered for surgical treatment with either C1 osteosynthesis or arthrodesis
      (C1–C2 or occiput–C2). One fracture variant to be aware of that may result in late deformity and pain
      despite the presence of an intact TAL, is a unilateral sagittal split fracture involving the lateral mass of
      C1. This injury can lead to subsidence of the occipital condyle through the lateral mass and result in a
      "cock-robin" deformity.

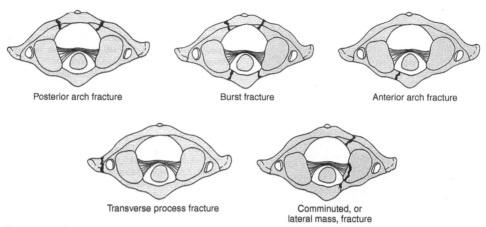

Posterior arch fracture   Burst fracture   Anterior arch fracture

Transverse process fracture   Comminuted, or lateral mass, fracture

Fig. 56.4 Classification of atlas fractures. (From Browner BD, Jupiter JB, Levine AM, editors. Skeletal Trauma. Philadelphia, PA: Saunders; 1998.)

15. What types of upper cervical traumatic injuries result in atlantoaxial instability?

Atlantoaxial instability is present when displacement of C1 in relation to C2 occurs in any direction. Translational, distractive, and rotational injury patterns have been described. Translational atlantoaxial instability may occur from traumatic injuries such as C1 fractures associated with TAL disruption, odontoid fractures, or isolated transverse ligament injuries. Atlantoaxial dissociation with distraction between C1 and C2 may occur with an occipitocervical dissociation or occipital condyle fractures due to disruption of the alar ligaments and tectorial membrane, which extend from the occiput to C2. Traumatic C1–C2 rotatory subluxation or C1–C2 dislocation are rare injuries but have been reported.

16. What are some criteria are used to assess the integrity of the TAL on imaging studies?

- The ADI should normally be less than 3 mm in adults and less than 5 mm in children and should be maintained on flexion–extension views.
- The dens should normally appear centered between the lateral masses of C1.
- If unilateral or bilateral overhang of the C1 lateral mass over the C2 lateral mass is present, this may or may not reflect loss of integrity of the TAL. Disruption of the TAL has been inferred in atlas fractures with bilateral lateral mass overhang of C1 over C2 in excess of 7 mm, but subsequent investigators have shown this parameter is unreliable and recommend assessment of TAL integrity with MRI.
- Based on MRI, TAL injuries have been differentiated into two types:
  - **Type 1 injuries:** Disruptions of the substance of the TAL
  - **Type 2 injuries:** Fractures and avulsions involving the tubercle for insertion of the TAL on the C1 lateral mass
    This distinction has treatment implications as type 1 injuries are not capable of healing and require surgical treatment while type 2 injuries have the potential for healing with immobilization if osseointegration of the avulsion fragment occurs.
- CT has utility for diagnosis of type 2 injuries as the avulsion fragment may be visualized but is not sensitive for diagnosis of type 1 injuries.
- Additional MRI findings that suggest C1–C2 instability include bilateral widening or increased signal in the C1–C2 joints, as well as increased signal involving the apical ligaments, tectorial membrane, or alar ligaments.

17. What surgical techniques are used for posterior stabilization of atlas fractures and TAL injuries?

A. C1–C2 fusion or O–C2 fusion

Historically, unstable atlas fractures and TAL injuries were treated by fusion of the C1–C2 motion segment utilizing **wire or cable fixation**. The Gallie technique placed 18-gauge wires under the posterior arch of C1 and around the C2 spinous process to secure a corticocancellous bone graft. The Brooks and Sonntag techniques placed wires or cables under the lamina of C1 and C2 to secure a structural bone graft between adjacent laminae. However, there are several limitations of these relatively simple and inexpensive techniques such as the presence of a fracture through the ring of C1, which render posterior cable or wire fixation useless, and the need for postoperative immobilization with a halo fixator due to the nonrigid fixation provided by wires or cables. Today, wire and cable techniques are rarely used as a stand-alone option due to the development of rigid segmental spinal instrumentation techniques.

Currently, when C1–C2 instrumentation and fusion are performed, the most widely used technique is **C1–C2 screw-rod fixation** (Fig. 56.8b). This construct relies on placement of lateral mass screws into the atlas and pedicle, pars or laminar screws in the axis, which are linked to longitudinal rods on each side. Bone graft is added between the joints and/or as an onlay to the lamina. This technique allows for intraoperative fracture reduction and can be extended rostrally or caudally for longer constructs as needed. C1–C2 screw-rod fixation has largely replaced use of **C1–C2 transarticular screws** directed from the inferior articular process of the axis into the lateral mass of the atlas. While elegant due to its simplicity, this technically challenging fixation method is limited by large patient size, medial vertebral artery location within the C2 segment, and the need for anatomic reduction of the atlantoaxial segment prior to screw insertion.

B. Osteosynthesis

An atlas osteosynthesis may be performed to repair an atlas ring fracture. This procedure involves open reduction and internal fixation of the C1 fracture and can be performed from a posterior approach using a C1 lateral mass screw on each side connected by a transverse rod. Surgery is limited to the atlas, preserves motion, and does not require the use of a bone graft. This procedure does not limit future treatment as it may be converted to an atlantoaxial fusion construct by removing the horizontal rod and inserting two additional screws in C2 and bilateral rods if inadequate healing or instability develops following the initial osteosynthesis procedure. Atlas osteosynthesis has also been described through an anterior transoral approach, as well as through combined approaches (Fig. 56.5).

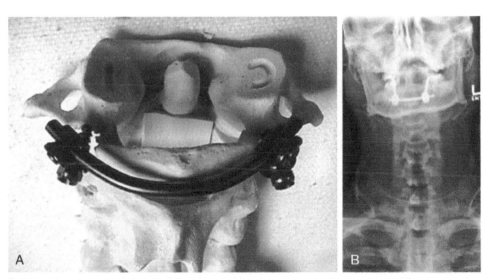

Fig. 56.5 (A) Saw bones demonstration using C1 lateral mass screws and transverse connection rod to reduce a Jefferson fracture, thus achieving direct fracture healing and avoiding a fusion. (B) Postoperative anteroposterior view of C1 osteosynthesis. (Jens R. Chapman. From Browner BD, Jupiter JB, Krettek C. et al., Craniocervical injuries. In: Browner BD, Jupiter JB, Krettek C, editors. Skeletal Trauma. Basic Science, Management, and Reconstruction. 5th ed. Philadelphia, PA: Saunders; 2015, pp. 813–874 e4, Fig. 33B-11.)

AXIS FRACTURES AND C2–C3 JOINT INJURIES

18. What is the usual mechanism of injury for an odontoid fracture?

Odontoid fractures typically occur secondary to forced extension or flexion of the head and neck during a fall or collision. Associated fractures of the atlas occur in 10%–15% of cases. Odontoid fractures are the most common cervical fracture in patients younger than 8 years, or older than 70 years. Odontoid fractures have reached epidemic proportions in the geriatric population and are the most common spine fracture in patients older than 80 years.

19. How are odontoid fractures classified?

The Anderson and D'Alonzo classification (Fig. 56.6) is widely used and is based on the location of the fracture line:

- **Type I:** Stable avulsion fracture occurring at the tip of the odontoid. This must be differentiated from an avulsion fracture associated with AOD or os odontoideum.
- **Type II:** Unstable transverse fracture involving the cortical bone of the waist of the odontoid.
- **Type III:** Unstable fracture extending into the cancellous portion of the C2 vertebral body.

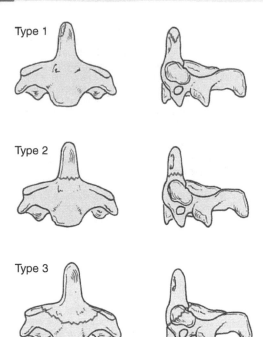

Type 1

Type 2

Type 3

Fig. 56.6 Anderson and D'Alonzo's classification of odontoid fractures. Type 1 fractures involve the tip of the odontoid process and are stable. Type 2 fractures penetrate the base of the odontoid. Type 3 fractures extend into the body of C2. (From Browner BD, Jupiter JB, Levine AM, editors. Skeletal Trauma. Philadelphia, PA: Saunders; 1998.)

Important fracture variables with potential therapeutic implications include segmental comminution, fracture displacement, and fracture obliquity. A more precise distinction between type II and type III fractures has been proposed. Type II fractures lack involvement of the superior articular facets of C2, whereas type III fractures involve the superior articular facet. Type II fractures have been subclassified based on fracture line orientation as type IIA (horizontal fracture line), type IIB (fracture line extends from superior–anterior to inferior–posterior), and type IIC (fracture line extends from superior–posterior to inferior–anterior).

Odontoid fractures may also be classified according to the AOSpine classification for axis and C2–C3 joint injuries which defines the following injury types: A (isolated bony injury, stable), B (ligamentous injury, stable or unstable) or C (displaced injury, unstable).

20. **How are odontoid fractures treated?**

Type I fractures are generally stable and nondisplaced and are treated with a cervical collar. It is important to evaluate the craniocervical junction to rule out concomitant ligamentous injuries, which require further evaluation and treatment.

Type II fractures are associated with a high incidence of nonunion, especially with nonoperative treatment (15%–85%). Risk factors associated with nonunion include initial fracture displacement greater than 5 mm, advanced age, posteriorly displaced or comminuted fractures, angulation greater than 11°, and inappropriate initial treatment. Treatment of type II fractures lacks consensus and is individualized based on a variety of factors, including patient age and comorbidities, initial fracture displacement, presence of associated cervical fractures, fracture comminution, fracture obliquity, and bone quality. Nondisplaced or minimally displaced fractures may be treated with a rigid collar for 8–12 weeks. Halo vest use is controversial but remains an option for younger patients, but is associated with increased morbidity and mortality in geriatric patients. Surgical treatment is generally recommended for displaced and unstable fractures. In geriatric patients, treatment algorithms remain controversial as odontoid fractures have been associated with high rates of morbidity and mortality regardless of whether operative or nonoperative treatment is recommended.

Type III fractures which are nondisplaced are treated with external immobilization. Severely comminuted or unstable fracture patterns are treated with posterior fusion and posterior stabilization.

21. **What are the options for surgical stabilization of odontoid fractures?**

1. **Anterior screw fixation:** Odontoid screw fixation offers the advantage of stabilization with preservation of motion at the C1–C2 joint. Single- or double-screw fixation can be considered for treatment of type IIA (horizontal fracture line) and type IIB (superior–anterior to inferior–posterior fracture line) injuries but not for type IIC (superior–posterior to inferior–anterior fracture line). Additional prerequisites include a fracture that is less than 3 weeks old, reducible, lacks comminution, and a patient without osteoporosis. Certain factors, such as a large

body habitus, may preclude this form of treatment. Anterior screw fixation in the elderly population is associated with a high complication rate including nonunion, fixation loss, and dysphagia and is not generally recommended (Fig. 56.8E).

2. **Posterior C1–C2 screw-rod fixation and fusion:** This is the most versatile and widely performed technique and can be used to treat all fracture types. The implant construct consists of C1 lateral mass screws and C2 screw fixation with pedicle, pars or laminar screws linked to a longitudinal rod on each side in combination with fusion. The disadvantage of this technique is loss of 50% of neck rotation due to fusion.

3. **Transarticular screw fixation:** Small fragment screws may be placed from the midpoint of the inferior articular processes of C2 across the pars of C2 into the lateral mass of C1. Although this technique is associated with a high rate of bony union, it is not applicable to all patients and is associated with risk of iatrogenic injury to the vertebral artery which passes laterally to the vertebral body of C2.

22. What is traumatic spondylolisthesis of the axis vertebra and what injury mechanisms are responsible for this condition?
Traumatic spondylolisthesis of the axis is defined as a bilateral separation of the C2 vertebral body from the posterior neural arch. The term hangman's fracture has been used to describe C2 traumatic spondylolisthesis due to perceived similarities to injury patterns associated with judicial hangings. Traumatic spondylolisthesis most often occurs due to bilateral fractures through the pars interarticularis, but fracture lines may alternatively involve the pedicle, facet joint, lamina, or posterior aspect of the vertebral body. Injury may occur due to variable combinations of extension, flexion, distraction, and axial loading. This injury is often accompanied by injury to the C2–C3 disc, as well as disruption of the anterior and/or posterior ligaments between C2 and C3. Concurrent soft tissue injuries heavily influence fracture stability and treatment.

23. How is traumatic spondylolisthesis of the axis classified?
The original Effendi classification, as modified by Levine and Edwards may be used (Fig. 56.7):

- Type I injuries consist of a fracture through the neural arch with no angulation and up to 3 mm of displacement. This injury type is due to combined hyperextension and axial load.
- Type II fractures have both significant angulation (>11°) and fracture displacement (>3 mm). This injury type is due to initial axial compression and extension forces followed by a rebound flexion force. Type II fractures are associated with injuries to the posterior longitudinal ligament and C2–C3 intervertebral disc.
- Type IIA injuries are minimally displaced (<3 mm) but are associated with severe angulation as a result of a flexion-distraction injury mechanism. This injury may not be recognized until a radiograph is obtained in traction. This injury type involves disruption of the intervertebral disc and posterior longitudinal ligament.
- Type III injuries combine severe angulation and displacement with a unilateral or bilateral facet dislocation between C2 and C3. This injury type is associated with disruption of the anterior and posterior longitudinal ligament and the intervertebral disc and is attributed to flexion and rebound extension mechanism.
- Atypical hangman's fractures involve the posterior aspect of the vertebral body, on one or both sides. These injuries most commonly consist of a unilateral pars interarticularis or lamina fracture on one side, in combination with a fracture line that cuts obliquely across the posterior vertebral body wall and may involve the foramen transversarium. These fractures are associated with neurologic injuries in up to one-third of patients versus a 3%–10% rate of neurologic injury with other subtypes as the fracture pattern may lead to spinal canal

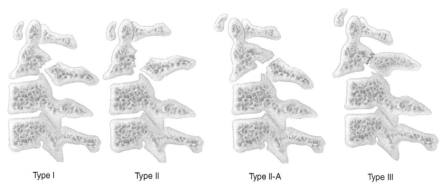

| Type I | Type II | Type II-A | Type III |

Fig. 56.7 Levine and Edwards classification. Type I, Fractures occur through the pars interarticularis bilaterally without angulation and up to 3 mm displacement. Type II. Fractures with both significant angulation and displacement of C2 with respect to C3. Type II-A. Fractures with severe minimal initial displacement but are associated with severe angulation which may not be evident until traction is applied. Type III. Fractures with severe angulation and displacement associated with unilateral or bilateral C2–C3 facet dislocations. (From Leventhal MR. Fractures, dislocations and fracture-dislocations of the spine. In: Crenshaw AH, editor. Campbell's Operative Orthopaedics. 8th ed. St. Louis: Mosby-Year Book; 1992.)

compromise if fracture displacement occurs. There is also potential for vertebral artery injury due to involvement of the foramen transversarium.

The AOSpine classification for axis and C2–C3 joint injuries is applicable to traumatic spondylolisthesis of the axis and defines the following injury types: A (isolated bony injury, stable), B (ligamentous injury, stable or unstable) or C (displaced injury, unstable).

24. How is traumatic spondylolisthesis of the axis treated?

Treatment options include nonsurgical treatment with a rigid cervical collar or halo fixator, C2–C3 or C1–C3 posterior fusion (PSF) and screw-rod instrumentation, C2–C3 anterior cervical discectomy and fusion (ACDF) in combination with plate fixation and rarely circumferential procedures or osteosynthesis. Treatment is based on the fracture type:

- Type I injuries are treated in a rigid neck collar
- Type II injuries are often initially treated nonoperatively. Reduction may be achieved with traction, followed by immobilization in a halo or a rigid collar. If significant disruption of the C2–C3 disc exists or if nonsurgical treatment is not adequate, anterior or posterior surgical stabilization is considered. Osteosynthesis with placement of posterior screws across the C2 fracture without fusion is an option for select type II fractures but is unable to address concomitant injury to the C2–C3 disc.
- Type IIA injuries may be treated with closed reduction by positioning in extension, followed by halo immobilization. If significant disruption of the C2–C3 disc exists or if alignment is not adequate, anterior or posterior surgical stabilization and fusion is performed. Traction is dangerous for this subtype and may lead to neurologic injury.
- Type III injuries require surgical treatment for open reduction of the facet dislocation and surgical stabilization. Open reduction of the facet dislocation and stabilization of the dislocation with C2–C3 or C1–C3 PSF and instrumentation or C2–C3 ACDF with plate fixation or a circumferential procedure are the options for surgical treatment (Fig. 56.8C, Fig. 56.8D).
- Atypical hangman's fractures without neurologic injury are usually treated nonoperatively (collar, halo). Fractures associated with neurologic injury are treated operatively. Surgical options include C2–C3 ACDF, C2–C3 or C1–C3 PSF, and occasionally combined approaches.

25. What are the different types of axis body fractures and how are they treated?

Axis body fractures may be classifed based on fracture line orientation:

- **Type 1:** Coronally oriented vertical fracture lines are present and pass through the posterior aspect of the vertebral body and may involve the pars interarticularis or intervertebral disc.
- **Type 2:** Sagittally oriented vertical fracture lines are present and pass through the vertebral body and may be associated with vertebral body compression.
- **Type 3:** Horizontally oriented vertebral body fractures lines are present. Proximal fractures correspond to Anderson type III odontoid fractures and are associated with C1–C2 instability while distal fractures may be associated with C2–C3 instability.

Type 1 and type 2 injuries are usually treated nonoperatively while type 3 injuries are often treated surgically.

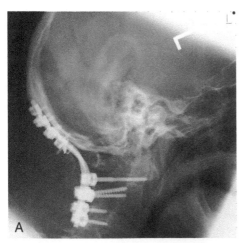
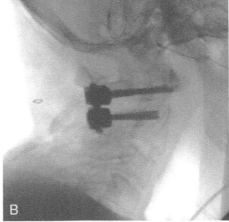

Fig. 56.8 Examples of various spinal implant constructs used in the treatment of upper cervical trauma. (A) Occipitocervical screw-rod fixation for treatment of a craniocervical dissociation. (B) C1–C2 posterior screw rod fixation for treatment of traumatic C1–C2 instability

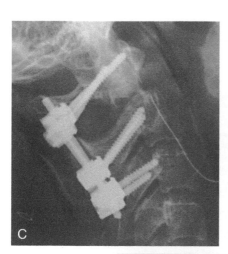

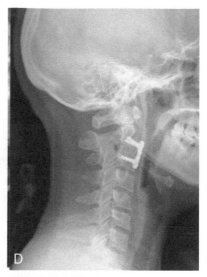

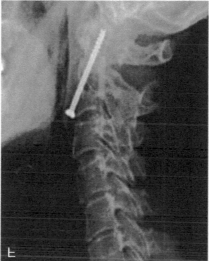

Fig. 56.8, cont'd (C) C1–C3 posterior screw rod fixation for treatment of Type III traumatic spondylolisthesis. (D) Anterior C2–C3 plate fixation for treatment of Type III traumatic spondylolisthesis. (E) Odontoid screw fixation for treatment of a Type II odontoid fracture. (D: From Li G, Yang Y, Liu H, et al. Residual deformity after cervical discectomy and fusion for unstable Hangman's fractures. World Neurosurg 2017;108:216–224, p. 220, Fig. 2D. E: From Kalantar SB: Fracture of the C1 and C2 vertebrae. Semin spine surg 2013;25: 23–35, p. 30, Fig. 13.)

KEY POINTS

1. The craniocervical junction consists of the osseous, ligamentous, and neurovascular structures that extend from the skull base to C2-C3 motion segment.
2. Injuries to the craniocervical junction are associated with a notable rate of mortality, neurologic deficits and associated injuries. Secondary deterioration is a danger when these injuries are missed or inappropriately treated.
3. Nonoperative treatment options include recumbent skeletal traction, cervical orthoses, and halo vest immobilization.
4. Direct fracture osteosynthesis is an option for surgical treatment of select type II odontoid fractures and C2 pars interarticularis fractures but is infrequently indicated due to the infrequent occurrence of suitable fractures and multiple associated patient factors.
5. Open reduction and fusion with stable segmental fixation is indicated for unstable craniocervical injury patterns. It is preferable to avoid inclusion of the craniocervical junction whenever possible.

Websites
1. AOSpine Injury Classification Systems: https://aospine.aofoundation.org/en/clinical-library-and-tools/aospine-classification-systems

BIBLIOGRAPHY

1. Bellabarba C, Mirza SK, West GA, et al. Diagnosis and treatment of craniocervical dislocation in a series of 17 consecutive survivors during an 8-year period. *J Neurosurg Spine* 2006;4:429–440.
2. Bellabarba C, Bransford RJ, Chapman JR. Occipitocervical and upper cervical spine fractures. In: Shen FH, Samaratzis D, Fessler RG, editors. Textbook of the Cervical Spine. Philadelphia, PA: Saunders; 2015, pp. 167–183.
3. Browner BD, Jupiter JB, Krettek C. Craniocervical injuries. In: Browner BD, Jupiter JB, Krettek C, editors. Skeletal Trauma: Basic Science, Management, and Reconstruction. 5th ed. Philadelphia, PA: Saunders; 2015, pp. 813–874.
4. Chapman JR, Smith JS, Kopjar B, et al. The AOSpine North America Geriatric Odontoid Fracture Mortality Study: A retrospective review of mortality outcomes for operative versus nonoperative treatment of 322 patients with long-term follow-up. *Spine* 2013;38:1098–1104.
5. Dickman CA, Greene KA, Sonntag VK. Injuries involving the transverse atlantal ligament: Classification and treatment guidelines based upon experience with 39 injuries. *Neurosurgery* 1996;38:44–50.
6. Dvorak MF, Johnson MG, Boyd M, et al. Long-term health-related quality of life outcomes following Jefferson-type burst fractures of the atlas. *J Neurosurg* 2005;2:411–417.
7. Grauer JN, Shafi B, Hilibrand AS, et al. Proposal of a modified treatment-oriented classification of odontoid fractures. *Spine J* 2005;5:123–129.
8. Levine AM, Edwards CC. Fractures of the Atlas. *J Bone Joint Surg* 1991;73:680–691.
9. Schleicher P, Scholz M, Pingel A, et al. Traumatic spondylolisthesis of the axis vertebra in adults. *Global Spine J* 2015;5:346–358.
10. Smith JS, Kepler CK, Kopjar B, et al. Effect of type II odontoid fracture nonunion on outcome among elderly patients treated without surgery: Based on the AOSpine North America geriatric odontoid fracture study. *Spine* 2013;38:2240–2246.

CHAPTER 57

LOWER CERVICAL SPINE INJURIES

Vincent J. Devlin, MD

INJURY CLASSIFICATION

1. **What are some criteria used to classify subaxial cervical spine injuries?**

   Many different classification systems have been proposed for subaxial cervical spine injuries based on a range of criteria, including radiographic instability, mechanism of injury, and injury morphology. While recognition of instability based on radiographic parameters such as relative sagittal plane translation >3.5 mm or relative sagittal plane angulation >11° is useful in clinical practice, classifications based on such criteria have not been widely accepted. Classifications based on mechanism of injury have been popularized but are limited by the challenges inherent in inferring injury type based on static imaging studies. Recent classification systems for subaxial cervical injuries assess injuries based on review of cervical computed tomography (CT), which may be supplemented by magnetic resonance imaging (MRI) and occasionally plain radiography, and consider a range of factors including injury morphology, disruption of the disco-ligamentous complex, neurologic status, and the status of the facet joints.

2. **How are subaxial cervical spine injuries classified on the basis of injury morphology?**

   The injury location and morphology are important factors to assess when classifying a subaxial cervical spine injury. The cervical spine has been conceptualized in terms of four columns: anterior column (anterior and posterior longitudinal ligaments, vertebral body, disc, uncinate processes, and transverse processes), right and left lateral columns (pedicle, superior and inferior facet joints, facet joint capsules, and lateral mass), and posterior column (lamina, spinous processes, ligamentum flavum, and the posterior ligament complex). (1) Injuries may be **isolated** (bony or ligamentous involvement of a single column) or **complex** (both bony and ligamentous involvement of single column or involvement of multiple columns). The **Cervical Spine Injury Severity Score** was developed to quantify the mechanical instability of subaxial cervical injuries and guide treatment. The severity of the bony or ligamentous injury to each column is graded on a scale from 0 to 5, with 0 being uninjured and 5 being the most severely injured. The sum of the scores for each of the four columns represents the Cervical Spine Injury Severity Score and may range from 0 to 20. Surgical treatment is generally indicated for injuries with severity scores greater than 7 while injuries with severity scores less than 5 are generally treated nonoperatively (Table 57.1).

Table 57.1 Subaxial Cervical Spine Fracture Morphology.

A. Injuries Involving the Anterior Column	
Isolated	Compression fracture Transverse process fracture Traumatic disc disruption
Complex	Burst fracture Disc distraction injury ± anterior avulsion fracture Flexion axial load fracture (Flexion-teardrop Injury)
B. Injuries Involving the Lateral Columns	
Isolated	Superior facet fracture Inferior facet fracture Lateral mass pedicle fracture
Complex	Fracture separation of the lateral mass Unilateral facet subluxation or dislocations ± fractures Bilateral facet subluxation or dislocation ± fractures
C. Injuries Involving the Posterior Column	
Isolated	Spinous process fractures Lamina fractures
Complex	Posterior ligamentous disruption ± fracture
D. Special Cases	
	Bilateral pedicle fractures with traumatic spondylolisthesis Spinal cord injury without radiographic abnormality Fractures in ankylosed spines

Adapted from Moore TA, Vaccaro AR, Anderson PA. Classification of lower cervical spine injuries. Spine 2006;31:37–43.

3. **What is the Subaxial Cervical Injury Classification scoring system?**

The Subaxial Cervical Injury Classification (SLIC) scoring system (Table 57.2) added neurologic status as a factor to consider in the classification of subaxial cervical spine injuries (10). The SLIC scoring system analyzes three injury characteristics to guide classification and treatment:

- **Injury morphology:** The injury pattern on imaging studies is classified as no injury, compression injury, burst injury, distraction injury, or rotational/translational injury.
- **Disco-ligamentous complex integrity:** The integrity of the spinal column soft tissue constraints, including the disc, annulus, anterior and posterior longitudinal ligaments, facet capsules, and posterior ligaments, is evaluated and described as none, indeterminate, or disrupted.
- **Neurologic status:** Neurologic status is assessed and described as no injury, root injury, complete cord injury, incomplete cord injury, or continuous cord compression. Incomplete neurologic injury in the setting of persistent neural compression is most likely to benefit from surgical intervention and is associated with the highest score.

Lack of consensus regarding nomenclature for injury morphology and identification of injury to the osteoligamentous complex led to additional classification efforts.

Table 57.2 Subaxial Cervical Spine Injury Classification (SLIC).

1. FRACTURE MORPHOLOGY	SCORE[a]
No injury	0
Compression	1
Burst	2
Distraction	3
Rotation/translation	4
2. DISCO-LIGAMENTOUS COMPLEX INJURY	
None	0
Indeterminate	1
Disrupted	2
3. NEUROLOGIC FUNCTION	
Intact	0
Root injury	1
Complete cord injury	2
Incomplete cord injury	3
Ongoing compression with deficit	+1
TOTAL SCORE (1 + 2 + 3)	**0–10**

[a]For a total score ≤3 nonoperative treatment is recommended, for a score = 4 either surgery or nonoperative treatment are options, and for a score ≥5 surgery is recommended.

From Vaccaro AR, Hulbert RJ, Patel AA, et al. The subaxial cervical injury classification system: A novel approach to recognize the importance of morphology, neurology and integrity of the disco-ligamentous complex. Spine 2007;32:2365–2374.

4. **How are lower cervical spine injuries stratified according to the AOSpine Subaxial Cervical Spine Injury Classification?**

The AOSpine Subaxial Cervical Spine Fracture Classification (2) builds on the classic AO-Magerl spine classification to address limitations of previous injury classifications. Injuries are stratified based on fracture morphology, facet joint injury, neurologic status, and case-specific modifiers. Injuries are first identified by injury level and morphology. The three main injury morphologies are: type A, compression injuries with an intact tension band; type B, anterior or posterior tension band injuries that occur through distraction; type C, injuries with translation along any axis. Type F is applied when the dominant injury pattern involves the facets. The injury level and type are used to identify the injury. When multiple injury types occur in the same patient, the injury with the highest severity determines the grade. Any additional injuries and any modifiers that are present are identified in parentheses (i.e., facet injury, neurologic status modifier, case-specific modifier).

A. Injury types

Type A injury: Compression injury with an intact tension band
- A0: Soft tissue injury or minor fracture involving the lamina, transverse process, or spinal cord injury without bony injury as often seen in a central cord syndrome

- A1: Compression fracture involving a single endplate without involvement of the posterior vertebral wall
- A2: Coronal split or pincer-type fracture involving both endplates without any involvement of the posterior wall of the vertebral body
- A3: Incomplete burst fracture involving a single endplate with involvement of the posterior vertebral body wall
- A4: Complete burst fracture or sagittal split involving both endplates with involvement of the posterior vertebral wall, but without disruption of the posterior tension band

Type B injury: Anterior or posterior tension band injury
- B1: Monosegmental osseous failure of the posterior tension band extending into the vertebral body
- B2: Posterior tension band injury affecting capsule/ligamentous structures (may involve any combination of bony, capsuloligamentous, or ligamentous structures)
- B3: Anterior tension band injury with disruption or separation of anterior structures (bone or disc) without translation, which is limited by intact posterior elements

Type C injury: Injury with translation in any axis

Type F injury: Dominant injury pattern involves the facet joints
- F1: Nondisplaced facet fracture with a fragment size of <1 cm, involving <40% of the lateral mass
- F2: Facet fracture with a fragment size of >1 cm in size, involving >40% of the lateral mass or any displaced fracture fragments
- F3: Floating lateral mass due to ipsilateral disruption of the pedicle and lamina, which dissociates the superior and inferior articular processes from the vertebral body
- F4: Facet subluxation or perched/dislocated facets

B. **Neurologic status modifiers**
- N0: Neurologically normal
- N1: Transient neurologic deficit
- N2: Radiculopathy or cranial nerve injury
- N3: Incomplete spinal cord injury
- N4: Complete spinal cord injury
- NX: Unexaminable patient
- N+: Ongoing spinal cord compression

C. **Case-specific modifiers**
- M1: Posterior capsuloligamentous complex injury without complete disruption
- M2: Critical disc herniation
- M3: Stiffening or metabolic bone diseases such as ankylosing spondylitis (AS), diffuse idiopathic skeletal hyperostosis (DISH), ossification of the posterior longitudinal ligament (OPLL) or ossification of the ligamentum flavum (OLF)
- M4: Signs of vertebral artery injury

(Fig. 57.1)

5. Describe the options for nonoperative care of subaxial cervical spine injuries.
Nonoperative care with an orthosis is appropriate for nondisplaced or minimally displaced subaxial cervical injuries that appear stable and are not associated with neurologic deficits, and for patients who are unable or unwilling to undergo surgery. The most common type of orthosis used for treatment of subaxial cervical injuries is a rigid cervical orthosis (CO). Rigid COs have a two-piece construction and current designs include apertures for ventilation, adjustable mandible and occipital components, and are ideally fitted by an orthotist. Trauma extrication collars or Philadelphia-type collars applied in emergency settings are not adequate for longer-term use postinjury. Soft cervical collars do not provide meaningful motion control and are not adequate for treatment of acute cervical injuries requiring motion restriction. Cervical thoracic orthoses (CTOs) are prescribed when greater motion restriction is desired in the lower cervical region and across the cervicothoracic junction. CTOs utilize chin and occipital supports attached to the trunk via straps or rigid circumferential supports. An alternative for providing increased stabilization of the lower cervical and upper thoracic regions is the attachment of a CO to a thoracic vest. CTOs are less well accepted by patients than COs due to lack of comfort and a high incidence of skin breakdown associated with their use. The most rigid orthosis available is a halo skeletal fixator, but it is poorly tolerated by patients and is infrequently used today. In patients in whom nonoperative treatment is initiated, it is important to obtain upright radiographs to assess spinal alignment after orthosis fitting. If spinal alignment is unchanged on upright radiographs, the patient remains comfortable, and no new neurologic symptoms are reported, a trial of physician-supervised orthotic treatment is initiated.

6. What is the role of cranial traction in the acute management of patients with cervical spine injuries?
Cranial traction applied using cervical tongs or a halo ring plays an important role in the closed reduction of subaxial fractures and dislocations in patients who are examinable, and provides a means of initial temporary stabilization of the injured cervical spine prior to surgery. Traction can restore spinal alignment and decrease or eliminate osseous cord compression in up to 80% of patients with cervical spine fractures or

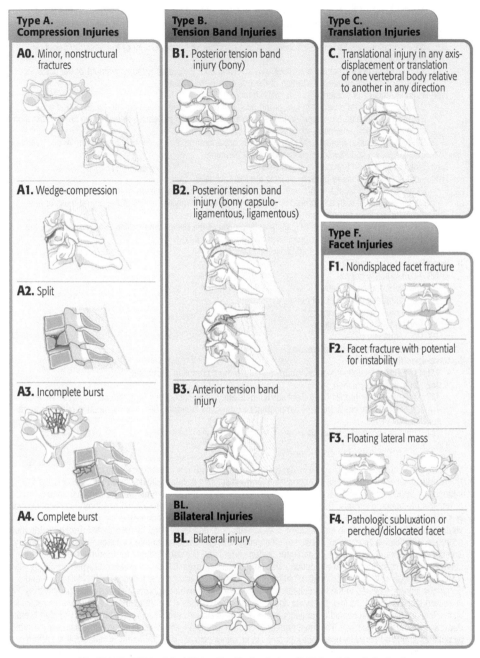

Type A.
Compression Injuries

A0. Minor, nonstructural fractures

A1. Wedge-compression

A2. Split

A3. Incomplete burst

A4. Complete burst

Type B.
Tension Band Injuries

B1. Posterior tension band injury (bony)

B2. Posterior tension band injury (bony capsulo-ligamentous, ligamentous)

B3. Anterior tension band injury

BL.
Bilateral Injuries

BL. Bilateral injury

Type C.
Translation Injuries

C. Translational injury in any axis-displacement or translation of one vertebral body relative to another in any direction

Type F.
Facet Injuries

F1. Nondisplaced facet fracture

F2. Facet fracture with potential for instability

F3. Floating lateral mass

F4. Pathologic subluxation or perched/dislocated facet

Fig. 57.1 The AOSpine Subaxial Injury Classification System. (© AO Foundation, Switzerland.)

cervical facet dislocations associated with spinal canal narrowing and acute spinal cord injury, and thus can improve neurologic outcomes. (3) For patients with head injuries or intoxication, a pre-reduction MRI is necessary before attempting a closed or open reduction of a cervical fracture-dislocation. Disrupted or herniated intervertebral disc material is present on MRI in one-third to one-half of patients with cervical fracture disloca-tions. However, these findings have not been shown to negatively impact outcome following closed reduction in awake patients. The overall rates of transient and permanent neurologic deficit following closed reduction have been estimated as 2%–4% and 1%, respectively. Closed reduction should not be attempted in patients with an ankylosed spine or those with a second proximal cervical spine injury.

7. What are the goals of surgical treatment of subaxial cervical spine injuries?
The goals of surgical treatment of subaxial cervical spine injuries include:
- Early decompression of the spinal cord and nerve roots when indicated
- Restoration of spinal alignment
- Stabilization of the spinal column
- Minimization and appropriate management of adverse events
- Early patient mobilization and rehabilitation

8. Describe the advantages and disadvantages of anterior, posterior, and combined surgical approaches for treatment of subaxial cervical spine injuries.
Surgical treatment options for subaxial cervical spine injuries include: 1) anterior decompression, fusion and plate fixation, 2) posterior segmental instrumentation with screw-rod systems and fusion with or without direct decompression, and 3) combined anterior-posterior surgical approaches. Selection of treatment is individualized based on the characteristics of the specific injury taking into account neurologic status, the severity and type of osseous and/or ligamentous disruption, the severity and cause of spinal cord compression, and patient-specific factors. (4)
- **Anterior cervical decompression, fusion, and plating:** Advantages of an anterior approach include surgery in the supine position, which avoids the necessity of turning patients with unstable injuries to the prone position, direct exposure of the ventral spinal canal for decompression, high arthrodesis rates, and the ability to restore segmental lordosis. Disadvantages of an anterior approach include biomechanical inferiority of anterior fixation compared with posterior fixation, approach-related adverse events, including dysphagia, and poor outcomes when anterior fixation is used without posterior stabilization in injuries with endplate compression fractures or with disruption of the posterior tension band or unreduced facet dislocations.
- **Posterior screw-rod instrumentation and fusion with or without decompression:** Advantages of posterior approaches include biomechanically superior implant constructs, the ability to directly reduce facet dislocations, and the opportunity to directly reconstruct the posterior tension band. Disadvantages of the posterior approach include use of the prone position, the inability to directly decompress anterior disc herniations, and a higher incidence of wound complications compared with anterior approaches.
- **Circumferential approaches for spinal decompression, stabilization, and fusion:** Combined approaches are indicated for treatment of complex injuries that result in severe instability due to disruption of the anterior spinal column and posterior tension band. Combined approaches are also indicated whenever there is residual instability or neural compression after completion of a first-stage anterior or posterior approach.

COMPRESSION SUBAXIAL CERVICAL SPINE INJURIES (AO TYPE A)

9. Discuss the treatment of the different types of compression injuries (AO Type A) involving the subaxial cervical spine.
Type A0 injuries most commonly consist of minor injuries such as isolated lamina or spinous process fractures, which are treated nonoperatively with a rigid CO. Uncommon variants include isolated lamina fractures with displacement into the spinal canal, which are treated with posterior decompression and stabilization. Transverse process fractures that extend into the foramen transversarium require screening for associated injury to the vertebral artery with magnetic resonance angiography or CT angiography. Central cord injuries with ongoing neural compression are evaluated for spinal decompression.

Type A1 (compression fracture, single endplate involvement) and A2 injuries (coronal split or pincer fracture involving both endplates) lack posterior vertebral body wall involvement. Patients with isolated injuries and less extensive osseous involvement may be treated initially with a rigid orthosis. Patients who fail nonoperative treatment or who present with extensive osseous involvement or traumatic disc herniation are treated with anterior cervical decompression, fusion, and plate stabilization.

Type A3 and A4 fractures are burst fractures involving one or both endplates with posterior vertebral body wall involvement but without disruption of the posterior tension band. Spinal cord compression and neurologic injury are common in A3 and A4 injuries. Surgical treatment is often required due to neurologic injury and/or extensive osseous disruption and most often consists of anterior corpectomy, placement of an anterior strut graft or vertebral body replacement device, and anterior plate fixation. In some cases, supplemental posterior fixation is considered. In neurologically intact patients with minimal retropulsion, an initial trial of nonoperative treatment with a rigid orthosis is an option. Burst fractures that occur in conjunction with posterior tension band injuries result from flexion-axial loading and are classified as type B injuries (Fig. 57.2).

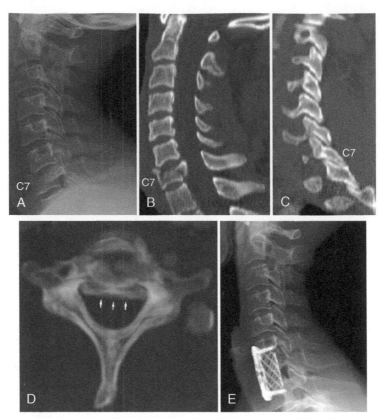

Fig. 57.2 C7 complete burst fracture (type A4 injury). This 32-year-old cyclist suffered an isolated C7 burst fracture when hit by a car. Plain radiograph (A) and sagittal computed tomographic reconstruction (B), show a C7 burst fracture with involvement of both end-plates and retropulsion of the posterior vertebral body into the spinal canal. Sagittal alignment is well maintained and no interspinous widening is present. (C) The facet joints are intact. (D) The axial computed tomography demonstrates the retropulsed posterior body of C7 *(arrows)*, which narrow the spinal canal. (E) The patient underwent a C7 corpectomy with titanium cage reconstruction and anterior cervical plating. (From Kwon BK, Anderson PA. Injuries to the lower cervical spine. In: Browner BD, Jupiter JB, Levine AM, et al, editors. Skeletal Trauma. 4th ed. Philadelphia, PA: Saunders; 2009.)

TENSION BAND SUBAXIAL CERVICAL SPINE INJURIES (AO TYPE B)

10. Discuss the treatment of the different types of tension band (AO Type B) subaxial cervical spine injuries.

Type B injuries affect either the posterior or anterior tension band in the subaxial cervical region. Type B injuries may be associated with vertebral body fractures. In these cases, the fracture remains classified as a B injury as this is the more severe injury component.

Type B1 injuries are distraction injuries through the posterior osseous structures. In the neurologically intact patient, nonoperative treatment with a rigid collar is an option for nondisplaced injuries. Surgical stabilization may be performed through either an anterior or posterior approach for displaced injuries, patients with neurologic deficits, and nonoperative treatment failures. B1 injuries in patients with stiff spines (M3 modifier) are highly unstable and surgical treatment is recommended in most patients.

Type B2 injuries are flexion-distraction injuries that disrupt the posterior tension band and involve capsular, ligamentous, or osseous structures and may extend anteriorly through the vertebral body or intervertebral disc. A spectrum of injuries are included in type B2 injuries. One variant, the flexion-teardrop fracture, occurs due to combined flexion-axial loading due to injury mechanisms, such as diving or motor vehicle injuries, and is associated with an extremely high rate of neurologic injury. A characteristic triangular or quadrangular fracture of the anteroinferior vertebral body occurs as the vertebra is cleaved into an anterior inferior segment (the teardrop

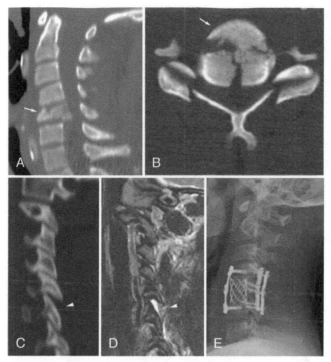

Fig. 57.3 Flexion-axial loading injury with tension band disruption (type B2 injury). This patient presented with a severe C5 flexion-axial loading injury and complete quadriplegia. Notice the large anterior fragment of the C5 vertebral body *(arrow)* on the sagittal (A) and axial (B) images. There is a sagittal split in the C5 vertebral body, bilaminar fractures, and facet disruption *(arrowheads)* as seen on sagittal computed tomography (C) and confirmed on T2-weighted magnetic resonance imaging (D). Due to the severe instability, a circumferential stabilization was performed (E). The autogenous bone from the C5 corpectomy was used to fill a titanium reconstruction cage, followed by anterior plating and posterior lateral mass fixation from C4 to C6. (From Kwon BK, Anderson PA. Injuries to the lower cervical spine. In: Browner BD, Jupiter JB, Levine AM, et al, editors. Skeletal Trauma. 4th ed. Philadelphia, PA: Saunders; 2009.)

segment) and the remaining portion of the vertebral body displaces posteriorly towards the spinal cord. Anterior cranial-caudal vertebral height loss is present in combination posterior tension band injury. Treatment involves realignment using traction followed by surgical treatment. Options for surgical treatment include anterior procedures with corpectomy, strut grafting and plate fixation, posterior procedures involving screw-rod constructs, or combined surgical approaches (Fig. 57.3).

Type B3 injuries disrupt the anterior tension band. These injuries often occur in mobile spines following trauma due to extension injury mechanisms. Surgical treatment varies based on the extent of injury and often consists of anterior fusion and plate fixation. Type B3 injuries also occur in younger patients with ankylosing spondylitis or DISH, as well as elderly patients with cervical spondylosis and stenosis following falls. Type B3 fractures in patients with spine stiffening due to AS or DISH are highly unstable and are most commonly treated with multilevel posterior screw-rod fixation. In elderly patients, type B3 fractures often present with central cord syndrome. Lack of consensus exists regarding timing of treatment and optimal surgical approach for B3 injuries associated with central cord syndrome, but the current trend is toward early decompression and stabilization.

TRANSLATIONAL SUBAXIAL CERVICAL INJURIES (AO TYPE C)

11. Discuss the treatment of translational (AO Type C) subaxial cervical spine injuries.
    Translational injuries are characterized by translation or displacement of one vertebral body relative to another along any axis in any direction (i.e., anterior, posterior, lateral, vertical). These are extremely unstable injuries and often occur in combination with other injury types including facet injuries, fractures through the pars interarticularis, or disruption of the intervertebral disc. These combined injuries are classified as translation type C injuries and the other injury subtypes are listed as associated injuries in parentheses. Surgical treatment is

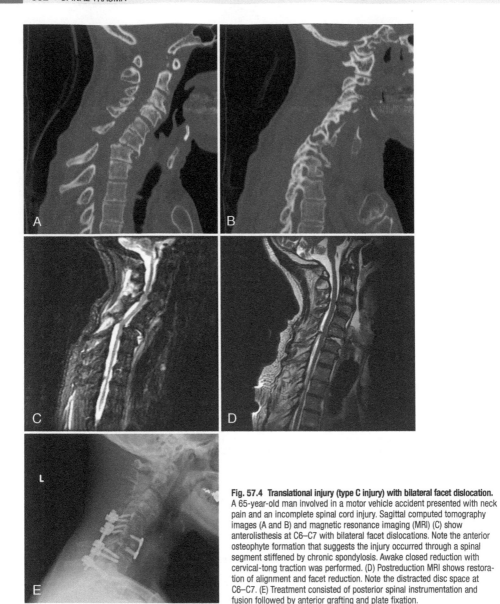

Fig. 57.4 Translational injury (type C injury) with bilateral facet dislocation.
A 65-year-old man involved in a motor vehicle accident presented with neck pain and an incomplete spinal cord injury. Sagittal computed tomography images (A and B) and magnetic resonance imaging (MRI) (C) show anterolisthesis at C6–C7 with bilateral facet dislocations. Note the anterior osteophyte formation that suggests the injury occurred through a spinal segment stiffened by chronic spondylosis. Awake closed reduction with cervical-tong traction was performed. (D) Postreduction MRI shows restoration of alignment and facet reduction. Note the distracted disc space at C6–C7. (E) Treatment consisted of posterior spinal instrumentation and fusion followed by anterior grafting and plate fixation.

dictated by the specifics of the injury and may involve anterior, posterior, or combined surgical approaches for decompression and stabilization (Fig. 57.4).

FACET INJURIES INVOLVING THE SUBAXIAL CERVICAL SPINE (AO TYPE F)

12. Discuss the treatment of the different types of facet injuries (AO Type F) involving the subaxial cervical spine.

Facet injuries may occur as the primary component of an injury or in association with other A, B, or C injury types. Type F injuries are classified separately in specific circumstances such as unilateral facet joint fracture, fracture-separation of the lateral mass, or bilateral facet dislocations. Bilateral facet injuries are identified using a modifier, BL, and list the right-sided injury before the left-sided injury. When facet injuries occur in association with other A, B, or C injuries, the facet injury type is listed after the main injury type.

Type F1 facet injuries are unilateral, nondisplaced facet fractures involving either the superior or inferior facet with a fragment size of <1 cm or involving <40% of the lateral mass. In the absence of radiculopathy, listhesis, or fracture comminution, these injuries may be treated initially with a rigid collar and observed. If subluxation or radiculopathy develop, patients may be treated with either an anterior or posterior single-level instrumented fusion. (5)

Type F2 injuries are unilateral facet injuries that are displaced or have a fracture fragment size >1 cm, or involve >40% of the lateral mass. Nonoperative treatment of these injuries is associated with a higher risk for failure than F1 injuries, and operative treatment is most commonly recommended. Either an anterior or posterior surgical approach can be utilized when a disc herniation causing neural compression is ruled out by MRI.

Type F3 injuries involve ipsilateral disruption of the pedicle and lamina that dissociates the superior and inferior articular processes from the vertebral body and is referred to as a fracture separation of the lateral mass. This injury creates potential instability at two adjacent motion segments with the possibility of anterior subluxation at both the cranial and caudal levels. This injury type is also associated with an increased risk of vertebral artery injury. Surgical treatment is generally indicated for type F3 injuries and consists of anterior or posterior instrumentation and fusion over two motion segments (Fig. 57.5).

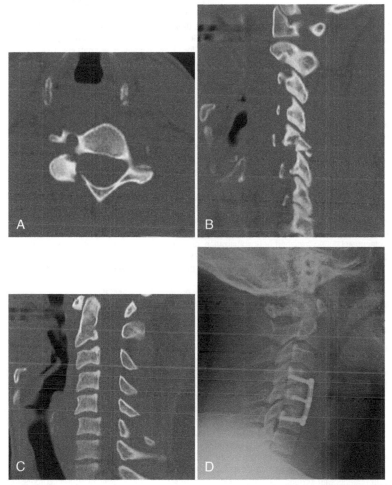

Fig. 57.5 Fracture separation of the lateral mass (F3 Injury). (A) Axial computed tomography (CT) shows ipsilateral pedicle and lamina fractures, which create a free-floating lateral mass. (B) Sagittal CT image shows rotational deformity of the fractured lateral mass. (C) CT image shows associated anterolisthesis at C5–C6. (D) Treatment consisted of anterior reduction and two-level discectomy and fusion combined with anterior plate fixation.

Type F4 injuries involve subluxed, perched, or dislocated facets and may occur unilaterally or bilaterally. Unilateral facet joint dislocations present with up to 25% anterolisthesis; bilateral facet joint dislocations present with 25%–50% or even greater anterolisthesis; and perched facets demonstrate increased segmental kyphosis with minimal translation on midsagittal CT or a lateral radiograph. Surgical treatment is generally indicated for treatment of facet subluxations, perched facets, and facet dislocations with treatment strategies dependent on neurologic status, injury pattern, and severity, as well as patient-specific factors.

The role of closed reduction of facet subluxations and dislocations and the necessity for prereduction cervical MRI has been debated because of the risk of spinal cord injury from displacement of intervertebral disc during closed reduction. Closed reduction requires an awake, cooperative patient. In patients with *incomplete spinal cord injuries* who can be reliably examined, immediate closed reduction with traction and Gardner-Wells tongs has been shown to be safe. For patients with *complete spinal cord injuries* who can be reliably examined, closed reduction immediately preceding an MRI is reasonable. For patients who are unable to be examined, open reduction is performed following an MRI. For *neurologically intact patients* who can be reliably examined, options include immediate closed reduction or MRI to assess for the presence of a traumatic disc herniation which, if present, would require treatment with anterior cervical discectomy, fusion, and plate stabilization.

In all patients with a facet dislocation, a cervical MRI should be obtained following attempted closed reduction and prior to surgical treatment. If an acute disc herniation is noted on the postreduction or preoperative MRI, an anterior approach with anterior discectomy, fusion, and anterior plate fixation is indicated. If a vertebral endplate fracture is noted, a posterior stabilization or combined procedure is performed. In patients with reduced facet dislocations without associated disc herniations or vertebral endplate fractures, either an anterior or posterior approach may be utilized. Combined anterior and posterior procedures are indicated for dislocations not completely reducible from an anterior approach, and for highly unstable injury patterns. Open reduction is required for injuries that fail closed reduction, and techniques for reduction have been described using both anterior and posterior surgical approaches.

INJURIES IN SPECIAL CIRCUMSTANCES

13. **What unique features are associated with subaxial cervical spine injuries in patients with AS and DISH?**
Patients with AS and DISH who present for evaluation following trauma require special consideration:
   - Diagnosis may be difficult, especially with nondisplaced fractures in patients with osteopenia and spinal deformity. AS and DISH patients complaining of neck pain are presumed to have a cervical fracture until ruled out with advanced imaging studies.
   - Fracture patterns are frequently three-column spinal injuries and are highly unstable due to the long, rigid lever arms created by fused spinal segments proximal and distal to the level of injury.
   - Multiple noncontiguous spine fractures or *skip fractures* may be present
   - Neurologic injury is common and may result from initial fracture displacement, subsequent fracture displacement during transport or hospitalization, or associated epidural hematoma (surgical emergency).
   - When such a fracture is recognized, immobilization of the cervical spine in its preinjury position is necessary. In the patient with preexisting kyphotic deformity, this requires placing bolsters underneath the occiput to maintain prefracture alignment.
   - Surgical treatment consists of expedient multilevel posterior instrumentation (three levels above and below the injury if possible). Fusion of the fracture site may not be necessary due to the bony proliferative disease in these patients. Supplemental anterior fusion and plate fixation is indicated in the presence of a significant anterior column osseous defect (Fig. 57.6).

14. **What incomplete spinal cord injury syndrome is commonly associated with a hyperextension injury mechanism in patients with preexistent cervical spondylosis?**
Traumatic central cord syndrome is the incomplete spinal cord injury syndrome most commonly associated with a hyperextension injury mechanism in older patients with cervical spondylosis and a narrow spinal canal. A spectrum of neurologic deficits ranging from weakness limited to the hands to complete quadriparesis may occur. More severe neurologic involvement is noted in the upper extremities compared with the lower extremities. Early surgical treatment is indicated for patients with associated fractures, spinal instability, major neurologic deficits, or deterioration in neurologic status. Evidence exists to support the safety of decompression during the initial hospital admission and <2 weeks after injury, although nonoperative treatment may be considered for patients who demonstrate rapid neurologic recovery following injury. Factors considered in surgical decision making include cervical alignment, cervical stability, location of neural compression, and the number of stenotic levels. In patients with lordotic or neutral spinal alignment and multiple levels of neural compression, a laminoplasty or laminectomy and fusion are treatment options. In patients with anterior neural compression limited to one or two spinal levels or kyphotic deformity, an anterior decompression and plate fixation with or without additional posterior fixation is considered. (3)

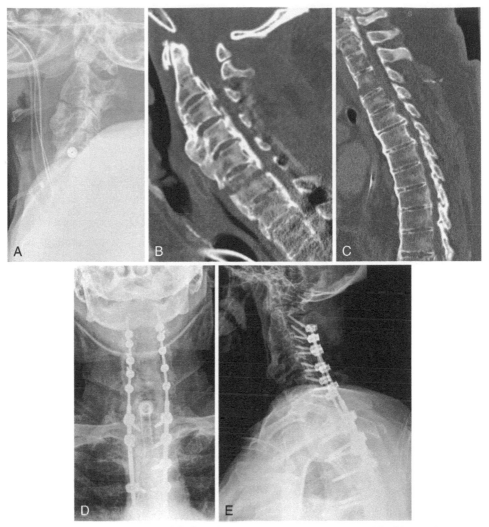

Fig. 57.6 Noncontiguous anterior distraction injuries in a stiffened spine. A 07-year old man with diffuse idiopathic skeletal hyperostosis was an unrestrained driver in a motor vehicle accident and presented with a complete spinal cord injury (American Spinal Injury Association class A) at the C4 level. (A) Lateral cervical spine radiograph reveals a transverse fracture through C3. (B) Sagittal cervical computed tomography (CT) reveals an additional transverse fracture through C6. (C) Sagittal thoracic CT reveals another transverse fracture through T3. (D and E) The patient was subsequently treated with posterior stabilization and fusion from C2 to T6. (From Amorasa LF, Vaccaro AR. Subaxial cervical spine trauma. In: Browner BD, Jupiter JB, Krettek C, et al, editors. Skeletal Trauma: Basic Science, Management, and Reconstruction. 5th ed. Philadelphia, PA: Saunders; 2015, Fig. 34.24, p. 897.)

KEY POINTS

1. Appropriate management of subaxial cervical spine injuries is dependent on injury morphology, neurologic status, and patient-specific factors.
2. Following both nonsurgical and surgical treatment, it is necessary to assess spinal alignment on a regular basis with upright radiographs.
3. The goals of surgical treatment of subaxial cervical spine injuries include early decompression of neural compression, restoration of spinal alignment and stability, avoidance of adverse events, and early patient mobilization.

Websites
1. Subaxial Cervical Spine Injury Classification: https://aospine.aofoundation.org/clinical-library-and-tools/aospine-classification-systems
2. Lower cervical spine fractures and dislocations: https://emedicine.medscape.com/article/1264065-overview#showall
3. Guidelines for the management of acute cervical spine and spinal cord injury: https://www.cns.org/guidelines/browse-guidelines-detail/16-treatment-of-subaxial-cervical-spinal-injuries

REFERENCES

1. Moore TA, Vaccaro AR, Anderson PA. Classification of lower cervical spine injuries. *Spine* 2006;31:37–43.
2. Schnake KJ, Schroeder GD, Vaccaro AR, et al. AOSpine classification systems (subaxial, thoracolumbar). *J Orthop Trauma* 2017;31:14–23.
3. Gelb DE, Hadley MN, Aarabi B, et al. Initial closed reduction of cervical spinal fracture-dislocation injuries. *Neurosurgery* 2013;72:73–83.
4. Dvorak MF, Fisher CG, Fehlings MG, et al. The surgical approach to subaxial cervical spine injuries: An evidence-based algorithm based on the SLIC classification system. *Spine* 2007;32:2620–2629.
5. Pehler S, Jones R, Staggers JR, et al. Clinical outcomes of cervical facet fractures treated nonoperatively with hard collar or halo immobilization. *Global Spine J* 2019;9:48–54.

BIBLIOGRAPHY

1. Anderson PA. Lower cervical spine injuries. In: Garfin SR, Eismont FJ, Bell GR, et al, editors. *Rothman-Simeone and Herkowitz's The Spine*. 7th ed. Philadelphia, PA: Elsevier; 2018, pp. 1311–1332.
2. Anderson PA, Moore TA, Davis KW, et al. Cervical spine injury severity score: Assessment of reliability. *J Bone Joint Surg* 2007;89:1057–1065.
3. Anderon KK, Tetreault L, Shamji MF, et al. Optimal timing of surgical decompression for acute traumatic central cord syndrome: A systematic review of the literature. *Neurosurgery* 2015;77:15–32.
4. Divi AN, Schroeder GD, Oner FC, et al. AOSpine—Spine Trauma Classification System: The value of modifiers: A narrative review with commentary on evolving descriptive principles. *Global Spine J* 2019;9:77–88.
5. Dvorak MF, Fisher CG, Fehlings MG, et al. The surgical approach to subaxial cervical spine injuries: An evidence-based algorithm based on the SLIC classification system. *Spine* 2007;32:2620–2629.
6. Gelb DE, Hadley MN, Aarabi B, et al. Initial closed reduction of cervical spinal fracture-dislocation injuries. *Neurosurgery* 2013;72:73–83.
7. Moore TA, Vaccaro AR, Anderson PA. Classification of lower cervical spine injuries. *Spine* 2006;31:37–43.
8. Pehler S, Jones R, Staggers JR, et al. Clinical outcomes of cervical facet fractures treated nonoperatively with hard collar or halo immobilization. *Global Spine J* 2019;9:48–54.
9. Schnake KJ, Schroeder GD, Vaccaro AR, et al. AOSpine classification systems (subaxial, thoracolumbar). *J Orthop Trauma* 2017;31:14–23.
10. Vaccaro AR, Hulbert RJ, Patel AA, et al. The subaxial cervical injury classification system: A novel approach to recognize the importance of morphology, neurology and integrity of the discoligamentous complex. *Spine* 2007;32:2365–2374.

CHAPTER 58

THORACIC AND LUMBAR SPINE FRACTURES

Vincent J. Devlin, MD

GENERAL

1. **How does regional spinal anatomy influence the characteristics and distribution of thoracic and lumbar spine fractures?**

   The thoracic and lumbar spinal fractures occur in three distinct anatomic regions: the thoracic (T1–T9), thoracolumbar (T10–L2), and low lumbar (L3–L5) regions.

   The **thoracic region** is aligned in kyphosis, has limited mobility except for rotation due to coronal orientation of the facet joints, and is stabilized by the rib cage, sternum, and thickened ligaments. The spinal canal is narrowest in the thoracic region and occupied by the spinal cord, which is poorly vascularized and susceptible to injury with high-energy injury mechanisms.

   The **thoracolumbar junction** is neutrally aligned in the sagittal plane and serves as a transition area between the stiff thoracic region and the mobile lower lumbar region, which increases susceptibility to injury compared with adjacent regions. Facet joint orientation changes to a more sagittal alignment, which favors flexion-extension motion and limits rotation. The contents of the spinal canal in the thoracolumbar region vary with a transition from spinal cord to conus medullaris and cauda equina at L1–L2. Over 50% of vertebral body injuries and more than 40% of all spinal cord injuries occur in this spinal region. Injuries to the lower part of the spinal cord, the conus medullaris, are often associated with permanent impairment of bowel and bladder function.

   The **lower lumbar region** is highly mobile and possesses a wide range of flexion-extension but limited rotation as a consequence of the sagittal orientation of the facet joints. Sagittal alignment is lordotic and any degree of kyphosis in this region is poorly tolerated. The spinal canal has a larger diameter than in the thoracic or thoracolumbar regions and is occupied by the cauda equina and exiting nerve roots, which are less susceptible to injury and have a better prognosis for recovery compared with injuries to the spinal cord or conus medullaris.

2. **Why is it important to image the entire spinal axis when a significant spine fracture is identified in one region of the spine?**

   There is a 5%–20% chance that a patient has a second fracture in a different region of the spine. Factors that increase the risk of missed spine fractures on initial evaluation include head injuries, intoxication, drug use, and polytrauma.

3. **Discuss the current role of plain radiography, CT, and MRI in the initial assessment of thoracic and lumbar spine fractures.**

   Plain radiography plays a lesser role in the initial imaging evaluation of the potentially injured spine patient than in past years and has been largely replaced by multidetector computed tomography (CT). Adequate sagittal and coronal reconstructions of the spine can be obtained from CT scans of the chest, abdomen, and pelvis performed during an initial trauma evaluation and are more sensitive for the detection of osseous spinal injuries compared with radiographs. Plain radiography continues to play a role in monitoring nonoperatively and operatively treated patients and provides the ability to image the spine in the weight-bearing position. Magnetic resonance imaging (MRI) plays a complementary role in the evaluation of spine trauma and is used to assess patients with neurologic deficits and to evaluate specific injury types including ligamentous injuries, traumatic disc herniations, and pathologic fractures. (6)

INJURY CLASSIFICATION

4. **How are thoracic and lumbar spine fractures classified?**

   Various classification systems have evolved over time based on a range of injury parameters, including assessment of spinal stability, presumed mechanism of injury, and fracture morphology. More recent classification systems have incorporated neurologic status and clinical factors considered to play an important role in treatment decision making.

5. Explain what is meant by spinal instability.
   Clinical instability of the spine has been defined as the loss of the spine's ability to maintain its patterns of displacement under physiologic loads so that no initial or additional neurologic deficit, major deformity, or incapacitating pain occurs. (1) This definition is difficult to apply to clinical practice. **Mechanical instability** refers to the inability of the injured spine to maintain alignment under physiologic loads due to the onset of significant pain or deformity. The presence of mechanical instability may be inferred from injury morphology on static imaging studies or assessed more directly based on upright radiographs, but remains challenging to precisely define. **Neurologic instability** is defined by the presence of neurologic findings at the time of postinjury evaluation. Injuries sufficiently severe to cause neurologic injury are usually mechanically unstable. Neurologic status is considered the most important clinical factor influencing treatment of a thoracic or lumbar spine fracture. (2)

6. How is neurologic status classified following thoracic and lumbar spine fractures?
   A detailed neurologic examination consistent with the International Standards for Neurological Classification of Spinal Cord Injury (ISNCSCI) is performed and includes testing of sensory, motor, and reflex function, as well as a rectal examination. Neurologic status is reported using the **American Spinal Injury Association (ASIA) Impairment Scale (AIS)**. For fractures that occur at the level of the spinal cord, neurologic status is graded as **complete neurologic injury** (ASIA A, complete lack of motor and sensory function below the level of injury, including the anal area), **incomplete neurologic injury** (ASIA B, sensory incomplete; ASIA C, motor incomplete with presence of voluntary anal contraction or half of muscles below the neurologic level of injury rated less than grade 3; ASIA D, at least half of muscles below the neurologic level of injury rated grade 3 or greater), or **normal neurologic status** (ASIA E). For fractures associated with neurologic injury at the level of the conus medullaris of the spinal cord, neurologic status is graded as complete or incomplete depending on neurologic findings that are present, which may include an areflexic bowel and bladder, lower extremity sensory loss, and incomplete paraplegia. For fractures associated with cauda equina injury, variable lower extremity motor and sensory function, bowel and bladder dysfunction, and saddle anesthesia may be present and require detailed neurologic assessment.

7. How are thoracic and lumbar spine fractures classified using the three-column model of the spine as described by Denis?
   Denis proposed a **three-column model** of the thoracic and lumbar spine (Fig. 58.1):
   - The **anterior column** is composed of the anterior longitudinal ligament, anterior half of the vertebral body, and anterior half of the disc.
   - The **middle column** is composed of the posterior half of the vertebral body, the posterior half of the disc, and the posterior longitudinal ligament.
   - The **posterior column** includes the pedicles, facet joints, laminae, and posterior ligament complex.

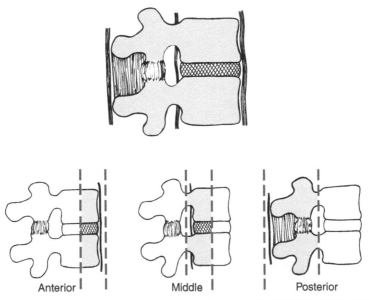

Anterior   Middle   Posterior

Fig. 58.1 The Denis three-column model of the spine. The middle column is made up of the posterior longitudinal ligament, the posterior annulus fibrosis, and the posterior aspects of the vertebral body and disc. (Lee YP, Templin C, Eismont F, et al. Thoracic and upper lumbar trauma. In: Browner BD, Jupiter JB, Levine AM, et al., editors. Skeletal Trauma. 4th ed. Philadelphia, PA: Saunders; 2008.)

Fractures were classified as minor or major. **Minor fractures** included fractures of the transverse processes, articular processes, pars interarticularis, or spinous processes. **Major fractures** were defined based on mechanism of injury and classified into four main fracture types: compression, seat belt, burst, and fracture-dislocations, and further subclassified into more than 16 injury subtypes. The complexity of this classification and the recognition that the middle spinal column was not the primary determinant of spinal instability led to additional research regarding thoracolumbar fracture classification.

8. **What are the six most common patterns of thoracolumbar fractures described according to the classification system proposed by McAfee?**
The **McAfee Classification** expanded Denis's concepts and classified thoracic and lumbar spine fractures into six patterns according to the mechanism and morphology of injury based on CT scan analysis. Six injury patterns were identified based on the forces (compression, axial distraction, or translation) that disrupt the middle spinal column: wedge compression fracture, stable burst fracture, unstable burst fracture, Chance fracture, flexion-distraction injury, and translational injury. These injury pattern descriptors have become widely adopted.
- **Compression fracture:** Isolated failure of the anterior column due to flexion loading. Also referred to as a wedge compression fracture.
- **Stable burst fracture:** Anterior and middle column failure due to compressive loading without loss of integrity of the posterior column.
- **Unstable burst fracture:** Anterior and middle column failure in compression and posterior column disruption due to compression, lateral flexion, or rotation.
- **Chance fracture:** Horizontal fracture around an axis anterior to the anterior longitudinal ligament, which results in tensile failure of the anterior, middle, and posterior columns, and disruption of bone, ligamentous structures and/or the intervertebral disc.
- **Flexion-distraction injury:** An injury due to flexion around an axis located posterior to the anterior longitudinal ligament, which results in compressive failure of the anterior spinal column and tensile failure of the middle and posterior columns.
- **Translational injury:** An injury that results in malalignment of the neural canal due to vertebral displacement in the transverse plane. Injury pattern includes dislocations and fracture-dislocations (Fig. 58.2).

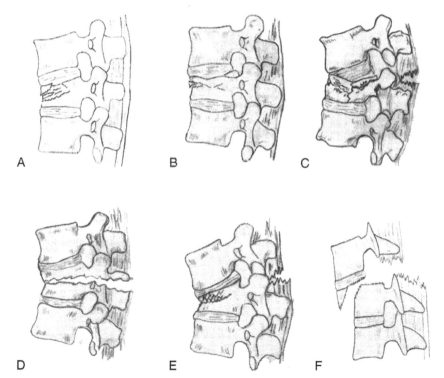

Fig. 58.2 McAfee classification of thoracic and lumbar fractures. (A) Compression fracture. (B) Stable burst fracture. (C) Unstable burst fracture. (D) Chance fracture. (E) Flexion-distraction injury. (F) Fracture-dislocation or translational injury.

9. **What is the AO/Magerl classification of thoracolumbar fractures?**
The **AO/Magerl classification** identifies three major injury patterns according to the primary injury mechanism assessed from radiographs: Type A: compression injuries, type B: distraction injuries, and type C: torsional injuries. Type A fractures are due to anterior column failure in compression and include compression fractures and stable burst fractures. Type B fractures include unstable burst fractures, Chance fractures, flexion-distraction injuries, and extension injuries. Type C fractures consist of translational injuries. A limitation of this original classification was the subdivision of primary injury types into more than 50 distinct injury patterns, which limited its applicability to clinical practice.

10. **What is the Thoracolumbar Injury Classification and Severity Score (TLICS)?**
The **Thoracolumbar Injury Classification and Severity Score (TLICS)** was introduced to address limitations of previous spine injury classifications, including failure to consider neurologic injury status, define spinal instability, incorporate MRI data, or provide guidelines for nonoperative versus operative treatment. TLICS provides a composite injury severity score derived from **three critical injury components** based on assessment of imaging studies (radiographs, CT, and MRI), as well as neurologic status:
(1) injury morphology,
(2) neurologic status, and
(3) integrity of the posterior ligamentous complex (PLC).
    The classification system assigns between 1 and 4 points to each critical injury component, which are combined to determine the **total composite injury severity score**. A score of 3 or less suggests nonoperative treatment; a score of 4 suggests either nonoperative or operative treatment; and a score of 5 or greater suggests operative treatment. Limitations of this classification related to lack of agreement regarding precise definitions of injury morphology and PLC integrity and led to efforts to develop a consensus-based classification (Table 58.1).

Table 58.1 Thoracolumbar Injury Classification and Severity Score (TLICS).

	POINTS
Injury Morphology	
Compression fracture	1
Burst fracture	2
Translational-rotational injury	3
Distraction injury	4
Neurologic Status	
Intact	0
Nerve root injury	2
Incomplete spinal cord or conus injury	3
Complete spinal cord or conus injury	2
Cauda equina injury	3
Posterior Ligamentous Complex Integrity	
Intact	0
Indeterminate	2
Disrupted	3

Adapted from Vaccaro AR, Lehman RA Jr, Hurlbert RJ, et al. A new classification of thoracolumbar injuries: The importance of injury morphology, the integrity of the posterior ligamentous complex, and neurologic status. Spine 2005;30:2325–2333.

11. **Explain how fractures are evaluated using the AOSpine Thoracolumbar Spine Injury Classification.**
The AOSpine Thoracolumbar Spine Injury Classification (3) builds on the classic AO/Magerl spine classification to address limitations of previous injury classifications. Injuries are stratified based on fracture morphology, neurologic status, and case-specific modifiers. The **three main injury morphologies** are: **Type A**, compression injuries with an intact tension band; **Type B**, anterior or posterior tension band injuries that occur through distraction; **Type C**, injuries associated with translation along any axis. The injury level and type are used to classify the injury. When multiple injury types occur in the same patient, the injury with the highest severity determines the grade.

Any additional injuries and any modifiers that are present are identified in parentheses. Multilevel injuries are classified separately and recorded in order of declining severity. Note that type A and B1 injuries affect a single vertebral body level while type B2, B3, and C injures involve at least one motion segment.

A. Injury types
Type A injury: Compression injury with an intact tension band
- A0: Soft tissue injury or minor fracture involving the lamina or transverse process
- A1: Compression fracture involving a single endplate without involvement of the posterior vertebral wall
- A2: Coronal split or pincer-type fracture involving both endplates without any involvement of the posterior wall of the vertebral body
- A3: Incomplete burst fracture involving a single endplate with involvement of the posterior vertebral body wall
- A4: Complete burst fracture or sagittal split involving both endplates with involvement of the posterior vertebral wall, but without disruption of the posterior tension band.

Type B injury: Anterior or posterior tension band injury
- B1: Monosegmental osseous failure of the posterior tension band extending into the vertebral body (Chance fracture)
- B2: Posterior tension band injury affecting capsule/ligamentous structures. It may involve any combination of bony, capsuloligamentous, or ligamentous structures. Associated type A fractures are classified separately.
- B3: Anterior tension band injury with disruption or separation of anterior structures (bone or disc) without translation, which is limited by intact posterior elements. Most commonly occurs in an ankylosed spine due to a hyperextension injury.

Type C injury: Injury with translation in any axis.

B. Neurologic status modifiers
- N0: Neurologically normal
- N1: Transient neurologic deficit that has resolved
- N2: Radiculopathy
- N3: Incomplete spinal cord injury or any degree of cauda equine injury
- N4: Complete spinal cord injury
- NX: Unexaminable patient
- N+: Ongoing spinal cord compression

C. Case-specific modifiers
- M1: Indeterminate injury to the posterior tension band based on clinical exam or imaging studies (i.e., MRI)
- M2: Patient-specific comorbidities that influence surgical decision making such as metabolic bone diseases (osteoporosis), ankylosing disorders (ankylosing spondylitis [AS], Diffuse Idiopathic Skeletal Hyperostosis [DISH]), or burns or abrasions involving skin across the injured spinal levels (Fig. 58. 3).

OVERVIEW OF TREATMENT OPTIONS

12. Describe the indications and methods for nonoperative treatment for thoracic and lumbar fractures.

Minor nonstructural fractures, vertebral body compression fractures, and burst fractures without disruption of the PLC, which occur in neurologically intact patients, are treated without surgery. Based on AOSpine Thoracolumbar Spine Injury Classification, A0, A1, A2, and A3 injuries are generally treated nonoperatively in neurologically intact patients. Contraindications to orthotic treatment include intracranial injury, polytrauma, neurologic deficits, fracture-dislocations, ligamentous injuries, morbid obesity, impaired mental status, impaired skin sensation and noncompliant patients. Treatment consists of an orthosis to provide stability across the injured spinal segments. A custom thoracolumbosacral spinal orthosis (TLSO) is commonly used to treat injuries between T6 and L3. For injuries above T6, a neck extension is added to the TLSO to immobilize the upper thoracic region. For injuries below L3, addition of a thigh cuff is required for immobilization of the lumbosacral region but is poorly tolerated by patients. Upright spinal radiographs in the brace are obtained to confirm adequate immobilization of the injured spinal levels. The brace is generally worn for 3–4 months whenever the patient is out of bed. During follow-up visits, in-brace radiographs are obtained to assess fracture stability and healing. Limited literature exists regarding the use of an orthosis for treatment of these injuries, and available evidence suggests similar clinical and radiological outcomes for patients with stable injuries treated with and without an orthosis.

13. Discuss the indications, timing, and surgical treatment options for thoracic and lumbar fractures.

Operative treatment is indicated for thoracic and lumbar spine fractures associated with neurologic deficit and/or instability, as well as patients who are unable to tolerate or fail brace treatment. In patients with intact neurologic status, the extent of spinal canal compromise is not considered an indication for surgery. The goals of surgical treatment include decompression, realignment, and stabilization of the injured spinal segments. Common injury patterns treated operatively include unstable burst fractures, Chance fractures, flexion-distraction injuries,

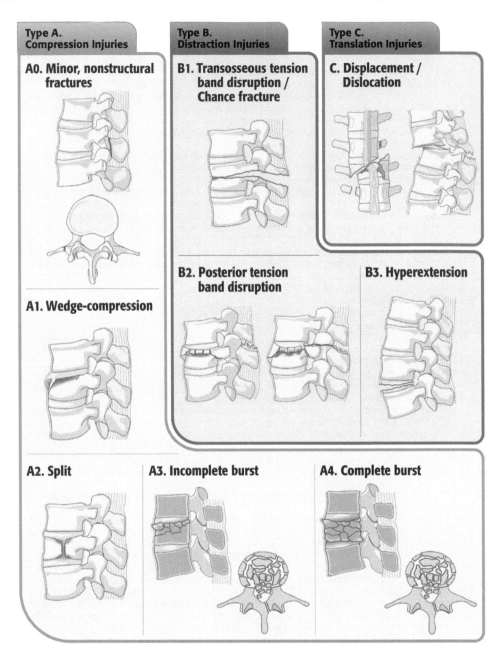

Fig. 58.3 AOSpine Thoracolumbar Classification. (© AO Foundation, Switzerland.)

hyperextension injuries, and translational injuries (fracture-dislocations). Based on the AOSpine Thoracolumbar Spine Injury Classification, A4, B1, B2, B3, and C injuries are treated surgically. Lack of consensus exists regarding precise recommendations for timing of surgery for thoracic and lumbar injuries. In general, early surgery is recommended in a well-resuscitated patient to optimize the potential for neurologic recovery in patients with neurologic deficits and to decrease perioperative complications, intensive care unit days, and length of hospital stay across all injury types. Options for surgical treatment include posterior approaches, anterior approaches, combined approaches, and minimally invasive approaches.

The **posterior surgical approach** is the most common approach used for treatment of thoracic and lumbar fractures. Decompression (indirect or direct), fracture reduction by postural reduction and ligamentotaxis, stabilization through use of pedicle screw-rod systems with or without fusion, can be efficiently performed through a single posterior approach and may be followed by staged anterior procedures as indicated. Short segment implant constructs limit fixation to one level above and below the injured spinal levels. Long segment constructs include fixation at least two to three levels above and below the injured level(s) and may include use of hook fixation or sublaminar fixation in conjunction with pedicle screw-rod systems.

An **anterior surgical approach** is an alternative option for surgical decompression, stabilization, and reconstruction of thoracic and lumbar injuries. An anterior approach is most commonly used for treatment of thoracolumbar burst fractures with high-grade spinal canal compromise at the level of the spinal cord or conus medullaris or extensive vertebral body comminution as it provides direct access to the spinal canal for ventral decompression and allows restoration of anterior column load sharing through placement of an anterior strut graft or vertebral body replacement device. In the absence of major posterior spinal column injury, the combination of anterior spinal decompression, anterior column reconstruction, and anterior spinal instrumentation provides a single-stage treatment option for select thoracic and lumbar fractures.

Combined anterior and posterior surgical approaches are occasionally indicated for treatment of fractures associated with significant anterior and posterior column disruption associated with spinal cord or cauda equina compression. Combined approaches are also indicated for treatment of patients with persistent anterior neural compression following posterior decompression and stabilization. Due to advances in surgical technique and spinal implants, separate anterior and posterior surgical approaches are less commonly performed today as similar outcomes may be obtained through a single-stage posterior-based circumferential surgical approach, which allows for posterior stabilization, spinal canal decompression, corpectomy, and anterior column reconstruction, and is associated with lesser surgical morbidity compared with separate anterior and posterior approaches.

Minimally invasive surgical approaches have been applied to the treatment of thoracic and lumbar fractures. Posterior stabilization using percutaneous minimally invasive pedicle-screw fixation and stabilization with or without fusion can minimize the physiologic burden of surgery, minimize muscle injury and blood loss, and facilitate early rehabilitation. Minimally invasive approaches to the anterior spinal column can also be utilized to reduce the surgical morbidity associated with anterior decompression and stabilization. (2)

14. What is the role of posterior spinal stabilization without fusion in the treatment of thoracic and lumbar spine fractures?
Percutaneous minimally invasive pedicle-screw fixation and stabilization without fusion provides a technique for spinal stabilization that enables fracture healing without permanent stiffening of the spine associated with spinal fusion. Due to the decreased surgical morbidity associated with minimally invasive posterior fracture stabilization without fusion, such techniques have been increasingly utilized for treatment of multiply injured trauma patients, morbidly obese patients, and patients with compromised lung function. Injury patterns amenable to minimally invasive posterior fracture stabilization without fusion include fractures through ankylosed spinal segments as seen in patients with AS or DISH, distraction injuries with osseous failure of the posterior tension band, burst fractures, and multilevel fractures. Potential disadvantages associated with posterior fracture stabilization without fusion include loss of deformity correction over time, recurrence of deformity following implant removal, facet arthrosis, and the potential need for additional spinal procedures. The role of posterior fracture stabilization without fusion in the overall spectrum of operative spine fracture treatment is currently evolving, with available studies demonstrating similar outcomes in patients treated with spinal instrumentation and fusion compared with those in which no fusion was performed.

15. What are the surgical goals for treatment of thoracic or lumbar fractures?
- **Decompression:** Spinal canal decompression is indicated for patients with neurologic deficits, especially progressive or incomplete deficits.
- **Realignment:** Spinal realignment is achieved through use of spinal instrumentation
- **Stabilization:** The combination of spinal instrumentation and spinal fusion can restore long-term stability to injured spinal segments. In select fracture types, instrumentation without fusion offers an option that minimizes the physiologic burden of surgery and potentially limit loss of motion compared with fusion.
- **Minimization of surgical morbidity:** Limit spinal implant construct length and number of fused spinal levels. Consider minimally invasive approaches and avoid fusion for appropriate fracture types.
- **Minimization of complications:** Preoperative patient optimization, appropriate and timely surgery, and meticulous postoperative management can decrease the rate of complications and allow for early recognition and treatment of complications that occur.

TREATMENT OF SPECIFIC INJURIES

COMPRESSION FRACTURES

16. Describe the mechanism, injury pattern, and treatment of thoracic and lumbar compression fractures.

Compression fractures represent an isolated failure of the anterior spinal column due to a combination of flexion and axial compression loading (Fig. 58.4). Because the structural stability of the spine is not compromised by this single-column injury, treatment consists of early patient mobilization with or without brace immobilization. Injuries located above T11 may be treated without an orthosis, as support to the injured level is provided by the thoracic cage, although an orthosis may be prescribed for patient comfort. Thoracolumbar and lumbar fractures are commonly treated with an orthosis (e.g., Jewett brace, thoracolumbosacral orthosis [TLSO]) until back pain resolves, although evidence to support this practice is limited. Radiographic and clinical follow-up is recommended during the first 3 months following injury.

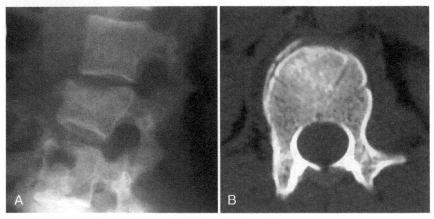

Fig. 58.4 Compression fracture. (A) Lateral radiograph. (B) Axial computed tomography scan. A compression fracture represents an injury of the anterior spinal column. Note the loss of anterior vertebral height. Treatment with an orthosis led to complete resolution of symptoms within 2 months.

17. What are some pitfalls related to assessment of compression fractures?
- In a patient with a vertebral body fracture resulting from significant trauma such as a motor vehicle accident or fall from a height, posterior tenderness or a palpable gap at the level of injury on physical examination suggests a more complex injury pattern. It is estimated that approximately 25% of burst fractures are misdiagnosed as compression fractures if radiographs alone are evaluated. For this reason, it is important to evaluate traumatic thoracic and lumbar spine fractures with CT. MRI has been suggested to evaluate a clinical concern regarding PLC disruption, but is associated with low specificity.
- Multiple adjacent compression fractures may lead to a symptomatic kyphotic deformity, which requires surgical treatment.
- When a compression fracture is encountered in a patient less than age 50 with no history of trauma, workup to rule out a pathologic fracture due to an underlying malignancy or previously undiagnosed metabolic bone disease should be considered.
- Imaging findings that suggest a possible pathologic fracture secondary to a tumor or infection include loss of the pedicle shadow on the anteroposterior (AP) radiograph or coronal CT, presence of a paravertebral or epidural soft tissue mass on MRI, and loss of height of two adjacent vertebral bodies accompanied by narrowing of the intervertebral disc space with endplate erosions.

18. Outline the treatment of compression fractures secondary to osteoporosis.

Osteoporotic compression fractures may occur spontaneously or as the result of low-energy trauma, and may be asymptomatic or symptomatic. The incidence of osteoporotic vertebral compression fractures increases with age in both males and females, and vertebral fracture risk is highest in postmenopausal females over 65 years of age. Osteoporotic compression fractures are associated with an increased mortality rate and an increased risk for future fractures. Multiple fractures may occur and may lead to significant spinal deformities and/or pain. It is important to rule out pathologic fracture due to tumor (e.g. multiple myeloma, metastatic disease) or metabolic bone disease (e.g. osteomalacia). Symptomatic fractures may be treated initially with pain management, analgesic medications, activity modification, physical therapy and bracing. It is important to diagnose and treat the underlying osteoporosis with appropriate medications in addition to treating the fracture. Baseline bone mineral density testing should be performed. Minimally invasive surgical procedures such as vertebroplasty and kypho-plasty are considered for the treatment of select symptomatic acute and subacute compression fractures. These procedures attempt to relieve pain by supplementing the structural integrity of the collapsed vertebral body via the injection of polymethylmethacrylate (PMMA) bone cement. Open surgical treatment with spinal canal decompres-sion combined with stabilization and fusion is reserved for fractures associated with neurologic deficit.

STABLE BURST FRACTURES

19. Describe the characteristics of a stable burst fracture.

Burst fractures result from an axial compression injury of the vertebral body. Key features that identify a stable burst fracture (Fig. 58.5) include:

- The fracture involves both the anterior and middle spinal columns resulting in loss of vertebral height.
- The fracture may involve the posterior vertebral cortex but there is minimal retropulsion of middle column bony fragments
- Posterior column integrity is maintained (i.e., absence of widening between the spinous processes and facet joints at the fractured level when compared with adjacent spinal levels; facet joints and lamina do not demon-strate displaced fractures; the PLC is not disrupted on MRI).
- The patient has intact neurologic status.

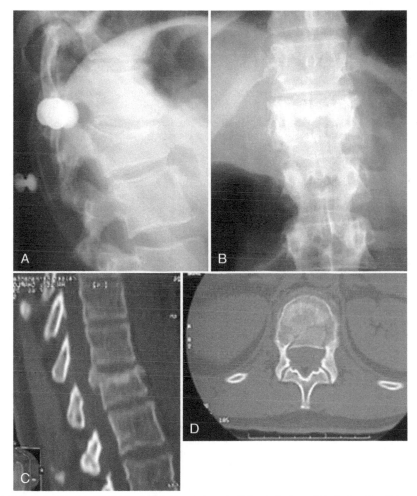

Fig. 58.5 Stable L1 burst fracture. This fracture involves the anterior and middle spinal columns. Note the disruption of the posterior vertebral body cortex. The posterior spinal column is not disrupted. (A) Lateral radiograph. (B) Anteroposterior radiograph. (C) Sagittal computed tomography (CT). (D) Axial CT. Treatment with a thoracolumbosacral orthosis led to resolution of symptoms.

20. What are the treatment options for a stable burst fracture?

Stable burst fractures are usually treated by nonoperative techniques. Treatment methods include closed reduction and immobilization in a body cast or custom-molded TLSO. A cervical extension is added for fractures above T6, and a thigh cuff is considered for low lumbar fractures (L4, L5). Upright radiographs in the cast or brace are obtained following application to assess fracture alignment. The cast or brace is generally worn for 3 months, during which time the patient is assessed clinically and radiographically for increasing symptoms or changes in alignment that would indicate the need for surgery.

UNSTABLE BURST FRACTURES

21. Describe the mechanism and injury pattern of an unstable burst fracture.

Unstable burst fractures result from axial compression forces that disrupt all three columns of the spine. The anterior and middle columns fail in compression with loss of vertebral body height and disruption of the posterior vertebral body cortex with variable degrees of retropulsion of the posterior vertebral body into the spinal canal. The AP radiograph or coronal CT reconstruction shows widening of the distance between the pedicles at the level of fracture. The lateral radiograph or sagittal CT reconstruction shows decreased vertebral height, loss of the normal contour of the vertebral body with retropulsion of the posterior cortex towards the spinal canal, and evidence of posterior column disruption such as segmental kyphosis, increased interspinous distances, facet joint disruption, or spinous process or lamina fractures.

22. What nonspinal injuries are commonly associated with burst fractures?

Calcaneus fractures, long bone fractures, chest injuries, and closed head injuries.

23. What is the major concern regarding a burst fracture associated with a laminar fracture?

Patients with a lumbar burst fracture and a lamina fracture may have incarceration of the dura or neural elements in the fracture site. At the time of injury, lateral splay of the posterior elements under axial loading occurs and may result in a complete or incomplete (greenstick) fracture of the lamina, which can entrap dura or elements of the cauda equina and cause a dural tear with cerebrospinal fluid (CSF) leakage. Recognition of these types of lamina fractures is important to allow fracture site exploration, repair of dural tears, and extrication of entrapped neural elements prior to spinal realignment.

24. When is surgery considered for treatment of thoracic and lumbar burst fractures?

In general, surgical treatment is considered for burst fractures associated with neurologic deficit or instability. (8) Some specific surgical indications include:
- Burst fractures associated with neurologic deficit.
- Burst fractures associated with major disruption of the posterior column—for example, due to facet subluxation or significant disruption of the PLC. Note that minor posterior column injuries such as minimally displaced facet joints, spinous process or vertical lamina fractures, do not disrupt the integrity of the PLC.
- Unstable burst fractures in patients who are unable to be treated with a brace due to associated injuries or body habitus.

25. What are three options for achieving decompression of spinal canal stenosis resulting from a burst fracture in a patient with a neurologic deficit?

- **Indirect decompression:** Distraction applied to the fracture through the use of posterior spinal instrumentation has the potential to reduce the fracture fragments and decompress the spinal canal through *ligamentotaxis*. This technique is most likely to be successful if performed within the first 48 hours after the fracture occurs.
- **Direct posterolateral decompression:** The fragments impinging on the neural elements are pushed away anteriorly to decompress the ventral dural sac after exposure of the spinal canal is achieved through a laminectomy or transpedicular approach. This procedure is performed in conjunction with posterior spinal instrumentation and fusion and allows for removal of the fractured vertebral body (corpectomy) and implantation of a vertebral body replacement device (fusion cage) from the posterior approach.
- **Direct anterior decompression:** The fracture may be exposed directly through an anterior approach, and the entire vertebral body may be removed to decompress the spinal canal. A bone graft or vertebral body replacement device is implanted to reconstruct the anterior spinal column. Spinal stability is restored by placement of anterior spinal instrumentation, posterior spinal instrumentation, or a combination of both anterior and posterior spinal implants.

26. What are the advantages and disadvantages of posterior versus anterior surgical approaches for treatment of thoracic and lumbar burst fractures?

Similar radiographic and functional outcomes may be achieved when thoracic and lumbar burst fractures are treated with either anterior or posterior surgical approaches.

Posterior approaches: Advantages of posterior approaches include their versatility and familiarity to surgeons. Posterior approaches allow surgeons to efficiently perform fracture reduction, indirect and direct spinal canal decompression, and either short- or long-segment pedicle screw-rod constructs with or without anterior column reconstruction through a single surgical approach. Disadvantages of posterior approaches include wound complications and reoperations for implant-related complications (Fig. 58.6).

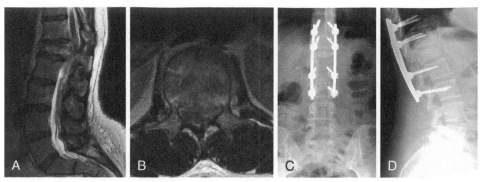

Fig. 58.6 Unstable burst fracture using a posterior approach. (A) Sagittal and (B) axial views of the T2-weighted magnetic resonance image of a 51-year-old woman who fell after completing a ski jump and sustained a severe burst fracture of L1 with disruption of both endplates, 20° of local kyphosis, and 65% canal compromise caused by bony retropulsion. She was neurologically intact. Postoperative (C) anteroposterior and (D) lateral radiographs show restoration of sagittal alignment with fixation and posterolateral fusion from T11 to L3. (From Phan P, Osler P, Wood KB. Treatment of thoracolumbar burst fractures. In: Browner BD, Jupiter JB, Krettek C, et al., editors. Skeletal Trauma: Basic Science, Management, and Reconstruction. 5th ed. Philadelphia, PA: Saunders; 2015, pp. 920–934, Fig. 35B-4, p. 924.)

Anterior approaches: Advantages of anterior approaches include access for direct decompression of the ventral spinal canal and anterior column reconstruction for significant kyphotic deformities and when restoration of anterior load sharing is indicated. In addition, fewer complications and reoperations have been reported following anterior procedures when compared with posterior procedures. Disadvantages of anterior approaches include difficulties when performing instrumentation below L3 due to local anatomic constraints, including the proximity of the aorta, vena cava, and iliac vessels and approach-related morbidity. Caution is necessary in injuries with significant disruption of the posterior column and in patients with osteoporosis as anterior instrumentation may not provide adequate stability in these scenarios. Also, it is not possible to explore lamina fractures for potential neural element incarceration from an anterior approach (Fig. 58.7).

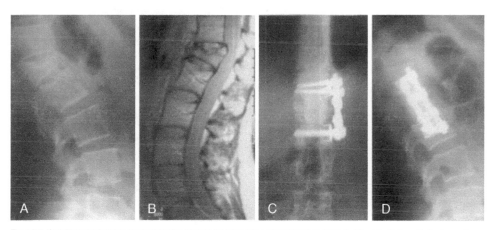

Fig. 58.7 Unstable burst fracture treatment using an anterior approach. L1 burst fracture treated with corpectomy, anterior femoral allograft, and anterior screw-rod construct (Kaneda instrumentation). (A) Preoperative lateral radiograph. (B) Preoperative sagittal magnetic resonance image. Postoperative (C) anteroposterior and (D) lateral radiographs. (From Devlin VJ, Pitt DD. The evolution of surgery of the anterior spinal column. Spine State Art Rev 1998;12:493–527.)

27. When are combined anterior and posterior surgical procedures indicated for treatment of thoracic and lumbar burst fractures?
    Combined anterior and posterior surgery may be necessary for treatment of fractures with significant anterior and posterior column disruption associated with severe spinal cord or cauda equina compression or kyphotic deformity. A combined approach may also be required for treatment of patients with persistent anterior neural

compression following posterior decompression and stabilization. Circumferential surgery can be performed either through separate anterior and posterior surgical approaches or through a single-stage posterior-based circumferential surgical approach, which allows for posterior stabilization, spinal canal decompression, corpectomy, and anterior column reconstruction.

CHANCE FRACTURES

28. **Describe the mechanism and injury pattern of a Chance fracture.**

Chance fractures result from a flexion injury mechanism, most commonly in a lap belt–restrained car passenger. Imaging studies show an injury to all three spinal columns in which transverse failure occurs due to distraction. The axis of rotation for this injury is anterior to the vertebral body. The disruption of the spine may progress through bone (vertebral body, pedicle, and spinous process), soft tissue (disc, facet joint, and interspinous ligament), or a combination of bone and soft tissue structures.

29. **What nonspinal injuries are associated with Chance fractures?**

Intraabdominal injuries (bowel, liver, spleen), vascular injuries (intimal vascular tears, aortic injuries) and neurologic injuries.

30. **What are the options for treatment of a Chance fracture?**

In general, patients with Chance fractures are treated with posterior spinal instrumentation with or without fusion (Fig. 58.8). A short-segment posterior instrumentation construct, which applies compression forces across the fracture, is appropriate. Chance fractures entirely through bone are reasonable candidates for treatment with posterior stabilization using percutaneous minimally invasive pedicle screw fixation and stabilization without fusion. The pattern of injury determines the minimum number of levels requiring instrumentation. If the injury to the middle column involves the posterior disc, MRI is indicated to identify a disc herniation that may require excision prior to application of posterior compression forces. Treatment with extension casting or a TLSO is an option for patients who sustain injuries entirely through bone without concomitant abdominal or neurologic injuries.

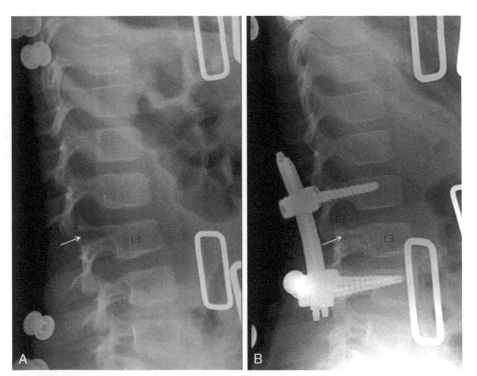

Fig. 58.8 Chance fracture. (A) Lateral preoperative radiograph showing L3 Chance fracture *(arrow)*. (B) Lateral postoperative radiograph following fracture stabilization performed 1 week after abdominal and aortic repair. (From West CA Jr, Johnson LW, Doucet L, et al. Acute aortic occlusion in a child secondary to lap-belt injury treated with thromboendarterectomy and primary repair. J Vasc Surg 2011;54:515–518, Fig. 3, p. 517.)

FLEXION-DISTRACTION INJURIES

31. Describe the mechanism and injury pattern of a flexion-distraction injury.
Flexion-distraction injuries are due to high-energy injury mechanisms such as motor vehicle accidents, falls from a height, and sports injuries. Such injuries result in tensile failure of the posterior spinal column and compressive failure of the anterior column and possibly the middle column. Posterior column injuries include separation of the spinous processes and facet joints. The vertebral body is wedged anteriorly. Bony fragments from the middle column may be retropulsed into the spinal canal. The axis of rotation for a flexion-distraction injury is within the vertebral body, in contrast to a Chance fracture where the axis of rotation is located anterior to the vertebral body. A flexion-distraction injury may be misdiagnosed initially as a compression fracture if the disruption of the posterior spinal column is unrecognized. Similar to Chance fractures, flexion-distraction injuries are associated with intraabdominal injuries.

32. What are the treatment options for a flexion-distraction injury?
These unstable injuries are treated with posterior spinal instrumentation with or without posterior fusion. Fracture variants associated with neurologic deficit, spinal canal comprise, or severe vertebral body comminution require decompression and reconstruction of the anterior spinal column (Fig. 58.9).

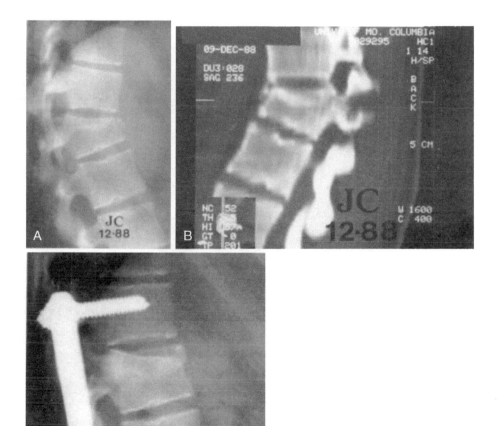

Fig. 58.9 Flexion-distraction injury. (A) Preoperative lateral radiograph. (B) Preoperative computed tomography scan. (C) Postoperative lateral radiograph. (From Holt BT, McCormack T, Gaines RW Jr. Short-segment fusion: Anterior or posterior approach? Spine State Art Rev 1993;7:277–286.)

EXTENSION INJURIES

33. Describe the mechanism and injury pattern of an extension injury.
Extension injuries involving the thoracic and lumbar spine are most commonly encountered in patients with ankylosed spines due to AS or DISH and may occur following minor trauma. These injuries are often missed on initial evaluation but are highly unstable despite their often benign appearance on imaging studies due to the long, rigid lever arms created by fused spinal segments proximal and distal to the level of injury. Neurologic injury is common and may be due to initial fracture displacement, subsequent fracture displacement during transport or hospitalization, or as a result of associated epidural hematoma. Extension injuries may also occur in young healthy trauma patients with normal spines due to high-energy hyperextension injury mechanisms, and an association with aortic and abdominal injuries has been reported.

34. Describe the surgical treatment of a thoracic or lumbar extension injury.
Surgical treatment of extension injuries is fraught with complications. Care in transfer and positioning on the operating room table is essential as fracture displacement and neurologic injury can occur. Fracture reduction is challenging and requires extreme caution to avoid displacement of the injured segment. Treatment consists of multilevel posterior screw-rod instrumentation with or without posterior decompression. If inadequate fracture reduction persists following posterior reduction and instrumentation, fusion of the anterior column is considered to reconstruct the anterior column defect (Fig. 58.10).

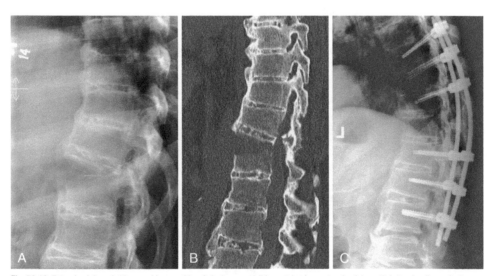

Fig. 58.10 Extension injury. A 45-year-old man with ankylosing spondylitis sustained an extension injury. (A) Lateral radiograph shows anterior distraction between T11 and T12. (B) Sagittal computed tomography scan shows the severe distraction injury. (C) The patient was treated by closed reduction using postural reduction and bolstering to achieve reduction and then percutaneous instrumentation three levels above and below the fracture. (From Belin EJ, Neal JVI, Tannous O, et al. New concepts in the management of thoracolumbar fractures. In: Browner BD, Jupiter JB, Krettek C, et al., editors. Skeletal Trauma: Basic Science, Management, and Reconstruction. 5th ed. Philadelphia, PA: Saunders; 2015, pp. 972–979, Fig. 35E-3, p. 975.)

TRANSLATIONAL INJURIES (FRACTURE-DISLOCATIONS)

35. Describe the mechanism and injury pattern of a translational injury (fracture-dislocation).
Fracture-dislocations result from high-energy injuries and are the most unstable type of spine injuries. The structural integrity of all three spinal columns is disrupted and is associated with displacement of the spine in one or more planes. Severe neurologic deficits generally accompany this injury pattern.

36. What are the treatment options for a translational injury (fracture-dislocation)?
These injuries require surgical stabilization regardless of the patient's neurologic status. These injuries are best treated initially from a posterior approach to realign the spine and restore spinal stability by fixation two or three levels above and below the injury. Anterior column reconstruction may be indicated if there is severe comminution precluding achievement of construct stability with isolated posterior instrumentation or if spinal canal decompression is required, especially for patients with incomplete neurologic deficits (Fig. 58.11).

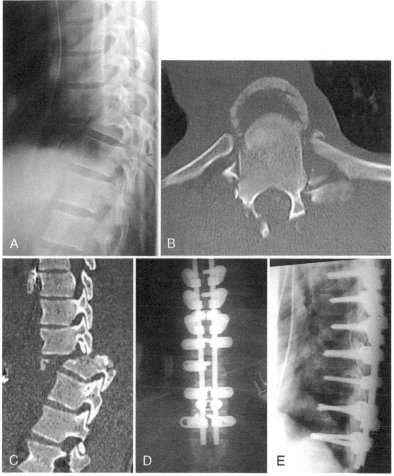

Fig. 58.11 Translational injury. (A) Preoperative lateral radiograph. (B) Axial computed tomography (CT) image. (C) Sagittal CT image. (D) Postoperative anteroposterior radiograph. (E) Postoperative lateral radiographs.

GUNSHOT INJURIES TO THE SPINE

37. Outline the key points regarding treatment of thoracolumbar injuries due to gunshot wounds.

Gunshot injuries involving the thoracic and lumbar spinal column are the third most common cause of spinal injury, trailing behind falls from a height and motor vehicle accidents. Two main types of injuries are encountered: low-velocity injuries (muzzle velocity <2000 ft/second) and high-velocity injury (muzzle velocity >2000 ft/second). Although most civilian gunshot injuries are low velocity and cause injuries due to direct contact, high-velocity injuries are increasingly encountered and cause injuries not only from direct contact but also from shock wave and cavitation effects. Initial evaluation and management requires a multidisciplinary approach that follows Advanced Trauma Life Support (ATLS) protocols as injuries to other organ systems occur in up to 80% of cases of high-velocity injuries. While the majority of civilian low-velocity gunshot wounds are managed nonoperatively, high-velocity gunshot wounds such as rifle injuries require operative debridement. Treatment of low-velocity civilian spinal gunshot wounds includes tetanus prophylaxis, initial broad-spectrum antibiotics for 2–3 days and a longer course of antibiotics for up to 7–14 days for transcolonic gunshot wounds involving the spine, although consensus is lacking in this area. Indications for surgery include spinal infections, CSF leaks, progressive neurologic deficits, and spinal instability.

KEY POINTS

1. The goals of surgical treatment for thoracic and lumbar fractures include decompression of symptomatic neurologic compression, spinal stabilization, spinal realignment, and minimization of surgical morbidity and complications.
2. Computed tomography (CT) is an integral part of the initial assessment of thoracic and lumbar spine fractures.
3. Comprehensive assessment of a thoracic or lumbar fracture includes a description of the injury morphology, neurologic status, and integrity of the posterior ligamentous complex (PLC).
4. Compression fractures and burst fractures without neurologic deficit are usually treated nonoperatively.
5. Abdominal visceral injuries are frequently associated with spinal injuries that occur as a result of distraction.
6. Unstable burst fractures, Chance fractures, flexion-distraction injuries, hyperextension injuries, and translational injuries (fracture-dislocations) are generally treated surgically.

Websites
1. AOSpine Thoracolumbar Classification System: https://aospine.aofoundation.org/clinical-library-and-tools/aospine-classification-systems

---

REFERENCES

1. White AAIII, Panjabi MM, editors. Clinical Biomechanics of the Spine. 2nd ed. Philadelphia, PA: JB Lippincott; 1990.
2. Mirza SK, Mirza AJ, Chapman JR, et al. Classifications of thoracic and lumbar fractures: Rationale and supporting data. *J Am Acad Orthop Surg* 2002;10:364–377.
3. Schnake KJ, Schroeder GD, Vaccaro AR, et al. AOSpine classification systems (subaxial, thoracolumbar). *J Orthop Trauma* 2017;31:14–23.

BIBLIOGRAPHY

1. Jakoi A, Iorio J, Howell R, et al. Gunshot injuries of the spine. *Spine J* 2015;15:2077–2085.
2. Gjolaj J, Williams SK. Thoracic and lumbar spinal injuries. In: Garfin SR, Eismont FJ, Bell GR, et al, editors. Rothman-Simeone and Herkowitz's the Spine. 7th ed. Philadelphia, PA: Elsevier; 2018, pp. 1333–1363.
3. Grossbach AJ, Dahdaleh NS, Abel TJ, et al. Flexion-distraction injuries of the thoracolumbar spine: Open fusion versus percutaneous pedicle screw fixation. *Neurosurg Focus* 2013;35:E2.
4. McAfee PC, Yuan HA, Fredrickson BE, et al. The value of computed tomography in thoracolumbar fractures. An analysis of one hundred consecutive cases and a new classification. *J Bone Joint Surg* 1983;65:461–473.
5. Mirza SK, Mirza AJ, Chapman JR, et al. Classifications of thoracic and lumbar fractures: Rationale and supporting data. *J Am Acad Orthop Surg* 2002;10:364–377.
6. Oner FC, van Gils AP, Faber JA, et al. Some complications of common treatment schemes of thoracolumbar spine fractures can be predicted with magnetic resonance imaging: Prospective study of 53 patients with 71 fractures. *Spine* 2002;27:629–636.
7. Schnake KJ, Schroeder GD, Vaccaro AR, et al. AOSpine classification systems (subaxial, thoracolumbar). *J Orthop Trauma* 2017;31:14–23.
8. Wood KB, Butterman GR, Phukan R, et al. Operative compared with nonoperative treatment of thoracolumbar burst fracture without neurological deficit: A prospective randomized study with follow-up at sixteen to twenty-two years. *J Bone Joint Surg* 2015;97:3–9.
9. Vaccaro AR, Baron EM, Sanfilippo J, et al. Reliability of a novel classification system for thoracolumbar injuries: The Thoracolumbar Injury Severity Score. *Spine* 2006;31:62–69.
10. White AAIII, Panjabi MM, editors. Clinical Biomechanics of the Spine. 2nd ed. Philadelphia, PA: JB Lippincott; 1990.

CHAPTER 59

SACRAL FRACTURES

Jens R. Chapman, MD, Thomas A. Schildhauer, MD, PhD, and Robert Hart, MD

1. **Describe the important anatomic features and functions of the sacrum.**

   The sacrum is located at the junction between the pelvis and spinal column and functions as a keystone between the iliac crests. The sacrum is formed by the coalescence of five vertebral segments (S1–S5) and is attached to the caudal lumbar spine and posterior pelvic ring through broad, well-developed ligamentous structures. The sacrum transmits load from the lumbar spine through the sacroiliac joints to the pelvis and distally to the hip joints. Of biomechanical importance is the fact that the main weight transmission of the lumbosacral junction is borne by the S1 segment, while the S2–S5 segments provide minimal additional support. The sacrum also serves as a protective conduit for major neurovascular structures, including the lumbosacral and sacral plexuses, iliac vessels and their bifurcations, and the organs within the lesser pelvis. The kyphotic alignment of the sacrum in the sagittal plane predetermines lumbar lordosis through inclination of its upper sacral endplate relative to the horizon line. Upwards of 10% of patients have a segmentation anomaly of the lumbosacral junction with either an assimilation of the L5 vertebra to the sacrum (sacralization), or an S1 vertebra, which transitions to a lumbar morphology (lumbarization). Failure to recognize such transitional anomalies can have significant clinical implications.

2. **What injury mechanisms and patient groups are most commonly associated with sacral fractures?**

   There are two distinct injury mechanisms and patient groups associated with sacral fractures:
   1. **High-energy injury mechanisms:** These fractures usually occur in younger, mostly male patients as result of motor vehicle accidents, falls from a height, and crush injuries.
   2. **Low-impact, insufficiency or stress fractures:** This patient group is generally older and more commonly female. Etiologies include low-energy injury mechanisms such as a ground level fall on the buttocks, insufficiency fractures, and stress fractures. Insufficiency fractures may occur in patients with osteoporosis, other metabolic bone diseases, or previously undiagnosed neoplastic disorders. A sacral stress fracture may arise following instrumented lumbosacral fusions surgery. Another subgroup of patients who develop sacral stress or insufficiency fractures includes endurance sports athletes, especially younger females with amenorrhea.

3. **How are patients at risk for sacral fractures evaluated clinically?**

   Clinical symptoms may be vague or non-specific and diagnosis of sacral fractures is often delayed or missed. Common symptoms include low back and buttock pain. A detailed patient history including mechanism of injury and associated injuries is critical. Patients with sacral insufficiency fractures describe intolerance to being upright, even when sitting, and are much more comfortable in a recumbent position. Physical examination with inspection and palpation of the patient's backside and thorough examination of neurologic function is important. In patients with high-energy injury mechanisms, clinical inspection, palpation and percussion of the posterior pelvic ring may reveal focal tenderness, ecchymosis, swelling, and discoloration. Crepitus with manipulation of the hip joints may be noted depending upon the type of injury and its acuity. Suspicion of an acute posterior pelvic ring injury usually should prompt rectal examination and inspection of the vaginal vault in female patients (with chaperone present) to assess for occult soft tissue injuries, blood products, and integrity of sphincters. Any disruption of the dorsal integument or rectal or vaginal cavities in the presence of a sacral fracture of any acuity is suspicious for an open fracture, which profoundly changes surgical treatment.

4. **Describe the components of a complete neurologic examination for patients with a sacral fracture.**

   Regardless of the patient's cognitive status, an evaluation consistent with the *Guidelines of the American Spinal Injury Association* is performed. Neural structures potentially affected by a sacral fracture include the lumbosacral plexus (L4, L5, and S1 roots on either side) and the sacral plexus (S2–S4 bilaterally), as well as the sacral sympathetic nerves (superior and inferior hypogastric plexus). Injury mechanisms include compression, crush, traction, and transection.

   Lumbosacral plexus assessment includes examination of motor, sensory, and reflex function. In addition, pain reproduction with straight leg raises and hip manipulation can help identify nerve root entrapment.

   Sacral plexus evaluation is more limited in its direct clinical findings. It is important to evaluate light touch and pinprick sensation in the S2–S4 dermatomes on either side along the buttocks, the perineum, and include the perianal and genital area. External bladder sensation and internal bladder wall sensation, as applied through a Foley catheter, for instance, usually implies at least partial integrity of the upper sacral plexus. Integrity of perianal sensation on either side and presence of a baseline anal sphincter tone, as well as strong voluntary anal contraction, are helpful to identify integrity of the lower sacral plexus. Presence of a bulbocavernosus reflex is a key determinant in identifying the conclusion of spinal shock following spinal cord injury. A **complete rectal examination** should document:

1. Presence of spontaneous anal sphincter tone
2. Maximum voluntary anal sphincter contractility
3. Perianal sensation to light touch and pinprick
4. Presence of anal wink and bulbocavernosus reflex

In a postacute setting, **postvoid residuals on bladder ultrasound scan** can be used as a follow-up test for patients with a neurogenic bladder to assess for reinnervation. A bladder scan and establishing postvoid residuals can be very helpful in the diagnosis and long-term follow-up of patients with a neurogenic bladder.

5. **What imaging tests are used to assess sacral fractures?**
   The basic radiographic assessment starts with an *anteroposterior (AP) pelvis radiograph*. It is important to realize that the naturally curved kyphotic shape of the sacrum partially obscures visualization of the entire sacrum on the AP pelvic radiograph. Subtle details, such as disruption of the fine cortical lines of the sacrum and especially its foramina, aid as a screening tool. Abnormal pelvic projections, such as seeing a pelvic inlet view on a standard AP pelvic radiograph are other important pointers toward detection of a major sacral fracture. Suspicion based on radiographic findings, clinical findings, or injury mechanism should prompt ordering of a computed tomography (CT) scan, which remains the single most useful test for diagnosis of a sacral fracture. More specific plain radiographs that can reveal posterior pelvic ring and sacral injuries include pelvic inlet and outlet views and a lateral sacral radiograph. While these are helpful, initial radiographic studies for evaluation of sacral alignment, the three-dimensional complexities of sacral and posterior pelvic ring pathology require assessment with CT, including sagittal and coronal reformatted images. In cases associated with bleeding in the region of the sacrum and sciatic notch, CT-angiography is an essential tool for assessment of vascular injury. Magnetic resonance imaging (MRI) is not routinely necessary but is helpful for diagnosis of sacral insufficiency or stress fractures, metastatic disease, and to evaluate unclear neurologic injuries. MRI neurography can localize known root or plexus injury in a subacute setting. For diagnosis of insufficiency fractures and as screening tool for neoplastic and infectious diseases, technetium bone scans with single-photon emission CT (SPECT) images can reveal abnormal osseous activity. This test, however, has little or no role in the assessment of acute injuries.

6. **What other diagnostic tests play a role in the evaluation of patients with sacral injuries?**
   There are a number of tests that can help delineate neurologic injuries and also measure recovery:
   - Electromyogram (EMG) of L5 and S1 innervated muscles (lumbosacral plexus function)
   - Anal sphincter EMG (S2–S4 function)
   - Somatosensory-evoked potentials (SSEPs) of tibial and peroneal nerves
   - Pudendal sensory-evoked potentials (pudendal SEPs)
   - Cystometrography (CMG) in combination with cystoscopy
   - Direct visualization of urethral sphincter function during cystoscopy
   - Postvoid residuals on bladder ultrasound scan

   Use of conventional EMG is limited to assessment of the L5 and S1 roots and usually requires waiting for at least 2–3 weeks before injury-related changes are detectable. Anal sphincter EMG and CMG-EMG can diagnose lower sacral root damage but are usually not useful in the immediate postinjury period. CMG-EMG has been used as a follow-up study for patients with neurogenic bladder and may demonstrate bladder reinnervation. Assessment of postvoid residuals on a bladder ultrasound scan is the most commonly used test to determine sacral plexus recovery in an outpatient setting.

7. **What are some of the main obstacles to timely diagnosis of sacral fractures?**
   Sacral fractures are commonly overlooked on presentation and diagnosis is delayed in up to one-half of patients. The reasons for this include a low clinical index of suspicion, failure to order appropriate imaging, and incomplete understanding of intricacies related to interpretation of diagnostic imaging of this region. The sacrum intersects between two surgical specialties, spine surgery and trauma surgery, and has historically been considered to exist in a "no man's land." Direct clinical challenges may be present, which impede diagnosis in patients with morbid obesity, prior lumbosacral fusions, slow growing neoplastic diseases, lumbosacral transition zone anomalies, and osteopenia. In multiply-injured patients, resuscitation-related activities and evaluation of active hemorrhage, brain injuries, and extremity injuries may divert attention away from sacral injuries and interfere with otherwise well-established diagnostic algorithms, leading to a delay in diagnosis. Systematic evaluation protocols for posttraumatic patients and a heightened sense of awareness in at-risk patients can effectively help decrease the occurrence of missed sacral injuries. Patients with delay in diagnosis of sacral injuries may present with one or more of the following symptoms:
   - Reproducible pain with weight bearing
   - Progressive lumbopelvic malalignment in sagittal and/or coronal plane

- Secondary neurologic deficits, including bowel/bladder/sexual dysfunction from progressive fracture displacement and/or neural element impingement
- Posterior soft tissue breakdown from progressive sacral kyphosis

8. **How have sacral fractures been classified historically?**

The wide range of sacral fracture patterns and their frequent association with pelvic fractures has led to development of many different fracture classification systems based on parameters such as fracture line orientation, pattern of neurologic deficit, and the effect of injury on posterior pelvic and spino-pelvic instability.

The **Denis classification** has been widely used as a general classification of sacral fractures because of its significant implications regarding incidence and type of associated neurologic injury. It uses *fracture location* to distinguish three types of fractures:

- **Zone I fractures** remain lateral to the sacral foramina. This is the most frequent fracture type and is associated with the lowest rate of neurologic injury (6%). Neurologic injury in Zone I fractures is primarily limited to the L5 nerve root.
- **Zone II fractures** extend through the sacral foramina. These are the second most frequent fracture type. Associated lumbosacral nerve root injuries (L5, S1) occur in approximately one-quarter of patients.
- **Zone III fractures** involve the central sacral spinal canal. These are the least common injury type but have the highest rate of neurologic injuries (>50%) ranging from sacral root deficits to cauda equina injuries with associated bowel and bladder control deficits.

The **Roy-Camille classification** stratifies *transverse sacral fractures* based on the pattern of sacral vertebral body involvement. It differentiates fractures with kyphotic angulation without translation (type 1), fractures with kyphotic angulation and posterior translation of the upper sacrum relative to the lower sacrum (type 2), anterior displacement of the upper sacrum relative to the lower sacrum without angulation (type 3), and segmentally comminuted fractures (type 4, as subsequently described by Strange-Vognsen).

The **Isler classification** stratified longitudinal fractures based on their *location relative to the L5–S1 facet joint*. Fractures lateral to the L5–S1 facet joint were not associated with lumbosacral instability, while fractures through or medial to the L5–S1 facet joint potentially destabilize the lumbosacral junction. Three injury types were identified: type 1 (lateral to the facet joint), type 2 (fracture line passes through the L5–S1 facet joint), and type 3 (fracture line passes medial to the L5–S1 facet joint).

Descriptive classifications of sacral fractures are frequently used and simply describe the coronal sacral fracture pattern based upon letters including "U," "H," "Y," lambda, and other radiographic phenotypes.

Sacral fractures associated with pelvic ring injuries require additional classification strategies. Standard pelvic injury classifications (e.g., Tile classification, Young-Burgess classification, AO pelvic fracture classification) have been utilized to assess stability, injury mechanism, and associated injuries.

9. **How are sacral injuries stratified according to the AOSpine Sacral Fracture Classification?**

The AOSpine Sacral Fracture Classification is a hierarchical tripartite system, which progresses from least to most unstable injuries. Three main groups of fractures are identified based on injury morphology: type A, lower sacrococcygeal injuries; type B, posterior pelvic injuries; and type C, spino-pelvic injuries (Fig. 59.1).

Type A injuries involve the lower sacrococcygeal region below the level of the SI joint and do not impact posterior pelvic or spino-pelvic stability. However, some type A injuries may have adverse outcomes due to associated pain and neurologic dysfunction.

- Type A1 injuries are coccygeal and ligamentous avulsion injuries.
- Type A2 injuries are nondisplaced fractures below the SI joint and involve the S2–S4 segments.
- Type A3 injuries are displaced fractures below the SI joint. In contrast to the previous subtypes, type A3 injuries are often associated with injury to the cauda equina. A common injury mechanism is a fall from height with buttock impact.

Type B Injuries impact posterior pelvic ring stability but do not impact spino-pelvic stability. These are osteoligamentous injuries that unilaterally disrupt the posterior pelvic ring in a longitudinal fashion but do not impact spino-pelvic instability as the ipsilateral superior S1 facet is continuous with the medial portion of the sacrum. These injuries occur as a result of an external rotation or vertical shear mechanism of a hemipelvis relative to the axial trunk.

- Type B1 injuries are due to a longitudinal fracture line medial to the neural foramina where the most medial part of this fracture courses through the spinal canal. These injuries are rare with a low likelihood of neurologic injury and correspond to an injury in Denis Zone III.
- Type B2 injuries are due to a longitudinal fracture lateral to the neural foramina and are associated with a 5% chance of neurologic injury, most commonly involving the L5 nerve root. This fracture subtype corresponds to an injury in Denis Zone I.
- Type B3 injuries are due to longitudinal fractures that involve the neural foramina but not the spinal canal. Type B3 injuries are associated with neurologic injury in up to 25% of patients and correspond to an injury in Denis Zone II.

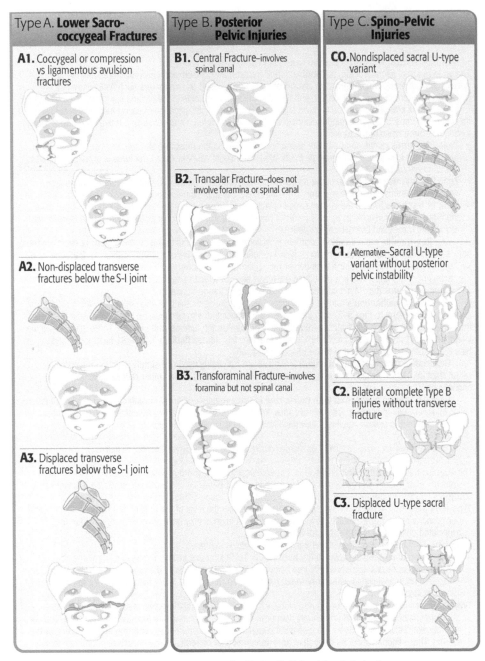

Type A. Lower Sacro-coccygeal Fractures

A1. Coccygeal or compression vs ligamentous avulsion fractures

A2. Non-displaced transverse fractures below the S-I joint

A3. Displaced transverse fractures below the S-I joint

Type B. Posterior Pelvic Injuries

B1. Central Fracture–involves spinal canal

B2. Transalar Fracture–does not involve foramina or spinal canal

B3. Transforaminal Fracture–involves foramina but not spinal canal

Type C. Spino-Pelvic Injuries

C0. Nondisplaced sacral U-type variant

C1. Alternative–Sacral U-type variant without posterior pelvic instability

C2. Bilateral complete Type B injuries without transverse fracture

C3. Displaced U-type sacral fracture

Fig. 59.1 AOSpine Sacral Fracture Classification. (© AO Foundation, Switzerland.)

Type C injuries are injuries that result in spino-pelvic instability. Successive worsening of lumbopelvic junction stability and neurologic compromise occur with higher numeric ranking.

- Type C0 injuries are nondisplaced fractures of the sacrum with some vertical and horizontal components that resemble a sacral "U," "T," or similar fracture type. These are inherently stable injuries with little risk of neurologic injury and can be expected to remain stable in most cases. These injuries commonly occur due to low-energy injury mechanisms or as insufficiency fractures.

- Type C1 injuries are a diverse group of injuries and include any unilateral B-subtype where the ipsilateral superior S1 facet is discontinuous with the medial portion of the sacrum. These injuries incorporate vertical and horizontal fractures lines but do not result in posterior pelvic ring disruption.
- Type C2 injuries are bilateral complete type B injuries without a transverse component. Instability and risk of neurologic injury are greater than type C1 and less than type C3 injuries.
- Type C3 injuries are displaced vertical and horizontal fractures of the sacrum which may be of a "U," "H," or lambda or similar pattern. This injury type is unstable and associated with a high likelihood of neurologic injury.

10. **How are neurologic injuries described when using the AOSpine Sacral Classification System?**
Neurologic status is classified as:
- N0: No neurologic injury
- N1: Transient neurologic injury
- N2: Nerve root injury
- N3: Cauda equina syndrome
- NX: Cannot be examined
- +: Continued neural compression
    Note that bladder or bowel sphincter dysfunction and sexual dysfunction are not separately listed in this classification system, although they affect patient outcomes substantially. Impairment in these categories would be described as N3. Based on sacral tumor resection studies, it is believed that even unilateral preservation of sacral roots S2–S4 will preserve anal and bladder sphincter function.

11. **What important case-specific injury modifiers (M) are considered when sacral injuries are classified according to the AOSpine Sacral Classification System?**
Case-specific injury modifiers are used to supplement the sacral injury classification to ensure the most complete injury representation, and may be used singularly or in combination:
- M1: Soft tissue injury. This identifies any form of soft tissue, ranging from simple contusions to severe closed lumbodorsal degloving injuries (Morel-Lavallée injury) and any form of open fracture.
- M2: Metabolic bone disease. Impaired bone stock can impact treatment. For example, use of additional fixation points may be considered in such patients.
- M3: Anterior pelvic ring injury. This component is an important observation as it may substantially affect the overall pelvic ring stability and may alter the surgical sequence or surgical approach.
- M4: Sacroiliac joint injury. A substantial injury component affecting the sacroiliac joint(s) may exert a deleterious impact on posterior pelvic ring integrity.

12. **What are the nonoperative treatment options for sacral fractures?**
Nonsurgical treatment of sacral fractures can be successful if a number of conditions are met. This usually implies a single-system injury, predominately osseous in nature with minimal displacement, and absence of an associated neurologic deficit. Nonsurgical management options include:
- Early, protected weight bearing
- Immobilization with a thoracolumbosacral orthosis (TLSO) with a unilateral or bilateral thigh extension or pantaloon spica cast
- Prolonged bed rest with recumbent skeletal traction
    The duration of nonoperative treatment varies depending upon a number of factors, but ranges from 6 to 12 weeks and beyond. Complications associated with nonoperative management include secondary displacement of the posterior pelvic ring leading to posttraumatic pelvic obliquity or impingement on the birth canal in women of child-bearing age, progressive painful sacral kyphosis, incomplete neurologic recovery or secondary neurologic decline, and adverse consequences related to immobility including decubiti and thromboembolic complications.

13. **When is surgical intervention indicated for sacral fractures?**
Surgical interventions may be classified as (1) decompression procedures, (2) procedures that provide sacral fracture reduction and stabilization, and (3) procedures to treat open fractures and related soft tissue injuries. In the presence of lumbosacral or sacral nerve deficits or sacral radicular pain, surgical decompression is considered after taking into account the potential benefits of surgery versus the surgical risks for each patient. In general, sacral fracture displacement of 1 cm or greater has been used as a criterion to define fracture instability and consideration of surgical treatment, especially for injuries that involve the neural foramina, lumbosacral facet joints, or for type C3 injuries. Expedient surgery is undertaken for open fractures with direct communication to the skin, rectum, or vagina to perform irrigation and debridement, bladder drainage with cystostomy, and bowel diversion with colostomy. Extensive soft tissue injuries, including the fascial degloving injury known as the Morel-Lavallée lesion, are treated with surgical debridement and drainage as indicated.

14. **How is surgical decompression of a sacral fracture performed?**
Surgical decompression of sacral fractures may be performed using direct or indirect surgical techniques. Lumbosacral or sacral nerve deficits or sacral radicular pain may benefit from direct surgical decompression

performed preferably within 2 weeks of injury. This surgical approach is most commonly performed through a dorsal midline laminotomy and foraminotomy as needed. Fluoroscopic guidance can aid in intraoperative localization and limit the surgical exposure required. In some cases, neural decompression can be achieved with indirect techniques through fracture disimpaction or fracture reduction and stabilization.

Surgical decompression is ineffective in presence of traumatic sacral neural transection. Unfortunately approximately 35% of displaced sacral fractures with neural canal or foraminal displacement are associated with transected sacral roots, a circumstance which cannot be reliably predicted preoperatively. Surgeons performing sacral decompression surgery must be prepared to manage dural tears with cerebrospinal fluid leakage and have familiarity with the management of complex wound healing issues that are common to posterior sacral procedures. While an isolated sacral laminectomy in itself is not destabilizing, when this procedure is performed for trauma indications usually some form of additional stabilization is preferable.

15. What are the currently preferred methods for surgical stabilization of a sacral fracture?
Surgical stabilization of sacral fractures is most commonly performed using two main techniques:
1. Percutaneous iliosacral or transiliac-transsacral screw fixation
2. Unilateral posterior spino-pelvic fixation (triangular osteosynthesis) or bilateral posterior spino-pelvic fixation

Depending on the injury type, supplemental stability can be accomplished by anterior pelvic ring stabilization either with external fixation or direct plate and screw fixation. However, when used in isolation these supplemental methods have a limited biomechanical effect on the posterior pelvic ring. Historically, several other procedures were described for repair of sacral fractures and sacroiliac joint disruptions using plates and screws but these techniques have largely fallen by the wayside. One exception is the occasional use of plate fixation in the treatment of type A3 sacral fractures. Surgical care has been recommended to commence as early as possible after medical clearance to optimize chances for neurologic recovery and encourage return to mobility. Sacral trauma surgeries delayed for more than 2–3 weeks may have less chance for neurologic recovery and become increasingly difficult to perform due to increased scarring and distorted fracture anatomy (Fig. 59.2A–C).

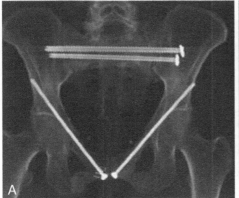

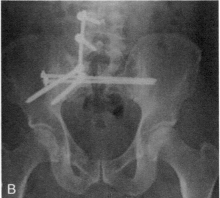

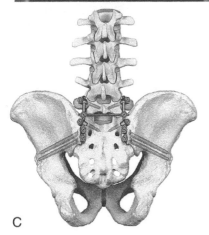

Fig. 59.2 Options for surgical stabilization of sacral fractures. (A) Iliosacral screw fixation, (B) triangular fixation, and (C) spino-pelvic fixation. (A and B: From Bellabarba C, Schildhauer TA, Chapman JR. Management of sacral fractures. In: Quinones-Hinojosa A, editor. Schmidek and Sweet's Operative Neurosurgical Techniques. Philadelphia, PA: Saunders; 2012, pp. 2035–2045, Fig. 179-6D, p. 2039, Fig. 179-8D, p. 2041. C: Courtesy Jens R Chapman, MD.)

16. **When is iliosacral or transiliac-transsacral screw fixation indicated and how is this stabilization technique performed?**

Percutaneous iliosacral or transiliac-transsacral screw fixation provides a method for improving posterior pelvic ring stability and are most commonly utilized for treatment of minimally or nondisplaced longitudinal sacral fractures. Indications include type B sacral fractures and minimally displaced type C injuries. Attention to detail in terms of patient selection, radiographic visualization, and technical execution are key elements for success using these techniques. One or more large caliber cannulated screws with washers are inserted under fluoroscopy and anchored in the sacral vertebral bodies or contralateral ilium. Lag screws of sufficient length can be used if there is no sacral ala comminution; otherwise two or more static screws without lag effect that are positioned in the uninvolved side of the sacrum are preferred. These techniques can be performed supine or prone and can be combined with decompression surgery if needed. Limitations include the challenge of achieving closed reduction for more displaced injuries and the requirement for a period of protected weight bearing, due to the limited stability provided by these techniques. These techniques may also be used in combination with spino-pelvic fixation (Fig. 59.2A).

17. **What is the role of triangular osteosynthesis?**

The term *triangular osteosynthesis* describes a unilateral, usually temporary, implant construct that combines longitudinal vertebro-pelvic fixation (i.e., pedicle screw-rod fixation between the lower lumbar pedicles and iliac column or sacral ala) with horizontal fixation using an iliosacral screw for clearly unilateral posterior pelvic injuries. Such a triangular osteosynthesis provides greater stability than isolated iliosacral screw constructs. It is intended to facilitate early progressive weight bearing for patients with vertically unstable sacral fractures where isolated sacroiliac screws would be prone to fail. The unilateral fixation can be removed after sacral fracture healing has been established thereby avoiding a lumbopelvic fusion (Fig. 59.2B).

18. **When is spino-pelvic fixation indicated and how is this stabilization technique performed?**

The most stable method of fixation for displaced sacral fractures is achieved by spino-pelvic fixation. For fractures not amenable to indirect reduction through ligamentotaxis, direct open reduction and stabilization with spino-pelvic fixation is preferable. This technique can be performed unilaterally (triangular fixation) or bilaterally, and requires pedicle screw fixation of the fifth and possibly fourth lumbar vertebra and iliac fixation. If the S1 segment is intact, additional pedicle screws are placed into this segment. The iliac screw starting point is selected approximately 2 cm inferior to the posterior superior iliac spine and a drill is aimed toward the anterior inferior iliac spine. The thickened portion of the ilium within 2–3 cm above the sciatic notch provides a predictable conduit for pelvic anchors, which can be up to 130 mm in length and 8 mm or larger in diameter. On obturator oblique imaging this bony passage can be recognized by its typical "teardrop" appearance. An iliac oblique fluoroscopic image can confirm proper screw placement between the inner and outer iliac tables with avoidance of the sciatic notch and acetabulum. Percutaneous iliosacral screws can aid with holding a reduction of a repositioned hemipelvis while performing spino-pelvic fixation. Complications associated with this fixation method include increased blood loss, wound healing problems, implant prominence or loosening, and rod breakage. Multiple rod constructs may be used to bridge the lumbo-pelvic junction and decrease the rate of rod breakage in injuries associated with high-grade instability. The stability provided by properly performed spino-pelvic fixation usually permits early, full weight-bearing mobilization.

19. **What are the functional outcomes following treatment of displaced sacral fractures?**

"Return to normal" is unfortunately not a realistic expectation for most displaced sacral fractures due to associated injuries and impairment of neurologic function. Return to weight bearing is related to completion of bone healing or achievement of stable fibrous ankylosis through the pelvic ring and its ligamentous structures. When the patient's medical condition and associated injuries do not preclude intervention, surgical stabilization to facilitate early mobilization to avoid the complications associated with prolonged recumbency is preferable.

KEY POINTS

1. A high index of clinical suspicion, targeted physical examination, and appropriate imaging studies are required for timely diagnosis of sacral fractures.
2. Sacral fractures may result in posterior pelvic ring instability, spino-pelvic instability, or combined instabilities.
3. Surgical treatment is indicated for sacral fractures associated with neurologic deficit, displacement, or instability.

Websites
1. AOSpine Sacral Classification System: https://aospine.aofoundation.org/en/clinical-library-and-tools/aospine-classification-systems
2. Classification of sacral fractures: https://radiopaedia.org/articles/classification-of-sacral-fractures?lang=us

BIBLIOGRAPHY

1. Bellabarba C, Schroeder GD, Kepler CK, et al. The AOSpine sacral fracture classification. *Global Spine J* 2017;6(Suppl. 1):s-0036-1582696-s-0036-1582696.
2. Denis F, Davis S, Comfort T. Sacral fractures: An important problem: Retrospective analysis of 236 cases. *Clin Orthop Relat Res* 1988;227:67–81.
3. Nork SE, Jones CB, Harding SP, et al. Percutaneous stabilization of U-shaped sacral fractures using iliosacral screws: Technique and early results. *J Orthop Trauma* 2001;15:238–246.
4. Rodrigues-Pinto R, Kurd MF, Schroeder GD, et al. Sacral fractures and associated injuries. *Global Spine J* 2017;7:609–616.
5. Schildhauer TA, Bellabarba C, Nork SE, et al. Decompression and lumbopelvic fixation for sacral fracture-dislocations with spino-pelvic dissociation. *J Orthop Trauma* 2006;20:447–457.
6. Schildhauer TA, Josten C, Muhr G. Triangular osteosynthesis of vertically unstable sacrum fractures: A new concept allowing early weight-bearing. *J Orthop Trauma* 2006;20:44–51.
7. Schildhauer TA, McCulloch P, Chapman JR, et al. Anatomic and radiographic considerations for placement of transiliac screws in lumbopelvic fixations. *J Spinal Disord Tech* 2002;15:199–205.
8. Schroeder GD, Kurd MF, Kepler CK, et al. The development of a universally accepted sacral fracture classification: A survey of AOSpine and AOTrauma members. *Global Spine J* 2016;6:686–694.

CHAPTER 60

SPINAL INJURIES IN ATHLETES

Robert G. Watkins, IV, MD and Robert G. Watkins, III, MD

CERVICAL SPINE INJURIES

1. **What sports are associated with the highest risk of head and neck injuries?**
   The organized sports with the highest risk of head and neck injuries are football, gymnastics, wrestling, and ice hockey. Football is associated with the highest risk of such injuries. Head and neck injuries also occur in a variety of nonorganized sports activities, including diving, skiing, surfing, and trampoline use.

2. **What types of cervical injuries are considered in the differential diagnosis of an injured athlete?**
   Sports-related cervical injuries can involve the muscles, tendons, ligaments, intervertebral discs, osseous structures, and neural elements. Common athletic cervical injuries include muscular strains, intervertebral disc injuries, major and minor cervical spine fractures, stinger or burner injuries, and cervical cord neuropraxia. In addition, preexisting cervical conditions may predispose an athlete to neurologic injury and be discovered during subsequent evaluation. These include congenital cervical stenosis, Klippel-Feil syndrome, and os odontoideum.

3. **When performing an on-field assessment of an athlete's cervical spine, how does the presence of neck pain versus extremity symptoms help guide differential diagnosis?**
   See Fig. 60.1.

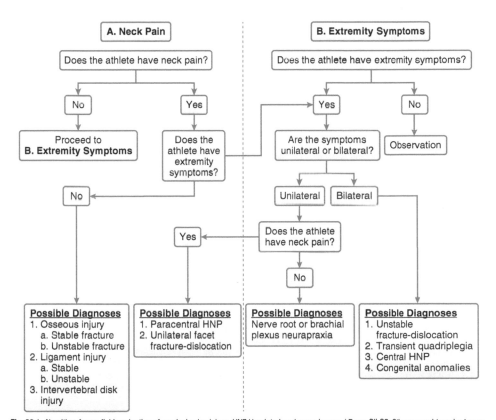

Fig. 60.1 Algorithm for on-field evaluation of cervical spine injury. *HNP,* Herniated nucleus pulposus. (From Gil SS. Stingers and transient paresis. In: Shen FH, Samartzis D, Fessler RG, editors. Textbook of the Cervical Spine. Philadelphia, PA: Saunders; 2015, Fig. 21.9, p. 209.)

4. **What is the most common mechanism responsible for catastrophic sports-related cervical spine injuries?**
Catastrophic cervical spine injuries result in injury to the spinal cord that causes temporary or permanent neurologic injury. The primary mechanism responsible for catastrophic sports-related cervical spine injuries is axial loading resulting from head contact while the neck is in a slightly flexed position. When the cervical spine is in lordotic alignment, it is capable of absorbing applied loads. However, when the neck is flexed, force applied directly along the axis of the spine results in axial loading of the cervical spine.

5. **What is the most common sports-related injury of the cervical spine?**
The most common sports-related injury involving the cervical spine is a soft tissue injury involving muscles, tendons, or ligaments in the cervical region. Despite the frequency of these injuries, careful evaluation is warranted to rule out a more serious injury. The athlete may return to sports if neck pain is resolved, neck strength is normal, full functional cervical range of motion is present without pain, and cervical radiographs are normal.

6. **Explain what is meant by a "hidden flexion injury" of the cervical spine?**
This term refers to a purely ligamentous injury associated with three-column disruption of the spine, in the absence of osseous injury. Such injuries may be missed on plain radiographs. Persistent posterior cervical tenderness following an acute injury should raise concern about the possibility of this injury pattern. The lateral cervical radiograph should be carefully evaluated for a subtle increase in the distance between adjacent spinous processes. Cervical magnetic resonance imaging (MRI) is useful to evaluate posterior cervical ligamentous disruption. Physician-supervised flexion-extension lateral radiographs are considered only for alert, cooperative, and neurologically intact patients, and are not advised or considered useful in the immediate postinjury period. Criteria for defining instability between adjacent motion segments in the subaxial cervical region are 11° or greater angulation or 3.5 mm or greater translation of one vertebra relative to an adjacent vertebra.

7. **Describe the clinical presentation of a traumatic cervical disc herniation?**
The clinical presentation of a traumatic cervical disc herniation is variable. Patients may present with isolated neck pain, radiculopathy, or an anterior cord syndrome with paralysis of the upper and lower extremities. In contrast to adults in whom cervical disc herniations occur most commonly at C5–C6 and C6–C7, immature athletes most commonly develop disc herniations at C3–C4 and C4–C5. Disc injury is associated with axial loading and hyperflexion during activities such as wrestling, diving, and football.

8. **What is spear tackler's spine?**
Spearing refers to contact the crown of the head while the neck is maintained in a flexed posture. In this posture, the normal cervical lordosis is no longer present, and the cervical spine is predisposed to injury. Injuries due to this mechanism have been described in football, diving, and hockey. Spear tackler's spine was defined by analysis of injured football players and is considered to be a contraindication to participation in contact sports. Criteria for diagnosis of spear tackler's spine include:
- Developmental narrowing of the cervical spinal canal
- Persistent straightening or reversal of cervical lordosis on erect lateral cervical radiographs
- Posttraumatic radiographic changes on cervical radiographs
- History of use of spear-tackling techniques during athletics

9. **What is a stinger or burner?**
A stinger or burner (burner syndrome) is a peripheral nerve injury involving individual cervical nerve roots or a portion of the brachial plexus. It is associated with unilateral burning arm pain or paresthesias and may be accompanied by weakness, most often in the muscle groups supplied by the C5 and C6 nerve roots (deltoid, biceps, supraspinatus, infraspinatus) on the affected side. Although pain may resolve spontaneously in minutes, it is not uncommon to have trace abnormal neurologic findings for several months. Bilateral symptoms suggest a different etiology, such as a neuropraxic injury of the spinal cord. Injury mechanisms responsible for stingers include: (1) head contact leading to hyperextension, compression, and rotation toward the involved arm, thereby closing the neural foramen and causing a nerve root contusion (essentially a replication of the Spurling maneuver); and (2) head abduction and lateral neck flexion combined with shoulder depression on the affected side, resulting in brachial plexus stretch. Three grades of injury have been described:
- **Grade 1:** neuropraxia. This is the most common injury type. All nerve structures remain intact. Complete resolution of symptoms typically occurs in minutes, but may take as long as 6 weeks.
- **Grade 2:** axonotmesis. Axonal disruption and Wallerian degeneration occur distal to the injury site. Recovery is complete, but may take months. An intact epineurium allows axonal regrowth at a rate of approximately 1 mm/day.
- **Grade 3:** neurotmesis. There is complete disruption of axons, endoneurium, perineurium, and epineurium. The prognosis varies, and complete loss of function is common.

Most stingers resolve within minutes. For an athlete's first episode, with only brief transitory symptoms, treatment is conservative and no special testing is required. Neck and shoulder muscle strengthening programs can have a positive effect on recovery and help reduce recurrences. If the symptoms have not resolved by 3 weeks, electromyography (EMG) may be considered to define the specific pattern of nerve root involvement but is not useful to guide return to play as abnormal EMG findings lag behind motor recovery. An athlete should not return to play until there is pain-free and unrestricted neck and shoulder range of motion; resolution of paresthesias; normal motor strength; and provocative tests are negative, including the Spurling test, brachial plexus stretch test, and axial compression test.

10. **What is cervical cord neuropraxia?**
Cervical cord neuropraxia is a temporary neurologic episode following cervical trauma and is characterized by the presence of sensory symptoms with or without motor changes involving at least two extremities in the absence of cervical instability. The most commonly described mechanism of injury is axial compression with a component of either hyperflexion or hyperextension. Neurologic findings are classified according to severity as plegia (complete loss of motor function), paresis (motor weakness), or paresthesia (sensory symptoms only) and graded by duration as grade I (<15 minutes), grade II (15 minutes–24 hours), and grade III (>24 hours). The anatomic distribution of neurologic symptoms is variable and may involve all four extremities, both arms, both legs, or an ipsilateral arm and leg. Neurologic symptoms are transient and typically last between 15 minutes and 36 hours. Neck pain is often absent.

11. **Describe initial management of an episode of cervical cord neuropraxia.**
Initial management following an episode of cervical cord neuropraxia consists of immobilization, clinical assessment, and triage. Immediately following an episode of transient quadriparesis, the athlete should be prohibited from continuing to participate in the sport for that particular event, even if a full recovery occurs soon after the episode. A thorough history of all events leading up to and following the episode should be carefully documented. A complete onsite physical examination including a complete neurologic examination should be performed. The athlete should be considered to have a fracture until proven otherwise, especially if the patient complains of persistent or significant neck stiffness or pain or if a neurologic deficit is present. Depending on the results of the initial evaluation, a decision is made whether the patient should be transported for further medical treatment and imaging studies. Initial imaging evaluation includes plain cervical radiographs and/or computed tomography (CT) to evaluate cervical osseous anatomy and spinal alignment, and MRI to evaluate for the presence of intrinsic spinal cord abnormalities or spinal cord or nerve root compression. Cervical spinal stenosis is often diagnosed during the workup of patients following an episode of cervical cord neuropraxia and is associated with an increased risk of a recurrent episode of cervical cord neuropraxia.

12. **What factors should be considered in making a return-to-play decision for an athlete after the first episode of cervical cord neuropraxia?**
Return-to-play guidelines following a single episode of cervical cord neuropraxia permit return to contact sports if there is complete resolution of symptoms, unrestricted cervical range of motion, normal cervical alignment, absence of spinal instability, and absence of cervical stenosis or spinal cord parenchymal injury on cervical MRI. Return-to-play decisions are made on an individual basis after considering a range of factors, including the severity of symptoms during the initial episode of cervical cord neuropraxia, the specific sport involved, career and economic considerations, and patient preferences. Contraindications to return to sports include instability, deformity, and severe stenosis.

13. **What types of cervical stenosis affect athletes?**
The types of cervical stenosis that affect athletes are the same as found in the general population: developmental or congenital stenosis (typified by short pedicles and decreased sagittal diameter of the spinal canal) and acquired stenosis (associated with osteophytes and degeneration at the level of the disc space).

14. **How is cervical stenosis diagnosed?**
Imaging studies that play a role in the diagnosis of cervical stenosis include radiographs, MRI, and CT-myelography. Criteria used to diagnose cervical stenosis include:
- **Radiographic sagittal diameter of the spinal canal:** Sagittal canal width (C3–C7) measured between the posterior vertebral margin and the nearest point on the spinolaminar line that is greater than 15 mm is considered normal and less than 13 mm is considered stenotic. However, diagnosis of cervical stenosis based on measurements from plain radiographs is inadequate as such measurements are affected by radiographic technique and are unable to assess the relationship between neural, soft tissue and osseous structures within the spinal canal. MRI is the most reliable way to identify cervical stenosis. (Fig. 60.2, measurement "a")
- **Torg-Pavlov ratio:** Measured as the sagittal diameter of the spinal canal (a) divided by the anteroposterior vertebral body diameter (b) (Fig. 60.2). This ratio method avoids the potential for measurement error secondary to radiographic magnification. A normal ratio is 1.0. A ratio less than 0.8 suggests a diagnosis of cervical spinal stenosis. The Torg-Pavlov ratio is a highly sensitive method of determining cervical stenosis (93% sensitivity) but has an extremely low positive predictive value for determining future injury (0.2%). It is not a useful screening method for determining athletic participation in contact sports and should not be used as the sole

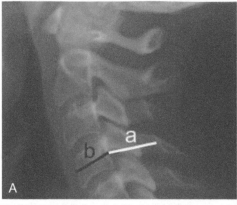
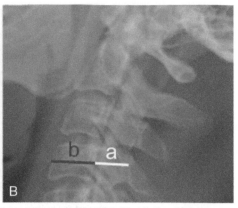

Fig. 60.2 The Torg-Pavlov ratio is the distance from the midpoint of the posterior aspect of the vertebral body to the nearest point on the corresponding spinolaminar line *(distance a)* divided by the anteroposterior width of the vertebral body *(distance b)*. (A) Normal cervical spine with the ratio a/b greater than 1. (B) Cervical spine with developmental stenosis of the spinal canal with the ratio a/b less than 0.8. (From Tyrakowski M, Nandyala SV, Marquez-Lara A, et al. Congenital and developmental anomalies of the cervical spine in athletes—current concepts. Oper Tech Sports Med 2013;21:159–163, Fig. 1, p. 160.)

criterion for the diagnosis of cervical stenosis in an athlete. Although an athlete may have the same size spinal canal as a nonathlete, the athlete's vertebral body may be larger, thus falsely lowering the Torg-Pavlov ratio and implying stenosis. In addition, the Torg-Pavlov ratio has not been correlated with the development of permanent quadriparesis in athletes. The Torg-Pavlov ratio should not be used as the sole criterion in making a return-to-play decision after an episode of transient quadriplegia.

- **Functional reserve of the spinal cord:** Axial MRI or CT-myelography images are the most reliable way to identify cervical spinal stenosis. The most important parameter is the presence of an adequate protective cushion (functional reserve) of cerebrospinal fluid (CSF) around the spinal cord in a nonstenotic spinal canal. The term *functional spinal stenosis* is used to refer to loss of CSF signal surrounding the spinal cord (Fig. 60.3).
- **Dynamic stenosis:** Extremes of extension may lead to compression of the spinal cord between the posterior inferior aspect of the superior vertebral body and the proximal and anterior border of the lamina of the inferior vertebra. This type of dynamic combined anterior and posterior cord compression is referred to as a *pincer mechanism*. In some patients, extreme neck positions may lead to combined anterior and posterior

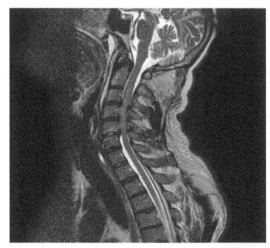

Fig. 60.3 Sagittal T2-weighted magnetic resonance imaging demonstrates severe central spinal stenosis from C3 to C6 with loss of the functional reserve of cerebrospinal fluid around the spinal cord. (From Lamothe G, Muller F, Vital JM, et al. Evolution of spinal cord injuries due to cervical stenosis without radiographic evidence of trauma: A prospective study. Ann Phys Rehab Med 2011;54:213–224, Fig. 1, p. 215.)

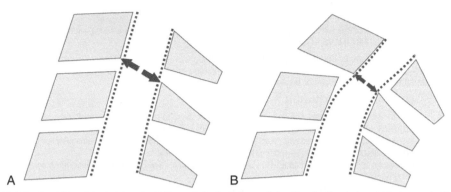

Fig. 60.4 Functional (dynamic) spinal stenosis. (A) The cervical spine is in a neutral position. A wide spinal canal *(black arrows)* with a normal spinal cord is depicted *(dotted lines)*. (B) Hyperextension of the cervical spine with relative hypermobility causing dynamic or functional narrowing of the spinal canal *(black arrows)* and compression to the spinal cord *(dotted lines)*. (From Tyrakowski M, Nandyala SV, Marquez-Lara A, et al. Congenital and developmental anomalies of the cervical spine in athletes—current concepts. Oper Tech Sports Med 2013;21:159–163, Fig. 2, p. 160.)

cord impingement between invaginated ligamentum flavum and bulging of the margin of the intervertebral disc. Dynamic flexion-extension MRI may be used to evaluate this mechanism (Fig. 60.4).

15. **When should an athlete be allowed to return to play following cervical injury?**
    There are no universally accepted guidelines for determining when an athlete may return to play after a cervical injury. Basic principles guiding decision making include:
    - The athlete should be asymptomatic with respect to neck pain.
    - Unrestricted and pain-free cervical motion should be present.
    - Neurologic evaluation should be normal.
    - Full muscle strength should be present.
    - There should be no evidence of radiographic instability, abnormal spinal alignment, functional cervical stenosis, or other high-risk spinal abnormalities after radiographic and MRI evaluation.

    Specific guidelines for return to play following cervical injury have been defined based on expert opinion (Table 60.1) and are modified based on individual clinical factors. It is helpful to divide athletes into three general groups:
    1. No contraindication to return to play. Such conditions are considered to permit return to contact sports without restriction after comprehensive patient assessment.
    2. Relative contraindication to return to play. Such conditions are associated with a possibility for recurrent injury, despite the absence of any absolute contraindication. The athlete, family, and coach must be counseled that recurrent injury is a possibility and the degree of risk is uncertain.
    3. Absolute contraindication to return to play. Such conditions are associated with clear increased risk of serious injury.
       Literature supports return to all levels of sporting activities following successful single-level anterior cervical discectomy and fusion or single level laminotomy. Two-level cervical fusion is considered a relative contraindication and three-level cervical fusion is generally considered as an absolute contraindication to return to play. However, there is a lack of adequate quality data to guide return to play decisions following other types of cervical surgeries including artificial disc replacement and laminoplasty.

Table 60.1 Summary of Cervical Spine Return to Play Criteria.

NO CONTRAINDICATION

- Healed C1–C7 fracture that meets general criteria[a] and without sagittal malalignment, asymptomatic clay shoveler's (C7) fracture
- Congenital conditions including single-level Klippel-Feil not involving occiput-C1, spina bifida occulta
- Degenerative conditions following successful nonoperative treatment
- Postsurgical following single-level ACDF ± instrumentation, single- or multiple-level posterior laminotomy
- Less than three stingers with symptoms less than 24 hours that meets general criteria[a]
- One episode of transient quadriparesis that meets general criteria[a]

(Continued on following page)

Table 60.1 Summary of Cervical Spine Return to Play Criteria. *(Continued)*

RELATIVE CONTRAINDICATION

- Prolonged symptomatic burner/stinger or transient quadriparesis lasting longer than 24 hours
- Three or more stingers or two episodes of transient quadriparesis that meet general criteria[a]
- Healed two-level ACDF or one or two-level PCF ± instrumentation

ABSOLUTE CONTRAINDICATION

- Previous transient quadriparesis with cervical myelopathy or failure to meet general criteria[a] after cervical surgery
- C1–C2 fusion, cervical laminectomy, or three-level ACDF or PCF
- Soft tissue injury: asymptomatic ligamentous laxity defined as >11° kyphosis, C1–C2 hypermobility with ADI >3.5 mm (adult) or >4 mm (child), symptomatic cervical disc herniation
- Spear-tackler's spine, multilevel Klippel-Feil, healed subaxial fracture with sagittal malalignment, coronal plane abnormality, cord encroachment
- Ankylosing spondylitis or RA with spinal abnormalities
- Spinal cord abnormality, Arnold-Chiari, basilar invagination, occiput-C1 assimilation, C1–C2 fusion

[a]General criteria for return to sport include no pain, full range of motion, full strength, no evidence of functional spinal stenosis, no instability, and no neurologic injury.

ACDF, Anterior cervical discectomy and fusion; *ADI,* atlantodens interval; *PCF,* posterior cervical fusion.

Data from Cantu R, Li YM, Abdulhamid M, et al. Return to play after cervical spine injury in sports. Curr Sports Med Rep 2013;12:14–17.

THORACIC SPINE INJURIES

16. What types of athletic injuries involve the thoracic spinal region?

Athletic injuries involving the thoracic region are less common than either cervical or lumbar injuries due to the increased stability provided to this region by the thoracic cage. Thoracic injuries reported in association with athletic activities include musculoligamentous injuries, stress fractures of the spinous or transverse processes, vertebral body compression fractures, high-energy fracture patterns with or without associated spinal cord injuries (burst fractures, fracture-dislocations), and thoracic disc herniations.

17. What guidelines are available for return to play following athletic injuries involving the thoracic spinal region?

There are no published guidelines for return to play following thoracic injuries. In general, it is reasonable for patients to return to play following nonsurgical treatment if symptoms have resolved, neurologic status is intact, and strength and range of motion are normal. Return to play following thoracic decompression or fusion is more controversial. Patients who undergo midthoracic decompression or fusion can often return to play if they are pain-free, neurologically intact, and spinal imaging confirms that the goals of surgery have been reached. Patients with fusions that cross the cervicothoracic or thoracolumbar junction or fusions that terminate at a transitional zone are generally prohibited from returning to contact sports.

LUMBAR SPINE INJURIES

18. What conditions are considered in the differential diagnosis for an injured athlete who presents with symptoms of low back pain with or without radiculopathy?

- Muscle strain/ligament sprain
- Overuse syndrome
- Lumbar disc injury (annular tear, discogenic pain syndrome, disc herniation)
- Apophyseal ring injury (adolescents)
- Stress fracture (e.g., spondylolysis, sacral stress fracture)
- Spondylolysis or spondylolisthesis
- Minor lumbar fracture (e.g., transverse process fracture)
- Major lumbar fracture (± instability, neurologic deficit)
- Disc degeneration
- Lumbar spinal stenosis
- Serious underlying spinal condition (discitis/osteomyelitis, neoplasm)
- Nonspinal conditions that mimic spinal pathology

19. What are the most common lumbar athletic injuries in adolescents and adults?

In adolescents, the most common conditions diagnosed following an athletic-related injury are lumbar strain, spondylolysis/spondylolisthesis, lumbar disc injuries, and overuse syndromes. In adults, the most common conditions diagnosed following an athletic-related injury are lumbar strain, discogenic pain syndromes, disc herniations, and spinal stenosis.

20. Are certain lumbar spinal injuries associated with specific sports activities?

Yes. Certain lumbar disorders have been associated with specific sports activities, and this information may be helpful in evaluation of an injured athlete. Some common associations include:

- Spondylolysis—football, gymnastics, diving, wrestling, weightlifting, hockey, soccer
- Lumbar disc herniation—weightlifting, football, ice hockey, soccer, basketball, baseball
- Vertebral ring apophyseal injury—wrestling, ice hockey, volleyball, gymnastics
- Lumbar strain—most common lumbar athletic injury across all types of sports
- Lumbar disc degeneration—gymnastics, weightlifting, soccer, baseball, swimming
- Lumbar fractures—skiing, snowboarding
- Sacral stress fracture—running

21. Describe the workup for an athlete with symptoms of low back pain with or without radiculopathy.

A detailed patient history, physical examination, and diagnostic workup are performed to characterize the presenting clinical syndrome and identify the pain generator.

Key points to assess from the history include:
- The cause of the injury and duration of symptoms
- The time of day when the pain is worse
- A comparison of pain levels during different activities (walking, sitting, standing)
- The effect of a Valsalva maneuver, coughing, and sneezing on pain
- The percentage of back versus leg pain (axial vs. radicular pain)
- The presence of any bowel or bladder dysfunction

Key points to assess during the physical examination include:
- Maneuvers and positions that reproduce pain (flexion vs. extension ± rotation)
- The presence of sciatic nerve tension signs
- The presence of neurologic deficit
- Back and lower extremity stiffness or loss of range of motion
- The exact location of tenderness or radiation of pain or paresthesias

Diagnostic workup must always consider the possibility of a tumor, infection, and impending neurologic crisis.

- If the main complaint is **leg pain**, after initial plain x-rays are obtained, an MRI of the lumbar spine is performed to diagnose nerve root compression due to disc, soft tissue, or osseous structures. A CT or CT-myelogram is an option if the etiology of pain remains unclear or if MRI is not possible. EMG and nerve conduction velocity (NCV) studies may be considered to distinguish a peripheral nerve lesion from a radiculopathy.
- If **back pain** is the predominant symptom, workup is initiated with plain x-rays. If radiographs are negative, then advanced imaging studies are indicated. In the adolescent and young adult athlete, lack of consensus exists regarding selection of the next imaging study after plain radiographs. Traditionally, a single-photon emission computed tomography (SPECT) bone scan is obtained, but is associated with substantial radiation exposure. If the SPECT scan is positive and thus suspicious for a pars fracture, a CT scan with thin cuts may be ordered to evaluate the abnormal area. If the SPECT scan is negative, MRI is indicated. Some experts prefer MRI as the initial screening test after plain radiography due to lack of ionizing radiation exposure and ability to visualize stress reactions, while other experts recommend a localized lumbar CT as the initial advanced imaging study in the pediatric athlete. In adult athletes, low back pain is rarely due to acute spondylolysis and more commonly due to soft tissue injury, lumbar degenerative disorders, or idiopathic causes. If initial radiographs do not show a significant osseous injury, treatment is initiated for acute low back pain according to adult protocols, and further imaging studies are deferred pending the outcome of standard treatment algorithms.

The goal of the workup is to **diagnose the clinical syndrome** responsible for symptoms and to localize the pain generator. Commonly encountered clinical syndromes include:

- **Nonmechanical back pain or leg pain:** Minimally; affected by activity; usually worse at night or early morning.
- **Mechanical back or leg pain:** Made worse by activity; relieved by rest.
- **Sciatica:** Predominantly radicular pain; positive sciatic stretch signs, with or without neurologic deficits.
- **Neurogenic claudication:** Radiating leg or calf pain; negative sciatic stretch signs; made worse with standing and spinal extension; relieved by flexion or sitting.

22. What are the most common types of lumbar fractures reported in athletes?

Minor fractures are the most common types of lumbar spine fractures reported in athletes. Minor fractures occur as a result of low-energy impact or chronic repetitive spinal loading and do not lead to spinal instability. Minor fractures may involve the pars interarticularis, articular processes, transverse processes, or spinous processes. Most minor fractures are treated nonoperatively. Major fractures are less common in athletes and result from high-energy injury mechanisms. Major fractures most commonly involve the thoracolumbar junction (T11–L2). Major fractures that are unstable or associated with neurologic deficits are treated operatively, while stable major fractures are treated nonoperatively.

23. What is the prognosis for an athlete who develops a symptomatic lumbar disc herniation following a sports injury?

The overall prognosis for an athlete diagnosed with a symptomatic lumbar disc herniation is favorable. Most athletes are able to return to contact sports following successful completion of an appropriate physical therapy and rehabilitation program, including athletes treated operatively. When surgery is indicated, microscopic lumbar discectomy is the preferred surgical treatment. A study of North American professional athletes reported return to professional sports 82% of the time without a statistically significant difference in return to play rates or career length for nonoperatively and operatively treated athletes. However, sports-specific differences were noted, with Major League Baseball players demonstrating a significantly higher return to play rate and National Football League (NFL) athletes demonstrating a lower return to play rate than players of other sports. (1)

24. How prevalent is spondylolysis in athletes compared with the general population?

The prevalence of spondylolysis is 3%–7% in the general population. Spondylolysis is one of the most common causes of low back pain in adolescent athletes. Injuries are diagnosed along a spectrum, which includes impending or incomplete pars defects, unilateral pars defects, and bilateral pars defects. Studies have documented higher rates of spondylolysis in Olympic divers (43%), wrestlers (30%), weightlifters (23%), and gymnasts (16%). Studies have shown increased rates in football interior linemen (15%–50%). Thus clinical suspicion in athletes should be high, especially in athletes with persistent low-grade back pain that has been unresponsive or aggravated by physical therapy or local modalities.

25. Describe a treatment plan for an athlete with spondylolysis.

The treatment plan starts with rest or restriction of sufficient activity to relieve or improve symptoms. This plan may require merely stopping the sport or immobilization in a lumbosacral corset. No specific immobilization method has been proven scientifically to heal an athlete's spondylolysis. A neutral-position trunk stabilization program is initiated after a period of activity restriction or immobilization. A skilled therapist or trainer is important. Starting flexion, extension, or rotation exercises will exacerbate symptoms, whereas neutral isometric core stabilization exercises are less likely to increase symptoms. Nonoperative treatment for acute spondylolysis is successful in over 80% of athletes regardless of evidence of healing of the pars defect. In patients with persistent low back pain symptoms despite a proper core stabilization program, surgery may be considered. In skeletally immature patients, either repair of the pars interarticularis defect or single-level fusion is an option, while adult patients require treatment with spinal fusion.

26. Can athletes diagnosed with spondylolysis and isthmic spondylolisthesis continue participation in their sport?

Athletes with spondylolysis and spondylolisthesis require evaluation on an individual basis to assess their ability to continue sports participation as evidence-based criteria are limited. Indirect evidence that supports continued participation by athletes with spondylolysis and spondylolisthesis is partly based on the high incidence of spondylolysis and low-grade spondylolisthesis (grades 1 and 2) observed in athletes. Semon and Spengler (12) noted that 21% of college football players presenting with back pain had spondylolysis. In these symptomatic football players, there was no difference in time lost from sports between athletes with spondylolysis and those with back pain and negative findings on radiographs. A subsequent study by Brophy (2) showed that spondylolisthesis did not significantly reduce the chance of playing in the NFL for any position, while a history of acute spondylolysis did have a significant effect for running backs. Patients with high-grade spondylolisthesis (grades 3 and 4) are not likely to participate in high-level sporting activity over long time periods. Return-to-play recommendations for contact and collision sports following surgical treatment with pars repair or instrumented spinal fusion performed for spondylolysis and spondylolisthesis vary among surgeons, and range from recommendations against sports participation to recommendations to return to contact and collision sports without restriction.

27. What are some general recommendations for returning to sports after lumbar spinal decompression procedures?

General criteria for return to sports following lumbar decompression procedures include resolution of preoperative symptoms, full range of motion, normal neurologic status and successful completion of a structured rehabilitation program. Most patients treated with lumbar discectomy are permitted to return to sports. A minimum of 6 to 12 weeks is allowed for healing of the annulus fibrosus to prevent recurrent disc herniation. Many surgeons allow athletes to return to all sports following treatment of lumbar stenosis with lumbar laminectomies or laminotomies, although some surgeons will limit sports participation.

28. What are some general recommendations for returning to sports after lumbar and thoracolumbar spinal fusion procedures?

Limited data are available to assist with decision making for return to play after lumbar and thoracolumbar spinal fusions. According to a survey of North American Spine Society members about sports participation after spinal fusions, 80% returned to high school sports, 62% returned to collegiate sports, and only 18% returned to professional sports. Some of the criteria used to determine return to play included the presence of a solid fusion based on clinical assessment and imaging studies and full recovery as determined by near normal range of motion with normal muscular strength. Return-to-play decisions must be made on a case-by-case basis, and various factors, such as the number of levels fused, must be taken into account. For example, after a multilevel fusion, as for scoliosis or kyphosis, return to gymnastics or contact sports would not be advised by some experts because of the risk of injury due to increased stress at levels adjacent to the fusion. In contrast, after a limited fusion for spondylolysis or spondylolisthesis, return to contact sports may be a consideration after the fusion has healed and a comprehensive rehabilitation program has been completed.

29. What type of rehabilitation is recommended for athletes after a spinal injury or following spinal surgery?

A neutral-position, isometric coordinated core stabilization program is initiated shortly after surgery. The key to the core stabilization program is to use balance and coordination exercises to train the core muscles to dynamically protect the spine while performing the functions necessary for the sports activity. This program helps decrease the risk of future spine injury. The stabilization program has five levels of proficiency based on the ability of the athlete to perform exercises in eight categories: (1) dead bug, (2) partial sit-up, (3) bridging, (4) prone, (5) quadruped, (6) wall slide, (7) ball, and (8) aerobics. This program begins with the athlete finding a neutral pain-free position for the spine and holding this position while performing the exercises. Once the athlete has established the proper technique at level 1 of the program, they are advanced through successive levels of increasing difficulty with the goal of reaching level 5. After reaching the highest level of the training program that is appropriate for the athlete's status, the athlete begins a series of sports-specific exercises (Fig. 60.5).

30. What objective factors can guide an athlete's return to play after a spinal injury or following spinal surgery?

Return-to-play decisions are complex and must be individualized on a case-by-case basis. Factors such as patient age, spinal pathology, type of surgery (fusion vs. decompression), radiographic factors, and type of sport activity enter into decision making. Objective factors that can guide the physician in determining an athlete's readiness for full return to play are as follows:

- Completion of an appropriate level in the trunk stabilization program (professional athletes: level 5, recreational athletes: level 3)
- Completion of a course of sport-specific exercises
- Attainment of an appropriate level of aerobic conditioning for their sport
- Practicing their sport fully
- Successful slow return to the sport with some limit on minutes played
- Commitment to continue to do the stabilization exercises after return to play

INJURIES INVOLVING THE SACRUM

31. Describe the clinical presentation, workup, and treatment of a sacral stress fracture.

A sacral stress fracture presents with nonspecific low back pain, buttock pain, or hip pain. The onset of pain may be acute or insidious. This injury most commonly develops in running athletes (e.g., marathon runners) and is more common in females. Tenderness is often present over the sacroiliac region. Provocative maneuvers that stress the sacroiliac region may be painful. One-legged stance on the affected side is typically painful. Plain x-rays are not sufficiently sensitive to diagnose early stress fractures. MRI is the preferred imaging modality for diagnosis of sacral stress fractures. Nuclear medicine studies are sensitive for areas of increased bone turnover and may be used for diagnosis but are not as specific as MRI. CT is less sensitive than MRI. Treatment is activity restriction, including a period of protected weight bearing or non–weight bearing, followed by a rehabilitation program. Basic laboratory tests to assess for metabolic bone disease may be considered, including serum calcium, phosphate, alkaline phosphatase, parathyroid hormone, vitamin D, and thyroid-stimulating hormone. Treatment is nonoperative with a period of rest followed by return to low-impact activity and progression to usual athletic activity. This injury has a good prognosis with athletes returning to sports after 8 weeks.

Back Doctor by Dr. Robert Watkins

	Level 1	Level 2	Level 3	Level 4	Level 5
Dead Bug	Supported Arms, Marching Legs, 2 Min. or Supported Legs, Extended Arms, 2 Min.	Unsupported Alternate Opposite Arms & Legs, 3 Min.	Unsupported Alternate Opposite Arms & Legs, 7 Min.	Unsupported Alternate Opposite Arms & Legs, 10 Min. May Add Weights.	Unsupported Alternate Opposite Arms & Legs, 15 Min. May Add Weights.
Partial Sit-up	Forward, Hands on Chest, 10 Reps.	Forward, Hands on Chest, 3 Sets × 10 Reps.	Hands Behind Head: Forward, Right, Left: 3 Sets × 10 Reps.	Weight on Chest: Forward, Right, Left: 3 Sets × 20 Reps.	Weights Overhead: Forward, Right, Left: 3 Sets × 30 Reps.
Bridging	Double Leg Supported, 2 Sets × 10 Reps.	Double Leg Supported 2 Sets × 20 Reps. May Add Weights to Hips	Single Leg Supported, Alternate Opposite Leg Extended, 3 Sets × 20 Reps, Each Side.	On Ball, Single Leg Extended, 4 Sets × 20 Reps, Each Side.	On Ball, Single Leg Extended, 5 Sets × 20 Reps, Earh Side. With Ankle Weights.
Prone	Alternating Arm or Leg Lifts, 1 Set × 10 Reps, Hold 2 Sec.	Alternating Opposite Arm and Leg Lifts, 2 Sets × 10 Reps, Hold 5 Sec. Each Side.	On Ball: Flys, Swim, Supermans: 2 Sets × 20 Reps, Hold 5 Sec.	On Ball: Flys, Swim, Supermans w/ Weights, 2 Sets × 20 Reps. Walkout/pushups 3 Sets × 5 Reps.	On Ball: Flys, Swim, Supermans w/ Weights, 4 Sets × 20 Reps. Walkout/pushups 4 Sets × 10 Reps.
Quadruped	Alternate Arm or Leg, 1 Set × 10 Reps, Hold 2 Sec. Each Side.	Alternating Opposite Arm and Leg, 2 Sets × 10 Reps, Hold 5 Sec. Each Side.	Alternating Opposite Arm and Leg, 2 Sets × 20 Reps, Hold 5 Sec, Each Side.	Alternating Opposite Arm and Leg, 3 Sets × 20 Reps, Hold 5 Sec., w/ Weights.	Alternating Opposite Arm and Leg, 3 Sets × 20 Reps, Hold 15 Sec., w/ Weig hts.
Wall Slide	45 Degrees, 10 Reps, Hold 5 Sec.	90 Degrees, 10 Reps × 20 Sac.	90 Degrees, 10 Reps × 30 Sec. Lunges 1 Min.	90 Degrees, Weights at Side, 10 Reps × 30 Sec. Lunges w/ Weights at Side 3 Min.	90 Degrees, Weights with Arms Extended, 10 Reps × 30 Sec. Lunges w/ Weights in Front 5 Min.
Ball	Dooble Supported Leg Press, Arms at Side, 10 Reps, Hold 2 Sec.	Double Supported Leg Press, Arms Overhead, 10 Reps, Hold 2 Sec.	Arms on Chest, Ball Sit-ups, 20 Reps. Hold 2 Sec: Forward, Right, Left.	Weight on Chest, Ball Sit-ups, 30 Reps, Hold 5 Sec: Forward, Right, Left.	Weight in Extended Arms, 30 Reps, Hold 5 Sec: Forward, Right, Left. May Add: Pulleys, Weighted Stick.
Aerobic	Walk: Land or Water.	10–20 Min: Walk, Bike , Elliptical, Swim.	20–30 Min: Run, Bike, Elliptical, Swim.	45 Min: Run, Bike, Elliptical, Swim.	60 Min: Run, Bike , Elliptical, Swim.
Sports	None	Rotator Cuff Exercises, Scapular Stabilization, Light Throw, Flat Foot Shoot, Skate.	Rotational Exercises, Swinging, Shooting, Throwing, Striding on Field. Weight Room (Protected).	Sport-Specific Exercises, Short Sprints, Cutting, Practice with Team.	Gradual Return to Sport.

Check out **WatkinsSpine.com** for HD video guides

Fig. 60.5 Spinal exercise program-core stabilization program.

KEY POINTS

1. During on-field evaluation of the injured athlete, a significant cervical spinal injury should be suspected until proved otherwise.
2. In the absence of special circumstances, such as respiratory distress combined with inability to access the patient's airway, the helmet should not be removed during the prehospital care of the injured athlete with potential head or neck injury. However, the face mask should be removed at the injury scene to permit airway access.
3. A stinger or burner represents a neuropraxia of cervical nerve roots or brachial plexus, and typically presents with unilateral symptoms.
4. Cervical cord neuropraxia is characterized by an acute transient episode of bilateral sensory and/or motor abnormalities involving the arms, legs, or both.
5. In adolescent athletes, the most common causes of low back pain are lumbar strain, spondylolysis/spondylolisthesis, lumbar disc injuries, and overuse syndrome.
6. In adult athletes, the most common causes of low back pain are lumbar strain, degenerative disc disorders, disc herniations, and spinal stenosis.
7. Patients with lumbar strain, lumbar disc herniation, and spondylolysis can anticipate successful return to sports activities if they are able to successfully complete an appropriate trunk-stabilization rehabilitation program.
8. Limited data exist to assist with decision making for return to play after lumbar and thoracolumbar spinal fusions, and return-to-play decisions are determined on a case-by-case basis.

Websites

1. Sports injuries: https://www.spine.org/KnowYourBack/Conditions/Injuries/Sports-Injuries
2. Brachial plexus injury: https://emedicine.medscape.com/article/91988-clinical
3. Cervical spine injuries in sports: https://emedicine.medscape.com/article/1264627-overview
4. Lumbar disc problems in the athlete: https://emedicine.medscape.com/article/93419-overview
5. Lumbar spine injuries in athletes: https://www.medscape.com/viewarticle/553959
6. Trunk and pelvic stabilization program: https://www.marinahospital.com/blog/trunk-stabilization-program

---

REFERENCE

1. Hsu WK, McCarthy KJ, Savage JW, et al. The Professional Athlete Spine Initiative: Outcomes after lumbar disc herniation in 342 elite professional athletes. *Spine J* 2011;11:180–186.

BIBLIOGRAPHY

1. Ball JR, Harris CB, Lee J, et al. Lumbar spine injuries in sports: Review of the literature and current treatment recommendations. *Sports Med Open* 2019;5:26–36.
2. Brophy RH, Lyman S, Chehab EL, et al. Predictive value of prior injury on career in professional American football is affected by player position. *Am J Sports Med* 2009;37:768–775.
3. Cantu RC, Li YM, Abdulhamid M, et al. Return to play after cervical spine injury in sports. *Curr Sports Med Rep* 2013;12:14–17.
4. Cook RW, Hsu WK. Return to play after lumbar spine surgery. *Clin Sports Med* 2016;35:609–619.
5. Hecht AC, editor. Spine Injuries in Athletes. Philadelphia, PA: Wolters Kluwer, 2017.
6. Hsu WK, McCarthy KJ, Savage JW, et al. The Professional Athlete Spine Initiative: Outcomes after lumbar disc herniation in 342 elite professional athletes. *Spine J* 2011;11:180–186.
7. Huang P, Anissipour A, McGee W, et al. Return-to-play recommendations after cervical, thoracic, and lumbar spine injuries: A comprehensive review. *Sports Health* 2016;8:19–25.
8. Menzer H, Gill GK, Paterson A. Thoracic spine sports-related injuries. *Curr Sports Med Rep* 2015;14:34–40.
9. Rosenthal BD, Boody BS, Hsu WK. Return to play for athletes. *Neurosurg Clin N Am* 2017;28:163–171.
10. Watkins RGIV, Watkins RG III. Lumbar spondylolysis and spondylolisthesis in athletes. *Semin Spine Surg* 2010;22:210–217.
11. Li Y, Hresko MT. Lumbar spine surgery in athletes: Outcomes and return-to-play criteria. *Clin Sports Med* 2012;31:487–498.
12. Semon RL, Spengler D. Significance of lumbar spondylolysis in college football players. *Spine* 1981;6:172-4.

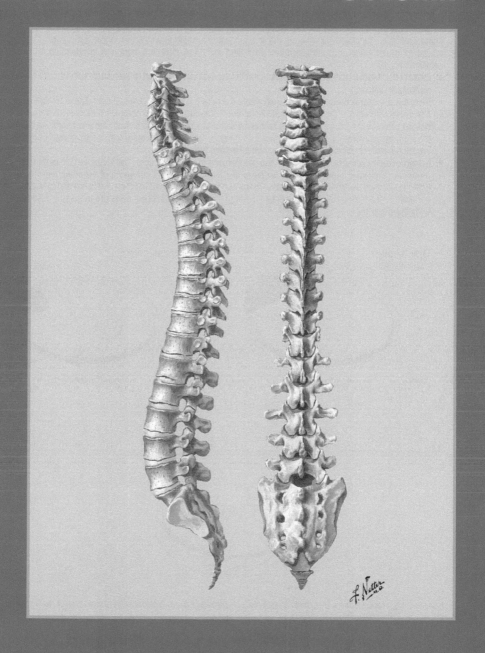

CHAPTER 61

DISORDERS OF THE SPINAL CORD AND RELATED STRUCTURES

Benjamin D. Elder, MD, PhD and Vincent J. Devlin, MD

SPINAL CORD TUMORS

1. **How does one describe the anatomic location of a spine tumor?**

   Spine tumors are localized according to the anatomic compartment in which they occur: *extradural, intradural-extramedullary,* or *intramedullary* (Figs. 61.1 and 61.2). Certain tumors may invade multiple anatomic planes.

   - **Extradural tumors** may be *primary* spinal tumors (benign or malignant) or *secondary* tumors (due to metastatic disease).
   - **Intradural-extramedullary tumors** arise within the dura but outside the spinal cord. These tumors *displace the spinal cord* toward the contralateral side of the thecal sac. The most common tumors arise from the sheath cells covering the spinal nerve root (schwannoma, neurofibroma) or from the arachnoid cap cells in the dura (meningioma). If the tumor arises as the nerve root leaves the dural sac, it may possess both an intradural and extradural component (dumbbell-shaped tumor).
   - **Intramedullary tumors** originate from the parenchyma of the spinal cord. The characteristic pattern on magnetic resonance imaging (MRI) is *widening of the spinal cord* and narrowing of the cerebrospinal fluid (CSF) space over several vertebral levels. These tumors are located within the spinal cord and typically enhance with administration of gadolinium. Syringomyelia and perilesional cysts are frequently associated with these lesions.

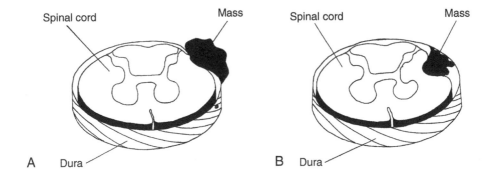

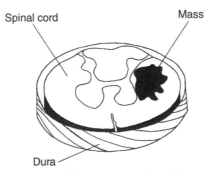

Fig. 61.1 Location of spinal tumors. (A) Extradural. (B) Intradural-extramedullary. (C) Intramedullary. (From Rolak LA. Neurology Secrets. 4th ed. Philadelphia, PA: Mosby; 2005.)

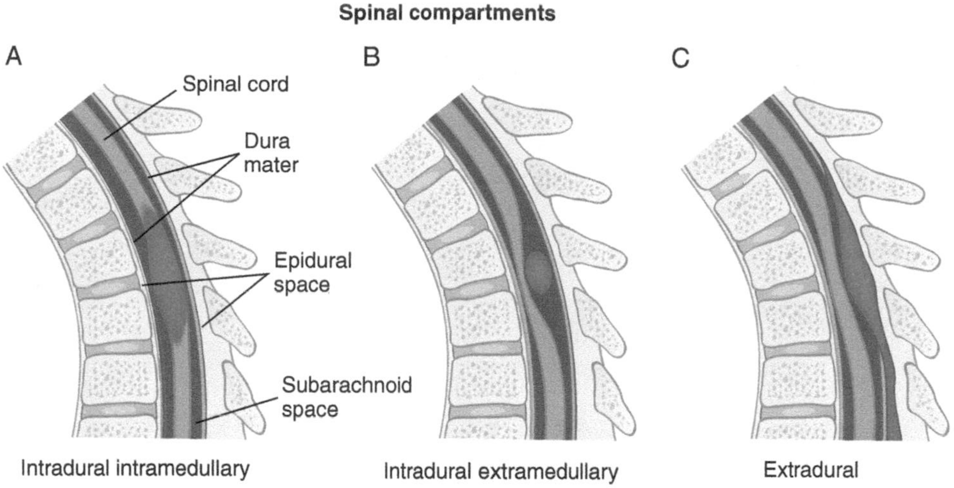

Spinal compartments

Fig. 61.2 Spinal compartments. (A) Intradural intramedullary. (B) Intadural extramedullary. (C) Extradural. (From Kollias SS, Capper DM, Saupe N, et al. Spinal Tumors. In: Naidich TP, Castillo M, Cha S, et al., editors. Imaging of the Spine. Philadelphia, PA: Saunders; 2011.)

2. In what anatomic compartment do spinal tumors most commonly occur?
   The extradural anatomic compartment is the most common location for a spinal tumor. Approximately 60% of all spine tumors are extradural and 40% are intradural. Among intradural tumors, approximately 75% are extramedullary and 25% are intramedullary. Intradural-extramedullary tumors are more common in adults, while intramedullary tumors are more common in children. Intradural tumors are equally common in males and females, with the exception of meningiomas, which occur more frequently in females.

3. What are the most common types of extradural spinal tumors?
   Extradural tumors arise as primary tumors originating from the vertebra and adjacent soft tissues or develop secondary to metastatic disease. The most common extradural spinal tumor is a metastatic tumor. Primary bone tumors are uncommon. Myeloma is the most common primary spine neoplasm. Some common tumor types to consider in the differential diagnosis of an extradural spinal tumor are listed in Table 61.1.

Table 61.1 Extradural Spine Tumors.

PRIMARY SPINE TUMORS		METASTATIC SPINE TUMORS
Benign	Malignant	
Hemangioma	Myeloma	Breast
Osteoid osteoma	Lymphoma	Prostate
Osteoblastoma	Chordoma	Lung
Osteochondroma	Ewing sarcoma	Thyroid
Giant cell tumor	Chondrosarcoma	Renal
Aneurysmal bone cyst	Osteosarcoma	Melanoma
Langerhans cell histiocytosis		Gastrointestinal

4. What are the most common types of intradural-extramedullary spinal cord tumors?
   Eighty percent of the tumors in the intradural-extramedullary space are schwannomas, neurofibromas, or meningiomas (Fig. 61.3). Tumors of the intradural-extramedullary space account for approximately 60% of all intradural spinal tumors in adults but occur less commonly in children. Nerve sheath tumors (schwannomas, neurofibromas) arise from sheath cells covering the spinal nerve roots, while meningiomas arise from arachnoid cap cells, dural fibroblasts, or pial cells localized at the spinal cord surface. Approximately 5% of intradural-extramedullary tumors have both an intradural and extradural component (dumbbell tumors).

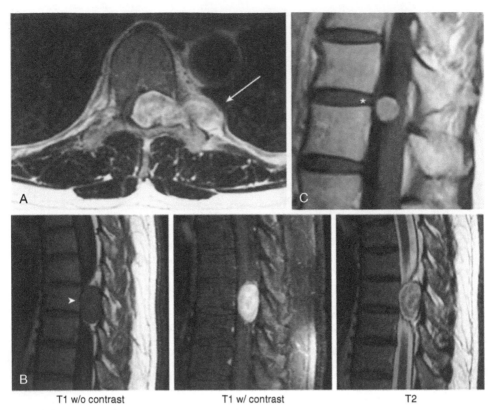

T1 w/o contrast   T1 w/ contrast   T2

Fig. 61.3 Examples of intradural-extramedullary spinal cord tumors. (A) Axial view on T2-weighted magnetic resonance imaging (MRI) showing a "dumbbell"-shaped schwannoma *(arrow)*. (B) Schwannoma *(arrowhead)* typically enhances with contrast on T1-weighted MRI and is hyperintense on T2-weighted MRI. (C) Meningioma *(asterisk)* similarly enhances with contrast on T1-weighted imaging. *w/*, With; *w/o*, without. (Copyright © 2015 Ziya L. Gokaslan, Published by Elsevier Inc. All rights reserved.)

Schwannomas are the most common type of nerve sheath tumor. These benign encapsulated nerve sheath tumors are comprised of proliferating Schwann cells and usually occur as a solitary lesion. The presence of multiple spinal schwannomas warrants evaluation for schwannomatosis, a rare genetic disorder that is recognized most often in patients over 30 years of age.

Neurofibromas are benign, unencapsulated nerve sheath tumors comprised of proliferating Schwann cells mixed with fibroblasts and occur less commonly than schwannomas. Over half of these tumors occur in patients with neurofibromatosis type 1 (NF1) and occasionally may undergo malignant degeneration to malignant peripheral nerve sheath tumors (MPNSTs).

Meningiomas occur most frequently in females between 40 and 80 years of age, and typically present as isolated lesions, except in patients with neurofibromatosis type 2 (NF2). These tumors are slow-growing, encapsulated tumors that are most commonly located in the thoracic region along the dorsolateral aspect of the spinal cord, but may occasionally occur in the cervical region or along the anterior aspect of the spinal cord.

Other tumor types may occur in the intradural-extramedullary space but are less common (Table 61.2).

5. **What are the most common types of intramedullary spinal cord tumors?**
The most common types of intramedullary tumors are ependymomas, astrocytomas, and hemangioblastomas (Table 61.3, Fig. 61.4). In adults ependymomas are the most common tumor type, while in children astrocytomas are most common.

Ependymomas arise from the cuboidal ependymal cells that surround the ventricular system and central canal of the spinal cord. As the tumor enlarges in the central canal, the flow of CSF is obstructed and cystic cavities frequently develop above and below the lesion.

Table 61.2 Intradural–Extramedullary Spinal Tumors.	
Schwannoma	Ependymoma
Neurofibroma	Paraganglioma
Meningioma	Epidermoid and dermoid cysts
Hemangiopericytoma	Subarachnoid seeding of metastatic disease
Lipoma	

Table 61.3 Intramedullary Spinal Tumors.	
Ependymoma	Neuroblastoma
Astrocytoma	Gliomas (malignant oligodendroglioma, ganglioglioma)
Hemangioblastoma	Epidermoid and dermoid cysts
Lipoma	Spinal cord metastasis

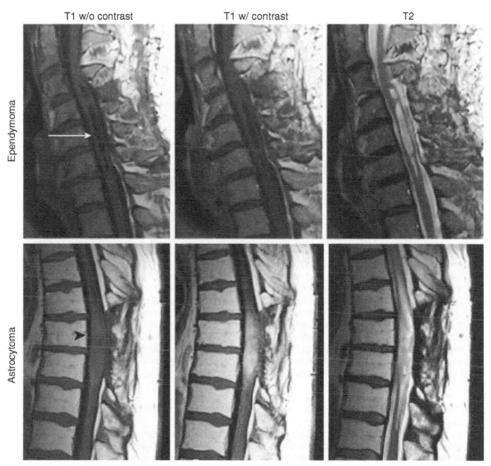

Fig. 61.4 Examples of intramedullary spinal cord tumors. Magnetic resonance imaging of a cervical ependymoma *(arrow)* and thoracic astrocytoma *(arrowhead)* shows contrast enhancement with the astrocytoma but not with the ependymoma. Ependymomas are typically hyperintense on T2-weighted imaging. *w/,* With; *w/o,* without. (Copyright © 2015 Ziya L. Gokaslan, Published by Elsevier Inc. All rights reserved.)

Astrocytomas result from malignant transformation of astrocyte cells, which are glial cells that provide nutritional support to neurons and axons. The majority of tumors are low grade, but more aggressive and infiltrating types such as glioblastoma multiforme (GBM) may occur and are associated with a very poor prognosis.

Hemangioblastomas are the most common intramedullary spinal cord tumor of nonglial origin. These are highly vascular lesions that often have a very large syrinx compared with the size of the tumor. Hemangioblastomas of the spine typically occur as solitary lesions, but may also present as multiple lesions in patients with von Hippel-Lindau (VHL) disease, an autosomal dominant disorder associated with the development of tumors in different organs.

6. **What is the differential diagnosis of a tumor located in the region of the conus medullaris or cauda equina?**
The most common intradural tumors presenting in the region of the conus medullaris or cauda equina include myxopapillary ependymoma, schwannoma, meningioma, and lipoma. Metastatic tumors may also occur but are less common.

7. **Describe common clinical presentations and best methods for diagnosis of intradural spinal tumors.**
In general, most intradural tumors present with an insidious onset of symptoms, although occasionally, intradural tumors may present with acute neurologic deterioration secondary to intratumoral or extramedullary hemorrhage. Because of the slow-growing nature of many intradural spinal tumors, symptoms tend to precede diagnosis for periods ranging from months to years. Pain is often the earliest symptom and is typically reported as occurring at night. The clinical signs and symptoms associated with an intradural spinal tumor are related to the *level of the lesion* along the spinal column (cervical, thoracic, lumbar, sacral), *tumor location*, and the *rate of tumor growth*. Motor dysfunction, sensory dysfunction, reflex abnormalities, long tract signs, and autonomic dysfunction (bowel, bladder, and/or sexual dysfunction) may occur. *Cervical tumors* may present with occipitocervical pain, upper extremity pain, and myelopathy with sensory changes or clumsiness and/or balance/gait dysfunction. *Thoracic tumors* may present with thoracic radicular pain, sensory changes involving the trunk and/or lower extremities, and myelopathy involving the lower extremities. *Tumors involving the conus medullaris* may present with a mixture of upper and lower motor neuron (LMN) findings involving the lower extremities and often are accompanied by bowel and/or bladder dysfunction. *Tumors involving the cauda equina* often present with radicular symptoms involving the lower extremities. Notably, back and leg pain are often worse with lying down and relieved with erect posture. An LMN syndrome may develop and include flaccid paraparesis, loss of reflexes, segmental sensory loss, and sphincter dysfunction, although this is an uncommon acute presentation due to the typical slow-growing nature of cauda equina tumors. MRI with and without gadolinium enhancement is the imaging modality of choice for diagnosis of intradural tumors. Consideration should be given to performing a screening MRI of the entire neural axis as subarachnoid seeding of tumor is possible, particularly with ependymomas. Histologic evaluation of tumor tissue after biopsy or surgical resection is used to establish a definitive diagnosis.

Extramedullary tumors frequently cause unilateral symptoms due to their eccentric location (i.e., unilateral radicular pain, unilateral spastic weakness, Brown-Séquard syndrome). For tumors of nerve sheath origin such as schwannomas and neurofibromas, radicular pain and sensory changes are the most common initial presentation, as these tumors typically develop in the dorsal sensory roots. Myelopathic signs develop later as the tumor increases in size and causes spinal cord compression. The initial presentation of spinal meningiomas is variable and may include pain, unilateral or bilateral numbness, and/or weakness, and myelopathy.

Intramedullary tumors most commonly present with pain. Pain is often described as burning, poorly localized, and involving large areas of the body. Tumors may disrupt the spinothalamic tracts but spare the dorsal columns, which are relatively resistant to tumor infiltration and cause a dissociated sensory loss (loss of pain and temperature sensation without loss of position and vibration sensation). Additional presentations include motor dysfunction, reflex abnormalities, long tract signs, gait abnormalities, or autonomic dysfunction (bowel, bladder, and/or sexual dysfunction). Children may present with clumsiness, frequent falls, progressive scoliosis, or torticollis.

8. **Discuss and contrast the general approach to treatment of intradural-extramedullary spinal cord tumors versus intramedullary spinal cord tumors.**
Intradural-extramedullary spinal cord tumors tend to be histopathologically benign and can be successfully resected in the majority of patients, most commonly through a posterior surgical approach. Tumors in an anterior location and dumbbell-shaped tumors are more challenging to treat surgically as these tumors generally require more extensive surgical exposures to facilitate safe access for tumor resection. Radiotherapy or chemotherapy is generally reserved for tumors with malignant histologic characteristics and for recurrent tumors.

Intramedullary spinal cord tumors are typically treated with open surgical resection. Advances that have transformed the surgical treatment of these lesions include MRI, microscopic surgical techniques, improved surgical instrumentation, intraoperative ultrasound, the ultrasonic aspirator, and intraoperative neurophysiologic monitoring. A posterior midline surgical approach is most commonly utilized. Following laminectomy, a midline myelotomy is made in the posterior aspect of the spinal cord to minimize injury to the posterior columns of the cord. The midline is located by identifying the midpoint between the dorsal root entry zones, identifying where blood vessels enter into the spinal cord or by dorsal column mapping using neurophysiologic monitoring. However, this can be challenging in many cases due to distortion of normal anatomy by the tumor. The aggressiveness of surgical resection is dependent on the histologic diagnosis based on intraoperative frozen section and the ability to locate and maintain a surgical plane. Well-circumscribed tumors such as ependymoma and hemangioblastoma are typically amenable to gross total resection. Well-differentiated astrocytomas are amenable to resection, but infiltrative and high-grade types are impossible to completely resect and their treatment remains controversial. Radiotherapy and chemotherapy are reserved for high-grade malignant lesions and for lesions that are not surgically resectable.

9. Describe the expected postoperative neurologic function following resection of intramedullary spinal cord tumors.
Due to the midline myelotomy approach to intramedullary tumors, nearly all patients have postoperative dorsal column sensory abnormalities, particularly with proprioception, that may take at least several months to resolve or improve. Many patients also have additional significant neurologic deficits in the immediate postoperative period due to spinal cord manipulation that will often improve over time, unless there has been permanent damage to the motor tracts. Some surgeons have found that intraoperative neuromonitoring with motor evoked potentials and epidural D-wave monitoring may be predictive of postoperative neurologic function.

SYRINGOHYDROMYELIA AND CHIARI MALFORMATION

10. What is syringohydromyelia?
A **syrinx** is a cystic dilatation or cavitation that develops within the substance of the spinal cord. **Hydromyelia** refers to a dilatation of the central canal with an ependymal-cell lining. **Syringomyelia** is an eccentric cavitation that is not lined by ependyma. Although hydromyelia and syringomyelia are described as distinct entities, it is not possible to separate these entities in practice and these lesions are most appropriately referred to as **syringo-hydromyelia**. A syrinx extending into the brainstem is called **syringobulbia**.

11. What are some causes of syringohydromyelia?
Syringohydromyelia may be idiopathic or arise as the result of spinal cord trauma, tumors, spinal cord infarction, postradiotherapy, hemorrhage, or developmental anomalies (e.g., Chiari malformation, basilar invagination), or spinal cord tethering.

12. Describe classic clinical features associated with syringohydromyelia.
- **Dissociated sensory loss:** A centrally located syrinx disrupts the decussating spinothalamic tracts (loss of pain and temperature sensation), while dorsal column function remains intact (position and vibration sensation is preserved). When this pattern of sensory loss involves the shoulders and upper trunk it is described as a "cape-like" pattern.
- **Dysesthetic pain:** Severe pain may develop and most commonly involves the trunk and upper extremities.
- **LMN lesions:** Involvement of the anterior horn cells leads to atrophy, weakness, and absent reflexes below the level of the lesion. Lesions that involve the cervical cord lead to muscle atrophy, which begins distally in the hands and progresses to involve more proximal musculature.
- **Bulbar lesions:** Syringobulbia can manifest as tongue fasciculations, hoarseness, facial anesthesia, and dysphagia.
- **Autonomic system involvement:** Horner syndrome, impaired bowel or bladder function.
- **Musculoskeletal manifestations:** Scoliosis, Charcot arthropathy (classically the shoulder joint is involved), basilar invagination, Klippel-Feil anomaly.

13. What are the treatment options for a symptomatic syrinx?
Syringohydromyelia has been classified into two main types:
- Communicating (associated with Chiari malformation, basilar arachnoiditis)
- Noncommunicating (associated with spinal cord trauma, spinal cord tumor, or spinal arachnoiditis)
    Surgical treatment of communicating syringohydromyelia initially involves suboccipital decompression if a Chiari malformation is present. Placement of a ventriculoperitoneal (VP) shunt may also be indicated if hydrocephalus is present.
    Surgical treatment options for noncommunicating syringohydromyelia vary and include syringostomy, expansile duraplasty (to create a path for CSF flow around the lesion), syringosubarachnoid or syringopleural shunting, or lysis of adhesions. Despite treatment, outcomes in patients with arachnoiditis are often less than satisfactory.

14. What is the Chiari malformation?
The spectrum of Chiari malformations consists of four hindbrain abnormalities that share a common entity of impaired CSF flow around the brainstem and through the foramen magnum. These disorders may be congenital or

acquired. The tonsillar herniation is usually greater than 5 mm, but this is not essential or diagnostic of the disorder. Treatment of symptomatic Chiari malformations usually requires surgery. Exact surgical indications and procedures remain controversial.

15. **What are the types of Chiari malformations and their respective features?**
    Chiari types I and II are the commonly encountered forms, while types III and IV are exceedingly rare.
    Type I
    - Caudal descent of the cerebellar tonsils below the foramen magnum (>2–5 mm) results in crowding of the subarachnoid space at the craniocervical junction
    - Usually occurs in adults or adolescents without myelomeningocele
    - Classic symptom is suboccipital headache brought on by Valsalva or neck extension
    - May be associated with scoliosis, hand weakness, craniovertebral osseous anomalies, Klippel-Feil anomaly, syringomyelia, or hydrocephalus
    Type II
    - Caudal descent of the brainstem, cerebellar vermis, and fourth ventricle through the foramen magnum (Fig. 61.5)
    - Occurs almost exclusively in children with myelomeningocele
    - Associated with hydrocephalus (90%), syringomyelia (20%–95%), kinking of the medulla, Klippel-Feil, atlantoaxial abnormalities, and various brain abnormalities.
    Type III
    - Dorsal protrusion of a craniocervical sac containing posterior fossa contents (cerebellum, brainstem) is seen externally
    - Rare, frequently fatal during infancy
    Type IV
    - Crowded posterior fossa associated with hypoplastic cerebellum and brainstem without hindbrain herniation
    - Rare, some authors have removed this from the Chiari classification

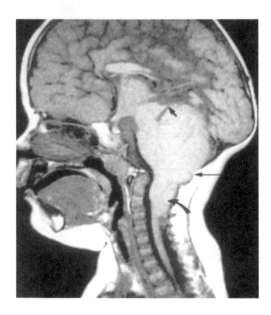

Fig. 61.5 Magnetic resonance image of a patient with Chiari II malformation. Note the upward herniation of the cerebellum as indicated by the *short arrow*. The *curved arrow* indicates downward herniation of the brainstem through the foramen magnum. The *thin long arrow* marks the foramen magnum. (From Fleisher LA, editor. Anesthesia and Uncommon Diseases. 5th ed. Philadelphia, PA: Saunders; 2005.)

16. **What are the indications for surgical decompression in Chiari malformations?**
    Indications remain controversial, but most authors agree that any Chiari malformation with an associated symptomatic syrinx would portend surgery. Additionally, any signs of brainstem compression or cerebellar dysfunction are indications for surgical intervention. In Chiari I malformation patients, surgical decompression is most commonly performed for treatment of suboccipital headaches. In Chiari II malformation patients with associated hydrocephalus, it is critical to ensure that the patient's VP shunt is functional prior to considering any additional surgical intervention. Controversy exists regarding the exact surgical procedure, if any, required to decompress the cervicomedullary junction and restore CSF circulation across the foramen magnum.

SPINAL DYSRAPHISM

17. Define spinal dysraphism.

Spinal dysraphism refers to a spectrum of congenital spinal anomalies due to failure of fusion of midline structures. The anomalies may involve the osseous vertebral elements, spinal cord, nerve roots, bladder, rectum, and genitalia.

18. What is spina bifida?

The neural tube usually closes between days 24 and 28 following conception during a process called *neurulation.* Spina bifida is a descriptive term applied to a group of neural tube defects associated with the disruption of neurulation leading to failure of posterior fusion of vertebral osseous elements (Fig. 61.6). Spina bifida is classified into two main types:

- **Spina bifida occulta:** Intact skin overlies the underlying anomaly, which ranges from an osseous defect involving the posterior lamina without associated structural or neurologic significance to clinically significant involvement of neural and meningeal structures with significant neurologic sequelae (e.g., diastematomyelia, lipomyelomeningocele, anterior sacral meningocele, tethered filum terminale).
- **Spina bifida cystica:** A mass extrudes through the defect and overlying skin. The mass may contain meninges and CSF (meningocele), or meninges, CSF, and spinal neural tissue (myelomeningocele). The spectrum of conditions may be detectable with prenatal imaging, are visible at birth, and may be associated with severe neurologic sequelae. These sequelae may include hydrocephalus, neurogenic bowel and bladder dysfunction, and varying degrees of lower extremity paralysis.

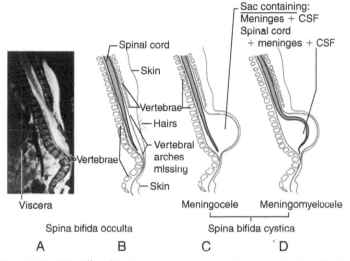

Fig. 61.6 Sagittal views of spina bifida malformations. Magnetic resonance image and corresponding views showing spina bifida occulta (A and B). Spina bifida cystica (C, meningocele and D, meningomyelocele). *CSF,* Cerebrospinal fluid. (From Haines DE. Fundamental Neuroscience for Basic and Clinical Applications. 3rd ed. Philadelphia, PA: Churchill Livingstone; 2006.)

19. Describe the clinical features of spina bifida occulta.

In spina bifida occulta the underlying spinal and/or neural defect is covered by intact skin and thus may not be grossly evident on examination. External signs may include a lumbosacral hair tuft *(faun tail)*, skin-covered lipoma, cutaneous hemangioma, or a lumbosacral skin dimple. If the defect is limited to failure of fusion of the vertebral arch, the finding has little clinical significance. However, more complex types are associated with neurologic, urologic, and/or orthopedic abnormalities. The majority of more complex cases will require surgical intervention to prevent progression of neurologic deficits.

Associated neurologic findings may include lower extremity atrophy, weakness, radicular pain, or numbness. Urologic signs may include an abnormal voiding pattern in an infant, new incontinence after toilet training, or a urinary tract infection in a child of any age. Orthopedic findings may include cavovarus foot deformities, claw toes, leg-length discrepancy, and scoliosis. Diagnosis is often delayed until adolescence or adulthood, due to absent initial neurologic or urologic findings. Early identification is paramount because prophylactic surgery is usually indicated to preserve neurologic function. Initial workup involves spinal MRI and cranial ultrasound evaluation to rule out the presence of hydrocephalus.

20. **What is diastematomyelia?**
    Diastematomyelia is a congenital spinal anomaly in which splitting of the spinal cord is identified. Two separate *hemicords* divided by a septum are present. Variations include two separate hemicords separated by a septum (osseous or cartilaginous) and contained in separate dural coverings, or two separate hemicords (fibrous septum) in one dural covering. There is a female predominance and the condition most commonly presents in the lower thoracic or upper lumbar spine. Patients present with a tethered cord syndrome. Spinal deformities are commonly associated with diastematomyelia. Surgical intervention is indicated for patients with progressive neurologic deficits. If surgical correction of coexistent spinal deformity is planned, surgery to untether the spinal cord by removal of the septum may be performed either prior to the surgical procedure to correct spinal deformity or during this procedure.

21. **What is the tethered cord syndrome?**
    During fetal development the conus medullaris ascends from its position in the sacral region to a location between the T12 and L2 vertebra due to the differential growth rates of the spinal cord and spinal column. The spinal cord is normally suspended freely within the spinal canal and is able to accommodate vertebral growth and adjust for movements associated with daily activities. Tethering of the spinal cord develops when the spinal cord becomes abnormally attached to the spinal column. Stretch-induced neurologic dysfunction of the spinal cord may occur due to hypoxic stress and vascular insufficiency and is referred to as a tethered cord syndrome. Spinal tethering may result from congenital or acquired causes which include thickening of the filum terminale, lipoma, meningocele, split cord malformations, spinal injuries or infections and prior surgery including myelomeningocele repair. Although symptoms often develop early in life, an initial presentation may not occur until adulthood. Signs and symptoms may include neurologic deficits, back pain, cutaneous abnormalities, spinal deformities, bowel and bladder dysfunction, gait abnormalities, and orthopedic deformities. MRI including dynamic imaging is the primary diagnostic modality. Surgical intervention is directed toward release of tethering structures to relieve chronic tension in the spinal cord.

22. **What is a lipomyelomeningocele?**
    A **lipomyelomeningocele** is a common congenital spinal anomaly in which herniation of a lipoma into the conus medullaris or the dorsal aspect of the spinal cord occurs through an osseous defect and communicates with an adjacent subcutaneous fatty mass. It is a common cause of tethered cord syndrome. Symptoms may include constipation, urinary urgency, dyspareunia, lumbar pain, or cephalgia (headache) with defecation. The term lipomyelomeningocele is actually a misnomer, because abnormal neural tissue does not extend outside of the spinal canal. Surgical treatment of this anomaly is extremely challenging.

23. **Describe the presentation of an anterior sacral meningocele.**
    An **anterior sacral meningocele** is a rare congenital spinal anomaly in which herniation of dura mater and/or neural elements through a defect in the ventral spine is identified. The anomaly contains CSF and may contain neural elements. Unlike the myelomeningocele, this anomaly is not associated with hydrocephalus or Chiari malformation. Associated findings include the triad of sacral bony anomalies, a presacral mass and anorectal anomalies (Currarino syndrome). Symptoms may include constipation, urinary urgency, dyspareunia, lumbar pain, or cephalgia with defecation. Examination findings include a smooth pelvic mass palpable on pelvic or rectal examination. This entity is most commonly found at the sacral level and is more common in females.

24. **Define myelomeningocele and describe the scope of this problem in the United States and worldwide.**
    Myelomeningocele is a neural tube defect in which the dorsal neural structures are open through the skin due to failure of the neural tube closure. It is the most common major spinal birth defect. In the United States, approximately 3000 pregnancies are affected by neural tube defects each year. Worldwide, it is estimated that more than 300,000 infants are born with neural tube defects each year. Prevalence has diminished since the 1980s in some regions due to utilization of the B vitamin folic acid, which significantly decreases the risk of having an infant born with a neural tube defect.

25. **What is the etiology of myelomeningocele?**
    Embryologically, the defect occurs around day 28 following conception when the posterior neuropore fails to close or reopens due to distention of the central canal from CSF. This event has been associated with multiple factors including genetic factors, maternal nutritional factors (folic acid deficiency), season of conception, and environmental factors (socioeconomic status, degree of urbanization).

26. **How is myelomeningocele diagnosed and treated in the prenatal period?**
    Fetal diagnosis can be made prenatally by amniocentesis (increased amniotic fluid alpha-fetoprotein and acetylcholinesterase levels), maternal serum alpha-fetoprotein testing, and high-resolution ultrasound, with high accuracy. Ultrafast fetal MRI imaging may be safely performed to further characterize the location of the lesion and assess the presence of hydrocephalus or Chiari II malformation. This can inform prenatal counseling and decision-making regarding termination of pregnancy, fetal closure, or elective cesarean section. Patients require careful evaluation for associated cardiac and renal defects. When the condition is identified prenatally, cesarean section is usually recommended.

A recent treatment option for select patients is prenatal repair of spinal bifida. A prospective, randomized study, the Management of Myelomeningocele Study (MOMS), compared the outcomes of prenatal and postnatal repair and showed that fetal surgery prior to 26 weeks gestation may reduce the incidence and severity of neurologic deficits, reverse the hindbrain component of the Arnold-Chiari II malformation, and reduce the need for a VP shunt. However, this prenatal procedure is associated with significant risks including premature birth and complications related to the uterine incision.

27. What is the management for a newborn patient with myelomeningocele?

Upon birth, the baby should be placed prone and the lesion covered with moist nonadherent dressing (Telfa). The trendelenburg position may prevent CSF accumulation at the lesion site. If the lesion is open and CSF leakage is noted, prophylactic antibiotics to prevent meningitis are administered. A detailed neurologic examination is documented prior to surgery. Surgical closure should be performed within 24–48 hours of birth (Fig. 61.7). The surgical procedure for closure of the defect involves resection of the *zona epitheliosa* and recapitulation of the *neural placode* into a tube. The dura and fascia are then closed over the closed placode in a watertight fashion. The skin is then carefully closed over the repair. A rotational flap or a *Z-plasty* may be required to adequately cover the repair without tension.

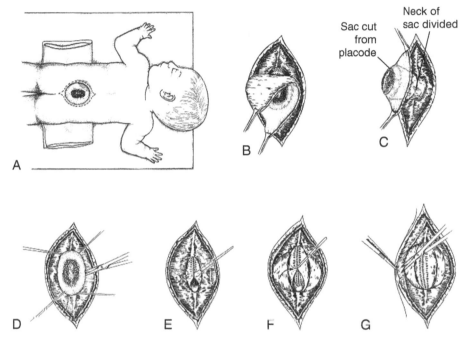

Fig. 61.7 Technique for closure of a myelomeningocele. (A) The infant is placed prone with towel rolls under the hips. An elliptical incision is outlined just outside the zona epithelioserosa, which may be oriented on a vertical or horizontal axis. (B) The incision is to the level of the lumbodorsal fascia. The apices of the island of skin within the incision are grasped with clamps, and the skin is under-mined medially until the dural sac is seen to funnel through the fascial defect. The skin is then excised from the placode and discarded, allowing the placode to fall into the spinal canal. (D) The everted dura is undermined and reflected medially to envelop the placode. The placode itself may be folded medially and sewn into a tube at this point. (E) The dural layer is closed with nonabsorbable suture, using a running stitch. (F) The fascia is incised to the muscle, undermined, and reflected medially to create a second layer of closure. (G) The skin is undermined using blunt techniques to permit closure. (From Sutton LN, Schwartz DM. Congenital anomalies of the spinal cord. In: Herkowitz HN, Garfin SR, Eismont FJ, et al., editors. Rothman-Simeone The Spine. 5th ed. Philadelphia, PA: Saunders; 2006.)

28. What are the clinical sequelae of myelomeningocele?

The clinical sequelae involve multiple body systems and may include:
- **Neurologic:** 90% of patients develop clinically significant hydrocephalus, requiring CSF diversion procedures (e.g., VP shunt). Children will frequently have some degree of lower extremity motor, sensory, and/or autonomic dysfunction correlating to the level of the lesion. Cognitive deficits are common.
- **Urologic:** Nearly all patients have abnormalities in urologic function.
- **Gastrointestinal:** Neurogenic bowel dysfunction is present in a high percentage of patients.

- **Musculoskeletal deformities:** Spinal deformities are common and include scoliosis, kyphosis, and deformities associated with congenital osseous anomalies. A spectrum of lower extremity deformities may develop depending on the level of the lesion and may include hip dislocation, hip and knee contractures, and foot deformities.

MISCELLANEOUS DISORDERS INVOLVING THE SPINAL CORD

29. Define the terms myelopathy and myelitis.

    Myelopathy is a broad term that refers to any pathologic process affecting the spinal cord and is responsible for neurologic dysfunction. Myelopathy usually indicates a compressive, toxic, vascular, or metabolic etiology. **Myelitis** indicates an inflammatory process, most often due to infectious or autoimmune causes.

30. What are some causes of myelopathy and myelitis?
    A. Idiopathic transverse myelitis (TM)
    B. Demyelinating diseases
       1. Multiple sclerosis
       2. Neuromyelitis optica (NMO) or Devic syndrome
       3. Acute disseminated encephalomyelitis (ADEM)
    C. Postvaccination myelitis
    D. Infectious myelopathies
       1. Viral (HIV, human T-lymphotropic virus 1 [HTLV-1], varicella-zoster virus [VZV], cytomegalovirus [CMV], Epstein-Barr virus [EBV], enteroviruses)
       2. Bacterial (syphilis, tuberculosis)
       3. Fungal
       4. Parasitic
    E. Connective tissue diseases related to myelitis
       1. Rheumatoid arthritis
       2. Sjögren disease
       3. Systemic lupus erythematosus
       4. Antiphospholipid antibody syndrome
    F. Sarcoidosis
    G. Metabolic and nutritional (deficiencies of vitamin B12, folic acid, copper, vitamin E)
    H. Paraneoplastic syndromes
       1. Small cell carcinoma of the lung
       2. Radiation myelopathy
       3. Intrathecal methotrexate
       4. Hodgkin disease/lymphomas
    I. Toxins
       1. Spinal anesthesia—epidural or intrathecal
       2. Spinal angiography
       3. Intrathecal steroids
    J. Electrical injury (high-tension current, lightning, electroshock therapy)
    K. Barotrauma (caisson work, scuba diving, flying)
    L. Familial disorders (hereditary spastic paraplegia, Friedreich ataxia)
    M. Spinal cord compression (extradural or intradural tumor, infection, trauma, cervical spondylosis)
    N. Vascular disorders involving the spinal cord
       1. Spinal cord infarct
       2. AVMs
       3. Arteriovenous fistulas
       4. Cavernous malformations

31. What is the most common cause of myelopathy in adults over 55 years of age?

    Cervical spondylotic myelopathy is the most common cause of myelopathy after age 55.

32. What are some considerations in the initial evaluation and workup of a patient suspected of having myelopathy or myelitis?

    A **comprehensive medical history and detailed physical examination** are the initial steps towards establishing the diagnosis. The time course of myelopathies is variable, and onset may be acute, subacute, or chronic. Some myelopathies present as a single event, while others present in phases or with recurrent symptoms. Back pain and/or neck pain, the presence of a sensory level or dysesthesia, saddle anesthesia, bilateral upper or lower extremity weakness, and autonomic dysfunction (bladder, bowel, cardiovascular or thermoregulatory dysfunction) suggest the presence of a lesion involving the spinal cord. Acute onset with rapid progression over hours to days suggests a spinal cord infarct, hemorrhage, acute transverse myelitis, or a compressive myelopathy. Early identification of compressive myelopathies is critical to allow for early surgical intervention prior to irreversible cord injury. Clinical features that suggest a compressive myelopathy include: radicular and vertebrogenic pain, early upper motor neuron (UMN) signs, ascending paresthesias, and the presence of a Brown-Séquard syndrome. Clinical features that suggest a noncompressive myelopathy include: dysesthetic pain, dissociated sensory loss, descending sensory loss with sacral sparing, initial LMN signs followed by later onset of UMN signs, and sphincter dysfunction. Longitudinal localization of the spinal cord lesion is estimated based on the level of dermatomal involvement. Transverse localization of the spinal cord lesion based on the extent and type of cord involvement (i.e., complete cord lesion, Brown-Séquard syndrome, posterior cord syndrome, central cord syndrome, or tract-specific dysfunction).

MRI of the **entire spine** with and without contrast is the initial step in the diagnostic process. Cord lesions will show a different signal intensity from the normal cord and demonstrate increased signal intensity on T2-weighted images. The size of the spinal cord may increase, decrease, or remain normal. The longitudinal extent of lesions on sagittal MRI images, as well as the extent of the lesion on axial MRI images (i.e., involvement of the entire cross section of the cord vs. central cord involvement vs. tract-specific involvement) are important findings. If spinal cord compression is not present, additional workup includes a **brain MRI** to look for coexistent or prior lesions, which can inform diagnosis.

If MRI is unrevealing, or an inflammatory or infectious cause is suspected, a **lumbar puncture** is performed and samples sent for cell count and differential, total protein, glucose, gram stain, cultures, immunoglobulin (Ig) G index, oligoclonal bands, and cytology.

Initial **blood tests** are performed for the workup of suspected myelitis and include serum erythrocyte sedimentation rate, C-reactive protein, free T4, 25-OH vitamin D, thyroid stimulating hormone (TSH), syphilis serologies, HIV antibodies, methylmalonic acid, and serum vitamin B12 levels.

Depending on the clinical situation and initial findings, additional blood tests (serum aquaporin-4 antibody [also known as NMO antibody], antinuclear antibodies, rheumatoid factor, antiphospholipid antibodies, antineutrophil cytoplasmic antibodies, serum copper and ceruloplasmin, serum vitamin E), assessment of somatosensory-evoked potentials, electrodiagnostic testing or neuro-ophthalmologic consultation may be considered.

33. Describe the clinical picture of a patient presenting with transverse myelitis.
Transverse myelitis is a heterogeneous inflammatory disorder that results in acute or subacute spinal cord inflammation and causes motor, sensory, and autonomic dysfunction. Etiologies include infection, inflammation postvaccination, demyelinating diseases, paraneoplastic syndromes, drugs and toxins, connective tissue or granulomatous diseases, and vasculitis. The cause is unknown in up to one-third of cases. The initial presentation is variable and may manifest as a complete or incomplete spinal cord syndrome, which evolves over hours to days, but not generally beyond 4 weeks. Lower extremity weakness, sensory abnormalities, pain and bowel and bladder dysfunction are seen with acute complete transverse myelitis. A variety of incomplete cord syndromes or tract-specific dysfunction are noted with acute partial transverse myelitis. If the cervical cord is involved, upper extremity symptoms are also present. Lhermitte phenomenon (lightning-like electric shock pain radiating into the extremities and down the spine with neck flexion) may be elicited with cervical involvement. Initial treatment is with intravenous steroids, but response to this treatment is highly variable. Plasma exchange is performed for cases that fail to respond to initial steroid treatment. If an underlying disorder is identified, treatment is directed to address this condition.

34. What is multiple sclerosis?
Multiple sclerosis is a disorder in which the myelin sheath within the central nervous system is destroyed by a poorly understood inflammatory process. Genetic and environmental factors have been implicated as triggers for the disease. The disease is more common in women (2:1 ratio) and onset is most common between ages 18 and 50 years. Diagnosis is challenging and requires documentation of damage in at least two separate areas of the central nervous system and ruling out other possible diagnoses through careful medical history, neurologic examination, MRI, visual evoked potentials, and CSF analysis. Symptoms associated with multiple sclerosis are variable and wide-ranging. These may include numbness, fatigue, gait problems, ataxia, bowel/bladder dysfunction, cognitive dysfunction, and spasticity. Spinal lesions are typically limited in length to one or two spinal levels and demonstrate increased T2 signal intensity. No cure is available, but a variety of medications are used in an attempt to limit disease activity and progression.

35. What is amyotrophic lateral sclerosis?
Amyotrophic lateral sclerosis (ALS) is a progressive degenerative disorder of motor neurons in the spinal cord, brainstem, and motor cortex manifested clinically by muscular weakness, atrophy, and corticospinal tract involvement. Clinical presentation typically includes atrophic weakness of hands and forearms, spasticity of the legs, and generalized hyperreflexia. Other findings may include hand and finger stiffness, cramping, fasciculations, and atrophy and weakness of tongue, pharyngeal, and laryngeal muscles. There is no sensory loss. The disease is characterized by middle-life presentation and death is usually within 2–6 years. Diagnosis is made on the basis of history and neurologic examination and electromyography (EMG)/nerve conduction studies. Riluzole is a medication to treat ALS and may improve the neurologic function and survival. Its mechanism is not well understood. Physical therapy, occupational therapy, and speech therapy are necessary treatments. Symptomatic treatment for depression, secretion control, pain, fatigue, muscle spasms, and constipation are supportive measures.

The disease is also called *Lou Gehrig disease*, named for the New York Yankee's baseball player who died from this disorder.

36. **How is ALS differentiated from cervical myelopathy?**
Cervical myelopathy and myeloradiculopathy may mimic the symptoms of ALS. However, ALS should be differentiated by the lack of sensory abnormalities and the presence of facial symptoms.

37. **Describe the various types of vascular lesions of the spinal cord that may cause myelopathy.**
Cavernous malformations are vascular lesions with irregular sinusoidal vascular channels within the spinal cord, without intervening parenchyma. They typically are occult on angiography and diagnosed on MRI, due to the appearance of surrounding microhemorrhages. Patients may present with subacute symptoms similar to intramedullary spinal cord tumors, or may present with more acute neurologic deficits due to hemorrhages around the lesions. Surgical treatment is indicated for symptomatic lesions.

    Spinal dural arteriovenous fistulas (dAVFs) and **arteriovenous malformations (AVMs)** are vascular lesions with abnormal connections between arteries and veins. Spinal dAVFs are supplied by meningeal vessels, while spinal AVMs are supplied by branches that normally supply the neural tissue. Most patients present with stepwise neurologic decline manifested by progressive lower extremity weakness and sensory deficits. Treatment typically involves endovascular embolization, microsurgical resection, or a combination of both treatments.

    Spinal cord infarction may also present as an acute myelopathy and may result from mechanical disruption of spinal cord blood supply or as a consequence of a period of prolonged hypotension and cord hypoperfusion. The pattern of neurologic deficit depends on the site and extent of disruption of the blood supply to the cord and may present as an anterior, posterior, or complete cord syndrome.

38. **What is a spinal cord herniation and what commonly presenting symptoms are associated with this condition?**
Spinal cord herniation is a herniation of the spinal cord through a dural defect. Spinal cord herniation may be idiopathic, postsurgical, or posttraumatic, and most commonly occurs in the ventral thoracic spine. Patients typically present with progressive myelopathy or Brown-Séquard syndrome. Diagnosis is made with MRI and/or CT myelography. Treatment involves careful microdissection of the neural elements from the defect, often complicated by the location of the anterior spinal artery in the defect, followed by closure of the dural defect to prevent reherniation.

KEY POINTS

1. The differential diagnosis of a spinal cord tumor is determined by the anatomic compartment in which it occurs (i.e., extradural, intradural-extramedullary, or intramedullary).
2. Syringohydromyelia is an abnormal fluid cavity within the spinal cord, which may cause progressive neurologic dysfunction.
3. Spinal dysraphism is broadly classified into two forms: spina bifida occulta and spina bifida cystica.
4. Myelomeningocele is the most common major spinal birth defect and results from disruption of the process of neurulation between days 24 and 28 following conception.

Websites
1. Chiari malformation: http://emedicine.medscape.com/article/1483583-overview
2. Intramedullary spinal cord tumors: http://emedicine.medscape.com/article/251133-overview
3. Neural tube defects: http://emedicine.medscape.com/article/1177162-overview
4. Spinal cord disorders: http://neuromuscular.wustl.edu/spinal.html
5. Spinal dysraphism and myelomeningocele: http://emedicine.medscape.com/article/413899-overview
6. Syringomyelia: http://emedicine.medscape.com/article/1151685-overview
7. Maternal-fetal surgery for myelomeningocele: https://www.acog.org/Clinical-Guidance-and-Publications/Committee-Opinions/Committee-on-Obstetric-Practice/Maternal-Fetal-Surgery-for-Myelomeningocele

BIBLIOGRAPHY
1. Abd-El-Barr MM, Huang KT, Scott RM, et al. Congenital anomalies of the spinal cord. In: Garfin SR, Eismont FJ, Bell GR, editors. Rothman-Simeone and Herkowitz The Spine. 7th ed. Philadelphia, PA: Saunders; 2018, pp. 641–659.
2. Aydin AL, Sasani M, Erhan B, et al. Idiopathic spinal cord herniation at two separate zones of the thoracic spine: The first reported case and literature review. *Spine J* 2011;11:9–14.

3. Gebauer GP, Farjoodi P, Sciubba DM, et al. Magnetic resonance imaging of spine tumors: Classification, differential diagnosis, and spectrum of disease. *J Bone Joint Surg* 2008;90:146–162.

4. Minagar A, Rabinstein A, editors. Spinal cord diseases. *Neurol Clin* 2013;31:1–341.

5. Rangel-Castilla L, Russin JJ, Zaidi HA, et al. Contemporary management of spinal AVFs and AVMs: Lessons learned from 110 cases. *Neurosurg Focus* 2014;37:14.

6. Raudenbush BL, Selioutski O, Samkoff L, et al. Medical myelopathies. In: Garfin SR, Eismont FJ, Bell GR, et al., editors. Rothman-Simeone and Herkowitz The Spine. 7th ed. Philadelphia, PA: Saunders; 2018, pp. 689–703.

7. Samartzis D, Gillis CC, Shih P, et al. Intramedullary spinal cord tumors: Part I—Epidemiology, pathophysiology, and diagnosis. *Glob Spine J* 2015;5:425–435.

8. Samartzis D, Gillis CC, Shih P, et al. Intramedullary spinal cord tumors: Part II—Management options and outcomes. *Glob Spine J* 2016;6:176–185.

9. Shah AH, Johnson JN, Green BA. Intradural tumors. In: Garfin SR, Eismont FJ, Bell GR, et al., editors. Rothman-Simeone and Herkowitz The Spine. 7th ed. Philadelphia, PA: Saunders; 2018, pp. 1627–1640.

CHAPTER 62

PRIMARY SPINE TUMORS

Benjamin D. Elder, MD, PhD and Vincent J. Devlin, MD

1. **What types of tumors arise in the spine?**
   Primary tumors and secondary tumors.

2. **What is the difference between primary and secondary tumors of the spine?**
   Primary tumors of the spine arise de novo in the osseous, cartilaginous, neural, or ligamentous structures of the spine. They may be classified as extradural or intradural. **Secondary tumors** are either metastatic to the spine from distant origins or grow into the spine from adjacent structures, such as a Pancoast tumor from the upper lobe of the lung. Primary spine tumors are extremely rare. Metastatic lesions involving the spine are the most common type of spinal tumor and account for over 90% of all spinal tumors. To put these numbers in perspective, estimates are that one person per million has a primary spine tumor compared with 85 persons per million with a metastatic spinal tumor. Primary bone tumors of the spine are the emphasis of this chapter.

3. **How are primary tumors of the spine classified?**
   Multiple classifications have been proposed for primary spine tumors. One method for classifying primary spine tumors is **based on histology**. The World Health Organization (WHO) developed a classification of bone tumors based on histomorphologic features, which was initially published in 1972 and has been updated periodically (Table 62.1).
   Benign tumors are nonaggressive tumors that may be asymptomatic or may cause pain, local symptoms, or local tissue destruction. However, these lesions do not aggressively invade adjacent structures, have limited ability to recur, and do not metastasize (e.g., osteoid osteoma).
   Intermediate tumors may be categorized as *locally aggressive* (e.g., osteoblastoma, grade 1 chondrosarcoma) or *locally aggressive with the capacity for distant metastases*, most commonly to the lung (e.g., giant cell tumor [GCT] of bone).
   Malignant tumors of bone (also termed *bone sarcomas*) cause local destruction, recur locally, and have the capacity to metastasize to other organs. These are life-threatening tumors by their fundamental nature (e.g., osteosarcoma, Ewing sarcoma).
   Other categories of bone tumors in the WHO classification include *tumors of undefined neoplastic nature* and *miscellaneous tumors*.

4. **Is there a relationship between age, location, and whether a spine tumor is benign or malignant?**
   Yes. There is a relationship between **age at diagnosis** and whether a tumor is benign. In patients younger than 18 years, 68% of all tumors are benign. If age at presentation is older than 18 years, more than 80% of all tumors are malignant. There is also a relationship between **tumor location** and whether a tumor is benign. Benign lesions tend to occur more frequently in the posterior elements (e.g., osteoblastoma, osteoid osteoma), whereas malignant lesions tend to involve the vertebral body.

5. **What are some common spine tumor diagnoses according to patient age?**
   - **10–30 years:** Langerhans cell histiocytosis (eosinophilic granuloma), osteoid osteoma, osteoblastoma, osteochondroma, GCT, aneurysmal bone cyst (ABC), osteosarcoma, Ewing sarcoma
   - **30–50 years:** chordoma, chondrosarcoma, hemangioma
   - **Older than 50 years:** metastatic tumors, myeloma, lymphoma

6. **What are some common spine tumor diagnoses according to location?**
   - **Posterior spinal elements:** osteoid osteoma, osteoblastoma, osteochondroma, ABC
   - **Vertebral body:** chordoma, GCT, myeloma, hemangioma, Langerhans cell histiocytosis (eosinophilic granuloma), ABC, Ewing sarcoma, metastatic disease
   - **Involvement of both anterior and posterior spinal elements:** osteosarcoma, chondrosarcoma, osteoblastoma, ABC, myeloma
   - **Involvement of adjacent vertebra:** ABC, chondrosarcoma, chordoma, GCT, myeloma, metastatic disease
   - **Involvement of multiple vertebra:** metastatic disease, Langerhans cell histiocytosis, myeloma

Table 62.1 World Health Organization Classification of Bone Tumors and Tumor-Like Lesions.

I. Osteogenic Tumors

1. **Benign**
   - Osteoma
   - Osteoid osteoma
2. **Intermediate (locally aggressive)**
   - Osteoblastoma
3. **Malignant (osteosarcoma)**
   - Low-grade central osteosarcoma
   - Conventional osteosarcoma (chondroblastic, fibroblastic, osteoblastic, and secondary types)
   - Telangiectatic osteosarcoma
   - Small cell osteosarcoma
   - Parosteal osteosarcoma
   - Periosteal osteosarcoma
   - High-grade surface osteosarcoma

II. Chondrogenic Tumors

1. **Benign**
   - Osteochondroma
   - Chondroma (enchondroma, periosteal chondroma)
   - Osteochondromyxoma
   - Subungual exostosis
   - Bizarre parosteal osteochondromatous proliferation
   - Synovial chondromatosis
2. **Intermediate (locally aggressive)**
   - Chondromyxoid fibroma
   - Atypical cartilaginous tumor/chondrosarcoma grade I
3. **Intermediate (rarely metastasizing)**
   - Chondroblastoma
4. **Malignant**
   - Chondrosarcoma grade II, grade III
   - Dedifferentiated chondrosarcoma
   - Mesenchymal chondrosarcoma
   - Clear-cell chondrosarcoma

III. Fibrogenic Tumors

1. **Intermediate (locally aggressive)**
   - Desmoplastic fibroma of bone
2. **Malignant**
   - Fibrosarcoma of bone

IV. Fibrohistiocytic Tumors

- Benign fibrous histiocytoma/nonossifying fibroma

V. Hematopoietic Neoplasms

1. **Malignant**
   - Plasma cell myeloma
   - Solitary plasmacytoma of bone
   - Primary non-Hodgkin lymphoma of bone

VI. Osteoclastic Giant Cell Rich Tumor

1. **Benign**
   - Giant-cell lesion of the small bones
2. **Intermediate (locally aggressive, rarely metastasizing)**
   - Giant-cell tumor of bone
3. **Malignant**
   - Malignancy in giant-cell tumor of bone

VII. Notochordal Tumors

1. **Benign**
   - Benign notochordal tumor
2. **Malignant**
   - Chordoma, NOS
   - Chondroid chordoma
   - Dedifferentiated chordoma

VIII. Vascular tumors

1. **Benign**
   - Hemangioma
2. **Intermediate (locally aggressive, rarely metastasizing)**
   - Epithelioid hemangioma
3. **Malignant**
   - Epithelioid hemangioendothelioma
   - Angiosarcoma

IX. Myogenic Tumors

1. **Malignant**
   - Leiomyosarcoma of bone

X. Lipogenic Tumors

1. **Benign**
   - Lipoma of bone
2. **Malignant**
   - Liposarcoma of bone

XI. Tumors of Undefined Neoplastic Nature

1. **Benign**
   - Simple bone cyst
   - Fibrous dysplasia
   - Osteofibrous dysplasia
   - Chondromesenchymal hamartoma
   - Rosai-Dorfman disease
2. **Intermediate (locally aggressive)**
   - Aneurysmal bone cyst
   - Langerhans cell histiocytosis (monostotic, polyostotic)
   - Erdheim-Chester disease

XII. Miscellaneous Tumors

- Ewing sarcoma
- Adamantinoma
- Undifferentiated high-grade pleomorphic sarcoma of bone

NOS; Not otherwise specified

Data from Schajowicz F, McDonald DJ. Classification of tumors and tumor lesions of the spine. Spine State Arts Rev 1998;10:1–11; Fletcher CDM, Bridge JA, Hogendoorn P, et al. WHO Classification of tumours of soft tissue and bone. 4th ed. Lyon Cedex: International Agency for Research on Cancer; 2013, pp. 240–242.

7. **What is the most common clinical presentation of a primary spinal tumor?**

Pain is the most common presenting symptom. Pain is frequently described as persistent, progressive, and not typically associated with activity. Pain at night is a characteristic symptom. Subjective weakness, radiculopathy, objective neurologic deficit, and bladder or bowel dysfunction may develop over time. Occasionally patients may present with a palpable mass, pathologic fracture or a painful spinal deformity. Pelvic girdle malignancies, including chordoma, osteosarcoma, chondrosarcoma, and malignant fibrous histiocytomas, may present with back pain and sciatica. Always remember to evaluate the pelvis if the spine appears normal or the degenerative lesion does not fit the patient's degree of pain or neurologic involvement.

8. **What are the initial steps in the evaluation of a patient with a newly diagnosed bone lesion involving the spinal column?**

New bone lesions identified on plain radiographs have a long list of differential diagnoses, ranging in severity from developmental abnormalities or benign lesions to malignancies. The patient should be evaluated with a detailed and comprehensive medical history, family history, review of systems, physical examination, and radiographs. Patient history should include details regarding pain (if present), including its intensity, duration, and pattern. The examiner should inquire about any changes in bowel or bladder control, as well as any complaints of extremity pain, weakness, sensory changes, and gait or balance problems. Family history should address whether there is any history of benign or malignant tumors, common cancer risk factors, or conditions that alter bone development and/or metabolism. Physical examination should include a general survey and detailed neurologic examination. Initial lab tests to consider include a complete blood count (CBC), erythrocyte sedimentation rate (ESR), and C-reactive protein (CRP) to rule out infection.

Plain radiographs are the recommended initial imaging modality. Review of plain radiographs by a fellowship-trained musculoskeletal radiologist can be used to initially triage lesions as nonaggressive/indolent versus other lesions that require additional imaging studies and referral. For example, for an asymptomatic patient diagnosed with a lesion that has all of the imaging characteristics of a benign lesion (e.g., vertebral hemangioma), observation is appropriate and no further workup or treatment is indicated. Lesions that are symptomatic or lesions with aggressive features on initial radiographs require further evaluation. Magnetic resonance imaging (MRI) is indicated if diagnostic uncertainty remains. Computed tomography (CT) may be considered if MRI is contraindicated.

If the patient with a painful bone lesion is less than 40 years old and initial lab tests and spinal MRI are not consistent with spinal infection, referral to an orthopedic oncologist to rule out a primary bone tumor is recommended.

If the patient is greater than age 40 years, metastatic carcinoma involving the spine is the most likely diagnosis. Workup for metastatic disease includes lab tests (CBC, ESR, CRP, comprehensive metabolic panel [CMP], serum protein electrophoresis [SPEP]), urine protein electrophoresis [UPEP], prostate-specific antigen [PSA] for males), CT of the chest, abdomen, and pelvis with contrast, technetium-99m (^{99}Tc) bone scan, mammogram in females, and CT-guided biopsy of the spinal lesion.

9. **What workup is required to stage a primary malignant tumor of the axial skeleton?**

A **comprehensive imaging evaluation** and a **biopsy of the lesion** are required. In addition to plain radiography and MRI of the spine, additional imaging modalities that may be considered include CT (spine, chest), ^{99}Tc bone scanning, 18-fluorine fluorodeoxyglucose (^{18}F-FDG), positron emission tomography (PET), and angiography.

Spine CT provides information regarding the extent of bone destruction and osseous architecture. Chest CT is used to assess for lung metastases. The presence of extrapulmonary bone metastases may be assessed with a whole body ^{99}Tc bone scan. Alternative options for whole body screening include ^{18}F-FDG, PET/CT, and whole body MRI. Angiography is useful in specific situations, for example, to identify the anatomy and vascular supply to a tumor as an aid to surgical planning. In addition, preoperative angiography and embolization are used to reduce intraoperative blood loss and blood transfusion volume during the surgical treatment of highly vascular tumors such as GCT, ABC, osteoblastoma, chondroblastoma, and chondrosarcoma.

Biopsy is required to reach a histologic diagnosis and assess the tumor grade. Options for biopsy included CT-guided fine-needle aspiration, CT-guided core needle biopsy, incisional biopsy, and excisional biopsy. CT-guided fine-needle or core-needle biopsy are most commonly utilized for spinal lesions. The advantages of core-needle biopsy versus fine-needle biopsy include a larger sample of tissue and preservation of tissue architecture. Oncologic principles require that the biopsy technique minimize local contamination and the biopsy tract should be marked to allow for later excision if a definitive surgical resection is required.

10. **Explain why oncologic staging is performed for a primary spine tumor and what staging systems are used?**

An oncologic staging system creates a framework to guide treatment decision making and provides insight into prognosis, including the risks for tumor recurrence and metastasis. It integrates the data obtained from the patient history, physical examination, imaging studies, and biopsy and considers the histopathologic diagnosis and grade, local extent of the lesion, and whether metastases are present. Two staging systems are used for bone sarcomas, the Musculoskeletal Tumor Society Staging System for Bone Sarcomas (MSTS), also known as the Enneking Classification, and the American Joint Committee on Cancer (AJCC) staging system.

11. **What factors are considered in the AJCC staging system?**
The AJCC uses a TGNM system in which T (tumor) refers to the size of the tumor, G (grade) refers to the histo-pathologic grade, N (nodes) refers to the presence of lymph node involvement, and M (metastasis) refers to the spread of tumor to distant organs. While originally proposed for staging soft tissue sarcomas, the AJCC has been updated to address staging of bone sarcomas. In the eighth edition of the AJCC Cancer Staging Manual, defini-tions for primary bone tumors of the spine and pelvis were introduced as part of the T component of the staging system and include designation of tumor extent as: T1= one to two adjacent vertebral segments, T2 = three adjacent segments, T3 = four or more adjacent vertebral segments or nonadjacent segments, and T4 = extension into the spinal canal (T4a) or great vessels (T4b).

12. **Explain how the MSTS classifies benign and malignant primary bone tumors.**
MSTS (Enneking) staging combines three factors: surgical grade (G), site (T), and the presence/absence of metastases (M).
All benign tumors are surgical grade G_0 and are divided into three stages using Arabic numbers:
- **Stage 1**: Latent lesions, which are generally asymptomatic and surrounded by a well-defined margin
- **Stage 2**: Active lesions, which grow slowly and are bordered by a thin capsule
- **Stage 3**: Aggressive lesions, which grow rapidly to invade surrounding structures
Malignant tumors are also divided into three stages using Roman numerals. All low-grade malignancies (based on histology, imaging and clinical features) are stage I; all high-grade malignancies are stage II, and any malignancy with evidence of metastatic disease is stage III. Malignant tumors are further subdivided into A and B subgroups depending on whether the tumor is intracompartmental (T1) or extends beyond the compartment of origin (T2).
- **Stage IA:** G1—Low grade; T1—intracompartmental; M0—no metastasis
- **Stage IB:** G1—Low grade; T2—extracompartmental; M0—no metastasis
- **Stage IIA:** G2—High grade; T1—intracompartmental; M0—no metastasis
- **Stage IIB:** G2—High grade; T2—intracompartmental; M0—no metastasis
- **Stage III:** Any grade (G); any (T); M1—presence of regional or distant metastases

13. **How does oncologic staging guide surgical tumor treatment?**
The oncologic stage of a tumor determines the type of spine procedure that is indicated and determines the surgical margin required to adequately treat the tumor. The surgical margin is defined in relation to the reactive zone at the periphery of the tumor, also termed the "pseudocapsule" or "capsule." The **four types of surgical margins** are:
- **Intralesional:** The plane of dissection is within the lesion (intracapsular) and may leave tumor at the margin of the lesion or inside the tumor capsule.
- **Marginal:** The plane of dissection is within the reactive zone surrounding the tumor, and may leave satellite tumor at the periphery of the lesion and beyond the reactive zone. This type of margin is not adequate for the treatment of intermediate or malignant tumors.
- **Wide:** The plane of dissection is through normal tissue beyond the reactive zone surrounding the tumor. How-ever, "skip" lesions may persist beyond a wide surgical margin and potentially leave microscopic tumor behind. This type of resection is often challenging for spinal tumors due to the proximity of the neural elements, which may be adherent or encased by tumor.
- **Radical:** The plane of dissection includes removal of the tumor and the entire compartment of tumor origin. A radical margin cannot be achieved for spine tumors even if the spinal cord is sectioned above and below the lesion because the epidural space forms a continuous compartment from the skull to the sacrum
In practice, surgical procedures performed for primary spine tumors can be considered as either intralesional/curettage or *en bloc* excision.
- **Curettage** refers to the piecemeal removal of tumor and is always an intracapsular (intralesional) procedure. This type of procedure is appropriate for stage 1 and 2 benign tumors.
- ***En bloc* excision** refers to an attempt to remove the entire tumor in a single piece, together with a surround-ing cuff of normal healthy tissue. The surgical specimen requires gross and microscopic assessment to deter-mine whether the surgical margin achieved was intralesional, marginal, or wide. This type of procedure is appropriate for some stage 3 benign aggressive tumors and stage I and II malignant tumors.

14. **What is the WBB (Weinstein, Boriani, Biagini) surgical staging system for spinal tumors?**
The WBB surgical staging system for spinal tumors correlates principles of oncologic surgery with the unique anatomy of the spine and provides a guide for treatment. The vertebra is divided into 12 radiating **zones** in clock-wise order. Note that zones 4 and 9 define the left and right pedicles, respectively (Fig. 62.1).
The spine is also divided into five **tissue layers** extending from the paravertebral extraosseous area to the dura:
A. Extraosseous soft tissue
B. Intraosseous superficial
C. Intraosseous deep
D. Extraosseous extradural
E. Extraosseous intradural

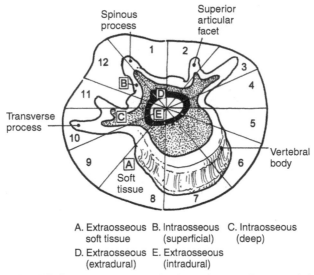

A. Extraosseous   B. Intraosseous   C. Intraosseous
   soft tissue   (superficial)   (deep)

D. Extraosseous   E. Extraosseous
   (extradural)   (intradural)

Fig. 62.1 WBB (Weinstein, Boriani, Biagini) surgical staging system for primary spine tumors. Tumor extent is described by dividing the involved vertebra into 12 sections in a clockface arrangement. Five tissue layers are defined, moving from the superficial paraspinal soft tissue *(layer A)* to the dural compartment *(layer E)*. The longitudinal extent of the tumor is recorded according to the levels involved. (From Hart RA, Weinstein JN. Primary benign and malignant musculoskeletal tumors of the spine. Semin Spine Surg 1995; 7:288–303, with permission.)

In the cervical region, an additional layer "F" is used to identify involvement of the vertebral artery/intervertebral foramen by tumor.

Based on the WBB surgical staging system, various types of *en bloc* tumor excisions are defined including resection of the posterior arch, vertebrectomy, and sagittal resection which may be performed using a range of surgical strategies.

15. **When is resection of the posterior arch indicated according to the WBB staging system?**
   When a tumor is localized between zones 3 and 10, an *en bloc* excision can be achieved from a posterior approach (Fig. 62.2). A laminectomy is performed to expose the dural sac at the levels above and below the tumor. The pedicles are sectioned at the level of the tumor and the posterior arch is removed *en bloc*. The stability of the spine is restored with posterior spinal instrumentation and fusion. Note that if tumor extends into tissue layer D it may not be possible to obtain a negative margin unless a layer of healthy tissue is present between the tumor and the dura.

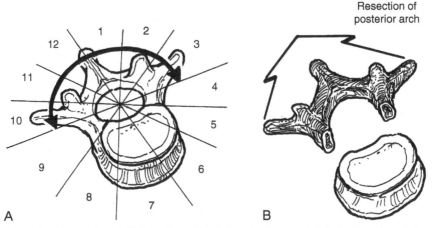

Fig. 62.2 Resection of the posterior arch. (A) The *en bloc* excision of a tumor to achieve an oncologically appropriate surgical margin is possible if tumor extent is limited between zones 3 and 10. The pedicles must be uninvolved by tumor. (B) Surgery is performed through a posterior approach.

16. When is a vertebrectomy indicated according to the WBB staging system?

Marginal or wide *en bloc* excision of the vertebral body can be performed if the tumor is confined to zones 4–8 or 5–9 (Fig. 62.3). In this situation, the tumor is located centrally and at least one pedicle is free from tumor. The posterior elements are removed first without entering the tumor. Subsequently the vertebral body is removed. The decision whether to remove the vertebral body from the posterior surgical approach or via a separate anterior approach depends on several factors, including the location of the spinal level(s) involved by the tumor and the anterior extent of the tumor in relation to tissue layer A. Spinal reconstruction following tumor excision consists of placement of an anterior column allograft or structural spacer (fusion cage) combined with posterior spinal instrumentation. If the vertebral body is removed from an anterior surgical approach, anterior spinal instrumentation may be used to provide additional stabilization.

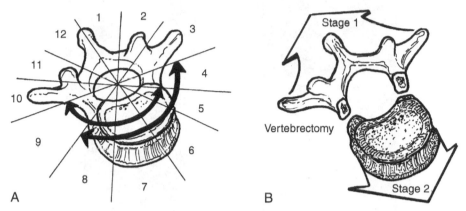

Fig. 62.3 Vertebrectomy. (A) *En bloc* excision with oncologically appropriate margin for a tumor located in the vertebral body is possible if at least one pedicle is uninvolved by tumor. (B) A posterior approach is performed to remove the posterior spinal structures (spinous process, lamina, pedicles), transect the posterior longitudinal ligament, and separate the anterior surface of the dura from the posterior vertebral margin. An anterior approach is essential to maintain an oncologically appropriate margin if the tumor extends outside the vertebra.

17. When is a sagittal resection indicated according to the WBB staging system?

Sagittal resection to achieve a marginal or wide *en bloc* excision is indicated if the tumor is confined to zones 3–5 or 8–11 (Fig. 62.4). In this situation, the tumor is located eccentrically in the vertebral body, pedicle, or transverse process. As in vertebrectomy, the first step is removal of the uninvolved posterior spinal structures. Then, through a separate surgical approach, the vertebra is cut with an osteotome, Tomita saw, or ultrasonic bone cutting device remote from the tumor to permit *en bloc* excision. Spinal reconstruction is performed in a similar fashion to reconstruction following vertebrectomy (Fig. 62.5).

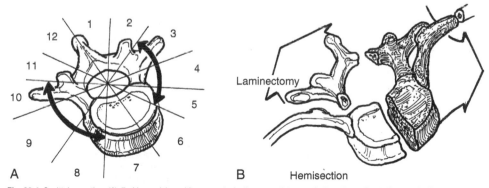

Fig. 62.4 Sagittal resection. (A) *En bloc* excision with an oncologically appropriate margin for a tumor located eccentrically in the body, pedicle, or transverse process is possible when the tumor is confined to zones 3–5 or 8–11. (B) A posterior approach is performed to excise the posterior spinal structures uninvolved by tumor. A combined posterior and anterior approach is required to complete the *en bloc* excision safely with an oncologically appropriate margin.

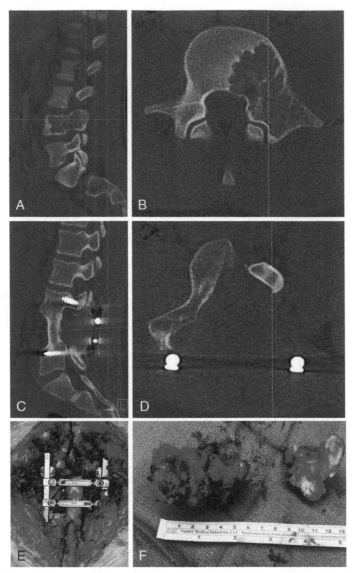

Fig. 62.5 Case of L4 osteoblastoma resected in an *en bloc* fashion. (A) Sagittal and (B) axial computed tomography (CT) images demonstrating lesion involving the left L4 transverse process, superior articulating process, pedicle, and hemivertebrae. (C) Sagittal and (D) axial CT images demonstrating sagittal cut through the L4 vertebrae leaving the right pedicle intact, performed through an all posterior approach with preservation of the bilateral L4 nerve roots, followed by reconstruction with tricortical iliac crest autograft and pedicle screw fixation. (E) Intraoperative image demonstrating reconstruction and preservation of the L4 nerve roots. (F) Gross pathology image showing the hemivertebrae specimen *(left)* and posterior element specimen *(right)*.

18. **Does the presence of neurologic structures within or adjacent to a primary malignant tumor influence the choice of surgical treatment?**
    Yes and no. Sacrifice of the neural elements that may be required for *en bloc* resection can result in significant neurologic deficits and should be discussed extensively with the patient preoperatively. However, the treatment associated with the best chance of survival is complete resection of an aggressive spinal sarcoma according to oncologic surgical principles, even if neural elements that course through the tumor must be sacrificed. An alternative option is to plan a limited tumor violation (planned limited tumor transgression) to protect adjacent neural and vascular structures, which is associated with a lower rate of local recurrence compared with intralesional excision.

19. **How is the appropriate surgical approach selected for treatment of sacral tumors?**
The appropriate surgical approach for treatment of sacral tumors depends on the extent of sacral involvement. Tumors that involve only the distal portion of the sacrum (S3 and below) can be treated with a single procedure from a posterior surgical approach. Tumors that involve the S1 and S2 segments or those that involve the entire sacrum generally require a combined anterior and posterior resection, though recent case series have demonstrated the feasibility of posterior-only techniques for high and total sacral amputations (Fig. 62.6).

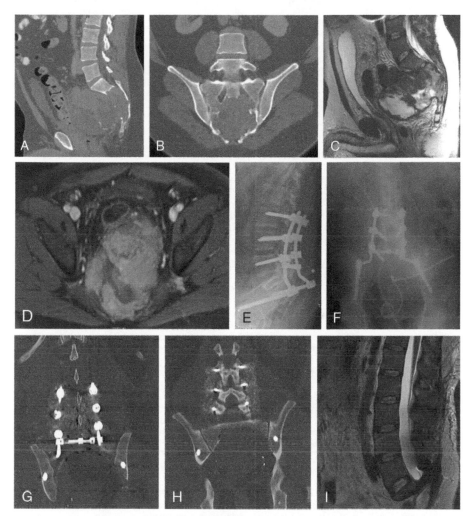

Fig. 62.6 Case of giant cell tumor involving the sacrum. (A) Preoperative sagittal and (B) coronal nonenhanced computed tomography (CT) scans demonstrating 13.3 × 8.5 cm osteolytic S2–S4 sacral mass with invasion of the sacral foramina and anterior displacement of the sigmoid colon and bladder. (C) Preoperative sagittal T2-weighted magnetic resonance imaging (MRI) demonstrating heterogeneous-appearing mass arising from the sacrum. (D) Preoperative axial gadolinium-enhanced T1-weighted MRI demonstrating sacral mass extending into the pelvis and abutting the rectum. Postoperative (E) lateral and (F) anteroposterior radiographs demonstrating L3-pelvis instrumentation. Postoperative coronal nonenhanced CT scan demonstrating (G) instrumentation and (H) extent of *en bloc* resection. (I) Postoperative sagittal T2-weighted MRI demonstrating extent of tumor resection. (Reproduced, with permission, from Elder BD, Sankey EW, Goodwin CR, et al. Surgical outcomes in patients with high spinal instability neoplasm score secondary to spinal giant cell tumors. Global Spine J 2016;6:21–28.)

20. **What is the relationship between the level of nerve root preservation and continence following sacral resection procedures?**
Sacral resection procedures have been classified (1) by the level at which sacral roots are preserved as: low sacrectomy (S3 roots preserved bilaterally), middle sacrectomy (S2 roots preserved bilaterally), high sacrectomy (S1 root preserved unilaterally), and total sacrectomy (no sacral roots preserved). Bilateral preservation of the

S3 roots is associated with normal bladder, bowel, and sexual function. Preservation of one S3 root generally results in near normal bowel and bladder function. Bilateral preservation of S2 roots is required for satisfactory bladder, bowel, and sexual function. In patients with unilateral preservation of an S2 root, functional urinary and fecal continence is often achievable. In patients treated with high sacrectomy or total sacrectomy, unilateral/bilateral sacrifice of S1 roots and bilateral sacrifice of the S2, S3, and S4 roots results in loss of bowel, bladder, and sexual function and variable ankle plantarflexion weakness. These patients will require self-catheterization and a bowel regimen (constipating diet and nightly suppositories), and some may require external support for ambulation.

For unilateral sacral tumors appropriate for treatment with hemisacrectomy, if all sacral nerve roots can be preserved unilaterally, the patient will have near normal bowel, bladder, and sexual function.

21. What vascular structures require control during the anterior approach for a complete sacrectomy?
The posterior divisions of the internal iliac vessels and the middle and lateral sacral vessels should be ligated during the anterior preparation for a complete sacrectomy. As the posterior resection is completed, the pelvis will hinge on the symphysis pubis. If the internal iliac vessels are not controlled, a tear of these vessels may lead to catastrophic bleeding.

22. In a complete sacrectomy, what other considerations must be taken into account during the anterior resection?
The patient is left incontinent by such a resection. Therefore, a diverting colostomy and ureterostomy should be performed during the anterior preparation. Staging the anterior preparation separately from the posterior resection should be considered. A myocutaneous vascularized flap is frequently used for posterior wound coverage. Success of this complex surgical procedure requires the support of a multidisciplinary surgical team.

23. How does one stabilize the spine to the pelvis after sacral resection?
With preservation of the sacroiliac (SI) joints in mid and low sacral amputations, no reconstruction is typically required. With high and total sacral amputations, spinopelvic fixation is required with iliac fixation or S2 alar-iliac fixation distally, to anchor the lumbar spine to the pelvis. In some cases that require partial resection of the ilium, more extensive reconstruction with a trans-iliac strut or bar is required.

24. Name the most frequently encountered nonmalignant primary spine tumors and describe key characteristics and treatments for each tumor type.
Nonmalignant primary spine tumors include hemangioma, osteoid osteoma, osteoblastoma, Langerhans cell histiocytosis, osteochondroma, GCT, and ABC. Benign tumors are staged according to the MSTS system as S1 (latent, inactive), S2 (active, slow growing), and S3 (aggressive, rapid growth). S1 lesions are observed unless there is an indication for decompression and/or stabilization. S2 lesions may be treated with intralesional resection or *en bloc* resection. S3 lesions are treated with *en bloc* resection when feasible. Additional treatments, depending on tumor type include medication, selective arterial embolization, radiofrequency (RF) ablation, and rarely radiation therapy.
Hemangioma
- This vascular tumor is the most common benign primary spine tumor.
- Most hemangiomas are asymptomatic and usually located within the vertebral body.
- Symptoms occur in less than 1% of patients secondary to bone erosion, bone expansion, or pathologic fracture.
- Radiographs demonstrate coarse vertical striations in the vertebral body, axial CT demonstrates a punctate appearance, MRI shows increased signal on T1 and T2 images.
- Treatment options for symptomatic lesions includes vertebroplasty, kyphoplasty, radiotherapy, alcohol injection, embolization, and surgery (Fig. 62.7).
Osteoid osteoma
- Benign bone-forming tumor <2 cm, common in posterior spinal elements, age <30 years
- Symptoms include severe night pain (relieved with nonsteroidal antiinflammatory drugs [NSAIDs]) and scoliosis
- Appear as radiolucent lesions with peripheral sclerosis and central nidus
- Treatment options include NSAIDs, surgical excision, or RF ablation (Fig. 62.8).
Osteoblastoma
- Intermediate bone-forming tumor >2 cm in posterior spinal elements, age <30 years
- Symptoms include dull, aching pain, little relief with NSAIDs, not worse at night
- Imaging shows a bone-forming destructive lesion often with cortical breach
- *En bloc* resection is preferred as intralesional resection is associated with recurrence
Langerhans cell histiocytosis
- Most common form of Langerhans cell histiocytosis is eosinophilic granuloma
- Lytic vertebral lesion may lead to vertebral flattening (vertebra plana), age <20 years
- Often a self-limiting condition with spontaneous vertebral height reconstitution
- Biopsy if diagnosis unclear or surgery indicated for decompression or stabilization (Fig. 62.9)
Osteochondroma
- Presents in third and fourth decades as benign cartilage-capped bony projection on the surface of a bone with a marrow cavity that is continuous with the underlying bone.

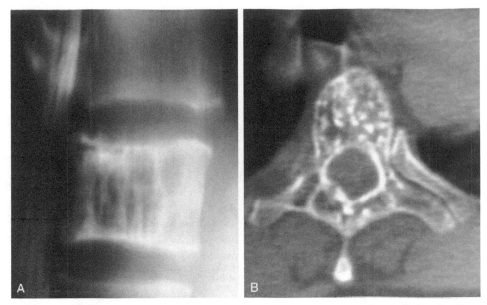

Fig. 62.7 Hemangioma. (A) Lateral computed tomography (CT) view shows corduroy-like appearance of vertebral body produced by thickening of vertical bone trabeculae traversing hemangioma. (B) Axial CT view. (From Czerniak B. Vascular Lesions. In: Czerniak B, editor. Dorfman and Czerniak's Bone Tumors. 2nd ed. Philadelphia, PA: Saunders; 2016, Fig. 13.3.)

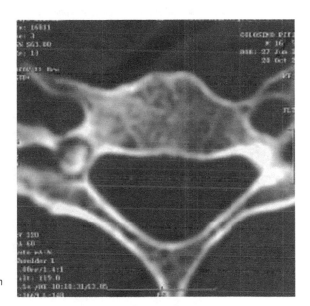

Fig. 62.8 Osteoid osteoma of the cervical spine. Axial computed tomography. (From Gasbarrini A, Cappuccio M, Donthineni R, et al. Management of benign tumors of the mobile spine. Orthop Clin N Am 2009; 40:9–19, Fig. 3.)

- Occur in posterior spinal elements; solitary or multiple lesions may be present
- Treatment is observation for incidental lesions without pain or size increase
- If surgery is performed, complete excision *(en bloc)* is preferred due to potential for tumor recurrence.

Giant cell tumor (GCT)
- Presents in third and fourth decades and is most commonly located in sacrum or vertebral body
- Expansile lytic lesion composed of osteoclastic giant cells mixed with spindle cells
- Tumor is locally aggressive and may metastasize to the lungs
- If surgery is planned, preoperative embolization recommended due to tumor vascularity

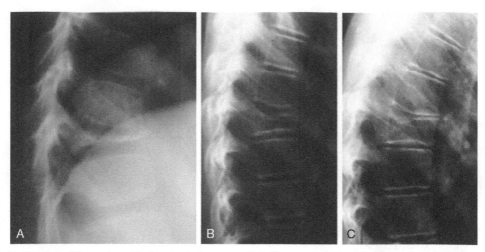

Fig. 62.9 Eosinophilic granuloma of the thoracic spine in a young patient with progressive healing and restoration of vertebral height. (A) Vertebra plana at onset, (B) after 6 months, and (C) after 12 months. (From Gasbarrini A, Cappuccio M, Donthineni R, et al. Management of benign tumors of the mobile spine. Orthop Clin N Am 2009;40:9–19, Fig. 1.)

- Treatment of choice is *en bloc* resection with wide margin. When this is not feasible consider adjuvant treatment (phenol, polymethylmethacrylate [PMMA]) to extend the surgical margin following intralesional resection.
- Denosumab, a human monoclonal antibody, has demonstrated effectiveness in decreasing tumor size.

Aneurysmal bone cyst (ABC)

- Presents in second and third decades as a primary tumor, but may also occur as secondary lesion associated with another tumor (e.g., GCT, osteogenic sarcoma).
- Locally aggressive expansile lytic lesion composed of multiloculated blood-filled cystic spaces surrounded by thin layers of reactive cortical bone.
- Most commonly involve the posterior elements but may extend into the vertebral body.
- Treatment options include intralesional resection, cryotherapy, radiotherapy, embolization, and *en bloc* resection.
- Selective arterial embolization is associated with similar recurrence rates as surgery (Fig. 62.10).

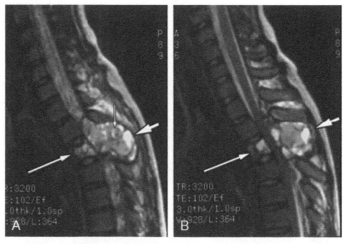

Fig. 62.10 Aneurysmal bone cyst involving T3 vertebra. (A) T2-weighted left parasagittal magnetic resonance image. (B) Midsagittal image. The aneurysmal bone cyst predominantly involves the posterior vertebral arch of T3 *(short arrow)*. The lesion contains multiple ovoid areas of heterogeneous signal intensity that has replaced the left posterior vertebral arch and left posterolateral aspect of the vertebral body *(long arrow)*. At least one loculation *(thin arrow in image A)* contains a fluid/fluid level, which is vertical on the image with the patient supine. The lesion extends into the epidural space causing cord compression. The lesion was largely cystic in nature at surgery, containing multiple loculated cystic collections of bloody liquid. (From Czervionke LF. Aneurysmal bone cyst. In: Czervionke LF, Fenton DS. Imaging Painful Spine Disorders. Philadelphia, PA; Saunders; 2011, Fig. 7.1.)

25. Name the most frequently encountered malignant primary spine tumors and describe key characteristics and treatment options for each tumor type.

Malignant primary spine tumors include myeloma, chordoma, osteosarcoma, Ewing sarcoma, and chondrosarcoma. Myeloma is the most common primary spine neoplasm and chordoma is the second most common primary spine neoplasm. Ewing sarcoma is the most common primary malignant tumor of the spinal column in children. Osteosarcoma is the most common primary sarcoma of bone.

Myeloma
- Multiple myeloma is a multifocal plasma cell malignancy in adults (sixth and seventh decades).
- Workup includes CBC, serum and/or urine immunoglobulin studies, bone marrow biopsy, and imaging (skeletal survey, MRI, CT, PET).
- Symptoms are due to hypercalcemia, renal failure, anemia, and bone lesions (CRAB).
- Bone scan may be negative due to limited osteoblastic activity.
- Plasmacytoma is a solitary lesion and most commonly involves the vertebral body.
- Plasmacytoma occurs in fifth decade, >50% of patients develop multiple myeloma.
- Treatment is with radiation and chemotherapy unless surgery is required for neurologic deterioration or spinal instability (Fig. 62.11).

Chordoma
- Slow-growing, locally aggressive tumor, arises from embryonic notochordal remnants
- Midline, lytic lesion, most frequently in anterior sacrum or base of skull (sixth to seventh decades)
- Tumor contains physaliphorous cells, positive for keratin and S-100 protein
- Treatment is *en bloc* excision and postoperative radiation therapy (proton beam) (Fig. 62.12)

Osteosarcoma
- Aggressive intraosseous malignant neoplasm in which tumor cells produce woven bone
- Bimodal age distribution (second and fourth decades)
- Tumor may arise *de novo* or from a secondary lesion (i.e., Paget disease, after radiation)
- Imaging: mixed lytic and sclerotic lesion, cortical destruction, and soft tissue calcification
- Treatment is neoadjuvant chemotherapy and wide *en bloc* excision (Fig. 62.13)

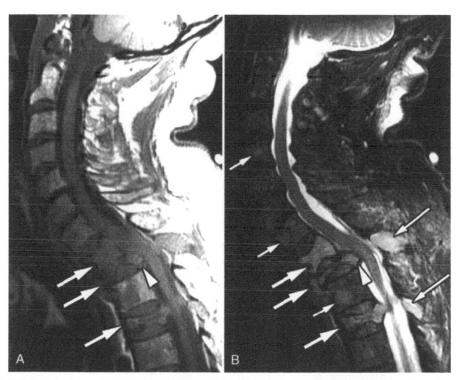

Fig. 62.11 Multiple myeloma. (A) Sagittal T1-weighted image. (B) Fat-saturated, T2-weighted image. Several compressed vertebral bodies with complete marrow replacement *(large arrows)*, as well as several ovoid regions of marrow signal intensity *(small short arrows)*. Posterior elements are also involved *(small, long arrows;* image B). Abnormal epidural soft tissue from collapsed vertebral body *(arrowhead)* compresses the spinal cord. (From Fenton DS. Multiple myeloma. In: Czervionke LF, Fenton DS. Imaging Painful Spine Disorders. Philadelphia, PA: Saunders; 2011, Fig. 48.1.)

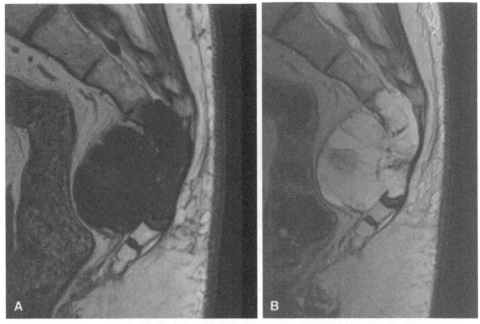

Fig. 62.12 Chordoma. (A) T1- and (B) T2-weighted magnetic resonance imaging shows the chordoma destroying the distal sacrum and involving anterior soft tissue. (From Rieth JD. Bone and joints. In: Goldblum JR, Lamps LW, McKenney, et al., editors. Rosai and Ackerman's Surgical Pathology. 11th ed. Philadelphia, PA: Elsevier, 2018, Fig. 40.52.)

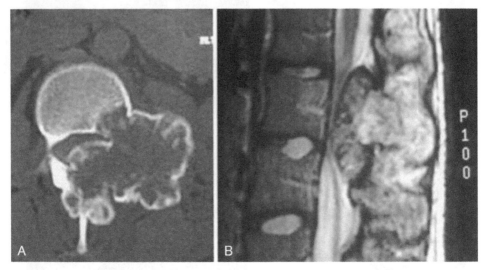

Fig. 62.13 Osteosarcoma. (A) Axial computed tomography and (B) T2-weighted magnetic resonance imaging of lumbar osteosarcoma. (From Sundaresan N, Rosen G, Boriani S. Primary malignant tumors of the spine. Orthop Clin N Am 2009;40:21–36, Fig. 5.)

Ewing Sarcoma
- Small, round cell tumor of neuroectodermal origin, age typically <30 years
- Destructive lytic vertebral body lesion associated with a paravertebral mass
- Presentation often includes systemic symptoms and may be misdiagnosed as infection
- Approximately 20% of patients present with metastatic disease
- Treatment is multimodality chemotherapy and radiation therapy
- *En bloc* excision is considered when feasible or for neurologic deficit and/or instability

Chondrosarcoma
- Group of cartilage matrix–producing tumors that includes both locally aggressive and malignant types
- May occur de novo or by sarcomatous transformation of a benign cartilage tumor
- Imaging shows a destructive spinal lesion or paraspinal mass with calcification
- Primary treatment is wide or marginal *en bloc* excision as tumor is resistant to chemotherapy and conventional radiotherapy
- Adjuvant radiation therapy (proton beam, conventional) is used when *en bloc* excision is not possible or tumor margins are positive (Fig. 62.14)

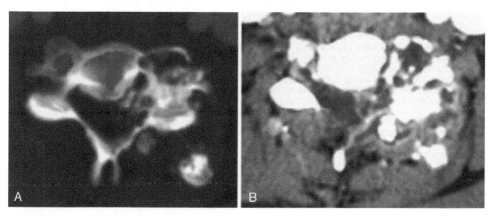

Fig. 62.14 Chondrosarcoma; cervical spine computed tomography images. (A) Bone window, and (B) soft tissue window. These show paraspinal, intraspinal, and intraforaminal extension of tumor, which is heavily calcified. (From Sundaresan N, Rosen G, Boriani S. Primary malignant tumors of the spine. Orthop Clin N Am 2009;40:21–36, Fig. 4.)

26. **What is denosumab and how is this medication used in the treatment of GCTs and other tumors of the spine?**
   Denosumab is a monoclonal antibody that functions as an inhibitor of the receptor of activator nuclear factor kappa-B ligand (RANKL), which is involved in bone resorption, and expressed in high levels in GCTs. It is currently US FDA-approved for treatment of adults and skeletally mature adolescents with GCT of bone that is unresectable or where surgical resection is likely to result in severe morbidity. It has been used as a pretreatment for up to 6 months prior to surgical resection, with significant decrease in tumor size prior to resection reported in some cases. It is also indicated for prevention of skeletal-related events in patients with multiple myeloma, and in patients with bone metastases from solid tumors. It is also used for treatment of hypercalcemia of malignancy refractory to bisphosphonate therapy.

27. **What primary tumors of the spine are amenable to kyphoplasty or vertebroplasty?**
   Marrow-based tumors, such as multiple myeloma and plasmacytoma, as well as hemangiomas.

KEY POINTS

1. Biopsy for primary spine tumors is a critical diagnostic step and may lead to an adverse outcome unless performed according to strict oncologic principles.
2. *En bloc* resection with tumor-free surgical margins provides the best possible local control for malignant primary tumors of the spinal column and is the procedure of choice when technically feasible, though it can often be associated with high morbidity.

Websites
1. Comprehensive bone tumor information: http://www.bonetumor.org/foot%20tumors/intro.htm
2. Spinal tumors: http://emedicine.medscape.com/article/1267223-overview
3. *En bloc* vertebrectomy: http://www.medscape.com/viewarticle/465369
4. Diagnostic imaging of solitary tumors of the spine: what to do and say: https://pubs.rsna.org/doi/10.1148/rg.284075156

REFERENCES

1. Fourney D, Rhines L, Hentschel S, et al. En bloc resection of primary sacral tumors: Classification of surgical approaches and outcome. *J Neurosurg Spine* 2005;3:111–122.

BIBLIOGRAPHY

1. Batista N, Dea N, Fisher CG. Assessment and treatment of primary tumors of the axial skeleton. In: Winn HR, editor. Youmans and Winn Neurological Surgery. 7th ed. Philadelphia, PA: Elsevier, 2016, pp. 2421–2427.
2. Boriani S. (2018). En bloc resection in the spine: a procedure of surgical oncology. *J Spine Surg* 4(3):668-676.
3. Bydon M, De la Garza-Ramos R, Wolinsky JP, et al. Assessment and treatment of benign tumors of the axial skeleton. In: Winn HR, editor. Youmans and Winn Neurological Surgery. 7th ed. Philadelphia, PA: Elsevier; 2017, pp. 2414–2420.
4. Clarke MJ, Dasenbrock H, Bydon A, et al. Posterior-only approaches for en bloc sacrectomy: Clinical outcomes in 36 consecutive patients. *Neurosurgery* 2012;71:357–364.
5. Dea N, Gokaslan Z, Choi, Fisher C (2017). Spine oncology-primary spine tumors. *Neurosurgery* 80:S124-S130.
6. Donthineni R, Ofluoglu O, editors. Spine oncology. *Orthop Clin N Am* 2009;40:1–177.
7. Fourney D, Rhines L, Hentschel S, et al. En bloc resection of primary sacral tumors: Classification of surgical approaches and outcome. *J Neurosurg Spine* 2005;3:111–122.
8. Gasbarrini A, Bandiera S, Amendola L, et al. Management of primary malignant tumors of the osseous spine. In: Quinones-Hinojosa A, editor. Schmidek and Sweet Operative Neurosurgical Techniques. 6th ed. Philadelphia, PA: Saunders; 2012, pp. 2169–2176.
9. Ishida W, Elder BD, Lo SL, et al. Spinopelvic reconstruction following lumbosacral tumor resection. *World Spinal Col J* 2016;7:25–30.
10. Kelley SP, Ashford RU, Rao AS, et al. Primary bone tumors of the spine: A 42-year survey from the Leeds Regional Bone Tumour Registry. *Eur Spine J* 2007;16:405–409.
11. Metkar U, Kurra S, Lavelle WF. Tumors of the spine. In: Garfin SR, Eismont FJ, Bell GR, editors. Rothman-Simeone The Spine. 7th ed. Philadelphia, PA: Saunders; 2018, pp. 1503–1525.
12. Shah AA, Nuno R, Pereira P, Pedlow FX, Wain JC, Yoon SS, Hornicek FJ, Schwab JH. (2017). Modified en bloc spondylectomy for tumors of the thoracic and lumbar spine. *J Bone Joint Surg Am* 99(17):1476-1484.
13. Zoccali C, Skoch J, Patel AS, et al. Residual neurological function after sacral root resection during en-bloc sacrectomy: A systematic review. *Eur Spine J* 2016;25:3925–3931.

CHAPTER 63

METASTATIC SPINE TUMORS

Nickul S. Jain, MD, Scott C. McGovern, MD, Winston Fong, MD, and Jeffrey C. Wang, MD

1. **What is the most common tumor of the spine?**
   Metastatic lesions are the most common tumors of the spine. Metastatic lesions account for over 90% of all spinal column tumors. Spine metastases are the most common type of skeletal metastases.

2. **What percentage of spinal metastases result in spinal cord compression?**
   Spinal cord compression occurs in 20% of patients who develop spinal metastases.

3. **Which malignancies most commonly metastasize to the spine?**
   In descending order of frequency: breast (21%), lung (14%), prostate (7.5%), renal (5%), gastrointestinal (GI) (5%), and thyroid (2.5%).

   A useful mnemonic to aid recall of common malignancies that metastasize to the spine is "P T Barnum Loves Kids" (prostate, thyroid, breast, lung, kidney).

4. **Where are metastatic spinal lesions most commonly located?**
   Within the vertebra, metastatic lesions first involve the vertebral body, followed by subsequent invasion of the pedicles and surrounding tissues. The disc space remains relatively uninvolved by metastatic tumor.
   Within the spinal column, metastatic lesions are found most commonly in the lumbar region, less commonly in the thoracic region, and least commonly in the cervical region.
   With respect to tumor type, breast and lung tumors most commonly metastasize to the thoracic spine. Prostate tumors tend to metastasize to the lumbar spine, pelvis, and sacrum.

5. **What are the pathways by which metastatic disease spreads to the spine?**
   Potential pathways for spread of metastatic disease to the spinal column include:
   1. Hematogenous spread (venous or arterial route)
   2. Direct tumor extension
   3. Lymphatic spread
      The most common pathway for spread of metastatic disease is the hematogenous route. Batson plexus, a thin-walled system of veins that extend along the entire spinal column, provides a connection between the spinal column and the major organ systems and is a common pathway for tumor migration and metastases. Alternatively, tumor cells may spread via the segmental arteries to the vertebral body.

6. **What is the most common presenting complaint of a patient with a metastatic spinal tumor?**
   Progressive and unrelenting pain is the most common presenting complaint. The pain is often unrelieved with rest and is worse at night. Constitutional symptoms may be present and include unintended weight loss, fatigue, and anorexia. Other presentations include mechanical pain, radicular pain, motor and/or sensory deficits, bladder dysfunction, sphincter dysfunction, and symptomatic spinal fracture. Occasionally patients may present with spinal deformity or a palpable mass.

7. **What causes pain in patients with metastatic tumors of the spine?**
   Many causes of pain are possible: hyperemia and edema secondary to tumor, expansion of tumor into the periosteum of the vertebra and surrounding tissues, direct compression or invasion of nerve roots, spinal cord compression, and osseous destruction leading to segmental spinal instability or pathologic spinal fracture with associated mechanical pain.

8. **What radiographic signs are suggestive of a metastatic spinal lesion?**
   Radiographic signs suggestive of a metastatic lesion include an absent pedicle, vertebral cortical erosion/expansion, and loss of vertebral body height.

9. **When are metastatic spinal tumors detectable on plain radiographs?**
   Most tumors of the spine are osteolytic. They are not demonstrated on plain films until more than 30%–50% destruction of the vertebral body has occurred. An exception is prostate cancer, which tends to be osteoblastic.

10. What is the "winking owl" sign?

This sign refers to the loss of one of the pedicle shadows on an anteroposterior (AP) spine radiograph. The cause for this radiographic finding is most frequently a metastatic vertebral lesion that has extended into the pedicle region and caused destruction of the pedicle.

11. What are the steps in evaluating a patient with a suspected metastatic spinal lesion?

Evaluation should occur in an organized and comprehensive fashion, as outlined below:

- **Patient history** should assess the pain pattern, sphincter control, neurologic symptoms, and pertinent factors such as baseline and current ambulatory status, use of assistive devices, and ability to perform activities of daily living. Risk factors for pyogenic osteomyelitis should also be assessed as this condition is included on the initial list of differential diagnoses.
- **Physical examination** should be comprehensive and include a full neurologic assessment with rectal examinatio, as well as examination of the breasts, thyroid, abdomen, prostate, and regional lymph nodes.
- **Laboratory studies** should include routine tests such as complete blood count, erythrocyte sedimentation rate, C-reactive protein, electrolytes, calcium, phosphate, and liver function tests including alkaline phosphatase. Additional special tests such as prostate-specific antigen, serum and urine protein electrophoresis, thyroid function tests, and nutritional indices are obtained as indicated.
- **Imaging studies** are critical for diagnosis and planning treatment. AP and lateral **spinal radiographs** are used to assess spinal anatomy, bony destruction, and alignment. **Magnetic resonance imaging (MRI)** is the primary imaging study for defining the anatomic extent of metastatic spine tumors. Metastatic lesions generally demonstrate low signal intensity on T1 and high signal intensity on T2 and enhance when gadolinium contrast is administered. MRI also provides information on the extent of neurologic compression. As metastatic disease involving the spine may be multicentric, the entire spinal column should be evaluated with MRI. **Radioisotope studies** are valuable to survey the skeleton for metastatic lesions. Technetium total body bone scans are highly sensitive but nonspecific, and their ability to detect osseous metastases depends on tumor type. Osteoblastic metastases are readily detected on bone scans, whereas osteolytic lesions such as multiple myeloma and hypernephroma may not be detectable. Positron emission tomography is an alternative radioisotope study that is highly sensitive and specific for cancer cells. Fluorine-18-labeled fluorodeoxyglucose undergoes rapid uptake by tumor cells due to their increased metabolic activity. **Computed tomography (CT)** plays a role in the localization and quantification of bony vertebral destruction and allows for surgical planning in regard to fixation strategies. If the primary tumor remains unknown, CT scans with intravenous and oral contrast should be obtained to assess the chest, abdomen, and pelvis in an attempt to locate the primary tumor. Female patients may require mammography.
- **Biopsy** is performed if the diagnosis remains in question at this point. CT-guided biopsy is generally preferred. Thoracic and lumbar lesions are generally approached posterolaterally, cervical lesions are approached anterolaterally, and for sacral lesions a direct posterior approach is used. If there is a possibility of infection, cultures should be obtained at the time of biopsy. Bone marrow biopsy is performed if multiple myeloma is in the differential diagnosis.

12. What is the goal for treatment of a metastatic spinal lesion?

The goal of treatment is generally palliation and not cure. Metastasis indicates that regional disease has progressed to a systemic illness that is generally incurable. Treatment is directed toward maximizing quality of life by providing pain relief, structural stabilization, and maintaining or restoring neurologic function via adequate neural decompression. Accordingly, surgery generally involves intralesional tumor resection (piecemeal removal). An exception to this treatment strategy is the patient with a solitary metastasis and potential for long-term survival with *en bloc* spondylectomy (removal of tumor in a single, intact piece encased by a continuous shell of healthy tissue called a "margin").

13. What are the options for treatment of a metastatic spinal lesion?

Potential treatment options include orthotic treatment, medication (bisphosphonates, steroids, and analgesics), radiotherapy, chemotherapy, hormonal therapy, kyphoplasty and/or vertebroplasty, surgical decompression and stabilization, tumor resection with spinal reconstruction, or a combination of these options.

14. What factors are important in determining a treatment plan for patients with a spinal metastatic lesion?

- Tumor type, grade, and location
- Tumor radiosensitivity
- Extent/pattern of spinal metastases
- Metastases to major internal organs
- Life expectancy
- Neurologic status
- Comorbid medical conditions
- Nutritional status

- Performance status and activity level
- Patient and family preferences

15. What classifications have been proposed to guide decision-making for patients with metastatic spinal disease?

Various classifications for patients with metastatic spinal disease have been proposed to:
- Guide treatment (Harrington classification)
- Determine the most appropriate surgical procedure (Tomita classification)
- Determine prognosis, life expectancy, and treatment (Tokuhashi classification, modified Bauer score)
- Determine the most appropriate multimodal therapeutic option (NOMS algorithm)

The **Harrington classification** stratifies patients with spinal metastases into five groups based on *spinal stability* and *neurologic status*:
- Class 1: No significant neurologic dysfunction
- Class 2: Bone involvement without collapse or instability, minimal neurologic involvement
- Class 3: Major neurologic dysfunction without significant bone involvement or instability
- Class 4: Vertebral collapse or instability causing pain, no significant neurologic compromise
- Class 5: Vertebral collapse or instability with major neurologic impairment

Surgery is recommended in the presence of spinal instability or mechanical pain (class 4 and 5). Radiotherapy is considered for class 3 patients, as well as class 1 or 2 patients who fail to obtain pain relief from other nonsurgical treatments.

The **Tomita classification** is a prognostic scoring system that considers the growth rate of the primary tumor, presence of visceral metastases, and number of bone metastases to guide decision making. A prognostic score based on these factors is used to determine the goal of treatment as surgery for long-term local control (wide or marginal excision), surgery for middle-term control (marginal or intralesional excision), surgery for short-term palliation (spinal cord decompression with stabilization), or nonoperative care.

The **Tokuhashi classification** system provides a scoring system for prognosis and incorporates six components. Five criteria are scored from 0 to 2 each, with higher scores being better.
- General condition: good (2), moderate (1), and poor (0)
- Number of extraspinal metastases: 0 (2), 1–2 (1), >3 (0)
- Number of vertebral body metastases: 0 (2), 1–2 (1), >3 (0)
- Major visceral organ metastases: none (2), removable (1), unremovable (0)
- Severity of motor deficit due to spinal cord compression: none (2), incomplete (1), complete (0)

In the revised version of the Tokuhashi scoring system, the primary tumor type is scored 0–5 based on the average survival of surgically treated patients, with higher scores representing increased survival:
- (0) lung, osteosarcoma, stomach, bladder, esophagus, pancreas
- (1) liver, gallbladder, unidentified
- (2) others (colon, ovary, ureter, melanoma, germinoma, liposarcoma, leiomyosarcoma)
- (3) kidney, uterus
- (4) rectum
- (5) breast, prostate, thyroid, carcinoid

Patients with scores below 9 were suggested to undergo nonoperative treatments (apy, chemotherapy, hormonal therapy, analgesics), those with scores between 9 and 11 were treated with   ve surgery (spinal cord decompression and stabilization), and those with scores between 12 and 15 were t   th excisional surgery.

As now treatment algorithms and more modern treatment options for metastatic spine disease evolve, alternative classification systems have been proposed. **A decision framework (NOMS)** based on neurologic (N), oncologic (O), mechanical instability (M), and systemic diseases and medical comorbidity (S) has been developed. An additional classification to identify neoplastic spinal instability and identify patients who could benefit from surgical consultation, the **Spine Instability Neoplastic Score (SINS)**, has been proposed. The Skeletal Oncology Research Group (SORG) has developed and validated a nomogram to estimate survival for patients with metastatic spinal disease.

16. How does the NOMS treatment algorithm guide treatment?

The NOMS algorithm is an evidence-based multimodal therapeutic algorithm aimed at improving local tumor control, pain relief, neurologic function, and reducing patient morbidity. It facilitates communication and decision making among members of a multidisciplinary spine oncology team comprised of surgery, radiation oncology, medical oncology, interventional radiology, and internal medicine specialists.

Neurologic (N) considers the presence or absence of myelopathy and/or radiculopathy, as well as the degree of epidural cord compression. **Oncologic (O)** considers whether the primary tumor is radiosensitive, radioresistant, or previously radiated. **Mechanical (M)** factors simply assess whether the spine is stable or unstable. **Systemic (S)** factors consider the patient's ability to tolerate surgery.

This algorithm is used to guide decision making regarding a range of treatment options, including conventional external-beam radiation, stereotactic radiosurgery, conventional open surgical intervention, separation surgery, and percutaneous vertebral body augmentation procedures (Table 63.1).

Table 63.1 NOMS Decision Framework.

NEUROLOGIC	ONCOLOGIC	MECHANICAL	SYSTEMIC	DECISION
Low-grade ESCC + no myelopathy	Radiosensitive	Stable		cEBRT
	Radiosensitive	Unstable		Stabilization followed by cEBRT
	Radioresistant	Stable		SRS
	Radioresistant	Unstable		Stabilization followed by SRS
High-grade ESCC + myelopathy	Radiosensitive	Stable		cEBRT
	Radiosensitive	Unstable		Stabilization followed by cEBRT
	Radioresistant	Stable	Able to tolerate surgery	Decompression/stabilization followed by SRS
	Radioresistant	Stable	Unable to tolerate surgery	cEBRT
	Radioresistant	Unstable	Able to tolerate surgery	Decompression/stabilization followed by SRS
	Radioresistant	Unstable	Unable to tolerate surgery	Stabilization followed by cEBRT

cEBRT, Conventional external beam radiation therapy; *ESCC,* epidural spinal cord compression; *SRS,* spinal stereotactic radiosurgery.
Low-grade ESCC is defined as grade 0 or 1 on Spine Oncology Study Group scoring system; high-grade ESCC is defined as grade 2 or 3 on the ESCC scale.
Adapted from Laufer I, Rubin DF, Lis E, et al. The NOMS framework: Approach to the treatment of spinal metastatic tumors. Oncologist 2013;18(6):744–751.
Reprinted from Lavelle WF, Ramakrishnan R, Simpson VM. Thoracic and thoracolumbar spinal tumors-regional challenges. In: Steinmetz MP, Benzel EC, editors. Benzel's Spine Surgery. 4th ed. Philadelphia, PA: Elsevier; 2017, pp. 1048–1060, Table 120.2.

17. **What scale is commonly used to describe the severity of epidural spinal cord compression diagnosed on MRI in a patient with metastatic spinal disease?**
    The **Epidural Spinal Cord Compression (ESCC) scale** was developed by the Spinal Oncology Study Group to describe the severity of epidural spinal cord compression in patients with metastatic disease based on axial T2-weighted MRI images at the most severely involved level. (1) The **components of the ESCC scale** are:
    • Grade 0: Tumor is contained within bone
    • Grade 1: Epidural impingement by tumor
    • Grade 2: Spinal cord compression, with cerebral spinal fluid (CSF) visible around the spinal cord
    • Grade 3: Spinal cord compression, no CSF visible around the cord.
      Grade 1 ESCC is subdivided into three groups:
    • Grade 1a: Epidural impingement without deformation of the thecal sac
    • Grade 1b: Deformation of the thecal sac, without spinal cord abutment
    • Grade 1c: Deformation of the thecal sac, with spinal cord abutment, without spinal cord compression
      Low grade compression is defined as grade 0 or 1. **High grade compression** is defined as grade 2 or 3. Literature demonstrates that the severity of epidural spinal cord compression on MRI according to the ESCC scale does not always correlate with the severity of neurologic deficit. Additional factors merit consideration, including the location of the compressive lesion in the transverse plane, and the spinal level and region involved.

18. **How is spinal instability defined in a patient with a metastatic spinal lesion?**
    According to the Spinal Oncology Study Group, **neoplastic spinal instability** is defined as "...loss of spinal integrity as a result of a neoplastic process that is associated with movement-related pain, symptomatic or progressive deformity, and/or neural compromise under physiologic loads". (3)
    A comprehensive classification system, the **Spine Instability Neoplastic Score (SINS)**, was developed to aid in the diagnosis of neoplastic spinal instability and guide patient referral and treatment. The SINS is determined by adding six individual component scores: global spinal location of tumor, pain, bone lesion quality, spinal alignment, vertebral body collapse, and posterior spinal element involvement, to determine a composite score ranging from 0 to 18. A score of 0–6 is considered "stable," 7–12 is considered "potentially unstable," and 13–18 is considered "unstable." Surgical consultation is advised for patients with a SINS ≥7 (Table 63.2).

Table 63.2 The Spinal Instability Neoplastic Score (SINS).

COMPONENT	SCORE
1. Spine Location	
Junctional (Occiput–C2, C7–T2, T11–L1, L5–S1)	3
Mobile spine (C3–C6, L2–L4)	2
Semirigid (T3–T10)	1
Rigid (S2–S5)	0
2. Mechanical or Postural Pain	
Yes	3
Occasional pain but not mechanical	1
Pain-free lesion	0
3. Bone Lesion Quality	
Lytic	2
Mixed (lytic/blastic)	1
Blastic	0
4. Radiographic Spinal Alignment	
Subluxation/translation present	4
De novo deformity (kyphosis/scoliosis)	2
Normal alignment	0
5. Vertebral Body Involvement	
>50% collapse	3
<50% collapse	2
No collapse with >50% of body involved	1
None of the above	0
6. Posterior Spinal Element Involvement (facet, pedicle, costovertebral joint)	
Bilateral	3
Unilateral	1
None of the above	0

Data derived from Fisher CG, DiPaola CP, Ryken TC, et al. A novel classification system for spinal instability in neoplastic disease: An evidence-based approach and expert consensus from the Spine Oncology Study Group. Spine 2010;35(22):1221–1229.

19. What is the role of bisphosphonates in treatment of metastatic spinal disease?
Bisphosphonates are useful for controlling bone pain due to metastatic tumor bony destruction and decrease the incidence of skeletal-related complications such as pathologic fracture and hypercalcemia of malignancy. Metastatic tumor cells secrete cellular modulators, including parathyroid hormone-related protein receptor activator for nuclear factor κB ligand (RANKL), and serine protease urokinase, which exert their effect through stimulation of osteoclasts. Bisphosphonates function by binding to bone matrix and lead to osteoclast dysfunction and apoptosis.

20. What is the role of steroid treatment for metastatic spinal lesions?
Steroids (usually dexamethasone) play a role in the initial treatment of edema associated with neural compression prior to definitive treatment. Complications associated with use of steroids include psychosis, diabetes, infection, avascular necrosis of the hip, and GI bleeding.

21. What are the indications for radiation therapy as the primary form of treatment for metastatic spinal lesions?
Radiation therapy plays a role in the treatment of malignancies by promoting reossification of the vertebral body and reducing tumor load. Pain relief has been reported in up to 80% of patients receiving radiation. Use of a spinal orthosis for 3 months following radiation therapy is recommended to prevent development of spinal fracture and instability. Tumors are defined as radiosensitive or radioresistant based on response to conventional external beam radiation therapy. Tumors that are sensitive to radiation therapy include lung, breast, prostate, and ovarian cancer, as well as lymphoma, myeloma, seminoma, and neuroendocrine carcinoma. Radioresistant tumors include GI adenocarcinoma, metastatic melanoma, thyroid carcinoma, renal cell carcinoma, hepatocellular carcinoma, non–small-cell lung carcinoma, and sarcoma. Potential indications for radiation therapy as the primary form of treatment for metastatic spinal lesions include radiosensitive tumors with stable or slowly progressive neurologic

symptoms, spinal canal compromise secondary to soft tissue tumor lesions, and patients who are not candidates for surgery due to medical comorbidities.

Radiation therapy is not indicated as an initial treatment for patients with spinal canal compromise secondary to bone or for patients with spinal instability due to metastatic spinal disease. Patients with metastatic disease and epidural compression who are surgically treated with spinal cord decompression and reconstruction followed by radiation have demonstrated more favorable outcomes (improved neurologic function and pain relief) than patients treated with radiation alone.

22. **What complications are associated with the use of radiation therapy for metastatic spine lesions?**
Complications associated with radiation therapy include bone marrow suppression, impaired wound healing, radiation myelopathy, neoplasia, and impaired healing of bone grafts. When appropriate, surgical decompression prior to radiation is preferred because this approach is associated with improved neurologic outcomes and decreased rates of postsurgical wound complications. In children, radiation therapy may lead to skeletal growth arrest, scoliosis, and neoplasia. The radiation sensitivity of the spinal cord and cauda equina limit the dose of radiation that can be safely administered with conventional external beam radiation therapy. New techniques such as intensity modulated radiation therapy (IMRT) and three-dimensional conformal radiation therapy (3D-CRT) have been developed to provide a higher radiation tumor dose without increasing damage to surrounding tissues.

23. **What is spinal stereotactic radiosurgery and how does it differ from conventional external beam radiation therapy?**
Treatment with conventional external beam radiation therapy involves targeting the tissue volume containing the metastatic lesion, as well as adjacent tissue uninvolved by tumor. Nonconventional radiation therapy modalities such as spinal stereotactic radiosurgery (SRS) allow for delivery of high-dose radiation focused at a smaller target site with decreased toxicity to surrounding tissues as compared with conventional external beam radiation therapy, and are effective in treating tumors that are resistant to conventional external beam radiation therapy.

24. **What is the role of chemotherapy in the treatment of a metastatic spinal lesion?**
Chemotherapy is used in patients with documented spinal metastases, patients at risk of developing spinal metastases, and patients with spinal lesions not amenable to surgical excision. The response to chemotherapy is determined by the tumor type. Tumors that are highly sensitive to chemotherapy include small-cell carcinoma of the lung, Ewing sarcoma, thyroid carcinoma, breast carcinoma, lymphoma, germ cell tumors, and neuroblastoma. Tumors that are relatively resistant to chemotherapy include adenocarcinoma of the lung and GI tract, squamous cell carcinoma of the lung, metastatic melanoma, and renal cell carcinoma.

25. **What are the indications for surgical intervention for metastatic spinal lesions?**
Patients who are advised to undergo surgery for metastatic lesions of the spine should be predicted to survive the proposed procedure and must demonstrate adequate nutritional parameters to permit wound healing. The patient's expected lifespan should be greater than 3 months. Indications for surgical intervention in such patients include:
- Need for a biopsy to obtain a definitive histologic diagnosis
- Impending pathologic fracture
- Spinal instability
- Pathologic fracture with bone in the spinal canal
- Increasing neurologic deficit despite steroid administration or during radiation therapy
- Neurologic compromise at a previously irradiated level
- Radioresistant tumors associated with high-grade ESCC

26. **What are the relative contraindications to surgical reconstruction for patients with metastatic spinal disease?**
- Widespread visceral or brain metastases
- Severe nutritional depletion
- Immunosuppression
- Significant metastases in all three spinal regions
- Active infection
- Expected survival less than 3 months
- Inability to survive the proposed procedure

27. **For patients with symptomatic spinal cord compression, what is the most important prognostic factor?**
The most important prognostic factor is the severity and latency of the neurologic deficit prior to treatment. Profound weakness lasting more than 48 hours generally fails to respond to radiation or surgical treatment. Epidural spinal cord compression is an oncologic emergency requiring prompt diagnosis and treatment.

28. What is the role of embolization in the treatment of metastatic spinal disease?
    Preoperative embolization of spinal tumors can be used to reduce operative blood loss in hypervascular tumors such as renal cell carcinoma, thyroid carcinoma, and Ewing sarcoma. Embolization is typically performed within 48 hours of the proposed procedure to prevent revascularization of the tumor, and some authors advocate for surgical procedures on the same day as embolization for reduced blood loss.

29. What surgical approaches have been described for treating metastatic spinal lesions?
    Surgical approaches described for treatment of metastatic lesions include:
    1. Posterior
    2. Anterior
    3. Combined anterior and posterior
    4. Posterolateral
    5. Minimally invasive (e.g., kyphoplasty, vertebroplasty, percutaneously placed rod-screw constructs)

30. What surgical options are used to treat spinal instability due to a metastatic spinal lesion?
    Surgical options for treatment of neoplastic spinal instability include percutaneous cement augmentation procedures, percutaneous pedicle screw-rod instrumentation, and conventional open surgical procedures for implantation of spinal instrumentation.

31. Why is laminectomy usually an inadequate procedure for treatment of a metastatic spinal lesion?
    In patients with neurologic deficit due to metastatic spinal lesions, 70% have anterior tumors compressing the dural sac, 20% have lateral compression of the dural sac, and only 10% have posterior neural compression by tumor mass. The anterior spinal canal is inadequately decompressed by posterior laminectomy. Furthermore, the destabilization of the spinal column created by a laminectomy increases the risk of postoperative spinal cord compression and neurologic deterioration due to the development of a postoperative kyphotic deformity and increased spinal instability. The primary indication for laminectomy as a stand-alone procedure is the relatively uncommon presentation of posterior epidural compression by metastatic tumor in a patient without anterior spinal column involvement by tumor.

32. What factors determine the choice of surgical approach for metastatic spinal lesions?
    The approach to the spine depends on the location of the tumor, the presence/absence of spinal instability, and the presence/absence of neural compression/neural deficit. Because most metastases involve the vertebral body, reconstruction of the anterior and middle spinal columns is often indicated. An anterior approach provides direct access for removal of the affected vertebral body, decompression of the dural sac, and reconstruction of the anterior and middle spinal columns with an intracolumnar spacer and anterior spinal instrumentation. A single-stage posterolateral approach for decompression and stabilization is an acceptable alternative surgical approach, and may be advantageous for patients with circumferential epidural spinal cord compression, patients who cannot tolerate an anterior or combined anterior-posterior approach due to medical comorbidities, and for tumors located in the upper thoracic region that are difficult to approach through a thoracotomy. Lateral approaches to the thoracolumbar spine have also been popularized for tumor resection and anterior column reconstruction in the thoracolumbar spine. If two or more vertebral bodies require removal, or if bone quality is poor, posterior spinal instrumentation is generally required.

33. What are the options for reconstruction of the anterior and middle spinal columns after resection of a metastatic lesion involving the vertebral body?
    Options for reconstruction of the anterior and middle spinal columns include bone graft (autograft or allograft), methylmethacrylate, titanium mesh cages, and carbon fiber or polyether ether ketone (PEEK) cages. Expandable cages have been popularized for use in this setting. All of the above intracolumnar implants are used in combination with anterior spinal instrumentation (plate systems, rod systems) and/or posterior segmental spinal fixation.

34. Define separation surgery and its role in the surgical management of spinal metastatic disease?
    Separation surgery is a minimally invasive treatment strategy involving concomitant surgical stabilization and surgical dissection of neural elements from the metastatic tumor, with limited intralesional epidural tumor resection to decompress the thecal sac and nerve roots, followed by stereotactic radiation of nonepidural tumor. This procedure avoids significant anterior column and vertebral body resection. It requires an integrated multidisciplinary team for success. Advantages of this treatment strategy include significantly less operative morbidity and blood loss. However, long-term outcomes on this treatment strategy are still being studied.

35. What is the role of kyphoplasty and vertebroplasty in the treatment of spinal metastatic disease?
    Kyphoplasty and vertebroplasty provide a minimally invasive approach for spinal stabilization and reduction of pain associated with pathologic spine fractures resulting from metastatic disease. The injected cement does not interfere with radiation therapy. The most common complication associated with these techniques is local cement extrusion.

Contraindications to these procedures include: vertebral body height loss exceeding 75%, posterior vertebral body cortex destruction, and significant spinal canal compromise due to epidural tumor.

36. A 50-year-old woman with a history of breast cancer has been treated with a right mastectomy, radiation therapy, and chemotherapy. The patient presents with a several-week history of unrelenting back pain and increasing weakness in both lower extremities. The patient remains ambulatory and has intact bowel and bladder function. The patient has normal nutritional indices and has no other major medical problems. Plain radiographs (Fig. 63.1), axial MRI (Fig. 63.2), sagittal MRI (Fig. 63.3), and axial CT (Fig. 63.4) are shown below. What treatment should be advised?

If the patient is willing to undergo surgery, this is the best treatment option. Two-level anterior thoracic spinal cord compression is most directly treated through a transthoracic anterior surgical approach. A kyphotic deformity due to multilevel tumor involvement and pathologic fracture is a classic indication for a combined approach with anterior and posterior spinal reconstruction. In this case, an initial anterior approach was used to decompress the spinal cord and place an expandable cage and bridging anterior plate. Subsequent posterior segmental spinal instrumentation was used to correct the kyphotic deformity and supplement the anterior spinal construct (Fig. 63.5). A single-stage posterior approach with posterolateral decompression and posterior placement of an expandable cage combined with posterior segmental spinal instrumentation is an alternative treatment option.

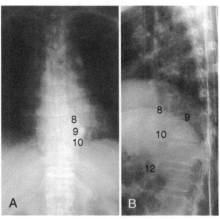

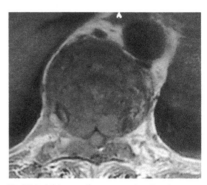

Fig. 63.1 (A) Anteroposterior and (B) lateral radiographs show pathologic fractures involving the T9 and T10 vertebral bodies with associated loss of vertebral body height and kyphotic deformity.

Fig. 63.2 Axial magnetic resonance imaging shows tumor infiltration of all three spinal columns with tumor extension into the epidural space.

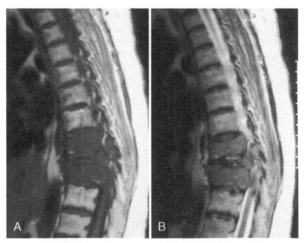

Fig. 63.3 (A) T1- and (B) T2-weighted sagittal magnetic resonance imaging depicts two-level vertebral body destruction and severe spinal cord compression.

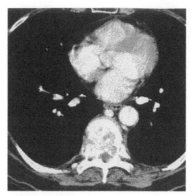

Fig. 63.4 Axial CT image at the level of pathologic fracture shows infiltrative osseous destruction and narrowing of the spinal canal.

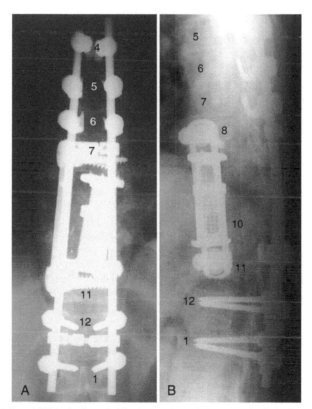

Fig. 63.5 (A) Anteroposterior and (B) lateral radiographs following two-stage spinal reconstruction. In the first stage, an anterior trans-thoracic exposure was performed to permit T9 and T10 corpectomies and placement of an expandable cage and anterior plate. In the second stage, posterior segmental spinal instrumentation, and posterior decompression were performed.

KEY POINTS

1. Back pain is the most common presenting symptom in patients with metastatic spinal disease.
2. Treatment of metastatic spinal disease is directed toward maximizing quality of life by providing pain relief and maintaining or restoring neurologic function.
3. Treatment strategies for metastatic spine tumors include orthoses, bisphosphonates, steroids, analgesics, radiotherapy, chemotherapy, hormonal therapy, vertebroplasty, kyphoplasty, surgical decompression and stabilization, separation surgery, tumor resection with spinal reconstruction, or a combination of these options.

Website

1. Spinal metastasis: https://emedicine.medscape.com/article/1157987-overview

---

REFERENCES

1. Bilsky, M. H., Laufer, I., Fourney, D. R., Groff, M., Schmidt, M. H., Varga, P. P., et al. (2010). Reliability analysis of the epidural spinal cord compression scale. *J Neurosurg Spine, 13*(3), 324–328.
2. Fisher, C. G., DiPaola, C. P., Ryken, T. C., Bilsky, M. H., Shaffrey, C. I, Berven, S. H., et al. (2010). A novel classification system for spinal instability in neoplastic disease: an evidence-based approach and expert consensus from the Spine Oncology Study Group. *Spine, 35*(22), 1221–1229.

BIBLIOGRAPHY

1. Lewandrowski, K., Anderson, M. W., & McLain, R. F. (2011). Tumors of the spine. In R. H. Rothman & F. A. Simeone (Eds.), *The Spine* (6th ed., pp. 1480–1512). Philadelphia, PA: Saunders.
2. Laufer, I., Rubin, D. G., Lis, E., Cox, B. W., Stubblefield, M. D., Yamada, Y., et al. (2013). The NOMS Framework: Approach to the treatment of spinal metastatic tumors. *Oncologist, 18*(6), 744–751.
3. Bilsky, M. H., Laufer, I., Fourney, D. R., Groff, M., Schmidt, M. H., Varga, P. P., et al. (2010). Reliability analysis of the epidural spinal cord compression scale. *Journal of Neurosurgery. Spine, 13*(3), 324–328.
4. Fisher, C. G., DiPaola, C. P., Ryken, T. C., Bilsky, M. H., Shaffrey, C. I., Berven, S. H., et al. (2010). A novel classification system for spinal instability in neoplastic disease: An evidence-based approach and expert consensus from the Spine Oncology Study Group. *Spine, 35*(22), E1221–E1229.
5. Ibrahim, A., Crockard, A., Antonietti, P., Boriani, S., Bünger, C., Gasbarrini, A., et al. (2008). Does spinal surgery improve the quality of life for those with extradural (spinal) osseous metastases? An international multicenter prospective observational study of 223 patients. *Journal of Neurosurgery. Spine, 8*(3), 271–278.
6. Lavelle, W. F., Ramakrishnan, R., & Simpson, V. M. (2017). Thoracic and thoracolumbar spinal tumors-regional challenges. In M. P. Steinmetz & E. C. Benzel (Eds.), *Benzel's Spine Surgery* (4th ed., pp. 1048–1060). Philadelphia, PA: Elsevier.
7. Patchell, R. A., Tibbs, P. A., Regine, W. F., Payne, R., Saris, S., Kryscio, R. J., et al. (2005). Direct decompressive surgical resection in the treatment of spinal cord compression caused by metastatic cancer: A randomized trial. *Lancet, 366*(9486), 643–648.
8. Tokuhashi, Y., Matsuzaki, H., Oda, H., Oshima, M., & Ryu, J. (2005). A revised scoring system for preoperative evaluation of metastatic spine tumor prognosis. *Spine, 30*(19), 2186–2191.
9. Tomita, K., Kawahara, N., Kobayashi, T., Yoshida, A., Murakami, H., & Akamaru, T. (2001). Surgical strategy for spinal metastases. *Spine, 26*(3), 298–306.
10. Sciubba, D. M., De la Garza Ramos, R., Goodwin, C. R., Xu, R., Bydon, A., Witham, T. F., et al. (2016). Total en bloc spondylectomy for locally aggressive and primary malignant tumors of the lumbar spine. *European Spine Journal, 25*(12), 4080–4087.
11. Wang, J. C., Boland, P., Mitra, N., Yamada, Y., Lis, E., Stubblefield, M., et al. (2004). Single-stage posterolateral transpedicular approach for resection of epidural metastatic spine tumors involving the vertebral body with circumferential reconstruction: Results in 140 patients. *Journal of Neurosurgery. Spine, 1*(3), 287–298.
12. Moussazadeh, N., Laufer, I., Yamada, Y., & Bilsky, M. H. (2014). Separation surgery for spinal metastases: Effect of spinal radiosurgery on surgical treatment. *Cancer Control, 21*(2), 168–174.
13. Kato, S., Hozumi, T., Takaki, Y., Yamakawa, K., Goto, T., & Kondo, T. (2013). Optimal schedule of preoperative embolization for spinal metastasis surgery. *Spine, 38*(22), 1964–1969.

CHAPTER 64

METABOLIC BONE DISEASES OF THE SPINE

Paul A. Anderson, MD, Vincent J. Devlin, MD, and Preston Phillips, MD

BONE BASICS—STRUCTURE, FUNCTION, AND HOMEOSTASIS

1. What are some major functions of bone?

Major bone functions include:

- Mineral storage (i.e., calcium, phosphorus, magnesium)
- Protection of internal organs from injury (i.e., brain, spinal cord, viscera)
- Provide support to the body by serving as a framework for tissue attachment
- Facilitate movement including locomotion by serving as an attachment for muscles
- Hematopoiesis

2. Describe the two major types of bone tissue.

The skeleton is composed of two types of bone tissue:

1. Cortical (compact) bone (80%)
2. Cancellous (trabecular) bone (20%)

Cortical bone provides skeletal strength and rigidity, especially under torsional and bending loads. Cancellous bone serves two major functions: resistance to compressive loads and facilitation of bone remodeling by providing a high surface area for metabolic activity. Both types of bone adapt throughout life to mechanical effects according to Wolff's law, which states that bone will adapt to the loads under which it is placed (i.e., bone under load hypertrophies, while absence of load is associated with bone mass loss).

3. Describe the composition of bone tissue.

Bone tissue is composed of cells and matrix.

The **cellular components** of bone include:

1. Osteoblasts
2. Osteocytes
3. Osteoclasts

The **matrix** is composed of:

1. Organic components (40%)
2. Inorganic components (60%)

The organic components include type 1 collagen, proteoglycans, noncollagenous matrix proteins (e.g., osteocalcin, osteonectin), and growth factors. The inorganic component, predominantly calcium hydroxyapatite [$Ca_{10}(PO_4)_6(OH)_2$], provides mineralization of the matrix and is responsible for the hardness and rigidity of bone tissue. Uncalcified bone matrix, known as osteoid, is pathologic and is a hallmark of rickets and osteomalacia.

4. Describe the cellular components of bone tissue.

- **Osteoclasts** develop from the myeloid hematopoietic stem cells of monocyte/macrophage lineage. These multinucleated giant cells are located in cavities along bone surfaces called *Howship lacunae* and are responsible for bone resorption.
- **Osteoblasts** develop from the pluripotential mesenchymal stem cells of bone marrow and perform various functions, including synthesis of osteoid, bone mineralization, and regulation of calcium and phosphate flux.
- **Osteocytes** arise from osteoblasts that have undergone terminal cell division and become surrounded by mineralized bone matrix. They possess extensive cell processes that communicate with other osteocytes and osteoblasts.
- **Osteoprogenitor cells** are derived from bone marrow mesenchymal stem cells and have capacity under certain conditions to differentiate into osteoblasts.

5. What is meant by bone remodeling?

Bone remodeling is the coupled process of bone resorption and subsequent formation through which skeletal repair, adaption to change in biomechanical stress, and release of calcium into the systemic circulation occurs. The basic multicellular unit of bone remodeling involves osteoclasts, osteoblasts, bone lining cells, and osteocytes. Osteocytes function as mechanoreceptors, which detect skeletal stress and initiate bone remodeling at a specific site. Osteoclasts attach to the bone surfaces and secrete acid and enzymes that dissolve away underlying bone. Osteoblasts migrate into these resorption pits (cancellous bone) and tunnels (cortical bone) and secrete osteoid, which is subsequently mineralized. Normal skeletal homeostasis requires a balance between bone formation by osteoblasts and resorption by osteoclasts, which is achieved by *coupling*. Coupling of bone formation and resorption is regulated by direct interaction between osteoblasts and osteoclasts, by local interactions between the immune system and bone cells, and by neuroendocrine mechanisms involving a range of mediators including sex hormones, growth hormones, osteocalcin, and leptin (Fig. 64.1).

Bone Remodeling Cycle

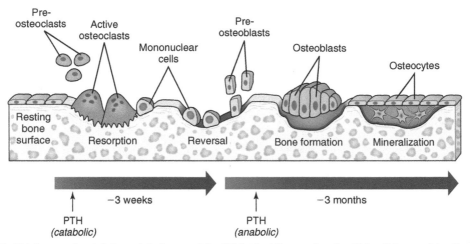

Fig. 64.1 Sequence of events that occur during bone remodeling. *PTH*, Parathyroid hormone. (From Garg AK. Bone biology, osseointegration, and bone remodeling. In: Garg AK, editor. Implant Dentistry. 2nd ed. Philadelphia, PA: Mosby; 2010, pp. 193–211.)

6. **What are some of the known pathways involved in bone remodeling that regulate the interactions between osteoblasts and osteoclasts?**
   Pathways that influence the balance between bone formation and resorption include the Wnt pathway (bone formation) and the receptor **a**ctivator of **n**uclear factor **k**appa (κ) beta (β) (RANK) and RANK ligand (RANKL) pathway.
   Interactions between RANK, RANKL, and osteoprotegerin (OPG) play an important role in the pathophysiology of osteoporosis. Osteoclast precursor cells are derived from bone marrow hematopoietic progenitor cells and have surface receptors for RANK. Under the influence of parathyroid hormone (PTH), osteoblasts express RANK ligand, which binds to the RANK receptor on preosteoclasts and causes signaling changes promoting osteoclastogenesis and bone resorption. Osteoblasts also secrete OPG, a soluble decoy receptor that inhibits bone resorption by binding to RANKL which prevents it from binding to RANK (Fig. 64.2).

7. **What factors are responsible for regulation of bone mineral balance?**
   Bone mineral balance is tightly regulated by the interaction of vitamin D metabolites (25-hydroxyvitamin D and 1,25-dihydroxyvitamin D), PTH, and calcitonin. Calcium homeostasis depends on the interaction of these factors with various organ systems, including the liver, kidney, and gastrointestinal tract, as well as the thyroid and parathyroid glands.
   PTH acts directly on bone and the kidney, and indirectly at intestinal sites. The direct actions of PTH include activation of osteoblasts and stimulation of reabsorption of calcium and loss of phosphate in the distal renal tubule. PTH acts indirectly at intestinal sites through the vitamin D pathway by increasing the conversion of inactive 25-hydroxyvitamin D (25-OH vitamin D) into the active form, 1,25-dihydroxyvitamin D in the kidney. The active form of vitamin D binds to intestinal vitamin D receptors to promote calcium and phosphorous absorption.
   Vitamin D is available in two natural forms: cholecalciferol (D3) and ergocalciferol (D2). Humans acquire vitamin D by two routes: endogenous synthesis in the skin during sunlight exposure (D3) and dietary intake (D2 and D3). Vitamin D from either source is converted in the liver by 25-hydroxylase to 25-OH vitamin D and then by 1-alpha-hydroxylase in the kidney to the active form, 1,25-dihydroxy vitamin D (Fig. 64.3).

8. **What is peak bone mass?**
   Peak bone mass (PBM) is defined as the highest level of bone mass achieved as a result of normal growth. Bone mineral density (BMD) increases rapidly during adolescence until PBM is reached between 16 and 25 years of

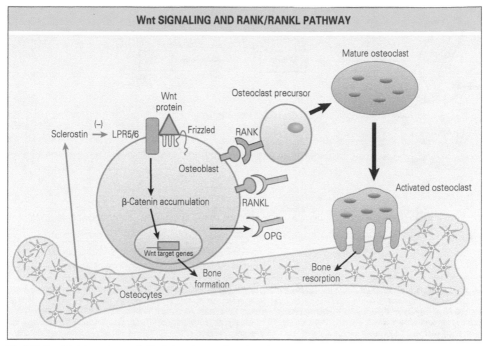

Fig. 64.2 Crosstalk between bone cells. The balance between bone formation and resorption is largely regulated by the Wnt pathway (bone formation), receptor activator of nuclear factor κB *(RANK)*/RANK ligand *(RANKL)* pathway (osteoclast activation), and sclerostin (negative regulation of bone formation). Osteoblasts express the cell surface receptors RANKL and also secrete a soluble decoy receptor, osteoprotegerin *(OPG)*, a member of the superfamily of tumor necrosis factor receptors. Wnt protein binds the coreceptors Frizzled and low-density lipoprotein receptor–like proteins 5 and 6 *(LRP5/6)*, which leads to stabilization of β-catenin and its translocation to the nucleus to regulate target genes, resulting in increased bone formation. In the absence of OPG, RANKL on the osteoblast surface is available to bind the RANK present on osteoclast precursors. Binding of RANK/RANKL leads to osteoclast maturation and resorption of bone. Sclerostin, secreted by osteocytes, inhibits Wnt from binding LRP5. (From Strocton EA, Sarada J, Hochberg MC. Pathophysiology of osteoporosis. In: Hochberg MC, Gravallese EM, Silman AJ, et al., editors. Rheumatology. 7th ed. Philadelphia, PA: Elsevier; 2019, pp. 1656–1660.)

age. After age 30, men normally lose bone at a rate of 0.3% per year. After age 30, women normally lose bone at a rate of 0.5% per year until menopause, at which time the rate of bone loss accelerates to 3%–5% per year over a 5- to 7-year period before returning to the previous rate of bone loss. The greater the PBM, the better the chance of avoiding osteoporosis later in life. This explains why increasing age is an important risk factor for osteoporosis (Fig. 64.4).

9. What common metabolic bone diseases cause significant problems relating to the spinal column?
Metabolic bone diseases are a diverse group of disorders characterized by abnormalities in calcium metabolism and/or bone cell physiology. Osteoporosis, Paget disease, osteomalacia, and renal osteodystrophy are some common metabolic bone diseases that affect the spinal column. In developed countries, the most common metabolic bone disease is osteoporosis.

OSTEOPOROSIS

DEFINITION, TYPES, AND RISK FACTORS

10. What is osteoporosis?
Osteoporosis is the most prevalent metabolic bone disease. It affects 10% of adults in the United States over age 50 years. Osteoporosis leads to decreased **bone mass** and **bone quality,** resulting in reduced bone strength. A reduction in the amount of normally mineralized bone per unit volume occurs as a result of an imbalance in the cellular activity responsible for maintaining the bony microarchitecture. Such structural alteration increases bone fragility and hence, the risk of fracture. Osteoporosis is diagnosed by the presence of a fragility fracture or by measurement of BMD in the absence of fracture (Fig. 64.5).

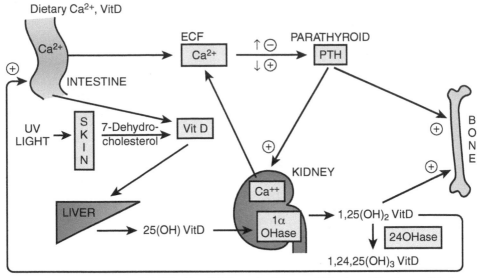

Fig. 64.3 Regulation of extracellular fluid *(ECF)* calcium *(Ca²⁺)* by parathyroid hormone *(PTH)* action on kidney, bone, and intestine. The calcium-sensing receptor senses a decrease in ECF Ca²⁺, and leads to an increase in PTH secretion, which acts directly on kidney and bone that express the PTH/PTHrP (PTH-related peptide) receptor. The skeletal effects of PTH are to increase *(+)* osteoclastic bone reabsorption via the RANK-RANKL pathway. In the kidney, PTH stimulates *(+)* 1α hydroxylase *(1αOHase)* to increase the conversion of 25-hydroxy vitamin D *(25[OH]D)* to the active metabolite 1,25-dihydroxy vitamin D *(1,25[OH]₂ D)*, which is subsequently inactivated by 24-hydroxylase. In addition, PTH increases *(+)* the reabsorption of Ca²⁺ from the renal distal tubule and inhibits the reabsorption of phosphate from the proximal tubule, thereby leading to hypercalcemia and hypophosphatemia. PTH also inhibits Na⁺ –H⁺ antiporter activity and bicarbonate reabsorption, thereby causing a mild hyperchloremic acidosis, and it reduces expression of two sodium-dependent phosphate cotransporters, NPT2a and NPT2c, thereby increasing urinary phosphate excretion. The elevated 1,25[OH]₂ D acts on the intestine to increase *(+)* absorption of dietary calcium and phosphate, and it is important to note that PTH does not appear to have a direct action on the gut. Thus in response to hypocalcemia and the increase in PTH secretion, all of these direct and indirect actions of PTH on the kidney, bone, and intestine will help to increase ECF Ca²⁺, which in turn will act via the calcium-sensing receptor to decrease PTH secretion. (From Thakker RV, Bringhurst R, Juppner H. Regulation of calcium homeostasis and genetic disorders that affect calcium metabolism. In: Jameson LJ, De Groot LJ, de Kretser DM, et al., editors. Endocrinology: Adult and Pediatric. 7th ed. Philadelphia, PA: Saunders; 2016, pp. 1063–1089.)

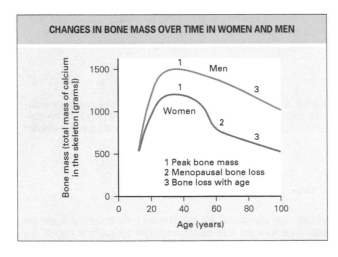

Fig. 64.4 Changes in bone mass over time in men and women. (From Holroyd CR, Dennison E, Cooper C. Epidemiology and classification of osteoporosis. In: Hochberg MC, Gravallese EM, Silman AJ, et al., editors. Rheumatology. 7th ed. Philadelphia, PA: Elsevier; 2019, pp. 1639–1646.)

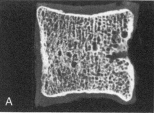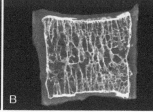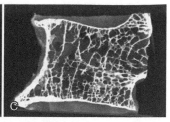

Fig. 64.5 Specimen radiographs of 2 mm slices through the vertebral body of T2. (A) The first specimen represents normal bone texture, density, and pattern. (B) The second specimen shows a moderate degree of osteopenia, with accentuation of the vertical trabeculae and selective loss of the horizontal trabeculae. (C) The third specimen shows severe osteoporosis, with irregular thin trabeculae and partial central collapse of the superior endplate. (From Bullough PG. Orthopaedic Pathology. 5th ed. Philadelphia, PA: Mosby; 2010.)

11. What are fragility fractures?
Fragility fractures occur spontaneously or following minimal trauma such as falling from standing height, and most commonly involve the thoracic and lumbar vertebral bodies, proximal femur, and distal radius. Fragility fractures may also involve the proximal humerus, pelvis, ribs, and odontoid process. Approximately 2 million fractures are attributed to osteoporosis annually in the United States. The lifetime risk of an osteoporotic fracture is estimated as 40% in women and 13% in men. Not all fragility fractures are associated with clinical symptoms. For example, up to two-thirds of osteoporotic vertebral fractures are asymptomatic. History of fragility fracture is among the strongest risk factors for future fracture.

12. What are the risk factors for development of osteoporosis?
See Table 64.1.

Table 64.1 Risk Factors for Osteoporotic Fractures.

NONMODIFIABLE RISK FACTORS	POTENTIALLY MODIFIABLE RISK FACTORS
• Advanced age • Female gender • History of fracture in a first-degree relative • Patient history of fracture during adulthood • Ethnicity (white, Asian) • Menopause or hysterectomy • Long-term glucocorticoid therapy • Rheumatoid arthritis • Primary or secondary hypogonadism in men • Dementia • Poor health or frailty	• Low calcium or vitamin D intake • Alcohol excess • Smoking • Low body mass index • Poor nutrition or eating disorder • Estrogen deficiency (menopause before age 45 years, bilateral ovariectomy, prolonged premenopausal amenorrhea >1 year) • Impaired eyesight despite correction • Recurrent falls • Inadequate physical activity • Poor health or frailty • Excess caffeine intake • Poor health or frailty

13. What are the different types of osteoporosis?
Osteoporosis has been classified into two major types: primary and secondary.
- **Primary osteoporosis** is further subdivided into type 1 or postmenopausal osteoporosis and type 2 or senile osteoporosis.
  - **Type 1** osteoporosis is due to estrogen deficiency and typically occurs in women 5–10 years after menopause. It predominantly affects trabecular bone and is associated with vertebral fractures, intertrochanteric hip fractures, and distal radius fractures.
  - **Type 2** osteoporosis occurs secondary to aging and calcium deficiency and is seen in both women and men after age 70 years. It affects both cortical and trabecular bone and is associated with vertebral fractures, femoral neck fractures, and pelvic fractures, as well as proximal tibia and humerus fractures.
- **Secondary osteoporosis**, also called **type 3** osteoporosis, occurs as a result of endocrinopathies, miscellaneous disease states, and medications.

14. What are some of the common causes of secondary osteoporosis?
- **Endocrine disorders:** Cushing disease, hypogonadism, hyperthyroidism, hyperparathyroidism, diabetes mellitus
- **Hematologic disorders:** lymphoma, multiple myeloma, metastatic disease, chronic alcohol use

- **Genetic diseases:** osteogenesis imperfecta, Marfan syndrome, hypophosphatasia
- **Gastrointestinal disorders:** malabsorption, celiac disease, inflammatory bowel disease, liver disease
- **Hypogonadal states:** androgen insensitivity, premature menopause, athletic amenorrhea
- **Neurologic disorders:** spinal cord injury, Parkinson disease, multiple sclerosis
- **Medications:** glucocorticoids, thyroid replacement therapy, anticonvulsants, chemotherapy agents, aluminum-containing antacids, thiazolidinediones, selective serotonin reuptake inhibitors, and proton pump inhibitors
- **Rheumatologic and autoimmune diseases:** rheumatoid arthritis, systemic lupus, ankylosing spondylitis
- **Lifestyle factors:** smoking, excess alcohol and inactivity, poor nutritional intake
- **Other:** chronic renal failure, chronic metabolic acidosis, idiopathic scoliosis

15. Explain some important ways osteoporosis in men differs from osteoporosis in women.

Similar to women, the risk of fragility fractures in men increases with age. However, the peak incidence of fracture occurs approximately 10 years later in men compared with women. The consequences of fragility fractures are greater in men compared with women. For example, the 1-year mortality rate for men following hip fracture is approximately twice the rate of mortality in women. The majority of men diagnosed with osteoporosis have an identifiable secondary cause of osteoporosis such as hypogonadism, glucocorticoid use, smoking, excessive alcohol consumption, low calcium intake, or vitamin D deficiency. Treatment of osteoporosis in men is similar to women except that testosterone hormone replacement (intramuscular injection or transdermal patch) is used for treatment of hypogonadism in men.

16. What is the most common cause of drug-related secondary osteoporosis?

Glucocorticoid use is the most common cause of drug-related secondary osteoporosis. Glucocorticoids impair bone formation and increase bone resorption. More than 10% of patients treated with long-term glucocorticoids are diagnosed with a fracture, and 3%–4% of patients have radiographic evidence of vertebral fractures. A rapid decrease in BMD is noted within the initial 3–6 months of glucocorticoid use and peaks around 6 months, followed by a less rapid decline with continued use. Data suggest that patients receiving glucocorticoids may experience fractures at higher (better) BMD than patients with other types of osteoporosis (T-score < -1). Increased risk of fracture has been reported with doses of prednisone or its equivalents as low as 2.5–7.5 mg daily. Men taking glucocorticoids may experience lowering of testosterone levels and may require treatment with testosterone in addition to medication for osteoporosis.

DIAGNOSIS, EVALUATION, AND PREVENTION

17. How is BMD measured?

The most widely accepted method of determining BMD is **dual-energy x-ray absorptiometry (DEXA)** performed at a central skeletal site (hip or lumbar spine). BMD measurements may also be performed at peripheral sites (distal radius, calcaneus, hands) and have utility when central measurements are not possible but are less accurate. Additional methods for BMD measurement include computed tomography (CT) and ultrasound.

A bone densitometry report describes BMD in relative terms (T-score, Z-score) and absolute terms (grams of mineral per centimeter squared, g/cm^2). Because BMD varies depending on the scanner, statistical scores are used to classify patients and estimate fracture risk using the formula:

$$T \text{ or } Z \text{ score} = \left(BMD\,(subject) - BMD\,(reference)\right)/SD\,(reference)$$

- **T-score** reports the patient's BMD as the number of units of standard deviation (SD) above or below the mean value of a young (30-year-old) normal (PBM) subject of the same sex. One SD is equal to a 10%–12% decrease in bone mass. The T-score is used to define bone health according to World Health Organization (WHO) standards as *normal* (T-score between $+1$ and -1 SD of the mean), *low bone mass (osteopenia)* (T-score between 1 and 2.5 SD below the mean), or *osteoporosis* (T-score > -2.5 SD below the mean). *Severe osteoporosis* is defined as a T-score less than -2.5 and the presence of one or more fragility fractures. The T-score may be used to estimate fracture risk. Each one-point decrease in T-score is estimated to increase fracture risk twofold.

T-Score	Percentage Bone Loss	Increased Fracture Risk
-1	12%	Twofold
-2	24%	Fourfold
-3	36%	Eightfold

- **Z-score** reports the patient's BMD as the number of units of SD compared with age-, sex-, and ethnicity-matched controls. A Z-score more than 1.5 SDs below the mean value should prompt an evaluation for secondary causes of osteoporosis.
- **Absolute BMD** is reported as grams of mineral per centimeter squared (g/cm^2). Absolute BMD is used to assess change in bone density over time. Knowledge of the minimum BMD change that should be considered significant (least significant change, LSC) for a specific DEXA machine is needed for accurate interpretation of serial measurements of BMD (Fig. 64.6).

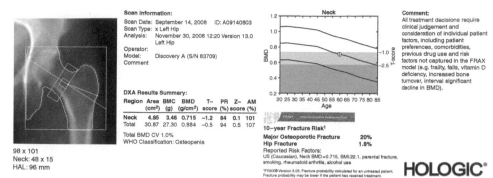

Fig. 64.6 Printout of dual-energy x-ray absorptiometry (DEXA) scan of the hip. (From Duncan WE. Measurement of bone mass. In: McDermott MT, editor. Endocrine Secrets. Philadelphia, PA: Saunders; 2013, pp. 102–109.)

18. What is the Fracture Risk Assessment (FRAX) tool?

DEXA scans do not convey all the necessary information to predict a specific patient's fracture risk. This is high-lighted by the finding that up to half of all osteoporotic-related fractures occur in patients with BMD values classified as low bone mass (osteopenia). Thus, factors in addition to BMD require consideration in the assessment of fracture risk. **The Fracture Risk Assessment** (FRAX) tool (http://www.sheffield.ac.uk/FRAX/) has been developed by the WHO to integrate important clinical risk factors and bone density measurements to determine the 10-year probability of major osteoporotic fracture (defined as clinical vertebral, hip, forearm, or proximal humerus fracture). The risk factors included in the FRAX model include age, sex, weight, height, previous fracture in adult life, parent with hip fracture, current smoking, glucocorticoid use, rheumatoid arthritis, secondary osteoporosis, alcohol use, and femoral neck BMD (if available). Based on the FRAX model, postmenopausal women and men over age 50 with low bone mass (T-score between -1 and -2.5 at the femoral neck or spine) and a 10-year probability of hip fracture $\geq 3\%$ or a 10-year probability of major osteoporosis-related fracture $\geq 20\%$, are candidates for antiosteoporotic medication.

19. How are clinical factors incorporated into the diagnosis of osteoporosis?

Based on criteria from the National Bone Health Alliance, a diagnosis of osteoporosis may be made in post-menopausal women or men over age 50 who are at an elevated risk for fracture due to any of the following factors:
- T-score less than or equal to -2.5 at the spine or hip
- Hip fracture with or without BMD testing
- Vertebral fractures, proximal humeral fractures, pelvic fractures, and specific types of distal forearm fractures in patients with osteopenia by BMD
- FRAX score with 10-year risk for hip fracture $\geq 3\%$ or for major osteoporosis-related fracture $\geq 20\%$ in patients with osteopenia.

20. Explain what is meant by vertebral fracture assessment and trabecular bone score.

Vertebral fracture assessment (VFA) refers to the use of the bone densitometer to scan the entire thoracic and lumbar spine at the time of BMD measurement. VFA evaluates vertebral height and can diagnose vertebral frac-tures that are often silent. This technique is attractive as it can screen the entire thoracic and lumbar spine and may avoid the need for spinal radiographs in some cases.

Trabecular bone score (TBS) is a noninvasive analytical method that estimates the trabecular microarchi-tecture of bone through the use of gray-level textural measurements extracted from DEXA images. TBS provides skeletal information that is not captured on standard BMD measurements and can complement data provided by lumbar DEXA measurements, as patients with similar BMD may vary in TBS. TBS scores can be entered into the FRAX risk calculator and may alter treatment by increasing the 10-year fracture risk.

(Figs. 64.7A,B and 64.8)

21. What is an opportunistic CT scan?

CT is frequently performed and contains information regarding bone status that can be used in an opportunistic manner to screen for osteoporosis, without additional cost. CT is based on determination of x-ray attenuation in each voxel of irradiated tissue. The x-ray attenuation is normalized to zero for water and -1000 for air and is called a Hounsfield unit (HU). This quantity can be measured on any CT for any region of interest using picture archiving and communication system (PACS) tools. An ellipse is drawn in an area of bone and the mean HU is

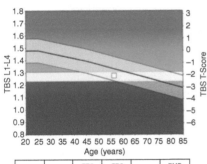

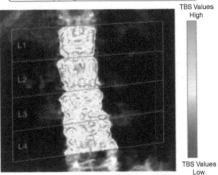

A

AP Spine Bone Density

USA (Combined NHANES/Lunar) AP Spine: L1-L4 (BMD)

COMMENTS:

	BMD (g/cm²)	Young-Adult T-score	Age-Matched Z-score
Region			
L1	0.892	−2.0	−1.5
L2	0.873	−2.7	−2.2
L3	0.957	−2.0	−1.5
L4	0.988	−1.8	−1.3
L1-L4	0.932	−2.1	−1.6

Densitometry: USA (Combined NHANES/Lunar)

TBS reference graph
Reference population: USA (NHANES / Medimaps)

TBS L1-L4: 1.2.78

TBS Mapping

B

Region	TBS	TBS T-Score	TBS Z-Score	BMD	BMD T-Score
L1	1.244	---	---	0.892	−2.0
L2	1.190	---	---	0.873	−2.7
L3	1.399	---	---	0.957	−2.0
L4	1.281	---	---	0.988	−1.8
L1-L4	1.278	−2.1	−0.6	0.932	−2.1
L1-L3	1.278	−2.3	−0.7	0.909	−2.2
L1-L2	1.217	−2.9	−1.2	0.882	−2.4
L2-L3	1.295	−2.4	−0.6	0.916	−2.4
L2-L4	1.290	−2.0	−0.5	0.943	−2.1
L3-L4	1.340	−1.3	−0.1	0.973	−1.9

FRAX

The 10 year probability of fracture, adjusted for TBS:
  Major Osteoporotic Fracture: 16.9 %
  Hip Fracture: 4.0 %

FRAX web site:https://www.shef.ac.uk/FRAX/?lang=en

Fig. 64.7 (A) A 58-year-old female who had a lumbar dual-energy x-ray absorptiometry (DEXA) scan prior to planned L4–L5 decompression and fusion for synovial cyst and grade 1 degenerative spondylolisthesis. Her DEXA scan shows low bone mass of L1–L4 (T-score −2.1). (B) Trabecular bone score *(TBS)* from L1 to L4 was obtained in the same patient and showed degraded bone microarchitecture (TBS: 1.28). An adjusted Fracture Risk Assessment (FRAX) predicts a 10-year hip and 10-year all fracture risk of 4.0% and 16.9% respectively. These values exceed the threshold for treatment and thus she was given 3 months of teriparatide before surgery. *BMD,* Bone mineral density.

measured. Cortical bone ranges from 250 to 500 HU while normal cancellous bone is 150–300 HU. Thresholds for L1 vertebral body have been determined: HU >160 is likely normal, HU <135 suggests osteopenia or osteoporosis, and HU <110 indicates likely osteoporosis. It is also possible to derive quantitative CT BMD measurements from opportunistic CT images obtained for another purpose and calculate T-scores using specialized software and image processing techniques (Fig. 64.9).

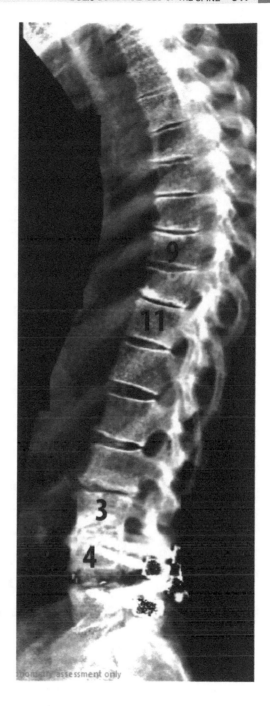

Fig. 64.8 A 64-year-old female who is 2 years after instrumented L4–5 fusion. She now has adjacent segment degeneration and is being considered for L3–L4 decompression and fusion. Dual-energy x-ray absorptiometry (DEXA) with vertebral fracture assessment (VFA) was obtained. The VFA shows moderate occult T10 fracture. This finding combined with low bone mass found on DEXA indicates she has clinical osteoporosis and was treated with teriparatide before surgery.

22. What workup should be performed following a diagnosis of osteoporosis?

   The physician should perform a complete history and physical examination with attention to specific risk factors for osteoporosis (see Table 64.1). In older adults, the risk of falling should be assessed by screening for visual, auditory, or cognitive impairment, use of sedatives, orthostatic hypotension, and the presence of obstacles to ambulation in the home. Physical examination should include assessment of height loss by performing annual measurements, assessment of thoracic kyphosis, and palpation for spinous process tenderness. Laboratory tests are

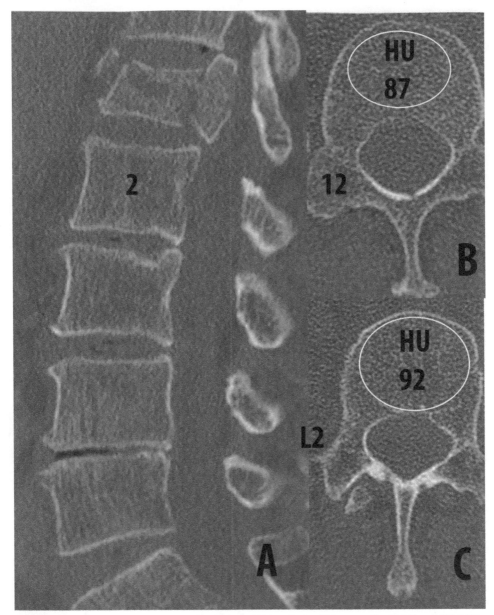

Fig. 64.9 Computed tomography of 78-year-old male who sustained L1 burst fracture (A) from ground level fall. Hounsfield Unit (HU) values of 87 and 92 are found on regions of interest *(circle)* at T12 (B) and L2 (C) consistent with osteoporosis.

not required for the diagnosis of osteoporosis. However, baseline lab tests are recommended, including serum calcium, albumin, phosphate, and 25-OH vitamin D levels. Biochemical bone marker assays may be considered to evaluate the balance between bone resorption and bone formation. Common bone formation markers include serum bone-specific alkaline phosphatase and osteocalcin. Common bone resorption markers include urine or serum amino-terminal-telopeptides (NTX) and serum carboxy-terminal-telopeptides (CTX).

In cases where secondary osteoporosis is suspected based on age, clinical findings, or Z-scores, additional evaluation is pursued. For example:

- **To rule out endocrinopathy:** Assess serum calcium and phosphate, PTH, thyroid function tests (TSH, T3, free T4), blood glucose, testosterone level (men) and LH, FSH, and estrogen (women).

- **To rule out gastrointestinal disorders:** Erythrocyte sedimentation rate (ESR), C-reactive protein (CRP), celiac disease antibody tests, colonoscopy.
- **To rule out liver disease:** Liver function tests, antimitochondrial antibody, and antibody testing for hepatitis A, B, and C.
- **To rule out bone marrow abnormality:** Perform complete blood count with differential, ESR, serum protein electrophoresis, and urinary protein electrophoresis.
- **To rule out renal failure:** Blood urea nitrogen (BUN), creatinine.
- **To rule out local bone tumor:** Perform radiographs, magnetic resonance imaging (MRI), CT, and/or bone scan.
- **To rule out osteomalacia:** Assess serum calcium, phosphate, alkaline phosphatase, PTH, 25(OH) vitamin D, and 24-hour urine calcium level; consider a bone biopsy.

23. Summarize the universal recommendations for physicians in relation to osteoporosis screening, prevention, and treatment.
    - Counsel postmenopausal women and men aged 50 and older about risk factors for osteoporosis and related fractures as it is a silent disease process that is generally preventable and treatable.
    - Advise all patients to maintain adequate dietary calcium and vitamin D intake.
    - Recommend a routine of weight-bearing and muscle-strengthening exercise to reduce the risk of falls and fractures.
    - Counsel patients to avoid smoking and limit alcohol and caffeine intake.
    - Assess risk factors for falls and recommend appropriate modifications.
    - Utilize the FRAX tool for screening and treatment decisions.
    - Recommend BMD testing, VFA, and assessment of biochemical markers of bone turnover based on an individual's fracture risk profile, skeletal health assessment, and in accordance with current clinical practice guidelines.
    - Recommend pharmacologic therapy for osteoporosis prevention and treatment when appropriate (Fig. 64.10).

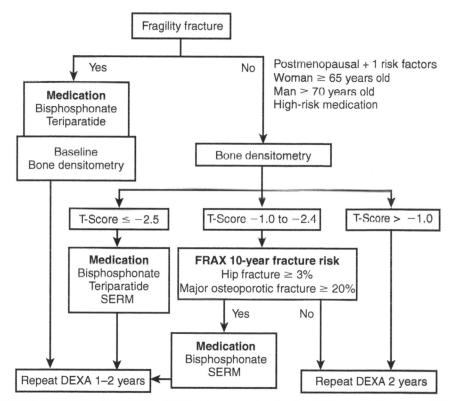

Fig. 64.10 Osteoporosis management algorithm. *DEXA,* Dual-energy x-ray absorptiometry; FRAX, Fracture Risk Assessment; *SERM,* selective estrogen receptor modulator. (From McDermott MT. Osteoporosis. In: McDermott MT, editor. Endocrine Secrets. Philadelphia, PA: Saunders; 2013, pp. 90–98.)

24. **What are the daily recommended vitamin D and calcium requirements?**

Recommendations regarding daily requirements vary based on patient age and are frequently updated to reflect the current state of scientific knowledge. Currently, the daily adult requirement for vitamin D is 800 to 1000 IUs (international units). Vitamin D deficiency is common in adults and is diagnosed by measuring the blood level of 25-OH vitamin D, the major circulating form of vitamin D. A sufficient 25-OH vitamin D level is defined as 30 ng/mL. Adults with vitamin D deficiency are treated with 2000 IU/day of vitamin D2 or D3, or 50,000 IU of vitamin D2 or D3 once weekly for 8 weeks, reassessment of 25-OH vitamin D levels, followed by maintenance therapy of 1500 to 2000 IU/day to maintain 25-OH vitamin D levels above 30 ng/mL.

The daily adult requirement for calcium is 1000 mg for men aged 50–70; 1200 mg for women aged 51 and older and men aged 71 and older. A balanced diet, including low-fat dairy products, fruits, and vegetables, is the best sources of calcium. Calcium supplements, most commonly calcium citrate or calcium carbonate, should be added when target dietary intake is not achieved. Advantages of the use of calcium citrate include that it does not lead to renal stones and it is absorbed in patients who take proton pump inhibitors or H2 receptor blockers. PTH levels can be measured to assess adequacy of calcium intake. PTH levels greater than 50 pg/mL suggest inadequate calcium intake, while PTH levels less than 25 pg/mL suggest oversupplementation of calcium.

25. **What are the indications for BMD testing with DEXA?**

BMD testing with DEXA is suggested based on guidelines from the National Osteoporosis Foundation for:
- Women age ≥65 years and men ≥70 years regardless of risk factors
- Women in menopausal transition, postmenopausal women, and men aged 50–69 with clinical risk factors for fracture
- Adults with a fracture at age ≥50 years
- Adults with a condition (e.g., rheumatoid arthritis) or taking a medication (e.g., glucocorticoids) associated with low bone mass or bone loss

26. **What are the indications for performing VFA?**

VFA is recommended based on guidelines from the National Osteoporosis Foundation for:
- All women aged >70 and men >80 years if BMD T-score ≤−1.0
- Women aged 65–69 and men aged 70–79 if BMD T-score ≤−1.5
- Postmenopausal women and men aged 50 and older with specific risk factors:
  - Low-energy fracture in adulthood
  - Historical height loss of 4 cm or more
  - Prospective height loss of 2 cm or more
  - Recent or ongoing long-term glucocorticoid treatment

27. **What strategies can be utilized to mitigate the risk of falls?**

Strategies which have been demonstrated to reduce falls include:
- Regular weight-bearing and muscle-strengthening exercise
- Balance training
- Performing a home safety assessment
- Prescribing walking aids and assistive devices as needed
- Correcting visual impairment
- Minimizing or discontinuing sedative medication
- Ensuring adequate protein intake

PHARMACOLOGIC TREATMENT

28. **When is pharmacologic treatment advised for patients with osteoporosis?**

Current indications for pharmacologic treatment in postmenopausal females or males age 50 or greater include:
- Presence of hip or vertebral fractures (with or without clinical symptoms)
- T-score of −2.5 or lower at the hip or spine by DEXA
- Patients with low bone mass (T-score −1 to −2.5 at the hip or spine) and a 10-year probability of hip fracture ≥3% or a 10-year probability of any major osteoporosis-related fracture ≥20% (fracture probabilities are determined by FRAX)

29. **What pharmacologic therapies are currently available for osteoporosis?**

Two classes of medications for osteoporosis prevention and treatment are approved by the US Food and Drug Administration (FDA). These are antiresorptive and anabolic.

1. **Antiresorptive medications**
   - **Oral bisphosphonates** (e.g., alendronate, risedronate, ibandronate): These antiresorptive agents are analogs of pyrophosphates and are absorbed onto the surface of hydroxyapatite crystals in bone. They alter bone remodeling by decreasing osteoclast-mediated bone resorption and cause apoptosis of osteoclasts. Short-term potential side effects include gastrointestinal reflux, esophageal irritation, and adverse effects on renal function. Longer-term potential side effects include osteonecrosis of the mandible and adynamic fragile bone, which can lead to atypical femur fractures. A "drug holiday" or time off bisphosphonate

therapy is considered after 5 years of use based on individual patient circumstances and fracture to mitigate the chance of atypical femur fractures.

- **Intravenous bisphosphonates** (e.g., ibandronate, zoledronic acid): Provide an alternative medication for patients who are unable to tolerate an oral bisphosphonate. These are given by infusion annually for 2–3 years. These drugs are typically more effective than oral but are associated with increased risk of atypical femur fracture and osteonecrosis of the mandible due to suppression of bone turnover.
- **Denosumab:** This monoclonal IG2 antibody inhibits the RANK ligand. This action inhibits osteoclast formation, function, and survival. Denosumab has similar risk of atypical femur fracture and osteonecrosis of the jaw as bisphosphonates.
- **Estrogen/hormone replacement therapy** (ERT/HRT): Estrogen-only (for women without an intact uterus) versus estrogen-progestin hormone replacement (for women with an intact uterus) are used to counteract the increased rate of bone loss noted during the period after the onset of menopause and for treatment of postmenopausal symptoms. Contraindications to estrogen use include a history of breast cancer, uterine cancer, or thromboembolism. It is considered a second-line therapy and use is recommended in the lowest effective dose for the shortest duration within the first few years of menopause.
- **Selective estrogen receptor modulators** (SERMs): This drug class was developed in an attempt to provide the beneficial effects of estrogen therapy in patients unable to take estrogen due to a history of breast or uterine cancer.
- **Calcitonin:** This peptide hormone functions by reducing osteoclastic bone resorption. It is considered to be less effective than bisphosphonates or hormone replacement. It also provides an analgesic effect in patients with acute osteoporotic fractures. It may be administered by nasal spray or injection. Concern with an increased risk of neoplasm and lower efficacy has decreased use of calcitonin.

2. **Anabolic medications**
- **PTH and PTH-related peptide analogs:** Teriparatide (Forteo) is a recombinant human PTH analog (1–34), [rhPTH (1–34)] that, when administered in pulsed dosages, increases new bone formation. It is indicated for treatment of (1) postmenopausal women with osteoporosis at high risk for fracture, (2) men with primary or hypogonadal osteoporosis at high risk for fracture, and (3) men and women with osteoporosis associated with sustained systemic glucocorticoid therapy at high risk for fracture. It mimics the action of PTH at bone, kidney, and intestinal sites (activates osteoblasts, stimulates renal tubular reabsorption of calcium and loss of phosphate, and indirectly increases intestinal calcium absorption via its effect on vitamin D metabolism). It is administered by injection via a prefilled delivery device. Because of the risk of osteogenic sarcoma, teriparatide can only be administered for a lifetime maximum of 24 months and is contraindicated in patients with history of cancer or irradiation. Abaloparatide (Tymlos) is a human PTH-related peptide analog [PTHrP (1–34)] indicated for treatment of postmenopausal women with osteoporosis at high risk for fracture, and its label contains similar warnings as teriparatide. After treatment by either anabolic agent, it is recommended to maintain BMD improvement by using antiresorptive agents.
- **Sclerostin inhibitor:** Romosozumab-aqqg (Evenity) is a monoclonal antibody that blocks the effects of sclerostin and works mainly by increasing new bone formation, and to a lesser extent, by decreasing bone resorption. It is indicated for treatment of osteoporosis in postmenopausal women at high risk for fracture, or patients who have failed or are intolerant to other available therapies.

30. What are some recommendations regarding prevention and treatment of glucocorticoid-induced osteoporosis?
All patients receiving glucocorticoid medications should be counseled to have adequate intake of calcium and vitamin D. Treatment decisions are based on risk stratification (high, medium, low) using the FRAX tool (with adjustment for glucocorticoid dose and BMD, if available), the lowest T-score value, history of fragility fracture, and age ≥40 versus <40 years. Recent guidelines recommend all patients treated with glucocorticoids be assessed for fracture risk within 6 months of starting these medications. Clinical fracture risk assessment is repeated every 12 months during drug treatment. Oral bisphosphonates are considered as the first-line treatment option. Second-line treatments (IV bisphosphonates, teriparatide, denosumab) are considered when oral bisphosphonates are not appropriate.

BONE HEALTH OPTIMIZATION AND SECONDARY FRACTURE PREVENTION

31. What are some factors to consider regarding optimization of bone health prior to spinal surgery?
- **Check vitamin D levels and correct abnormal vitamin D levels prior to spine surgery**. Hypovitaminosis D is extremely common in patients undergoing spinal surgery and is correlated with delayed fusion, decreased fusion rates, and increased disability. Patients undergoing spine surgery are optimized when serum vitamin D concentration is >30 ng/mL.
- **Screen for osteoporosis risk factors and obtain DEXA as indicated based on current guidelines, including use of WHO criteria and the FRAX tool**. Osteopenia and osteoporosis are associated with an increased rate of implant-related complications such as screw loosening, subsidence of anterior column implants, junctional kyphotic deformities, adjacent-level fractures, and nonunion.
- **For patients diagnosed with osteoporosis or severe osteopenia, consider pharmacologic intervention prior to spine surgery**. Based on expert opinion, patients evaluated for elective spine fusion who present with

T-scores between −2 and −3 are considered for treatment for a minimum of 6 weeks with an anabolic agent (teriparatide, abaloparatide) prior to elective surgery. For patients with T-scores between −3 and −4, an anabolic agent is initiated and elective surgery is delayed until repeat DEXA shows improved BMD. If T-score is < -4 or bone density is <0.6 g/cm^3, in addition to initiation of pharmacologic intervention, use of techniques to augment pedicle screw fixation are considered.

- **Currently, no guidelines exist regarding when to initiate or discontinue bisphosphonates before or after spinal fusion procedures.** Based on expert opinion it may be reasonable to hold these medications for a period of time around spinal fusion procedures to limit potential negative effects on bone remodeling and spinal fusion, with the knowledge that these medications may still have beneficial long-term effects with respect to improving BMD and decreasing vertebral fracture risk.

32. What is secondary fracture prevention?

Secondary fracture prevention, also commonly called a *fracture liaison service*, is a comprehensive program to provide evaluation and treatment of bone health after fragility fracture. The goal is to make the first fragility fracture the last fracture. Secondary fracture prevention programs vary in intensity and therefore effectiveness, with the best performing programs consisting of a coordinator imbedded into the orthopedic treatment team. This can be a bone health specialist such as a rheumatologist, endocrinologist, or an advanced practice provider. The American Orthopaedic Association created a national program to encourage orthopedic surgeons to assume care of bone health called *Own the Bone*. This program is highly effective at increasing the number of patients with fragility fractures who receive proper secondary fracture prevention.

OSTEOMALACIA

33. What are the causes of osteomalacia?

The causes of osteomalacia are varied. To arrive at the correct diagnosis, all of the causes must be considered during an appropriate workup, including:

1. Nutritional deficiency
   - Vitamin D deficiency
   - Calcium deficiency due to dietary chelators (e.g., phytates, oxalates)
   - Phosphorus deficiency (e.g., secondary to aluminum-containing antacids)
2. Gastrointestinal malabsorption
   - Intestinal disease
   - Following intestinal surgery
3. Renal tubular acidosis
4. Renal tubular defects causing renal phosphate leak (e.g., vitamin-dependent rickets, type 1 and 2; Fanconi syndrome)
5. Renal osteodystrophy
6. Miscellaneous causes
   - Anticonvulsants (induce hepatic P450 microsomal system, thereby increasing degradation of vitamin D metabolites)
   - Oncogenic
   - Heavy metal intoxication
   - Hypophosphatasia

34. Compare and contrast important findings that aid in distinguishing osteomalacia and osteoporosis.

- **Symptoms:** Osteoporosis is generally asymptomatic until a fracture occurs. Osteomalacia is frequently associated with generalized bone pain and tenderness most commonly localized to the appendicular skeleton.
- **Radiographs:** Osteoporosis and osteomalacia have many similar features but axial involvement predominates in osteoporosis, and appendicular findings predominate in osteomalacia. Findings consistent with osteomalacia include pseudofractures, Looser zones, and biconcave (codfish) vertebrae.
- **Laboratory tests:** Laboratory tests are generally normal in osteoporosis. Osteomalacia is associated with decreased or normal serum calcium, low serum phosphate, increased serum alkaline phosphatase, and increased urine phosphate.
- **Bone biopsy:** In osteoporosis, a biopsy reveals a decreased quantity of normally mineralized bone. In contrast, osteomalacia is characterized by delayed or impaired mineralization of bone matrix. A hallmark of osteomalacia is increased width and extent of osteoid seams.

PAGET DISEASE

35. What is Paget disease?

Paget disease is named after Sir James Paget, who described its clinical and pathologic aspects in 1876. Paget disease is the second most common metabolic bone disease. It has been found in up to 5% of northern European adults older than 55 years. However, most affected individuals are asymptomatic. The cause is unknown, but viral infection and genetic factors are believed to be responsible. The disease causes focal enlargement and deformity of the skeleton. The pathologic lesion is abnormal bone remodeling. The disease progresses through three phases: lytic, lytic-blastic, and blastic. Radiographs are characteristic and show osteosclerosis with bone enlargement. Elevated alkaline phosphatase levels are typical. The wide spectrum of clinical presentation depends on the extent and site of skeletal involvement. Paget disease commonly affects the skull, hip joints, pelvis, and spine. Back pain in the lumbar or sacral region is common. Neurologic deficits may occur due to the compression of the spinal cord or nerve roots from enlarging vertebrae. Spinal stenosis is common when the lower lumbar spine is involved. Treatment options include medication to suppress osteoclastic activity (bisphosphonates, calcitonin), as well as surgical treatment for spinal stenosis, fracture, or degenerative joint disease. Approximately 1% of patients develop malignant degeneration within a focus of Paget disease. This complication usually develops in the peripheral skeleton and rarely involves the spine.

KEY POINTS

1. Osteoporosis is the most prevalent metabolic bone disease and is characterized by a decreased amount of normally mineralized bone per unit volume.
2. Osteoporosis may be diagnosed based on dual-energy x-ray absorptiometry (DEXA) using the WHO criteria as a T-score less than or equal to -2.5.
3. As many as half of all osteoporotic-related fractures occur in patients with bone mineral density (BMD) values classified as low bone mass (osteopenia). Assessment of the probability for fracture using the Fracture Risk Assessment (FRAX) tool can be used to determine the 10-year probability of major osteoporotic fracture and identify patients with low bone mass who might benefit from pharmacologic treatment.
4. Osteomalacia is a metabolic bone disease characterized by delayed or impaired mineralization of bone matrix.
5. Paget disease is the second most common metabolic bone disease.

Websites
1. Osteoporosis and bone physiology: http://courses.washington.edu/bonephys/index.html
2. Clinician's guide to prevention and treatment of osteoporosis (2014): https://link.springer.com/article/10.1007/s00198-014-2794-2
3. International Society for Clinical Densitometry: https://www.iscd.org/about/
4. National Osteoporosis Foundation. Bone Source: https://www.cme.nof.org/Resources.aspx
5. Paget's disease: https://www.nof.org/pagets/
6. World Health Organization Fracture Risk Assessment Tool (FRAX): https://www.sheffield.ac.uk/FRAX/index.aspx

---

BIBLIOGRAPHY

1. Buckley L, Guyatt G, Fink H, et al. American College of Rheumatology Guideline for the prevention and treatment of glucocorticoid-induced osteoporosis. *Arth Rheumatol* 2017;69:1521–1537.
2. Cosman F, deBeur SJ, LeBoff MS, et al. Clinician's guide to prevention and treatment of osteoporosis. *Osteoporos Int* 2014;25:2359–2381.
3. Dell RM, Greene D, Anderson D, et al. Osteoporosis disease management: What every orthopaedic surgeon should know. *J Bone Joint Surg* 2009;91:79–86.
4. Lane JM, Cohn MR, Kreitz T, et al. Metabolic bone disorders of the spine. In: Garfin SR, Eismont FJ, Bell GR, editos. Rothman-Simeone The Spine. 7th ed. Philadelphia, PA: Elsevier; 2018, pp. 1585–1609.
5. McDermott MT. Osteoporosis. In: McDermott MT, editor. Endocrine Secrets. Philadelphia, PA: Saunders; 2013, pp. 90–98.
6. Menga E, Webb AJ, Mesfin A. Do bisphosphonates affect fusion rates? How to manage these medications in the perioperative time frame. *Semin Spine Surg* 2018;30:46–48.
7. Pickhardt PJ, Pooler BD, Lauder T, et al. Opportunistic screening for osteoporosis using abdominal computed tomography scans obtained for other indications. *Ann Intern Med* 2013;158:588–595.
8. Warriner AH, Saag KG. Osteoporosis diagnosis and medical treatment. *Orthop Clin N Am* 2013;44:125–135.
9. Zeytinoglu M, Jain RK, Vokes TJ. Vertebral fracture assessment: Enhancing the diagnosis, prevention, and treatment of osteoporosis. *Bone* 2017;104:54–65.

CHAPTER 65

TREATMENT OPTIONS FOR OSTEOPOROTIC VERTEBRAL COMPRESSION FRACTURES

R. Carter Cassidy, MD

1. **What is the incidence of osteoporotic vertebral compression fractures?**
   Vertebral compression fractures are the most common fractures due to osteoporosis. Vertebral fractures are two to three times more prevalent than hip or wrist fractures. It is estimated that a vertebral fracture due to osteoporosis occurs every 22 seconds worldwide in men and women over age 50. In the United States alone, an estimated 700,000 new osteoporotic vertebral compression fractures occur each year. A 50-year-old white female is estimated to have a 16% lifetime risk of developing a vertebral fracture compared with 5% risk in a male. As only one-third of osteoporotic vertebral compression fractures are recognized clinically, underdiagnosis of vertebral fractures is an important problem.

2. **What is the economic impact of osteoporotic vertebral compression fractures on the health care system?**
   The estimated annual cost of treatment for vertebral compression fractures is 5–10 billion dollars in the United States. Hospital admissions for vertebral compression fractures exceed 150,000 each year, with an average cost of $12,000 per admission.

3. **Who is at greatest risk of developing an osteoporotic vertebral compression fracture?**
   The incidence of osteoporotic vertebral compression fractures increases with age in both males and females. In a large cohort of middle-aged individuals studied with serial radiographs over two decades, 24% of women and 10% of men sustained a vertebral fracture during the study. Although the rate of fracture for men and women over age 50 is not significantly different, the prevalence of fractures is higher in females due to longer life span.

   An important risk factor for development of a vertebral compression fracture is a history of osteoporotic fracture. A person who experiences a vertebral compression fracture is five times more likely to experience an additional fracture, when compared with a control with no fracture.

   Additional risk factors include genetics, race, physical inactivity, smoking, high alcohol intake, prolonged use of glucocorticoids, and low body weight. The risk factors for vertebral compression fractures mirror those for osteoporosis and are classified as modifiable or nonmodifiable:

   Potentially Modifiable Risk Factors
   - Smoking
   - Low body weight
   - Estrogen deficiency
   - Low calcium or vitamin D intake
   - Alcohol excess
   - Caffeine excess
   - Impaired eyesight despite correction
   - Recurrent falls
   - Inadequate physical activity
   - Poor health or frailty
   - Glucocorticoid use

   Nonmodifiable Risk Factors
   - History of fracture during adulthood
   - History of fracture in a first-degree relative
   - Early or surgical menopause
   - Race (White, Asian)
   - Advanced age
   - Female sex
   - Dementia
   - Poor health or frailty

4. **What is the biomechanical explanation for the increased risk of additional osteoporotic vertebral body compression fractures following an initial fracture?**
   Following an initial compression fracture, the loss of vertebral body height leads to kyphotic deformity as the anterior spinal column load-bearing capacity is compromised. As kyphosis at the fracture site increases, the posterior elements of the spine are unloaded, which further increases the load on the compromised anterior spinal column. A vicious cycle develops, which leads to progressive spinal deformity and additional fractures.

5. What is the effect of an osteoporotic vertebral compression fracture on health-related quality of life and longevity?

Osteoporotic vertebral compression fractures have a significant impact on health-related quality of life (HRQOL) measures. A review of 600 patients with various osteoporotic fractures demonstrated that after 2 years from injury, those with vertebral fractures improved slightly from baseline, but still had significant impairment in both physical and mental domains on HRQOL as measured with the 36-Item Short Form Survey (SF-36). In contrast, those with wrist or shoulder fractures returned to normal function after 2 years. Studies have documented an increased mortality risk following osteoporotic vertebral compression fractures compared with a control group. The increased risk of death following vertebral fracture is higher for men (72% survival) than women (84% survival) at 5 years.

6. In which spinal region do osteoporotic vertebral compression fractures most commonly occur?

Osteoporotic vertebral compression fractures occur most commonly at the thoracolumbar junction and the mid-thoracic region but may occur at any location along the spinal column. Cervical osteoporotic fractures are less prevalent than thoracic or lumbar fractures. Fractures above the T5 level are considered as suspicious for a possible spinal tumor.

7. Describe key points to consider in the evaluation of a patient with a suspected osteoporotic compression fracture.

Vertebral compression fractures may present as *acute*, *subacute*, or *chronic* deformities. Statistics show that approximately one-third of radiographically detectable vertebral compression fractures are recognized clinically.

Patient evaluation begins with a detailed history and physical examination. Important elements of the **history** include acuity of pain onset, antecedent trauma, height loss, and prior fractures. Query of medical conditions that affect bone mineral metabolism, such as renal failure, hypogonadism, or chronic steroid use, is important. The onset of symptoms may be insidious, with a specific inciting event reported only in 40% of patients. Pain is often described over the posterior spinal region near the level of the fracture. In some cases, pain may radiate along the chest or abdominal wall, or to proximal or distal spinal regions. Symptoms of back, flank, sacral, or abdominal pain in a patient with risk factors for osteoporosis should prompt consideration of a vertebral compression fracture.

On **physical examination**, the entire spine should be palpated to identify areas of tenderness because the level of the fracture often exhibits point tenderness with palpation or percussion over the posterior spinous process. Although usually normal, a thorough evaluation of motor strength, sensation, and reflexes in the upper and lower extremities should be documented.

Plain radiographs of the spine are recommended as an initial imaging study and are evaluated for the characteristic loss of vertebral height associated with a fracture. Advanced imaging is helpful. **Magnetic resonance imaging (MRI)** or a **combination of a computed tomography (CT) and technetium-99m bone scan** are valuable when the acuity of the fracture is in question or when metastatic disease is a consideration (Fig. 65.1). If CT is performed, bone mineral density can be estimated by measuring the Hounsfield units against established norms using software.

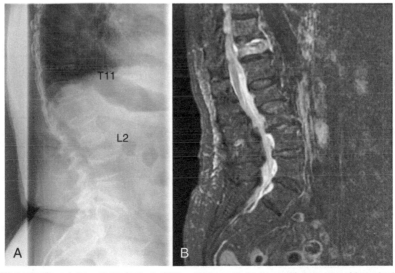

Fig. 65.1 (A) Lateral radiograph demonstrates fractures of T11 and L2 in an elderly woman with acute onset of thoracolumbar pain. (B) T2 sequence magnetic resonance imaging shows increased signal in T11, while the L2 body has no increased signal compared with the surrounding vertebral bodies. This signifies the T11 fracture as acute and the L2 fracture as chronic and healed.

Dual-energy x-ray absorptiometry (DEXA) scanning to determine bone density is recommended for women aged ≥65 and men aged ≥70 years, men and postmenopausal women aged 50–69 years with clinical risk factors for fracture, adults with a fracture at age ≥50 years, as well as adults with a condition (e.g., rheumatoid arthritis) or taking a medication (e.g., glucocorticoids) associated with low bone mass or bone loss. The bone densitometer can also be used to perform a **vertebral fracture assessment** and screen the entire thoracic and lumbar spine for fractures.

Laboratory tests play a role when infection, malignancy, or metabolic bone disease is suspected. Tests to order include a complete blood count, comprehensive metabolic panel, C-reactive protein level, erythrocyte sedimentation rate, serum and urine protein electrophoresis, and 25-hydroxyvitamin D level.

8. What are important features to assess on plain radiographs that demonstrate a compression fracture?
   - **Loss of vertebral height** is assessed and described in terms of a percentage of normal height. Loss of height is described as mild (<25%), moderate (25%–40%), or severe (>40%). *Vertebrae plana* is a term used to describe extreme loss of vertebral body height that occurs when the vertebral body is reduced to a thin, flat shape.
   - **Kyphotic deformity** may be determined by measuring deformity at the level of the fractured vertebra or with reference to adjacent vertebrae: (1) **vertebral wedge angle** (angle between the superior and inferior endplates of the fractured vertebra) and (2) **local kyphotic deformity** (angle between the vertebral endplates above and below the level of fracture).
   - **Vertebral body fracture morphology** is described as a wedge (anterior height loss exceeds posterior height loss), crush (symmetric loss of height), or biconcave deformity. Wedge fractures are more common in the thoracic spine, while biconcave fractures are most common in the lumbar spine. Rarely, burst fractures may occur and result in retropulsion of bone into the spinal canal and may be associated with neurologic deficit.
   - **Discontinuity of the posterior vertebral body wall** is suspected in fractures with pedicle widening or loss of height exceeding 50%. CT and/or MRI are the best tests to assess integrity of the posterior vertebral body cortex.
   - **Dynamic mobility** is detected by comparing a supine cross-table lateral radiograph with a standing lateral radiograph centered at the level of fracture. Increased vertebral body height or decreased kyphotic deformity on a supine radiograph in comparison with findings on an upright radiograph suggest that vertebral height may be partially restored with a vertebral body augmentation procedure.
   - **Intravertebral clefts** (gas-filled cavities) within compression fractures may be present and represent fracture nonunion or ischemic necrosis of the vertebral body (Kümmell disease) and imply dynamic mobility at the level of fracture.
   - **Fracture acuity** is difficult to determine from a single plain radiograph. Change in fracture configuration over time with loss of height supports the diagnosis of an acute or subacute fracture. Acute fractures are often defined as less than 3 months of age, while chronic fractures are defined as greater than 3 months of age.

9. What is the role of MRI in the diagnosis and treatment of osteoporotic vertebral compression fractures?
   MRI is the single best imaging study for evaluating a vertebral body compression fracture. MRI is useful to distinguish between acute and chronic fractures when a patient presents with a spinal fracture on plain radiographs. An area of increased signal on T2 images or short-tau inversion recovery (STIR) sequences and low or isointense signal on T1 sequences is indicative of an acute fracture. MRI is helpful in determining the integrity of the posterior vertebral body wall. MRI is also helpful in evaluating the patency of the spinal canal, especially if there is retropulsion associated with the fracture or in patients with preexisting spinal stenosis. MRI can also identify atypical cases where a tumor or infection is the cause of the vertebral fracture.

10. What is the role of a technetium bone scan in the diagnosis and treatment of compression fractures?
   Increased vertebral body uptake on a bone scan occurs 48–72 hours following a vertebral fracture. However, bone scans can be positive for up to 18 months following a compression fracture, even if a vertebral fracture is healed and asymptomatic. Therefore, the role of bone scanning in an acute vertebral compression fracture is limited. However, it does play a role in evaluating vertebral fractures in patients who are unable to undergo MRI (e.g., due to a pacemaker).

11. What are the treatment options for osteoporotic vertebral compression fractures?
   The goal of treatment is rapid return to baseline functional status, while limiting possible complications. Traditionally, osteoporotic compression fractures were treated nonoperatively except in unusual cases where the fracture was associated with neurologic compromise or extreme spinal instability. Rationale for this approach included the finding that a certain percentage of these fractures were associated with mild symptoms that improved over time. In addition, surgical treatment in this population is complicated by surgical morbidity due to associated medical comorbidities and implant complications due to poor fixation in osteoporotic bone using traditional surgical techniques.

Table 65.1 Treatment Options for Osteoporotic Vertebral Body Compression Fractures.

MEDICAL TREATMENT OPTIONS	SURGICAL TREATMENT OPTIONS
Analgesic medication	Minimally invasive vertebral body augmentation • Vertebroplasty • Kyphoplasty

Spinal orthoses	Traditional maximally invasive spine surgery
	• Anterior approach
	• Posterior approach
	• Combined anterior and posterior approach
	  • Single incision
	  • Separate anterior and posterior incisions

Rehabilitation approaches • Weight-bearing exercise • Fall prevention program	Hybrid approaches • Vertebral body augmentation combined with laminectomy • Vertebral body augmentation combined with laminectomy and posterior spinal instrumentation

Osteoporosis medications
• Calcium
• Vitamin D
• Anticatabolics
  • Bisphosphonates
  • Hormone replacement
  • Selective estrogen modulators
  • Denosumab
  • Calcitonin
• Anabolics
  • Teriparatide
  • Abaloparatide
  • Romosozumab
	Special procedures
	• Pedicle subtraction osteotomy
	  • Burst fractures with canal compromise
	• Vertebral column resection
	  • Salvage revision for complex deformity

Studies have shown that although some patients with compression fractures improve without intervention, up to two-thirds may experience intense pain 1 year after injury. This led to current treatment approaches including analgesics, spinal orthoses, and medications (calcium, vitamin D, bisphosphonates, denosumab, teriparatide, abaloparatide, romosozumab) to prevent the next compression fracture by treating the underlying cause of osteoporosis. Administration of nasal calcitonin (200 IU [International Units]) for 4 weeks following an acute fracture has shown benefit in reducing pain. Minimally invasive vertebral augmentation using polymethyl methacrylate (PMMA) is a treatment option in select patients. Decision making is based on fracture-related factors (i.e., acuity, morphology) and patient-related factors, including medical comorbidities, pain level, ability to comply with treatment, and patient preference. Selection of a specific treatment option is tempered by realistic expectations and goals regarding the specific intervention in the context of the best available medical evidence regarding treatment effectiveness and outcomes (Table 65.1)

12. What are potential complications associated with orthotic treatment of osteoporotic vertebral body compression fractures?
Orthotic treatment of osteoporotic spine fractures is challenging. There is a paucity of data to support the role of orthotic treatment to enhance fracture healing, mobility, or pain relief following osteoporotic spinal fracture. Lack of compliance with treatment due to brace discomfort frequently leads to abandonment of treatment. If not monitored closely, skin breakdown can occur, especially in patients of poor health and questionable mental status. The most common types of orthoses prescribed are a limited contact orthoses such as a Jewett extension brace or an elastic brace.

13. What is vertebroplasty?
Vertebroplasty is the percutaneous injection of PMMA into a vertebral body to provide stabilization and relief of pain. The procedure was introduced in the 1980s, initially for treatment of vertebral hemangiomas. Currently, the procedure is most commonly used to treat acute and subacute osteoporotic vertebral body compression fractures. The procedure is performed with local anesthetic, with or without intravenous sedation, or with general anesthesia. The patient is placed prone on a radiolucent table and positioned to optimize fracture alignment. High-quality, high-resolution fluoroscopy is required and biplane fluoroscopy is preferable. Following placement of a needle into the vertebral body through either a pedicular or extrapedicular approach, bone cement mixed with barium contrast is introduced into the vertebral body with fluoroscopic monitoring. Multiple small syringes

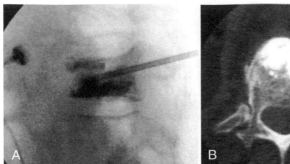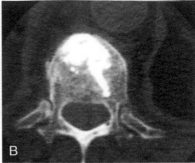

Fig. 65.2 Vertebroplasty. (A) Lateral fluoroscopic view during procedure. (B) Postoperative computed tomography demonstrating cement placement. (From Resnick D, Kransdorf MJ. Bone and Joint Imaging. 3rd ed. Philadelphia, PA: Saunders; 2005.)

are commonly used to introduce the PMMA into the access needle. Alternatively, use of a remote cement delivery system permits the operator to stand away from the fluoroscope and needle to decrease radiation exposure. The typical amount of cement injected varies from 2 to 4 mL for thoracic vertebrae and 4 to 8 mL for lumbar vertebrae (Fig. 65.2).

14. **What is kyphoplasty?**
    Kyphoplasty is a minimally invasive vertebral augmentation technique developed in the 1990s for treatment of painful vertebral body compression fractures. The procedure is intended to provide a method for achieving reduction of vertebral body compression fractures prior to injection of PMMA. It permits injection of high-viscosity cement under low pressure, which is intended to minimize complications related to inadvertent cement leakage. The procedure is most commonly performed under general anesthesia. A Jamshidi needle is placed into the vertebral body through a pedicular or extrapedicular approach. A guidewire is used to place a working cannula into the vertebral body. If a biopsy is planned, it is performed at this time. Next, a balloon tamp is placed and inflated with visible radiocontrast medium. Inflation of the balloon tamp reduces the fracture and creates a cavity for cement insertion. The balloon tamps are removed and cement is introduced under fluoroscopic visualization. Approximately 2–6 mL of cement per side can be accepted at a single vertebral level (Fig. 65.3).

15. **Compare and contrast the minimally invasive methods of vertebral augmentation, vertebroplasty, and kyphoplasty.**
    Vertebroplasty and kyphoplasty are methods of stabilizing fractured vertebral bodies. Both techniques utilize a percutaneous approach to the vertebral body. A cannulated needle is inserted into the body, under fluoroscopy, through one or both pedicles at the level of fracture.
    • Vertebroplasty is performed by injecting liquid PMMA containing barium contrast into the body. The cement fills the voids within the osseous trabeculae to stabilize the fractured vertebra. This is typically less viscous cement than is used in kyphoplasty, which theoretically is more likely to not only fill the trabecular bone but also leak out of the vertebral body. Fracture reduction occurs due to dynamic mobility at the fracture site and from patient positioning on the fluoroscopy table.
    • In kyphoplasty, a balloon is introduced into the body through the working cannula. The balloon is then inflated to create a cavity. A more viscous cement than is used in vertebroplasty is then placed into the void created by the balloon tamp and is less likely to leak from the vertebra. Theoretically, the balloon aids in reducing the fracture by distracting the vertebral endplates relative to one another (Fig. 65.4).

16. **Explain how to safely access the thoracic and lumbar spine with a Jamshidi needle to perform a vertebroplasty or kyphoplasty.**
    The most common approach utilized is the transpedicular approach. Anteroposterior (AP) and lateral fluoroscopy is mandatory, and use of two C-arms is ideal, to permit simultaneous AP and lateral views of the target vertebra. The level of the fracture is localized on the AP view. The skin is marked at the lateral border of the pedicle on the AP view. A small incision is made and the needle is advanced to contact bone at the 10 o'clock position on the left pedicle and 2 o'clock position on the right pedicle on the AP view. Next, the lateral view is examined to guide needle trajectory in the sagittal plane. The needle is advanced into the vertebral body while monitoring its path on AP and lateral fluoroscopic images. To avoid violation of the medial pedicle wall and unintended entry into the spinal canal, *the needle should not cross the medial pedicle border on the AP fluoroscopic view until the needle has passed the posterior cortex of the vertebral body on the lateral view.*
    In the thoracic spine, a modification of the standard approach, the lateral extrapedicular approach, may be used when the pedicles are small and difficult to cannulate. In the lumbar spine, a posterolateral extrapedicular approach is also an alternative to the standard transpedicular approach.

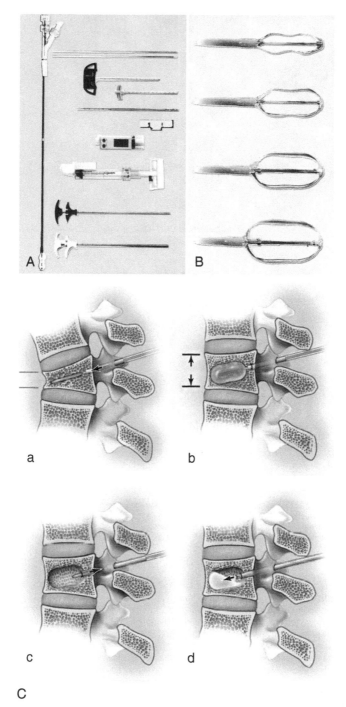

Fig. 65.3 (A) Instruments used in kyphoplasty, including large-bore trocars, drill, syringe for injecting cement with attached pressure monitor, cement delivery device, and bone tamp. (B) Inflation of balloon tamp is demonstrated. (C) Steps in the kyphoplasty procedure: *(a)* needle and cannula insertion, *(b)* placement of balloon tamp, *(c)* creation of cavity, and *(d)* cement insertion. (A and B: From Majd ME, Farley S, Holt RT. Preliminary outcomes and efficacy of the first 360 consecutive kyphoplasties for the treatment of painful osteoporotic vertebral compression fractures. Spine J 2005;5[3]: 244–255. C: From Canale ST, Beaty JH, Phillips BB. Campbell's Operative Orthopaedics. 11th ed. Philadelphia, PA: Mosby; 2007.)

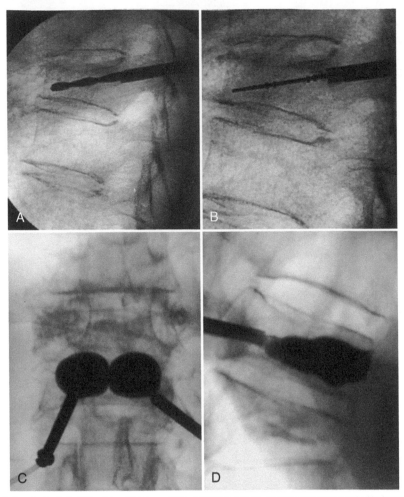

Fig. 65.4 Balloon kyphoplasty, T12 vertebra. (A) A 3-mm drill is directed through the anterior extent of the vertebral body after initial placement of 11-gauge needles and subsequent placement of a working cannula. (B) Insertion of the balloon tamp before inflation. (C) Inflation of the balloon tamp filled with sterile saline and radiocontrast dye, anteroposterior view. (D) Deposition of bone cement following cavity creation and vertebral height restoration. (From Haaga JR, Vikran SD, Michael F, et al. CT and MRI of the Whole Body. 5th ed. Philadelphia, PA: Mosby; 2008.)

17. **When are vertebroplasty or kyphoplasty indicated for treatment of osteoporotic vertebral compression fractures?**

Minimally invasive vertebral augmentation procedures are indicated for the treatment of pain related to acute and subacute osteoporotic vertebral compression fractures following failure to control pain with medical management. No consensus exists regarding how long to wait to perform these procedures following an acute fracture. Early intervention can be considered after 1–2 weeks in patients who have become nonambulatory due to progressive vertebral body compression fractures and for patients who are hospitalized due to pain and functional impairment. In ambulatory patients with adequate pain control, intervention may be deferred for 4–6 weeks. Certain fracture patterns are less likely to improve with standard medical management: burst fractures, wedge fractures with more than 30° of kyphotic deformity, fractures at the thoracolumbar junction, fractures with intravertebral clefts, and fractures with progressive height loss on serial radiographs. Ideal candidates for vertebral augmentation report pain that is sufficiently severe to limit daily activities, demonstrate bone edema at the level of fracture on MRI, and have focal tenderness at the level of fracture on physical examination. In general, chronic vertebral compression fractures are not an indication for vertebral augmentation procedures. Also, vertebral augmentation can be considered in those for whom orthoses are contraindicated. Typically, use of a spinal orthosis is unnecessary after vertebral augmentation.

18. **What are contraindications to minimally invasive vertebral augmentation?**
    - Vertebral fractures associated with a high-energy injury mechanism
    - Vertebral fractures associated with retropulsed bone and/or discontinuity of the posterior vertebral body cortical margin
    - A fracture associated with neurologic deficit
    - Pain unrelated to vertebral body collapse
    - Vertebral osteomyelitis in the vertebra considered for injection
    - Severe vertebral collapse (vertebra plana) that makes injection technically impossible
    - Inability to adequately visualize vertebral anatomy
    - Patients with coagulopathy
    - Severe cardiopulmonary difficulties
    - Chronic fractures
    - Allergy to PMMA or opacification agents
    - Lack of surgical backup to treat adverse events

19. **What complications have been reported in association with vertebroplasty and kyphoplasty?**
    Reported complications include persistent pain, nerve root injury, spinal cord compression due to cement extravasation, cement embolism, infection, hypotension secondary to bone cement monomer, medical complications, and death. Rib fractures, pedicle fractures, and transverse process fractures may occur during the procedure. New vertebral fractures may occur following the procedure at adjacent levels, remote spinal levels, and previously treated vertebral levels. Although vertebral body cement augmentation procedures are usually well tolerated and associated with overall low complication rates, serious neurologic complications due to cement leakage may result in compression of adjacent neural structures and necessitate emergency decompressive surgery (Fig. 65.5). Cement injection into the paravertebral vessels may lead to pulmonary emboli with serious sequelae.

20. **Does kyphoplasty or vertebroplasty increase the risk of an adjacent level fracture?**
    This complication has been reviewed in multiple studies, and the data are conflicting as to whether placing cement in a vertebral body poses an independent increased risk of fracture in the adjacent bodies. Following kyphoplasty, the risk of adjacent-level fracture seems to be highest in the first 2 months following the procedure (Fig. 65.6). Evidence suggests that patients with steroid-induced osteoporosis are more likely to refracture than

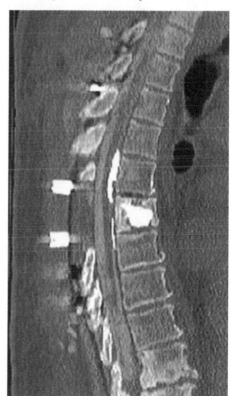

Fig. 65.5 Sagittal computed tomography reconstruction demonstrating a clinically significant cement leak along the posterior longitudinal ligament. This reinforces the importance of careful fluoroscopic monitoring while injecting cement, and ensuring that radiographic visualization of the target level is optimized.

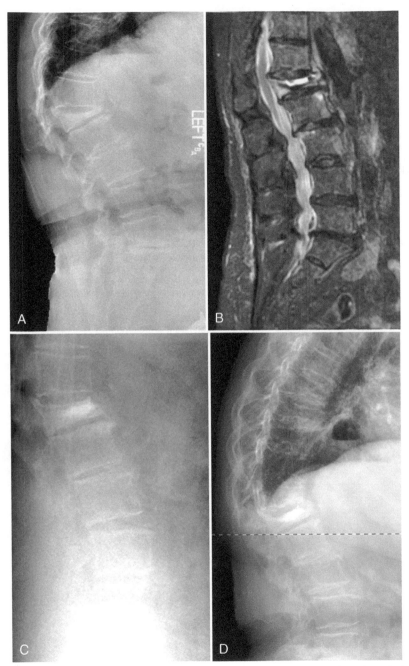

Fig. 65.6 An 80-year-old woman with no antecedent trauma presented with 2 months of back pain, despite bracing and pain medication. (A) Lateral radiograph demonstrating significant collapse of L1. (B) T2 magnetic resonance imaging of the same patient, with high signal intensity present at the L1 fracture. This is an intravertebral cleft, which implies dynamic mobility at the fracture site. (C) Radiograph immediately following kyphoplasty. Notice the adjacent vertebral body morphology. (D) Radiograph at 6 weeks after kyphoplasty. Patient reported excellent pain relief immediately after surgery, but more pain at week 5. Notice the deformity of the inferior endplate at T12, signifying acute adjacent-level vertebral fracture.

patients with primary osteoporosis. It is important to realize that certain adjacent level fractures may reflect the natural history of osteoporosis rather than the consequence of cement augmentation. In patients with osteoporotic compression fractures treated without kyphoplasty or vertebroplasty, the annual incidence of an additional vertebral compression fracture is approximately 20%. A meta-analysis of treatment of fractures with PMMA augmentation versus nonoperative care by Anderson and colleagues showed that the rate of new fractures following either non-operative treatment or PMMA augmentation was similar (around 20%). Appropriate medical therapy for osteoporosis can decrease the risk of new fractures.

21. Is vertebral augmentation an effective treatment for osteoporotic compression fractures?
Multiple studies have reported that vertebral body augmentation with PMMA leads to rapid diminution of pain and improvement in HRQOL measures that persist in the short and medium term in appropriately selected patients. There have been some trials directly comparing kyphoplasty and vertebroplasty but the results of these investigations are mixed. In one meta-analysis of these techniques, adverse events were rare, but short-term adverse events were more common with vertebroplasty, specifically cement leakage. Publication of results from two randomized clinical trials in the *New England Journal of Medicine* in 2009 questioned the efficacy of vertebroplasty. Subsequent studies by Wardlaw and colleagues (kyphoplasty) and Farrokhi and colleagues (vertebroplasty) countered these arguments. Results of a meta-analysis by Anderson and colleagues showed greater pain relief, functional recovery, and improved HRQOL with cement augmentation using either vertebroplasty or kyphoplasty compared with controls at early (<12 weeks) and late (6–12 month) time points.

22. What other materials, besides PMMA, have been investigated for use in vertebral body augmentation?
Additional materials that have been investigated to augment vertebral bodies include calcium phosphate, calcium sulfate, and allograft bone. Unlike PMMA, calcium-based cements are biologically active. The osteoconductive nature of these products theoretically allows for the vertebral body to heal and integrate the cement, unlike PMMA.

23. When is spinal instrumentation and fusion considered for the treatment of osteoporotic vertebral body compression fractures?
Major reconstructive spinal surgery consisting of instrumentation and fusion for osteoporotic spine fractures has a high rate of complications and is reserved for patients with significant neurologic deficits, spinal instability, or severe spinal deformities. Reconstructive spinal surgery is rarely indicated for patients with osteoporosis and multiple compression fractures in the absence of neurologic deficit.

24. What potential complications are associated with spinal instrumentation and fusion in the osteoporotic patient? Compare and contrast the limitations of anterior, posterior, and circumferential surgical approaches.
Spinal instrumentation and fusion for treatment of osteoporotic spine fractures, although not common, remains a necessary procedure in some instances. General complications associated with spine surgery include blood loss, neurologic injury, dural tear, and infection, as well as perioperative anesthetic and medical complications. Problems specific to spinal instrumentation in osteoporotic bone include an increased risk of implant failure, loss of correction, and adjacent-level fractures.
- Anterior surgical approaches are often poorly tolerated in elderly patients. Anterior rod-screw constructs provide poor purchase in osteoporotic bone. Anterior bone grafts and cages tend to subside and telescope into adjacent vertebral bodies leading to implant construct failure. It can be difficult to obtain and maintain correction of kyphotic deformities via an isolated anterior surgical approach.
- Isolated posterior spinal instrumentation and fusion procedures are insufficient for correction of kyphotic spinal deformity in patients with osteoporosis. Anterior spinal column load sharing is impaired in this setting, resulting in increased stress on posterior spinal implants. As posterior implants loosen and fail, kyphotic deformity recurs and the implant construct fails. An additional problem that can occur following posterior instrumentation and fusion in the osteoporotic patient is the development of a fracture at the cranial or caudal fixation point or at the level above the construct, which leads to junctional kyphosis and the need for additional surgery.
- Circumferential surgical approaches provide a method for restoration of anterior column load sharing and improve arthrodesis rates, thereby decreasing the risk of implant construct failure. However, extensive anterior and posterior procedures are not well tolerated in elderly patients with osteoporotic compression fractures and are associated with significant morbidity.

25. What surgical procedure has developed as an alternative to a combined anterior and posterior procedure for treatment of patients with kyphotic deformities and neurologic deficits secondary to osteoporotic compression fractures?
A posterior closing-wedge osteotomy procedure (pedicle subtraction osteotomy [PSO]) is an effective procedure in this setting and can be accomplished in a shorter operative time and with less morbidity than a combined AP procedure. Pedicle screws are placed at multiple levels above and below the fractured vertebra and a wide laminectomy is performed. Under direct visualization, the pedicles and lateral vertebral body are removed. Next, the portion of the

posterior vertebral body wall compressing the dural sac is removed. The kyphotic deformity is corrected by closing the osteotomy by connecting the screws to precontoured rods and by changing the patient's position on the operating table. Sagittal alignment and anterior spinal column load sharing are restored through a single surgical approach.

26. **What techniques can be considered to limit spinal instrumentation–related complications in osteoporotic bone?**
    - Use multiple points of fixation (segmental fixation) to distribute stress over many spine segments
    - Use large-diameter screws that fill the pedicle
    - Supplement screws with sublaminar wires or hooks
    - Reinforce screws with PMMA (this indication for use is not approved by the U.S. Food and Drug Administration and represents "off-label" use)
    - Use cross-links to connect rods on each side of the spine to increase stability of the implant construct
    - Perform a supplemental anterior fusion to restore anterior column load sharing
    - Accept fewer degrees of spinal deformity correction to decrease loads on spinal implants
    - Avoid ending implant constructs at kyphotic spinal segments or at transitional areas of the spine
    - Consider PMMA augmentation of vertebra at the proximal level of screw fixation and at the next adjacent vertebra to decrease the risk of junctional fractures (this indication for use is not approved by the U.S. Food and Drug Administration and represents "off-label" use)

27. **What are some emerging techniques for treatment of osteoporotic fractures?**
    Innovative techniques include use of bioactive cements, implantation of devices in combination with PMMA into the fractured vertebral body to maintain vertebral height and limit cement leak (e.g., polyetheretherketone [PEEK] implants), and use of radiofrequency energy for vertebral body cavity creation. Hybrid surgical procedures have been reported that combine vertebral body augmentation procedures with traditional open surgical techniques. In patients with kyphotic deformity, posterior pedicle screw-rod fixation has been performed in combination with posterior surgical decompression and cement augmentation. Although compromise of the posterior vertebral body cortex was originally considered an absolute contraindication to vertebral augmentation due to risk of cement leakage into the spinal canal, intraoperative visualization of the posterior vertebral body wall during open surgical decompression combined with cement augmentation has been described in the treatment of patients with symptomatic neurologic compression related to fractures. This technique permits immediate detection and treatment of cement extravasation and allows for optimal cement placement, as well as immediate spinal canal decompression if a critical cement leak occurs. This technique has been applied to osteoporotic vertebral fractures, as well as vertebral defects resulting from metastatic tumors. Use of cement products not receiving U.S. Food and Drug Administration clearance specifically for vertebroplasty or kyphoplasty represents off-label use.

KEY POINTS

1. Vertebral compression fractures are the most common type of fracture due to osteoporosis.
2. Kyphoplasty and vertebroplasty provide pain relief and improvement in quality of life measures in appropriately selected patients with acute and subacute osteoporotic vertebral body compression fractures.
3. When placing a needle into the vertebra during a kyphoplasty or vertebroplasty procedure, the needle should not cross the medial pedicle border on the AP fluoroscopic view until the needle has passed the posterior cortex of the vertebral body on the lateral view.
4. Major reconstructive spinal surgery for osteoporotic spine fractures has a high rate of complications and is reserved for patients with significant neurologic deficits, spinal instability, or severe spinal deformities.

Websites
1. International Osteoporosis Foundation Facts and Statistics: https://www.iofbonehealth.org/facts-statistics
2. National Osteoporosis Foundation Professional Learning Center: https://www.cme.nof.org/
3. Treatments for compression fractures: kyphoplasty and vertebroplasty: http://www.spineuniverse.com/display-article.php/article1525.html

---

BIBLIOGRAPHY

1. Anderson, P. A., Froyshteter, A. B., & Tontz, Jr., W. L. (2013). Meta-analysis of vertebral augmentation compared to conservative treatment for osteoporotic spinal fractures. *Journal of Bone and Mineral Research, 28*(2), 372–382.
2. Ballane, G., Cauley, J. A., Luckey, M. M., & Fuleihan, G. E. (2017). Worldwide prevalence and incidence of osteoporotic vertebral fractures. *Osteoporosis International, 28*(5), 1531–1542.
3. Buchbinder, R., Osborne, R. H., Ebeling, P. R., Wark, J. D., Mitchell, P., Wriedt, C., et al. (2009). A randomized trial of vertebroplasty for painful osteoporotic vertebral fractures. *New England Journal of Medicine, 361*(6), 557–568.

4. Burval, D. J., McLain, R. F., Milks, R., & Inceoglu, S. (2007). Primary pedicle screw augmentation in osteoporotic lumbar vertebrae: Biomechanical analysis of pedicle fixation strength. *Spine, 32*(10), 1077–1083.
5. Farrokhi, M. R., Alibai, E., & Maghami, Z. (2011). Randomized controlled trial of percutaneous vertebroplasty versus optimal medical management for the relief of pain and disability in acute osteoporotic vertebral compression fractures. *Journal of Neurosurgery: Spine, 14*(5), 561–569.
6. Hallberg, I., Rosenqvist, A. M., Kartous, L., Löfman, O., Wahlström, O., & Toss, G. (2004). Health-related quality of life after osteoporotic fractures. *Osteoporosis International, 15*(10), 834–841.
7. Kallmes, D. F., Comstock, B. A., Heagerty, P. J., Turner, J. A., Wilson, D. J., Diamond, T. H., et al. (2009). A randomized trial of vertebroplasty for osteoporotic spinal fractures. *New England Journal of Medicine, 361*(6), 569–579.
8. Klazen, C. A., Lohle, P. N., de Vries, J., Jansen, F. H., Tielbeek, A. V., Blonk, M. C., et al. (2010). Vertebroplasty versus conservative treatment in acute osteoporotic vertebral compression fractures (Vertos II): An open-label randomised trial. *Lancet, 376*(9746), 1085–1092.
9. Lee, M. J., Dumonski, M., Cahill, P., Stanley, T., Park, D., & Singh, K. (2009). Percutaneous treatment of vertebral compression fractures: A meta-analysis of complications. *Spine, 34*(11), 1228–1132.
10. Patel, A. A., Vaccaro, A. R., Martyak, G. G., Harrop, J. S., Albert, T. J., Ludwig, S. C., et al. (2007). Neurologic deficit following percutaneous vertebral stabilization. *Spine, 32*(16), 1728–1734.
11. Singh, K., Heller, J. G., Samartzis, D., Price, J. S., An, H. S., Yoon, S. T., et al. (2005). Open vertebral cement augmentation combined with lumbar decompression for the operative management of thoracolumbar stenosis secondary to osteoporotic burst fractures. *Clinical Spine Surgery, 18*(5), 413–419.
12. Suk, S. I., Kim, J. H., Lee, S. M., Chung, E. R., & Lee, J. H. (2003). Anterior-posterior surgery versus posterior closing wedge osteotomy in posttraumatic kyphosis with neurologic compromised osteoporotic fracture. *Spine 28*(18), 2170–2175.
13. Taylor, R. S., Taylor, R. J., & Fritzell, P. (2006). Balloon kyphoplasty and vertebroplasty for vertebral compression fractures: A comparative systematic review of efficacy and safety. *Spine, 31*(23), 2747–2755.
14. Wardlaw, D., Cummings, S. R., Van Meirhaeghe, J., Bastian, L., Tillman, J. B., Ranstam, J., et al. (2009). Efficacy and safety of balloon kyphoplasty compared with nonsurgical care for vertebral compression fracture (FREE): A randomized controlled trial. *Lancet, 373*(9668), 1016–1024.

CHAPTER 66

SPINAL INFECTIONS

Vincent J. Devlin, MD and John C. Steinmann, DO

1. How are spinal infections classified?
   - **Host immune response:** Pyogenic versus granulomatous
   - **Anatomic location:** Vertebral body, disc, epidural space, subdural space, facet joint, paraspinous soft tissue
   - **Infectious route:** Hematogenous, local extension, direct inoculation
   - **Host age:** Pediatric versus adult
   - **Duration:** Acute versus chronic spinal infection

PYOGENIC INFECTIONS

PYOGENIC VERTEBRAL OSTEOMYELITIS

2. What are the three most frequent routes by which bacterial infection spreads to the spinal column?
   The most common method for bacteria to spread to the spine is by the **hematogenous** route. Common sources of infection include infected catheters, urinary tract infection (UTI), dental caries, intravenous drug use, and skin infections.
   The second most common route is direct inoculation via trauma, puncture, or following spine injections or surgery.
   The third most common route is local extension from an adjacent soft tissue infection or paravertebral abscess.
   The disc is nearly always involved in pyogenic vertebral infections. The nucleus pulposus is relatively avascular in adults, providing little or no immune response, and thus is rapidly destroyed by bacterial enzymes. Bacterial infection may begin in the vertebral body and extend into the disc space or initially develop in the disc and spread to adjacent vertebrae. In contrast, granulomatous infections typically do not involve the disc space.

3. Define risk factors for developing pyogenic vertebral osteomyelitis.
   Risk factors for development of pyogenic vertebral osteomyelitis (PVO) include advanced age, diabetes, individuals on hemodialysis, intravenous drug use, immune compromise, individuals with HIV, recent or concurrent extraspinal infection (UTI, pneumonia, endocarditis, soft tissue infection), long-term steroid use, recent surgical procedures, and history of malignancy.

4. Describe the clinical presentation of pyogenic vertebral infection.
   The most consistent symptom at presentation is spinal pain, which is noted in 90% of patients. Pain generally has an insidious onset. Pain is often exacerbated by activity, although it may be variably affected by recumbency or worse at night. Paravertebral muscle tenderness, spasm, and limited spinal motion are common physical findings. Fever is documented in approximately 50% of patients. Neurologic deficits are noted in up to one-third of patients at initial presentation. Weight loss is often present and occurs over a period of weeks to months. Spinal deformity is a late presenting finding. A delay in diagnosis is common, with 50% of patients reporting symptoms for more than 3 months before diagnosis. The lumbar region is the most common site of PVO (50%), followed by the thoracic region (35%), and cervical region (15%).

5. What is the most common pyogenic organism responsible for spinal infection?
   Staphylococcus aureus is the most common organism and has been identified in over 50% of cases. However, infections due to a diverse group of gram-positive, gram-negative, and mixed pathogens may occur. Gram-negative organisms (*Escherichia coli, Pseudomonas* spp., *Proteus* spp.) are associated with spinal infections following genitourinary infections or procedures. Intravenous drug abusers have an increased incidence of *Pseudomonas* infections. Anaerobic infections are common in people with diabetes and following penetrating trauma. Antibiotic-resistant organisms are noted with increasing frequency, including methicillin-resistant *S. aureus* (MRSA), vancomycin-resistant *S. aureus* (VRSA), and vancomycin-resistant *Enterococcus* (VRE).

6. When pyogenic vertebral infection is suspected, what diagnostic tests are indicated?
An algorithm for evaluation of a suspected spinal infection includes:
   - **Laboratory tests:** Complete blood count (CBC), erythrocyte sedimentation rate (ESR), C-reactive protein (CRP), aerobic and anaerobic blood cultures
   - **Imaging studies:** Magnetic resonance imaging (MRI) is the imaging study of choice. If MRI is unavailable or contraindicated, next best options include technetium bone scan with or without a gallium scan, positron emission tomography (PET), or computed tomography (CT)
   - **Biopsy:** CT-guided or open biopsy
   - **Echocardiogram:** Indicated for patients with cardiac risk factors, history of intravenous drug use, or failure to improve with initial treatment

7. Discuss the relative value of different laboratory tests in the diagnosis of pyogenic vertebral infection.
The white blood cell count on a CBC is not a sensitive test for diagnosis of PVO as it is elevated in fewer than half of patients. The ESR is elevated in more than 90% of patients with infection but is nonspecific and may be normal in the presence of low-virulence organisms. CRP is typically elevated in pyogenic infections and is considered more specific than ESR, and is helpful for monitoring treatment as it normalizes more quickly than ESR following adequate infection treatment. Blood cultures, although helpful if positive, yield the causative organism in only one-quarter to one-half of cases.

8. Describe the roles of the various imaging studies in the diagnosis of pyogenic vertebral infection.
Radiographs: Positive radiographic findings are not evident for 2–4 weeks after the onset of symptoms. The earliest detectable radiographic finding is disc space narrowing, followed by localized osteopenia, and finally destruction of the vertebral endplates. Radiographs remain valuable to rule out other noninfectious etiologies responsible for back pain symptoms and to follow-up nonoperative and operative treatment. Upright radiographs are used to evaluate spinal alignment and stability.

 MRI: Considered the imaging modality of choice for diagnosis of vertebral infection. It provides detailed assessment of the vertebral body, disc space, spinal canal, and surrounding soft tissue not provided with any other single test. The typical findings associated with pyogenic vertebral infection are decreased signal in the vertebral body and adjacent discs on T1-weighted sequences and increased signal intensity noted in these structures on T2-weighted images. Paravertebral abscess, if present, also demonstrates increased uptake on T2-weighted images. Gadolinium contrast is a useful adjunct in diagnosing infection because the disc and involved regions of adjacent vertebral bodies enhance in the presence of contrast (Fig. 66.1A,B).

 Radionuclide studies: Technetium-99m bone scanning is informative in the early diagnosis of PVO as it demonstrates positive findings before the development of radiographically detectable changes. It has utility as a screening study if MRI is unavailable or contraindicated and may be performed in conjunction with a gallium scan. PET with 18F-fluoro-2-deoxy-2D-glucose (FDG) is another alternative diagnostic study when MRI is not possible. However, radionuclide studies do not provide sufficiently detailed information for surgical planning.

 CT: Plays a role in defining the extent of bony destruction and localization of lesions for biopsies.

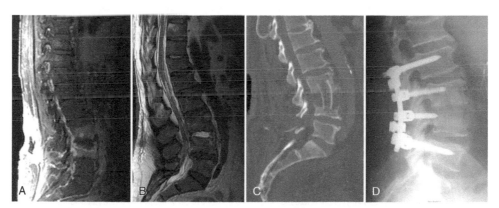

Fig. 66.1 A 60-year-old man with severe low back pain. (A) T1-weighted magnetic resonance imaging (MRI) and (B) T2-weighted MRI images reveal findings consistent with discitis/osteomyelitis at L3–L4. Treatment consisted of anterior debridement and fusion with iliac autograft (C) followed by posterior instrumentation and fusion (D).

9. **What is the role of biopsy in the diagnosis of pyogenic vertebral infections?**
In the absence of positive blood cultures, biopsy of the site of presumed vertebral osteomyelitis or discitis is essential to provide a definitive diagnosis, identify the causative organism, and guide treatment. The biopsy ideally should be performed before initiation of antibiotics. If antibiotics have been given, they should be discontinued for 3 days before the biopsy. Exceptions to this practice include patients with sepsis or impending spinal cord compression. CT-guided needle biopsy needle biopsy is safe and effective and yields the etiologic organism in 70% of cases. If a closed biopsy is negative after two attempts, an open biopsy is an option.

10. **What tests should be done on tissue samples from an open biopsy?**
Tissue samples should be sent for Gram stain, aerobic and anaerobic cultures, and acid-fast stain. Mycobacterial, fungal, and brucellar cultures are recommended in patients with suspected spinal infection based on epidemiologic factors, host risk factors, or characteristic radiographic findings. Bacterial cultures should be observed for at least 10 days to detect low-virulence organisms. Tuberculosis (TB) cultures may take weeks to grow. Histology studies should also be performed to detect neoplastic processes and to differentiate acute versus chronic infection.

11. **What are the goals of treatment of pyogenic vertebral infection?**
The goals in treating PVO include early definitive diagnosis, eradication of infection, relief of axial pain, prevention or reversal of neurologic deficits, preservation of spinal stability, and correction of spinal deformity (if present).

12. **Describe the nonoperative treatment of pyogenic vertebral infection.**
Nonoperative treatment includes antibiotic administration, treatment of underlying disease processes, nutritional support, and spinal immobilization with an orthosis. Antibiotic selection is based on identification and sensitivity testing. If cultures are negative, treatment with broad spectrum antibiotics is recommended. Consultation with an infectious disease specialist is recommended. Intravenous antibiotics generally should be continued for 6 weeks, provided that satisfactory clinical results and reduction in ESR and CRP occur. In the setting of a broadly sensitive organism and rapid clinical resolution, intravenous antibiotics may be replaced with a highly bioavailable oral antimicrobial therapy regimen after several weeks.

13. **What are the results of nonoperative treatment of pyogenic vertebral infections?**
Nonoperative treatment is reported as successful in up to 75% of appropriately treated patients when criteria for success focus on infection cure, absence of recurrent infection, and neurologic status following treatment. Quality of life data suggest less favorable success rates with 31% of patients reporting unfavorable outcomes and only 14% of patients free of pain following treatment. Contemporary mortality rates resulting from PVO range from 2% to 17%.

14. **What factors suggest a successful outcome with nonoperative treatment for PVO?**
The ideal patient for nonoperative treatment is a neurologically intact patient with primarily disc space involvement, minimal involvement of adjacent vertebrae, absence of kyphotic deformity, and absence of systemic disease or immune suppression. The most consistent predictors of success for nonoperative treatment include:
- Patients younger than 60 years
- Patients who are immunocompetent
- Infections with methicillin-sensitive *S. aureus*
- Decreasing ESR and CRP with antibiotic treatment

15. **When is operative intervention indicated for the treatment of pyogenic spinal infection?**
- To perform an open biopsy (when closed biopsy is negative or considered unsafe)
- Following failure of appropriate nonsurgical management as documented by persistently elevated ESR or CRP or refractory severe back pain
- To drain a clinically significant abscess (e.g., associated with sepsis)
- To treat neurologic deficit due to spinal cord, cauda equina, or nerve root compression
- To treat progressive spinal instability (e.g., secondary to extensive vertebral body or disc space destruction)
- To correct a progressive or unacceptable spinal deformity

16. **What are the goals of surgical management in pyogenic spinal infection?**
Surgery of PVO should achieve complete debridement of nonviable and infected tissue, adequate decompression of neural elements, and long-term stability through fusion (use of autogenous graft material is considered as the gold standard). Surgical treatment generally includes anterior spinal column debridement and grafting followed by a staged or simultaneous posterior spinal stabilization procedure (Fig. 66.1C,D).

17. **What principles guide the selection of the appropriate surgical approach for a spinal infection?**
The *location of the infection, presence/absence of abscess, extent of bone destruction,* and *need for stabilization* are the critical decision-making factors. Spinal discitis/osteomyelitis is a disease process that predominantly affects the anterior spinal column. Anterior approaches or combined anterior and posterior approaches are indicated in the majority of spinal infections. Circumferential surgery through a single posterior approach is favored by some surgeons and combines anterior column debridement performed from a posterior approach with posterior spinal

stabilization. Various minimally invasive surgical approaches including anterior column debridement in combination with percutaneous stabilization have also been described. CT-guided percutaneous drainage is an option for treatment of patients with PVO and a secondary psoas abcess. Laminectomy alone is not recommended due to its destabilizing effect and association with deformity progression, worsening spinal instability, and neurologic deterioration.

18. **Can posterior spinal instrumentation be utilized in the setting of an acute spinal infection without an increased rate of infection-related complications?**
Yes. Experimental and clinical evidence supports the concept that bone infections are better controlled with antibiotics and bone stabilization than with antibiotics alone in an unstable osseous environment. In this setting, advantages of posterior spinal instrumentation include:
    1. Preservation of spinal alignment and restoration of spinal stability following radical debridement
    2. Increased fusion rates
    3. Ability to correct kyphotic deformities
    4. Avoidance of graft collapse or dislodgement
    5. Rapid patient mobilization and early rehabilitation without the need for an external orthosis
    The use of implants comprised of titanium alloys is preferable to stainless steel due to increased bacterial adherence to stainless steel implants.

19. **Are foreign bodies applied to the anterior spinal column such as structural allografts, cages, and anterior spinal instrumentation safe and effective in the setting of acute infection?**
Case series report the use of structural allograft, static titanium mesh cages, and expandable titanium cages in osteomyelitic vertebrae without adverse effects on eradication of spinal infection. Successful use of anterior cervical and thoracolumbar plate fixation, as well as anterior thoracic and lumbar screw rod instrumentation, have been reported following anterior debridement of discitis/osteomyelitis.

20. **Are infection-related complications increased if combined anterior and posterior surgical procedures are performed under the same anesthetic versus performing the procedures in separate stages on different days?**
Evidence does not support the superiority of staged anterior and posterior surgery versus single-stage (same day) surgery for pyogenic discitis/osteomyelitis. Decision making can be individualized based on patient-specific factors such as the presence/absence of systemic sepsis, patient response under anesthesia during an anterior procedure (hemodynamic stability), medical comorbidities, and inherent stability of the anterior spinal column construct following debridement and anterior reconstruction.

SPINAL EPIDURAL ABSCESS

21. **Describe the clinical presentation and evaluation of a patient with a suspected pyogenic spinal epidural abscess.**
Spinal epidural abscess (SEA) due to a pyogenic infection leads to accumulation of purulent material in the epidural space. It may result from hematogenous spread, local extension from disc space infection/vertebral osteomyelitis, or direct inoculation following spinal surgery or spinal injections. This condition is usually found in adults. Risk factors include intravenous drug abuse, diabetes mellitus, immunodeficiency, prior spine trauma, renal failure, localized or systemic infections, spinal injections, and pregnancy. The initial presentation is variable and delayed diagnosis is common. The most common early findings are spinal pain and local spinal tenderness. Fever and neurologic symptoms are present in less than 50% of patients. The classic clinical triad of back pain, fever, and neurologic deficit is present in less than 15% of patients. ESR, CRP, and leukocyte counts are elevated and blood cultures are positive in 60% of patients. Definitive diagnosis of SEA is with spinal MRI, preferably with gadolinium. Without prompt recognition and treatment of an SEA, significant neurologic deficits predictably develop as the clinical condition progresses through four stages: (1) back pain, (2) radicular pain, (3) motor deficit and bowel/bladder dysfunction, and (4) paralysis. Epidural abscesses occur most frequently in the thoracic and lumbar regions, and least frequently in the cervical region. Clinicians should be aware that patients may present with concurrent noncontiguous epidural abscesses involving different spinal regions and that MRI of the entire spine is required for diagnosis of this condition.

22. **What is the most common pyogenic organism responsible for an SEA?**
S. aureus is the most common organism and has been identified in over 60% of cases of SEA. Infections due to a range of gram-positive, gram-negative, and mixed pathogens may occur. Antibiotic-resistant organisms such as MRSA, VRSA, and VRE are increasingly common.

23. **What is the prognosis for neurologic recovery for a patient with an epidural abscess associated with neurologic deficit?**
Significant neurologic recovery is observed in patients with mild neurologic deficits or paralysis of less than 36 hours' duration who undergo surgical decompression. Complete paralysis of greater than 36 to 48 hours' duration has not shown recovery. The death rate associated with epidural abscess has been reported as 12%.

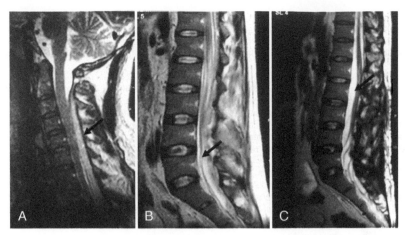

Fig. 66.2 Epidural abscess in a 36-year-old man with a history of fever and severe neck pain due to infection with gram-positive coccus. The epidural abscess extended from C2 to the sacral region. (A) The epidural abscess *(arrow)* is located posterior to the spinal cord in the cervical region. (B, C) The epidural abscess *(arrow)* circumferentially surrounds the neural elements in the lumbar region. (From Urrutia J, Rojas C. Extensive epidural abscess with surgical treatment and long-term follow-up. Spine J 2007;7:708–711.)

24. What operative approach is recommended for an epidural abscess?

The surgical approach is determined by the location of the SEA. An abscess located posteriorly and extending over multiple levels is best treated by multiple-level laminotomies or laminectomy, taking care to preserve the facet joints. Alternatively, debridement of the spinal canal through fenestrations with the ligamentum flavum and portions of adjacent laminae in combination with the use of catheters to evacuate material from beneath laminae to avoid laminectomy is an option. An abscess located anteriorly and associated with vertebral osteomyelitis is most directly treated with an anterior surgical approach. If an abscess involves both the anterior and posterior epidural space, an anterior and posterior approach combined with spinal stabilization may be necessary (Fig. 66.2).

25. Is nonoperative management of an epidural abscess ever indicated?

Nonoperative management of an SEA is considered only in exceptional circumstances. A symptomatic epidural abscess is considered a medical and surgical emergency. The combination of surgical and antibiotic treatment is required for successful treatment of a symptomatic epidural abscess in most cases. Nonoperative management may be considered in patients who are extremely high-risk surgical candidates and in patients with an established complete neurologic deficit for greater than 72 hours. Also, neurologically intact patients without sepsis with positive culture results may be considered for a trial of culture-specific antibiotic therapy under close clinical supervision. However, it has been reported that medical management is associated with a greater than 40% risk of failure, and that delayed operative intervention after failed medical management is associated with worse neurologic outcomes compared with early surgical treatment. Risk factors predictive of failure of medical management of SEAs include diabetes mellitus, white blood cell count greater than $12.5 \times 10^9/L$, positive blood cultures, and CRP levels greater than 115 mg/L.

PEDIATRIC DISC SPACE INFECTION AND OSTEOMYELITIS

26. Describe the presentation and management of a child with discitis.

The presentation of pediatric discitis is highly variable. Infants are more likely to become systemically ill, whereas nonspecific findings are more common in children older than 5 years. Spinal infection should be suspected when children present with back pain, refusal to bear weight, or a flexed position of the spine. Less commonly, children may present with nonspecific abdominal pain complaints. Less than 50% present with fever. After several weeks, radiographs may demonstrate disc space narrowing, which is the earliest detectable radiographic finding. Endplate erosions, bony destruction, and paravertebral soft tissue swelling may occur later. The ESR and CRP are usually elevated. Blood cultures are usually negative, and the leukocyte count is usually normal. Initial treatment includes bedrest, immobilization, and administration of an antistaphylococcal antibiotic (initially parenteral but may be changed to oral medication after resolution of symptoms). Treatment failure or abscess formation requires biopsy and/or surgical intervention.

GRANULOMATOUS INFECTIONS

TUBERCULOSIS

27. Describe the presentation of a patient with a tuberculous spinal infection.

TB is the most common granulomatous infection of the spine. The presentation of TB spondylitis is highly variable. Mild back pain is the most common symptom. Patients with TB spondylitis may present with malaise, fevers, night sweats, and weight loss. Paravertebral abscesses and neurologic deficits develop in up to half of patients. Acute TB spondylitis may present with neurologic deficits due to neural compression by an epidural abscess, retropulsed bone or disc material, or pathologic vertebral subluxation. Chronic TB spinal infections may result in cutaneous sinuses or neurologic deficits due to progressive kyphotic spinal deformity or disease reactivation.

28. What are the risk factors for contracting tuberculosis of the spine?

People from countries with a high incidence of TB, such as Southeast Asia, South America, Africa, China, and Russia are considered at risk and are most commonly affected by TB in the first three decades of life. In Western countries, adults are most commonly affected by TB, and high-risk populations include adults who live in confinement with others, such as homeless centers and prisons, chronic alcoholics, HIV-positive individuals, and persons with a family member or a household contact with tuberculosis.

29. Discuss the value of laboratory tests and biopsy in the diagnosis of tuberculous vertebral infection.

The leukocyte count may be normal or mildly elevated. The ESR is mildly elevated (typically <50 mm/hour) but may be normal in up to 25% of cases. CRP is elevated in the majority of patients and is a more specific test than ESR. Although the tuberculin skin test (TST) can detect active infection or past exposure, skin testing is unreliable because false-negative results may occur in malnourished and immunocompromised patients and false-positive tests may occur in bacille Calmette-Guerin (BCG)-vaccinated patients. An interferon gamma release assay (IGRA) blood test addresses the limitations associated with skin testing and results can be available in 24 hours, but it does not help differentiate latent tuberculosis infection from tuberculosis disease. Urine cultures, sputum specimens, and gastric washings may be helpful for diagnosis if the primary source is unknown. A definitive method for diagnosis of tuberculous vertebral infection is CT-guided biopsy to confirm the presence of acid-fast bacilli (AFB) on smear, culture, or histopathology. A characteristic finding on histology is a granuloma, which is described as a multinucleated giant-cell reaction surrounding a central region of caseating necrosis. Molecular detection of mycobacterium DNA or RNA is useful and provides a method for rapid diagnosis and for determining drug resistance.

30. What is the value of imaging studies in the diagnosis of tuberculous vertebral infection?

Radiographs: A clue to diagnosis of TB spondylitis is the presence of extensive vertebral destruction out of proportion to the amount of pain. Typically, the intervertebral discs are preserved in the early stages of this disease. Chest radiographs can be useful in demonstrating pulmonary involvement.

Radionuclide studies: These are not helpful because of the high false-negative rate in TB.

MRI: The imaging modality of choice for diagnosis of spinal TB (Fig. 66.3).

CT: Plays a role in defining the extent of bony destruction and localization for biopsies.

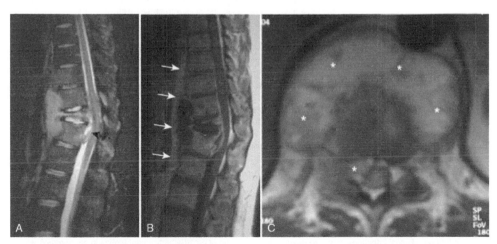

Fig. 66.3 Spinal tuberculosis (Pott disease). (A) The sagittal T2-weighted (T2W) magnetic resonance (MR) image *(left)* confirms single-level vertebral collapse with absence of disc space involvement. There is a large anterior high-signal intensity paravertebral soft tissue abscess. Also, an epidural abscess extends behind the T12 vertebra compressing the spinal cord *(broken arrow)*. (B) Nonenhancing fluid collections are seen on the T1W MR image *(center)* obtained after administration of a contrast agent, which also shows extensive enhancing soft tissue inflammatory disease *(white arrows)*. The prominent superior and inferior spread is typical of TB. (C) The large abscess collection *(asterisks)* is also seen on the axial T2W MR image *(right)*. (From Waldman SD, Campbell RSD. Pott disease. In: Waldman SD, Campbell RSD, editors. Imaging of Pain. Philadelphia, PA: Saunders; 2011, pp. 147–148, Fig. 58.1.)

31. **What are the three patterns of spinal involvement associated with TB?**
    The three main patterns of spinal involvement in TB spondylitis are peridiscal, central, and anterior. The most common form, **peridiscal**, occurs adjacent to the vertebral endplate and spreads around a single intervertebral disc as the abscess material tracks beneath the anterior longitudinal ligament. The intervertebral disc is usually spared in distinct contrast to pyogenic infections. **Central** involvement occurs in the middle of the vertebral body and eventually leads to vertebral collapse and kyphotic deformity. This pattern of involvement can be mistaken for a tumor. **Anterior** infections begin beneath the anterior longitudinal ligament, causing scalloping of the anterior vertebral bodies, and extend over multiple levels. In rare cases, TB may involve only the posterior spinal column or the spinal canal without adjacent osseous lesions.

32. **What are some features noted on MRI that help distinguish tuberculous spondylitis from PVO?**
    MRI features that favor a diagnosis of PVO include:
    - Lumbar spinal involvement (most common location)
    - Intervertebral disc involvement with narrowing and destruction
    - Vertebral endplate destruction
    - Vertebral involvement limited to regions adjacent to a single disc space
    - Paraspinal abscess wall is thickened and has irregular rim enhancement
    - Poorly defined paraspinal signal abnormality (postcontrast)
    - Presence of paraspinal or intraosseous abscess in up to 50% of cases
        MRI features that favor a diagnosis of TB spondylitis include:
    - Thoracic or thoracolumbar spinal involvement (most common location)
    - Intervertebral discs with normal height and signal intensity
    - Involvement of more than two vertebral bodies with extensive bony involvement
    - Involvement of the anterior aspect of several adjacent vertebral bodies
    - Involvement of the central portion of a vertebral body
    - Involvement of the posterior spinal elements
    - Well-defined paraspinal signal abnormality (postcontrast)
    - A thin, smooth, abscess wall
    - Presence of large paraspinal or intraosseous abscess

33. **Discuss the nonsurgical treatment of TB spondylitis.**
    Medical treatment is effective for TB spondylitis. Multidrug combination therapy and brace immobilization are the initial treatment except in patients presenting with surgical indications such as neurologic deficit or progressive deformity. An initial four-drug regimen, for a minimum 2-month duration, includes isoniazid, rifampin, pyrazinamide, and ethambutol. This is followed by an additional 4-month treatment with isoniazid and rifampin, although longer courses of chemotherapy are prescribed by some practitioners. Multidrug-resistant TB spondylitis and TB spondylitis in HIV-positive patients have a worse prognosis and require treatment with second-line chemotherapeutic agents.

34. **Discuss the surgical treatment of spinal tuberculosis.**
    The indications for surgery and the principles of surgical reconstruction for TB spondylitis are similar to those recommended for pyogenic spinal infections—drainage of abscesses, debridement of nonviable bone and disc material, spinal decompression, spinal stabilization, and correction of spinal deformity. Radical anterior debridement and insertion of a strut graft, termed the Hong Kong operation, was initially developed for treatment of TB spondylitis. Subsequently, the addition of anterior and/or posterior spinal instrumentation, including the use of vertebral body replacement devices, has been adopted to improve spinal implant construct stability. Posterior and posterolateral surgical approaches have been developed, which combine anterior column debridement or resection and posterior spinal stabilization through a single surgical approach for treatment of acute and chronic spinal instability and deformity.

NONTUBERCULOUS GRANULOMATOUS SPINAL INFECTIONS

35. **Which organisms are associated with nontuberculous granulomatous spinal infections?**
    Atypical mycobacteria (*Actinomyces*, *Nocardia*, and *Brucella* spp.), as well as fungal infections (coccidioidomycosis, blastomycosis, cryptomycosis, candidiasis, aspergillosis), are potential pathogens. Patients from endemic regions and immunocompromised patients are at increased risk for developing atypical mycobacterial and fungal infections. Fungal infections may also develop following use of broad-spectrum antibiotics in combination with central venous catheters for parenteral nutrition. Sarcoidosis, an inflammatory disease characterized by formation of granulomas, often involves the spine and should be included in the differential diagnosis.

36. **What treatment is advised for nontuberculous granulomatous spinal infections?**
    Basic principles of treatment include correction of host factors, specific drug therapy, and surgical treatment following the general principles for treatment of spinal infections.

KEY POINTS

1. Spinal infection should be suspected in patients who present with nonmechanical back pain symptoms and risk factors for infection including diabetes, immunosuppression, advanced age, intravenous drug use history, or recent surgical procedure history.
2. Identification of the responsible organism through cultures and determination of antibiotic sensitivities are necessary to guide nonoperative treatment of adult spinal infections.
3. Spinal MRI with gadolinium contrast is the most reliable imaging study for diagnosis and determination of the extent of a spinal infection.
4. Surgical treatment of spinal infection is indicated for persistent or recurrent infection despite medical management, drainage of abscesses, debridement of nonviable bone and disc material, neurologic deficits, spinal instability, and spinal deformity.
5. The disc is nearly always involved in pyogenic vertebral infections. In contrast, granulomatous infections typically do not involve the disc space.

Websites
1. Spinal infections: https://emedicine.medscape.com/article/1266702-overview
2. Wheeless' Textbook of Orthopaedics, vertebral osteomyelitis: http://www.wheelessonline.com/ortho/vertebral_osteomyelitis
3. Spinal conditions: http://www.spine-health.com/conditions/pain/osteomyelitis-a-spinal-infection

BIBLIOGRAPHY

1. Berbari EF, Kanj SS, Kowalski TJ, et al. Infectious Diseases Society of America Clinical Practice Guidelines for the diagnosis and treatment of native vertebral osteomyelitis in adults. *Clin Infect Dis* 2015;61:26–46.
2. Butler JS, Shelly MJ, Timlin M, et al. Nontuberculous pyogenic spinal infection in adults: A 12-year experience from a tertiary referral center. *Spine* 2006;31:2695–2700.
3. Carragee EJ, Lezza A. Does acute placement of instrumentation in the treatment of vertebral osteomyelitis predispose to recurrent infection: Long-term follow-up in immune-suppressed patients. *Spine* 2008;33:2089–2093.
4. Cornett CA, Vincent SA, Crow J, et al. Bacterial spine infection in adults: Evaluation and management. *J Am Acad Orthop Surg* 2016;24:11–18.
5. Eck JC, Kim CW, Currier BL, et al. Infections of the spine. In: Garfin SR, Eismont FJ, Bell GR, editors. Rothman-Simeone the Spine. 7th ed. Philadelphia, PA: Saunders; 2018, pp. 1526–1583.
6. Dimar JR, Carreon LY, Glassman SD, et al. Treatment of pyogenic vertebral osteomyelitis with anterior debridement and fusion followed by delayed posterior spinal fusion. *Spine* 2004;29:326–332.
7. Hadjipavlou AG, Mader JT, Necessary JT, et al. Hematogenous pyogenic spinal infections and their surgical management. *Spine* 2000;25:1668–1679.
8. Patel AR, Alton TB, Bransford RJ, et al. Spinal epidural abscesses: Risk factors, medical versus surgical management, a retrospective review of 128 cases. *Spine J* 2014;14:326–330.
9. Ruf M, Stoltze D, Merk HR, et al. Treatment of vertebral osteomyelitis by radical debridement and stabilization using titanium mesh cages. *Spine* 2007;32:275–280.

CHAPTER 67

RHEUMATOID ARTHRITIS

Ronald Moskovich, MD, FRCS Ed and Michael J. Moses, MD

1. **What is rheumatoid arthritis?**
   Rheumatoid arthritis (RA) is a chronic, systemic inflammatory disorder of uncertain etiology that affects the synovium of joints. It is an immunologically mediated systemic disorder that affects articular and nonarticular organ systems. The articular involvement is a symmetrical peripheral joint disease affecting large and small joints. Axial involvement predominantly affects the cervical region, especially the upper cervical spine. The extraarticular involvement may affect the skin, eyes, and larynx, as well as the pulmonary, cardiovascular, hematologic, renal, neurologic, and lymphatic systems. Prevalence of RA is estimated to be 1%–2% of the global population. RA is the most common inflammatory disorder affecting the spine.

2. **Describe the pathogenesis of RA.**
   The exact pathogenesis of RA is unknown. It is hypothesized that RA is due to a complex interplay of genetic, epigenetic, and environmental factors, which ultimately act in conjunction to generate a destructive synovial response in selective targets. According to current theories, an unknown antigen triggers the body to produce rheumatoid factor (RF), which is an immunoglobulin M (IgM) molecule directed against the Fc portion of immunoglobulin G (IgG). Antigen-activated CD4+ T cells amplify the immune response by stimulating monocytes, macrophages, T-cells, B-cells, and synovial fibroblasts to produce the proinflammatory cytokines interleukin-1, interleukin-6, and tumor necrosis factor α (TNF-α), as well as matrix metalloproteinases. Interleukin-1, interleukin-6, and TNF-α are the key cytokines that drive synovial inflammation. This synovial inflammation results in the production of *synovial pannus*, which is the major site of immune activation in RA. Synovial pannus has the capacity to invade and destroy the substructure of joints. Synovitis initially manifests as joint swelling, stiffness, palpable warmth, and joint pain. Juxta-articular osteopenia occurs in early stages of RA, followed by erosion of bone at the margins of small joints. Disease progression leads to destruction of adjacent cartilage and bone, as well as weakening of joint capsules, ligaments, and tendons leading to various types of skeletal deformities.

3. **How is RA diagnosed?**
   A comprehensive **history and physical examination** is performed. RA is a symmetrical, erosive polyarthritis of small and large joints that often involves the cervical spine. The most common joints initially involved are the metacarpophalangeal joints (MCP), proximal interphalangeal (PIP) joints, wrist joints, and metatarsophalangeal joints. Involvement of the distal interphalangeal joints of the hand, thoracolumbar spine, or sacroiliac joints is rare and suggests a different diagnosis. Patients typically complain of significant morning stiffness. Rheumatoid nodules are common. Neck pain may or may not be present. Cervical radiographs are characterized by C1–C2 instability, facet joint erosions without sclerosis, and disc space narrowing without osteophyte formation.
   Characteristic abnormalities on **laboratory testing** include:
   - Elevated erythrocyte sedimentation rate (ESR) and C-reactive protein (CRP)
   - RF is present in 70%–80% of patients but is a nonspecific finding
   - Anticyclic citrullinated peptide (anti-CCP) antibody positivity (57%–66%) and is highly specific for RA
   - Antinuclear antibody (ANA) antibodies are positive in 30% of RA patients
   - Synovial fluid analysis has a nonspecific or inflammatory profile
   - Anemia and hypergammaglobulinemia may be present

   Various **classification criteria** have been proposed for RA and also may be used to aid in diagnosis. The **American College of Rheumatology 1987 criteria** focused on differentiation between patients with established RA and patients with other rheumatologic diagnoses, and defined RA by the presence of late-stage features. Patient were required to meet four of seven criteria to classify as RA, and criteria 1 through 4 must have been present for a minimum of 6 weeks:
   1. Morning stiffness ($\geq$1 hour)
   2. Soft tissue swelling involving $\geq$ three joints
   3. Soft tissue swelling of hand joints (PIP, MCP, wrist)
   4. Symmetrical soft tissue swelling
   5. Subcutaneous nodules
   6. Serum RF
   7. Erosions and/or periarticular osteopenia in hand or wrist joints on x-rays

   With the recognition that early therapeutic intervention could improve clinical outcome and reduce or even prevent joint damage in many patients, there has been a paradigm shift to early diagnosis and treatment of RA.

Table 67.1 The 2010 American College of Rheumatology/European League Against Rheumatism Classification Criteria for Rheumatoid Arthritis.

		SCORE[a]
1. Joint involvement (0–5 points)	1 large joint[b]	0
	2–10 large joints	1
	1–3 small joints[c] (large joints not counted)	2
	4–10 small joints (large joints not counted)	3
	>10 joints (at least 1 small joint)	5
2. Serology (0–3 points)	Negative RF *and* negative ACPA	0
	Low positive RF *or* low positive ACPA	2
	High positive RF *or* high positive ACPA	3
3. Acute phase reactants (0–1 point)	Normal CRP *and* normal ESR	0
	Abnormal CRP *or* abnormal ESR	1
4. Duration of symptoms (0–1 point)	<6 weeks	0
	≥6 weeks	1

[a]Patients with a total score of ≥6 points may be classified as having rheumatoid arthritis.
[b]Large joints include shoulders, elbows, hips, knees, and ankles.
[c]Small joints include metacarpophalangeal joints, proximal interphalangeal joints, second to fifth metatarsophalangeal joints, thumb interphalangeal joints, and wrists.
ACPA, Anticitrullinated peptide antibodies; *CRP,* C-reactive protein; *ESR,* erythrocyte sedimentation rate; *RF,* rheumatoid factor.
Data from Aletaha D, Neogi T, Silman AJ, et al. 2010 Rheumatoid Arthritis Classification criteria: An American College of Rheumatology/European League Against Rheumatism collaborative initiative. Ann Rheum Dis 2010;69:1580–1588.

The **American College of Rheumatology (ACR)/European League Against Rheumatism (EULAR) criteria** were introduced to improve early classification of RA and for use in clinical trials (Table 67.1).

4. List some of the extraarticular manifestations associated with RA that may impact spine care.
   Skin: Subcutaneous nodules, pyoderma gangrenosum, fragility
   Eyes: Keratoconjunctivitis sicca (dry eyes), scleritis, Sjögren syndrome
   Ears, nose, throat: Cricoarytenoid arthritis, tracheal pain, dysphonia, stridor, dysarthria, tinnitus, decreased hearing
   Pulmonary: Chronic diffuse interstitial fibrosis, pleural effusion, rheumatoid nodules, bronchiolitis obliterans, active tuberculosis
   Cardiovascular: Pericarditis, valve disease, coronary vasculitis, conduction abnormalities, atherosclerosis
   Hematologic: Anemia, thrombocytopenia, Felty syndrome (RA, splenomegaly, neutropenia), lymphadenopathy
   Renal: Amyloidosis, decreased renal function, vasculitis
   Neurologic: Peripheral neuropathy, mononeuritis multiplex, peripheral nerve entrapment neuropathy
   Infectious: Increase infection risk secondary to immunosuppressive medication
   Osseous: Osteoporosis

5. What pharmacotherapy is recommended for patients with RA?
   - Drug treatment is targeted to achieve remission or very low disease activity
   - Treatment is usually initiated with a synthetic, conventional disease-modifying antirheumatic drug (DMARD), most commonly methotrexate, accompanied by a short-term course of corticosteroids. Methotrexate in combination with corticosteroids has been shown to induce disease remission in up to 50% of patients with early RA. Nonsteroidal antiinflammatory drugs (NSAIDs) may also be considered, though these do not alter the underlying disease process.
   - In patients who continue to show high or moderate disease activity, addition of a biologic agent such as a TNF-α blocker (e.g., infliximab, etanercept, adalimumab) is considered.
   - Additional approaches to drug treatment include janus kinase inhibition (tofacitinib), T-cell costimulatory blockade (abatacept), B-cell depletion (rituximab), and interleukin-6 antagonists (tocilizumab).
   - Biologic DMARDs have a greater efficacy when used in conjunction with first-line DMARDs, as opposed to use as a monotherapy
   - It is highly advisable to manage RA patients in conjunction with a rheumatologist. For RA patients undergoing spine surgery, it is important to develop an individualized plan for perioperative medication management. Prior to surgery, aspirin and NSAIDs are discontinued due to concerns regarding bleeding. Patients using DMARDs

and biologic agents require consultation regarding advisability and timing of a drug holiday due to the adverse impact of these medication on wound healing and infection risk. The need for perioperative stress-dose steroids should also be assessed due to concerns regarding potential for perioperative adrenal crisis.

6. **How does RA affect the spine?**

RA may involve all spinal regions, but cervical spine involvement is most common and leads to the most severe complications. The cervical spine is composed of 32 synovial joints. The occiput–C1 and C1–C2 articulations rely on soft tissue integrity for stability. In the subaxial cervical spine, the facet joints are true synovial joints. Rheumatoid pannus produces enzymes that destroy cartilage, ligaments, tendons, and bone. This synovitis may lead to spinal instability, subluxation, and spinal deformity. Secondarily, the discs in the subaxial spine degenerate, which may contribute to additional facet joint subluxations and/or ankylosis. Spinal cord and brainstem compression may develop secondary to static or dynamic cervical spinal deformities or from direct pressure by synovial pannus.

Three types of cervical deformities may develop secondary to rheumatoid disease, and may present singularly or in combination:

1. **Atlantoaxial (C1–C2) subluxation (AAS):** Most common type, responsible for 65% of cervical rheumatoid deformities. AAS arises due to compromise of the integrity of the transverse and alar ligaments due to synovial proliferation, and limits the ability of these ligaments to keep the odontoid in contact with the anterior arch of C1. Anterior, lateral (rotatory), and posterior (less common) subluxations can occur, and may be reducible or fixed.

2. **Atlantoaxial impaction (AAI):** Also termed superior migration of the odontoid, cranial settling, or pseudobasilar invagination. It is the second most common type (20%) of cervical rheumatoid deformity, and arises due to compromise of the integrity of the occipitoatlantal and atlantoaxial articulations, leading to cephalad migration of the odontoid into the foramen magnum, where it may compress the brainstem.

3. **Subaxial subluxation (SAS):** Responsible for 15% of cervical rheumatoid deformities and arises due to destruction of facet joint, ligaments, and intervertebral discs. Subluxations may occur at multiple levels and lead to development of a staircase type deformity as the cephalad vertebra subluxes anteriorly in relation to the caudad vertebra. Subluxations may be fixed or mobile (Figs. 67.1 and 67.2).

7. **What are some disorders included in the differential diagnosis of RA of the cervical spine?**
   - **Systemic lupus erythematosus (SLE),** a chronic, inflammatory autoimmune disorder, may involve the cervical region. However, most often the axial disease in SLE is secondary to vertebral collapse resulting from systemic use of corticosteroids or due to osteoporosis.

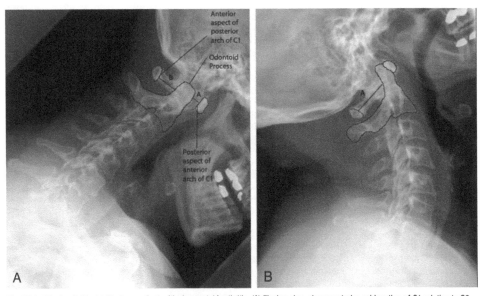

Fig. 67.1 Atlantoaxial instability in a patient with rheumatoid arthritis. (A) Flexion view shows anterior subluxation of C1 relative to C2 with increase in the anterior atlantodental interval (AADI) to 7 mm *(line A)* and decrease in the posterior atlantodental interval (PADI) to 13 mm *(line B)*. Note the break in the spinolaminar line at C1–C2. (B) Extension radiograph shows reduction of the subluxation with a normal AADI (<3.5 mm) and a normal PADI which is greater than 14 mm.

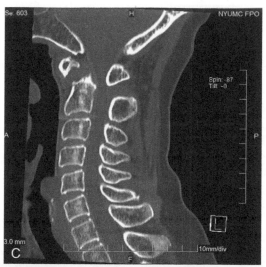

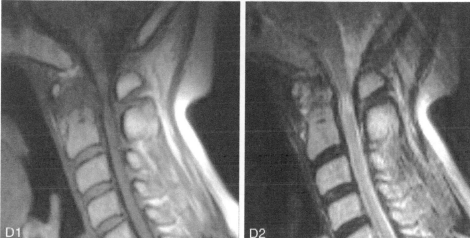

Fig. 67.1, cont'd (C) Severe erosion of the odontoid is seen on the sagittal computed tomography reconstruction. (D) T1 *(1)* and T2 *(2)* magnetic resonance imaging sequences of the craniocervical junction. The florid pannus has eroded the dens and, combined with the subluxation, contributes to the degree of stenosis seen at the C1–C2 level. Abnormally increased signal in the spinal cord is evident in the T2 image. (A and B: Hohl JB, Grabowski G, Donaldson III WF. Cervical deformity in rheumatoid arthritis. Semin Spine Surg 2011;23:181–187.)

- **Seronegative spondyloarthropathies** (includes ankylosing spondylitis, psoriatic arthritis, reactive arthritis) may initially behave in a similar fashion to RA and can be distinguished by serologic testing and the radiographic pattern of osseous involvement. In seronegative spondyloarthropathies, the cervical abnormalities are associated with ligamentous calcification or new bone formation, which is not typical for RA.
- **Ankylosing spondylitis (AS)** results in progressive ankylosis of the entire spine associated with marked sacroiliac joint disease. The classic bamboo spine results from calcification of ligamentous attachments at the marginal areas of the vertebral body (enthesitis) with maintenance of disc height and shape. AAS has been reported in up to 20% of AS patients.
- **Psoriatic spondylarthritis** may present with calcification of the perivertebral structures and premature degenerative disc changes but is rarely associated with instability.
- **Reactive arthritis** and **enteropathic arthritis** rarely involve the cervical spine.

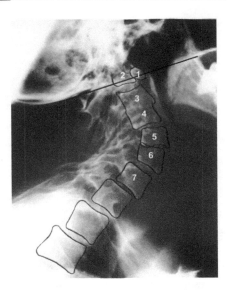

Fig. 67.2 Atlantoaxial impaction (AAI) and subaxial subluxation (SAS) due to rheumatoid arthritis. Note (1) the presence of AAI with proximity of the base of the odontoid to the McGregor line and the paradoxically small AADI; (2) C3–C4 ankylosis; and (3) multilevel subluxations (C4–C5, C6–C7, C7–T1) giving rise to the characteristic staircase appearance.

8. What clinical findings may be present in patients with rheumatoid involvement of the cervical spine?
   • Pain (neck pain, occipital neuralgia, facial and ear pain)
   • Lhermitte sign (electric shock-like sensation in the limbs and trunk when the neck is flexed)
   • Symptoms and signs of myelopathy or radiculopathy
   • Symptoms and signs of vertebrobasilar insufficiency (transient weakness, vertigo, visual disturbance, loss of equilibrium, dysphagia)

9. List some of the clinical signs and symptoms that suggest the diagnosis of cervical myelopathy in the RA patient.
   • Loss of endurance
   • Gait disturbance
   • Loss of dexterity
   • Paresthesia
   • Change in walking ability
   • Bowel and bladder dysfunction
   • Weakness
   • Spasticity
   • Loss of proprioception
   • Brisk reflexes
   • Babinski sign
   • Hoffmann sign

10. What are some of the pitfalls in evaluating neurologic status in rheumatoid patients?
    • Chronic polyarthritis and deformity interfere with motor and reflex testing. For example, the Babinski response may be absent in patients with severe forefoot deformity, hallux valgus, or ankylosis of these joints. Similarly, tendon reflexes and the Hoffmann reflex may be difficult to elicit.
    • Patients may have had prior operations to fuse joints, which interfere with muscle and reflex testing.
    • Muscle atrophy is common in chronic deforming arthritis and may not be due to neural compression.
    • Nerve root symptoms may be confused with nerve entrapment and polyneuropathy.

11. What are some options for reporting and scoring neurologic function in patients with RA, which are commonly used by spine specialists?
    A complete neurologic evaluation should document the assessment of sensory, motor, and reflex function in the upper and lower extremities, as well as bowel and bladder function. It is often helpful to score neurologic function using a scale such as the **Ranawat Classification of Neurologic Function**:
    • **Class 1:** No neural deficit
    • **Class 2:** Subjective weakness with hyperreflexia and dysesthesia

- **Class 3:** Objective findings of weakness and long-tract signs
- **Class 3A:** Able to walk
- **Class 3B:** Quadriparetic and not ambulatory

Another commonly used scale is the **modified Japanese Orthopaedic Association (mJOA) score**, which is specifically intended to assess the severity of clinical symptoms in patients with cervical compressive myelopathy. This scale assesses motor dysfunction of the upper and lower extremities, sensory changes in the upper extremities, and bladder dysfunction. Severity of myelopathy is defined as mild if mJOA ≥15, moderate 12–14, and severe <12.

12. Is there evidence that cervical collars protect patients with cervical subluxation?

No. There is no evidence that cervical collars positively influence the natural history of rheumatoid cervical disease. An orthosis may be considered for patients with minor occipitocervical pain symptoms but is often poorly tolerated.

13. When are plain radiographs of the cervical spine indicated in patients with RA?

All patients with RA should be evaluated at initial presentation with cervical radiographs, because half of patients with radiographic instability are asymptomatic. Cervical radiographs are also advised prior to surgical procedures requiring endotracheal intubation. Additional indications for radiographs include new onset of cervical pain or neurologic signs or symptoms. Radiographs should include standard anteroposterior (AP) and lateral views, as well as lateral flexion and extension views. Radiographic findings that merit cervical magnetic resonance imaging (MRI) and referral to a spine surgeon include:

- AAS with a posterior atlantodens interval (ADI) ≤14 mm or anterior ADI ≥9 mm
- SAS with a sagittal diameter of the spinal canal ≤14 mm
- Any degree of AAI

14. Which radiologic measurements are useful to evaluate AAS?

- **Anterior atlantodental interval (AADI) or ADI.** This is the distance from the posterior aspect of the anterior ring of the atlas to the anterior aspect of the odontoid. In normal adults, this distance should not exceed 3.5 mm.
- **Posterior atlantodental interval (PADI) and space available for the cord (SAC).** The PADI is measured from the posterior surface of the odontoid to the anterior aspect of the C1 lamina. This measurement represents the SAC defined by the osseous elements. The PADI has been demonstrated to be a more reliable predictor of neurologic symptoms than the AADI. PADI of 14 mm or less is associated with an increased risk of cord compression and myelopathy. The SAC as determined on MRI may actually be less than estimated on plain radiographs due to the presence of soft tissue pannus, causing a narrowing of the spinal canal.

15. Which radiologic measurements are useful to evaluate AAI?

Multiple radiographic measures have been proposed to assess AAI. However, it may be challenging to clearly identify anatomic landmarks on radiographs due to bone erosion and superimposition of the skull on adjacent spinal structures. It has been suggested that screening for AAI with a combination of the Clark stations, Ranawat criterion, and the Redlund-Johnell criterion is optimal. If plain radiographic measurements or clinical findings suggest AAI, advanced imaging with MRI or computed tomography (CT) with or without contrast are suggested to definitively evaluate spinal anatomy (Figs. 67.3 and 67.4, Table 67.2).

16. Which radiologic measurements are useful to evaluate SAS?

Subluxations greater than 20% or more than 3.5 mm on plain radiographs are significant. The subaxial spinal canal diameter should be measured from the posterior aspect of the vertebral body to the ventral lamina. A sagittal canal diameter of less than 14 mm suggests an increased risk of developing a neurologic deficit. MRI is indicated because the actual canal diameter may be less than suggested by osseous measurements due to the presence of pannus.

17. What is the natural history of rheumatoid cervical disease?

Understanding of the natural history of rheumatoid cervical disease is incomplete. Neck pain is common and can be present in up to 80% of patients. The most common early instability pattern is AAS, which is estimated to develop in 33% to 50% of patients within 5 years of diagnosing RA. However, up to half of patients with cervical radiographic instability are asymptomatic. Between 2% and 10% of patients with AAS develop myelopathy over the next 10 years. Disease progression may cause the AAS to become fixed. Erosion of the C1–C2 and occiput–C1 joints may lead to superior migration of the odontoid and result in brainstem compression (AAI). Once diagnosed with myelopathy, up to 50% of patients may die within a year. SAS is less common than the other deformity patterns and typically develops after AAI or following C1–C2 fusion or occipitocervical fusion. Early treatment with DMARDs and biologic agents may prevent the development of cervical disease but may not prevent progression of preexisting cervical involvement.

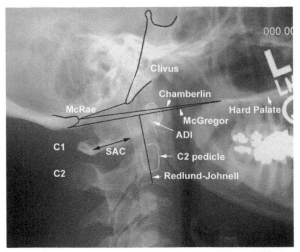

Fig. 67.3 Radiologic landmarks and lines in the occipitocervical region. (see Table 67.2)

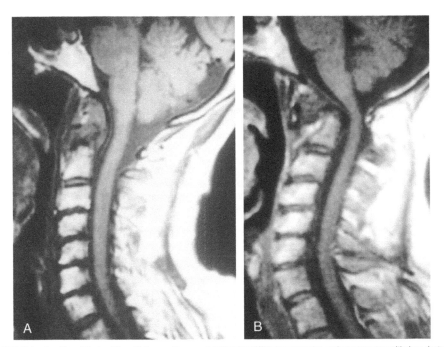

Fig. 67.4 Extension (A) and flexion (B) sagittal magnetic resonance imaging (MRI) demonstrating exuberant pannus with dens destruction and severe atlantoaxial instability. The high-grade subluxation and its effect on the craniocervical junction may have been missed if the flexion view had been omitted. These images were acquired using standard MRI equipment.

18. What are the indications for surgical treatment for RA involving the cervical spine?
    Indications for surgical treatment include neck pain, neurologic dysfunction, or abnormal imaging parameters (instability). Often patients present with a combination of these factors:
    1. **Pain:** Neck pain or occipital pain has multiple etiologies. If pain is secondary to spinal instability or associated with symptomatic neurologic compression (e.g., radiculopathy, myelopathy), surgery is recommended.
    2. **Neurologic dysfunction:** Cervical myelopathy is an indication for surgery to prevent neurologic deterioration and facilitate recovery.

Table 67.2 Evaluation of atlantoaxial impaction.

Measurement	Description	Diagnostic Criteria
McRae line	Line from basion (anterior rim of foramen magnum) to opisthion (posterior rim of foramen magnum)	Protrusion of the tip of the dens above this line indicates AAI
Chamberlain line	Line from posterior aspect of the hard palate to the opisthion	Protrusion of the tip of the dens >3 mm above this line indicates AAI
McGregor line	Line from posterosuperior aspect of the hard palate to the most inferior cortical margin of the occiput	Protrusion of the tip of the dens >4.5 mm above this line indicates AAI
Redlund-Johnell measurement	Distance from McGregor line to midpoint of the inferior margin of C2 body	Positive if <34 mm in males and <29 mm in females
Ranawat index	Vertical distance from the midpoint of the C2 pedicle to a horizontal line through the transverse axis of C1 on a lateral x-ray	Positive if <15 mm in males or <13 mm in females
Stations of the Atlas (Clark)	Divide odontoid height into thirds (called "stations") on a lateral radiograph. The anterior ring of the atlas normally lies adjacent to the upper third of the odontoid (station 1).	AAI is present if odontoid lies at mid-third (station 2) or lower third (station 3) of the odontoid
Multiplanar CT	Optimal for evaluation of bone detail and craniocervical anatomy	Used mainly for surgical planning
MRI	The CMA is determined on a sagittal MRI by drawing a line along the anterior aspect of the cervical spinal cord and a second line along the brainstem longitudinally. This angle is normally between 135° and 175°.	As the odontoid migrates proximally and compresses the brainstem, the CMA decreases. An angle of <135° correlates with AAI

AAI, Atlantoaxial impaction; *CMA*, cervicomedullary angle; *CT*, computed tomography; *MRI*, magnetic resonance imaging.

3. **Abnormal Imaging parameters**:
   A. **Atlantoaxial subluxation (AAS)**
      - PADI ≤14 mm or less
      - AADI ≥9 mm
      - Spinal cord diameter <6 mm in neutral or flexed position (MRI)
      - Spinal canal diameter <10 mm in flexed position (MRI)
      - Inflammatory tissue behind the dens >10 mm
   B. **Atlantoaxial impaction (AAI)**
      - Cervicomedullary angle <135° on sagittal MRI
      - Cranial migration distance <34 mm in males or <29 mm in females (Redlund-Johnell measurement)
      - Ranawat index <15 mm in males or <13 mm in females
      - Clark station 2 or 3
      - Migration of odontoid >5 mm above McGregor line
      - Surgery is generally recommended following development of AAI due to risk of neurologic injury
   C. **Subaxial subluxation (SAS)**
      - Subaxial canal diameter of ≤14 mm
      - SAS associated with neurologic deficit

19. **What are the surgical treatment options for AAS?**
    Surgical treatment options are guided by whether AAS is **reducible** or **nonreducible**.
       Options for **reducible atlantoaxial subluxations** include:
    - Screw-rod fixation: C1 lateral mass screws and C2 pedicle, pars, or translaminar screws and rods can be used to reduce subluxations and achieve excellent fixation (Fig. 67.5A,B)
    - Transarticular screw fixation ± supplemental posterior wiring is an option but requires reduction of the subluxation prior to screw placement (Fig. 67.6)

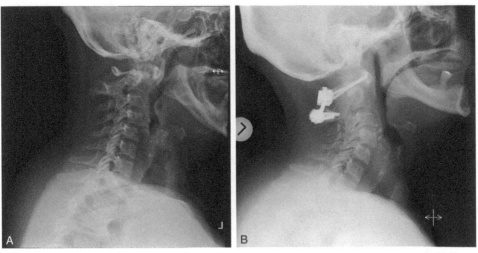

Fig. 67.5 (A) Lateral radiograph of a 61-year-old patient with chronic rheumatoid arthritis who developed anterior atlantoaxial subluxation and superior migration of the odontoid with myelopathy. (B) Surgery included intraoperative traction to reduce the deformity. Structural allografts were inserted into the C1–C2 facet joints to maintain the vertical reduction. Stabilization and fusion included posterior C1–C2 screw-rod fixation with C1 lateral mass screws and translaminar C2 screws and autograft. (Courtesy T. Protopsaltis, MD, NYU Langone Health.)

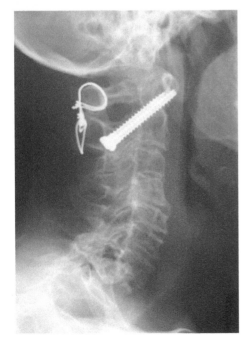

Fig. 67.6 Treatment of rheumatoid atlantoaxial subluxation with C1–C2 posterior fusion with autograft and instrumentation using transarticular screws and modified Gallie wiring.

- Posterior Brooks or Gallie wiring with autograft is rarely used today in as a stand-alone fixation technique given its relatively high failure rate due to poor control of rotation and translation. Supplemental halo vest use may increase the success rate but is poorly tolerated by patients.
- Interlaminar clamps (e.g., Halifax clamp) with structural autograft
  Options for **nonreducible atlantoaxial subluxations** include:
- Posterior spinal fusion and posterior instrumentation (C1 lateral mass screws and C2 pedicle or translaminar screws and rods) combined with C1 laminectomy
- Occipitocervical fusion and posterior instrumentation combined with C1 laminectomy
- Resection of the odontoid

20. What is the fate of retrodental rheumatoid pannus after successful posterior atlantoaxial or occipitocervical arthrodesis?

Achievement of a solid posterior fusion results in reduction of the volume of atlantoaxial rheumatoid pannus in most patients. Instability resulting from the inflammatory process is considered to play a critical role in the development of retrodental pannus. Direct anterior decompression is indicated for patients with symptomatic persistent anterior cord compression following posterior decompression and fusion.

21. What are the surgical treatment options for AAI?

For patients with mild to moderate cervicomedullary compression, preoperative halo traction may be used in an attempt to reduce the degree of AAI and potentially avoid the need for posterior decompression of the foramen magnum or odontoid resection. If adequate decompression is achieved with traction, the patient may be treated with posterior occipitocervical fusion and instrumentation. If traction is unsuccessful, C1 laminectomy and posterior occipitocervical fusion and instrumentation or odontoid resection, combined with posterior instrumentation and fusion, are options. Odontoid resection in patients with AAI is necessary when there is irreducible severe ventral compression of the cervicomedullary junction by pannus or a superiorly migrated odontoid. Odontoid resection may be performed via microscopic transoral, endoscopic transoral, or transnasal approaches and may be assisted by neuronavigational technology. An alternative technique, which has been advocated by some experts, is atlantoaxial joint distraction using bone grafts or spacers in combination with screw-rod fixation for treatment of select patients with combined atlantoaxial instability and vertical migration of the odontoid.

22. What airway management techniques are used when transoral surgery is performed on a rheumatoid patient?

- Nasotracheal intubation (commonly)
- Tracheostomy (rarely)
- Elective postoperative intubation for 24–48 hours to allow pharyngeal swelling to resolve

23. Discuss some methods for occipitocervical fixation that have proven successful in patients with RA.

- Occipitocervical fixation using screw-rod systems is the most commonly utilized method for stabilization of rheumatoid cervical deformities and instabilities. Modular systems provide a variety of options for linkage of occipital screws, cervical screws, and thoracic screws, to longitudinal rods (Fig. 67.7).
- Occipitocervical fixation, using a contoured rod (i.e., Hartshill-Ransford loop) and sublaminar wires with or without bone grafting, is a well-validated technique with a high success rate and low morbidity. Sublaminar wires should not be placed in the setting of an irreducible C1–C2 subluxation or severely stenotic canal.
- A recent development is the option for use of occipital condyle screws as the sole cranial anchor for a posterior screw-rod construct.

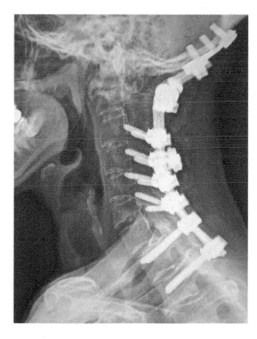

Fig. 67.7 Posterior occiput to T2 fusion and stabilization with a modular midline occipital plate and screws linked to a dual-rod construct with cervical lateral mass screw and thoracic pedicle screw fixation. Surgery was performed for treatment of atlanto-axial impaction and atlantoaxial instability due to long-standing rheumatoid arthritis. (From Bonic EE, Stockwell CA, Kettner NW. Brain stem compression and atlantoaxial instability secondary to chronic rheumatoid arthritis in a 67-year-old female. J Manip Physiol Ther 2010;33:315–320.)

24. What are the surgical treatment options for SAS?
- Anterior decompression (discectomy or corpectomy) and arthrodesis with a structural graft or spacer and anterior plate fixation. However, due to osteoporosis and the inflammatory process, anterior grafts and cages are prone to subsidence and pseudarthrosis, and anterior screw purchase is often poor. Concomitant posterior fixation should be strongly considered if an anterior fusion procedure is planned
- Posterior cervical arthrodesis with screw-rod fixation provides rigid fixation and a high rate of successful arthrodesis.

25. Describe the management of an elderly Ranawat IIIb patient who is bedbound or has severe chronic spinal cord compression.
The prognosis for surgical management is poor. Supportive management rather than an operation may be preferable due to the unfavorable benefit-risk profile and poor prognosis for neurologic recovery.

KEY POINTS

1. Three types of cervical deformities develop secondary to rheumatoid disease: atlantoaxial subluxation (AAS), atlantoaxial impaction (AAI), and subaxial subluxation (SAS).
2. Once patients with rheumatoid arthritis are diagnosed with cervical myelopathy, operative treatment is indicated due to the risks of neurologic deterioration, pain, and sudden death.
3. Radiographic findings that merit cervical MRI and referral to a spine surgeon include AAS with a posterior atlantodens interval of 14 mm or less, SAS with a sagittal diameter of the spinal canal of 14 mm or less, and any degree of AAI.

Websites
1. Rheumatoid arthritis clinical presentation: http://www.hopkins-arthritis.org/arthritis-info/rheumatoid-arthritis/rheum_clin_pres.html
2. Rheumatoid arthritis: http://www.nlm.nih.gov/medlineplus/rheumatoidarthritis.html
3. Rheumatoid arthritis in the cervical spine: what you need to know: http://www.amjorthopedics.com/html/5points/archives/5points0807.pdf

---

BIBLIOGRAPHY

1. Aletaha D, Smolen JS. Diagnosis and management of rheumatoid arthritis. A review. *JAMA* 2018;320:1360–1372.
2. Boden SD, Dodge LD, Bohlman HH, et al. Rheumatoid arthritis of the cervical spine: A long term analysis with predictors of paralysis and recovery. *J Bone Joint Surgery* 1993;75:1282–1297.
3. Cui S, Daffner SE, Emery SE. Surgical management of rheumatoid arthritis. In: Garfin SR, Eismont FJ, Bell GR, et al., editors. Rothman-Simeone the Spine. 7th ed. Philadelphia: Saunders; 2018, pp. 1467–1485.
4. Casey A, Crockard HA, Bland JM, et al. Surgery on the rheumatoid cervical spine for the bed-bound, non-ambulant myelopathic patient—too much, too late? *Lancet* 1996;347:1004–1007.
5. Crockard HA, Calder I, Ransford AO. One-stage transoral decompression and posterior fixation in rheumatoid atlanto-axial subluxation. *J Bone Joint Surg* 1990;72, 682–685.
6. Goel A, Sharma P, Dange N, et al. Techniques in the treatment of craniovertebral instability. *Neurology* 2005;53:525–533.
7. Joaquim AF, Ghizoni E, Tedeschi H, et al. Radiological evaluation of cervical spine involvement in rheumatoid arthritis. *Neurosurg Focus* 2015;38:1–7.
8. Kim DH, Hilibrand AS. Rheumatoid arthritis in the cervical spine. *J Am Acad Orthop Surg* 2005;13:463–474.
9. Moskovich R, Crockard HA, Shott S, et al. Occipitocervical stabilization for myelopathy in patients with rheumatoid arthritis: Implications of not bone grafting. *J Bone Joint Surg* 2000:82;349–365.

CHAPTER 68

ANKYLOSING SPONDYLITIS AND DIFFUSE IDIOPATHIC SKELETAL HYPEROSTOSIS

José H. Jiménez-Almonte, MS, MD, R. Carter Cassidy, MD, and Vincent J. Devlin, MD

1. **What is ankylosing spondylitis?**
   Ankylosing spondylitis (AS) is a seronegative inflammatory rheumatic disease that affects the sacroiliac joints, spine, and peripheral joints. Eponyms for AS include Marie-Strümpell disease and von Bechterew disease. AS is a subtype of a group of interrelated disorders termed *seronegative spondyloarthritides*, which includes AS, psoriatic arthritis, reactive arthritis, and arthritis in association with ulcerative colitis or Crohn disease. These conditions are grouped under an umbrella term as axial spondyloarthritis (axSpA) due to predominant involvement of the axial skeleton and distinguished from peripheral spondyloarthritis (pSpA). Onset of symptoms due to AS commonly occurs between 15 and 35 years of age (mean age of onset, 28 years) and rarely after age 45. AS is more common in males than in females (3:1). AS presents in its early stages with inflammatory arthritic pain that initially involves the sacroiliac joints and later may involve other spinal regions. The classic feature of AS is enthesopathy (inflammation at the attachments of ligaments, tendons, and joint capsules to bone). Initially, range of motion is normal or mildly limited. Disease progression leads to spinal ossification, osteoporosis, and altered spinal biomechanics. The spine may eventually fuse in a kyphotic posture, leading to severe spinal deformities in some patients. The lack of spinal flexibility causes the spinal column to be vulnerable to fractures following minor trauma. Other skeletal manifestations include dactylitis (sausage-shaped digits), heel pain (enthesopathy involving the Achilles tendon insertion), and hip arthritis. Extraskeletal manifestations occur and commonly involve the eyes (anterior uveitis), as well as cardiac, pulmonary, renal, and neurologic systems (Fig. 68.1).

2. **What is the incidence, prevalence, and role of genetics in AS?**
   The incidence of AS in the US is estimated as 7.2 per 100,000 adults. The overall prevalence of AS in the general US population is 0.5%. Heredity plays an important role in AS, as twin studies show that over 90% of the susceptibility to AS is attributed to genetic factors. The prevalence of AS worldwide roughly parallels the prevalence of the Human Leukocyte Antigen (HLA)-B27 gene, which is high in northern latitudes (approaches 15% in Scandinavia) and low near the equator (<1% in Asians and African blacks). However, only 2% of HLA-B27-positive individuals develop AS over their lifetimes. A family history is reported by 7%–36% of AS patients. For individuals who are first degree relatives of patients with AS, the rate of developing AS is approximately 15%–20% if the individual is positive for HLA-B27, and less than 1% if the individual is HLA-B27 negative.

3. **What criteria are used to diagnose AS?**
   - Inflammatory pain and stiffness beginning in the sacroiliac joints, which may subsequently spread to other spinal regions. Inflammatory back pain differs from mechanical back pain and is characterized by insidious onset in patients <45 years of age, alternating buttock pain, awakening in the second half of the night by pain, morning stiffness (>30 minutes), improvement with exercise and nonsteroidal antiinflammatory drugs (NSAIDs), and lack of improvement with rest.
   - Limitation of spinal motion in the coronal and sagittal planes
   - Decreased chest expansion relative to normative values for age and sex
   - Laboratory testing is negative for rheumatoid factor (RF) and antinuclear antibodies (ANA). Nonspecific elevation of erythrocyte sedimentation rate (ESR) and C-reactive protein (CRP) are common.
   - HLA-B27 antigen test positivity. This finding must be interpreted with caution. Although up to 90% of white patients with AS have HLA-B27, the gene is present in up to 8% of the white population, and <1% of persons in the United States develop AS.
   - Imaging studies. Arthritic changes in the sacroiliac joints have traditionally been considered the hallmark for diagnosis of AS. Recent studies have shown that evidence of sacroiliitis on plain radiographs is a late finding and occurs 5–10 years following disease onset. Evidence of sacroiliitis on magnetic resonance imaging (MRI) and thoracic MRI evidence of costovertebral joint inflammation are thought to represent the earliest detectable changes of AS on imaging studies. Spinal imaging hallmarks include marginal erosions at the anterior vertebral corners at the attachment sites of the anterior longitudinal ligament (Romanus lesion), marginal

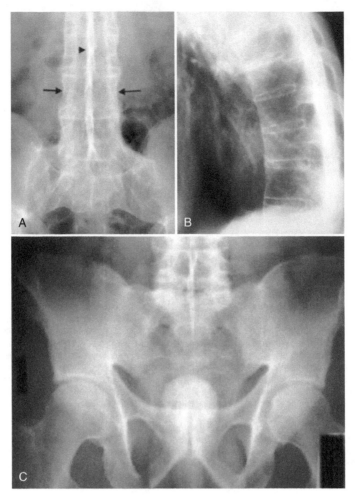

Fig. 68.1 Ankylosis of the lumbar spine in a patient with ankylosing spondylitis. (A) Anteroposterior radiograph of the lumbar spine demonstrates ossification of the interspinous ligament, known as the dagger sign *(arrowhead).* One can also see ankylosis of the facet joints resulting in the tram track sign *(arrows)* paralleling the dagger sign. (B) Lateral radiograph of the thoracic spine in the same patient reveals the bamboo spine appearance owing to ossification of the outer fibers of the annulus fibrosus and resultant fusion of the thoracic spine. (C) Grade 4 sacroiliitis (using the modified New York criteria) in a patient with ankylosing spondylitis. The radiograph readily demonstrates bilateral ankylosis of the sacroiliac joints. (From Bennett DL, Ohashi K, El-Khoury GY. Spondyloarthropathies: Ankylosing spondylitis and psoriatic arthritis. Radiol Clin North Am 2004;42:121–134.)

    syndesmophytes, spondylodiscitis (Andersson lesion), insufficiency fractures, arthritis of the apophyseal and costovertebral joints, enthesopathy involving the interspinal ligaments and kyphotic deformities."
- The Assessment of SpondyloArthritis International Society (ASAS) classification criteria (7) include MRI for identification of active inflammation to aid in earlier diagnosis of axial spondyloarthritides without radiographic sacroiliitis (Table 68.1; Fig. 68.2).

4. What are the accepted treatments for patients with AS?
    Treatment of AS is based on current disease manifestations and level of symptoms. Many patients are able to control joint and spine pain/stiffness with NSAIDs, while other patients require stronger agents, such as a tumor necrosis factor α (TNF-α) inhibitor or secukinumab (interleukin [IL]-17A antagonist). Up to 30% of patients develop uveitis, which may be treated with medications such as corticosteroid eye drops, mydriatic agents, topical NSAIDs, systemic steroids, immunosuppressive agents, and TNF-α inhibitors. Regular exercise and group physical therapy have proven helpful. Total hip arthroplasty is considered for severe hip joint involvement. Spinal surgery is of value in select patients. (6)

Table 68.1 The Assessment of Spondylo Arthritis International Society Classification Criteria for Axial Spondyloarthritis.[a]

Sacroiliitis on imaging	OR	HLA-B27
and		and
≥1 SpA Feature		≥2 SpA Features

- **SpA features:** inflammatory back pain, arthritis, enthesitis (heel), uveitis, dactylitis, psoriasis, Crohn disease/ulcerative colitis, good response to NSAIDs, family history for SpA, HLA-B27, elevated CRP.

- **Sacroiliitis on imaging:** active (acute) inflammation on MRI showing sacroiliitis OR definite radiographic sacroiliitis (modified New York criteria[b])

[a]In patients with back pain >3 months and age at onset <45 years.
[b]Modified New York Criteria (unilateral grade 3 or 4 or bilateral grade 2–4 sacroiliitis where 0= normal, 1= suspicious, 2= minimal, 3= moderate, 4= ankyloses for radiographic grade).
ASAS, Assessment of SpondyloArthritis International Society; *CRP,* C-reactive protein; *HLA,* human leukocyte antigen; *MRI,* magnetic resonance imaging; *NSAIDs,* nonsteroidal antiinflammatory drugs; *SpA,* spondyloarthritis.
Modified from Rudwaleit M, van der Heijde D, Landewé R, et al. The development of Assessment of SpondyloArthritis International Society classification criteria for axial spondyloarthritis (part II): Validation and final selection. Ann Rheum Dis 2009;68:777–783.

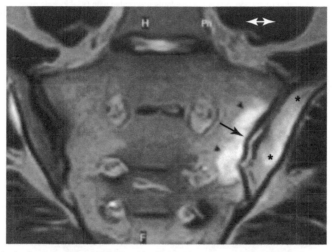

Fig. 68.2 Coronal fat saturation fast-spin echo (FSE) T2-weighted image shows increased periarticular signal about the left sacroiliac joint *(arrowheads and asterisks)* consistent with bone marrow edema and increased signal within the sacroiliac joint *(black and white arrows).* These findings correlated with active left sacroiliitis in this patient with ankylosing spondylitis. (From Bennett DL, Ohashi K, El-Khoury GY. Spondyloarthropathies: Ankylosing spondylitis and psoriatic arthritis. Radiol Clin North Am 2004;42:121–134.)

5. **What problems associated with AS should be considered in relation to patients undergoing surgical treatment?**
   The disease manifestations of AS may involve multiple organ systems. Consideration must be given to a wide range of issues in patients undergoing surgical treatment including the following:
   - **Cardiac issues:** Valve insufficiency, aortitis, conduction abnormalities, ventricular dysfunction, pericarditis. Echocardiogram and cardiology consults are recommended.
   - **Pulmonary issues:** Fibrobullous lung disease, decreased chest expansion, diaphragmatic contribution to ventilation. Consider pulmonary function testing and consultation with a pulmonologist. Do not disrupt the diaphragm during an anterior thoracolumbar surgical approach.
   - **Airway issues:** Difficult intubation due to temporomandibular and cricoarytenoid arthritis, as well as cervical deformity. Awake intubation under fiber-optic visualization is recommended.
   - **Positioning issues:** Kyphotic deformities and atlantoaxial instability require careful consideration to safely position patients for surgical treatment.
   - **Renal issues:** Renal dysfunction may be present secondary to chronic use of NSAIDs, amyloidosis or immunoglobulin A (IgA) nephropathy.
   - **Osteoporosis:** Pedicle screw anchor points may provide less than optimal fixation due to reduced bone density and quality.

6. **What is diffuse idiopathic skeletal hyperostosis and how is this condition different from AS?**

Diffuse idiopathic skeletal hyperostosis (DISH), also known as Forestier disease or senile ankylosing hyperostosis, is a proliferative bone disease that affects ligaments along the anterior spinal column. The etiology and pathogenesis of DISH are unknown. The radiographic hallmark of DISH is the presence of asymmetric *nonmarginal syndesmophytes* (i.e., the new bone formation is located outside the margin of the intervertebral disc), which appear as flowing anterior ossification originating from the anterior longitudinal ligament, typically involving four or more vertebrae in the thoracic region. These nonmarginal syndesmophytes are more prominent on the right side of the spine and project horizontally from the vertebral column. The intervertebral discs, facet joints, and sacroiliac joints are typically not involved in DISH. In contrast, in AS there are *marginal syndesmophytes* (i.e., the new bone formation is contained within the margin of the intervertebral disc), which appear thin, vertically oriented, closely apposed to the spinal column and the facet joints, and the disc spaces are typically involved. Peripheral joint involvement by DISH may coexist with osteoarthritis (OA) and cause heterotopic ossification involving joints that are not commonly involved by OA, including the metacarpophalangeal joints, elbows, shoulders, and ankles. Other entheses involved by DISH include the calcaneus, patella, and olecranon.

DISH typically presents after age 50 and has a slight male predominance. DISH is quite common, with reported prevalence rates in males of 10%–25% compared with 5%–15% in females over the age of 50 years. DISH has been linked to metabolic and constitutional factors as it has a higher association with type 2 diabetes, hypertension, heart disease, dyslipidemia, hyperuricemia, and obesity. It is a seronegative disease and has no affiliation with HLA B27 tissue type. Patients may be asymptomatic or may experience symptoms related to spinal involvement, including pain and motion restriction. Additional problems associated with DISH include dysphagia (secondary to cervical osteophytes), spinal stenosis, heterotopic ossification, enthesopathy, and peripheral joint involvement. Loss of spinal mobility leads to altered spinal biomechanics and predisposes patients to spine fractures following minor trauma. The long, rigid lever arms of stiff spine segments above and below the level of injury increase instability and make fracture treatment challenging. In patients undergoing surgery, limitation of neck motion can lead to difficulties with intubation and an increased risk of aspiration pneumonia has been reported postoperatively.

There are no specific treatments for DISH beyond the use of antiinflammatory agents and physical therapy modalities for pain. Patients should be screened for cardiovascular and metabolic risk factors and treated as appropriate (Fig. 68.3).

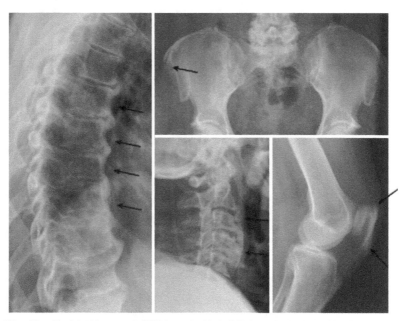

Fig. 68.3 Diffuse idiopathic skeletal hyperostosis (DISH) is seen in older individuals, predominantly, involving the thoracic spine with flowing anterior ossification (at least four levels) and associated with enthesophytes elsewhere (especially pelvis). Patients are at increased risk for heterotopic bone formation after joint replacement. Differentiated from ankylosing spondylitis by age (older); location (C, T spine > L spine, no sacroiliac involvement); and morphology (loosely flowing ossification on lateral view). *Left image,* lateral thoracic radiograph shows classic osteophyte pattern seen in DISH. *Upper right image,* anteroposterior pelvis radiograph shows pelvic enthesophyte. *Center image,* lateral cervical radiograph shows classic osteophyte pattern noted in DISH. *Lower right image,* lateral knee radiograph shows patella enthesophyte. (From Morrison W, Sanders T. Problem Solving in Musculoskeletal Imaging. 1st ed. Philadelphia, PA: Mosby; 2008.)

Table 68.2 Distinguishing Features of AS and DISH.

	AS	DISH
Cause	Autoimmune	Idiopathic
Age of symptom onset	2nd to 3rd decade	>50 years
Sex ratio (M/F)	3:1	2:1
Clinical features	Inflammatory back and SI pain, spine fractures, postural abnormalities, involvement of large peripheral joints	Variably painful, spine fractures, dysphagia, spinal stenosis
Radiologic features	Marginal syndesmophytes, ossification of disc spaces and facet joints, "bamboo spine," bilateral sacroiliitis, ossification progresses from lumbar spine proximally	Nonmarginal syndesmophytes, preserved disc spaces and facet joints, large flowing osteophytes connect atleast four thoracic vertebrae
Laboratory tests	Increased ESR, CRP; negative for RF and ANA; association with HLA-B27	Nonspecific, association with HLA-B8
Associated conditions	anterior uveitis, osteoporosis; cardiac, pulmonary, renal, and neurologic conditions	Type 2 diabetes, hypertension, heart disease, dyslipidemia, hyperuricemia, obesity
Medical treatment	NSAIDs, TNF-α inhibitors, IL-17A antagonist	NSAIDs, treat cardiac and metabolic risk factors
Surgical treatment	Fractures, spondylodiscitis, spinal osteotomies, C1–C2 instability, hip arthroplasty	Fractures, dysphagia secondary to cervical osteophytes, spinal stenosis

ANA, antinuclear antibody; *AS,* ankylosing spondylitis; *CRP,* C-reactive protein; *DISH,* diffuse idiopathic skeletal hyperostosis; *ESR,* erythrocyte sedimentation rate; *HLA,* human leukocyte antigen; *IL-17A,* interleukin 17A; *NSAID,* nonsteroidal antiinflammatory drug; *RF,* rheumatoid factor; *SI,* sacroiliac, *TNF,* tumor necrosis factor.

7. **What spinal problems may require surgical treatment in patients with AS or DISH?**
   In **patients with AS**, spine surgeons may need to intervene for treatment of:
   - Fractures
   - Sagittal plane spinal deformities
   - Atlantoaxial instability
   - Spondylodiscitis
       In **patients with DISH**, spine surgery is most commonly indicated for treatment of:
   - Fractures
   - Dysphagia due to anterior cervical osteophytes
   - Spinal stenosis (Table 68.2)

8. **What are the causes of dysphagia and airway obstruction in patients with DISH?**
   - Direct mechanical compression of the larynx, pharynx, and esophagus. Patients with large anterior osteophytes at C2–C3 may develop respiratory difficulties, since these osteophytes can compress the posterior pharyngeal wall and larynx and obstruct breathing. Osteophytes from C4 to C7 can press on the posterior esophagus and cause compression and dysphagia (see Fig. 68.3).
   - Combination of extrinsic compression from large anterior cervical osteophytes and internal obstruction from a reactive inflammatory mass.
   - Cricopharyngeal spasm
   - Disturbances of the normal epiglottis tilt over the laryngeal inlet by the osteophytes at the C3-C4 level

9. **When is resection of anterior cervical osteophytes in DISH indicated?**
   DISH as a cause of dysphagia and/or airway obstruction may be an underappreciated phenomenon. Surgical excision of osteophytes through the Smith-Robinson approach, usually without fusion, is considered in the presence of dysphagia and airway obstruction if conservative support fails. The spine surgeon should team with head and neck surgeons to ensure that both intrinsic and extrinsic compression of the pharynx and esophagus are addressed. Recent studies indicate that ossification may reoccur several years after successful initial surgical resection.

10. **How does instability of the cervical spine develop in patients with AS in the absence of a traumatic injury?**
    Although AS results in ossification of the cervical region, spinal instability may still develop. Ossification occurs from the lumbar region and progresses proximally and can stiffen the lower cervical region while sparing the

upper cervical region. This can result in increased stress concentration at the craniocervical junction and lead to instability. In addition, inflammation may result in attritional effects on the transverse ligament due to hyperemia at its bony attachments. As these changes progress, atlantoaxial subluxation or dislocation may occur.

11. **What is ankylosing spondylodiscitis?**
Spinal lesions in AS patients which involve the intervertebral disc, vertebral body or discovertebral junction in the absence of spinal infection are referred to by various terms such as spondylodiscitis, Andersson lesions, destructive spinal lesions or pseudarthrosis. Such lesions occur in up to 25% of AS patients, most commonly in the lower thoracic and upper lumbar regions or near the apex of a rigid kyphosis. Lesions which develop early in the disease process suggest an inflammatory etiology, while mechanical factors including stress fracture and incidental trauma are considered responsible for the majority of cases. Surgical treatment consists of posterior spinal instrumentation and decompression and often includes spinal osteotomy. Supplemental anterior spinal column bone grafting is infrequently needed due to the predilection of AS patients to form bone (2).

12. **What are some common pitfalls and recommendations regarding the evaluation and management of fractures in patients with an ankylosed spine due to DISH or AS?**
Some important considerations in the management of fractures in patients with ankylosed spines include the following:
- A high rate of associated neurologic injury is associated with fractures in ankylosed spines
- A low-energy injury may lead to a highly unstable three-column fracture whose diagnosis may be delayed and lead to secondary neurologic deterioration.
- Radiographs may not adequately provide the initial diagnosis of a fracture. Computed tomography (CT) and/or MRI should be obtained if a fracture is suspected and should image the entire spine.
- Nonoperative management is associated with a high complication rate and prompt, aggressive surgical management is the preferred treatment for most injuries.
- Posterior instrumentation extending multiple levels above and below the level of fracture, with or without surgical decompression is recommended in most cases.
- Addition of anterior surgery may be necessary for cases with incomplete apposition of the anterior spinal elements or anterior spinal cord compression.
- Postoperative complications, including epidural hematoma, pneumonia, respiratory insufficiency, deep vein thrombosis, and wound infection are common, and mortality occurs in up to one-third of patients. (9)

13. **Discuss key points to consider in the initial assessment of a patient with AS following a traumatic spinal injury.**
Spinal pain in the AS patient represents a spinal fracture until proven otherwise. A spine fracture in an AS patient is a high-risk injury with an associated mortality rate reported as high as 30%. These fractures are frequently three-column spinal injuries and are highly unstable due to the long, rigid lever arms created by fused spinal segments proximal and distal to the level of injury. Neurologic injury is common and may be due to initial fracture displacement, subsequent fracture displacement during transport or hospitalization, or as a result of associated epidural hematoma. Multiple noncontiguous spine fractures or skip fractures may be present. Special care must be taken during initial evaluation at the injury scene. Patients with kyphotic deformities are at risk of neurologic deterioration with supine positioning on a rigid spine board or application of a cervical collar. The spine-injured AS patient should be splinted in the position of injury with pillows and use of a scoop stretcher instead of a spine board. If a cervical collar does not fit the shape of the neck, immobilization can be achieved with blankets or sandbags. Supportive ventilation with adjuvants is recommended because intubation can be very challenging in this population and is best achieved with fiber-optic visualization in the emergency department setting (Fig. 68.4).

14. **What treatment is recommended for a cervical fracture in a patient with AS?**
Expeditious surgical stabilization is generally preferred, although immobilization in a halo vest is an option is select circumstances. Unstable injuries (e.g., translational shear fractures, extension-distraction injuries) are highly unstable and are treated with multisegmental posterior instrumented fusion or combined anterior and posterior instrumented fusion.

15. **Is a previously undiagnosed cervical spine fracture a common cause of chronic flexion deformity in patients with AS?**
Yes. Chronic flexion deformity of the cervical spine may result from a previously undiagnosed fracture that heals in a displaced position. The site of injury is usually in the lower cervical spine or at the cervicothoracic junction. The fracture is generally a transversely oriented shear-type fracture. This injury may not be obvious on plain radiographs; CT scans and MRI are required for diagnosis.

16. **What treatment is recommended for a thoracic or lumbar fracture in a patient with AS?**
Thoracic and lumbar fractures are most commonly treated with posterior spinal instrumentation and fusion. The goal is to stabilize the spine in its *preinjury alignment* and perform a posterior decompression if indicated. Supplemental anterior procedures are indicated when there is significant disruption of the anterior spinal column

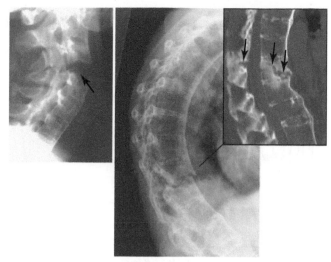

Fig. 68.4 Fractures associated with ankylosing spondylitis (AS) typically involve the disc space and run obliquely through the fused segments. *Left image,* lateral cervical radiograph depicts an extension-distraction injury resulting in extreme cervical instability. *Center image,* lateral thoracic radiograph shows a three-column fracture typical for AS. *Right image,* magnified view depicting the three-column thoracic fracture. (From Morrison W, Sanders T. Problem Solving in Musculoskeletal Imaging. 1st ed. Philadelphia, PA: Mosby; 2008.)

(e.g., burst fractures, distractive extension injuries) or when neurologic deficit is secondary to anterior compressive pathology. Attempts to improve on the preinjury sagittal spinal alignment (e.g., osteotomy) are not advised in an acute fracture setting.

17. What are the indications for spinal osteotomy in patients with AS?

Cervicothoracic osteotomy is indicated for symptomatic fixed flexion deformity of the cervical region. In the most extreme cases, a chin-on-chest deformity is present. Cervical deformities may impair the ability to maintain a forward gaze, limit ambulation, cause difficulty with personal hygiene, and adversely impact oral intake and cause dysphagia. Because cervicothoracic osteotomy is a high-risk procedure, diligent presurgical screening and assessment are paramount, and patients should have an earnest desire to accept the risks and rehabilitative measures required for surgical correction. (4,5,8)

Thoracic osteotomy is performed less commonly than cervical or lumbar osteotomies due to concerns regarding the risk of thoracic spinal cord injury due to the narrow thoracic spinal canal and limited vascular supply to thoracic cord levels, as well as the limiting effect of the rib cage and fused costovertebral joints on deformity correction. The diaphragm must not be violated if surgical reconstruction includes a transthoracic anterior surgical approach because the diaphragm plays an important role in respiration in AS patients due to limited chest wall motion resulting from fusion of the costovertebral and costotransverse joints.

Lumbar osteotomy is commonly performed for AS patients with fixed flexion deformities due to thoracolumbar or lumbar deformity. Indications for osteotomy include inability to stand upright, difficulty with forward gaze, and inability to lay flat. If both cervicothoracic deformity and thoracolumbar/lumbar deformities are present and require treatment, lumbar osteotomy is most commonly performed first, unless the magnitude of the cervical deformity precludes prone positioning for lumbar osteotomy. (3)

Treatment decision-making is complex as hip joint disease, loss of lumbar lordosis and progressive cervical and thoracic kyphosis may coexist and contribute to the stooped forward posture characteristic of AS. Patients with fixed flexion deformities secondary to arthrosis involving the hip joints should be considered for **total hip arthroplasty**. As some patients require both spinal osteotomy and hip replacement, it is important to consider which procedure should be performed first. Previous recommendations were to perform hip arthroplasty prior to spinal osteotomy in AS patients, but more recently it has been recommended to perform spinal osteotomy first to avoid changes in acetabular cup position following correction of spinopelvic malalignment which can increase the risk of hip instability and hip component dislocation.

18. How does the surgeon determine the osteotomy location and degree of correction that is necessary when performing a cervical or lumbar osteotomy?

A detailed clinical and imaging evaluation is necessary to determine the optimal osteotomy location and degree of correction that is required. (1) Clinical assessment involves examination of the patient in the standing, seated, and supine positions to identify the major contributing component(s) to the overall spinal deformity. A cervicothoracic deformity will be unchanged in the standing, seated, and supine positions. In contrast, a deformity that is present

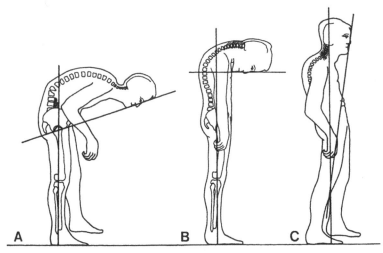

Fig. 68.5 The chin-brow to vertical angle is used to measure the degree of flexion deformity of the spine in ankylosing spondylitis. (A) For thoracolumbar deformity. (B) For cervical deformity. (C) For postoperative assessment. The chin-brow to vertical angle is the angle between a line connecting the brow to the chin and a vertical line with the patient standing with the hips and knees extended and the neck in a fixed or neutral position. (From Simmons Jr ED, Simmons EH. Ankylosing spondylitis. Spine State Art Rev 1994;8:589–604.)

on standing and sitting and corrects with supine positioning, suggests that the major component of the deformity is in the thoracic, thoracolumbar, or lumbar region. A deformity that corrects with transition from a standing to a seated position suggests that the major component of the deformity arises from the hip joints or lumbar spine, and directs attention to further evaluation of the hip joints to assess whether the patient is a candidate for total hip arthroplasty.

Imaging evaluation should include full-length standing anteroposterior and lateral radiographs with the knees in full extension to allow measurement of global sagittal balance, cervical lordosis, thoracic kyphosis, lumbar lordosis, pelvic parameters, and the chin-brow line to vertical angle (CBV angle). Cross-sectional imaging (i.e., MRI, CT) is helpful to characterize distorted anatomy, evaluate the presence and extent of spinal stenosis that may require decompression, and evaluate the position of the vertebral arteries when surgery involves the cervical region.

Multiple techniques are used to assess the degree of correction required. One method is to measure the CBV angle on a full-length lateral spinal radiograph. The measured angle is transposed onto a radiograph and used to estimate how much bone resection is needed to achieve the desired correction. In patients with fused cervical spines, it is important to avoid overcorrection of the CBV angle and a minimally flexed (10°–15°) posture is optimal. Additional techniques to assess the desired degree of correction include use of tracing paper to outline the spinal osteotomy or the use of preoperative computer modeling software (Fig. 68.5).

19. **What are the preferred spinal levels for an osteotomy for treatment of cervicothoracic deformity due to AS?**
The osteotomy is usually carried out at the C7 or T1 levels. This site is below the entry point of the vertebral arteries, which typically enter at the foramen transversarium at C6. The spinal canal at C7–T1 is relatively capacious, and injury to the C8 or T1 nerve roots would cause less disability than injury to other cervical nerve roots.

20. **What are the different types of cervical osteotomy procedures for treatment of a cervicothoracic deformity due to AS?**
The two main types of cervical osteotomies used to treat cervicothoracic deformity caused by AS are the Smith-Petersen osteotomy (SPO) and the pedicle subtraction osteotomy (PSO). A cervical SPO is an opening wedge osteotomy which lengthens the anterior spinal column. A cervical PSO is a closing wedge osteotomy which involves removal of the pedicles, a wedge of vertebral body, and posterolateral vertebral body walls.

21. **What are the key steps involved in performing a cervicothoracic SPO for treatment of cervicothoracic deformity due to AS?**
- According to the initial procedure description, a halo cast is applied prior to surgery. The procedure is carried out under local anesthesia, with the patient awake and seated in a dental chair with halo traction in place to stabilize the head. This protocol allows active spinal cord monitoring and immediate assessment of vital functions and neurologic status. A Doppler device is fixed to the patient's chest to detect air embolism.

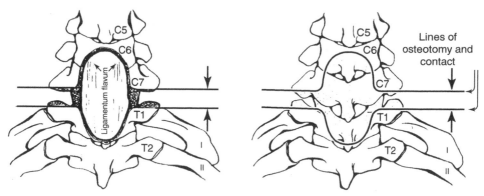

Fig. 68.6 Outline of area of bony resection for a cervical osteotomy in the coronal plane. The lines of resection of the laterally fused facet joints are beveled slightly away from each other, extending posteriorly so that the two surfaces will be parallel and in apposition following correction. The pedicles must be undercut to avoid impingement on the C8 nerve roots. The midline resection is beveled on its deep surface above and below to avoid impingement against the dura following extension correction. (From Simmons Jr ED, Simmons EH. Ankylosing spondylitis. Spine State Art Rev 1994;8:589–604, with permission.)

Fig. 68.7 Preoperative and postoperative depiction of Smith-Petersen cervical osteotomy, sagittal plane. (From Lo V, Hsieh J, Bergey DL, et al. Deformity surgery for ankylosing spondylitis. In: Steinmetz MP, Benzel EC, editors. Benzel's Spine Surgery. 4th ed. Philadelphia, PA: Elsevier; 2017, pp. 1347–1352, Fig. 154.3.)

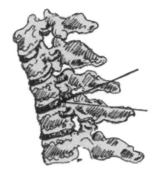

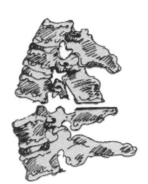

- The entire posterior arch of C7 with the inferior portion of C6 and the superior portion of T1 is removed. The eighth cervical nerve roots are identified at the C7–T1 neuroforamen and are widely decompressed through the lateral recess, removing the overlying bone at the foramen. The cervical pedicles are undercut with Kerrison rongeurs to allow ample room for the eighth cervical nerve roots when the osteotomy site is closed. The amount of bone to be resected is carefully assessed preoperatively and intraoperatively to avoid compression of the nerve roots during closure of the osteotomy. The residual portions of the laminae of C6 and T1 must be carefully beveled and undercut to avoid any impingement or kinking of the spinal cord on closure of the osteotomy site. A more recent modification of this technique includes wider resection of the lamina and complete removal of the C7 pedicles.
- After adequate removal of bone, the osteotomy is completed (osteoclasis). The patient is given an intravenous dosage of a short-acting barbiturate. The surgeon grasps the halo and brings the neck into an extended position. This maneuver closes the osteotomy posteriorly as osteoclasis occurs anteriorly. An audible snap and sensation of osteoclasis are noted. The lateral masses should be well approximated.
- The posterior elements of the spine are decorticated at the C7–T1 area and autogenous bone graft is packed on each side over the decorticated areas. The local bone removed from the posterior decompression is used as bone graft.
- With the surgeon holding the patient's head in the corrected position, the assistants attach the cast to the halo ring and the halo cast is worn for 3 months postoperatively (Figs. 68.6 and 68.7).

22. **What are some refinements of the original cervicothoracic SPO technique that have been introduced in recent years?**
    Some refinements of the originally described surgical technique include:
    - Performing the procedure with the patient in the prone position
    - Use of general anesthesia and intraoperative neurophysiologic monitoring

- Use of posterior segmental spinal instrumentation, most commonly rod-screw systems
- Avoidance of the use of a halo cast or halo brace

23. **What are the key steps involved in performing a C7 PSO for treatment of cervicothoracic deformity due to AS?**
    - After intubation and recording of baseline neuromonitoring signals (transcortical motor evoked potentials [MEPs], somatosensory-evoked potentials [SSEPs], electromyography [EMG]), the patient is placed in the prone position on the operating table after placement of a halo ring.
    - A standard posterior surgical exposure is performed from C2 through T3. If the occipitocervical joints are fused, consideration is given to including the occiput-C2 levels to increase the number of proximal fixation points.
    - Following spinal exposure, screw anchors are inserted (C2 pedicle screws, cervical lateral mass screws, thoracic pedicle screws).
    - Next, a C7 laminectomy is performed and the bone is saved as graft material. Next, the lateral masses of C7 are removed along with the caudal portion of the inferior articular process of C6 and the cranial portion of the superior articular process of T1. The C7 and C8 nerve are identified adjacent to the C7 pedicle and are traced out through their foramen, with removal of any overhanging bone.
    - Using the C7 pedicle as a conduit, bone is removed from the C7 vertebral body using a combination of curettes, spinal taps, and motorized tools to create a cavity in the posterosuperior portion of the C7 vertebral body to approximate a 30° wedge. Next, the C7 pedicle is removed and the lateral aspect of the C7 vertebral is partially removed under direct vision.
    - The osteotomy is closed by grasping the halo ring and extending the neck. Prebent rods are placed into the previously placed screws, and set screws are tightened to lock the instrumentation construct and maintain the spine in the corrected position (Figs. 68.8).

24. **What are some advantages and disadvantages of cervicothoracic SPO versus PSO for treatment of cervicothoracic deformity due to AS?**
    A similar degree of sagittal correction may be obtained with either technique. The SPO may be performed in either the seated or prone position, while the PSO is performed with the patient under general anesthesia in the prone position. The use of the SPO in the seated position can be advantageous for treatment of patients with extreme deformities, which create challenges related to positioning on an operating room table. Some disadvantages of the SPO include instability at the osteotomized level due to disruption of all three spinal columns, osteoclasis may inadvertently occur at a different spinal level other than C7, and elongation of the anterior spinal column may lead to complications such

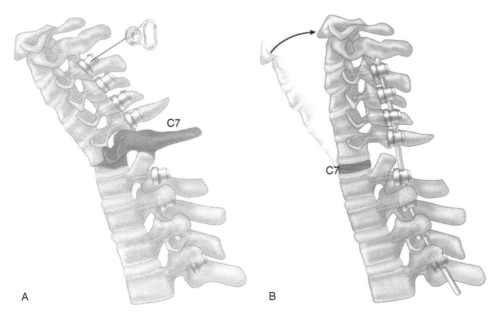

A   B

Fig. 68.8 (A) Note the shaded area, which represents bone that is resected for a C7 pedicle subtraction osteotomy. Before closure of the osteotomy, cervical and thoracic screws should be placed. (B) Closure of the osteotomy is performed by release of the cranial fixation and hyperextension of the cervical spine. After correction of the deformity, rods are inserted and locked. (From Link T, Jandial R, Sonntag V. Procedure 63: posterior cervicothoracic osteotomy. In: Jandial R, McCormick PC, Black PM, editors. Core Techniques in Operative Neurosurgery. Philadelphia, PA: Saunders; 2011, pp. 439–442, Figs. 63.5, 63.6.)

as dysphagia. In contrast, the PSO results in a more stable construct as it is a spinal shortening procedure but is associated with increased blood loss compared with an SPO. Both techniques are associated with potential for major complications including neurologic injury, inadequate or excessive deformity correction, and death.

25. **What types of osteotomies are used to treat thoracic, thoracolumbar, and lumbar sagittal plane spinal deformities in patients with AS?**
Commonly used types include the PSO and SPO. The **PSO** removes bone from all three spinal columns through a posterior approach. PSO involves a laminectomy, excision of the articular processes, pedicle resection, and resection of a wedge of bone from the vertebral body. A PSO hinges on the anterior column and shortens the middle and posterior spinal column. Although a PSO can be performed at any level of the thoracic or lumbar spine, when appropriate, performing the osteotomy at or below L2 helps to decrease neurologic and vascular complications, as this location places the osteotomy below the level of the conus medullaris and above the aortic bifurcation. In extremely severe kyphotic deformities, performing more than one PSO may be considered.

The **SPO** involves removal of a v-shaped wedge of bone from the posterior spinal column, which includes resection of the facet joints, portions of the lamina, and the ligamentum flavum. Closure of an SPO results in shortening of the posterior spinal column and elongation of the anterior spinal column.

Other osteotomies that have been described in AS patients include Ponte osteotomies, circumferential osteotomies, closing-opening wedge osteotomies, multisegmental closing-wedge osteotomies, multisegmental opening-wedge osteotomies, and vertebral column resection or decancellation procedures.

KEY POINTS

1. The classic feature of ankylosing spondylitis is inflammation at the attachments of ligaments, tendons, and joint capsules to bone, which is termed enthesopathy.
2. Diffuse idiopathic skeletal hyperostosis is a proliferative bone disease that affects ligaments along the anterior spinal column, most commonly in the thoracic region.
3. Patients with ankylosing spondylitis or diffuse idiopathic skeletal hyperostosis who sustain a low-energy spinal injury require evaluation with CT and/or MRI as they are prone to develop a highly unstable three-column injury whose diagnosis is often delayed and may lead to secondary neurologic deterioration if unrecognized.
4. Surgical intervention in patients with ankylosing spondylitis may be required for atlantoaxial instability, spondylodiscitis, fractures, correction of sagittal plane spinal deformities and total hip arthroplasty.
5. Surgical intervention in patients with diffuse idiopathic skeletal hyperostosis may be required for fractures, dysphagia caused by cervical osteophytes, and spinal stenosis.

Websites
1. Ankylosing spondylitis: http://emedicine.medscape.com/article/386639-overview
2. Ankylosing spondylitis: managing patients in an emergency setting—a primer for first responders: https://www.spondylitis.org/For-First-Responders
3. Diffuse idiopathic skeletal hyperostosis: http://emedicine.medscape.com/article/388973-overview

---

BIBLIOGRAPHY

1. Hu SS, Ananthakrishnan D. Ankylosing spondylitis. In: Garfin SR, Eismont FJ, Bell GR, et al., editors. Rothman-Simeone The Spine, 7th ed. Philadelphia, PA: Saunders; 2018, pp. 1487–1491.
2. Chang KW, Tu MY, Huang HH, et al. Posterior correction and fixation without anterior fusion for pseudoarthrosis with kyphotic deformity in ankylosing spondylitis. *Spine* 2006;31:408–413.
3. Chang KW, Chen YY, Lin CC, et al. Closing wedge osteotomy versus opening wedge osteotomy in ankylosing spondylitis with thoracolumbar kyphotic deformity. *Spine* 2005;30:1584–1593.
4. Chin KR, Ahn J. Controlled cervical extension osteotomy for ankylosing spondylitis utilizing the Jackson operating table—technical note. *Spine* 2007;32:1926–1929.
5. Etame AB, Than KD, Wang AC, et al. Surgical management of symptomatic cervical or cervicothoracic kyphosis due to ankylosing spondylitis. *Spine* 2008;33:559–564.
6. Kubiak EN, Moskovich R, Errico TJ, et al. Orthopaedic management of ankylosing spondylitis. *J Am Acad Orthop Surg* 2005;13:267–278.
7. Rudwaleit M, van der Heijde D, Landewé R, et al. The development of Assessment of SpondyloArthritis international Society classification criteria for axial spondyloarthritis (part II): Validation and final selection. *Ann Rheum Dis* 2009;68:777–783.
8. Simmons ED, DiStefano RJ, Zheng Y, et al. Thirty-six years' experience of cervical extension osteotomy in ankylosing spondylitis. *Spine* 2006;31:3006–3012.
9. Whang PG, Goldberg G, Lawrence JP, et al. The management of spinal injuries in patients with ankylosing spondylitis or diffuse idiopathic skeletal hyperostosis: A comparison of treatment methods and clinical outcomes. *J Spinal Disord Tech* 2009;22:77–85.

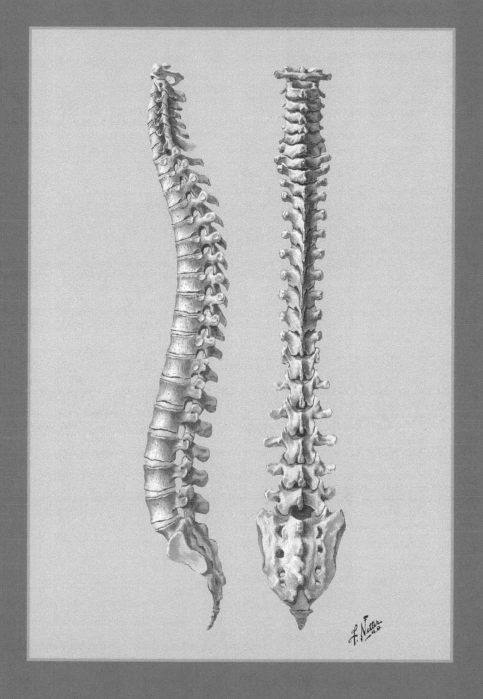

XII
EMERGING SPINAL TECHNOLOGIES

CHAPTER 69

SPINAL NAVIGATION, ROBOTIC SURGERY, AND THREE-DIMENSIONAL PRINTING

Terrence Kim, MD and Doniel Drazin, MD, MA

SPINAL NAVIGATION

1. Briefly outline the development of spinal navigation.

   Spinal navigation was introduced in the early 1990s as advances in computer-based technologies enabled a transition from frame-based systems developed for cranial surgery to frameless navigation systems. First-generation frameless systems involved a range of technologies, including two-dimensional (2D) fluoroscopy and wired navigation instruments. Second-generation systems involved passive reflective reference frames, point-by-point matching (PPM), self-registration, and relied on preoperative computed tomography (CT) datasets loaded onto an image postprocessing workstation. Current generation systems encompass and incorporate intraoperative three-dimensional (3D) CT (and CT-like) imaging with automatic registration and computer-guided software that allow the user to visualize 3D spinal anatomy and track instrumentation in real time.

2. What are the principles upon which intraoperative spinal navigation is based?

   Intraoperative spinal navigation is based on the principles of **stereotaxy**, which refers to localization of a specific point in space using a 3D coordinate system. Spinal imaging data and anatomic data from the surgical field are defined within separate 3D Cartesian coordinate systems and specific points within each dataset are matched using mathematical algorithms. Establishment of a spatial relationship between spinal imaging data and anatomic data from the surgical field is created through a process referred to as **registration**. Various registration methods have been described, including paired-point registration, surface-matching registration, and automatic registration. The aim of intraoperative spinal navigation is to track surgical instruments and spinal anatomy in the operative field in relation to a registered reference point. This is commonly performed using marker spheres attached to surgical instruments and a reference frame that is fixed to bony landmarks outside the immediate operative field. A camera is used to track the position of surgical instruments and spinal implants with respect to the reference frame and the resulting data is transmitted to the workstation where the data is processed for display.

3. What are the essential working components of an Intraoperative Spinal Navigation System?

   An Intraoperative Spinal Navigation System consists of four major components:
   - **Imaging modality:** Navigation may be based on use of an intraoperative imaging modality such as a 3D CT or CT-like scanner or 3D fluoroscopy scanner. Alternatively, imaging data obtained intraoperatively can be matched with preoperative CT data and used to guide surgery.
   - **Reference frame:** Provides a fixed point of reference to which navigated instruments are measured and displayed. Common sites for attachment of a reference frame (also referred to as a dynamic reference array) include the posterior spinal elements or ilium.
   - **Reflective light camera scanner:** Detects both the reference frame and the navigated instruments in a 3D grid, and sends the positional coordinates to the computer workstation.
   - **Marker spheres:** Reflective spheres are attached to the navigated instruments and are tracked by the reflective camera on the navigation station.
   - **Computer workstation** with appropriate software that integrates the intraoperative image and positional coordinates from the scanner to provide a real-time graphical representation of the navigated instruments in the spine (Figs. 69.1 and 69.2).

4. What are different options for reference frames in spinal navigation?
   - Spinous process clamp
   - Head holder attachments (Mayfield skull clamps)
   - Posterior superior iliac spine percutaneous pins
   - Surgical mask–based system (skin-adhesive cutaneous frame)
   - Pedicle screw clamps (for revision cases with screws in place or for second intraoperative navigation scans)

5. Is spinal navigation associated with improved accuracy of screw placement and decreased revision surgery rates due to malpositioned screws compared with alternative techniques?

   Yes. Spinal navigation has been shown in multiple meta-analyses, prospective randomized studies, and cadaveric studies to be more accurate for the insertion of pedicle screws and is associated with lower revision surgery rates

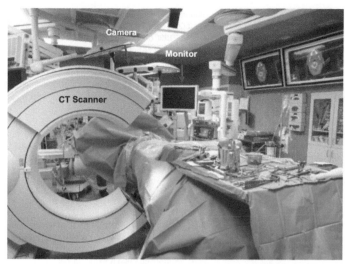

Fig. 69.1 Navigation setup. Imaging modality, reflective light camera scanner, monitor, and computer workstation. (From Freedman BA, Nassr A, Currier BL. Stereotactic navigation in complex spinal surgery: Tips and tricks. Oper Tech Orthop 2017;27:260–268, Fig. 1, p. 263.)

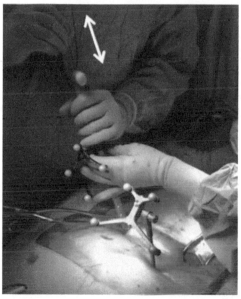

Fig. 69.2 Pedicle screw placement with spinal computed tomography navigation. Marker spheres are attached to the navigated instrument. Reference frame is attached to ilium. (From Oh T, Park P, Miller CA, et al. Navigation-assisted minimally invasive surgery deformity correction. Neurosurg Clin N Am 2018;29:439–451, Fig. 4, p. 442.)

compared with 2D fluoroscopy or freehand methods. On average, the reported radiographic accuracy rates are as follows: CT navigation, 97% (range: 86%–100%); 2D fluoroscopy, 90% (range: 80%–93%); freehand, 85% (range: 69%–94%). On average, the reported revision surgery rates are: CT navigation, <1%; 2D fluoroscopy, <2%; and freehand, <10%.

6. How is pedicle screw instrumentation accuracy measured?
   Accuracy rates of pedicle screw placement are commonly reported based on whether pedicle screws are located entirely within the pedicle. The amount of pedicle breach is commonly measured in millimeters and graded from A to E according to the Gertzbein-Robbins classification: Grade A (0 mm breach), B (<2 mm), C (<4 mm), D (<6 mm), E (≥6 mm). The clinical significance of a pedicle breach depends on several factors, including breach

direction, breach magnitude, spinal level, presence of a positive electromyography (EMG) response or neurologic deficit or other clinical sequalae. Medial breach is a concern due to the proximity of neural structures, while anterior breach of the vertebral body cortex endangers vascular and visceral structures. However, lateral breach in the thoracic spinal region may be contained within the posterior rib, and thoracic screw trajectories that involve intentional lateral pedicle penetration (the "in-out-in" technique) have been recommended to optimize thoracic fixation. It has been reported that less than 5% of misplaced pedicle screws are associated with symptoms. Medial pedicle breach >2 mm is considered significant in various literature reports. However, it is challenging to compare breach rates between studies due to variable verification methods and different definitions of breaches.

7. **What are the current indications for use of spinal navigation?**
Spinal navigation was initially used to guide placement of pedicle screws in the thoracic and lumbar regions. Subsequently, use of spinal navigation has expanded to all types of spinal surgery including cervical instrumentation, iliac and S2 alar-iliac screw placement, transoral procedures, spinal deformity surgery, revision surgery, corpectomy, interbody fusion, tumor resection, video-assisted thoracoscopic surgery, surgery involving congenital osseous anomalies, and minimally invasive surgery.

8. **How is the workflow for CT navigation different from other imaging modalities such as fluoroscopy?**
CT navigation in spinal surgery is a high-demand technologic advancement for the delivery of instrumentation. It relies heavily on input from multiple disciplines (radiology, anesthesia and nursing staff, surgical technologists, navigation technologists) to successfully implement image guidance in the operative room. Organization and management of this multidisciplinary team is more complex compared to use of fluoroscopy. Coordination of the movement of each individual during navigation, and emphasis of the importance of execution of each team member's role, is critical to maintaining a smooth workflow that is free of disruptions.

9. **What is the standard workflow for Spinal CT navigation?**
   - Patient setup
   - Exposure
   - Reference frame placement
   - Intraoperative image acquisition (CT spin)
   - Calibration of instruments
   - Navigated screw placement (point-drill-tap-screw)
   - Decompression, cage placement (if necessary)
   - Rod measurement and placement
   - Additional CT spins may be required when anatomy is altered, for multilevel implant constructs, or to confirm implant placement

10. **How is the accuracy of CT navigation affected by distance from the reference frame?**
Accuracy decreases after the distance from the reference frame exceeds 50 cm.

11. **How many levels are usually included in one imaging capture?**
One image capture (CT spin) translates into approximately 4–5 lumbar levels, 6–8 thoracic spine levels, and 1–7 cervical levels. Multilevel instrumentation cases that exceed the limits of a single image capture require more than one CT image acquisition due to the limits of the mobile scanner. Workflow efficiencies can be enhanced if multiple reference frames are placed and staggered CT spins are obtained.

12. **What are some common factors responsible for inaccurate Spinal CT navigation?**
   - Line-of-sight issues that prevent the light-emitting diode detectors in the reflective light camera scanner from detecting the navigated instruments
   - Intraprocedural movement of the reference frame
   - Workflow difficulties
   - Lack of coordination by team members
   - Equipment failure
   - Untrained or inadequately trained surgical teams
   - Movement of the reference frame after the CT image has been acquired
   - Changes in spinal position or intersegmental spinal alignment after the CT image has been acquired

13. **Comparing CT navigation and fluoroscopy, what are the equivalent radiation exposure times?**
Each CT imaging machine has a different radiation dosage level. According to manufacturer's data, in a medium-sized patient (70 kg), a single CT-navigation image capture is roughly equivalent to 35 seconds of fluoroscopy.

14. **How does the occupational radiation exposure to the surgeon and surgical team from CT navigation compare with use of fluoroscopy or portable x-ray?**
CT navigation and x-ray are associated with lower occupational radiation exposure to the surgeon and surgical team compared with fluoroscopy. During image acquisition, as the CT scan or x-ray is being performed, the

surgeon and surgical team are briefly able to exit the OR. This effectively eliminates any occupational risk of radiation exposure. The surgeon and surgical team return to the OR once the CT scan or x-ray is completed.

15. How does the radiation exposure delivered to the patient differ for CT navigation, fluoroscopy, and portable x-rays?

The radiation exposure delivered to the patient with CT navigation is definitely greater than with fluoroscopy or x-ray. It has been reported that one complete spin of a portable cone-beam CT is equivalent to approximately 38–51 C-arm fluoroscopy exposures and 1.3–2.4 x-ray exposures. (1) However, in the setting of morbid obesity, severe osteopenia, and difficult-to-image locations in the spine (i.e., occipitocervical junction, cervicothoracic junction, lumbosacral junction), where multiple fluoroscopic images are obtained, CT navigation can potentially deliver less radiation to the patient with far greater accuracy compared with fluoroscopy. In minimally invasive fusion surgery where fluoroscopy is heavily used, CT navigation has been shown to deliver up to a 1.9 times lower cumulative radiation exposure to the patient.

16. Why has CT navigation not become an accepted standard for use during instrumented spinal procedures?

Based on international surveys of spinal surgeons, high capital costs are the greatest barrier to increased acceptance of CT navigation in spine surgery. Additional factors identified as barriers to acceptance of CT navigation include lack of proper training and perceived increased surgical time. The acquisition costs and total equivalent annual costs for a CT-navigation system, including mobile CT scanner and workstation, are more than 3.5 times greater compared with a C-arm fluoroscopy unit. The cost-effectiveness of CT navigation is predominantly achieved by direct cost savings from reducing reoperation rates. When costs are economically justified based on reduction of reoperation rates in specific countries, (2) CT-guided navigation has been shown to be cost-effective for use in complex cases performed in high-volume spine centers.

ROBOT-ASSISTED SPINE SURGERY

17. What are the different types of surgical robotic systems?

A **surgical robot** is a powered computer-controlled manipulator with artificial sensing, which is capable of being reprogrammed to move and position tools to perform a variety of surgical tasks. (3) Robotic systems may be grouped into three types:

Teleoperated systems provide the surgeon with real-time full control of the robot from a remote location and allow the surgeon to perform telesurgery. An example is the da Vinci Surgical System (Intuitive Surgical).

Supervisory-controlled systems allow the surgeon to plan surgery offline, after which the robot performs the procedure autonomously under close supervision.

Shared-control systems allow the surgeon and robot to directly control surgical instruments simultaneously. This is the most common type of robot used in spine procedures and these systems are most commonly used for pedicle screw procedures. Examples include Mazor Renaissance (Mazor Robotics) and Mazor X Stealth Edition (Medtronic), ROSA ONE Spine System (Zimmer Biomet), and ExcelsiusGPS (Globus Medical, Inc.).

18. What are some potential advantages of using a robotic spine surgery system compared with CT navigation?

Robotic systems address some of the limitations associated with spinal navigation including the following:
- Line of sight issues that impede detection of navigated instruments
- Errors due to surgical instrument misregistration as the robot performs this function
- Human error and variability associated with pedicle cannulation by surgeons as the robot precisely and consistently places the drill cannula guide

19. Is spinal navigation necessary for robotic surgery?

No. A preoperative CT scan is utilized. Intraoperative localization with fluoroscopy is used as an initial step in registration.

20. What are the essential working components of a robotic surgery system for use in spine surgery?

Robotic surgery system for spine use consists of four major working parts:
1. Robot workstation/computer
2. Robotic guidance unit mount
3. C-arm
4. Optical camera tomography

21. What is the standard workflow for robotic spine surgery?
- Preoperative planning using CT
- Anatomic fixation of robotic mount
- Registration and image acquisition (fluoroscopy)
- Robot assembly

- Mount to frame and percutaneous fixation
- Pedicle cannulation (K-wire and screw insertion; Fig. 69.3)

22. Is robotic surgery more accurate than spinal navigation?
Yes. Published studies have reported that the accuracy of robotic surgical delivery of spinal instrumentation is higher than the accuracy with spinal navigation. The clinical impact on revision rates with high rates of accuracy with robotics has not been demonstrated.

3D-PRINTING APPLICATIONS FOR SPINE SURGERY

23. What is 3D printing?
Additive manufacturing techniques such as 3D printing use digital computer-aided design to create objects by sequentially building 2D layers that are joined to the layer below, rather than by subtractive manufacturing techniques. Recent technologic advances have led to rapid incorporation into the treatment paradigm for spinal disorders.

24. How is 3D printing currently being applied to spine surgery?
Some current applications of 3D printing to spine surgery include:
- Patient-specific anatomic models for preoperative planning, surgeon training, and patient education
- 3D-printed surgical guides
- Manufacture of various types of patient-specific spinal devices, including artificial discs, intervertebral body fusion devices, vertebral body replacement devices, and surgical tools
- Manufacture of spinal implants with complex geometries
- Future uses may include novel applications related to tissue-engineered biodegradable scaffolds and drug delivery devices

25. What is a 3D-printed surgical guide for use in spine surgery?
A 3D-printed surgical guide is a single-use, patient-specific navigation solution, which can substitute for other forms of intraoperative navigation. 3D-printed surgical guides are most commonly utilized to aid in spinal screw placement. The 3D guide is created based on a preoperative spine CT scan and used to create a 3D spine model. The navigational template is designed as the inverse of the vertebral surface to which it will be applied and incorporates optimal screw trajectories identified based on preoperative CT images. The surgeon reviews the surgical plan and approves the screw trajectories and screw sizes. The device is then sent to the hospital for use in surgery, where it is placed over the spine at the appropriate spinal level(s) and used to create pilot holes for screw placement. Use of 3D-printed surgical guides have been reported in placement of posterior spinal screws, anterior spinal screws, open-door laminoplasty procedures, and as cutting guides for spinal osteotomy procedures and oncologic resections (Fig. 69.4).

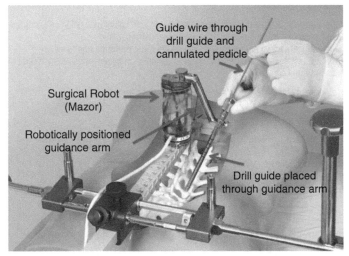

Fig. 69.3 Schematic of robot use in a spine model. (From Divi S, Pollster S, Ramos E, et al. The current role of robotic technology in spine surgery. Oper Tech Orthop 2017;27:275–282, Fig. 1, p. 277.)

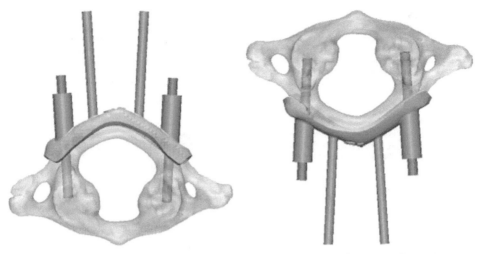

Fig. 69.4 3D-printed drill navigation guide for C1 screw placement. (From Pu X, Yin M, Ma J, et al. Design and application of a novel patient-specific three-dimensional printed drill navigational guiding in atlantoaxial pedicle screw placement. World Neurosurg 2018; 114:1–10, Fig. 1E,F, p. 3.)

26. What are some advantages associated with use of a 3D-printed surgical guide in spine surgery?
    Some advantages associated with the use of a 3D-printed spine surgical guide include the following:
    - Reported accuracy is comparable to navigation and robotics
    - Intraoperative radiation is not required
    - Allows for preoperative planning and modeling
    - Less expensive than surgical navigation
    - Decreased surgical time and blood loss

27. What are some disadvantages associated with use of a 3D-printed surgical guide in spine surgery?
    Some disadvantages associated with use of a 3D-printed spine surgical guide include:
    - Lack of immediate availability due to need for a preoperative CT and device production
    - Guide fit may be impaired by soft tissue or osseous structures
    - Inaccurate screw placement can occur if the guide is unstable or moves after it is positioned on the patient

KEY POINTS

- Intraoperative spinal navigation has demonstrated increased accuracy for insertion of pedicle screws and is associated with lower revision surgery rates compared with use of freehand methods and two-dimensional fluoroscopy.
- Use of intraoperative spinal navigation can decrease the radiation exposure to surgeons and operating room personnel. However, radiation to the patient is greater than with use of fluoroscopy or x-ray for routine surgical cases..
- Use of robotic systems in spine surgery can address some of the limitations associated with spinal navigation.
- Three-dimensional printing is a novel approach for increasing accuracy of spinal screw placement while minimizing radiation exposure and cost.

Websites
1. Navigation in minimally invasive spine surgery: https://www.ncbi.nlm.nih.gov/pmc/articles/PMC6626747/
2. Guidelines for the acquisition and application of imaging, navigation, and robotics for spine surgery: https://www.ncbi.nlm.nih.gov/pmc/articles/PMC6465454/
3. 3D-printed surgical guides: http://aoj.amegroups.com/article/view/4993/html

REFERENCES

1. Nelson, E. M., Monazzam, S. M., Kim, K. D., Seibert, J. A., & Klineberg, E. O. (2014). Intraoperative fluoroscopy, portable x-ray, and CT: patient and operating room personnel radiation exposure in spinal surgery. *Spine Journal* 14, 2985-2991.
2. Dea, N., Fisher, C. G., Batke, J., Strelzow, J., Mendelsohn, D., Paquette, S. J., et al. (2016). Economic evaluation comparing intraoperative cone beam CT-based navigation and conventional fluoroscopy for the placement of spinal pedicle screws: a patient-level data cost-effectiveness analysis. *Spine Journal* 16, 23-31.
3. Davies, B. (2000). A review of robotics in surgery. Proceedings of the Institution of Mechanical Engineers. Part H: *Journal of Engineering in Medicine* 214, 129-140.

BIBLIOGRAPHY

1. Davies B. A review of robotics in surgery. Proceedings of the Institution of Mechanical Engineers. *J Eng Med* 2000;214:129–140.
2. Dea N, Fisher CG, Batke J, et al. Economic evaluation comparing intraoperative cone beam CT-based navigation and conventional fluoroscopy for the placement of spinal pedicle screws: A patient-level data cost-effectiveness analysis. *Spine J* 2016;16:23–31.
3. Divi S, Pollster S, Ramos E, et al. The current role of robotic technology in spine surgery. *Oper Tech Orthop* 2017;27:275–282.
4. Freedman BA, Nassr A, Currier BL. Stereotactic navigation in complex spinal surgery: Tips and tricks. *Oper Tech Orthop* 2017;27:260–268.
5. Garg B, Mehta N. Current status of 3D printing in spine surgery. *J Clin Orthop Trauma* 2018;9:218–225.
6. Kochanski RB, Lombardi JM, Laratta JL, et al. Image-guided navigation and robotics in spine surgery. *Neurosurgery* 2019;84:1179–1189.
7. Larson AN, Santos ER, Polly Jr DW, et al. Pediatric pedicle screw placement using intraoperative computed tomography and 3-dimensional image-guided navigation. *Spine* 2012;37:188–194.
8. Malham GM, Wells-Quinn T. What should my hospital buy next? Guidelines for the acquisition and application of imaging, navigation, and robotics for spine surgery. *J Spine Surg* 2019;5:155–165.
9. Molliqaj G, Schatlo B, Alaid A, et al. Accuracy of robot-guided versus freehand fluoroscopy-assisted pedicle screw insertion in thoracolumbar spinal surgery. *Neurosurg Focus* 2017;42:14.
10. Nelson EM, Monazzam SM, Kim KD, et al. Intraoperative fluoroscopy, portable x-ray, and CT: Patient and operating room personnel radiation exposure in spinal surgery. *Spine J* 2014;14:2985–2991.
11. Wilcox B, Mobbs RJ, Wu AM, et al. Systematic review of 3D printing in spinal surgery: The current state of play. *J Spine Surg* 2017;3:433–443.

INDEX

Note: Page numbers followed by *f* indicate figures. Page numbers followed by *t* indicate tables.
Page numbers in **boldface type** indicate complete chapters.